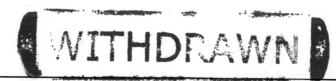

ANTIBODIES

Stimulation	Serology Saline / AHG		Comp. Binding	Immunoglobin Class IgM	IgG	Optimum Temperature	Clinical Significance HTR	HDN	Comments
RBC	occ	yes	no	occ	yes	warm	yes	yes	Very rarely IgA anti-D may be produced; however, this is invariable with IgG.
RBC	no	yes	no	occ	yes	warm	yes	yes	
RBC/NRBC	occ	yes	no	occ	yes	warm	yes	yes	Anti-E may often occur without obvious immune stimulation.
RBC	no	yes	no	occ	yes	warm	yes	yes	
RBC	no	yes	no	occ	yes	warm	yes	yes	Warm autoantibodies often appear to have anti-e like specificity.
RBC	no	yes	no	occ	yes	warm	yes	?	
RBC	no	yes	no	occ	yes	warm	yes	yes	
RBC/NRBC	occ	yes	no	occ	yes	warm	yes	yes	Anti-C^w may often occur without obvious immune stimulation.
RBC	no	yes	no	occ	yes	warm	yes	yes	
RBC	no	yes	no	occ	yes	warm	yes	yes	Antibodies to V and VS present problems only in the black population where the antigen frequencies are in the order of 20 to 25.
RBC	no	yes	no	occ	yes	warm	yes	yes	
RBC	occ	yes	some	occ	yes	warm	yes	yes	Some Antibodies to Kell system have been reported to react poorly in low ionic media.
RBC	no	yes	no	occ	yes	warm	yes	yes	
RBC	no	yes	no	occ	yes	warm	yes	yes	Kell system antigens are destroyed by AET and by ZZAP.
RBC	no	yes	no	occ	yes	warm	yes	yes	Anti-K1 has been reported to occur following bacterial infection.
RBC	no	yes	no	occ	yes	warm	yes	yes	
RBC	no	yes	no	occ	yes	warm	yes	yes	
RBC	no	yes	no	occ	yes	warm	yes	yes	The lack of Kx expression on RBCs and WBCs has been associated with the McLeod phenotype and CGD.
RBC	occ	yes	some	occ	yes	warm	yes	yes	Fy(a) and (b) antigens are destroyed by enzymes. Fy(a−b−) cells are resistant to invasion by *P. vivax* merozoites, a malaria causing parasite.
RBC	no	yes	some	occ	yes	warm	yes	yes	
RBC	occ	yes	?	occ	yes	warm	?	yes	Fy3, 4, and 5 are not destroyed by enzymes.
RBC	no	yes	some	occ	yes	warm			
RBC	no	yes	?	occ	yes	warm			Fy5 may be formed by interaction of Rh and Duffy gene products.
RBC	no	yes	?	?	yes	warm	?	?	Fy6 antibody reacts with most human red cells except Fy(a−b−) and is responsible for susceptibility of cells to penetration by *P. Vivax*.

(Continued on inside back cover)

Modern
Blood Banking
and Transfusion
Practices

Modern Blood Banking and Transfusion Practices

Third Edition

Editor-in-Chief

Denise M. Harmening, PhD, MT(ASCP), CLS(NCA)

Chair and Professor
Department of Medical and Research Technology
University of Maryland School of Medicine
Baltimore, Maryland

F. A. DAVIS COMPANY · Philadelphia

F. A. Davis Company
1915 Arch Street
Philadelphia, PA 19103

Printed in the United States of America

Last digit indicates print number: 10 9 8 7 6 5 4 3 2 1

Publisher: Jean-François Vilain
Developmental Editor: Ralph Zickgraf
Production Editor: Marianne Fithian
Cover Design By: Steven R. Morrone

Library of Congress Cataloging-in-Publication Data

Modern blood banking and transfusion practices / editor-in-chief,
　　Denise M. Harmening. — 3rd ed.
　　　　p.　　cm.
　　Includes bibliographical references and index.
　　ISBN 0-8036-4598-8
　　1. Blood banks. 2. Blood—Transfusion. I. Harmening, Denise.
　　[DNLM: 1. Blood Banks. 2. Blood Transfusion. 3. Blood—
immunology. 4. Blood Grouping and Crossmatching. WH 460 M688
1994]
RM172.M62 1994
615′.39—dc20
DNLM/DLC
for Library of Congress　　　　　　　　　　　　　　　94-3176
　　　　　　　　　　　　　　　　　　　　　　　　　　　CIP

Dedication

To all students, full-time, part-time, past, present, and future, who have touched and will continue to touch the lives of so many educators . . .

It is to you this book is dedicated in the hope of inspiring an unquenchable thirst for knowledge and love of mankind.

Foreword

Blood transfusion science is one of the newest branches of medical laboratory science. Blood groups were only discovered approximately 90 years ago, and most of them have only been recognized in the last 40 years. Although transfusion therapy was used soon after the ABO blood groups were discovered, it was not until after World War II that blood transfusion science really started to become an important branch of medical science in its own right. Thus, compared with many branches of medicine, or even pathology, blood transfusion science is an infant, growing fast, changing continually, and presenting a great potential for research and future development.

To be able to grow, our infant needs to be nurtured with a steady flow of new knowledge generated from research. This knowledge then has to be applied at the bench. To understand and best take advantage of the continual flow of new information being generated by blood transfusion scientists, and to apply it to everyday work in the blood bank, technologists (and pathologists) need to have a good understanding of basic immunology, genetics, biochemistry (particularly membrane chemistry), and the physiology and function of blood cells. To apply new concepts, they need technical expertise and enough flexibility to reject old dogma when necessary and to accept new ideas when they are supported by sufficient scientific data.

High standards are always expected and strived for by technologists who are working in blood banks or transfusion service. I very much believe that technologists should understand the principles behind the tests they are performing, rather than perform tasks as a machine does. Because of this, I do not think that "cookbook" technical manuals have much value in *teaching* technologists; they do have a place as reference books in the laboratory. Over the years (too many to put in print) that I have been involved in teaching medical technologists, it has been very difficult to select *one* book to cover all that technologists in training need to know about blood transfusion science, without confusing them. Classic texts used regularly in teaching SBB students and pathology residents often contain too much information for the average medical technologist, especially those in training. These texts contain certain sections that can, and perhaps should, be read, but sometimes even these sections may serve to confuse learners rather than help and stimulate them. Some of these texts are written to be encyclopedic reference tomes, and others contain a great deal of clinical material or esoterica that are unnecessary for medical technologists who are not yet experienced in blood transfusion practice.

Dr. Denise Harmening has produced a single volume that covers everything a student of medical technology needs to know about blood transfusion science. She has been involved in teaching medical technologists for most of her career. After seeing how she has arranged this book, I would guess that her teaching philosophies are close to those of my own. She has gathered together a group of experienced scientists and teachers who together with her cover all the important areas of blood transfusion science.

The chapters on the basic principles of cell preservation, genetics, and immunology provide a firm base for the learner to understand the practical and technical importance of the other chapters. The chapters on the blood groups and transfusion practice provide enough information for medical technologists, without overwhelming them with esoterica and clinical details.

Although this book was primarily designed for medical technologists, I believe it is admirably suited to pathology residents, hematology fellows, and others who want to review any aspect of modern blood transfusion science.

GEORGE GARRATTY, PhD, FIMLS, MRCPath
Scientific Director
American Red Cross Blood Services
Los Angeles, California

Preface

This book is designed to provide the medical technologist, blood bank specialist, or resident with a concise and thorough guide to transfusion practices and immunohematology. The book takes a practical and applied approach to the subject matter, in order to provide the practitioner with a working knowledge of modern, routine blood banking.

Twenty color plates provide a means for standardizing the reading of agglutination reactions. They also serve to foster the comprehension of difficult concepts not routinely illustrated in other texts.

Several features of this textbook offer great appeal to students and educators. Each chapter begins with comprehensive outlines and educational objectives and ends with study guide questions, complete with answers and cross-references to the relevant text pages. The blood group antibody characteristic chart on the inside cover of the book serves as an easy reference and guide to the characteristics of the blood group systems. A thorough glossary at the back of the book clearly defines all terms related to immunohematology.

Chapter 1 is an introduction to the historical aspects of blood transfusion and preservation that serves as a prelude to an overview of red cell and platelet metabolism as well as current and future approaches to blood storage. Basic concepts of genetics, blood group immunology, and routine serologic testing serve to introduce a thorough and current overview of blood group systems. The inheritance and synthesis of blood group antigens and the serologic activity of the associated antibodies are clearly presented with helpful illustrations, tables, and charts.

The next section of the book focuses on routine blood bank practices including donor selection and component preparation, detection and identification of antibodies, compatibility testing, transfusion therapy, and apheresis. A chapter on transfusion safety and federal regulations from the Division of Inspections and Surveillance of the Food and Drug Administration has also been included for clarification of the required quality assurance and inspection procedures. New to the third edition is a chapter devoted entirely to the issue of quality assurance.

The need to integrate and correlate the various laboratory procedures presented in previous chapters as they are performed on patient samples in the routine blood bank laboratory provides the conceptual basis for the chapter, "Orientation to the Routine Blood Bank Laboratory." This chapter introduces the student to the common organizational divisions of a routine blood bank laboratory, allowing the student to prepare for clinical rotations.

Certain clinical situations that are particularly relevant to blood banking are discussed in detail, including transfusion reactions, hemolytic disease of the newborn, autoimmune and drug-induced hemolytic anemia, transfusion-transmitted viruses, human leucocyte antigens (HLA), and paternity testing.

New to this edition is the chapter "Blood Bank Information Systems." Blood banks generate tremendous volumes of information relating to patients and blood products that must be maintained for extended periods of time. The ability to manage the information is crucial to efficiently providing quality patient care.

Unique to *Modern Blood Banking and Transfusion Practices* are the final two chapters, "Medicolegal and Ethical Aspects of Providing Transfusion Services" and "Technologic Advances and Future Trends in Blood Banking." Expansion of areas considered peripheral to the blood bank has necessitated the need for redefining the role and involvement of these areas within the structure of the modern blood bank laboratory. As a result, such specialized topics as genetic engineering and hybridoma technology, immunotherapy, bone marrow transplantation, bone marrow processing, bone grafts and procurement, and tissue banking are addressed in the final chapter. Both federal and American Association of Blood Banks regulations are cited throughout the text as well as referenced at the conclusion of each chapter for further consideration.

This book is a culmination of the tremendous efforts of a number of dedicated professionals who participated in this project by donating their time and expertise because they cared about the Blood Bank Profession. My thanks to the following educators and clinicians, who reviewed the manuscript of the third edition: Michael Coover, MS, MT(ASCP), Program Director, School of Medical Technology, Harbor Medical Center, University of California Los Angeles; Jane Elder, MS, MA, SCP, Hinds Community College; Patty Hanneman, MS, MT(ASCP)SBB, Duke University Medical Center; Lieta M. Maffei, MT(ASCP)SBB, Manager, Templin Management Associates; Arthur L. Paul, MT(ASCP), Program Coordinator, Medical Laboratory Technology, El Paso Community College; and special gratitude to Barbara Gorgone, MT(ASCP)SBB, Laboratory Director, AMI East Cooper Community Hospital, for her careful reading and insightful comments.

This book is intended to foster improved patient care by providing the reader with a basic understanding of the function of blood, the involvement of blood group antigens and antibodies, the principles of transfusion therapy, and the adverse effects of blood transfusion. It has been designed to generate an "unquenchable thirst for knowledge" in all medical technologists, blood bankers, and practitioners whose education, knowledge, and skills provide the public with excellent health care.

DENISE M. HARMENING, PhD, MT(ASCP), CLS(NCA)

Contributors

Margaret A. Brooks
Laboratory Administrator
Baltimore Rh Typing Laboratory
Baltimore, Maryland

Loni Calhoun, MT(ASCP)SBB
Senior Technical Specialist, Blood Bank
Educational Coordinator, Transfusion Medicine
University of California Los Angeles Medical Center
Los Angeles, California

Lloyd O. Cook, MD
Assistant Professor
Department of Pathology
Medical Director
Blood Bank and Transfusion Medicine
Medical College of Georgia
Augusta, Georgia

Estrellita Culotta, MHS, MT(ASCP)SBB
Manager, Transfusion Medicine
Department of Pathology
Southern Baptist Hospital
New Orleans, Louisiana

R. Ben Dawson, MD
Medical Director
The Therapeutic Apheresis Center
Baltimore Rh Typing Laboratory
Baltimore, Maryland

Felicia E. Dawson-Batcha, MT(ASCP)BB, CLS(NCA)
Technical Support Representative
Syva Company
San Jose, California

Deborah Firestone, MA, MT(ASCP)SBB
Clinical Assistant Professor
State University of New York at Stony Brook
Stony Brook, New York

Frankie Gillen Gibbs, MS, MT(ASCP)SBB
Red Cell Reference Laboratory
Associated Regional and University Pathologist, Inc.
Clinical Associate Professor
School of Medicine
University of Utah
Salt Lake City, Utah

Ralph E. B. Green, BAppSci, FAIMS, MACE
Principle Lecturer in Medical Laboratory Science
Acting Head of Department
Department of Medical Laboratory Science
Royal Melbourne Institute of Technology
Melbourne, Victoria, Australia

Denise M. Harmening, PhD, MT(ASCP), CLS(NCA)
Chair and Professor
Department of Medical and Research Technology
University of Maryland School of Medicine
Baltimore, Maryland

Chantal Ricaud Harrison, MD
Associate Professor of Pathology
University of Texas Health Science Center at San Antonio
San Antonio, Texas

Carmen Julius, MD
Fellow—Transfusion Medicine
The Ohio State University Hospitals
Columbus, Ohio

Melanie S. Kennedy, MD
Associate Director of Clinical Services
Associate Professor
Department of Pathology
The Ohio State University Hospitals
Columbus, Ohio

Patricia Joyce Larison, MT(ASCP)SBB, MA
Supervisor
Blood Bank
Associate Professor
Department of Medical Technology
Assistant Professor
Department of Pathology
Medical College of Georgia
Augusta, Georgia

Beth Lingenfelter, MS, MT(ASCP)SBB
Instructor
Department of Pathology
School of Medicine
University of Utah
Salt Lake City, Utah

Bonnie Lupo, MS, SBB(ASCP)
Director, Quality Assurance
New York Blood Center Laboratories
New York Blood Center
New York, New York

Sharon Martin, EdD, MT(ASCP)
Assistant Professor
Department of Medical Technology
Medical College of Georgia
Augusta, Georgia

JoAnn M. Moulds, PhD
Assistant Professor of Internal Medicine
University of Texas Health Science Center
Houston, Texas

Mary E. Paranto, MS, MT(ASCP)SBB
Instructor and Clinical Coordinator
Program in Medical Technology
Department of Laboratory Sciences
Thomas Jefferson University
Philadelphia, Pennsylvania

Donna L. Phelan, BA, CHS(ABHI), MT(HEW)
Technical Supervisor
HLA Laboratory
Barnes Hospital
St. Louis, Missouri

Herbert F. Polesky, MD
Director
Memorial Blood Centers of Minnesota
Minneapolis, Minnesota

Lee Ann Prihoda, BS, MT(ASCP)SBB
Manager, Education/SBB School
Gulf Coast Regional Blood Center
Houston, Texas

Linda T. Raichle, PhD, MT(ASCP)
Laboratory Training Advisor
Centers for Disease Control and Prevention
National Laboratory Training Network
Eastern Area Resource Office
Exton, Pennsylvania

Francis R. Rodwig, Jr., MD, MPH
Associate Medical Director, Blood Bank
Department of Pathology
Ochsner Medical Institutions
New Orleans, Louisiana

Kathleen Sazama, MD, JD, MT(ASCP)
Professor of Pathology and Laboratory Medicine
Medical College of Pennsylvania
Philadelphia, Pennsylvania

Chloe M. Scott, MT(ASCP), CLS(NCA)
Biomedical Computer Systems Officer
Regulatory Affairs
American Red Cross Blood Services
Philadelphia, Pennsylvania

Peggy Perkins Simpson, MT(ASCP)
MLT Program Director
Alamance Community College
Graham, North Carolina

Judith Ann Sullivan, BS, MT(ASCP)SBB
Independent Blood Bank Consultant
Silver Spring, Maryland

Mitra Taghizadeh, MS, MT(ASCP)
Clinical Assistant Professor
Department of Medical and Research Technology
University of Maryland School of Medicine
Baltimore, Maryland

Mary Ann Tourault, MA, MT(ASCP)SBB
Division of Inspection and Surveillance
Office of Compliance
Center for Biologics Evaluation and Research
Food and Drug Administration
Rockville, Maryland

Abdul Waheed, MS, MT(ASCP)SBB
Supervisor
Reference and Prenatal Laboratory
Transfusion Service
The Ohio State University Hospitals
Columbus, Ohio

Phyllis S. Walker, MS, MT(ASCP)SBB
Reference Laboratory Supervisor
Irwin Memorial Blood Centers
San Francisco, California

Merilyn A. Wiler, MA Ed, MT(ASCP)SBB
Quality Engineer
Belle Bonfils Memorial Blood Center
and
Clinical Instructor
Department of Pathology
Division of Medical Laboratory Sciences
University of Colorado
Denver, Colorado

Patricia A. Wright, BA, MT(ASCP)SBB
Assistant Administrative Director of Laboratories
and
Supervisor, Blood Bank
Maryland General Hospital
Department of Pathology
Baltimore, Maryland

Contents

PLATES 1 THROUGH 20

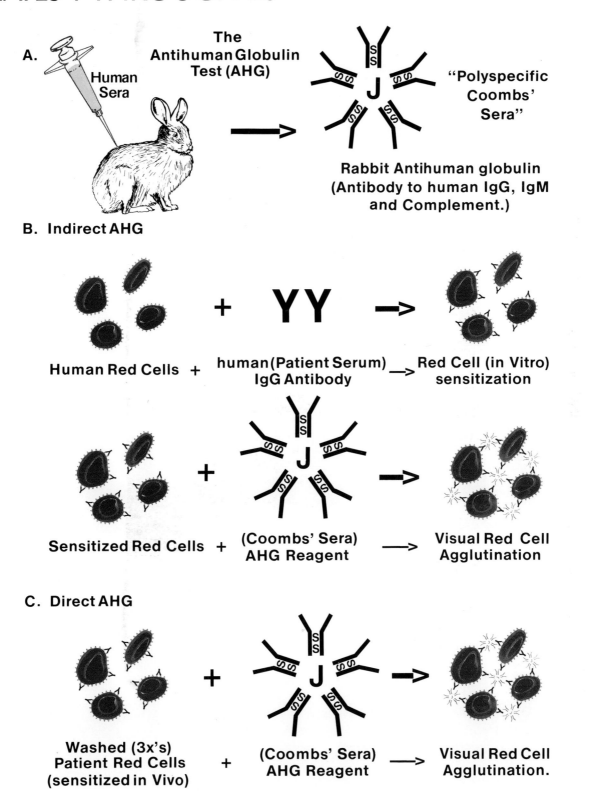

A. The Antihuman Globulin Test (AHG)

Human Sera

→

"Polyspecific Coombs' Sera"

Rabbit Antihuman globulin (Antibody to human IgG, IgM and Complement.)

B. Indirect AHG

Human Red Cells + human(Patient Serum) IgG Antibody → Red Cell (in Vitro) sensitization

Sensitized Red Cells + (Coombs' Sera) AHG Reagent ⟶ Visual Red Cell Agglutination

C. Direct AHG

Washed (3x's) Patient Red Cells (sensitized in Vivo) + (Coombs' Sera) AHG Reagent ⟶ Visual Red Cell Agglutination.

Plate 1.   The antihuman globulin (AHG) test (primary immunization). Note: The AHG reagents currently sold are the products of subsequent immunizations and contain primarily IgG rabbit antibody.

RED CELL ANTIGEN-
SEROLOGIC
MACROSCOPIC

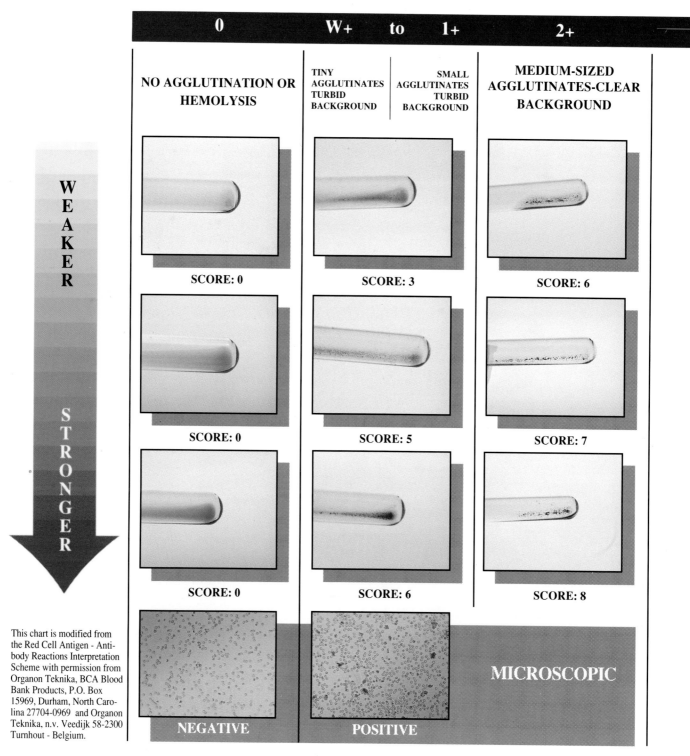

Plate 2. Red cell antigen-antibody reactions: serologic grading and macroscopic evaluation.

ANTIBODY REACTIONS
GRADING
EVALUATION

3+	4+
SEVERAL LARGE AGGLUTINATES-CLEAR BACKGROUND	**ONE SOLID AGGLUTINATE**

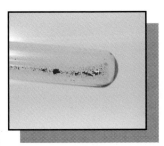

SCORE: 9

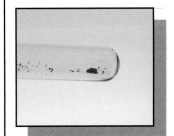

SCORE: 11

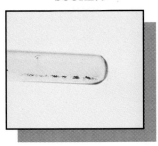

SCORE:10

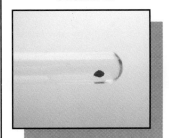

SCORE: 12

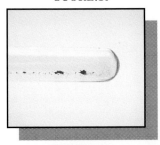

SCORE: 10

NOTE:
Partial or Complete Hemolysis is a Positive Reaction

NOTE: The scores utilized in this chart represent the Marsh Scoring System which is used in many reference laboratories during antibody identification and titrations. Numerical scores are assigned to the observed agglutination reactions using a scale from 0-12. Reference: Marsh, W.L. Scoring of hemag-glutination reactions. Transfusion 1972; 12: 352-3

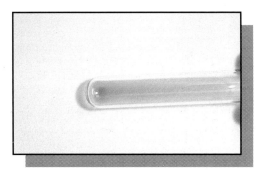

NEGATIVE: NO AGGREGATES

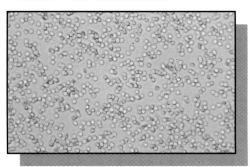

NEGATIVE: NO AGGREGATES (Microscopic)

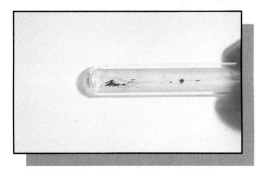

PSEUDOAGGLUTINATION OR STRONG ROULEAUX (2+)

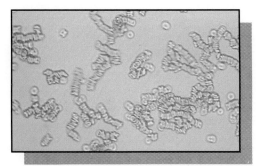

ROULEAUX:Microscopic (original magnification x10; enlarged 240%) NOTE: The "stack of coins" appearance of the agglutinates

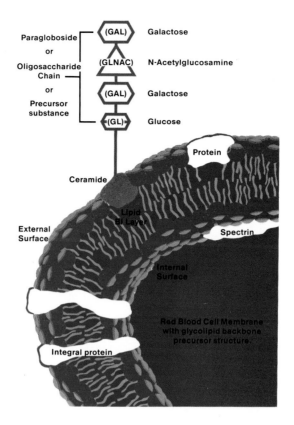

Plate 3. Red blood cell precursor structure (which represents a paragloboside).

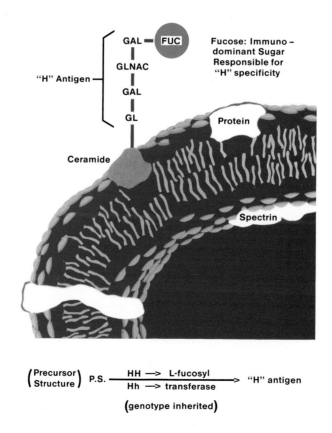

Plate 4. Formation of the H antigen.

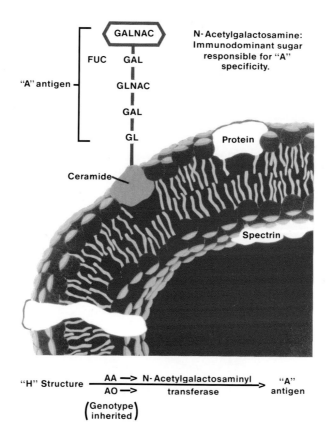

Plate 5.   Formation of the A antigen.

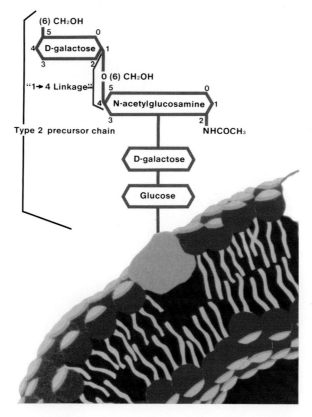

Plate 6.   Type-2 precursor chain.

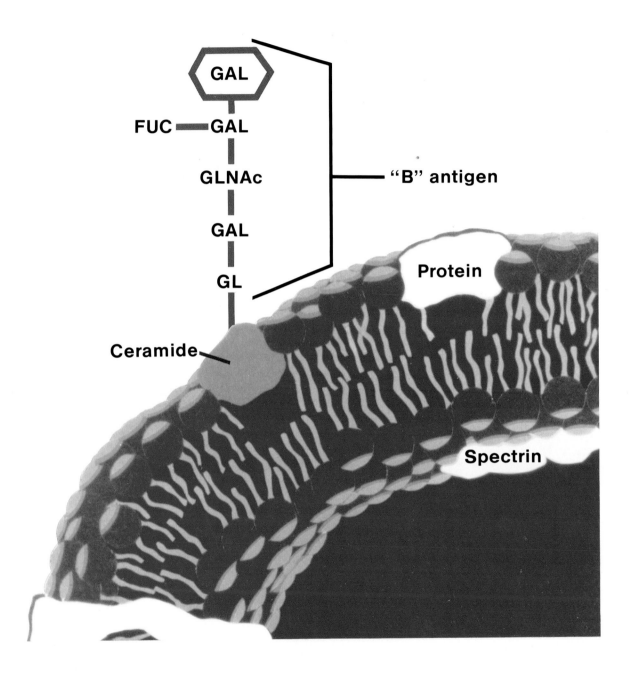

D-Galactose: Immunodominant Sugar responsible for "B" specificity

GAL

FUC — GAL

GLNAc

GAL

GL

"B" antigen

Protein

Ceramide

Spectrin

"H" structure $\xrightarrow[\text{BO} \longrightarrow \text{transferase}]{\text{BB} \longrightarrow \text{Galactosyl}}$ "B" antigen

$\left(\begin{array}{c}\text{Genotype} \\ \text{inherited}\end{array}\right)$

Plate 7. Formation of the B antigen.

Genotype: Se se
AB
HH

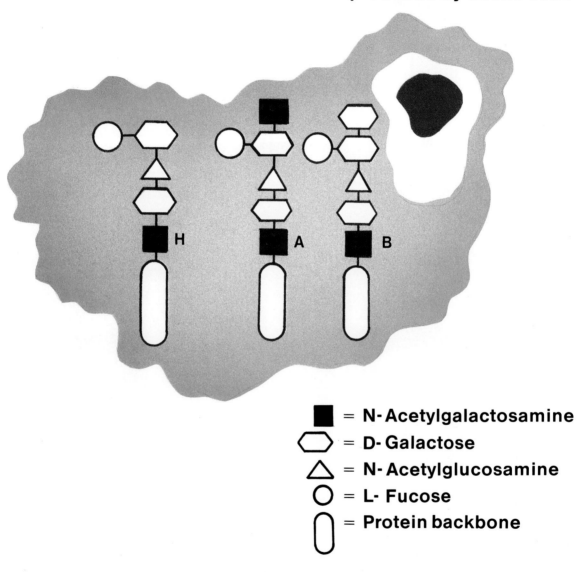

Plate 8. Secretor ABH glycoprotein substances.

A

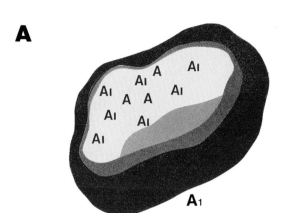

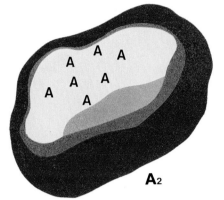

A₁

A₂

Reactions of Patient's Red Cells with

Blood Group	Antigens present	Anti A (from B sera)	Anti-A₁ lectin
A₁	A₁ A	+	+
A₂	A	+	neg

B

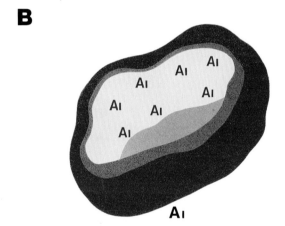

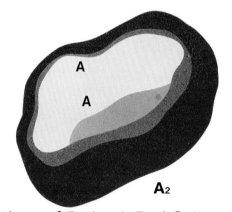

A₁

A₂

Reactions of Patient's Red Cells with

Blood Group	Antigens present	Anti-A (Anti-A plus Anti-A₁)	Anti A₁ lectin
A₁	A₁	+	+
A₂	A	+	neg

Plate 9.   (A) A₁ versus A₂ phenotypes. (B) A₁ versus A₂ phenotypes (alternative conceptual presentation).

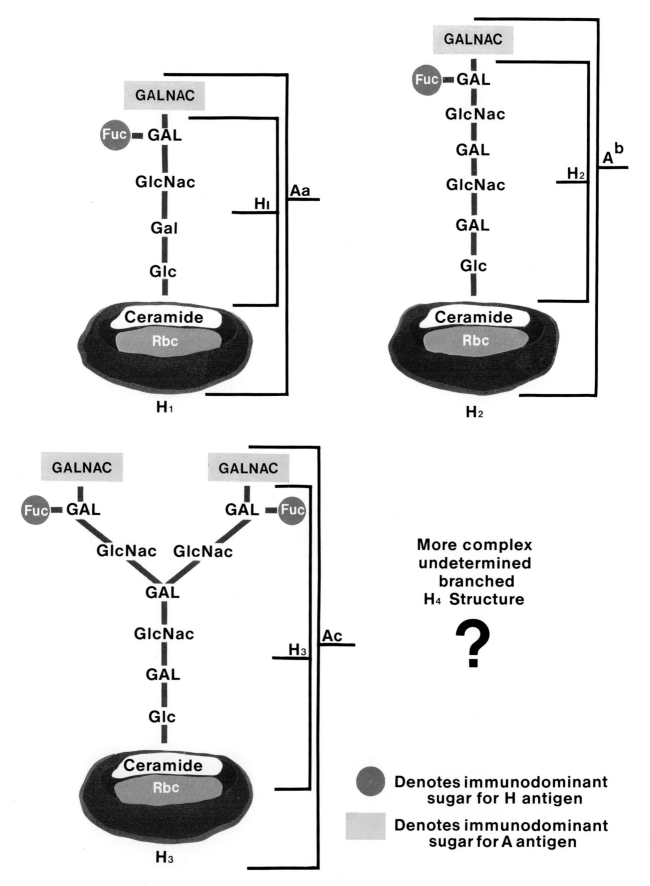

Plate 10. H-active antigenic structures.

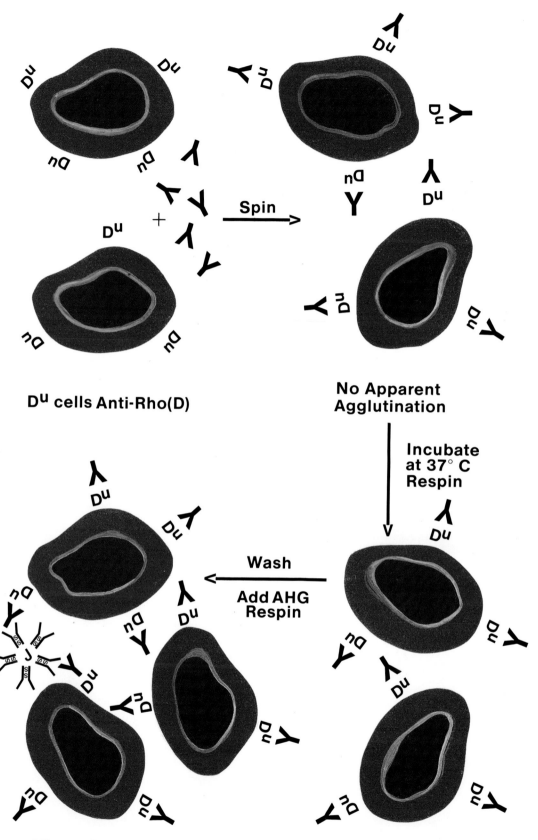

D^u cells Anti-Rho(D)

Spin

No Apparent
Agglutination

Incubate
at 37° C
Respin

Wash
Add AHG
Respin

Visual Agglutination (D^u Positive)

Plate 11.　D^u testing.

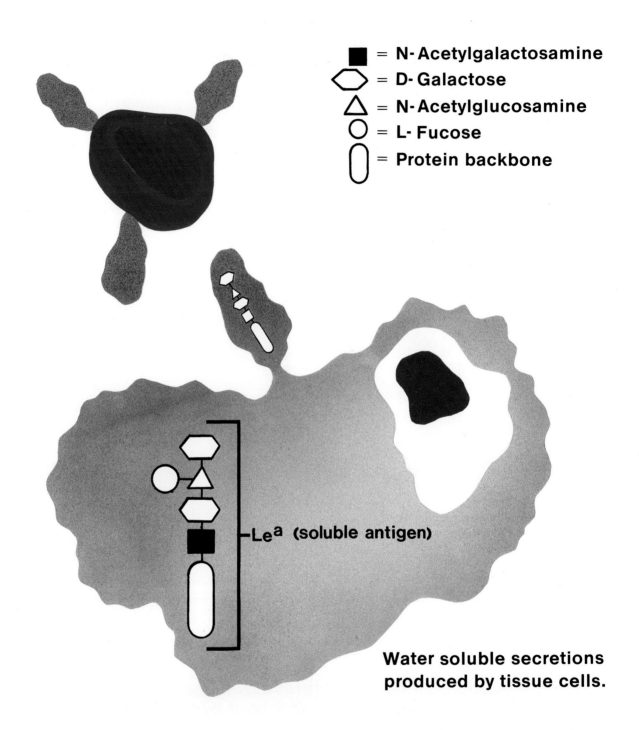

Genotype: **Le Le**
Le le

■ = **N-Acetylgalactosamine**
⬡ = **D-Galactose**
△ = **N-Acetylglucosamine**
○ = **L-Fucose**
▢ = **Protein backbone**

Le^a (soluble antigen)

Water soluble secretions produced by tissue cells.

P.S. $\xrightarrow{\text{Le Le} \atop \text{Le le}}$ $\xrightarrow{\text{fucosyl} \atop \text{transferase}}$ Le^a antigen

Plate 12.   Formation of Le^a substance.

Genotype: Le
H
Se

Water soluble secretions produced by tissue cells

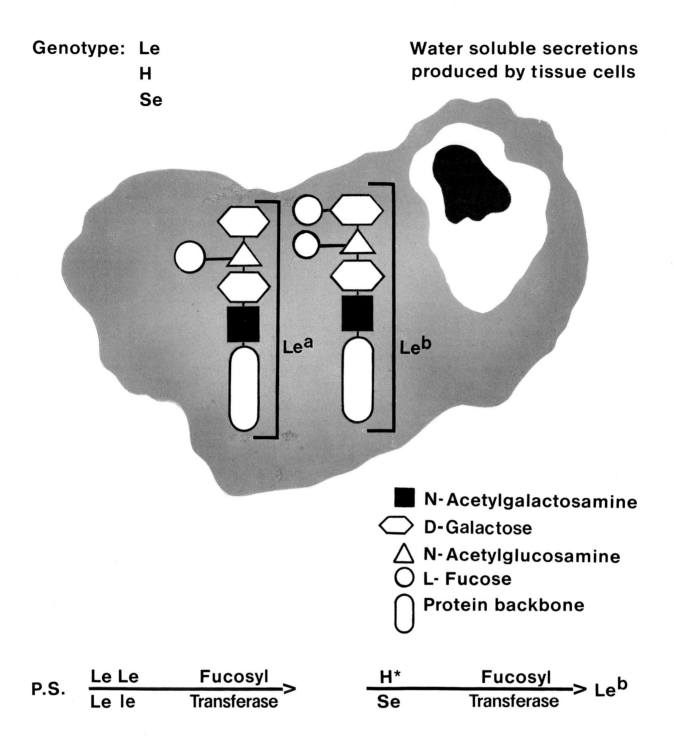

Le^a

Le^b

■ N-Acetylgalactosamine
⬡ D-Galactose
△ N-Acetylglucosamine
○ L-Fucose
▢ Protein backbone

P.S. $\dfrac{\text{Le Le}}{\text{Le le}} \xrightarrow[\text{Transferase}]{\text{Fucosyl}} \qquad \dfrac{\text{H}^*}{\text{Se}} \xrightarrow[\text{Transferase}]{\text{Fucosyl}} \text{Le}^b$

Le gene elicits L-fucosyl transferase which adds L-fucose to form Le^a (see Color Plate 13). H gene activated by Se gene elicits L-fucosyl transferase which adds L-fucose to the last sugar D-galactose forming Le^b.

Plate 13.   Formation of Le^b substance.

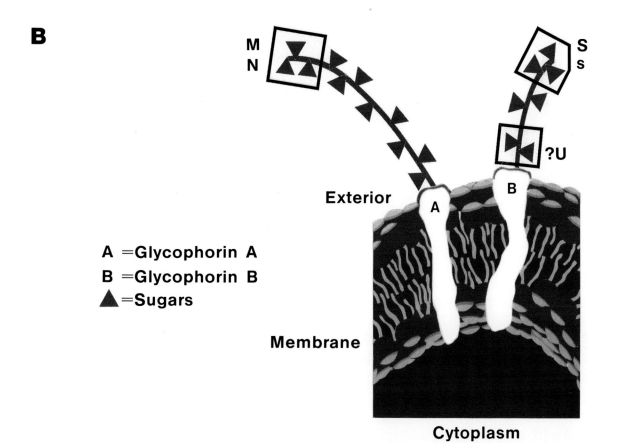

A

Carbohydrates

Exterior

A

C

Singer-Nicholson Model
A: Integral protein
C: Peripheral protein

Cytoplasmic Portion

B

MN

Ss

?U

Exterior

A

B

A =Glycophorin A
B =Glycophorin B
▲ =Sugars

Membrane

Cytoplasm

Plate 14.   Theoretical structure of the MNSs antigens.   (A) Singer-Nicholson model of the red blood cell membrane. (B) MNSsU red cell antigens.

Mother: Rh negative and Immunized
Baby: Rh positive

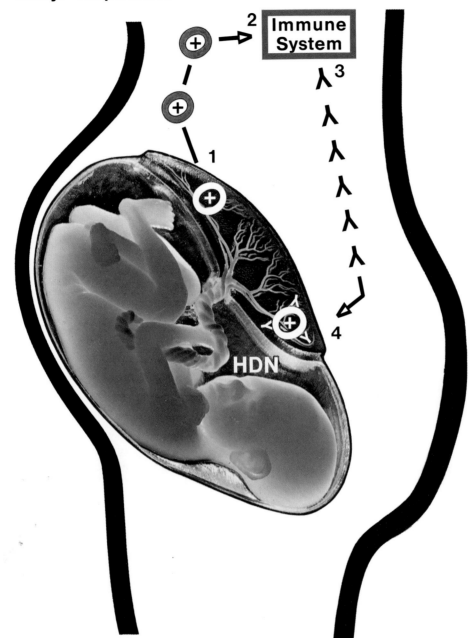

1. Fetal red cells enter maternal circulation at birth.
2. Red cells are recognized by the mother's immune system.
3. Mother is sensitized and produces antibody.
4. Antibody crosses the placenta and causes HDN.

Plate 15. Hemolytic disease of the newborn.

RhIG: Prevention of Antigenic Sensitization

Untreated:

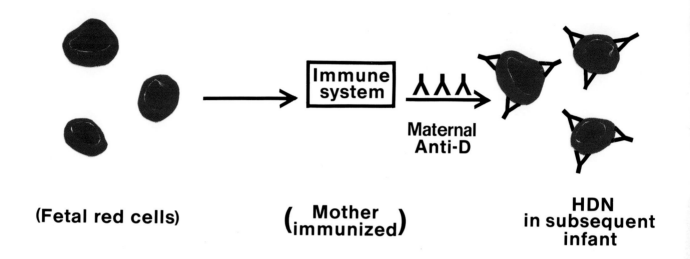

(Fetal red cells)   (Mother immunized)   HDN in subsequent infant

Treated:

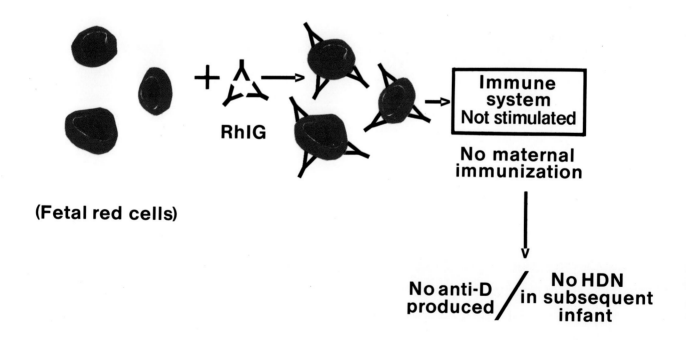

(Fetal red cells)

Plate 16.   Rh immune globulin (RhIG).

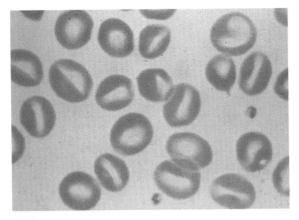

17

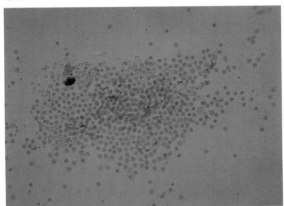

18(A)

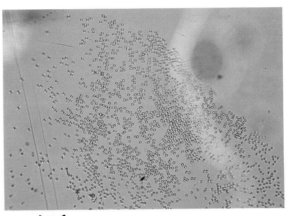

18(B)

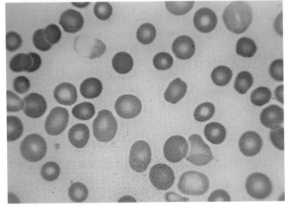

19

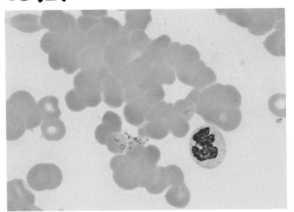

20

Plate 17.   Stomatocytosis (original magnification × 100; enlarged 230%).

Plate 18.   (A) Positive cytotoxic reaction. (B) Negative cytotoxic reaction.

Plate 19.   Autoimmune hemolytic anemia (peripheral blood). (From Pittiglio, DH and Sacher, RS: *Clinical Hematology and Fundamentals of Hemostasis,* FA Davis Company, Philadelphia, 1987, with permission.)

Plate 20.   Cold agglutinin disease (peripheral blood). (From Pittiglio, DH and Sacher, RS: *Clinical Hematology and Fundamentals of Hemostasis.* FA Davis, Philadelphia, 1987, with permission.)

CHAPTER 1

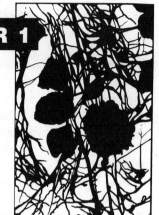

Blood Preservation: Historic Perspectives, Review of Metabolism, and Current Trends

Denise M. Harmening, PhD, MT(ASCP), CLS(NCA)
Chantal Ricaud Harrison, MD
R. Ben Dawson, MD

This chapter is dedicated to the memory of Charles E. Huggins, MD (1929–1990), the pioneer in red cell preservation by freezing and the first to demonstrate adverse effects of transfusion caused by low 2,3-diphosphoglycerate levels.

OBJECTIVES

Upon completion of this chapter, the learner should be able to:

1 List the areas of red cell metabolism that are crucial to normal red cell survival and functions.

2 Describe the chemical composition of the red cell membrane in terms of percentage of lipids, proteins, and carbohydrates.

3 List the two most important red blood cell membrane proteins and describe their function and the characteristics of deformability and permeability.

4 List the various metabolic pathways involved in red cell metabolism, stating the specific function of each one.

5 List the globin chains found in HbA, HbA$_2$, HbF, and glycosylated hemoglobin and their respective concentrations (in percent) found in vivo.

6 Describe hemoglobin function in terms of the oxygen dissociation curve.

7 Define P$_{50}$ and state normal in vivo levels.

8 List the approved preservative solutions and the blood storage time for each.

9 List five areas of blood preservation research.

10 Describe the following terms: red cell freezing, rejuvenation, and additive solutions.

11 State the storage temperature for red cell freezing.

12 List the advantages and disadvantages of red cell freezing.

13 Define autologous transfusion.

14 List the types of blood substitutes.

15 Define stroma-free hemoglobin solution (SFHS).

16 Define perfluorochemicals and their use as a blood substitute.

17 List the advantages and disadvantages of perfluorochemicals.

18 List the three structural zones of the platelet defined by transmission electron microscopy.

19 Describe the metabolism and function of platelets.

20 List the currently licensed storage times and temperatures for platelet concentrates.

Historic Aspects

People have always been fascinated by blood: ancient Egyptians bathed in it, aristocrats drank it, authors and playwrights used it as themes, and modern humanity transfuses it. The road to an efficient, safe, and uncomplicated transfusion technique has been rather difficult, but great progress has been made.

In 1492 blood was taken from three young men and was given to the stricken Pope Innocent VII in the hope of curing him; unfortunately, all four died. Although the outcome of this event was unsatisfactory, it is the first time a blood transfusion was duly recorded in history. The path to the successful transfusions so familiar today is marred by many reported failures, but our physical, spiritual, and emotional fascination with blood is primordial. Why did success elude experimenters for so long?

Clotting was the principal obstacle to overcome. Attempts to find a nontoxic anticoagulant began in 1869 when Braxton Hicks recommended sodium phosphate. This was perhaps the first example of blood preservation research. Karl Landsteiner in 1901 discovered the ABO blood groups and explained the serious reactions that occur in humans as a result of incompatible transfusions. His work, early in the century, won a Nobel prize.

Next came appropriate devices designed for performing the transfusions. Edward E. Lindemann was the first to succeed. He carried out vein-to-vein transfusion of blood by using multiple syringes and a special cannula for puncturing the vein through the skin. However, this time-consuming, complicated procedure required many skilled assistants. It was not until Unger designed his syringe-valve apparatus that transfusions from donor to patient by an unassisted physician became practical.

An unprecedented accomplishment in blood transfusion was achieved in 1914 when Hustin reported the use of sodium citrate and glucose as a diluent and anticoagulant solution for transfusions. Later, in 1915, Lewisohn determined the minimum amount of citrate needed for anticoagulation and demonstrated its nontoxicity in small amounts. Transfusions became more practical and safer for the patient.

The development of preservative solutions to enhance the metabolism of the red cell followed. Glucose was tried as early as 1916 when Rous and Turner introduced a citrate-dextrose solution for the preservation of blood. However, the function of glucose in red cell metabolism was not understood until the 1930s. Therefore, the common practice of using glucose in the preservative solution was delayed.

World War II stimulated blood preservation research because the demand for blood and plasma increased. The pioneer work of Dr. Charles Drew during World War II on developing techniques in blood transfusion and blood preservation led to the establishment of a widespread system of blood banks. In February 1941, Dr. Drew was appointed director of the first American Red Cross Blood Bank at Presbyterian Hospital. The pilot program Dr. Drew established became the model for the national volunteer blood donor program of the American Red Cross.[1] In 1943, Loutit and Mollison of England introduced the formula for the preservative acid-citrate-dextrose (ACD). Efforts in several countries resulted in the landmark publication of the July 1947 issue of the *Journal of Clinical Investigation*, which devoted nearly a dozen papers to blood preservation. Hospitals responded immediately, and in 1947 blood banks were established in many major cities of the United States; subsequently transfusion became commonplace. The daily occurrence of transfusions led to the discovery of numerous blood group systems. Antibody identification surged to the forefront as sophisticated techniques were developed. The interested student can review historic events during World War II in Kendrick's *Blood Program in World War II, Historical Note*.[2] In 1957, Gibson introduced an improved preservative solution, citrate-phosphate-dextrose (CPD), which was less acidic and eventually replaced ACD as the standard preservative used for blood storage.

Frequent transfusions and the massive use of blood soon resulted in new problems, such as circulatory overload. Component therapy has solved these problems. Before, a single unit of whole blood could serve only one patient. With component therapy, however, one unit may be used for multiple transfusions. Today, physicians can select the specific component for their patient's particular needs without risking the inherent hazards of whole blood transfusions. Physicians can transfuse only the required fraction in the concentrated form, without overloading the circulation. Appropriate blood component therapy now provides more effective treatment and more complete use of blood products. Extensive use of blood during this period, coupled with component separation, led to increased comprehension of erythrocyte metabolism and a new awareness of the problems associated with red cell storage. Today approximately 12 million units of packed red cells are transfused into 3.2 million recipients every year in the United States.[3]

Red Cell Biology and Preservation

Three areas of red blood cell (RBC) biology are crucial for normal erythrocyte survival and function: the RBC membrane, hemoglobin structure and function, and cellular metabolism. Defects or problems associated with any of these areas will result in impaired RBC survival. A thorough working knowledge of these areas of RBC physiology will ensure a basic understanding of the various complex erythrocyte functions.

RED CELL MEMBRANE

The red cell membrane represents a semipermeable lipid bilayer supported by a protein meshlike cytoskeleton structure (Fig. 1–1).[4] Phospholipids, the main lipid components of the membrane, are arranged in a bilayer structure comprising the framework in which globular proteins traverse and move. Proteins that extend from the outer surface and span the entire membrane to the inner cytoplasmic side of the RBC are termed "integral" membrane proteins. Beneath the lipid bilayer, a second class of membrane proteins, called "peripheral" proteins, is located and limited to the cytoplasmic surface of the membrane forming the red cell cytoskeleton (Table 1–1).[5] Both proteins and lipids are organized asymmetrically within the red cell membrane.[6] Lipids are not equally distributed in the two layers of the membrane. The external layer is rich in glycolipids and choline phospholipids—namely, sphingomyelin and phosphatidylcholine.[7] The internal cytoplasmic layer of the membrane is rich in phosphatidylserine, phosphatidylethanolamine (known as amino phospholipids), and phosphotidylinositol. The biochemical composition of the red cell membrane is approximately 52 percent protein, 40 percent lipid, and 8 percent carbohydrate.[8]

As mentioned previously, the normal chemical composition and the structural arrangement and molecular interactions of the erythrocyte membrane are crucial to the normal length of red cell survival in circulation of 120 days. In addition, they maintain a critical role in two important RBC characteristics: deformability and permeability.

Deformability

The loss of adenosine triphosphate (ATP) (energy) levels leads to a decrease in the phosphorylation of spectrin and, in turn, a loss of membrane deformability.[9] An accumulation or increase in deposition of membrane calcium also results, causing an increase in membrane rigidity and loss of pliability. These cells are at a marked disadvantage when they pass through the small (3 to 5 μm in diameter) sinusoidal orifices of the spleen, an organ that functions in extravascular sequestration and removal of aged, damaged, or less deformable RBCs or fragments of their membrane.[10] The loss of RBC membrane is exemplified by the for-

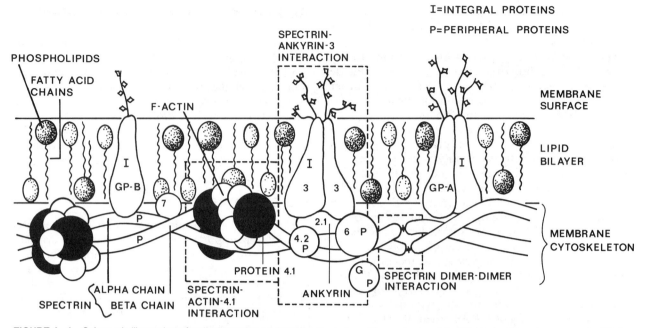

FIGURE 1–1 Schematic illustration of red cell membrane depicting the composition and arrangement of red cell membrane protein. GP-A = glycophorin A; GP-B = glycophorin B; G = globin. Numbers refer to pattern of migration on SDS (sodium, dodecylsulfite) polyacrylamide gel pattern stained with Coomassie brilliant blue. Relations of protein to each other and to lipids are purely hypothetical; however, the positions of the proteins relative to the inside or outside of the lipids bilayer are accurate. Note that proteins are not drawn to scale and that many minor proteins are omitted. (From Harmening,[4] p 4, with permission.)

TABLE 1–1 RED CELL MEMBRANE INTEGRAL AND PERIPHERAL PROTEINS

Integral Proteins	Peripheral Proteins
Glycophorin A	Spectrin
Glycophorin B	Actin (band 5)
Glycophorin C	Ankyrin (band 2.1)
Anion exchange channel protein (band 3)	Bands 4.1 and 4.2
	Band 6

From Wallace and Gibbs,[5] p 12, with permission.

trast, the RBC membrane is relatively impermeable to cations, with a half-time exchange of sodium (Na$^+$) and potassium (K$^+$) of more than 30 hours. It is primarily through the control of the sodium and potassium intracellular concentrations that the RBC maintains its volume and water homeostasis. The erythrocyte intracellular-to-extracellular ratios for sodium and potassium are 1:12 and 25:1, respectively. The passive influx of sodium and potassium is controlled by as many as 300 cationic pumps, which actively transport

mation of "spherocytes" (cells with a reduced surface-to-volume ratio) (Fig. 1–2) and "bite cells," in which the removal of a portion of membrane has left a permanent indentation in the remaining cell membrane (Fig. 1–3). The survival of these forms is also shortened.

Permeability

The RBC membrane is freely permeable to water and anions; chloride (Cl$^-$) and bicarbonate (HCO$_3^-$) traverse the membrane in less than a second. It is speculated that this massive exchange of HCO$_3^-$ and Cl$^-$ ions occurs through a large number of exchange channels formed by the integral membrane protein, band 3, a glycoprotein listed in Table 1–1.[5] In con-

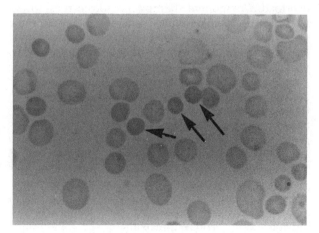

FIGURE 1–2 Spherocytes. (From Harmening,[4] p 7, with permission.)

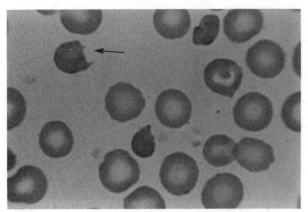

FIGURE 1–3 "Bite" cells. (From Harmening,[4] p 8, with permission.)

sodium out of the cell and potassium into the cell. Like other cationic pumps, these sodium-potassium pumps are energy dependent, requiring ATP. The functional active transport of these particular cations by these cationic pumps also requires the membrane enzyme, sodium-potassium adenosine triphosphatase (ATPase). It is interesting to note that full activation of the sodium-potassium ATPase pumps requires the presence of the RBC membrane aminophospholipid, phosphotidylserine.[11] Similarly, calcium (Ca^{++}) is also actively pumped from the interior of the RBC through the energy-dependent calcium-ATPase cationic pump. Calmodulin, a cytoplasmic calcium-binding protein, is speculated to control these calcium-ATPase pumps, preventing excessive intracellular calcium buildup, which is deleterious to the RBC, resulting in shape changes and loss of deformability. The permeability properties of the RBC membrane, as well as active cation transport, are crucial to preventing colloid osmotic hemolysis and controlling the volume of the red cell. In addition, ATP-depleted cells allow the accumulation of excess intracellular calcium and sodium, followed by potassium and water loss, resulting in a dehydrated, rigid cell subsequently sequestered by the spleen. The energy required for active transport and maintenance of membrane electrochemical gradients is provided by ATP. Any abnormality that increases membrane permeability or alters cationic transport may lead to a decrease in RBC survival.

METABOLIC PATHWAYS

Viability

Red cells generate energy almost exclusively through the breakdown of glucose because the metabolism of the anucleated erythrocyte is more limited than that of other body cells. The adult red cell possesses little ability to metabolize fatty acids and amino acids. Additionally, mature erythrocytes contain no mitochondrial apparatus for oxidative metabolism. The red cell's metabolic pathways are mainly anaerobic, as one expects, because the function of the red cell is to deliver oxygen, not to consume it. Red cell metabolism may be divided among the anaerobic glycolytic pathway and three ancillary pathways that serve to maintain the function of hemoglobin (Fig. 1–4). All of these processes are essential if the erythrocyte is to transport oxygen and to maintain those physical characteristics required for its circulation survival.

Ninety percent of the ATP needed by RBCs is generated by glycolysis, the erythrocyte's main metabolic pathway. Approximately 10 percent of the red cell's ATP is provided by the pentose phosphate pathway, which couples oxidative metabolism with pyridine nucleotide and glutathione reduction. The activity of this pathway increases following increased oxidation of glutathione or retardation of the glycolytic pathway.

When the pentose phosphate pathway is functionally deficient, the amount of reduced glutathione becomes insufficient to neutralize intracellular oxidants. This results in globin denaturation and precipitation as aggregates (Heinz bodies) within the cell. If this process results in sufficient membrane damage, cell destruction occurs.

Such oxidative destruction of the red cells usually occurs as a result of an increased oxidant load with a latent decrease in pathway capacity. It is clear, therefore, that some activity in this pathway is essential for normal function and red cell survival.

The methemoglobin reductase pathway is another important pathway of red cell metabolism. Two methemoglobin reductase systems are important in maintaining hemoglobin in a reduced functional state. Both pathways are dependent on the regeneration of reduced pyridine nucleotides and are referred to as NADH methemoglobin reductase and NADPH methemoglobin reductase. Of the two pathways, there is a physiologic preference of the NADH methemoglobin reductase activity. This pathway is necessary to maintain the heme iron of hemoglobin in the ferrous (Fe^{++}) functional state.

In the absence of the enzyme methemoglobin reductase and the reducing action of the pyridine nucleotide (NAD), methemoglobin, which results from the conversion of the ferrous iron of heme to the ferric form, accumulates. Methemoglobin represents a nonfunctional form of hemoglobin and a loss of oxygen transport capabilities, because the metheme portion cannot combine with oxygen. Normal efficiency of the methemoglobin reductase pathway is exemplified by the fact that usually no greater than 1 percent of methemoglobin exists in the erythrocytes of normal, healthy individuals. A defect in the methemoglobin reductase pathway is, therefore, significant to red cell posttransfusion survival and function.

Another pathway that is crucial to red cell function is the Luebering-Rapoport shunt. This pathway permits the accumulation of another important red cell organic phosphate, 2,3-diphosphoglycerate (2,3-DPG). A large amount of this compound is found in the red cell in a one-to-one molar relationship with hemoglobin, representing approximately 5 mM. The apparent reason for this extraordinary amount of 2,3-

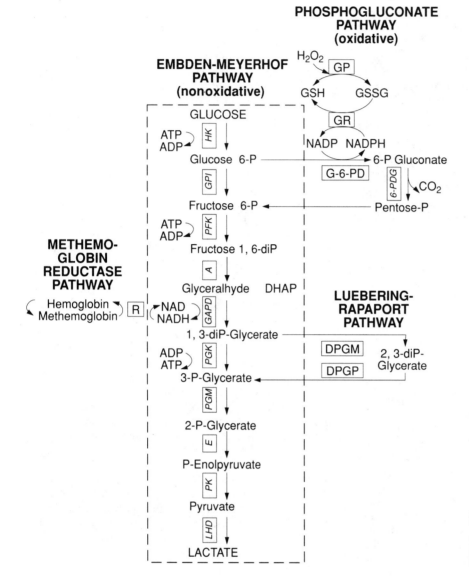

FIGURE 1–4 Pathways of red cell metabolism. (Modified from Hillman, RS and Finch, CA: Red Cell Manual, ed 6. FA Davis, Philadelphia, 1992, p 15, with permission.)

DPG lies in its profound effect on the affinity of hemoglobin for oxygen.

HEMOGLOBIN STRUCTURE AND FUNCTION

Hemoglobin makes up approximately 95 percent of the dry weight of a red cell or approximately 33 percent of its weight by volume.[6] Owing to its multichain structure, hemoglobin, which has a molecular weight of 68,000, is capable of considerable allosteric change as it loads and unloads oxygen. Normal hemoglobin consists of globin (a tetramer of two pairs of polypeptide chains) and four heme groups, each of which contains a protoporphyrin ring plus iron (Fe^{++}).

Hemoglobin Synthesis

Normal hemoglobin production is dependent on three processes:

1. Adequate iron delivery and supply
2. Adequate synthesis of protoporphyrins (the precursor of heme)
3. Adequate globin synthesis

All adult normal hemoglobins are formed as tetramers consisting of two alpha chains plus two (nonalpha) globin chains. Normal adult RBCs contain the following types of hemoglobin:

92 to 95 percent of the hemoglobin is HbA, which consists of two alpha and two beta ($\alpha_2\beta_2$) chains.

3 to 5 percent of the hemoglobin is HbA_{IC} (glycosylated), which consists of α_2(B-NH-glucose)$_2$ chains.

2 to 3 percent of the hemoglobin is HbA_2, which consists of two alpha and two delta ($\alpha_2\delta_2$) chains.

1 to 2 percent of the hemoglobin is fetal hemoglobin (HbF), which consists of two alpha and two gamma ($\alpha_2\gamma_2$) chains.

Each synthesized globin chain links with heme (ferroprotoporphyrin 9) to form hemoglobin, which normally consists of two alpha chains, two beta chains, and four heme groups.

The rate of globin synthesis is directly related to the rate of porphyrin synthesis, and vice versa: protoporphyrin synthesis is reduced when globin synthesis is impaired.

Hemoglobin Function

Hemoglobin's primary function is gas transport: oxygen delivery to the tissues and carbon dioxide (CO_2) excretion. One of the most important controls of hemoglobin affinity for oxygen is the RBC organic phosphate 2,3-DPG. The unloading of oxygen by hemoglobin is accompanied by widening of a space between beta chains and the binding of 2,3-DPG on a mole-for-mole basis, with the formation of anionic salt bridges between the chains. The resulting conformation of the deoxyhemoglobin molecule is known as the tense (T) form, which has a lower affinity for oxygen. When hemoglobin loads oxygen and becomes oxyhemoglobin, the established salt bridges are broken and beta chains are pulled together, expelling 2,3-DPG. This is the relaxed (R) form of the hemoglobin molecule, which has a higher affinity for oxygen.

These allosteric changes that occur as the hemoglobin loads and unloads oxygen, are referred to as the "respiratory movement." The dissociation and binding of oxygen by hemoglobin are not directly proportional to the partial pressure of oxygen (PO_2) in its environment but, instead, exhibit a sigmoid-curve relationship, the hemoglobin-oxygen dissociation curve is depicted in Figure 1–5. The shape of this curve is very important physiologically because it permits a considerable amount of oxygen to be delivered to the tissues with a small drop in oxygen tension. For example, in the environment of the lungs, where the PO_2 (oxygen tension), measured in millimeters of mercury, is nearly 100 mm Hg, the hemoglobin molecule is almost 100 percent saturated with oxygen. As the red cells travel to the tissues where the PO_2 drops to an average 40 mm Hg (mean venous oxygen tension), the hemoglobin saturation drops to approximately 75 percent saturation, releasing approximately 25 percent of the oxygen to the tissues.

This is the normal situation of oxygen delivery at basal metabolic rate. The normal position of the oxygen dissociation curve depends on three different ligands normally found within the red cell: H^+ ions, CO_2, and organic phosphates. Of these three ligands, 2,3-DPG plays the most important physiologic role. The dependence of normal hemoglobin function on 2,3-DPG levels in the red cell has been well documented.[12–14] In situations such as hypoxia, a compensatory "shift to the right" of the hemoglobin-oxygen dissociation curve occurs to alleviate a tissue oxygen deficit (Fig. 1–6). This rightward shift of the curve, mediated by increased levels of 2,3-DPG, re-

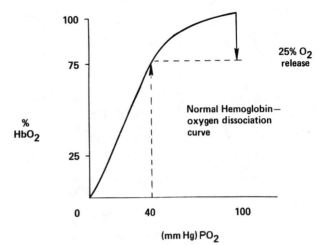

FIGURE 1–5 Hemoglobin-oxygen dissociation curve.

sults in a decrease in hemoglobin's affinity for the oxygen molecule and an increase in oxygen delivery to the tissues. Note in Figure 1–6 that the oxygen saturation of hemoglobin in the environment of the tissues (40 mm Hg PO_2) is now 50 percent; the other 50 percent of the oxygen is being released to the tissues. The RBCs thus have become more efficient in terms of oxygen delivery.

Therefore, a patient who is suffering from an anemia caused by loss of RBCs may be able to compensate by shifting the oxygen dissociation curve to the right, making the RBCs, although few in number, more efficient. Some patients may be able to tolerate anemia better than others because of this compensatory mechanism. A shift to the right may also occur in response to acidosis or a rise in body temperature. The shift to the right of the hemoglobin-oxygen dissociation curve is only one way in which patients may compensate for various types of hypoxia. Other ways include an increase in total cardiac output and an increase in erythropoiesis.

A "shift to the left" of the hemoglobin-oxygen dissociation curve results, conversely, in an increase in

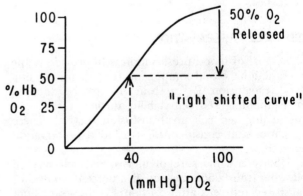

FIGURE 1–6 "Shift to the right" of the hemoglobin-oxygen dissociation curve.

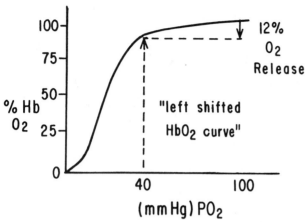

FIGURE 1-7 "Shift to the left" of the hemoglobin-oxygen dissociation curve.

hemoglobin-oxygen affinity and a decrease in oxygen delivery to the tissues (Fig. 1-7). With such a dissociation curve, RBCs are much less efficient because only 12 percent of the oxygen can be released to the tissues. Among the conditions that can shift the oxygen dissociation curve to the left are alkalosis; increased quantities of abnormal hemoglobins, such as methemoglobin and carboxyhemoglobin; increased quantities of hemoglobin F; or multiple transfusions of 2,3-DPG-depleted stored blood (attesting to the importance of 2,3-DPG in oxygen release).

Hemoglobin-oxygen affinity can also be expressed by P_{50} values, which designate the PO_2 at which hemoglobin is 50 percent saturated with oxygen under standard in vitro conditions of temperature and pH. The P_{50} of normal blood is 26 to 30 mm Hg. An increase in P_{50} represents a decrease in hemoglobin-oxygen affinity, or a shift to the right of the oxygen dissociation curve. A decrease in P_{50} represents an increase in hemoglobin-oxygen affinity, or a shift to the left of the oxygen dissociation curve. In addition to the reasons listed previously for shifts in the curve, inherited abnormalities of the hemoglobin molecule can result in either situation; these abnormalities are described by the P_{50} measurements. Abnormalities in hemoglobin structure or function can therefore have profound effects on the ability of the RBCs to provide oxygen to the tissues.

RED CELL PRESERVATION

The goal of blood preservation is to provide viable and functional blood components for patients needing blood transfusion. Research in this area has focused on maintaining red cell viability during storage and lengthening red cell posttransfusion survival. These are paramount considerations in blood preservation research.

Viability is a measure of in vivo red cell survival following transfusion. Seventy-five percent survival of transfused red cells after 24 hours is the lower limit for a successful transfusion. As storage time increases, red cell viability decreases. As a result, blood has always been stored between 1°C and 6°C with an assigned limited, predetermined shelf life.

The loss of red cell viability has been correlated with the "lesion of storage," which is associated with various biochemical changes. These changes include a decrease in pH, a buildup of lactic acid, a decrease in glucose consumption, a decrease in ATP levels, and a loss of red cell function, expressed as a shift to the left of the hemoglobin-oxygen dissociation curve or an increase in hemoglobin-oxygen affinity.

Viability is usually associated with both red cell ATP levels and membrane integrity. If viability can be maintained, the storage time of blood can be increased and the 70 percent posttransfusion survival of red cells ensured. Survival time of transfused red cells has been shown to correlate with ATP levels.[15] When ATP levels fall below approximately 1.5 μmol per gram of hemoglobin, viability is markedly impaired. In fact, Dern et al.[15] have established 1.5 μmol/g hemoglobin as the minimum acceptable ATP level for 70 percent posttransfusion survival of red cells stored in ACD and CPD preservatives. Therefore, any preservative that does not maintain ATP levels higher than approximately 1.5 μmol/g hemoglobin is unlikely to maintain adequate viability of stored red cells. However, many investigators feel that the relationship between ATP level and red cell survival is poorly defined and does not correlate well above and below certain established levels. A linear relationship between red cell survivals and ATP levels exists *only* in a certain range of values. Adequate ATP levels are necessary for maintenance of (1) red cell membrane integrity and deformability; (2) red cell volume, by sustaining the Na^+/K^+ ATPase pumps; (3) hemoglobin function; (4) adequate amounts of red cell–reduced pyridine nucleotides; and (5) red cell plasma-lipid exchange.

In 1954, Valtis and Kennedy[16] found that hemoglobin oxygen affinity increases during blood storage. The relationship of oxygen affinity to 2,3-DPG remained unclear until the works of Chanutin and Curnish[14] and Benesch and Benesch.[13] These investigators defined linear inverse relationship between 2,3-DPG concentrations and hemoglobin oxygen affinity.[14] As 2,3-DPG levels decrease, hemoglobin oxygen affinity increases. Akerblom and Kreuger[17] and Bunn et al.[18] confirmed these findings as they demonstrated that the increase in oxygen hemoglobin affinity correlates well with a decrease in 2,3-DPG concentrations during storage. A change of 0.43 mol/ml RBC of 2,3-DPG produces a change of 1 mm Hg in the P_{50}.[19] High concentrations of 2,3-DPG stabilize the hemoglobin molecule in the deoxygenated form, thereby decreasing hemoglobin affinity for oxygen and shifting the O_2 curve to the right.

DPG-depleted red cells may have an impaired capacity to deliver oxygen to the tissues because low 2,3-DPG levels profoundly influence the oxygen dissociation curve of hemoglobin. The rate of restoration of 2,3-DPG is influenced by the acid-base status of the recipient, phosphorus metabolism, and the degree of anemia.

Blood storage, however, is associated with low 2,3-DPG levels and a shift to the left of the hemoglobin-oxygen dissociation curve. A loss of red cell function, oxygen delivery to tissues, is also associated with this. Therefore, an effective blood preservative must be capable of maintaining both viability reflected in ATP levels and hemoglobin function reflected in 2,3-DPG levels.

APPROVED PRESERVATIVE SOLUTIONS

Both ACD and CPD are approved preservative solutions (Table 1–2). Owing to the lower pH in ACD preservative, most of the 2,3-DPG is lost early in the first week of storage. Therefore, a substitute preservative, CPD, came into widespread use in the United States because it was superior for preserving this organic phosphate. This effect is due to a higher pH (Table 1–3). Even in CPD, red cells become low in 2,3-DPG by the 2nd week. Subsequent studies led to the addition of various chemicals along with the currently approved anticoagulant CPD in pursuit of a means to stimulate glycolysis.[18,19]

One of the chemicals, adenine, was approved for addition to CPD by the Food and Drug Administration (FDA) in August 1978. The incorporation of adenine (CPDA-1) into blood storage seems to increase adenosine diphosphate (ADP) levels, thereby driving glycolysis toward the synthesis of ATP. CPDA-1 contains 0.25 mM of adenine plus 25 percent more glucose than is required in CPD (Table 1–3). Adenine-supplemented blood can be stored on the shelf for 35 days. The majority of blood now collected in the United States is drawn into CPDA-1 preservative solution. CPDA-2, containing 0.5 mM of adenine plus 75 percent more glucose than CPD, or 1.4 times more glucose than CPDA-1, was under consideration for future use but is currently not a licensed anticoagulant. However, blood stored in CPDA-1 also becomes depleted of 2,3-DPG by the 2nd week of storage.

TABLE 1–2 **APPROVED PRESERVATIVES**

Name	Abbreviation	Storage Time (d)
Acid-citrate-dextrose	ACD	21
Citrate-phosphate-dextrose	CPD	21
	CPDA-1	35
Adsol (AS-1) [Fenwal Laboratories]	AS-1	42
Nutricel (AS-2) [Cutter Biological]	AS-2	35
Nutricel (AS-3) [Cutter Biological]	AS-3	42

The reported pathophysiologic effects of the transfusion of red blood cells with low 2,3-DPG levels and increased affinity for oxygen include an increase in cardiac output or a decrease in mixed venous PO_2 tension, or a combination of these. The physiologic importance of these effects is *not* easily demonstrated. This is a complex mechanism, and there are numerous variables involved that are beyond the scope of this text.

Stored red cells do regain the ability to synthesize 2,3-DPG after transfusion, but levels necessary for optimal hemoglobin oxygen delivery are not reached immediately. It requires approximately 24 hours to restore normal levels of DPG after transfusion.[20] The 2,3-DPG concentrations after transfusion have been reported to reach normal levels as early as 6 hours posttransfusion.[21] Most of these studies have been performed on normal, healthy individuals. However, evidence suggests that in the transfused subject, whose capacity is limited by an underlying physiologic disturbance, even a brief period of altered oxygen hemoglobin affinity is of great significance.[22]

It is quite clear now that 2,3-DPG levels in transfused blood are important in certain clinical conditions. Several animal studies demonstrate significantly increased mortality associated with transfusing blood that is low in 2,3-DPG levels in individuals with persistent anemia, hypotension, hypoxia, and cardiac and

TABLE 1–3 **COMPARISON OF THE COMPOSITION OF ACID-CITRATE-DEXTROSE (ACD) AND PHOSPHATE-DEXTROSE (CPD) PRESERVATIVES**

	ACD	CPD	CPDA-1	CPDA-2
Tri-sodium citrate (g)	22.0	26.30	26.30	26.30
Citric acid (g)	8.0	3.27	3.27	3.27
Dextrose (g)	24.5	25.50	31.90	34.70
Monobasic sodium phosphate (g)	—	2.22	2.22	2.22
Adenine (g)	—	—	0.27	0.54
Water (ml)	1000	1000	1000	1000
Volume/100 ml blood (ml)	15	14	14	14
Approximate volume of preservative solution/bag (ml)	67.5	63.0	63.0	63.0
Initial pH of solution*	5.0	5.6	5.6	5.6
pH of blood on initial day drawn into storage bag*	7.0	7.2	7.4	7.3
pH of blood at day 28*	6.7	6.8	6.8	6.8
pH of blood at day 35*	—	—	6.8	6.8

*Indicates measurement at room temperature.

hemorrhagic shock. Human studies demonstrate that myocardial function improves following transfusion of blood with high 2,3-DPG levels during cardiovascular surgery.[23]

Several investigators suggest that the patient in shock who is transfused with 2,3-DPG–depleted erythrocytes may have already strained the compensatory mechanisms to their limits.[24] Perhaps for this type of patient the poor oxygen delivery capacity of 2,3-DPG–depleted cells makes a significant difference in recovery and survival.

It is apparent that factors other than ATP levels may limit the viability of transfused red cells. One of these factors is the plastic material used for the storage container. The plastic must be sufficiently permeable to carbon dioxide in order to maintain higher pH levels during storage. Glass storage containers are a matter of history in the United States. Currently all blood is stored in polyvinyl chloride (PVC) plastic bags. Another problem associated with PVC bags is the plasticizer diethylhepyl phthalate (DEHP), which is used in the manufacture of the bags. It has been found to leach into the blood from the plastic into the lipids of the plasma and cell membranes during storage. The accumulation of excessive amounts of acid from glucose use, even at low storage temperatures, is also a major problem in liquid preservation of red cells. Research, therefore, has been focused on the development of an improved plastic blood bag as well as better preservative solutions. In addition to blood preservation problems, adverse effects and risks associated with blood transfusion have created concern and caution among clinicians when determining the need for blood and blood components (see Chapter 18).

Current Trends in Blood Preservation Research

Research in blood preservation has developed in five directions: (1) chemical incorporation and additive solutions, (2) rejuvenation studies, (3) red cell freezing, (4) blood substitutes, and (5) the use of solid buffers.

CHEMICAL INCORPORATION AND ADDITIVE SOLUTIONS

Numerous chemical additives, after incorporation into stored blood, have been assessed for their ability to maintain the essential organic phosphates. Purine nucleosides were the first group to be evaluated, with adenosine the first substance investigated. These findings led to a more practical method for maintaining ATP levels: the addition of adenine to the preservative media.

In addition to glucose, other alternative sugars, such as mannose and fructose, have been examined. All three sugars share equal ability to sustain ATP levels during storage.[21]

Dihydroxyacetone (DHA) is a chemical used to maintain the other important organic phosphate in the red cell, 2,3-DPG. DHA enters directly into the glycolytic pathway as a three-carbon sugar. Red cells are able to metabolize DHA at a rate approximately equal to that at which glucose is metabolized. Dihydroxyacetone has also been shown experimentally to be essentially nontoxic. When added to the currently approved anticoagulants, DHA markedly enhances 2,3-DPG maintenance during red cell storage.[21]

Selected chemicals incorporated into the preservative medium can alter red cell metabolism, modifying the levels of various intermediates within the cell without directly being metabolized by the red cell. These modifiers include ascorbic acid, ascorbate-2-phosphate, and pyruvate.[21] Each of these chemicals, in combination with other additives, has been reported to maintain 2,3-DPG levels. However, research on ascorbate has demonstrated it to be a result of contamination by oxalate, which is nephrotoxic; therefore, it is no longer considered a potential additive to the preservative solution. Modifiers alone in the preservative medium produce only slight improvement. When used, however, in combination with other chemicals to improve 2,3-DPG levels, these mixtures may rapidly deplete red cell ATP.

Traditional anticoagulants and preservatives were developed and put into use when whole blood was the major blood product. With the advent of component therapy, red cell concentrate usage increased in the 1970s and several problems arose. Because approximately 40 percent of adenine and glucose present in standard anticoagulants is removed in the preparation of red cell concentrates, a decrease in viability was seen, particularly in the last 2 weeks of storage.[25,26] Red cell concentrates devoid of plasma were also more viscous and difficult to infuse in emergency situations.

In an effort to overcome these problems, blood centers began monitoring the hematocrits of their red cell units. In general, red cell concentrates were prepared with hematocrits of less than 80 percent to allow adequate plasma to remain for red cell nourishment and improved flow properties. This in turn resulted in lower plasma yields, affecting fresh frozen plasma and cryoprecipitate production as well as decreasing revenue from salvage plasma.

While blood centers in the United States were improving the quality of red cell concentrates by adjusting the hematocrit, a new additive system concept was developed by Lovric[27] in Australia and by Hogman et al.[28] in Sweden. This new blood collection system employed a primary bag containing standard anticoagulant and an accessory, or satellite, bag containing an additional nutrient solution. After the plasma is removed from a unit of whole blood, the additive solution is added to the cells, thus providing nutrients for improved viability.

Additive systems were routinely used in Sweden (Hogman) and in Australia (Lovric) before their introduction in the United States. In general, the additive solutions employed in the systems were composed of standard ingredients used intravenously: saline, dextrose, and adenine. The systems described by Hogman and Lovric differ only slightly in their approach. Hogman's system uses the standard CPD anticoagulant in the primary bag with an additive solution containing saline, adenine, and glucose (SAG). This system was modified further with the addition of mannitol (SAGM), which protected against spontaneous storage hemolysis.[29] Lovric doubled the dextrose concentration in the primary anticoagulant (CP2D) and used it in connection with an additive solution composed of saline, adenine, glucose, trisodium citrate, citric acid, and sodium phosphate.[27]

Based on these earlier formulations, two additive solutions were licensed in the United States in 1983: (1) Adsol (AS-1) (Fenwal Laboratories) was originally approved for 49 days of storage, and (2) Nutricel (AS-2) (Cutter Biological) was approved for 35 days of storage. Shortly afterward, Cutter Biological developed Nutricel (AS-3), which employs CP2D for the primary bag anticoagulant-preservative and 100 ml of buffered adenine glucose (AS-3) solution for RBC viability. This additive solution was approved for 42 days of storage. Both AS-1 and AS-3 are *currently* approved for 42 days.

Adsol (AS-1) (Fenwal Laboratories) solution contains buffered adenine, glucose, and mannitol to retard hemolysis. It is coupled with CPD as the primary bag anticoagulant. The formulations for each of these additive solutions appear in Table 1–4.[30,31]

In clinical trials, conflicting data regarding red cell survivals on Adsol-stored red cells resulted in the FDA convening a workshop on Adsol and other additive solutions in 1985. The consensus of the FDA Advisory Panel resulted in (1) changing the approval of Adsol from 49 days to 42 days, which is the storage limit for all additive solutions in the United States; and (2) raising the minimum average acceptable survival requirements for additive solutions from 70 percent to 75 percent. In clinical studies, red cells stored for 42 days in AS-3 or AS-1 demonstrated a mean posttransfusion survival greater than 75 percent.

Tables 1–5 and 1–6 show the mean results of in vitro testing and in vivo survival studies, respectively.[29,32] Poststorage survival rates of greater than 80 percent were demonstrated, safely above the minimum 75 percent level required, with less than 1 percent hemolysis. Additive system red cells are indicated

for use in the same patient population receiving standard red cell transfusions.

None of the additive solutions maintain 2,3-DPG, and one should be aware of the metabolic load the patient must handle in the blood stored in these additive solutions (see Table 1–5). Therefore, blood stored in additive solutions is *not* routinely given to newborn infants and should be evaluated in light of the patient's underlying condition.

With the ability to pack red cells to a higher hemocrit (85 to 90 percent), greater amounts of plasma may be harvested for use in the preparation of other blood components, or for salvage plasma. Saline in the additive solution also dilutes packed red cells to a transfusion-ready concentration. This eliminates the need for predilution and provides a product that flows rapidly during transfusion.

A further modification of the additive system was licensed in the United States; namely, the Leukotrap Red Cell Storage System (Cutter Biological) provides a means of producing and storing leukopoor red cells (Fig. 1–8).[33] Patterned after the circle pack developed by Lovric, the system contains an in-line leukocyte filter between the primary and additive bags. After removing plasma from a unit of whole blood, the additive solution is added to the red cells by passing it through the filter, thereby priming it. AS-3 red cells are then hung in an inverted position and passed through the filter, which renders them leukopoor. The Leukotrap system effectively removes 95 percent of the leukocytes while recovering 90 percent of the red cells. There is no microaggregate formation and the cells may be stored for 42 days. Such a product allows

TABLE 1–5 **ADDITIVE RED CELLS: IN VITRO PROPERTIES**

	AS-3	AS-1	CPDA-1
Storage period (d)	42.0	42.00	35.00
Hemolysis (%)	0.7	0.24	0.90
ATP μmol/g Hb	2.9	3.24	2.20
% of initial	67.0	69.00	53.00
2,3-DPG μmol/g Hb	0.9	0.65	0.54
% of day 0	6.0	6.00	5.00
Supernatant potassium (mEq/l)	46.0	46.00	36.00
Supernatant sodium (mEq/l)	121.0	123.00	104.00
Supernatant glucose (mg/dl)	522.0	604.00	97.00
pH	6.7	6.34	6.60

TABLE 1–4 **ADDITIVE SOLUTIONS**

	Lovric	SAGM	AS-1	AS-2	AS-3
Sodium chloride (mg)	718	880	900	718	718
Adenine (mg)	6.75	17	27	17	30
Dextrose	360 mg	990 mg	2.2 g	396 mg	1.1 g
Mannitol (mg)	—	525	750	—	—
Citric acid (mg)	42	—	—	42	42
Sodium citrate (mg)	588	—	—	588	—
Na$_2$HPO$_4$ (mg)	224	—	—	285	285

TABLE 1–6 **ADDITIVE RED CELLS: IN VIVO RED CELL SURVIVAL STUDIES**

	CPDA-1	AS-2	AS-1	AS-3
Storage period (d)	35.00	35.00	42.00	42.0
Storage hematocrit (%)	75–80	85.30	80.00	82.4
Samples (n)	19.00	19.00	10.00	9.0
24-hour survival* (%)	71.40	76.30	83.00	85.1
ATP (% initial)	45.70	63.00	62.00	60.5
Hemolysis (%)	0.60	0.58	0.32	0.7

*Survival studies reported are from selected investigators and do *not* include an average of all reported survivals.

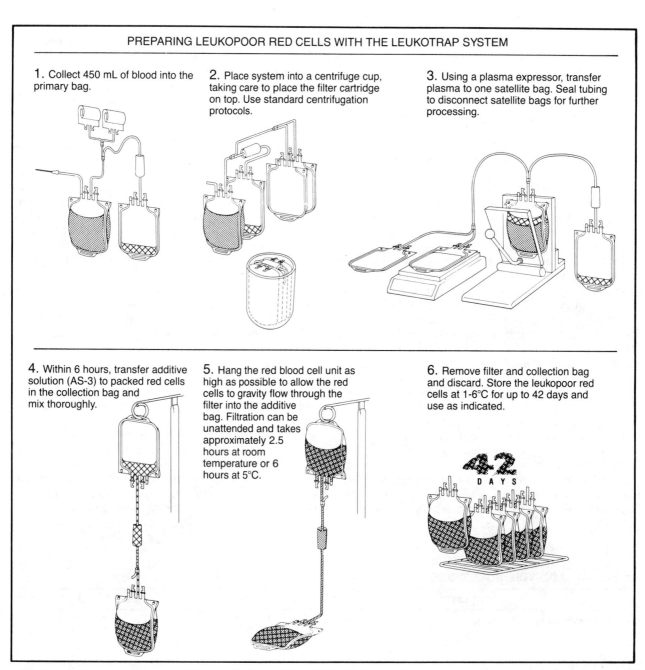

PREPARING LEUKOPOOR RED CELLS WITH THE LEUKOTRAP SYSTEM

1. Collect 450 mL of blood into the primary bag.

2. Place system into a centrifuge cup, taking care to place the filter cartridge on top. Use standard centrifugation protocols.

3. Using a plasma expressor, transfer plasma to one satellite bag. Seal tubing to disconnect satellite bags for further processing.

4. Within 6 hours, transfer additive solution (AS-3) to packed red cells in the collection bag and mix thoroughly.

5. Hang the red blood cell unit as high as possible to allow the red cells to gravity flow through the filter into the additive bag. Filtration can be unattended and takes approximately 2.5 hours at room temperature or 6 hours at 5°C.

6. Remove filter and collection bag and discard. Store the leukopoor red cells at 1-6°C for up to 42 days and use as indicated.

FIGURE 1–8 Preparing leukopoor red cells with the Leukotrap Red Cell Storage System. (Courtesy of Cutter Biological, Berkeley, California.)

for an inventory of leukopoor red cells to be available to reduce or prevent febrile transfusion reactions.

Formerly, the most commonly used methods for preparing "leukocyte-poor" red cells included the inverted spin procedure, or washing with automated equipment (see Chapter 10). However, the improved high-performance leukocyte adsorption filters developed in recent years can effectively remove 95 percent of the leukocytes in the original unit, although the filters do vary widely in the number of residual leukocytes in the product.

REJUVENATION STUDIES

Solutions containing phosphate, inosine, glucose, pyruvate, and adenine (PIGPA), incubated with outdated erythrocytes, can regenerate both ATP and DPG levels. Valeri[34] and coworkers have been the forerunners in these rejuvenation studies on outdated blood. Subsequent investigations have led to the removal of glucose from the original mixture, and the resulting solution is designated PIPA.[34] Generally, outdated blood can be rejuvenated by incubation for 1 to 4 hours at 37°C with these solutions. The red cells are washed before transfusion to remove the rejuvenation mixture and deleterious amounts of extracellular potassium. Because the blood bag has been open for the washing procedure, usually by mechanical devices, federal regulations require the unit to be used within 24 hours to minimize the risk of bacterial contamination. FRES, another rejuvenation solution, which was approved and sold by Fenwall Laboratories, contains inosine, pyruvate, and phosphate. This solution was used primarily to regenerate ATP and 2,3-DPG levels before freezing red cells. However, because of low market demand, FRES is no longer currently available for sale. A new approach to rejuvenation of ATP and 2,3-DPG levels is through the use of an acidic solution of phosphoenolpyruvate (PEP), which can cross the RBC membrane at a pH less than 6.5 after incubation with washed red cells at 37°C.[35] The practicality and efficiency of these solutions in routine blood banking are debatable. The procedures are time-consuming and require meticulous manipulation. Red cell rejuvenation procedures are currently reserved for use in salvaging rare or type O units that are close to the outdating period. PIPA is licensed and available (PIPA Laboratories, Inc., 4196 Washington Street, Boston, Massachusetts).

RED CELL FREEZING

Red blood cells stored by conventional methods have a shelf life of 21 to 35 days, depending on the preservative solution employed in the collection bag, or of 42 days using an additive solution. This storage period is usually quite satisfactory for the routine storage of bank blood. There are, however, occasions when a much longer shelf life is desirable and even necessary. Development of the technology for freezing

RBCs without subsequently hemolyzing them upon thawing has fulfilled this need and has also shown other advantages beyond long-term storage.

The procedure for freezing a unit of packed red cells is simple. Basically, it involves the addition of a cryoprotective agent to the red cells that are less than 6 days old. Glycerol is used most commonly and is added to the red cells slowly with vigorous shaking, thereby enabling the glycerol to permeate the red cells. The cells are then rapidly frozen and stored in a freezer. The usual storage temperature is below −65°C, although storage (and freezing) temperature depends on the concentration of glycerol used.

Transfusion of frozen cells must be preceded by a deglycerolization process, otherwise the thawed cells would hemolyze in vivo. Removal of glycerol is achieved by systematically replacing the cryoprotectant with decreasing concentrations of saline. The usual protocol involves washing with 12 percent saline, followed by 1.6 percent saline, with a final wash in normal saline.[36] A cell-washing system, such as those manufactured by COBE or Haemonetics, is used in the deglycerolizing process.

The final cell product, resuspended in the saline used for the last wash sequence, is used in transfusion. Excessive hemolysis is monitored by noting the hemoglobin concentration of the wash supernatant. Osmolality of the unit should also be monitored to ensure adequate deglycerolization. Because the unit of blood is entered to incorporate the glycerol (before freezing) or the saline solutions (for deglycerolization), the outdating period of thawed red cells is 24 hours. However, a sterile docking device developed by DuPont Corporation may lead to a method of sterile deglycerolization and possible extended storage at 4°C using an additive solution.

Advantages

Frozen red cells provide a method for long-term storage of blood. Currently, the FDA licenses frozen red cells for a period of 10 years from the date of freezing; that is, frozen red cells may be stored up to 10 years before thawing and transfusion. Once thawed, these cells demonstrate function and viability near those of fresh blood. Experience has shown that 10-year storage periods do not adversely affect viability and function. In fact, very rare blood types, such as Bombay or Tj(a-), have been transfused successfully during this storage period. These products are no longer licensed blood products, but to the patient with a very rare blood type they may be lifesaving. Hemolysis during the washing procedure must be closely examined before issuing these rare cells.

Studies have also shown that frozen-thawed red cells have several other advantages.[35] The final red cell product has very low quantities of residual leukocytes and platelets, often 1 to 5 percent of the original quantity. The washing procedure also removes significant amounts of plasma proteins. In accordance with these observations, deglycerolized red cells are often the product of choice for patients with histories of severe febrile or allergic transfusion reactions.

Disadvantages

The major disadvantages of red cell freezing are twofold: (1) the preparation of these red cells for both freezing and thawing is a time-consuming process; and (2) the cost of equipment, materials, and time of the technologist greatly inflates the cost of the product to the potential recipient.

These disadvantages, however, should be weighed against the potential benefits to the patient. Table 1–7 summarizes the advantages and disadvantages of red cell freezing.

Autologous Transfusion

Finally, autologous transfusion is another area in which red cell freezing allows an individual to donate blood for one's own (autologous) use in meeting transfusion needs (see Chapter 16). This "open-ended" autologous blood storage is usually reserved for a small percentage of patients who have a history of antibody problems and incompatibility with the general donor population. An overall recommendation of 5 units is considered a useful amount of blood that does not interfere with problems related to having enough freezer space.[36]

The use of autologous transfusion is now routine in many facilities because of the public fear of transfusion-transmitted acquired immunodeficiency syndrome (AIDS) (see Chapter 19). However, this "close-ended" autologous blood storage is usually reserved for patients undergoing elective surgery or complicated surgeries with predictable blood usage that has been defined for a predetermined time in the future, usually a 4- to 6-week lead time prior to surgery and a minimum hematocrit. Red cell freezing is not routinely used in this instance and a maximum number of 2 to 3 units is stipulated.[36] These patients are usually not expected to encounter any compatibility problems because they are being transfused with their own red cells. The use of autologous transfusion eliminates the possibility of transfusion-transmitted diseases (TTDs) such as AIDS, hepatitis, and alloimmunization to red cells, white cells, and plasma proteins.

TABLE 1–8 ADVANTAGES AND DISADVANTAGES OF STROMA-FREE HEMOGLOBIN SOLUTIONS

Advantages	Disadvantages
Long shelf life	Short intravascular half-life
Very stable	Toxicity
No antigenicity	High O_2 affinity
No requirement for blood-typing procedures	High oncotic effect

BLOOD SUBSTITUTES

Another area of blood research deals with the development of blood substitutes such as stroma-free hemoglobin solution (SFHS), the perfluorochemicals (PFCs), and hemoglobin encapsulation. A common feature among all of these products is their ability to carry oxygen in the absence of intact red cells. Advantages and disadvantages of blood substitutes are presented in Tables 1–8 and 1–9.

Despite more than 25 years of research for acceptable blood substitutes, an alternative to a unit of red cells is still not approved for human use. Originally developed to be used in trauma situations such as accidents, battlefield injuries, and surgery, blood substitutes have fallen short of meeting requirements for this application. Owing to major complicating side effects, blood substitutes are still not in use today, although four companies are in phase I of their clinical trials, and at least four other companies have products in the preclinical stages of development. Fluosol is currently approved by the FDA for use in percutaneous transluminal coronary angioplasty (PTCA) on patients with a high risk of ischemic complications.

Blood substitutes, however, are now demonstrating promise for other applications such as elective surgery, stroke, heart attack, septic shock, cancer therapy, and sickle cell anemia. One type of elective surgical procedure now being considered is acute normovolemic hemodilution (ANH). This procedure may be used in normal healthy patients to reduce the hematocrit before surgery by removing the patient's blood and replacing fluids. Surgery is then performed, and the patient's blood previously drawn is used if needed during the surgery, or returned to the patient at the end of surgery. During this process of ANH, the hematocrits can be safely reduced to approximately 25 percent and no long-term planning is required. The

TABLE 1–7 ADVANTAGES AND DISADVANTAGES OF RED CELL FREEZING

Advantages	Disadvantages
Long-term storage (10 years)	A time-consuming process
Maintenance of red cell viability and function	Cost of equipment and materials
Low residual leukocytes and platelets	Storage requirements (−65°C)
Removal of significant amounts of plasma proteins	Cost of product

TABLE 1–9 ADVANTAGES AND DISADVANTAGES OF PERFLUOROCHEMICALS

Advantages	Disadvantages
Biologic inertness	Adverse clinical effects
Lack of immunogenicity	High O_2 affinity
Easily synthesized	Retention in tissues
	Requirement for O_2 administration when infused
	Deep-freeze storage temperatures

majority of surgical patients may be candidates for this procedure, which can reduce the need for the 2 or 3 units of blood commonly used in most surgeries. Blood substitutes are ideal for this type of hemodilution in elective surgery by providing a product with no risk of TTDs and by reducing some of the demand on the blood supply.

Stroma-Free Hemoglobin Solution

Stroma-free hemoglobin solution (SFHS) has been considered for use as a medium to carry oxygen for many years.[37] These solutions are prepared by hemolyzing outdated red blood cells and removing all of the contaminating stroma, which is quite toxic to the kidney. These solutions have several shortcomings. One is their short intravascular persistence. Although *not* toxic to the kidney, SFHS is very quickly eliminated in the urine. The intravascular half-life of SFHS is approximately 2 to 4 hours.[38]

Another factor that poses problems is the high oxygen affinity of native SFHS. The hemoglobin-oxygen dissociation curve shows a shift to the left, and P_{50} values range from 12 to 17 mm Hg.[39] In unmodified SFHS, the hemoglobin tetramers dissociate into dimers and monomers and lose their relationship with 2,3-DPG.

High oncotic effect is the third problem associated with unmodified SFHS. Attempts to correct these deficiencies have been made by chemically modifying the SFHS.[39]

Intramolecular or intermolecular cross-linking will stabilize the hemoglobin tetramer, increasing the molecular weight and decreasing the number of molecules at a given concentration of hemoglobin. This will address the problems of both high oncotic pressure and short intravascular half-life. This cross-linking or polymerization has been attempted with a wide variety of agents.[40] Glutaraldehyde has been demonstrated as a successful polymerizing agent yielding cross-linked hemoglobin inside red cells. This modification, however, is not addressing the increased oxygen affinity. In addition, the cross-linking is not specific, and the resulting preparation contains molecules with an assortment of molecular weights. Batch-to-batch reproducibility is difficult. Another agent, 3,5-dibromosalicyl-fumarate (DBBF), which is capable of cross-linking hemoglobin at specific sites, was also evaluated.[39] This hemoglobin, cross-linked between the alpha subunits, cannot be excreted as filtered globin chains because it cannot break down into subunits within the circulation.

Another approach to the short intravascular half-life has been to link hemoglobin to larger molecules such as hydroxyethyl starch or dextran. The resulting preparation, however, has a high viscosity, which limits its administration. The increased oxygen affinity of SFHS has been addressed by modifying the molecule with 2,3-DPG analogs such as ATP or pyridoxal 5'-phosphate. The latter has successfully reduced the oxygen affinity of SFHS to a level comparable to whole blood. A combination of polymerization and pyridoxylation appears to yield preparations that have an acceptable oxygen dissociation curve, oncotic effect that permits administration at a concentration of 14 to 15 g/dl, and intravascular half-life of 20 to 25 hours.[39] Another agent, 2-nor-2-formyl-pyridoxal-5'-phosphate (NFPLP), can link the hemoglobin intramolecularly in the area that normally binds 2,3-DPG[41] and induce stabilization of the hemoglobin as a tetramer as well as a reduction of the oxygen affinity. Most of the early research on SFHS has been supported by the Army and Navy branches of the US Armed Forces.[40] However, recently research efforts have broadened in development of a clinically effective hemoglobin solution, and clinical trials in humans are encouraging.[42]

Finally, modern SFHS preparations have a long shelf life and are very stable. They may be stored as liquids or in the lyophilized form for up to 18 months. In addition, they do not appear to be antigenic, so that patient immunization is not likely to be a problem, as it is with blood products.[43] This would also eliminate the blood bank typing procedures normally performed prior to blood transfusion. The advantages and disadvantages of SFHS are summarized in Table 1–8.

Perfluorochemicals

Perfluorochemicals (PFCs) have experienced a tremendous amount of research and testing as well as publicity. Perfluorochemicals are hydrocarbon structures in which all the hydrogen atoms have been replaced with fluorine. They are chemically inert, are excellent gas solvents, and carry O_2 and CO_2 by dissolving them. Most PFCs can dissolve as much as 40 to 70 percent of oxygen per unit by volume, compared with whole blood, which can dissolve only about 20 percent.[44] The concentration of dissolved oxygen in the PFC solution is directly proportional to the concentration of oxygen in the environment. Because PFCs are immiscible with blood, these chemicals are injected as emulsions with albumin, fats, or other chemicals; otherwise, they may cause pulmonary embolism, asphyxia, and death.[44]

The ability of PFC to transport sufficient amounts of oxygen was first demonstrated when mice survived submersion in an oxygenated PFC. Shortly thereafter, Geyer[45] exchanged the blood of rats with PFCs to a hematocrit of 1 percent without any sign of complication. Reperfusion of the rats was also accomplished successfully. The advantages and disadvantages of PFCs are summarized in Table 1–9.

Advantages of PFCs as a red cell substitute include their biologic inertness, lack of immunogenicity, and the fact that they are easily synthesized from readily available materials. Because their mechanism of transport of oxygen and carbon dioxide is by dissolution and not chemical bond, they do not have the high affinity of hemoglobin for carbon monoxide and are particularly suitable in the therapy of patients with carbon monoxide poisoning. In addition, owing to the small size of the emulsion particles, PFCs can deliver oxygen to tissues distal to vascular occlusions and may hold beneficial effects in patients suffering from myocardial infarction, cerebral ischemia, or sickle cell crisis.

Developed in Japan, Fluosol-DA is the most widely studied PFC thus far.[46] This compound contains both perfluorodecalin and perfluorotripropylamine as well as hydroxyethyl starch (to maintain blood volume) and electrolytes (to maintain osmotic pressure). Fluosol-DA has been used successfully in Japan and under very limited circumstances in the United States when the patient absolutely refuses blood transfusion (usually for religious reasons), even in a life-threatening emergency.

Initial studies in Japan in 1970 indicated that 186 patients who received Fluosol-DA experienced no complication. Clinical trials began in the United States in 1980.[47] Fluosol-DA was marketed in the United States by Alpha Therapeutics and submitted to the FDA for licensure in 1983 as a treatment for anemia. The subsequent clinical trials were disappointing. Adverse clinical effects were noted, such as transient hypotension, reduction in white cell count, and pulmonary insufficiency. Activation of the complement system is suspected to be the cause of these complications.[47] In addition, owing to the linear dissociation curve of the compound, patients had to be placed in a high-oxygen environment to obtain any significant oxygen delivery to the tissues. There is some question regarding whether plasma alone in such a high-oxygen environment can deliver a comparable amount of oxygen to the tissues. In any event, a high oxygen environment is toxic when sustained for a long time. In view of the lack of adequate proof that the preparation was both effective and safe, the FDA disapproved the application for licensure.

One problem associated with PFCs is that some of these chemicals are retained in the tissues for very long periods of time. Accumulations of these chemicals have been shown in liver, spleen, and other organs. The long-term effects of these deposits need to be evaluated. Perfluorochemicals are also excreted unmetabolized in the urine and transpired through the lungs and to a small extent through the skin.

Another problem that has been observed involves the atmosphere under which Fluosol transfusions are carried out. Fluosol has required a simultaneous administration of 100 percent oxygen both during and after the transfusion. However, recent modifications by Japanese researchers have eliminated the need for oxygen administration, and such transfusions are now carried out under normal atmospheric conditions.

Another problem with PFCs that needs to be solved is that of storage requirements. Fluosol-DA must be maintained under deep-freeze storage temperatures. This aspect also puts constraints on its applicability as a blood substitute, but certain compounds now under

investigation have been freeze-dried successfully. Their capabilities as oxygen carriers are unknown.

Numerous PFCs have been studied, each with different characteristics as far as emulsification capacity, ability to dissolve oxygen, circulation half-life, and tissue half-life.[48] Emulsifying agents also vary. To be considered as a possible red cell substitute, a PFC should be nontoxic, chemically inert, stable to oxygen and carbon dioxide, rapidly excreted, and readily available.[49]

The particle size of the emulsion should be small — 0.1 to 0.2 μm.[50] Larger particle size emulsions are more rapidly removed from the circulation, increase the viscosity of the solution, and lessen the amount of oxygen dissolved. In addition, PFC emulsions of large size are unstable and may separate, thus causing embolization when transfused.

Research needs to focus on the production of a PFC that is very stable, does not have a prolonged tissue retention time, does not require oxygen administration for effectiveness, and has practical storage requirements.[51]

Hemoglobin Encapsulation

The third approach to produce a red cell substitute consists of encapsulation of hemoglobin inside a membranelike structure. This approach results in a close red cell analog. Inside the microcapsule, an environment could be created that would allow the normal relationship between the hemoglobin tetramer and 2,3-DPG.[52] Other investigators have succeeded in enclosing hemoglobin in liposomal vesicles at concentrations equal to those in erythrocytes.[53] The liposome capsule consists of a bilipid layer of phospholipid and cholesterol similar to a cellular membrane but without the incorporated protein or carbohydrate that would give most cellular membranes their immunogenicity. Although this approach is still in its infancy, some hemoglobin-containing liposomes have demonstrated an oxygen affinity similar to that of normal whole blood and a hemoglobin concentration similar to that of red cells. These preparations have been transfused in animals with very low apparent toxicity. However, their circulating half-life is very short. Three mechanisms are involved in this rapid disappearance of liposomes from the circulation: the irreversible binding of vesicles to tissues, the lysis by plasma lipoproteins, and the clearance of the liposomes by the reticuloendothelial system, particularly by the liver. In addition to the inconvenience of a short-circulating half-life term, there is some fear that this uptake by the reticuloendothelial system may cause an immunologic blockade that could decrease the resistance of the body to sepsis. Another approach to the encapsulation of hemoglobin, which uses polymerized hemoglobin as the membrane, is also being investigated.[54] These preparations, however, have higher oxygen affinity than the microcapsules prepared using liposomes.

Summary of Three Approaches to a Red Cell Substitute

Each of these three different approaches toward the development of a red cell substitute or synthetic oxygen carrier has its own inherent advantages and disadvantages. The PFCs are the only truly synthetic compounds that do not depend on a human or other animal protein as the substrate and thus are the only preparations that can be guaranteed not to transmit infectious diseases as well as be acceptable to those who, for religious reasons, refuse blood transfusion. Their inherent disadvantage is their requirement for a high-oxygen environment. The modified SFHS will prove to be a more practical oxygen-carrying resuscitation fluid but may maintain the risk of TTDs, and its availability will be restricted by the accessibility of the source material, hemoglobin, unless bovine hemoglobin proves to be a safe alternative. Research in encapsulated hemoglobin has just started and its limitations are yet unknown. Currently, all three approaches to red cell substitute have one drawback in common: their short-to-moderate intravascular half-life as compared with the normal 60-day half-life of red cells. Unless a solution to this problem is found, red cell substitutes, when available, will be restricted to the short-term therapy of the anemia secondary to acute hemorrhage in patients whose bone marrow is capable of replacing red cells as the red cell substitute is being cleared, as in elective surgery. Although a great proportion of red cells transfused does fulfill this role, and could conceivably be replaced by red cell substitutes, there is a growing need for red cell transfusions as a chronic or semichronic therapy for patients whose bone marrow is unable to produce red cells. This need could not be fulfilled by any of the red cell substitutes currently under investigation.

SOLID BUFFERS

The use of solid additive buffers represents yet another approach to the preservation of blood and blood products.

One system reported uses a solid Silastic block impregnated with calcium hydroxide for the absorption of carbon dioxide by the hydroxide in the block, which is located in the primary collection bag.[31] The addition of solution of bicarbonate buffer, adenine, glucose, phosphate, and mannitol (BAGPM) was also added to the red cells in the primary bag. A better maintained pH using this approach led to higher 2,3-DPG levels and acceptable ATP levels after 42 days of storage. However promising, this approach remains to be perfected because of developmental and inherent manufacturing challenges.

Research of a new concept in blood preservation using ion-exchange resins as a solid buffer with the storage container shows promise for better viability reflected in ATP levels and for functional ability re-flected in 2,3-DPG levels.[55] Ion-exchange resins as a solid buffering system may solve the problem of maintaining levels of both organic phosphates in stored red cells. An investigation during a 28-day storage period showed that the resin system yields high 2,3-DPG levels without an incorporation of any chemicals other than CPD preservative.[55]

Several types of ion-exchange resins were investigated, but Amberlite IR-45 anion-exchange resin seems to be most promising for future blood banking. These resin beads are approximately 400 μm large and completely filterable (removed) at the time of transfusion. The resins are biologically and chemically inert.

They are easily sterilized because they possess great thermal stability. IR-45 resin was pretreated and charged with dibasic phosphate to replace the hydroxyl functional group present on the commercially available bead. This replacement allows mobile phosphate ions to be slowly released to the blood in the free monomeric form. The phosphate ion, a normal constituent of blood, buffers best throughout the pH range of stored blood. This phosphate resin system, therefore, is tantamount to inserting a strong buffer into the closed blood storage bag, preventing a marked change in pH. The introduction of sufficiently strong buffers into a closed system, preventing pH change of stored blood, has been a research goal for many years. Regulation of pH significantly extends the shelf life of blood because deleterious amounts of lactic acid are made as the red cell metabolizes glucose. Ordinarily, hydrogen ion concentration, or pH, changes during storage. The pH has a great and complex influence on red cell metabolism and function. Thus, the answer to the blood preservation problems may lie in pH maintenance.

The resin system described slowly releases phosphate to the blood when needed. Its function is twofold: (1) as a buffer, it combines with H^+ to form H_2PO_4, thereby maintaining a narrower pH range; (2) as a source of inorganic phosphate, it maintains ATP levels and yields high 2,3-DPG levels by accelerating its synthesis owing to increases in the substrates needed for its production.

A follow-up study by Valeri et al.[56] using the baboon as the animal model reported comparable in vivo survivals between the control and resin-buffered stored blood after 28 days. Additionally, blood stored with the resin system did demonstrate improved hemoglobin function reflected in higher P_{50} and 2,3-DPG values, which were elevated 7 to 10 days beyond those levels observed for the CPD controls.

The use of this technology of solid buffers for the storage of platelet concentrates demonstrated that a higher pH and metabolic rate were observed in platelets stored with the resin system in comparison with the control, which led to an increased storage time.[57] Solid buffers represent a new technology that is useful in studying the metabolism of platelets and red cells, while also being effective in increasing the storage time of these components.

The resin solid-buffer system is associated with the following advantages:

1. An increase in initial pH promotes greater glucose use.
2. Inorganic phosphate is provided to maintain ATP and DPG simultaneously.
3. CO_2 can be bound by the resin molecule, and a narrow pH range is maintained to enhance enzyme activity.
4. The resin is inert, filterable, and uses no additional chemicals other than CPD.
5. Bacteria are absorbed, apparently irreversibly.

These research areas described are all working toward the common goal of not only providing functional and viable RBCs but also a practical blood preservation system.

Platelet Structure, Function, Metabolism, and Preservation

Platelets are intimately involved in "primary hemostasis," which is the interaction of platelets and the vascular endothelium in halting bleeding following vascular injury. Platelets are cellular fragments derived from the cytoplasm of megakaryocytes present in the bone marrow. Platelets are released and circulate approximately 9 to 12 days as small, disk-shaped cells with an average diameter of 2 to 4 μm. The normal platelet count ranges from 150,000 to 350,000, depending on the method employed. In the peripheral blood, approximately 30 percent of the platelets are sequestered in the microvasculature or in the spleen as functional reserves after their release from the bone marrow.

STRUCTURE

The platelet structure is quite distinct and is subdivided into three zones that possess unique functional capabilities (Table 1–10). These include (1) the peripheral zone (the stimulus receptor/transmitter region), (2) the sol-gel zone (the cytoskeletal/contractile region), and (3) the organelle zone (the metabolic/organellar region) (Table 1–10).[4]

Peripheral Zone

The peripheral zone is a complex region of the platelet consisting of the glycocalyx (an amorphous exterior coat), plasma membrane, numerous deeply penetrating surface-connecting channels known as the open canalicular system (OCS), and a submembranous area of specialized microfilaments.

The glycocalyx is considered an important component of the platelet membrane. A number of glycoproteins present in this area are responsible for blood

TABLE 1–10 PLATELET ULTRASTRUCTURAL ZONES

I. Peripheral zone (stimulus receptor/transmitter region)
A. Glycocalyx
B. Plasma membrane
C. Open canalicular system (OCS)
D. Submembranous region
II. Sol-gel zone (cytoskeletal/contractile region)
A. Circumferential microtubules
B. Microfilaments
C. Thrombosthenin
III. Organelle zone (metabolic/organellar region)
A. Granules
1. Alpha granules
2. Dense granules
3. Glycogen granules
B. Mitochondria
C. Dense tubular system (DTS)
D. Lysosomes and peroxisomes

From Harmening,[4] p 418, with permission.

group specificity (ABO), tissue compatibility (human leukocyte antigen [HLA]), and platelet-unique immunologic antigenicity. In addition, glycoproteins also serve as receptors and facilitate transmission of stimuli across the platelet membrane.

Similar to other plasma membranes, the platelet membrane represents a fluid lipid bilayer composed of glycoproteins, glycolipids, and lipoproteins. The membrane phospholipid portion of the activated platelet serves as a surface for the interaction of the plasma proteins involved in blood coagulation, which assemble in complexes on the platelet's surface. Coagulation factors V and VIII also are present on the surface of the platelet membrane, as are various platelet factors that participate in the formation of fibrin (i.e., PF 3, PF 4). In addition to containing receptors for various stimuli, the peripheral zone of the platelet also contains the mechanism for the development of "stickiness," which is essential for the platelet functions of adhesion and aggregation.

The membranous surface connecting system referred to as the open canalicular system (OCS) consists of tubular invaginations of the plasma membrane that articulate throughout the platelet, even though it is part of the peripheral zone. Platelet-stored products are released to the exterior through the OCS. The OCS also facilitates collection of plasma procoagulants that aid in fibrin formation by providing increased surface absorptive area.

Sol-Gel Zone

The aqueous sol-gel zone contains microtubules and microfilaments. Microfilaments are interwoven throughout the cytoplasm of the platelet and are composed of thrombosthenin, a microfibrillar "contractile" protein.

Thrombosthenin, together with microfilaments

actin and myosin, form the platelet's cytoskeleton, which contracts as the platelet's shape changes. The cytoskeleton is responsible for maintaining its normal discoid shape.

Organelle Zone

The organelle region is responsible for the metabolic activities of the platelet. Generally, the most numerous organelles are the platelet granules, which are heterogeneous in size and differentiated by their electron density and chemical contents. Two types of granules are considered unique to platelets: alpha granules and dense bodies. The alpha granules are more numerous (20 to 200 per platelet) and contain a number of different proteins. The physiologic role of these proteins present in the alpha granules of platelets has not been clearly defined. However, it is known that PF 4 does neutralize the anticoagulant heparin.

Dense bodies are fewer in number (2 to 10 per platelet) and represent densely opaque granules in transmission electron microscope (TEM) preparations. The intragranular concentration of ADP and ATP found in the dense bodies of the platelets is called the "storage pool" of adenine nucleotides. This contrasts with the metabolic pool of ATP and ADP that is found in the platelet cytoplasm.

The contents of both the alpha granules and dense bodies is released during the process called the "release reaction," which is energy dependent. As a result of ADP released from dense bodies during the "release reaction," additional platelets are drawn to the site of the vascular injury, resulting in the formation of platelet aggregates.

The dense tubular system (DTS) is another important structure present in the cytoplasm of the organelle zone of platelets. This complex of dense tubules is analogous to the sarcotubules in skeletal muscle.

The DTS is the site of prostaglandin synthesis and sequestration of calcium. It is primarily the release of calcium from the DTS that triggers contraction of thrombosthenin and subsequent internal activation of platelets.

FUNCTION

Platelets have specific roles in the hemostatic process that are critically dependent on an adequate number of circulating thrombocytes as well as on normal platelet function. The role of platelets in hemostasis includes (1) maintenance of vascular integrity, (2) initial arrest of bleeding by platelet plug formation, and (3) stabilization of the hemostatic plug by contributing to the process of fibrin formation.

Numerous stimuli can trigger a platelet response termed activation, which may be transient, reversible, or irreversible. Activation refers to several separate responses of platelet function, which include "stickiness," adhesion, shape change, aggregation, and release.

Maintenance of Vascular Integrity

Platelets are involved in the nurturing of endothelial cells lining the vascular system. When a platelet adheres to the endothelial cells, the amount of cytoplasm between platelet and cell is reduced, and the platelet may eventually become incorporated into the endothelial cell. This process has an effect of "nurturing" or "feeding" the tissue cells by releasing endothelial growth factor. In addition, through the release of this mitogen (platelet-derived growth factor) vascular healing is promoted by stimulating endothelial cell migration and medial smooth muscle cell migration in the vessel wall.

In the absence of platelets from the circulation, red cells migrate through the vessel walls in large numbers and enter the lymphatic drainage or appear as petechiae or purpura in the skin or mucous membranes. This process of maintenance of normal vascular integrity, involving nourishment of the endothelium by the platelet or actual incorporation of platelets into the vessel wall, requires less than 10 percent of the platelets in the circulation but is nevertheless an important function.

Platelet Plug Formation

Various steps or processes are involved in the initial formation of a platelet plug: platelet adhesion, platelet aggregation, and platelet release reaction.

Adhesion Exposure to subendothelial connective tissue, such as collagen fibers, initiates platelet adhesion. Adhesion is a reversible process whereby platelets stick to foreign surfaces. This process of platelet adhesion involves the interaction of platelet surface glycoproteins with the connective tissue elements of the subendothelium.

Adhesion of platelets to subendothelial fibers depends on a plasma protein called von Willebrand factor (vWF).

Platelets thus adhere to the area of injury at the endothelial lining or to each other when injured, acting to arrest the initial episode of bleeding.

Aggregation During platelet aggregation, the injured platelet changes shape from discoid to spheric, with pseudopod formation. Initial aggregation of platelets is caused by ADP, which is released from adherent platelets or endothelial cells. Adenosine diphosphate is a potent initiator of aggregation, resulting in the transformation of ambient discoid platelets to reactive spiny spheres. These spheres react with one another to form a mass of aggregated platelets. By binding specific membrane receptors, ADP induces further shape change of nearby circulating platelets, promoting additional aggregation. Both calcium and the plasma protein fibrinogen (coagulation factor I) are necessary for platelet aggregation.

The secondary wave of aggregation depends on the activation stimulus being strong enough to evoke the release of platelet granules as a consequence of stronger, more complete contraction.

Release Reaction   The release reaction from dense granules involves the secretion of ADP, serotonin (a vasoactive amine), and calcium. Adenosine diphosphate is responsible for further aggregation of more platelets. Thus, amplification of the initial aggregation of platelets (a reversible phenomenon) results in secondary aggregation of many other platelets into an irreversible aggregation of a mass of degenerative platelet material without membranes.

Stabilization of Hemostatic Plug

The last stage involved in arresting bleeding after vessel damage is the formation of a stable platelet plug. This stabilization is achieved through the formation and deposition of fibrin, the end product of coagulation. Fibrin is formed as a result of a sense of reactions that involve not only platelets but also various blood proteins, lipids, and ions.

Platelets provide an optimal environment for fibrin formation by exposing certain phospholipids on the platelet membrane surface during aggregation.

OVERVIEW OF PLATELET METABOLISM

Like other cells, platelets require energy in the form of ATP for cellular movement, active transport of molecules across the membrane, biosynthetic purposes, and maintenance of a hemostatic steady state. The study of ATP and ADP in platelets is complicated by the fact that adenine nucleotides are present in two pools.[58] The first is the metabolically active pool, which participates in metabolism and is found in the cytoplasm, mitochondria, and membranes. The second is the metabolically inactive storage pool, which is found in the dense granules and plays a role in the release reaction.

It is assumed that metabolic ATP undergoes continuous consumption in the platelets; its resynthesis is accomplished by the metabolism of glycogen and glucose to pyruvate and lactate through glycolysis, and by the metabolism of pyruvate and endogenous substances such as fatty acids and amino acids to carbon dioxide through the citric acid cycle and oxidative phosphorylation. A great deal of controversy exists, however, as to which metabolic pathway predominates. The relative contributions of glycolysis and oxidative phosphorylation to platelet energy requirements during preservation still need to be defined.[59] The glycolytic metabolism is estimated from the depletion of glycogen and glucose and the production of lactate, whereas aerobic oxidation is usually estimated from the rate of O_2 consumption. Under aerobic conditions, oxidative phosphorylation accounted for 55 percent of total ATP production with glucose and 90 percent without glucose. Under anaerobic conditions, however, ATP production was maintained by glycolysis alone when glucose was present but not when glycogen was the only available substrate.

Previously, platelets were considered to be primarily a glycolytic tissue.[60] Recently, however, several studies indicate that platelets have the capacity for aerobic metabolism. In fact, oxidative phosphorylation is critical for platelets because it will augment its production of lactic acid fivefold if it is deprived of oxygen.[61] This response, common to other cells, is known as the Pasteur effects. The platelet's capacity for gluconeogenesis has yet to be elucidated, and the role of the pentose phosphate pathway has not been clearly established.

PLATELET PRESERVATION

Preservative solutions, usually designed for maintenance of red cell function and viability, also have a direct influence on platelet function and viability.

Platelet concentrates (PCs) are effectively used to treat bleeding associated with thrombocytopenia as well as other disorders in which platelets are qualitatively or quantitatively defective.[62] In the 1950s, platelet transfusions were given as freshly drawn whole blood or platelet-rich plasma. Circulatory overload quickly developed as a major complication of this method of administering platelets. Today platelets are prepared as concentrates and still remain the only effective means of correcting thrombocytopenia, even though therapeutic responsiveness varies depending on the patient population and undefined consequences of platelet storage conditions.

Currently, two methods for PC preparation are available — centrifugation and hemapheresis, (see Chapter 10).[24] PCs are stored at 1°C to 6°C without agitation with a storage limit of 3 days if prepared in a closed system, or at 20°C to 24°C with continuous agitation for 5 days.

The last survey conducted by the American Red Cross indicated that 3.12 million PCs were collected in 1992, which represents approximately 50 percent of the units collected in the United States. In 1991 the total number of platelet concentrates transfused was 3.7 million units.[63] This increased demand for PCs generates a greater need to store viable platelets for longer periods in order to provide an acceptable component for clinical use.

By necessity, storage conditions do cause alterations in the metabolism and function of platelets. Initial pH, temperature of storage, total platelet count, volume of plasma, duration of storage, agitation during storage, and hydrogen ion accumulation are some of the controversial factors known to influence platelet metabolism and function.[64]

A number of other interrelated variables can also affect platelet viability and function during storage: the anticoagulant used for blood collection; the method used to prepare platelet concentrates; and the composition, surface area, and thickness of the walls of the storage container.

Several studies evaluating platelet storage at various temperatures reported that 20°C to 24°C was the optimal storage temperature for platelets, rather than

4°C.[65] Platelets stored at 4°C are associated with an irreversible disc-to-sphere transformation; when stored for several hours at 4°C, platelets do not return to their disc shape upon rewarming and are irreversibly sphered.[66] This loss of shape in platelets stored at 4°C is probably a result of microtubule disassembly, which may also be a major contributor to decreased survival of platelets stored at 4°C. The major objections to platelets stored at 4°C are their shortened life span after reinfusion and their marked decrease in survival after only 18 hours of storage.[65]

In light of these developments, PCs are now prepared and stored at 22°C. However, even storage at 22°C for platelets has several disadvantages. One major difficulty is the regulation of pH. Virtually all units of PC demonstrate a decrease in pH from their initial value of 7.0.[65] This decrease is primarily because of the production of lactic acid by platelet glycolysis and to a lesser extent to accumulation of CO_2 from oxidative phosphorylation. As pH falls from 6.8 to 6.0, the platelets progressively change shape from discs to spheres. In this pH range, the changes of shape are reversible if the platelets are resuspended in plasma with physiologic pH. However, if the pH falls below 6.0, a further irreversible change occurs that renders the platelets nonviable after infusion in vivo.[67]

The loss of platelet viability has been correlated with the "lesion of storage," which is associated with various biochemical changes. Because of this correlation, every effort is being made to understand the metabolic, morphologic, and functional changes that occur during platelet preservation. The ultimate goal is to increase the storage time of PCs while maintaining viability and function. Viability indicates the capacity of platelets to circulate after infusion without premature removal or destruction. Platelet viability is determined by measuring pretransfusion and multiple post-transfusion platelet counts or by determining the disappearance rate of transfused radiolabeled platelets.[68] Function is defined as the ability of viable platelets to respond to vascular damage in promoting hemostasis. The template bleeding time test represents the most important assay of the functional integrity of transfused platelets. However, no one in vitro test can predict the effectiveness of a particular PC before transfusion.

Maintenance of pH appears to prevent the deleterious changes associated with platelet storage. Apparently, oxygen supply to the platelets within the plastic bag is also intimately related to pH maintenance. If the supply is sufficient, glucose will be metabolized oxidatively, resulting in carbon dioxide production, which diffuses out of the walls of the plastic storage bag. If the supply of oxygen is insufficient, glucose will be metabolized anaerobically, resulting in the production of lactic acid, which must remain within the container and thus lowers the pH. The oxygen tension within the container is governed by several factors: the concentration of platelets, which consume oxygen; the permeability of the wall of the plastic PC bag; the

surface area of the container available for gas exchange; and the type of agitation used, inasmuch as this facilitates gas exchange.

Containers for platelet storage were originally constructed from PVC containing DEHP as a plasticizer.[65] Platelets stored in these "first-generation containers" had a pH below 6.0 after 3 days of storage.[69] Currently "second-generation containers" are available that allow 5 days of storage of platelets without a significant fall in pH.[70] The four containers that have been described include

1. Polyolefin (PL-732) bags, which do not contain a plasticizer
2. Cutter Biological's CLX containers, which are made of a new formulation of PVC with tri-2-ethylhexyltrimliate plasticizer (this plasticizer leaches in minimal amounts into the platelet suspension in comparison with DEHP used in the first-generation containers)
3. Fenwal's PL-1240 container, which is identical to the CLX container[65]
4. Teruflex XT-612, made of PVC and di-2-ethylhexyl phthalate, by Terumo Corporation, for 5-day storage of platelets.

The second-generation containers maintain a higher pH by facilitating gas transport, thereby allowing CO_2 escape and increased O_2 transport. The higher O_2 tension is thought to reduce the glycolytic rate by accelerating oxidative metabolism. Although these bags have the ability to store platelets for 7 days, the FDA allows storage for 5 days only because with room temperature storage, a high frequency of septicemia related to transfusion of contaminated platelets has been reported.

Current federal regulation licenses the storage of PCs for 5 days at 22°C and for 72 hours at 4°C.[71] Each PC must be resuspended in a sufficient volume of plasma to maintain a pH of 6.0 or greater and to maintain a minimum platelet count of 5.5×10^{10} platelets per bag (50 to 55 ml plasma).[71] Furthermore, when PCs are stored at 22°C, continuous gentle agitation must be used in order to facilitate gas exchange. This has also led to the controversial question regarding the type of agitator to be used. Platform, elliptical, and circular rotators are currently in use. In PL-732 bags, PCs may be stored for 5 days at 20°C to 24°C with circular or flatbed agitators. It should be noted that elliptical rotators are not recommended. In PVC (CLX) and PL1240 bags, PCs are stored for 5 days with either circular or elliptical agitators. If the PC bag is broken or opened, the unit must be used within 24 hours when stored at 1°C to 6°C and within 6 hours when stored at 20°C to 24°C.

A few investigators have also implicated the presence of large numbers of leukocytes present in PCs as precipitators of the fall in pH during storage.[72,73] Large numbers of contaminating white cells are proposed to affect deleteriously the metabolic activity of platelets by competing for glucose and increasing lactic acid production. Leukocyte contamination has also been implicated in transfusion reactions following platelet transfusions.

The effects of contaminating leukocytes in platelet concentrates have prompted increased preparation and use of leukopoor platelets. Methodologies to prepare such products include centrifugation, filtration, and a specially designed platelet pooling bag (Leukotrap Platelet Pooling System, Cutter Biological) (Fig. 1–9).[74-76] Efficiency of these methodologies ranges from 39 to 91 percent leukocyte removal.[77] As with leukopoor red cells, removal of white cells before storage is advocated for platelet preparation.[78]

Leukopoor platelets have been shown to prevent febrile transfusion reactions, and studies have been conducted to evaluate the efficacy in preventing HLA immunization[79-81] and transfusion-associated graft-versus-host disease (TA-GVHD). The storage lesion described for platelet concentrates has also been attributed to platelet activation.[82] In addition, complement activation in stored platelet concentrates has been implicated in platelet activation, which may be

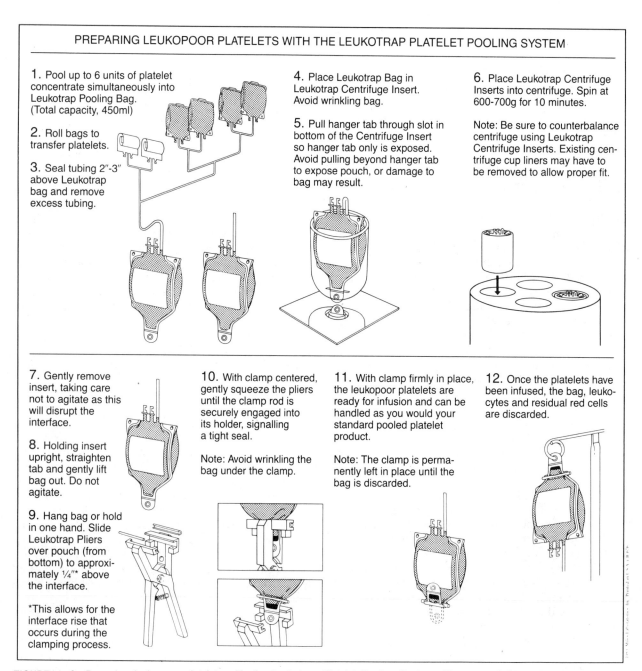

PREPARING LEUKOPOOR PLATELETS WITH THE LEUKOTRAP PLATELET POOLING SYSTEM

1. Pool up to 6 units of platelet concentrate simultaneously into Leukotrap Pooling Bag. (Total capacity, 450ml)

2. Roll bags to transfer platelets.

3. Seal tubing 2"-3" above Leukotrap bag and remove excess tubing.

4. Place Leukotrap Bag in Leukotrap Centrifuge Insert. Avoid wrinkling bag.

5. Pull hanger tab through slot in bottom of the Centrifuge Insert so hanger tab only is exposed. Avoid pulling beyond hanger tab to expose pouch, or damage to bag may result.

6. Place Leukotrap Centrifuge Inserts into centrifuge. Spin at 600-700g for 10 minutes.

Note: Be sure to counterbalance centrifuge using Leukotrap Centrifuge Inserts. Existing centrifuge cup liners may have to be removed to allow proper fit.

7. Gently remove insert, taking care not to agitate as this will disrupt the interface.

8. Holding insert upright, straighten tab and gently lift bag out. Do not agitate.

9. Hang bag or hold in one hand. Slide Leukotrap Pliers over pouch (from bottom) to approximately ¼"* above the interface.

*This allows for the interface rise that occurs during the clamping process.

10. With clamp centered, gently squeeze the pliers until the clamp rod is securely engaged into its holder, signalling a tight seal.

Note: Avoid wrinkling the bag under the clamp.

11. With clamp firmly in place, the leukopoor platelets are ready for infusion and can be handled as you would your standard pooled platelet product.

Note: The clamp is permanently left in place until the bag is discarded.

12. Once the platelets have been infused, the bag, leukocytes and residual red cells are discarded.

FIGURE 1-9 Preparing leukopoor platelets with the Leukotrap Platelet Pooling System. (Courtesy of Cutter Biological, Berkeley, California.)

related to the deleterious effects that occur during room temperature storage.[83]

In conclusion, all research is aimed at providing the highest quality blood product for cost-effective and efficient patient care.

Review Questions

1. The loss of ATP leads to:
   A. An increase in phosphorylation of spectrin and a loss of membrane deformability
   B. An increase in phosphorylation of spectrin and an increase of membrane deformability
   C. A decrease in phosphorylation of spectrin and a loss of membrane deformability
   D. A decrease in phosphorylation of spectrin and an increase of membrane deformability

2. Normal adult hemoglobin consists of:
   A. Two alpha chains and two beta chains
   B. Two alpha chains and two delta chains
   C. Two alpha chains and two gamma chains
   D. Four alpha chains

3. A major disadvantage of PFCs as a red cell substitute is:
   A. Dependence on human or animal protein
   B. Dependence on low O_2 atmosphere
   C. Dependence on high O_2 atmosphere
   D. High chance of disease transmission

4. When blood is stored, there is a "shift to the left." This means:
   A. Hemoglobin oxygen affinity increases owing to an increase in 2,3-DPG
   B. Hemoglobin oxygen affinity increases owing to a decrease in 2,3-DPG
   C. Hemoglobin oxygen affinity decreases owing to a decrease in 2,3-DPG
   D. Hemoglobin oxygen affinity decreases owing to an increase in 2,3-DPG

5. Which of the following is (are) the role(s) of platelets?
   A. Maintain vascular integrity
   B. Initially arrest bleeding
   C. Stabilize the hemostatic plug
   D. All of the above
   E. None of the above

6. Which of the following preservatives has the longest storage time?
   A. ACD
   B. Nutricel (AS-2)
   C. Adsol (AS-1)
   D. CPD

7. What is the currently licensed storage time and temperature for platelet concentrates?
   A. 10 days at 27°C
   B. 5 days at 27°C
   C. 5 days at 22°C
   D. 10 days at 22°C

8. All but which of these factors will influence platelet metabolism and function in a closed system?
   A. Total platelet count
   B. Duration of storage
   C. Temperature of storage
   D. Fibrinogen concentration

9. One of the major disadvantages of stroma-free hemoglobin solutions is:
   A. High oxygen affinity
   B. No antigenicity
   C. Long shelf life
   D. Long stability

10. Autologous blood storage is reserved for patients who:
    A. Are blood type AB negative
    B. Have no compatibility problems
    C. Are known to have a history of antibody problems
    D. Are not regular blood donors

Answers to Review Questions

1. C (p 3)
2. A (p 6)
3. C (p 16)
4. B (p 8)
5. D (p 19)
6. C (Table 1–2)
7. C (p 23)
8. D (p 20)
9. A (p 15)
10. C (p 14)

References

1. Parks, D: Charles Richard Drew, MD 1904–1905. J Natl Med Assoc 71:893–895, 1979.
2. Kendrick, DB: Blood Program in World War II, Historical Note. Washington Office of Surgeon General, Department of Army, Washington, DC, 1964, pp 1–23.
3. Wallace, EL, et al: Collection and transfusion of blood and blood components in the United States. Transfusion 33:139–144, 1993.
4. Harmening, DM: Clinical Hematology and Fundamentals of Hemostasis, ed 2. FA Davis, Philadelphia, 1992, p 4.
5. Wallace, ME and Gibbs, FL (eds): Blood Group Systems: ABH and Lewis. American Association of Blood Banks, Arlington, VA, 1986, p 12.
6. Wise, GE: Identification and function of transmembrane glycoproteins—the red cell model. Tissue Cell 16:665–676, 1984.

7. Yeasle, PL: Phospholipid-protein interactions and the structure of the human erythrocyte membrane, nuclear magnetic resonance studies. Prog Clin Biol Res 159:153–175, 1984.

8. Wolfe, LC: Red cell membrane storage lesions. Transfusion 25:185–202, 1985.

9. Sheetz, MP: Membrane skeletal dynamics: Role in modulation of red cell deformability, mobility of transmembrane proteins and shape. Semin Hematol 20:175–188, 1983.

10. Ferrant, A: The role of the spleen in hemolysis. Clin Hematol 12:489, 1983.

11. Schrier, SL: The red cell membrane and its abnormalities. In Hoffbrand, AV (ed): Recent Advances in Hematology, Vol 3. Blackwell Scientific Publications, Oxford, England, 1982.

12. Duhm, J, Deutikle, B, and Gerlach, E: Complete restoration of oxygen transport function and 2,3-diphosphoglycerate concentration in stored blood. Transfusion 11:147, 1971.

13. Benesch, R and Benesch, RE: The effect of organic phosphates from the human erythrocyte on the allosteric properties of hemoglobin. Biochem Biophys Res Commun 26:162, 1967.

14. Chanutin, A and Curnish, RF: Effect of organic and inorganic phosphates on the oxygen equilibrium of human erythrocytes. Arch Biochem Biophys 121:96, 1967.

15. Dern, RJ, Brewer, GJ, and Wiorkowski, JI: Studies on the preservation of human blood. II. The relationship of erythrocyte adenosine triphosphate levels and other in vivo measures to red cell storageability. J Lab Clin Med 69:968, 1967.

16. Valtis, DJ and Kennedy, AC: Defective gas-transport function of stored red blood cells. Lancet i:119, 1954.

17. Akerblom, O and Kreuger, R: Studies on citrate-phosphate-dextrose (CPD) blood supplemented with adenine. Vox Sang 29:90, 1975.

18. Bunn, HF, et al: Hemoglobin function in stored blood. J Clin Invest 48:311, 1969.

19. Oski, FA, et al: The effects of deoxygenation of adult and fetal hemoglobin on the synthesis of red cell 2,3-diphosphoglycerate and its in vivo consequences. J Clin Invest 49:400, 1970.

20. Beutler, E and Wood, LA: The in vivo regeneration of red cell–diphosphoglyceric acid (DPG) after transfusion of stored blood. J Lab Clin Med 74:300, 1969.

21. Beutler, E: Experienced blood preservatives for liquid storage. In Greenwalt, TJ and Jamieson, GA (eds): The Human Red Cell in Vitro. Grune & Stratton, New York, 1974, p 189.

22. Valeri, CR and Collins, FB: Physiological effects of 2,3-DPG depleted red cells with high affinity for oxygen. J Appl Physiol 31:823, 1971.

23. Dennis, RC, et al: Improved myocardial performance following high 2,3-diphosphoglycerate red cell transfusions. Surgery 77:741, 1975.

24. Maier, RV and Carrico, CJ: Developments in the resuscitation of critically ill surgical patients (Review). Adv Surg 19:271–328, 1986.

25. Zuck, TF, et al: The in vivo survival of red cells stored in modified CPD with adenine: Report of a multiinstitutional cooperative effort. Transfusion 17:374–382, 1977.

26. Widmann, FK (ed): Technical Manual, ed 9. American Association of Blood Banks, Arlington, VA, 1985.

27. Lovric, VA: Modified packed red cells and the development of the circle pack. Vox Sang 51:337, 1986.

28. Hogman, CF, Hedlund, K, and Zetterstrom, H: Clinical usefulness of red cells preserved in protein-poor mediums. N Engl J Med 299:1377–1382, 1982.

29. Hogman, CF: Additive system approach in blood transfusion birth of the SAG and Sagman systems. Vox Sang 51:337, 1986.

30. Cutter Biological Nutricel Additive System (AS-3), Technical Support Data. Cutter Publisher, Berkeley, CA 1984.

31. Miripol, J: ADSOL Preservation Solution. Fenwal Laboratories, Deerfield, IL.

32. Valeri, CR, et al: A clinical experience with ADSOL-preserved erythrocytes (Review). Surg Gynecol Obstet 166:33–46, 1988.

33. Cutter Biological Leukotrap Red Cell Storage System. Cutter Publisher, Berkeley, CA 1987.

34. Valeri, CR: Use of rejuvenation solutions in blood preservation. CRC Crit Rev Clin Lab Sci 17:299–374, 1982.

35. Minikami, S, Hamosaki, N, and Ikehara, Y: Rejuvenation of aged erythrocytes by incorporating phosphoenolpyruvate into the cells. Acta Med Ger 40:691, 1981.

36. Huggins, C: Preparation and usefulness of frozen blood. Annu Rev Med 36:499–503, 1985.

37. Biro, GP: Current status of erythrocyte substitutes. Can Med Assoc J 129:237–244, 1983.

38. Allen, RW, Kahn, RA, and Baldassare, JJ: Advances in the production of blood cell substitutes with alternate technologies. In Wallace, CH and McCarthy, LJ (eds): New Frontiers in Blood Banking. American Association of Blood Banks, Arlington, VA, 1986, pp 27–31.

39. Hess, JR, Wade, CE, and Winslow, RM: Filtration-assisted exchange transfusion using $\alpha\alpha$Hb, an erythrocyte substitute. J Appl Physiol 70:1639–1644, 1991.

40. Hedlund, BE, et al: Polymerized hemoglobins. In Murawski, K and Peetoom, F (eds): Transfusion Medicine: Recent Technological Advances. Alan R Liss, New York, 1986, pp 39–48.

41. Bakker, JC, Bleeker, WK, and van der Plas, J: Properties of hemoglobin interdimerically cross-linked with NFPLP. In Murashki, K and Peetoom, F (ed): Transfusion Medicine: Recent Technological Advances. Alan R Liss, New York, 1986, pp 49–55.

42. Dunlap, E and Farrell, L: New blood product: Diaspirin cross-linked hemoglobin as a blood substitute. V. Efficacy in a pig model of hemorrhagic shock. Transfusion 32:9S, 1992.

43. Kahn, RA, Allen, RW, and Baldassare, J: Alternate sources and substitutes for therapeutic blood components. Blood 66:112, 1985.

44. Lowe, KC: Perfluorocarbons as oxygen-transport fluids (Review). Comp Biochem Physiol [A] 87:825–838, 1987.

45. Geyer, RP: Substitutes for Blood-Experimental and Practical Considerations. In A Seminar of Blood Components: E Unum Plurbis. 30th Annual Meeting of the American Association of Blood Banks, Atlanta, GA, November 1977, pp 75–88.

46. Ohyanasi, H and Saitoh, Y: Development and clinical application of perfluorochemical artificial blood. Int J Artif Organs 9:363–368, 1986.

47. Tremper, KK and Anderson, ST: Perfluorochemical emulsion oxygen transport fluids: A clinical review. Ann Rev Med 36:309–313, 1985.

48. Lowe, KC and Bollands, AD: Physiological effects of perfluorocarbons blood substitutes (Review). Med Lab Sci 42:367–375, 1985.

49. Levine, EM and Tremper, KK: Perfluorochemical emulsions: Potential clinical uses and new developments (Review). Int Anesthesiol Clin 23:211–230, 1985.

50. Faithfull, NS: Fluorocarbons: Current status and future applications (Review). Anaesthesia 12:234–242, 1987.

51. Biro, GP and Blais, P: Perfluorocarbon blood substitutes (Review). CRC Crit Rev Oncol Hematol 6:311–374, 1987.

52. Farmer, MC and Gaber, BP: Encapsulation of hemoglobin in phospholipid: Surrogate red cells in vitro and in vivo. Biophys J 45:A201, 1984.

53. Djordjevich, L and Miller, IF: Synthetic erythrocytes from lipid encapsulated hemoglobin. Exp Hematol 8:584–592, 1980.

54. Davis, TA and Asher, WJ: Artificial red cells. US Patent No. 4,390,521, 1983.

55. Harmening, DM and Dawson, RB: The use of ion-exchange resins as a blood preservative system. Transfusion 18:358, 1978.

56. Valeri, CR, et al: Phosphate ion-exchange resin used in liquid preservation of baboon red blood cells. Transfusion 23:215–222, 1983.

57. Witkowska, L, Harmening-Pittiglio, D, and Schiffer, C: Storage of platelet concentrates using ion-exchange resin charged with dibasic phosphate: A preliminary report. J Am Soc Hematol 58:537–554, 1981.

58. Holmesen, H: Platelet metabolism and activation. Semin Hematol 22:219–240, 1985.

59. Heaton, AL: Enhancement of cellular elements. In Wallas, CH and McCarthy, LJ (eds): New Frontiers in Blood Banking. American Association of Blood Banks, Arlington, VA, 1986.

60. Rock, G, et al: An assessment of the requirements for plasma and oxygen. Transfusion 21:167–177, 1981.

61. Murphy, S and Gardner, FH: Platelet storage at 22°C: Role of gas transport across plastic containers in maintenance of viability. Blood 46:209–217, 1975.
62. Slichter, SJ: Poststorage platelet viability in thrombocytopenic recipients in reliably measured by radiochromium-labeled platelet recovery and survival measurements in normal volunteers (Review). Transfusion 26:8–13, 1986.
63. American Association of Blood Banks, Annual Report, Bethesda, MD, 1992.
64. Beutler, E and Kuhl, W: Platelet glycolysis in platelet storage. IV. The effect of supplemental glucose and adenine. Transfusion 20:97–100, 1980.
65. Murphy, S: PL-F-2-2, Evolution, Current State of Art, and Future Trends of Platelet Preservation. Cardeza Foundation for Hematologic Research, Philadelphia, 1986.
66. McGill, M: Temperature cycling preserves platelet shape and enhances in vitro test scores during storage at 4°C. J Lab Clin Med 92:971–982, 1978.
67. Murphy, S: Platelet storage for transfusion. Semin Hematol 22:165–177, 1985.
68. Snyder, EL: Effect of storage conditions on radiolabeling of stored platelet concentrates. Transfusion 26:6–8, 1986.
69. Solberg, C, Holme, S, and Little, C: Morphological changes associated with pH changes during storage of platelet concentrates. Beitr Infusionther Klin Ernahr 15:107–117, 1986.
70. Koerner, K: Platelet function of room temperature platelet concentrates stored in a new plastic material with high gas permeability. Vox Sang 47:406–411, 1984.
71. Code of Federal Regulation. Office of Federal Registrar. National Archives, Record Administration, February 8, 1992.
72. Savage, B: Platelet adenine nucleotide levels during room-temperature storage of platelets concentrates. Transfusion 2:288–291, 1982.
73. Beutler, E and Kuhl, W: Platelet glycolysis in platelet storage. The effect of supplemental glucose and adenine. Transfusion 20:97–100, 1980.
74. Dzik, MJ: Leukocyte poor platelet concentrates: Comparison of microaggregate blood filters. Transfusion 24:421, 1984.
75. Schiffer, CA, et al: Effective leukocyte removal from platelet preparations by centrifugation in Leukotrap pooling bags. Transfusion 25:416, 1985.
76. Cutter Biological Leukotrap Platelet Pooling System. Cutter Publisher, Berkeley, CA, 1986.
77. Rebulla, P, et al: White cell-reduced red cells prepared by filtration: A critical evaluation of current filters and methods for counting residual white cells. Transfusion 33:128, 1993.
78. Sweeney, JD, Holme, S, and Heaton, A: Preparation of leuko-depleted platelet concentrates from whole blood donations using an in-line filter. Transfusion 32:7S, 1992.
79. Dan, M and Stewart, S: Prevention of recurrent febrile transfusion reactions using leukocyte poor platelet concentrates. Prepared by the Leukotrap Centrifugation Method. Transfusion 26:569, 1986.
80. Stec, N, et al: Effectiveness of leukocyte (WBC) depleted platelets in preventing febrile reactions in multi-transfused oncology patients. Transfusion 26:569, 1986.
81. Sirchia, G: Platelet transfusion and HLA immunization. Vox Sang 51, 1986.
82. Bode, AP: Platelet activation may explain the storage lesion in platelet concentrates. Blood Cells 16:109–126, 1990.
83. Miletic, VD and Popovic, O: Complement activation in stored platelet concentrates. Transfusion 33:150, 1993.

Bibliography

Beal, RW and Isbister, JP: Blood Component Therapy in Clinical Practice. Blackwell Scientific Publications, Oxford, England, 1985.

Bolin, RB, Geyer, RP, and Nemo, GJ (eds): Advances in Blood Substitute Research. Alan R Liss, New York, 1983.

Brewer, GJ (ed): Progress in biological and clinical research: The red cell. Sixth Ann Arbor Conference. Alan R Liss, New York, 1984.

Edwards-Moulds, J and Lasky, LC (eds): Clinical Applications of Genetic Engineering Technical Workshop. American Association of Blood Banks, Arlington, VA, 1987.

Edwards-Moulds, J and Tregellas, WM (eds): Introductory Molecular Genetics. American Association of Blood Banks, Arlington, VA, 1986.

Hess, JR, Wade, CE, and Winslow, RM: Filtration-assisted exchange transfusion using $\alpha\alpha$Hb, an erythrocyte substitute. J Appl Physiol 70:1639–1644, 1991.

Long, MW: Current concepts in the development and regulation of the bone marrow megakaryocyte. J Med Tech 1:9, 1984.

Murawski, K and Peetoom, F (eds): Transfusion Medicine: Recent Technological Advances. Alan R Liss, New York, 1986.

Wallas, C and McCarthy, LJ (eds): New Frontiers in Blood Banking. American Association of Blood Banks, Arlington, VA, 1986.

Winslow, RM: Hemoglobin-Based Red Cell Substitutes. Johns Hopkins University Press, Baltimore, 1992.

Winslow, RM: Red cell substitutes current status. In Nance, DJ (ed): Blood Safety: Current Challenges. American Association of Blood Banks, Bethesda, MD, 1992.

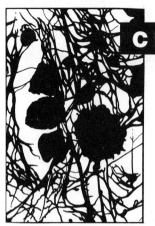

CHAPTER 2

Basic Genetics

JoAnn M. Moulds, PhD

OBJECTIVES

Upon completion of this chapter, the learner should be able to:

1 Describe the processes of mitosis and meiosis.

2 Discuss Mendel's laws of independent segregation and of dominance.

3 Correlate Mendel's law of dominance with specific examples of the inheritance of blood group antigens.

4 Correlate the Hardy-Weinberg principle with a specific example of the inheritance of blood group antigens.

5 Interpret the inheritance pattern of a trait or gene by examination of the pedigree analysis.

6 Distinguish between X-linked and autosomal inheritance.

7 Describe the processes of replication, transcription, and translation.

8 For each of the above processes, describe a specific example of how a mutation could occur.

9 Discuss the importance of restriction fragment length polymorphism analysis.

10 List the uses of polymerase chain reaction.

Today's study of blood group genetics requires not only an appreciation of classic mendelian genetics, but also an understanding of the structure of DNA and how it can be manipulated. The student of genetics must know how to interpret not only a familial inheritance pattern but also a Southern blot.

In this chapter 130 years of genetics is reviewed. Obviously, this must be nothing more than a brief overview. Interested readers are referred to the original references as well as selected books for more in-depth reading. However, these are only suggestions, and many other good books covering genetics alone are available for the reader who desires a deeper understanding of this complex topic.

Classic Genetics

MITOSIS AND MEIOSIS

Genetics is the study of inheritance—the transmission of characteristics from parents to offspring. The transmission of traits was first observed by the ancients and often led to bizarre theories on the mechanism of the hereditary process. Not until 1865, when Gregor Mendel did experimental matings with garden peas, did the science of genetics come into being. His studies led to the basic understanding of how genetic traits are passed to each generation.

Within each living human cell is a central organelle called a nucleus that contains most of the genetic material. Under a light microscope this appears as dark-staining bands known as heterochromatin and lighter bands called euchromatin. The chromatin coils up tightly to make structures called chromosomes. Humans have 46 chromosomes, whereas other species possess between 10 and 50 chromosomes. The chromosomes usually occur together in pairs (one from each parent), resulting in the diploid or 2N species. Humans have 22 pairs of autosomes and one set of sex chromosomes (XX and YY).

As a cell divides it must reproduce its chromosomes so that all the daughter cells are identical to the parent cell. This process is known as mitosis. The chromosomes are duplicated and one of each pair passes to the daughter. This process is illustrated in Figure 2–1.

Obviously, this process cannot explain the production of new individuals. If a diploid ovum and sperm combined, then the resulting cell would have 4N chromosomes; this is unacceptable. Therefore, the gamete must carry only one copy of each chromosome (haploid) so that when they fuse a diploid cell results. This type of cell division is unique to reproduction or the germinal tissues and is called meiosis (Fig. 2–2).

MENDEL'S LAWS

In his classic paper of 1865, Mendel demonstrated that the physical traits of an organism corresponded to some invisible "elementen" in the cell. We now know these "elementens" as genes. Furthermore, Mendel

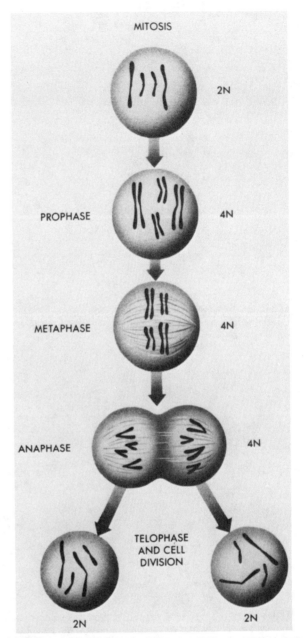

FIGURE 2–1 Cell division by mitosis leads to two daughter cells having the same number of chromosomes as the parent. (From Watson, JD, Tooze, J, and Kurtz, DT: Recombinant DNA: A Short Course. Copyright 1983 by James D. Watson, John Tooze, and David T. Kurtz. Reprinted by permission of W.H. Freeman and Company, New York, p 7.)

proposed that the genes occurred in pairs and that one of each gene was passed from parent to offspring.

In one set of experiments Mendel cultivated sweet peas until they bred offspring with flowers of all one color (e.g., red or white only). He then cross-bred these two plants and obtained a first filial generation that were all red flowered. When plants from this generation were bred with each other, they produced red and white flowers in a ratio of 3:1. This is illustrated in Figure 2–3, in which the parents are homo-

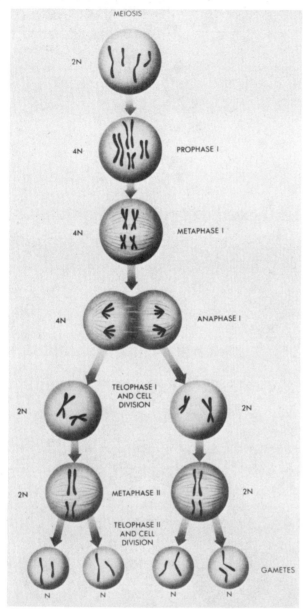

FIGURE 2-2 Sex-cell division, or meiosis, produces four gametes having half the number of chromosomes present in the parent cell. (From Watson, JD, Tooze, J, and Kurtz, DT: Recombinant DNA: A Short Course. Copyright 1983 by James D. Watson, John Tooze, and David T. Kurtz. Reprinted by permission of W.H. Freeman and Company, New York, p 7.)

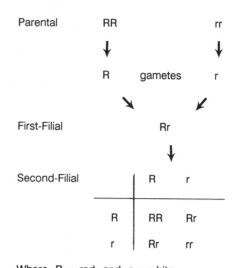

Where R = red and r = white

FIGURE 2-3 A schematic illustration of Mendel's law of separation.

zygous for the red trait (RR) or the white trait (rr). The first filial generation are heterozygous (Rr). They carry the dominant (expressed) gene R for red color as well as the recessive (nonexpressed) gene r. The second filial generation then results in one homozygous red plant (RR), two heterozygous red plants (Rr), and one homozygous recessive white plant (rr). This illustrates Mendel's law of independent segregation as well as his law of dominance.

A slight variation of this law can occur when one trait is not dominant over the other. When the traits are codominant, both are expressed equally. Thus, in the previous example, if the genes were codominant, the heterozygotes (Rr) would be pink, whereas RR plants would remain red and rr white. An example of codominantly inherited blood group genes is seen in Figure 2-4, wherein both the M and N antigens can be detected in the heterozygous family members.

Another of Mendel's laws is the law of independent assortment. Simply stated, this means that factors for different characteristics are inherited independently from each other (if they reside on different chromosomes). Mendel ascertained this by performing dihybrid crosses; that is, crosses between strains breeding true for two characteristics. For example, if seeds that were round or wrinkled and green or yellow were bred, the parental genotypes would be $RRYY$ and $rryy$. If the generations are bred as previously described, we would have gametes pairing as shown in Figure 2-5. The results of the dihybrid cross would yield the following phenotypes: round/yellow, round/green, wrinkled/yellow, and wrinkled/green in a ratio of $9:3:3:1$. Of course, there are exceptions to these rules. Sometimes the genes for different traits can be carried on the same chromosome, such as the genes for MN and Ss. Because they are so close to each other physically, they are inherited as a unit, or "travel" together. In addition, the expected gene ratios may not occur if recombination has happened during meiosis. This is caused by breaking of the DNA strand, followed by exchange of chromosomal material, which yields new hybrid genotypes.

Mendel's laws apply to all sexually reproducing diploid organisms. In combination, they demonstrate just how immense the genetic variations can become in just a few generations. Multiply this by thousands of genes in the human genome, and it is not surprising that each individual is unique.

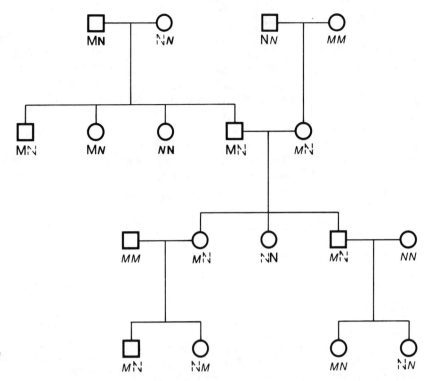

FIGURE 2-4 Independent segregation of the codominant genes *M* and *N*.

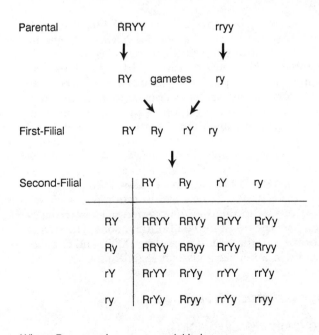

	RY	Ry	rY	ry

Parental   RRYY   rryy

RY   gametes   ry

First-Filial   RY   Ry   rY   ry

Second-Filial

	RY	Ry	rY	ry
RY	RRYY	RRYy	RrYY	RrYy
Ry	RRYy	RRyy	RrYy	Rryy
rY	RrYY	RrYy	rrYY	rrYy
ry	RrYy	Rryy	rrYy	rryy

Where R = round   r = wrinkled

Y = yellow   y = green

FIGURE 2-5 A schematic illustration of Mendel's law of independent assortment.

Population Genetics

HARDY-WEINBERG PRINCIPLE

Once the principles of mendelian inheritance gained acceptance, certain questions regarding recessive alleles persisted. The question of why a recessive trait would not be lost from the population was finally answered by a mathematician, G. H. Hardy, and a German physician, W. Weinberg, who produced the Hardy-Weinberg equation. Several basic premises, however, underlie this mathematical formula:

1. The population must be large and mating occur at random.
2. Mutations must not occur.
3. There must be no migration, differential fertility, or mortality of the genotype.

Obviously, these conditions are seldom met by human populations. Today there is a constant mixing of populations leading to "gene flow." All aside, the Hardy-Weinberg formula is the best estimate we can make for population genetics.

Genetic variability is widely divergent in large populations. To determine the frequency of each allele, we count the number of persons of each phenotype. Given two alleles D and d, the frequency of D would be the sum of D alleles in each phenotype divided by the total number of alleles. This will be p in the Hardy-Weinberg equation. Similarly, counting the number of an allele gives us the figure for q. P plus q must equal 1.0. Accordingly, the ratio of homozygotes and heterozygotes is represented by the formula $p^2 + 2pq + q^2 = 1$. This can also be visualized in the mating sequence, which we used in Figure 2–3.

	p	q
p	p²	pq
q	pq	q²

$\rightarrow p^2 + 2pq + q^2 = 1.0$

Let us look at an example using blood group gene frequencies. If we tested 1000 donors for the Rh factor and found that Rh positives (DD and Dd) represented 84 percent of the population and Rh negatives (dd) 16 percent, we could then calculate the gene frequencies as follows:

p = gene frequency of D
q = gene frequency of d

$$\left. \begin{array}{l} p^2 = DD \\ 2pq = Dd \end{array} \right\} 0.84$$

$$q^2 = dd = \frac{0.16}{1.00}$$

$q = \sqrt{0.16} = 0.4$
$p + q = 1$
$p = 1 - q$
$p = 1 - 0.4$
$p = 0.6$

This is only a simple example of the Hardy-Weinberg equation. Blood group systems with more codominant alleles require an expansion of the binomial equation. For example, a three-allele system would be calculated using the formula $p + q + r = 1$ or $p^2 + 2pq + 2pr + q^2 + 2qr + r^2 = 1$. The interested reader is referred to other genetic text books for these more complex equations.

INHERITANCE PATTERNS

In order to interpret pedigree analyses, we must first be familiar with some standard conventions. Males are denoted by squares and females by circles. A line joining a male and a female indicates mating, and the offspring are indicated by a vertical line. A consanguineous mating has a double line between the male and female. An abortion or stillbirth is shown as a small blackened circle; other deceased family members have a cross through them. When a particular individual is found who draws attention to the pedigree, he or she is called the propositus, or index case; this is indicated on the pedigree by an arrow. Figure 2–6 illustrates pedigrees and their inheritance patterns.

Example A is a pedigree demonstrating autosomal recessive inheritance. Autosomal means that the trait is not carried on the sex chromosomes. A recessive trait is carried by but not expressed in the parents. When two heterozygous individuals mate they can produce a child who inherits a recessive gene from each parent, thus he or she is homozygous recessive for that trait. An example of this can be found in the Rh blood group. The gene d can be carried by two Rh-positive parents (Dd), who both pass d to the child. The resulting genotype is dd, and the child's red cells type as Rh (D) negative.

In example B we see a dominant X-linked trait. If the father carries the trait on his X chromosome he has no sons with the trait (since he passed his Y chromosome to his sons); however, all his daughters will express the trait. If a female carries the X-linked gene she can be heterozygous or homozygous for the trait. In this case, transmission will be identical to an autosomal dominant inheritance pattern. The Xg^a blood group system is an example of this type of inheritance.

Finally, in example C, we see a case of X-linked recessive inheritance. Characteristically the trait is expressed in the father but is never passed from father to son. Instead, the father passes the trait to all his daughters, who then become carriers. These females then pass the trait on to half of their sons. The trait is expressed in the hemizygous state ($X'Y$), and less frequently in a homozygous female ($X'X'$).

Biochemical Genetics

DEOXYRIBONUCLEIC ACID

Human chromosomes are composed of linear strands of deoxyribonucleic acid (DNA) wound

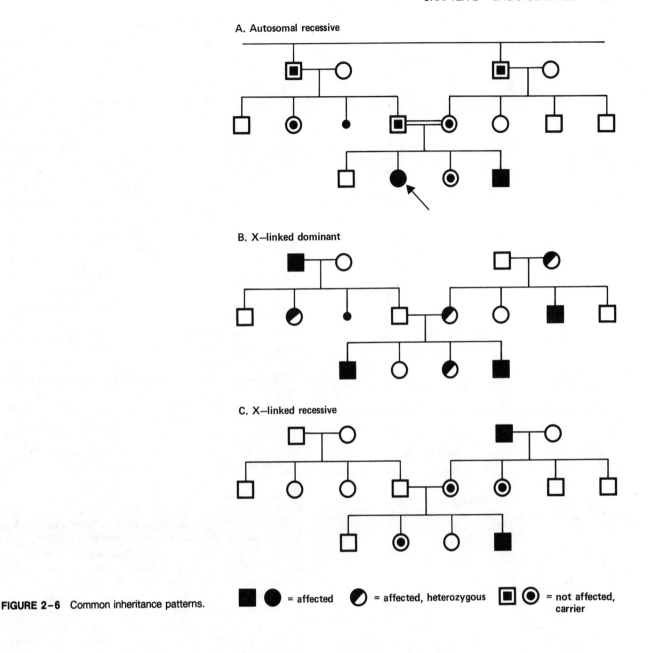

A. Autosomal recessive

B. X—linked dominant

C. X—linked recessive

FIGURE 2-6 Common inheritance patterns.

■ ● = affected   ◑ = affected, heterozygous   ▣ ◉ = not affected, carrier

around proteins called histones, as shown in Figure 2–7. This complex of DNA and proteins is called chromatin. It is this wrapping and condensing of DNA that allows so much genetic material to be stored in a small piece of the chromosome.

DNA is composed of four nitrogenous bases, a molecule of deoxyribose, and one phosphate group. The four nitrogen-containing bases (Fig. 2–8) are the purines adenine (A) and guanine (G) and the pyrimidines thymine (T) and cytosine (C). Each base can bind to a deoxyribose sugar to form a nucleoside; the addition of the phosphate group makes the compound a nucleotide. Hydrogen bonds can form between the A and T or the C and G bases of the nucleotide, as shown

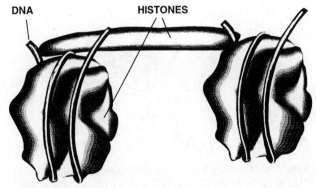

DNA   HISTONES

FIGURE 2-7 The nucleosome consists of a stretch of DNA wound around a group of proteins called histones.

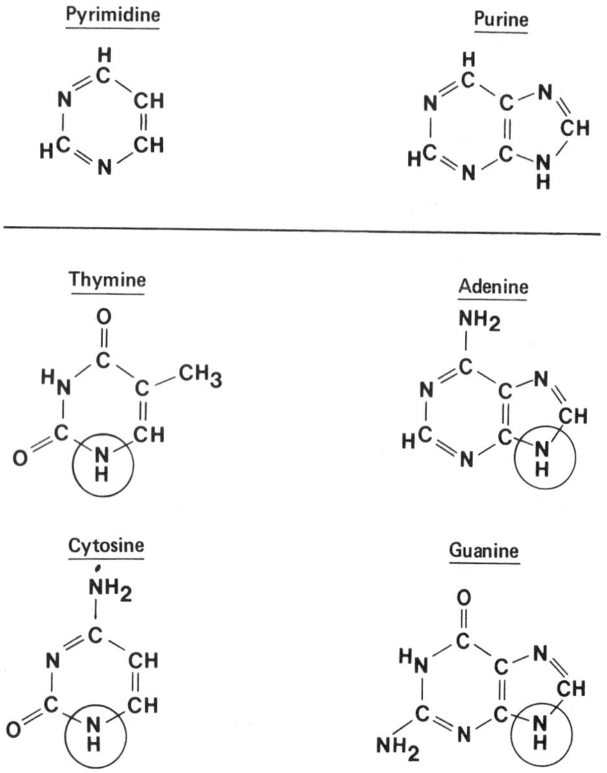

FIGURE 2-8 Pyrimidine and purine bases needed to build DNA.

in Figure 2–9. This binding together of two polymeric strands forms the DNA double helix, as first postulated by Watson and Crick.[1]

Phosphoric acid can attach to the deoxyribose sugar at either the third or the fifth carbon atom. The link-

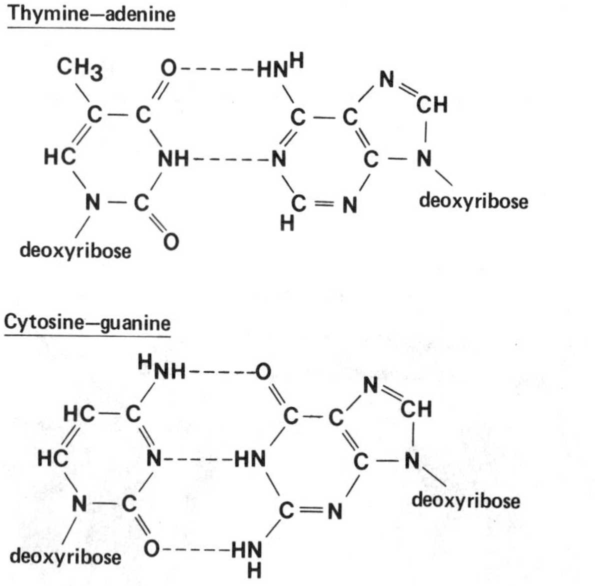

Dotted lines represent interatomic hydrogen bonds, which hold the base pairs together.

FIGURE 2-9 Base pairing in DNA.

age of the purine or pyrimidine base to the sugar is at carbon one. Thus, the two strands of the double helix are antiparallel; that is, one runs 5' to 3' while the other strand runs 3' to 5'. Usually the helix has a right-handed twist, but other studies have elucidated a left-handed configuration known as Z-DNA. In the case of DNA, only one strand of the double helix is transcribed; namely, the 3' to 5' (left-to-right) strand.

Because there are 20 amino acids, it is readily apparent that a single nucleotide cannot code for a single amino acid. Thus, DNA uses a triplet of nucleotides known as a codon to specify a single amino acid. Some amino acids have more than one codon, whereas other codons are signals for stopping transcription (discussed farther on). The genetic code is shown in Table 2–1.

Replication

Following mitoses, each cell must have the correct amount of DNA; therefore, synthesis of DNA must be integrated into the cell cycle. Most DNA replication is bidirectional as well as semiconservative. Simply stated, this means that replication occurs on both DNA strands, and the new DNA copies contain one each of the parent DNA strands.

Many enzymes and other factors participate in the replication process; the most important are shown in Figure 2–10. When DNA replicates, the two strands must unwind or separate from each other. This is accomplished by an enzyme known as helicase, which is driven by the energy produced from hydrolysis of ATP. DNA polymerase acts on the 5' to 3' parent strand to produce an anticomplementary duplicate strand. Replication of the 3' to 5' parent strand, also known as the lagging strand, is more complicated. A ribonucleic acid (RNA) primer is first produced by the enzyme primase, which must anneal to the parent strand to start the duplication process. This occurs at multiple sites along the DNA strand, producing what are called Okasaki fragments. These fragments are then joined together by a DNA ligase, resulting in the second identical copy of the DNA double helix. Finally the cell can proceed to divide.

Repair

With such a complex system for the replication of DNA, it is obvious that some errors may occur. Because the integrity of the DNA is vital to the cell, a system has evolved to correct the occasional replication error. The DNA polymerases themselves have an editing function and correct wrongly incorporated bases. A second system exists to correct the rare error missed by the polymerase editing. This correction system is called mismatch repair. In this system, the incorrect base is removed and DNA polymerase I again has a chance to fill in the blank with the correct base.

Many other alterations can occur in DNA when exposed to noxious chemicals, x-rays, ultraviolet (UV)

TABLE 2–1 **THE GENETIC CODE**

First Position	Second Position				Third Position
	U	C	A	G	
U	PHE	SER	TYR	CYS	U
	PHE	SER	TYR	CYS	C
	LEU	SER	Stop	Stop	A
	LEU	SER	Stop	TRP	G
C	LEU	PRO	HIS	ARG	U
	LEU	PRO	HIS	ARG	C
	LEU	PRO	GLN	ARG	A
	LEU	PRO	GLN	ARG	G
A	ILE	THR	ASN	SER	U
	ILE	THR	ASN	SER	C
	ILE	THR	LYS	ARG	A
	MET	THR	LYS	ARG	G
C	VAL	ALA	ASP	GLY	U
	VAL	ALA	ASP	GLY	S
	VAL	ALA	GLU	GLY	A
	VAL	ALA	GLU	GLY	G

light, etc. Chemicals known as alkylating agents can react with guanine, resulting in depurination. This observation has become a basis for cancer treatment. Ionizing radiation and chemicals such as peroxides can cause single-stranded breaks in the DNA. UV light can alter thymine bases, resulting in "thymine dimers." Some antibodies, such as mitomycin C, can form covalent linkages between bases in opposite strands, thus preventing strand separation during DNA replication. Each of these defects can be corrected by one of several repair systems.

The four major repair systems include photoreactivation (PR), excision repair, recombinational repair, and SOS repair. Photoreactivation enzymatically cleaves thymine dimers when the PR enzyme is activated by visible light. Thymine dimers can also be removed by the multiple enzyme process of excision repair where the bad section of DNA is cut out. Recombinational repair uses a DNA segment from the "good" strand to fill in the strand where the error has been excised. Polymerase I and DNA ligase then fill in the other dimer strand. Finally, SOS repair can be induced following cell (and DNA) damage.

Mutations

Even with all the proofreading and repair systems present, changes can occur in the DNA and hence in the messages contained in the genes. Mutation refers to any structural alteration of DNA in an organism (mutant) that is caused by a physical or chemical agent (mutagen). Some changes may occur in nature without

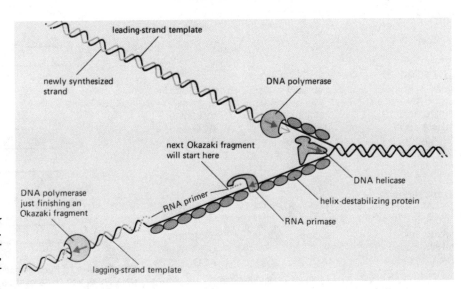

FIGURE 2–10 Some of the major proteins important for DNA replication. (From Alberts, B, et al: Molecular Biology of the Cell. Garland Publishing, New York, 1983, p 230, with permission.)

the presence of a mutagen, and this is referred to as spontaneous mutagenesis.

Mutations may involve only a single base or as much as an entire gene. Simple base changes are known as point mutations and include substitutions, insertions, and deletions. Although a base substitution will change the triplet code, it may not result in an amino acid change. For example, changing ACA to ACC still codes for threonine. A result of the redundancy in the genetic code, this is known as a "silent mutation." It may also refer to an amino acid substitution, which has no detectable effect on the phenotype. A change of a purine base to another purine is known as a transition (Fig. 2–11). When the mutation causes a purine to pyrimidine change, or vice versa, it is known as a transversion.

Other base substitutions may cause a change in the triplet code, which results in a change of the amino acid sequence. This may result in a protein that is incapable of performing its normal function. Many abnormal types of hemoglobin occur because of these "missense" mutations. Sometimes there is no amino acid that corresponds to the changed triplet code. These "nonsense" mutations may be referred to as amber, ochre, or opal mutations, depending on which particular base is mutated, causing the termination of polypeptide production.

Insertions and deletions always result in a change of the triplet code and usually of the resulting amino acid sequence. These types of mutations result in a change in the reading frame and are thus called frameshift mutations. Recent cloning of the A, B, and O genes has shown that the DNA sequence of the O gene is identical to the A allele, except for a single base deletion at position 258.[2] This deletion shifts the reading frame resulting in an entirely different but nonfunctional transferase protein.

Gross genetic changes occurring at a very low frequency can also be classified as mutations. These phenomena include duplications, recombinations, and large gene deletions. Duplications are fairly common in animal cells and may result from evolutionary pressures. Several examples are now known to exist in the world of blood groups. The glycophorin A and B genes, as well as the Rh genes *D* and *CcEe*, are thought to arise from gene duplication. The *C4* genes (the fourth component of complement) duplicated and evolved into *C4A* and *C4B*, which carry the Rodgers and Chido blood group antigens, respectively.

Recombination or crossing-over takes place during meiosis in sexually reproducing organisms. The process of recombination involves breaking two double-stranded homologous DNA molecules, exchanging of both strands at the break, and resolution of the two duplexes (Fig. 2–12). A number of such hybrids can be found in blood group genes, especially those of the MNSs blood group system. Single and double crossover events give rise to the genes for Stones (*St^a*), Dantu, and Mi V. Recombination is probably best observed in the splicing and joining of *V* and *J* genes to produce various types of immunoglobulins.

Deletion of large segments of DNA spanning several thousand base pairs are the final type of mutation to be discussed. Although some DNA mutations can revert to the original phenotype either spontaneously or

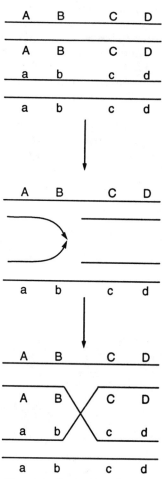

FIGURE 2–12 Recombination occurs when the two strands of DNA break and cross over as shown.

Transition

	S antigen	s̄ antigen
amino acid	methionine	threonine
mRNA code	AUG	ACG
DNA code	TAC	TGC

Transversion

	'N' antigen	He antigen
amino acid	leucine	tryptophan
mRNA code	UUG	UGG
DNA code	AAC	ACC

FIGURE 2–11 Types of DNA mutations.

induced by a mutagen, reversions are never observed in cases of gene deletions. Thus, the possibility of restoring function to a deleted gene is virtually zero. One such example is the Rodgers-negative phenotype. A deletion spanning approximately 30 kD removes the genes for both *C4A* (Rodgers) and 21-hydroxylase.[3] This deletion (in the homozygous state) results in Rodgers-negative phenotype owing to the complete loss of C4A protein.

RIBONUCLEIC ACID

Similar to DNA, ribonucleic acid (RNA) is composed of nucleotides but it usually exists as a single strand. Other differences include the substitution of ribose for deoxyribose and the nitrogenous base uracil for thymine. Ribose differs from deoxyribose by the presence of a hydroxyl group at the 1′ carbon. Uracil differs from thymine by its lack of a methyl group. Some viruses exist that use solely RNA to store their genetic information. In humans, however, RNA is used to translate the genetic code from DNA into protein.

There are three major classes of RNA molecules: messenger RNA (mRNA), ribosomal RNA (rRNA), and transfer RNA (tRNA). All are synthesized from DNA sequences but each has a very different function in protein synthesis. There are also significant differences in the RNA of prokaryotes versus eukaryotes.

Because we are interested in human genetics, our focus will be on the eukaryotic system.

Transcription

Messenger RNA accounts for only about 5 percent of the total RNA content of a cell; however, it has a primary role in protein production. This role is the transcription for DNA to RNA that can be translated into amino acid sequences. To begin transcription, an enzyme known as RNA polymerase II must bind to a specific region of the gene called the promoter. Promoters can be under the control of either positive or negative effectors that influence the rate of transcription. Transcription starts at the 3′ end of the coding DNA strand and proceeds to the 5′ end.

Shortly after initiation of transcription, the 5′ end of the mRNA is capped with a methyl residue. Capping may be needed to protect the mRNA from degradation by nucleases. Most mRNAs terminate at the 3′ end with a series of adenines called the poly A tail. Polyadenylation is thought to increase the stability of the mRNA.

Additional processing of the mRNA occurs in eukaryotes before it is translated (Fig. 2–13). Eukaryotic mRNA characteristically contains intervening sequences (introns) that are not translated. They must be removed from the mRNA by a process known as RNA splicing. The excision of the introns leaves a mature

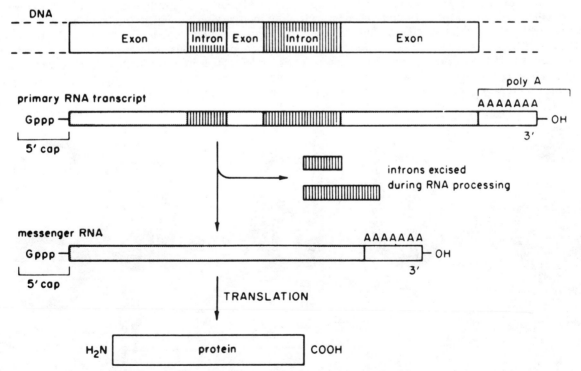

FIGURE 2–13 Transition of DNA to RNA and processing of the transcript to yield mRNA. (From Edwards-Moulds, J and Tregellas, WM: Introductory Molecular Genetics. American Association of Blood Banks, Arlington, VA, 1986, p 59, with permission.)

mRNA, which contains only coding regions (exons) of the gene. Once completed, the mRNA is transported to the cytoplasm, where it is translated.

Translation

Protein synthesis occurs on intracellular particles known as ribosomes composed of rRNA. Translation of mRNA in eukaryotes, unlike prokaryotes, is monocistronic; that is, only one ribosome reads the mRNA transcript at any point in time. The process of protein production involves three major steps: initiation, elongation, and termination.

As shown in Figure 2–14, the first event of the initiation sequence is the attachment of a free molecule of methionine to a specialized transfer RNA called tRNA^{Met}. This requires the additional presence of the high-energy molecule guanine triphosphate (GTP) and an initiation factor (IF2). In the presence of two other initiation factors, IF1 and IF3, the tRNA^{Met} binds to the small subunit (40S) of rRNA to form an initiation complex. A large ribosomal subunit (60S) then joins the complex hydrolyzing GTP and releasing the IFs in the process.

On the large rRNA subunit are two sites: the A and the P site. The tRNA^{Met} with its attached amino acid first occupies the P site. The empty and adjoining A site must next be filled with tRNA carrying the appropriately coded amino acid. There are many different tRNA molecules, but all display a similar structure (Fig. 2–15). This singlestrand of RNA contains two important regions. One of these is a sequence of three bases that can hydrogen-bond to the codon of the mRNA (i.e., the anticodon). The other major site is the area to which the amino acid is bound. Through a specific recognition region, a specific aminoacyl synthetase will attach the proper amino acid to the tRNA. Once charged, the tRNA can now transport its amino acid to the growing polypeptide chain. The incoming tRNA binds to the A site in the presence of an elonga-

tion factor (EF2). This complex hydrolyzes GTP to supply the energy so that the tRNA in the A site can move to the P site. At the same time the tRNA originally in the P site is removed from its amino acid and ejected. The ribosome continues to move down the codons on the mRNA one at a time.

When the ribosome arrives at the stop codon UAG, the translation is complete. With the aid of a termination factor the ribosomal units separate, and the polypeptide chain is ready for posttranslational processing such as glycosylation or sulfation. The mRNA may be rapidly degraded by enzymes at this point, or another 40S rRNA subunit may attach at the start site to begin the process again.

Modern Molecular Techniques

The past 25 years have witnessed an explosion not only in our knowledge of genetic material but also in how to manipulate it. Recombinant DNA techniques have made their way into the clinical laboratory and courtrooms alike. The project to sequence the entire human genome is well underway. Thus, it is appropriate that such discussions be presented here.

DNA TYPING

Restriction Fragment Length Polymorphism Analysis

One of the most-used methods in molecular genetics is the Southern blotting technique first described by Dr. E. M. Southern.[4] It has been a powerful tool in analyzing the eukaryotic genome, as a preliminary analysis before gene cloning, and for the typing of blood group genes including human leukocyte antigen (HLA). It is important, therefore, to have a basic understanding of the terminology as well as the technique.

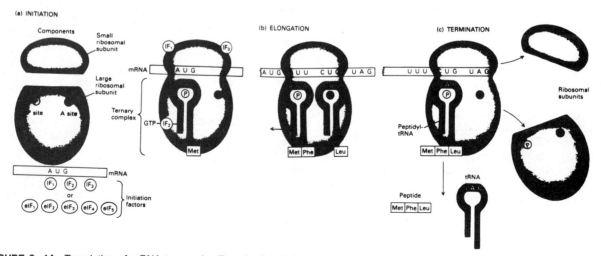

FIGURE 2–14 Translation of mRNA to protein. (From Lodish, Danrell, and Baltimore: Molecular Cell Biology. Copyright 1986 by W.H. Freeman, New York, pp 122–123, with permission.)

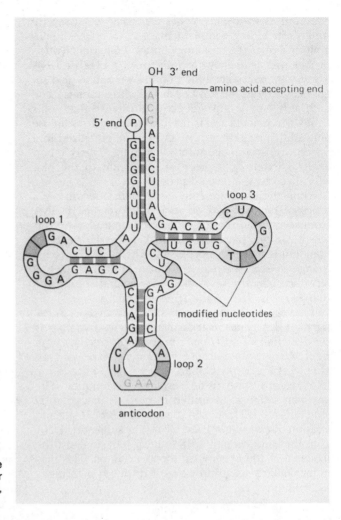

FIGURE 2–15 Schematic drawing of tRNA showing the base pairing and loop structures. (From Alberts, B, et al: Molecular Biology of the Cell. Garland Publishing, New York, 1983, p 109, with permission.)

The first step involved with Southern blotting is to obtain DNA for analysis. When RNA is substituted for DNA the procedure is called Northern blotting. Sources of DNA can be tissues in which the gene under study is expressed, bone marrow, peripheral leukocytes, or cell cultures, to name a few. Genomic DNA is usually prepared by a salting-out technique or a procedure that uses proteinase K digestion followed by phenol-chloroform extraction and ethanol precipitation.

Once the DNA is in hand it must be digested (cut into smaller pieces) by restriction enzymes. Restriction endonucleases (re) are enzymes found naturally occurring in various strains of bacteria. Each enzyme is named after its host organism (e.g., *Escherichia coli* produces an enzyme called *Eco* RI). Each enzyme cuts DNA of a specific length of base pairs and at a specific site. As shown in Figure 2–16, the cut may be either blunt or staggered. A blunt cut cuts the two pieces evenly into halves, whereas a staggered cut leaves overhanging edges. The latter is useful in cloning techniques.

The fragments that result from the digestion must now be separated by running them on agarose gel

Blunt Cut

5′ G T T ↓ A A C   <u>Hpa</u> I recognizes

3′ C A A ↑ T T G   6 base pairs

Staggered Cut

5′ G ↓ A A T T C   <u>Eco</u> RI recognizes

3′ C T T A A ↑ G   6 base pairs

FIGURE 2–16 Cutting of DNA by restriction techniques.

electrophoresis. Because the agarose gel is too bulky to be handled easily, the separated pieces are transferred to a solid support matrix, usually nitrocellulose, before detection. Once the replica of DNA is made, it can be probed.

A probe is a piece of DNA having a sequence for the

gene one is studying. Probes can come from several sources including complementary DNA (cDNA), genomic DNA, or oligonucleotides. Oligonucleotide probes are artificially manufactured pieces of DNA whose sequences are based on known amino acid sequences. The probe can be labeled with a radioisotope such as ^{32}P or a nonradioactive substance that emits light when reacted and hybridized to the nitrocellulose blot. Matching sequences can then be visualized in a procedure known as autoradiography. This method involves exposing a piece of x-ray film to the blot hybridized to the labeled probe.

When the blots are fully developed, one will see a series of bands based on molecular weight. If DNA from several individuals is analyzed, one may see different banding patterns (Fig. 2–17). These restriction fragment length polymorphisms (RFLPs) result from a change in the base pair sequence of DNA, which is recognized by the restriction enzyme and results in a change in the size of the DNA fragments.

One very useful application of RFLP analysis is typing for HLA genes in transplant patients. Another is the detection of an *O* gene in the heterozygous state (i.e., *AO* or *BO*). Because an *O* gene expressed no product it was impossible to detect its presence in the heterozygous state using serologic techniques. The base pair deletion identified in persons having an *O* gene (Fig. 2–18) results in the loss of a *BstE* II site and creation of a new *Kpn* I site.[2] Thus, by subjecting DNA from these individuals to Southern blot analysis, the presence of the *O* gene can be ascertained. This may be particularly useful in cases of disputed paternity.

Polymerase Chain Reaction and Allele-Specific Probes

Since the first report of DNA amplification using polymerase chain reaction (PCR), the number of different applications has grown steadily. Only the applications most pertinent to the field of immunogenetic and transfusion medicine are discussed here.

The PCR is an in vitro method for the enzymatic synthesis of specific DNA sequences, using two oligonucleotide primers that hybridize to opposite DNA strands and that flank the region of interest. Thus, as with most molecular techniques, one needs a source of DNA to amplify. One advantage to this technique is that only a small amount of DNA is necessary, as the

A or B Gene

5' G ↓ G T G A C C C

3' C C A C T G G ↑ G

BstE II restriction site

O Gene

deletion
#258

5' G G T - A C C ↓ C

3' C ↑ C A - T G G G

Kpn I restriction site

FIGURE 2–18 Identification of a blood group O gene by changes in restriction enzyme sites.

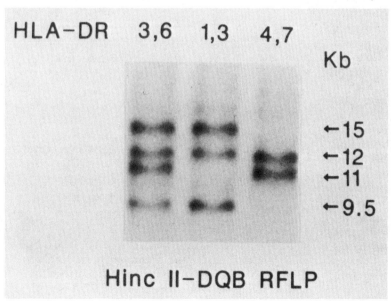

Hinc II-DQB RFLP

FIGURE 2–17 Southern blot analysis of genomic DNA to determine HLA-DR genotype.

reactions are typically done in small total volumes (50 to 100 μl).

The DNA is mixed with a reaction buffer, nucleotides, the appropriate oligonucleotide primers, and *Taq* enzyme. *Taq* is a thermal stable DNA polymerase obtained from the bacteria that live in hot springs (i.e., *Thermus aquaticus*). In the procedure, the target DNA is first denatured and the primers are allowed to base pair or anneal to the DNA. The *Taq* polymerase then fills in the remainder of the new DNA strand, resulting in two molecules of DNA where originally there had been one. Because these primer extension products can serve as templates in the next cycle, the number of target DNA copies double at each cycle. For example, after 20 PCR cycles there is a millionfold amplification of DNA. This entire process has been automated and has become a very useful technique in many settings.

Following the amplification process, the DNA samples can be blotted onto nitrocellulose. Because the thermocycler has 96 wells, a "dot blot" of all 96 samples can be made at one time. The blot is then hybridized to an allele-specific probe and interpreted following exposure to x-ray film (Fig. 2–19).

Polymerase chain reaction has already had an impact on the field of medicine. This new technique is now being used in place of RFLP analyses for the prenatal detection of sickle cell disease, β-thalassemia, etc. The ability to detect DNA polymorphisms in minute biologic evidence samples using PCR has revolutionized forensic testing. Probably the most significant applications in the practice of transfusion medicine will be the use of PCR to detect small amounts of viral DNA in donor blood samples and the ability to type more accurately for the HLA antigens that are so important in transplantations. Most of the hypervariable regions of the class II HLA genes have been sequenced, thus allowing allele-specific oligonucleotides to be produced. Because these oligonucleotides can be used to type individuals undergoing transplantation more accurately, it is highly likely that PCR and

allele-specific oligonucleotide typing will replace conventional serologic typing for all clinical purposes.[5]

Cloning and Sequencing

The field of blood group genetics is once again undergoing change. Recognition of blood group antigens was first performed serologically. Years later, biochemical analyses gave us new insights into antigenic structure and function. Today, we are attacking these questions at the gene level. Already the genes for ABO, Rh, MNSs, Gerbich, and Chido/Rodgers, to name a few, have been cloned. Thus, in order to understand the latest immunogenetics literature, one needs some knowledge of the basic terminology and techniques involved.

Just as with the crossmatch, many variations of gene cloning have evolved. It is impossible to discuss all of them here, so what follows is a general approach to cloning a blood group gene (Fig. 2–20). First one must obtain a source of RNA for the cloning process. In the case of blood group genes, this source is reticulocytes or the fetal liver. The mRNA is selectively separate from the total RNA by passing it over an oligo-dT column. The thymines will bind only to molecules of mRNA because only this type of RNA has the complimentary poly-A tail.

Next the single-stranded mRNA must be converted to double-stranded DNA. This procedure involves synthesis of the first strand of cDNA using the enzyme reverse transcriptase. Using this as a template, the second DNA strand can be generated using DNA polymerase I.

The double-stranded cDNA is then inserted into a cloning vector. A vector is a extrachromosomal genetic element that can carry a recombinant DNA molecule into a host bacterial cell. Vectors can be bacteriophages such as λgt11, plasmids such as pBR322, or cosmids. The cDNA is incubated with the vectors in

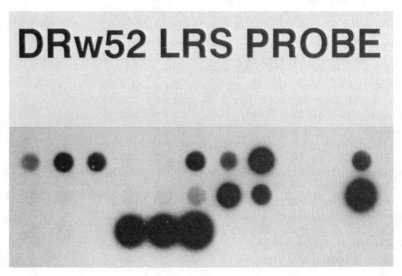

FIGURE 2–19 Dot-blot of PCR products hybridized to an allele-specific HLA probe.

Source total RNA

↓ Oligo dT columns

Selectively remove mRNA

↓ reverse transcriptase

Convert to cDNA

↓ DNA polymerase

Make double-stranded DNA

↓ bacteriophage, etc.

Insert into cloning vector

↓ <u>E. coli</u>

Transfect into bacterial host

↓ antibody or DNA probe

Screen for positive clones

↓

Propagate positives

FIGURE 2–20 Representative scheme for cloning of a blood group gene.

the presence of T4 ligase, which joins the two DNA molecules together.

The vector is then transfected or transferred into the bacterial host where it is replicated with each replication of the bacterium. Because each individual vector may contain a different mRNA, only a few vectors may contain the message of the gene being studied. This variety of vectors carrying many different mRNAs, propagated in a host bacteria, is called a cDNA library.

The blood group gene will be carried by those bacteria who have taken up the appropriate vector. These can be identified by screening a bacterial culture plate using a method very similar to that for Southern blotting. If the cDNA library is in an expression vector, the blood group antigen will be expressed, and the filter can be probed using a conjugated antibody to the antigen. Otherwise, the library can be screened with an oligonucleotide probe based on part of a known amino acid sequence. Positive clones are then picked out and propagated until a pure culture is obtained.

The cloned DNA is now ready to be purified and sequenced. Two basic methods are available for sequencing: the Maxam-Gilbert technique[6] and the Sanger dideoxy technique.[7] In the chemical degradation technique of Maxam and Gilbert,[6] a DNA fragment is first radiolabeled usually with ^{32}P. The DNA is then partially degraded in a set of base-specific chemical reactions, which result in removal of the derivative base and subsequent cleavage of the DNA. The set of labeled fragments is run side by side on an acrylamide gel electrophoresis followed by autoradiography. The pattern of bands on the x-ray film is read sequentially to determine the DNA sequence (Fig. 2–21).

In the enzymatic method of Sanger,[7] an oligonucleotide primer is hybridized to a single-strand DNA template. The strand is filled in using ^{32}P-labeled dATP, DNA polymerase, dideoxynucleotides, and normal deoxynucleotides. A series of labeled bands results, which can then be separated by electrophoresis as described previously. From the gene sequence it is a simple matter to deduce the amino acid sequence of its protein. In fact, today it is often easier to sequence the gene than to determine the amino acid structure.

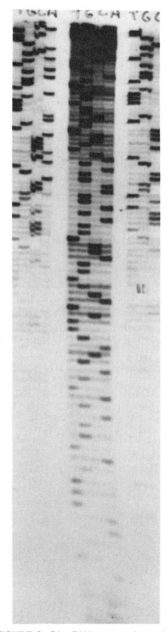

FIGURE 2–21 DNA sequencing gel.

Summary

This chapter gives the reader a basic introduction to both classic and modern genetics. By understanding the basic principles, we can better appreciate the complexity of today's knowledge regarding blood groups. In addition, knowledge of the molecular techniques used today will help us to assimilate them more rapidly into the ever-growing field of transfusion medicine.

Review Questions

1. Which of the following best describes mitosis?
   A. Genetic material is duplicated, equally divided among four daughter cells
   B. Genetic material is duplicated, equally divided between two daughter cells
   C. Genetic material is triplicated, equally divided between two daughter cells
   D. Genetic material is halved, equally divided between two daughter cells

2. When a recessive trait is expressed, it means that:
   A. One gene carrying the trait was present
   B. Two genes carrying the trait were present
   C. No gene carrying the trait was present
   D. The trait is present but difficult to observe

3. In a pedigree, the index case is another name for:
   A. Stillbirth
   B. Consanguineous mating
   C. Propositus
   D. Dizygotic twins
   E. Monozygotic twins

4. What four nitrogenous bases make up DNA?
   A. Adenine, leucine, guanine, thymine
   B. Alanine, cytosine, guanine, purine
   C. Adenine, cytosine, guanine, leucine
   D. Alanine, cytosine, guanine, thymine
   E. Adenine, cytosine, guanine, thymine

5. Proteins are formed on structures called:
   A. Golgi bodies
   B. Mitochondria
   C. Nuclei
   D. Ribosomes
   E. Azure bodies

6. Which phenotype could not result from the mating of a Jk(a+b+) female and a Jk(a+b+) male?
   A. Jk(a+b−)
   B. Jk(a+b+)
   C. Jk(a−b+)
   D. Jk(a−b−)

7. Exon refers to:
   A. The part of a gene that is excised when mRNA is produced
   B. The coding region of a gene
   C. The repetitive sequences at the end of the mRNA
   D. The enzymes used to cut DNA into fragments
   E. The control region of a gene

8. PCR technology can be used to:
   A. Amplify small amounts of DNA
   B. Clone fragments of RNA
   C. Digest genomic DNA into small fragments
   D. Repair broken pieces of DNA

9. Transcription can be defined as:
   A. Introduction of DNA into cultured cells
   B. Reading of mRNA by the ribosome
   C. Synthesis of RNA using DNA as a template
   D. Removal of intravening sequences to form a mature RNA molecule
   E. Production of many copies of genomic DNA

10. When a man possesses a trait that he passes to all his daughters and none of his sons, the trait is said to be:
    A. X-linked dominant
    B. X-linked recessive
    C. Autosomal dominant
    D. Autosomal recessive
    E. Balanced hemizygous

Answers to Review Questions

1. B (p 27)
2. B (p 28)
3. C (p 30)
4. E (p 31)
5. D (p 36)
6. D (p 28)
7. B (p 36)
8. A (p 38)
9. C (p 35)
10. A (p 30)

References

1. Watson, JD and Crick, FHC: Molecular structure of nucleic acids: A structure for deoxyribose nucleic acid. Nature 171:737, 1953.
2. Yamamoto, F, et al: Molecular genetic basis of the histo-blood group ABO system. Nature 345:229, 1990.
3. de Van Kim, C, et al: Molecular cloning and primary structure of the human blood group RhD polypeptide. Proc Natl Acad Sci USA 89:10925, 1992.
4. Southern, EM: Detection of specific sequences among DNA fragments separated by gel electrophoresis. J Mol Biol 98:503, 1975
5. Pollack, MS: Class II HLA antigens: HLA-D, -DR, -DQ, and DP. In Moulds, JM, Fawcett, KJ, and Garner, RJ (eds): Scientific and Technical Aspects of the Major Histocompatibility Complex. American Association of Blood Banks, Arlington, VA, 1989, p 47.

6. Maxam, AM and Gilbert, W: A new method for sequencing DNA. Proc Natl Acad Sci USA 74:560, 1977.
7. Sanger, R, Nicklen, S, and Coulson, AR: DNA sequencing with chain inhibitors. Proc Natl Acad Sci USA 74:5463, 1977.

Bibliography

Alberts, B, et al: Molecular Biology of the Cell. Garland Publishing, New York, 1983.
Edwards-Moulds, J and Tregellas, WM (eds): Introductory Molecular Genetics. American Association of Blood Banks, Arlington, VA, 1986.
Freifelder, D: Molecular Biology. A Comprehensive Introduction to Prokaryotes and Eukaryotes. Jones and Bartlett Publishers, Boston, 1983.
Giblett, ER: Genetic Markers in Human Blood. Blackwell Scientific Publications, Oxford, 1969.
Maxson, LR and Daugherty, CH: Genetics, A Human Perspective. Wm C Brown Publishers, Dubuque, IA, 1985.
Race, RR and Sanger, R: Blood Groups in Man, ed 6. Blackwell Scientific Publications, Oxford, 1975.

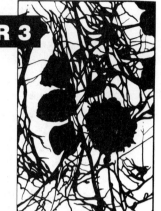

CHAPTER 3

Fundamentals of Immunology for Blood Bankers

Sharon Martin, EdD, MT(ASCP)

OBJECTIVES

Upon completion of this chapter, the learner should be able to:

1 Name and describe the characteristics and functions of cells involved in the immune response.

2 List cytokines according to their role in the immune response.

3 Explain how the major histocompatibility complex and human leukocyte antigen control the immune response.

4 Describe the characteristics of immunoglobulins in relation to structure, significance for blood banking, variations, and Fc receptors on effector cells.

5 Explain the activation sequence for the two major complement pathways, how complement is bound by red cell antibodies, and the preservation and destruction of complement in test systems and preserved blood products.

6 Characterize the immune response according to antigen-antibody reactions, host factors, suppression, and primary and secondary responses.

7 Discuss laboratory techniques for detecting antigen-antibody reactions.

8 Discuss factors affecting agglutination reactions.

9 Explain the significance of certain immune-mediated diseases for blood bank testing.

The immune response involves a highly complex network of tissues, organs, cells, and biologic mediators that function primarily to recognize and react to any substance regarded as foreign to the organism.[1-3] This response entails the discrimination of "self" from "nonself" (or foreign) in a process designed to eliminate those elements determined to be nonself.[3] Macrophages, T lymphocytes, B lymphocytes, and natural killer (NK) cells interact directly from cell to cell or indirectly by mediators through a complex system of cell markers and receptors. In laboratory testing, these cell surface molecules, which specify leukocyte definition and function, are designated as clusters of differentiation (CD), groups that are recognized by various monoclonal antibodies.[4] Many mediator substances such as cytokines, immunoglobulins, and proteins of the complement, kinin, clotting, and fibrinolytic systems represent cellular products that have effects on organ systems, cells, and other substances.[3,5] Additionally, immune response is genetically influenced by the genes of the major histocompatibility complex (MHC), which determine the human leukocyte antigen (HLA) found on cells. The HLA complex is important in antigen presentation and the cellular recognition processes that occur during immune reaction to a foreign substance.[6]

Although the blood banker is predominantly concerned with testing aimed at detecting blood group antigens and antibodies and preventing the formation of immune blood group antibodies, a basic knowledge of the overall immune response is helpful in understanding the performance and possible resolution of blood bank testing problems, especially those related to selection of test procedures and patient testing issues.

Cells of the Immune Response

Cells of the immune system are arranged in primary lymphoid organs such as the thymus and bone marrow, and secondary lymphoid organs such as lymph nodes and spleen. In the primary organs cells differentiate and mature into immune-competent cells; in the secondary organs, cells associate and communicate with each other and interact with antigens. Immune cells originate from pluripotential stem cells through two main lineages: the lymphoid and the myeloid. The myeloid cells consist of phagocytic cells such as monocytes and polymorphonuclear granulocytes, as well as other antigen-presenting cells (APCs) such as dendritic cells. The lymphoid cells include the various subpopulations of T cells, B cells, and NK cells.[7]

Myeloid precursors, which give rise to the cells of the mononuclear phagocytic system, originate in the bone marrow and differentiate into circulating blood monocytes and tissue macrophages. The primary function of these cells is phagocytosis and processing of antigen in order to prepare the antigen for further immune outcomes mediated by lymphocytes.[7] Phagocytic cells can be very effective in directly killing bacteria, fungi, and tumor cells.[8] Mononuclear phagocytes also serve as APCs, which present processed antigen to lymphocytes. Additionally, other cells that are not leukocytes can acquire the ability to become APCs under the proper immune stimulation. Examples of such cells include Langerhans' cells in the skin and follicular dendritic cells in the lymph nodes. Mononuclear phagocytes interact with other immune cells and antigens through a complex system of cellular receptors. When phagocytic cells function in antigen recognition and binding of antibody or of complement-coated (opsonized) antigen, or both, the principal receptors involved are those for the Fc portion of immunoglobulin G (IgG) and the CR1 receptor for the complement component C3b.[9] When the monocytes and macrophages function as APCs, they express the Ia antigens, the class II MHC antigens. Dendritic cells, however, although they express the Ia marker, lack the Fc receptor and some of the other distinctive monocyte-macrophage markers.[10]

Polymorphonuclear granulocytes originate in the bone marrow and account for approximately 70 percent of the circulating leukocytes. These cells are further classified as neutrophils, eosinophils, and basophils — mast cells based on the staining characteristics of their cytoplasmic granules. The main role of these cells is phagocytosis of microorganisms as they function primarily in acute inflammatory responses with antibody and complement.[11] All granulocytes possess receptors for the Fc portion of IgG (CD16) and complement receptors, C5a, CR1(CD35), and CR3(CD11b). Additionally, eosinophils possess low-affinity Fc receptors for IgE. Basophils and mast cells possess high-affinity Fc IgE receptors.

Lymphocytic cells generated in the thymus or bone marrow travel through the circulatory system to the lymph nodes and spleen. Lymphocytes account for approximately 20 percent of circulating leukocytes. In the primary organs, these cells acquire receptors that equip them to meet antigenic confrontations and to differentiate between self and nonself antigens. In the secondary organs, immune cells are provided with an interactive environment in which immune response information is exchanged and specific actions are initiated.[7]

The two primary classifications of lymphocytes are T cells and B cells. Although these cells may be similar in appearance, they may be distinguished by the presence of distinctive cell markers. The T cell has a T-cell antigen receptor (TCR) usually identified with the CD3 complex. The TCR associates in cell-to-cell contact and interacts with both antigenic determinants and MHC proteins.[12] The CD2 marker, which has the unique ability to bind with sheep erythrocytes, is also a distinctive molecule found on T cells. The two main subgroups of T lymphocytes are T-helper (TH) cells and T-suppressor or T-cytotoxic (TS/TC) cells. TH cells have the CD4 marker and recognize antigen together with the MHC class II molecules. TS/TC cells possess CD8 markers and interact with MHC class I molecules. T cells function in the initiation and regulation of the immune response by interceding in effector responses to specific antigens and secreting cellular mediator substances, such as interleukins and interferons.[13]

B cells are generally defined by the presence of immunoglobulin on their surface, although they also possess MHC class II antigens; complement receptors, CD35 and CD21; Fc receptors for IgG; and also CD19, CD20, and CD22 markers, which are commonly used to identify B cells. Immunoglobulin may act as an antigen receptor for binding simple structural antigens or those antigens having multiple repeating determinants (T-cell–independent antigens, not requiring the intervention of T-cell help). When T-cell–dependent antigens (structurally complex substances) are encountered, B cells require the intervention of T cells to assist in the production of antibody. When B cells become activated, they develop into plasma cells, which produce and secrete large quantities of soluble immunoglobulin into tissue or serum.[13] Immunoglobulin can neutralize toxic substances, facilitate phagocytosis by acting as an opsonin to coat antigens, kill microbes directly by causing cell lysis, and combine with antigens on cellular surfaces to cause destruction of antigen either extravascularly or intravascularly, in combination with complement.

Natural killer cells are sometimes referred to as third-population cells (TPCs) because, although they originate in the bone marrow, they have a distinct developmental line apart from those of T and B lymphocytes.[7] NK cells do not have surface immunoglobulin or secrete immunoglobulin; they do not have an antigen receptor like the TCR found on T lymphocytes. NK cells possess CD56 and CD16 markers and do not require the presence of an MHC marker in order to respond to an antigen. NK cells are capable of lysing virally infected cells and tumor cells. By possessing receptors for the Fc portion of an immunoglobulin molecule, NK cells may bind and lyse antibody-coated cells in a process known as antibody-dependent cellular cytotoxicity (ADCC).[14]

Cytokines

Cytokines are polypeptides that act as biologic mediators of immune and tissue cells. Cytokines are divided into lymphokines, which are produced by lymphocytes, and monokines, which are produced by monocytes and macrophages. Cytokines modulate the host response to antigens by regulating growth, mobility, and differentiation of leukocytes.[15] One cytokine may function alone to mediate one effect; several cytokines may have increased or decreased quantitative effects; or other cytokines may act in a synergistic manner, in which one cytokine requires the presence of a second cytokine to produce an effect.[16]

As a result of the various modes of action of cytokines, significant overlay in function may occur. Interleukins (ILs), colony-stimulating factors (CSFs), interferons (INFs), and tumor necrosis factors (TNFs) compose the major classifications of cytokines. Cytokines act by binding to target cell receptors. The number of receptors per cell dramatically increases as the cell is transformed from a resting to a response state. The initial sign for this transformation may be the binding of antigen or other cytokines to the cell receptor. IL-2, for example, requires this initial signal to be the antigen presented by an APC to a T cell. The production and response of receptor expression for

IL-2, therefore, is maximized by an antigen-activated T cell.[17] After binding, both the receptor and the cytokine is internalized by the cell to induce the target cell to produce various biologic responses such as cell growth and differentiation, as well as chemoattractive, antiviral, antiproliferative, and immunomodulating activities for other immune cells (Table 3–1).[15]

Genetic Control

The MHC is the region of the genome that encodes those proteins known as the HLAs. The MHC is very influential in immune recognition and regulation of antigen presentation in cell-to-cell interactions, as well as being significant in certain disease associations, transplantation, and paternity testing.[18,19]

Human leukocyte antigen molecules are categorized into three classes: class I, class II, and class III. Class I molecules are found on all nucleated cells. In order for antigen to be recognized by a cytotoxic (CD8) T cell, it must be recognized within the context of a class I molecule (Figs. 3–1 and 3–2). After recognition, the cytotoxic cell destroys the target cell bearing the antigen.[18] Class II molecules are found on immunocompetent cells such as B lymphocytes, APCs, and activated T cells.[20] A class II molecule on an APC is essential for presenting processed antigen to a TH (CD4) cell (Figs. 3–3 and 3–4). Class III molecules encode components such as C2, C4, and factor B (see Complement System).[18]

Characteristics of Immunoglobulins

Immunoglobulins are protein molecules that are produced in response to an immunogen or antigen. Immunoglobulins have specific antibody activity for the antigen that initially invoked their development.[21] As mentioned previously, immunoglobulins are found on the surface of B cells. B cells, on immune stimulation, mature into antibody-producing plasma cells. Immunoglobulins compose approximately 20 percent of the total plasma proteins that are disseminated in body fluids.[21] Although the main function of immunoglobulins is the binding of antigen, these molecules have other biologic functions, such as facilitating phagocytosis, neutralizing toxic substances, fixing complement, and killing microbes.[22]

Immunoglobulins have been classified as IgA, IgD, IgE, IgG, and IgM, corresponding to the chemical structure of the heavy chain of the molecule. In addition to the differences in heavy chain structure, immunoglobulin classes also vary in other features such as serum concentration, molecular weight, biologic activity, percentage of carbohydrate content, and plasma half-life, as illustrated in Table 3–2. The immunoglobulin found in greatest concentration in serum is IgG, which composes approximately 80 percent of the total

serum immunoglobulin; 13 percent is IgA (IgA, however, is the major immunoglobulin found in body secretions such as saliva); 6 percent is IgM; 1 percent is IgD; and IgE is present only in trace amounts.[23]

IMMUNOGLOBULIN STRUCTURE

All classes and subclasses of immunoglobulins have a common chemical structural configuration (Fig. 3–5). The basic immunoglobulin unit is composed of four polypeptide chains: two identical light chains (molecular weights of approximately 22,500 d) and two identical heavy chains (molecular weight from approximately 50,000 to 75,000 d). Both light and heavy chains are held together by covalent disulfide bonds. The heavy chains are interconnected by disulfide linkages in the hinge region of the molecule. Light and heavy chains are held together in a similar manner. The immunoglobulin classes are named according to the structure of their heavy chains, and the five types of heavy chains are designated alpha (IgA), delta (IgD), epsilon (IgE), gamma (IgG), and mu (IgM). Only two types of light chains, kappa and lambda, are found in all classes of immunoglobulins.[23]

The immunoglobulin molecule has two terminal regions, the carboxyl (-COOH) and amino (-NH2) terminal regions. The carboxyl region of the heavy chain has a comparatively constant amino acid sequence for any antibody class. This area of the heavy chain comprises the constant region. The light chain also has a constant region. Enzyme cleavage by papain splits the antibody molecule at the hinge region to give three fragments, two fragment antigen binding (Fab) fragments and one Fc fragment. The Fc fragment encompasses the portion of the immunoglobulin molecule from the carboxyl region to the hinge region. The Fc region is responsible for complement fixation, monocyte binding, and placental transfer (IgG only). The amino terminal regions are known as the variable regions of the light and heavy chains because they are structured according to the variations in antibody specificity against diverse antigens encountered in the immune response. The Fab fragments encompass the portions of the immunoglobulin from the hinge region to the amino terminal. The Fab portion is the region responsible for binding antigen[23] (Fig. 3–5).

Domains constitute regions of light and heavy chains, which are folded into compact globular loops (Fig. 3–6). Domains are held together by intrachain covalent disulfide bonds. V specifies the variable region, and C the constant region. One domain (V_L) is in the variable region and one domain (C_L) is in the constant region of each light chain. One variable domain (V_H) is also on each heavy chain. The immunoglobulin class determines the number of domains on the constant regions of each heavy chain. There are, therefore, four constant domains, C_H1 to C_H4, on the heavy chains of IgA, IgD, and IgG and five constant domains, C_H1 to C_H5, on the heavy chains of IgE and IgM. Antigen binding and idiotypic regions (which

TABLE 3–1 CYTOKINES

Cytokine	Source	Stimulatory Function
Interleukins		
IL-1	Mφ, fibroblasts	Proliferation activated B and T cells
		Induction PGE_2 and cytokines by Mφ
		Induction neutrophil and T-adhesion molecules on endothelial cells
		Induction IL-6, IFN-β1, and GM-CSF
		Induction fever, acute phase proteins, bone resorption by osteoclasts
IL-2	T	Growth activated T and B cells; activation NK cells
IL-3	T, MC	Growth and differentiation hemopoietic precursors
		Mast cell growth
IL-4	CD4, T, MC, BM stroma	Proliferation activated B, T, mast, and hemopoietic precursor
		Induction MHC class II and FcϵR on B cells, p75 IL-2R on T cells
		Isotype switch to IgG1 and IgE
		Mφ APC and cytotoxic function, Mφ fusion (migration inhibition)
IL-5	CD4 T, MC	Proliferation activated B cells; production IgM and IgA
		Proliferation eosinophils; expression p55 IL-2R
IL-6	CD4 T, Mφ, MC, fibroblasts	Growth and differentiation B- and T-cell effectors, and hemopoietic precursors
		Acute phase proteins
IL-7	BM stromal cells	Proliferation pre-B, CD4-, CD8-, T cells, and activated mature T cells
IL-8	Monocytes	Chemotaxis and activation neutrophils
		Chemotaxis T cells
Colony Stimulating Factors		
GM-CSF	T, Mφ, fibroblasts, MC, endothelium	Growth granulocyte and Mφ colonies
		Activates Mφ, neutrophils, eosinophils
G-CSF	Fibroblasts, endothelium	Growth mature granulocytes
M-CSF	Fibroblasts, endothelium, epithelium	Growth macrophage colonies
Tumor Necrosis Factors		
TNF-α	Mφ, T	Tumor cytotoxicity; cachexia
TNF-β	CD4 T	Induction acute phase proteins
		Antiviral and antiparasitic activity
		Activation phagocytic cells
		Induction IFN-γ, TNF-α, IL-1, GM-CSF, and IL-6
		Endotoxic shock
Interferons		
IFN-α	Leukocytes	Antiviral; expression MHC I
IFN-β	Fibroblasts	
IFN-γ	T (Mφ?)	Antiviral; Mφ activation
		Expression MHC classes I and II on Mφ and other cells
		Differentiation of cytotoxic T
		Synthesis IgG2a by activated B
		Antagonism several IL-4 actions
Other		
TGF-β	T, B	Inhibition IL-2R upregulation and IL-2 dependent T- and B-cell proliferation
		Inhibition (by TGF-β1) of IL-3 + CSF-induced hemopoiesis
		Isotype switch to IgA
		Wound repair (fibroblast chemotoxin) and angiogenesis
		Neoplastic transformation certain normal cells
CSIF	CD4 T	Inhibits IFNγ secretion
LIF	T	Proliferation embryonic stem cells without affecting differentiation
		Chemoattraction and activation of eosinophils

From Roitt, I: Essential Immunology, ed 7. Blackwell Scientific Publications, Oxford, 1991, with permission.
APC = antigen presenting cells; BM = bone marrow; CSIF = cytokine synthesis inhibitory factor; FcϵR = immunoglobulin Fc receptor for IgE; G-CSF = granulocyte colony stimulating factor; GM-CSF = granulocyte monocyte/macrophage colony stimulating factor; IFN = interferon; IL = interleukin; LIF = leukocyte inhibitory factor; MC = mast cell; M-CSF = monocyte colony stimulating factor; MHC = major histocompatibility complex; Mφ = macrophage; NK = natural killer cells; PGE_2 = prostaglandin E_2; T = T lymphocyte; TGF = transforming growth factor; TNF = tumor necrosis factor.

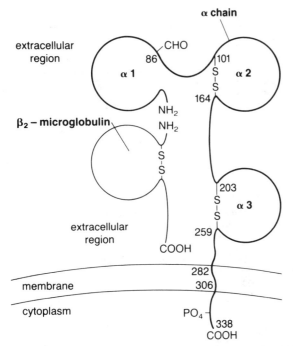

FIGURE 3–1   Class I HLA molecule. Molecule consists of an MW 44,000 polymorphic transmembrane glycoprotein, termed the α *chain*, which bears the antigenic determinant, in noncovalent association with an MW 12,000 nonpolymorphic protein termed β_2 *microglobulin*. The α chain has three extracellular domains termed α_1, α_2, and α_3. NH$_2$ = amino terminus; COOH = carboxy terminus; CHO = carbohydrate side chain; -SS- = disulfide bond; PO$_4$ = phosphate radical. (From Swartz,[20] p 47, with permission.)

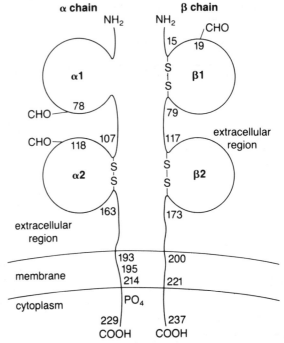

FIGURE 3–3   Class II (HLA-DR) molecule. The molecule consists of an MW 34,000 glycoprotein (the α chain) in a noncovalent association with an MW 29,000 glycoprotein (the β chain). (From Swartz,[20] p 49, with permission.)

distinguish one V domain from all other V domains) are located within the three-dimensional structures formed by the V_L and V_H domains. Heavy chain domains are associated with some of the biologic properties of immunoglobulins, especially those of IgG and IgM. Complement fixation, for example, is identified with the C_H2 domain. The C_H3 domain serves as an attachment site for the Fc receptor of monocytes and macrophages.[23]

IMMUNOGLOBULINS SIGNIFICANT FOR BLOOD BANKING

IgG and IgM are the immunoglobulins having the most significance for blood bankers. Most clinically significant antibodies are IgG, which react at body temperature, 37°C; clinically significant antibodies, therefore, are capable of destroying transfused antigen-positive red cells. IgM antibodies are found as naturally occurring antibodies in the ABO system. Other blood groups such as Lewis, Ii, P, and MNS may

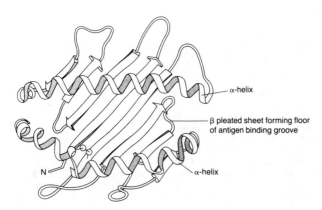

FIGURE 3–2   Top view of a crystalline structure of a class I HLA molecule. The molecule is shown as the T cell receptor would see it. The antigen-binding site formed by the α helices (ribbonlike structures) and β-pleated strands (broad arrows) is shown. N indicates the amino terminus. (From Swartz,[20] p 48, with permission.)

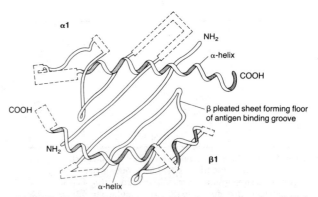

FIGURE 3–4   Top view of a crystalline structure of a class II HLA molecule. The molecule is shown as the T cell receptor would see it. The antigen-binding site formed by the α chain α_1 domain and β chain β_1 domain consists of the β-pleated sheet platform (thin strands) supporting two α helices (ribbonlike structures) and is very similar to that of the class I molecule (see Fig. 3–2). (From Swartz,[20] p 50, with permission.)

TABLE 3-2 **CHARACTERISTICS OF SERUM IMMUNOGLOBULINS**

Characteristic	IgA	IgD	IgE	IgG	IgM
Heavy chain type	Alpha	Delta	Epsilon	Gamma	Mu
Sedimentation coefficient(s)	7–15*	7	8	6.7	19
Molecular weight (d)	160–500	180	196	150	900
Biologic half-life (d)	5.8	2.8	2.3	21	5.1
Carbohydrate content (%)	7.5–9.0	10–13	11–12	2.2–3.5	7–14
Placental transfer	No	No	No	Yes	No
Complement fixation (classic pathway)	−	−	−	+	+++
Agglutination in saline	+	−	−	±	++++
Heavy chain allotypes	A_m	None	None	G_m	None
Proportion of total immunoglobulin (%)	13	1	0.002	80	6

*May occur in monomeric or polymeric structural forms.
− = absent; ± = weak reactivity; + = slight reactivity; +++ = strong reactivity; ++++ = very strong reactivity.

also produce IgM antibodies. The primary blood banking testing problem encountered with IgM antibodies is that they may interfere with the detection of clinically significant IgG antibodies by masking their reactivity. Because IgM exists in both a monomeric and a polymeric form with a pentameric configuration containing a J, or joining, chain, IgM can be dissociated through the cleavage of covalent bonds interconnecting the monomeric subunits and the J chain

(Fig. 3–7). The blood banker may use 2-mercaptoethanol (2-ME) or dithiothreitol (DTT) to accomplish the dissociation of the IgM molecule. By the use of these reagents, a mixture of IgM and IgG antibodies can be distinguished because only IgM antibodies will be removed by the use of such compounds.[23]

IgG antibodies are significant in the study of immunohematology because they denote the class of immunoglobulins formed in response to the transfusion

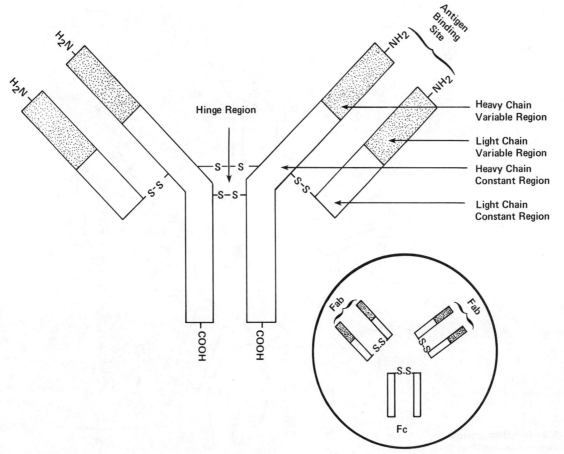

FIGURE 3-5 Schematic representation of basic immunoglobulin structure. The inset shows formation of Fab and Fc fragments after enzymatic cleavage of the IgG molecule by papain.

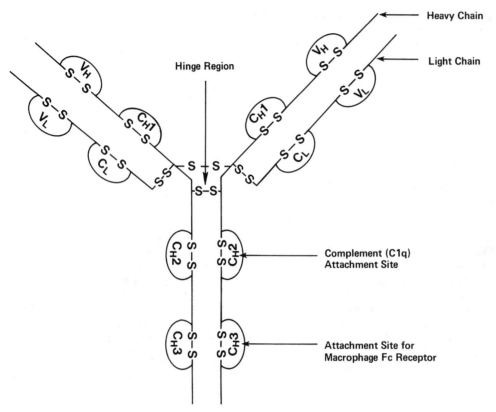

FIGURE 3-6 Schematic illustration of the domain structure within the IgG molecule.

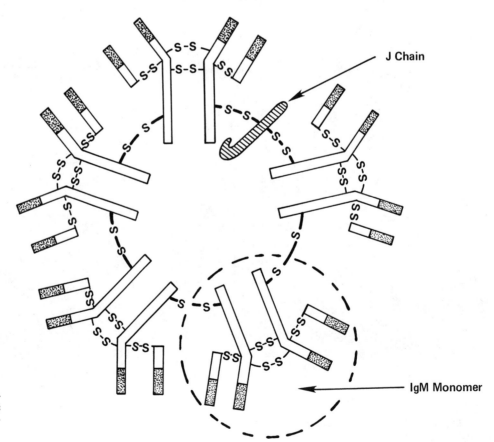

FIGURE 3-7 Schematic representation of the pentameric configuration of the IgM immunoglobulin.

of incompatible blood products. IgG antibodies are also important in hemolytic disease of the newborn (HDN). Maternal IgG immunoglobulins are formed in response to incompatible fetal red cells. Four different subclasses exist for IgG: IgG_1, IgG_2, IgG_3, and IgG_4. Small differences in chemical structure within the constant regions of the gamma heavy chains designate the various subclasses. The number of disulfide bonds between the two heavy chains in the hinge region of the molecule constitutes one of the main differences between subclasses. Subclasses also exhibit variations in electrophoretic mobility and biologic properties such as the ability to fix complement and cross the placenta[23] (Table 3–3).

IgG blood group antibodies of a single specificity may show immunoglobulins of all four subclasses or predominantly or exclusively one IgG subclass. Antibodies to Rh system antigens, for example, are mostly of the IgG_1 and IgG_3 subclasses. Anti-K (Kell) and anti-Fy^a (Duffy) antibodies, however, are usually of the IgG_1 subclass. Anti-Jk^a (Kidd) antibodies are mainly IgG_3. The purpose for the existence of biologic differences in subclass expression is unknown, but variations in immunologic responsiveness may possibly have underlying clinical significance, especially in HDN.[23] Severe HDN has been most often associated with IgG_1 antibodies.[24]

IgA, similar to IgM, exists in two main forms, a monomer and polymer form, with two immunoglobulin molecules in the polymer form joined by a J chain. Serum IgA is found in both monomeric and polymeric forms. Secretory IgA, usually found in the polymer form, also acquires a glycoprotein secretory component as it passes through epithelial cell walls of mucosal tissues and appears in saliva, tears, bronchial secretions, prostatic fluid, vaginal secretions, and the mucous secretions of the small intestine.[25]

IgA is important in the study of immunohematology

TABLE 3–3 BIOLOGIC PROPERTIES OF IgG SUBCLASSES

Characteristic	IgG$_1$	IgG$_2$	IgG$_3$	IgG$_4$
Proportion of total serum IgG (%)	65–70	23–28	4–7	3–4
Complement fixation (classic pathway)	++	+	+++	−
Binding to macrophage Fc receptors	+++	++	+++	±
Ability to cross placenta	+	±	+	+
Dominant antibody activities:				
Anti-Rh	++	−	+	±
Anti-factor VII	−	−	−	+
Anti-dextran	−	+	−	−
Anti-Kell	+	−	−	−
Anti-Duffy	+	−	−	−
Anti-platelet	−	−	+	−
Biologic half-life (days)	21	21	7–8	21

− = absent; ± = weak (or unusual) reactivity; + = slight (or usual) reactivity; ++ = moderate (or more common) reactivity; +++ = strong reactivity.

for several reasons. Approximately one third of anti-A and anti-B antibodies are of the IgA class (the other two thirds are IgM and IgG)[26] (Fig. 3–8). Anti-IgA antibodies sometimes form following the transfusion of plasma products to patients who are deficient in IgA. (See Chapter 18 for a discussion of anaphylactic shock in an IgA-deficient individual transfused with a plasma product.) Another reason for the importance of IgA is that secretory IgA antibodies may be found in patients who show autoimmune hemolysis because of multiple antibodies bound to the surface of red cells. IgA antibodies show an augmentation effect of IgG-induced red cell hemolysis.[27]

IgE is normally found only in monomeric form in very small concentrations in serum, composing only about 0.004 percent of total immunoglobulins. The Fc

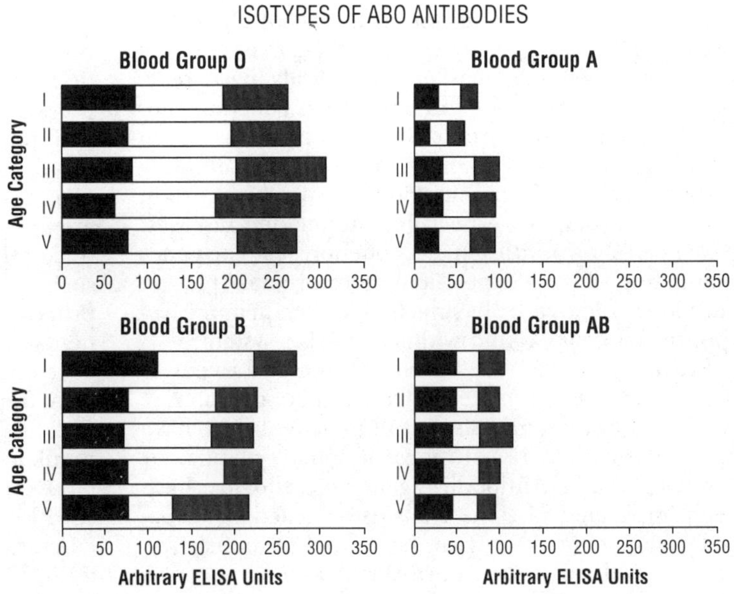

ISOTYPES OF ABO ANTIBODIES

FIGURE 3–8 Distribution of Anti-A IgM, IgG, and IgA antibodies by age categories. IgM (black), IgG (clear gray), IgA (gray), expressed as arbitrary ELISA units. Age categories: I = 20–30 years; II = 31–40 years; III = 41–50 years; IV = 51–60 years; V = 61–67 years. (Reprinted with permission from TRANSFUSION, published by The American Association of Blood Banks.)

portion of the molecule attaches to basophils and mast cells. When an allergen binds to the Fab portion of the molecule and cross-links with a second molecule on the cell surface, it triggers cellular release of biochemical mediators such as histamine, which is responsible for the manifestation of symptoms associated with the allergic reaction.

Transfusion reactions such as urticaria may occur because of the presence of IgE antibodies. Patients who have repeated allergic reactions to blood products may be given antihistamines to counteract the response when receiving blood products.[28]

IgD, present in only trace amounts (0.2 percent) in serum, has functions that probably relate primarily to the maturation of B cells into antibody-producing plasma cells. IgD may possibly perform some immunoregulatory roles during B-cell differentiation.[29]

IMMUNOGLOBULIN VARIATIONS AND PATERNITY TESTING

Immunoglobulin structures have genetic variability similar to inherited blood group differences. There exist three main types of antibody variation: isotype, allotype, and idiotype. Isotypic variation refers to variants present in all members of a species (e.g., the different immunoglobulin heavy and light chains and subclasses). All humans, therefore, have the same immunoglobulin classes and subclasses. Allotypic variation is present primarily in the constant region; not all variants occur in all members of a species. Idiotypic variation happens only in the variable region and is specific for each antibody molecule.[30] In the field of immunohematology, allotypic markers may be used in paternity testing, in studies of population genetics, and to ascertain the origin of antibody produced in patients who have had organ transplantations.[31]

Allotypic determinants have been defined as located on the C_L domains of kappa light chains (K_m markers), on the constant domains of IgA_2 (A_{2m} markers), and on the constant domains of IgG (G_m markers). Three K_m, two A_m, and 28 G_m markers have been described. G_m markers specifically have been typed in paternity cases and population genetics studies. Inheritance of certain G_m phenotypes may even define an individual's ability to mount an antibody response of a given immunoglobulin subclass. Certain disease associations, especially autoimmune diseases, have been shown with some G_m phenotypes. The genes that define allotype expression, therefore, may play an additional biologic role similar to other immune response (Ir) genes found within the HLA system.[32]

Pregnant women may become immunized to paternal allotypic determinants on fetal immunoglobulins.[33] Alloimmunization may also result in patients who have received multiple transfusions of blood, plasma, or gamma globulin. Antibodies against A_{2m} allotypes have been implicated in some transfusion reactions, especially in patients who may have an IgA deficiency. Patients with rheumatoid arthritis may spontaneously develop antiallotypic antibodies in the absence of a known sensitizing stimulus.[32]

IMMUNOGLOBULIN Fc RECEPTORS ON EFFECTOR CELLS

Mononuclear phagocytes, macrophages, and monocytes are equipped with receptors for the attachment of IgG immunoglobulin. These receptors bind to the C_H3 domain in the Fc portion of the IgG molecule. Only the IgG_1 and IgG_3 subclasses are capable of cytophilic attachment to the Fc receptors. Incompatible red cells, therefore, that are coated with IgG antibody will adhere to monocytes and macrophages, and phagocytosis of the antibody-coated cells will be promoted. Other cells with Fc receptors include neutrophils, NK cells (CD16), and mature B cells.

Complement System

The complement system denotes a group of approximately 25 serum and cell membrane proteins that have a variety of functions within the immune response. One role of the complement system is direct lysis of cells, bacteria, and enveloped viruses. Another capability of complement is the mediation of opsonization, whereby foreign substances are coated with complement in order to facilitate phagocytosis. A third function of the complement system is the production of split products, which are peptide fragments capable of directing certain inflammatory and immune response operations such as increased vascular permeability, smooth muscle contraction, phagocytic chemotaxis, migration, and adherence.[35,36]

Complement components circulate in inactive form (exception, factor D) and are sequentially activated through two main pathways, the classic pathway and the alternative pathway. The classic pathway is activated by the binding of antigen with antibody of the IgM class or IgG_1, IgG_2, or IgG_3 subclasses. The components are sequentially numbered C1 through C9, in order of their discovery, not necessarily their activation sequence. The alternative pathway is activated by polysaccharides and lipopolysaccharides, which may be found on the surfaces of certain target cells such as bacteria, fungi, parasites, and tumor cells. Four serum proteins are unique for the alternative pathway and are designated by letters: factor B, factor D, properdin (factor P), and initiating factor (IF). Divalent cations such as Ca^{++} and Mg^{++} are required in the activation process of some components. Complement components or complexes that have been stimulated and that have enzymatic activity are designated by a bar placed over the appropriate number or letter; for example, $C\overline{42}$ or factor $\overline{D}$. The complement system also contains regulatory or inhibitory proteins such as C1 inhibitor (C1INH), factor H, factor I, C4-binding protein (C4BP), anaphylatoxin inactivator, membrane attack complex (MAC) inhibitor, and C3 nephritic factor (NF).[37,38]

CLASSIC COMPLEMENT PATHWAY

The cascading activation of the classic complement pathway is initiated by the binding of C1 to the Fc fragment of IgM or an IgG subclass. The C1 component is composed of three C1 subunits: C1q, C1r, and C1s. The generation of $\overline{C1s}$ activates C4 and C2, forming a bimolecular complex. This activated complex, $\overline{C42}$, is a powerful cleaving esterase enzyme, which uses C3 as a natural substrate. Byproducts that result from the activation of the classic sequence include $C\overline{4b}$ and $C\overline{3b}$. Human red cells have CR1 receptors for $C\overline{4b}$ and $C\overline{3b}$, and some of the cleavage products will attach to the cell membrane. Later these fragments will be further degraded to $C\overline{4d}$ and $C\overline{3d}$ through the action of C4BP, factor H (which binds $C\overline{3b}$), and factor I (which degrades both $C\overline{4b}$ and $C\overline{3b}$)[38] (Fig. 3–9).

ALTERNATIVE COMPLEMENT PATHWAY

Factor $\overline{D}$ is analogous to $\overline{C1s}$ in the classic pathway, factor B is analogous to C2, and the cleavage product $C\overline{3b}$ is analogous to C4. Activation of the alternative pathway requires that a $C\overline{3b}$ molecule be bound to the surface of a target cell. Small amounts of $C\overline{3b}$ are generated continuously owing to the spontaneous hydrolytic cleavage of the C3 molecule. When $C\overline{3b}$ encounters normal cells, it is rapidly eliminated through the combined inactivating interactions of factors H and I. The accumulation of $C\overline{3b}$ on cell surfaces is associated with attachment of $C\overline{3b}$ to factor B. The complex of $C\overline{3b}$ and factor B (analogous to $\overline{C42}$) is then acted on by factor $\overline{D}$. As a result of this action, factor B is cleaved, yielding a cleavage product known as Bb. The C3bBb complex is stabilized by the presence of properdin (P), yielding C3bPBb. This complex acts as an esterase that cleaves C3 into additional $C\overline{3b}$. $C\overline{3b}$, therefore, acts as a positive feedback mechanism for driving the alternative pathway that bypasses the C142 sequence of the classic pathway (Fig. 3–9).[38]

MEMBRANE ATTACK COMPLEX

The terminal components of the complement sequence compose the MAC. In the classic pathway the MAC is initiated by the enzymatic activity of C4b2a3b on C5. In the alternative pathway C3bBbP has the ability to cleave C5. After C5 is split into C5a and C5b

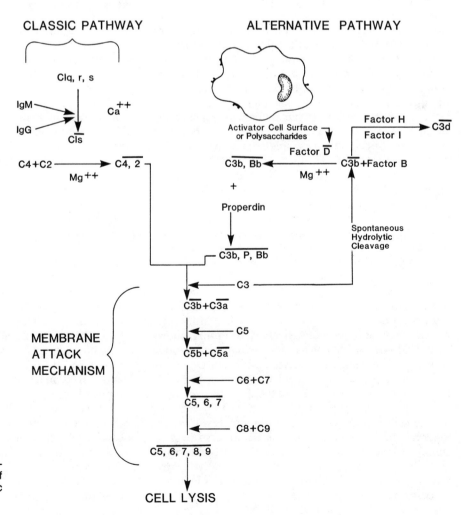

FIGURE 3-9 Schematic diagram illustrating the sequential activation of the complement system via the classic and alternative pathways.

by either the classic or the alternative pathway, C5b continues the complement cascade in initiating the membrane attachment of C6, C7, and C8. After the attachment of C9 to the C5b678 complex, a small transmembrane channel is formed, destroying the integrity of the cell membrane. Osmotic lysis eventually causes total cell destruction.[38,39]

BINDING OF COMPLEMENT BY RED CELL ANTIBODIES

Red cell antibody and complement can bring about the destruction of red cells. The effective activation of the classic pathway by C1q necessitates the binding of one C1 molecule to two adjacent immunoglobulin Fc regions. A pentameric IgM molecule provides two Fc regions side by side, thereby binding complement. A monomeric IgG molecule, however, binds C1q less efficiently and two IgG molecules are unlikely to align themselves side by side in order to bind complement. As many as 800 IgG anti-A molecules may need to attach to one adult A_1 red cell in order to bind a single C1 molecule.[38] Rh IgG antibodies usually do not bind complement because of the scarcity of Rh antigens on red cell surfaces, although there may be exceptions.[40] An interesting example of an efficient IgG hemolysin is found in patients with paroxysmal cold hemoglobinuria, who have antibodies directed against P blood group determinants. Antibodies to the Lewis blood group system are generally IgM, and they activate complement, sometimes causing hemolytic transfusion reactions.[41] With the exception of the ABO system, however, only very few antibodies activate the complement sequence that leads to complement-mediated intravascular hemolysis. Extravascular hemolysis most often occurs owing to antibody coating of red cells, but the split products of complement activation facilitate the activity of the reticuloendothelial system and cause anaphylatoxic effects.[42] Cells of the mononuclear phagocyte system, monocytes, macrophages, and the cells lining the hepatic and splenic sinusoids also play an important role in the clearance of antibody-coated red cells. These phagocytic cells are equipped with two biologically important types of surface receptors: complement receptors for C3b (CR1) and immunoglobulin Fc receptors (Fig. 3–10). Transfused red cells coated with C3b alone, without antibody, are sequestrated only transiently in the reticuloendothelial organs, and otherwise survive normally. Monocytes and macrophages do not have IgM receptors; therefore, IgM-coated red cells are not eliminated through Fc receptor-mediated phagocytosis. If erythrocytes are coated with IgG and complement, however, they will be cleared rapidly from circulation.[38]

Interestingly, the CR1 (C3b/C4b, CD35) receptor on red cells, which is important in immune adherence (attachment of immune complexes to erythrocytes, significant in the metabolism of immune complexes) is also a blood group antigen, Knops/McCoy, that generates high-titer low-avidity (HTLA) antibodies in immunized transfusion recipients.[43,44]

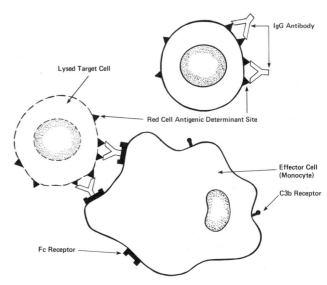

FIGURE 3–10 Schematic representation of the mechanism of antibody-dependent cell-mediated cytotoxicity (ADCC). Note the role of effector cell surface receptors for the Fc fragment of IgG.

COMPLEMENT PRESERVATION AND DESTRUCTION IN TEST SYSTEMS AND BLOOD SAMPLES REQUIRED FOR TESTING

Some blood banking tests require the use of serum in order to ensure that adequate amounts of viable complement are available for fixation by blood group antibodies. An anticoagulated sample, for example, would not be conducive to complement activation because anticoagulants bind Ca^{++} or Mg^{++}, or both, and inhibit complement activity. Adding 2 mg of Na_2H_2 ethylenediaminetetraacetic acid (EDTA) to 1 ml of serum will totally obstruct complement activation. Heparin will inhibit the cleavage of C4.[45] Using serum instead of plasma for most blood bank procedures ensures that viable complement is accessible for use in all methods; therefore, serum should be used for all antibody screening and compatibility testing. Serum should be removed as soon as possible from a clotted blood sample. If testing cannot proceed immediately after separation of serum and red cells, then serum should be removed and placed at 4°C for no longer than 48 hours. For longer periods of time, serum should be frozen at −4°C or lower in order to retain complement activity.

The lytic potential of complement may be abolished by heating serum at 56°C for 30 minutes. C1 and C2 are destroyed and C4 is damaged by this treatment. Factor B is inactivated by heating at 50°C for 20 minutes.[45]

Serum under normal circumstances has some natural complement inhibition. An inhibitor is present that blocks the action of activated C1 by binding to and removing C1s and C1r from the activated complex of C1qrs.[45]

The complement system may become activated during storage of preserved red cell products. In citrate-phosphate-dextrose-adenine (CPDA-1)–preserved red cells, for example, activation of C3 may be caused by activation of the alternate pathway of the complement system by contact of plasma with plastic surfaces.[46] This action may cause some hemolysis in the red cell product.

Immune Response

CHARACTERISTICS OF ANTIGENS

The immune response is initiated by the presentation of a provocation that takes the form of an immunogen or antigen. The difference between an immunogen and an antigen is associated with the body's reactivity to an immune stimulus. Even though immunogen and antigen are often used as equivalent terms, immunogen actually refers to any substance that can induce an immune response, whereas antigen implies the ability of an immunogenic substance to react with the products, such as antibodies, which result from an immune response.[47] The term "antigen" is more commonly used among blood bankers because their primary testing concern is the detection of antibodies to blood group antigens.

The immune reaction to an immunogen or antigen is determined by host response as well as several characteristics of the foreign substance. Properties such as size, complexity, conformation, charge, accessibility, solubility, digestibility, and chemical composition influence the amount and type of immune response (Table 3–4). A molecule having a small molecular weight (MW), less than 10,000 d, for example, is called a hapten and usually does not elicit an immune response by itself. When coupled with a carrier protein having a larger size than MW 10,000 d, however, the hapten can invoke a reaction.[47]

Chemical complexity is another property with implications for the type and extent of immune response generated upon exposure to a foreign substance. The more complex molecules generally produce a greater response. Antibody or cellular response is usually very specific for antigen conformation (e.g., linear versus globular molecules). Antibody response is also formed to the net charge of a molecule, whether it is to positive, negative, or neutral antigenic determinants. The accessibility of determinant groupings influences the immune response and subsequent antibody formation.

TABLE 3–4 CHARACTERISTICS OF ANTIGENS: PROPERTIES THAT INFLUENCE IMMUNE RESPONSE

Size
Complexity
Conformation
Charge
Accessibility
Solubility
Digestibility
Chemical composition

TABLE 3–5 RELATIVE IMMUNOGENICITY OF DIFFERENT BLOOD GROUP ANTIGENS

Blood Group Antigen	Blood Group System	Immunogenicity (%)*
D (Rh$_o$)	Rh	50.00
K	Kell	5.00
c (hr')	Rh	2.05
E (rh")	Rh	1.69
k	Kell	1.50
e (hr")	Rh	0.56
Fy^a	Duffy	0.23
C (rh')	Rh	0.11
Jk^a	Kidd	0.07
S	MNSs	0.04
Jk^b	Kidd	0.03
s	MNSs	0.03

Adapted from Williams, WJ, et al. (eds): Hematology. McGraw-Hill, New York, 1983, p 1491.
*Percentage of transfusion recipients lacking the blood group antigen (in the first column) who are likely to be sensitized to a single transfusion of red cells containing that antigen.

Insoluble substances are less likely to elicit an immune response. A molecule may be a protein, lipoprotein, polysaccharide, lipopolysaccharide, glycoprotein, polypeptide, or nucleic acid; the response will be generated according to the composition of the stimulus. Red cell antigens, for example, may be proteins (such as the Rh, M, and N blood group substances) or glycolipids (such as the ABH, Lewis, Ii, and P blood group substances). HLA antigens are glycoproteins. Because of structural, conformational, and molecular differences, not all blood group substances are equally immunogenic in vivo (Table 3–5). Fifty to 70 percent of Rh-negative recipients of Rh-positive blood would be expected to form antibodies if exposed to the D antigen; however, only approximately 5 percent of K-negative individuals would be likely to develop antibodies to the K antigen after being transfused with K antigen–positive blood. Varying immunogenicity for different blood group antigens has practical significance for blood bankers because red cells from donors need to be routinely typed only for ABO and D antigen groupings. Other blood group antigens, from a statistical standpoint, are unlikely to elicit an immune response in a recipient.[48]

ALLOANTIBODIES AND AUTOANTIBODIES

Antigens that initiate the immune cascade result in the formation of either alloantibodies or autoantibodies. Alloantibodies are produced after exposure to genetically different, or nonself, antigens of the same species. The implication for blood banking is that transfused components carrying nonself antigens are susceptible to immune attack by alloantibodies. Autoantibodies are antibodies produced in response to self antigens. Cold or warm autoantibodies that react specifically or nonspecifically with blood cell antigens may present both clinical problems for the patient and testing problems for the blood banker.

PROPERTIES OF ANTIGEN AND ANTIBODY REACTIONS

After the immune system has been stimulated and has produced antibody, many properties of antigen and antibody reactions influence the final response outcome. Intermolecular binding forces and antibody affinity, avidity, and specificity determine the extent of the reaction and resultant removal of the antigen. The antigen-binding site of the antibody molecule is uniquely designed to recognize a homologous antigen because of the structural arrangement of amino acid sequences in the variable regions of the light and heavy chains (see Immunoglobulin Structure). The extent of the reciprocal relationship or "fit" between the antigen-binding site of the immunoglobulin molecule and its corresponding antigen is somewhat controlled by the properties of antigen and antibody reactions.

Intermolecular binding forces such as hydrogen bonding, electrostatic forces, van der Waals' forces, and hydrophobic bonds compose those forces that do not involve the formation of covalent chemical bonds between antigens and their corresponding antibodies.[49] Antibody affinity is often defined as the strength of a single antigen-antibody bond produced by the summation of these attractive and repulsive forces. "Avidity" is the term often used to express the binding of a multivalent antigen with an antisera produced in an immunized individual. Avidity, therefore, is a measure of the functional affinity of an antiserum for the whole antigen.[49] HTLA antibodies may be annoying for blood bankers in that they exhibit low antigen-binding capacity but still show reactivity at high serum dilutions.[50]

Reaction strengths of antigens and antibodies are often quantified by affinity or avidity; however, the specificity of an antiserum is related to its relative avidity for antigen. Antibody specificity can be further classified as a specific reaction, cross-reaction, or no reaction. A specific reaction implies reaction between similar determinants. A cross-reaction results when some determinants of one antigen are shared by another antigen. No reaction results when there are no shared determinants (Fig. 3–11).[49]

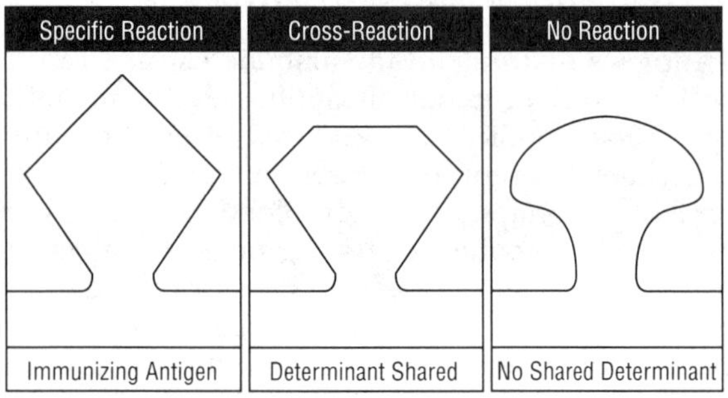

The forces of intermolecular binding that ultimately influence affinity, avidity, and specificity can often be manipulated by using various blood bank reagents and methods to enhance the reactivity of certain red cell antigens and antibodies (see Factors That May Influence Agglutination Reactions).

HOST FACTORS

The properties of antigens are not the only factors in determining the immunogenicity of blood group substances; host factors also play a key role in ascertaining an individual's ability to mount an immune response. The immune response can be influenced by such elements as nutritional status, hormones, genetic makeup, age, race, exercise level, and the occurrence of disease or injury. Severe malnutrition can lead to a 50 percent reduction in CD4 positive T cells and result in antibody responses of lower affinity. Hormone receptors are found on immunologic cells and both enhance and suppress immune response. Immune response can be genetically influenced by the genes of the MHC. Ir genes help control the type and extent of T- and B-cell response to individual antigens. Aging has an influence on immune response, as it is generally believed that immune function decreases as age increases.[51] For blood bankers, a decrease in antibody levels in older individuals may result in false-negative reactions. Race may be a factor in the susceptibility and nonsusceptibility to certain diseases. The majority of black individuals who do not inherit the Duffy blood system antigens (Fy^a or Fy^b) are resistant to malarial invasion with *Plasmodium knowlesi* and *P. vivax*. The absence of these antigens may make these individuals ideal donors for those who have developed Duffy system antibodies, because most individuals who make anti-Fy^a commonly have the Fy(a − b +) phenotype.

Extreme exercise, traumatic injury, and the presence of certain diseases are other factors that may have an immunosuppressive effect on the immune response.[51] Blood bankers may observe the consequences of these conditions by detecting negative or weak serum test results, especially on reverse ABO groupings (Table 3–6).[52]

FIGURE 3-11 Types of antigen/antibody reactions: specific reaction, cross reaction, and no reaction.

TABLE 3–6 **HOST FACTORS: PROPERTIES OF THE HOST THAT INFLUENCE IMMUNE RESPONSE**

Nutritional status
Hormones
Genetics
Age
Race
Exercise level
Disease
Injury

TOLERANCE AND IMMUNE UNRESPONSIVENESS

The concept of tolerance, or failure of the immune system to mount an immune response to an antigen, has important implications for blood bankers. Tolerance may be naturally or experimentally induced in an individual. Exposure to an antigen during fetal life may produce tolerance to that antigen. An example of this type of tolerance is found in the chimera, an individual who receives an in utero cross-transfusion of ABO-incompatible blood from a dizygotic (nonidentical) twin.[48,52,53] The chimera will never produce antibodies against the ABO group of the twin. Forward and reverse ABO grouping of such an individual may appear as a testing discrepancy to the blood banker.

Another blood banking implication involves the deliberate induction of immune unresponsiveness for Rh-positive cells in Rh-negative individuals. When an Rh-negative woman gives birth to an Rh-positive infant, she is exposed to Rh-positive red cells. From 50 to 70 percent of Rh-negative mothers will develop anti-D antibodies upon first exposure to Rh-positive cells. The formation of these antibodies can be prevented by the administration of IgG Rh immune globulin (RhIG) within 48 to 72 hours after the birth of the infant. Interestingly, 25 to 30 percent of Rh-negative individuals are nonresponders and will not produce anti-D antibodies, even when subjected to repeated exposure to Rh-positive cells.[48]

OVERVIEW

Nearly all immunogens, especially those that elicit the formation of blood group antibodies, need to be processed by an APC in order to initiate the immune response. After an immunogen, such as an incompatible red blood cell, has entered the bloodstream, it travels to the spleen or liver where it encounters an APC. The APC processes the foreign antigen in such a way as to present it to a T cell in the context of a class II MHC marker. T cells recognize antigens through the CD3/TCR complex.[12] The TCR contacts portions of both the MHC marker and the processed antigen peptide. This binding is assisted by the CD4 marker (for TH cells) or CD8 marker (for TS/TC cells). During and after antigen processing, cytokines are generated by source cells, APCs. Their receptors are expressed on recipient lymphocytes; for example, IL-1 is secreted by macrophages to activate lymphocytes by promoting the proliferation of T lymphocytes and enhancing production of IL-2 receptors on other T cells.[54] IL-2, a growth factor for other T cells, enhances the activity of TC cells and NK cells. Stimulated TH cells are also capable of producing IL-4 and IL-5 to promote the growth, proliferation, and differentiation of B cells, in a T-cell-dependent mechanism for antibody production. B cells are also capable of processing captured antigen through internalization of surface immunoglobulin, but this T-cell-independent mechanism is used only for very structurally simple molecules and does not produce immunologic memory. This mechanism is usually not involved in the formation of blood group antibodies. B cells that have been properly stimulated will differentiate into antibody-producing plasma cells. B cells will also activate other B cells by secretion of cytokines such as IL-6.[14] A foreign blood group antigen may initially elicit the production of IgM, but its production may terminate and IgG may then be produced with the same specificity as IgM. Most immune blood group antibodies are IgG$_1$ and IgG$_3$.[55]

IMMUNE SUPPRESSION

Regulatory and suppressive mechanisms must be present in the normal immune response in order to control the reaction at all levels of activity. Cytokines react to restrict immune activities through the techniques of competition, mutual suppression, and interaction in cycles regulated by positive and negative feedback routines. In addition, products of the kinin, complement, and lipoxygenase and cyclo-oxygenase pathways, and neuroendocrine hormonal peptides such as endorphins and corticosteroids regulate cytokine activities. Expression of cell membrane receptors also affects the activities of mediator substances.[56] Transforming growth factor (TGF) beta, for example, downregulates the expression of IL-2 receptors. IL-4 inhibits monocyte function by regulating monocyte adhesion through functional expression of adhesion structures, not necessarily through changes in the surface expression of cytokine receptors.[57]

CD8 positive T cells are generally considered to be the functional set of T cells that suppress immune responses through modulating cytotoxic T cells and antigen-specific T-cell proliferation. These suppressor cells, however, are produced in response to a CD4 subset of helper cells called suppressor-inducer cells.[58] Both subsets are antigen specific and may act to slow down immune response through an idiotypic transducing effect, similar to the effect of anti-idiotypic antibodies, which suppress specific antibody response. The suppressor cells may also release a soluble suppressor factor that acts on APCs, TH cells, and B cells.[6,58]

PRIMARY AND SECONDARY RESPONSE AND MEMORY CELLS

Because of the complexity of interactions required to mount an immune response to a foreign antigen, and because this response is influenced by antigen characteristics as well as a variety of host factors, a period extending from a few days to a few months may pass before realization of a full response to an antigenic stimulus. This time is sometimes referred to as the latency period, during which no antibody response

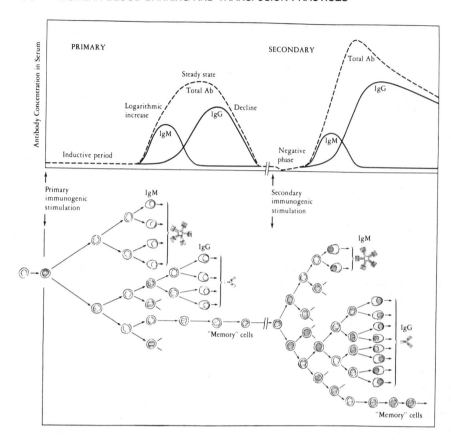

FIGURE 3-12 Schematic representation of primary and secondary antibody responses. Note the enhanced antibody production and expanded antibody-producing cell population during the secondary antibody response. (From Herscowitz, HB: Immunophysiology. In Bellanti, JA (ed): Immunology III. WB Saunders, Philadelphia, 1985, p 117, with permission.)

is detectable in the test serum. During the latency period, T- and B-cell response is occurring, and the first appearance of specific antibody constitutes the beginning of the primary response. Most of the antibodies produced in the beginning of the primary response are IgM, although they are later replaced by IgG antibodies (Fig. 3-12).[59] After elimination of the antigenic stimulus and the subsequent decline of antibody response, memory T and B cells are stored in organs of the immune system. When the same antigen is encountered again, these memory cells are responsible for the rapid production, higher intensity, and longer duration of secondary responses.[6] Secondary responses are characterized by the presence of large amounts of IgG antibodies. IgM antibodies are also formed at the beginning of the response but rapidly decline as they are replaced by IgG antibodies (Fig. 3-12). Secondary response antibodies have a higher avidity for antigen, are produced at significantly lower doses of antigen than antibodies formed during the primary response, and usually are formed more quickly, in 1 to 10 days. An Rh-negative individual, for example, may require a dose of at least 200 to 300 ml of Rh-positive red cells before mounting a primary response. A secondary exposure to Rh-positive cells, however, may require as little as 0.1 ml of Rh-positive red cells to induce a rapid antibody response.[59]

Laboratory Examination of Reactions Between Antigens and Antibodies

In vitro testing for the detection of antigens or antibodies may be accomplished by a variety of immunologic techniques. Such techniques as agglutination, precipitation, agglutination inhibition, and hemolysis are the most commonly used methods to detect the presence of blood group antigens or antibodies. Techniques such as radioimmunoassay (RIA), enzyme-linked immunosorbent assay (ELISA) or enzyme immunoassay (EIA), and immunofluorescence, which quantitate antigen or antibody with the use of a radioisotope, enzyme, or fluorescent label, may be used in automated or semi-automated blood banking instrumentation for detecting blood group antigens or antibodies but are routinely used in the serologic testing of blood products.

In blood bank testing, agglutination reactions are the major manifestation of the blood group antigen-antibody response. Typing for ABO, Rh, and other blood group antigens is accomplished by agglutination reactions. Agglutination can be shown to develop in two stages. In stage 1, known as sensitization, antibody binding occurs. Antigenic determinants on the red cell membrane combine with the antigen-combining site (Fab region) on the variable regions of the immunoglobulin heavy and light chains. Antigen and antibody are held together by noncovalent bonds, and no visible agglutination is seen at this stage. In stage 2, a lattice structure composed of multiple antigen-antibody bridges between antibodies and red cell antigens is formed. Visible agglutination is present during this stage.[60]

The development of a perceptible, insoluble antigen-antibody complex resulting from the mixing of equivalent amounts of soluble antigen and antibody is known as a precipitation reaction. The visible clumping depends on multiple binding sites on antibody and antigen. The generation of antigen-antibody complexes results in a lattice formation.

Agglutination inhibition is a method in which a positive reaction is the opposite of what is normally observed in agglutination. Agglutination, which usually occurs as a manifestation of an antigen-antibody reaction, is inhibited when an antigen-antibody reaction has previously occurred in a test system and, therefore, prevents agglutination. A blood bank test illustrating this method is the secretor study. To determine if soluble ABO substances are present in body fluids, saliva containing soluble ABO antigens is mixed with known ABO antisera and allowed to incubate. The antigen and appropriate antisera combine if the soluble ABO antigen is present in the saliva. If binding occurs, no free antibody is present to agglutinate reagent red cells. No agglutination, therefore, indicates that soluble antigen is present and the individual being tested is a secretor; if agglutination occurs, then no soluble antigen is present, the reagent antisera and red cells were available to react with each other, and the individual is a nonsecretor.

Hemolysis represents a positive result and indicates that an antigen-antibody reaction has occurred in which complement has been fixed. With the fixation of complement, red cell lysis occurs. The Lewis blood group antibodies, anti-Le[a] and anti-Le[b], may be regarded as clinically significant if hemolysis occurs as a result of an antigen, antibody, and complement reaction.

Radioimmunoassay, ELISA or EIA, and immunofluorescence are immunologic techniques based on quantitating antigen or antibody by the use of a radioisotope, enzyme, or fluorescent label. These techniques measure the initial interaction of the binding of antigen with antibody. Most of these techniques employ reagents that use either antigen or antibody, which is bound in a solid or liquid phase, in a variety of reaction systems ranging from plastic tubes or plates to microscopic particles. These methods also use a separation system to isolate bound and free fractions and a detection system to measure the amount of antigen-antibody interaction. The values of unknown samples are then calculated from the values of standards of known concentration.

Factors That May Influence Agglutination Reactions

Many factors influencing reactivity apply to all antigen-antibody reactions, but the main emphasis here is on agglutination reactions. The agglutination reaction is influenced by the concentration of both antigen and antibody as well as other factors such as pH, temperature, ionic strength, surface charge, antibody class, red cell antigen dosage, and the use of various enhancement media, antihuman globulin reagents, and enzymes.

CONCENTRATION OF ANTIGEN AND ANTIBODY

Under ideal reactive conditions, an equivalent amount of antigen and antibody bind in optimal proportions. An excess of either antigen or antibody, however, may lead to unbound immunoglobulin (prozone effect) or a surplus of antigen-binding sites (postzone effect) (Fig. 3–13). In either situation, the lattice formation and subsequent agglutination may not occur in the test system, leading to the assumption of false-negative results.[61] To correct the problem of excessive antibody, the serum may be diluted, with each serial dilution of serum tested against red cells. To correct the problem of excessive antigen, the serum-to-cell ratio in the test system may be increased, which will tend to increase the number of antibodies available to bind with each red cell.[62] Test systems, therefore, can be manipulated to overcome the effects of excessive antigen or antibody.

Dosage effect, another reason for lack of antigen sites on red cells, occurs as a result of the inheritance of genotypes, which give rise to heterozygous expression of red cell antigens. M+ cells from an individual having the genotype *MM*, for example, will have more M antigen sites than M+ cells from an individual having the *MN* genotype.[63] The Rh system is another blood group system that contains certain antigens that show the dosage effect.[63,64] The C, c, E, and e antigens show dosage depending on the inheritance of the homozygous versus the heterozygous expression of the genotype for these antigens. *DCe/DCe*, for example, may show a 3+ agglutination with specific antisera for C and e; *DCe/DcE*, however, may show only a 1+ reaction.[64] Some A subgroups such as A$_2$ may show a weaker reactivity with anti-A than will A$_1$ owing to fewer A antigen sites on the A$_2$, but this does not represent a true dosage effect.[63]

EFFECT OF pH

Agglutination reactions are also affected by pH. The ideal pH is between 6.5 and 7.5. Exceptions to this range include some examples of anti-M and some antibodies of the Pr(Sp$_1$) group, which show stronger reactivity below pH 6.5.[62]

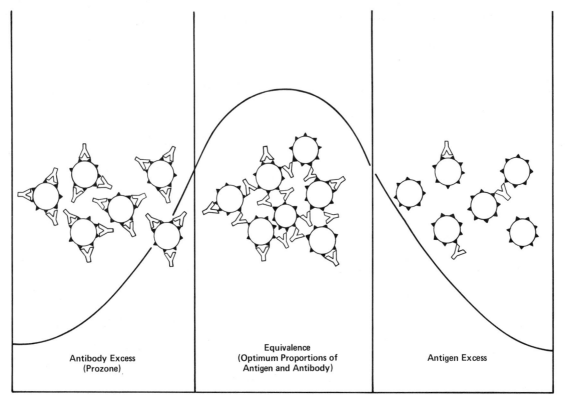

FIGURE 3–13 Schematic representation of the effects of varying concentrations of antigen and antibody on lattice formation.

EFFECT OF TEMPERATURE

Different types of antibodies may exhibit optimal reactivity at different temperatures. IgM antibodies, for example, usually react optimally at or below 22°C. IgG antibodies usually require 37°C temperatures.[61] By manipulating the temperature range, blood bankers are able to enhance detection of clinically significant antibodies (Fig. 3–14).

EFFECT OF IMMUNOGLOBULIN TYPE

IgM antibodies are generally capable of agglutinating red cells suspended in 0.85 percent saline media. The IgM antibody is approximately 750 times as efficient as IgG in agglutination reactions.[65] The IgM molecule easily bridges the distance between two red cells because it is 160 Å larger than an IgG molecule.[62] Another factor that may contribute to the difference in reactivity between the IgM and IgG molecules is the number of antigen-combining sites on each type of immunoglobulin. Theoretically, the IgM has the potential to bind 10 antigens; however, in reality this rarely happens owing to the size and spacing of antigens in relation to the size and configuration of the IgM molecule. When the IgM molecule attaches to two red cells, for example, probably two or three antigen-combining sites attach to each red cell.[62] An IgG molecule, however, has only two binding sites per molecule, which implies that an IgG molecule would have

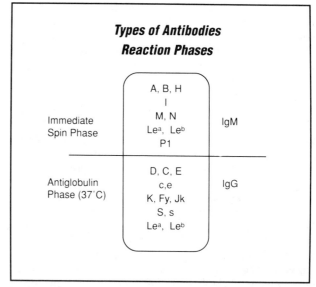

FIGURE 3–14 Types of antibodies reaction phases (From Kutt, et al,[68] p 10, with permission.)

to bind two red cells with only one binding site on each cell.[62] Of course, agglutination reactions involve more than one immunoglobulin molecule, but this example may be multiplied many times in order to represent its relevance in the agglutination reaction (Fig. 3–15).

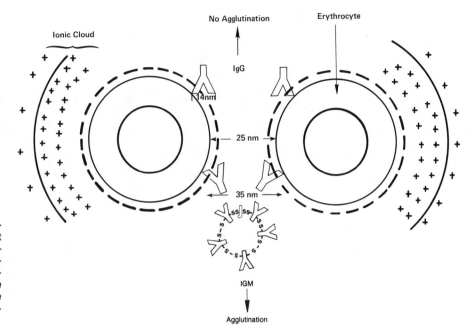

FIGURE 3-15 Schematic representation of the ionic cloud concept and its relevance to hemagglutination induced by IgM and IgG antibodies. Compare the size of the IgG antibody with the IgM molecule. The size of the IgG molecule is not large enough to span the distance between two adjacent red cells.

Examples of IgM antibodies that have importance in blood banking include those against the ABH, Ii, MN, Lewis (Le^a, Le^b), Lutheran (Lu^a), and P blood group antigens. IgG antibodies are those directed at Ss, Kell (Kk, Js^a, Js^b), Rh (DCEce), Lutheran (Lu^b), Duffy (Fy^a, Fy^b), and Kidd (Jk^a, Jk^b) (Fig. 3–14).

EFFECT OF ENHANCEMENT MEDIA AND POTENTIATORS

As stated previously, agglutination reactions for IgM antibodies and their corresponding red cell antigens are easily accomplished in saline medium. Detection of IgM antibodies, however, may not have the same clinical significance as the detection of most IgG antibodies because IgG antibodies, which react at body temperature, 37°C, are the type generally responsible for hemolytic transfusion reactions and hemolytic disease of the newborn. To discover the presence of IgG antibodies, the blood banker normally uses a variety of enhancement techniques (Table 3–7).

Several enhancement media are aimed at reducing the zeta potential of the red cell membrane. The net negative charge surrounding red cells is part of the force that repels red cells from each other. The zeta potential is an expression of the difference in electrostatic potential at the surface of the red cell and the ionic cloud of positive cations that are attracted to the negative charges on the surface (Fig. 3–15).[61,62] Reducing the zeta potential, therefore, should have the desired effect of allowing red cell agglutination by IgG molecules.

Protein Media

Various colloidal diluents such as albumin, polyethylene glycol (PEG), polybrene, polyvinylpyrrolidone (PVP), and protamine are used to enhance the aggluti-

TABLE 3-7 **POTENTIATORS**

Reagent	Action	Procedure	Type of Antibody ID
22% Albumin	Causes agglutination by adjusting zeta potential between red cells	Incubation at 37°C for 15–60 min; cell washing prior to indirect antiglobulin test (IAT)	IgG
LISS	Low ionic strength environment causes red cells to take up antibody more rapidly	Incubation at 37°C for 5–15 min; cell washing prior to IAT	IgG
Saline		4–22°C (IgM); 37°C (IgG); 45–60 min	Primarily IgM; IgG if incubated
Enzymes	Destroys or depresses some red cell antigens; enhances other red cell antigens	1. One-step: enzymes added directly to serum/red cell 2. Two-step: red cells pretreated with enzymes before addition of serum	Destroys Fy^a, Fy^b, MNS; enhances reactivity to Rh, Kidd, P$_1$, Lewis, and I antibodies
AHG	Cross links sensitized cells to give visible agglutination	1. DAT: AHG added directly to washed red cells 2. IAT: serum + screen cells incubated, washed, and AHG added	1. Polyspecific: IgG+ complement 2. IgG monospecific: IgG only

From Kutt, et al,[68] p 15, with permission.

nation of red cells coated with IgG molecules. These substances may accomplish this enhancement by increasing the dielectric constant (a measure of electrical conductivity), which consequently reduces the zeta potential of the red cell.[61]

Polyethylene Glycol and Polybrene

Polyethylene glycol and polybrene are macromolecule additives used within a low ionic strength solution (LISS) to bring sensitized red cells closer to each other in order to assist antibody cross-linking and enhancement of agglutination reactions. Use of these reagents offers some distinct advantages. Polybrene can detect ABO incompatibility as well as clinically significant IgG alloantibodies. PEG produces very specific reactions. Both PEG and polybrene are considered to be more effective than either albumin or LISS for detection of weak antibodies.[66] These reagents have been used in both automated and manual testing systems.

Low Ionic Strength Solution Media

Low ionic strength solutions media decrease the ionic strength of a reaction medium and, thus, reduce the zeta potential. With a reduction in zeta potential, there is an increased attraction between positively charged antibody molecules and negatively charged red cells. LISS media generally contain 0.2 percent sodium chloride. LISS is often used because it results in an increased rate of antibody uptake during sensitization, with an incubation period of 5 to 15 minutes instead of 30 to 60 minutes, which may be required when using a protein potentiator such as albumin.[61,62,64]

Enzymes

The reactions of certain blood group antigens and antibodies are selectively enhanced or suppressed by the use of certain enzymes. Some of the enzymes used in detection of blood group antibodies include ficin (from figs), papain (from papaya), trypsin (from pig stomach), and bromelin (from pineapple). Several theories have been proposed to explain the action of enzymes. One theory proposes that the treatment of red cells with enzymes results in the release of sialic acid from the membrane with the subsequent decrease in the negative charges of the red cells with a reduction of the zeta potential.[61,63] Another theory states that enzyme treatment removes hydrophilic glycoproteins from the membrane of red cells, causing the membrane to become more hydrophobic, thereby allowing the red cells to come closer together. Also, because of removal of glycoproteins from the membrane, antibody molecules may no longer be sterically obstructed from reacting with red cell antigens on the membrane surface.[63] The use of enzymes provides enhanced antibody reactivity to Rh, Kidd, P_1, Lewis, and I antigens and destroys or depresses reactivity to red cell antigens Fy^a, Fy^b, M, N, and S.[64]

Antihuman Globulin Reagents

The antihuman globulin (AHG) test is designed to detect red cells coated with antibody or complement or both. One type of antihuman globulin reagent, polyspecific AHG, is used to detect red cells that have been sensitized with IgG antibody or complement components C3b or C3d. Monospecific antihuman globulin reagent is used to detect red cells sensitized only with IgG antibody or only with complement.[64] Some AHG reagents are manufactured by injecting animals, usually goats or rabbits, with human globulin. The animals make an antibody response to the foreign human globulin and produce antihuman antibodies to the human globulin components. For the manufacture of polyspecific AHG, both gamma (IgG) and beta (C3b and C3d) globulin components are processed. For monospecific AHG, animals are injected only with IgG and produce antibodies directed against the gamma heavy chain. Monoclonal AHG reagents are also available. Monoclonals are produced by hybridoma technology (see Effect of Monoclonal versus Polyclonal Reagents).

AHG reagents act by cross-linking red cells already sensitized with antibody or complement, or both, thus bridging the gap among red cells. The agglutination reaction, therefore, is enhanced by the use of AHG reagents (Table 3–7).

Chemical Reduction of IgG and IgM Molecules

Blood bankers may sometimes discover mixtures of antibodies or the presence of autoantibodies in testing situations in which they must remove or enhance the reactivity of either IgG or IgM antibodies. DTT and 2-ME are sulfhydryl compounds that break the disulfide bonds of the J chain of the IgM molecule but leave the IgG molecule intact.[67,68] ZZAP reagent, consisting of a thiol reagent plus a proteolytic enzyme, causes the dissociation of IgG molecules from the surface of sensitized red cells as well as altering the surface antigens of the red cell.[69]

Chemical reduction of the disulfide bond of the IgG molecule is also used to produce chemically modified reagents that react with red cells in saline.[61,66] Sulfhydryl compounds reduce the disulfide bonds in the hinge region of the IgG molecule, rendering the Fab portions more flexible in facilitating agglutination reactions.[70]

EFFECT OF MONOCLONAL VERSUS POLYCLONAL REAGENTS

Traditional polyclonal antisera reagents to detect red cell antigens have been produced by immunizing donors and then collecting serum containing antibodies. AHG reagents have traditionally been made by injecting animals with human globulin components and then collecting the antihuman antibodies (see Antihuman Globulin Reagents). Polyclonal reagents, therefore, are directed against multiple epitopes or antigen-binding sites found on the original antigen used to stimulate antibody production in the host animal. Monoclonal reagents, however, are made by hybridoma technology whereby spleen lymphocytes from immunized mice are fused with rapidly proliferating myeloma cells. These hybrid cells, after extensive screening and testing, are selected and cultured to produce lines of immortal cell clones that manufacture a specific antibody directed against only a single epitope. Monoclonal reagents have some distinct advantages over polyclonal reagents. Because monoclonal reagents are produced from immortal clones, no batch variation exists, and high titers of antibodies can be produced. Monoclonal reagents react very specifically and often have higher affinities. For these reasons, monoclonal reagents are not subject to cross-reactivity and interference from nonspecific reactions and may even react strongly with very small quantities of antigen as may be found in subgroups (e.g., subgroups of A).[71,72] Disadvantages of monoclonal antisera include overspecificity, the fact that complement may not be fixed in the antigen-antibody reaction, and problems with sensitivity.[71,73] Some of the disadvantages of monoclonal reagents may be overcome by using blends of different monoclonal reagents or by using polyclonal reagents and monoclonal reagents together.[74] Monoclonal antisera have been used for typing red cell antigens, for AHG testing, and also for phenotyping lymphocyte antigens and HLA typing.

Immune-Mediated Diseases Important in Blood Bank Testing

IMMUNODEFICIENCY

Defects in either antibody-mediated immunity, cell-mediated immunity, phagocytosis, complement, or other mediator substances may result in immunodeficiency diseases. Immunodeficiencies may be congenital or acquired, may occur secondary to an embryologic abnormality or enzymatic defect, or may be of unknown origin (Table 3–8).[75] Blood bankers need a general knowledge of immunodeficiencies because these disorders may present laboratory and transfusion problems. An individual with a low immunoglobulin level, for example, may have a weak or negative test result for expected serum antibodies in reverse ABO grouping.[76]

HYPERSENSITIVITY

Many immune-mediated diseases with implications for blood banking can be classified as hypersensitivity reactions. Hypersensitivity is an inflammatory response to a foreign antigen and may involve antibody-mediated and cell-mediated reactions or only a cell-mediated reaction. The terms "hypersensitivity" and "allergy" are often used interchangeably, and allergic diseases are often classified according to the mechanisms involved in the response.[77] The Gell and

TABLE 3-8   CLASSIFICATION OF IMMUNODEFICIENCY DISORDERS

Antibody (B cell) Immunodeficiency Disorders

X-linked hypogammaglobulinemia (congenital hypogammaglobulinemia)
Transient hypogammaglobulinemia of infancy
Common, variable, unclassifiable immunodeficiency (acquired hypogammaglobulinemia)
Immunodeficiency with hyper-IgM
Selective IgA deficiency
Selective IgM deficiency
Selective deficiency of IgG subclasses
Secondary B cell immunodeficiency associated with drugs, protein-losing states
X-linked lymphoproliferative disease

Cellular (T cell) Immunodeficiency Disorders

Congenital thymic aplasia (DiGeorge's syndrome)
Chronic mucocutaneous candidiasis (with or without endocrinopathy)
T cell deficiency associated with purine nucleoside phosphorylase deficiency
T cell deficiency associated with absent membrane glycoprotein
T cell deficiency associated with absent class I or II MHC antigens or both (base lymphocyte syndrome)

Combined Antibody-Mediated (B cell) and Cell-Mediated (T cell) Immunodeficiency Disorders

Severe combined immunodeficiency disease (autosomal recessive, X-linked, sporadic)
Cellular immunodeficiency with abnormal immunoglobulin synthesis (Nezelof's syndrome)
Immunodeficiency with ataxia-telangiectasia
Immunodeficiency with eczema and thrombocytopenia (Wiskott-Aldrich syndrome)
Immunodeficiency with thymoma
Immunodeficiency with short-limbed dwarfism
Immunodeficiency with adenosine deaminase deficiency
Immunodeficiency with nucleoside phosphorylase deficiency
Biotin dependent multiple carboxylase deficiency
Graft-versus-host disease
Acquired immunodeficiency syndrome

Phagocytic Dysfunction

Chronic granulomatous disease
Glucose-6-phosphate dehydrogenase deficiency
Myeloperoxidase deficiency
Chédiak-Higashi syndrome
Job's syndrome
Tuftsin deficiency
Lazy leukocyte syndrome
Elevated IgE, defective chemotaxis, and recurrent infections

From Ammann,[75] p 319, with permission.

Coombs classification is useful to distinguish between disorders that may be involved with transfusion of blood products and those that may influence laboratory testing. A type I reaction, also known as anaphylactic or immediate hypersensitivity, involves mast cells or basophils with surface IgE antibody that cross-links allergen and causes release of histamine and other mediators responsible for the allergic reactions associated with the manifestation of the disease. IgA-deficient individuals, for example, who receive plasma products containing IgA may have an anaphylactic reaction to those products. Urticarial reactions may also result from transfusion and may be a response to a substance in donor plasma, such as drugs or certain food allergens.[78,79]

A type II reaction involves IgG or IgM antibody and complement, phagocytic cells, and proteolytic enzymes. HDN, transfusion reactions caused by blood group antibodies, and autoimmune hemolytic reactions are examples of type II reactions (see Autoimmune Disease and Hemolytic Disease of the Newborn).

Type III reactions also involve IgG and IgM antibodies, complement, and phagocytic cells. The main feature of this type of tissue-damaging reaction is the formation of immune complexes: aggregations of antibody, antigen, polymorphonuclear neutrophils (PMNs), and complement. Drug-induced antibodies, such as those to penicillin, may form complexes and eventually lead to hemolytic reactions.[80]

The type IV reaction is a T-cell–mediated response involving only T cells and their related cytokines. Antibody and complement are not involved in this reaction.[81] Graft-versus-host reaction is the primary clinical example of a type IV reaction that has significance for blood bankers. Transfusion of viable lymphocytes to an immune-suppressed recipient may result in the attack of those transfused lymphocytes against the recipient.

MONOCLONAL AND POLYCLONAL GAMMOPATHIES

Plasma cell neoplasms result in proliferation of abnormal immunoglobulin that is a product of a single clone of B cells (as in monoclonal gammopathies) or of multiple clones (as in polyclonal gammopathies).[82] The proliferation may be of a specific antibody class or only of a light or heavy chain. The increased amounts of immunoglobulin lead to increased viscosity of serum. This situation may present special testing problems for blood bankers. The increased concentrations of serum proteins cause nonspecific aggregation of RBCs. Rouleaux, or stacking of red cells like coins, may result from serum of individuals who have disorders such as multiple myeloma.[83] In some testing situations, special procedures such as saline dilution may be needed to distinguish true red cell agglutination from nonspecific aggregation caused by the presence of increased concentrations of abnormal immunoglobulins.

AUTOIMMUNE DISEASE

Autoantibodies are antibodies produced against an individual's own cells and tissues. Many theories have been proposed to explain why this breakdown in the normal immune response and why pathologic conditions develop. Cross-reactivity of the immune response between body tissues and foreign antigens, disturbance of the anti-idiotypic network, loss of self-tolerance, and aberrant presentation of antigen through MHC markers are among the theories for development of autoimmunity.[84] From a laboratory testing perspective, the autoimmune conditions that have the most significance for blood bankers are the autoimmune hemolytic anemias. These diseases may produce antibodies that cause red cell destruction and resultant anemia and also cause difficulties in red cell antigen testing because of antibody- or complement-coated red cells. A direct antiglobulin test (DAT) using anti-IgG/or anti-C3d, or both, is used to detect coated cells. Special procedures such as elutions or chemical treatment to remove antibody may be needed in order to prepare cells for antigen typing. Unbound serum autoantibodies may interfere with alloantibody detection and compatibility testing. In this situation, procedures such as adsorptions or chemical treatment to denature immunoglobulins may need to be performed to remove autoantibodies from serum so that they do not interfere with the testing for clinically significant antibodies.

HEMOLYTIC DISEASE OF THE NEWBORN

Immunoglobulins that can cross the placenta are responsible for conferring maternal immunity upon the fetus. In most situations this process is important for protecting the fetus and, after birth, the newborn infant until approximately 6 months of age, at which time infants begin to produce their own antibodies. HDN occurs when maternal antibody is directed toward foreign antigen on fetal red cells. If the mother is exposed to fetal red cells as a result of fetomaternal transfer of red cells during pregnancy or childbirth, then she will mount an immune response against those red cell antigens. Memory cells of this encounter will be stored in lymphatic organs. A subsequent pregnancy with a second exposure to the same red cell antigens will result in the production of fetal red cell antigen-specific antibodies. IgG_1, IgG_3, and IgG_4 are capable of crossing the placenta and attaching to fetal red cells.[85] Severe HDN, often requiring exchange transfusion, has been associated with IgG_1 antibodies more frequently than with antibodies of other subgroups such as IgG_3.[24] Transplacental antibodies may be focused on antigens A and B of the ABO system, antigens of the Rh system, or other blood group antigens such as those in the Kell system.

Summary

The immune response consists of an intricate system of many factors including tissues, organs, cells, and biologic mediators that act to defend an organism against intrusion by a foreign substance. The response functions under the genetic control of the HLA system to recognize and react to an immune stimulus. Immunoglobulins have special significance for blood bankers because blood bank testing is primarily focused on the prevention, detection, and identification of blood group antibodies. The complement system is important because of its interaction with the antibody response and the in vivo and in vitro effects of complement activation and resultant red cell destruction. Blood bankers need knowledge of the antigen characteristics and host factors that have an impact on the immune response to enable them to evaluate and solve testing problems. An immunologic viewpoint is essential in understanding the factors that affect agglutination reactions between red cells and red cell antibodies, especially in test media selection and testing conditions. Finally, in order to comprehend the consequences of certain immune-mediated disease conditions and their influences on blood bank testing, the blood banker should possess a basic knowledge of these disorders.

Review Questions

1. Which cell is identified primarily by the presence of immunoglobulin on its surface?
   A. TH cell
   B. NK cell
   C. B cell
   D. Macrophage

2. Which cell functions primarily in antigen processing and presentation?
   A. TC cell
   B. Macrophage
   C. Plasma cell
   D. NK cell

3. Which of the following would be a signal for the expression of IL-2 receptors on a TH cell?
   A. Antigen internalized by a B cell in a T-independent process
   B. Presentation of antigen by a monocyte to a TH cell
   C. Binding of immunoglobulin on surface of a macrophage
   D. Cross-linking of antigen on surface of a mast cell

4. Which class(es) of HLA marker(s) is (are) important in immune recognition of antigen in cell-to-cell interactions?
   A. Class II
   B. Class I
   C. Class III
   D. Class I and Class II

5. Which immunoglobulin class would be *most* important in the study of immune-mediated transfusion reactions due to the presence of alloantibodies?
   A. IgA
   B. IgM
   C. IgE
   D. IgG

6. Which immunoglobulins can activate the classic pathway of the complement system?
   A. IgA and IgM
   B. IgG (all subgroups) and IgA
   C. IgG_1, IgG_2, IgG_3, and IgM
   D. IgE and IgD

7. Which complement factor is common to both classic and alternative pathways?
   A. Factor B
   B. Factor C3
   C. Factor C1
   D. Factor C4

8. Which of the following patient samples for blood bank testing is *most likely* to contain complement?
   A. EDTA-anticoagulated sample
   B. Heparin-anticoagulated sample
   C. Serum sample at 4°C for 72 hours
   D. Serum sample drawn 2 hours ago

9. Which of the following statements is *true* concerning the formation of antibodies to blood group antigens?
   A. All blood group antigens are equally immunogenic.
   B. Only ABO and Rh blood group antigens are immunogenic.
   C. Antibodies may form to any foreign blood group antigen, but usually only ABO and Rh antibodies form in clinically significant numbers.
   D. Any blood group antigen may elicit an immune response, but only 50% of blood recipients will respond with antibody formation.

10. Which antibody is produced rapidly and in highest amounts during secondary response?
    A. IgG
    B. IgM
    C. IgA
    D. Both IgM and IgG are produced rapidly and in equal amounts.

11. Which of the following would *most likely* account for the failure of a visible red cell antigen-antibody reaction?
    A. Homozygous expression of antigen on red cell
    B. pH of 7.1
    C. Incubation at 37°C for suspected IgG antibody
    D. Excess antibody (prozone effect)

12. What is the main advantage of LISS media over other types of enhancement media such as albumin?
    A. Has rapid antibody uptake

B. Has increased saturation of antibody molecules

C. May be used for either manual or automated systems

D. Selectively enhances or suppresses certain blood group antigen-antibody reactions

13. What is the action of AHG reagent?
   A. Reduces the zeta potential of the red cell, allowing closer approach of red cells
   B. Cross-links red cells that have become sensitized with antibody or complement
   C. Renders the red cell membrane more hydrophobic, allowing red cells to come closer together
   D. Releases sialic acid from the red cell membrane, thereby decreasing negative charges between cells

14. A blood cell product is irradiated to prevent the transfusion of viable lymphocytes to an immunocompromised patient. What type of reaction is prevented by this action?
   A. Type I, anaphylactic shock
   B. Type II, transfusion reaction
   C. Type III, immune complex formation
   D. Type IV, graft-versus-host reaction

15. From a blood bank testing perspective, what is the main problem with a patient having an autoimmune hemolytic anemia?
   A. Large amounts of excess protein may coat red cells.
   B. Autoantibodies are formed rapidly and to many blood group determinants.
   C. Autoantibodies may interfere with the detection of clinically significant antibodies.
   D. Rouleaux of red cells makes antigen typing difficult.

Answers to Review Questions

1. C (p 45)
2. B (p 44)
3. B (p 45)
4. A (p 46)
5. D (p 51)
6. C (p 51)
7. B (p 54)
8. D (p 54)
9. C (p 55)
10. A (p 58)
11. D (p 56)
12. A (p 62)
13. B (p 62)
14. D (p 64)
15. C (p 64)

References

1. Miller, LE, et al: Manual of Laboratory Immunology, ed 2. Lea & Febiger, Philadelphia, 1991, p 1.
2. Bryant, NJ: Laboratory Immunology and Serology, ed 3. WB Saunders, Philadelphia, 1992, p 3.
3. Goodman, JW: The immune response. In Stites, DP and Terr, AI: Basic and Clinical Immunology, ed 7. Appleton & Lange, Norwalk, CT, 1991, p 34.
4. Kamani, NR and Douglas, SD: Structure and development of the immune system. In Stites, DP and Terr, AI: Basic and Clinical Immunology, ed 7. Appleton & Lange, Norwalk, CT, 1991, p 16.
5. Male, D and Roitt, I: Adaptive and innate immunity. In Roitt, I, Brostoff, J, and Male, D: Immunology, ed 2. CV Mosby, St Louis, 1989, pp 1.7–1.9.
6. Goodman, JW: The immune response. In Stites, DP and Terr, AI: Basic and Clinical Immunology, ed 7. Appleton & Lange, Norwalk, CT, 1991, pp 35–44.
7. Lydyard, P and Grossi, C: Cells involved in the immune response. In Roitt, I, Brostoff, J, and Male, D: Immunology, ed 2. CV Mosby, St Louis, 1989, pp 2.1–2.12.
8. Kamani, NR and Douglas, SD: Structure and development of the immune system. In Stites, DP and Terr, AI: Basic and Clinical Immunology, ed 7. Appleton & Lange, Norwalk, CT, 1991, p 24.
9. Waytes, AT, et al: Preligation of CR1 enhances IgG-dependent phagocytosis by cultured human monocytes. J Immunol 146:2694, 1991.
10. Kamani, NR and Douglas, SD: Structure and development of the immune system. In Stites, DP and Terr, AI: Basic and Clinical Immunology, ed 7. Appleton & Lange, Norwalk, CT, 1991, p 21.
11. Lydyard, P and Grossi, C: Cells involved in the immune response. In Roitt, I, Brostoff, J, and Male, D: Immunology, ed 2. CV Mosby, St Louis, 1989, pp 2.14–2.18.
12. Goverman, J and Parnes, JR: The T cell receptor. In Stites, DP and Terr, AI: Basic and Clinical Immunology, ed 7. Appleton & Lange, Norwalk, CT, 1991, pp 73–77.
13. Lanier, L: Cells of the immune response: Lymphocytes and mononuclear phagocytes. In Stites, DP and Terr, AI: Basic and Clinical Immunology, ed 7. Appleton & Lange, Norwalk, CT, 1991, p 65.
14. Lanier, L: Cells of the immune response: Lymphocytes and mononuclear phagocytes. In Stites, DP and Terr, AI: Basic and Clinical Immunology, ed 7. Appleton & Lange, Norwalk, CT, 1991, pp 68–70.
15. Oppenheim, JJ, Ruscetti, FW, and Faltynek, C: Cytokines. In Stites, DP and Terr, AI: Basic and Clinical Immunology, ed 7. Appleton & Lange, Norwalk, CT, 1991, pp 78–79.
16. Rook, G: Cell-mediated immune responses. In Roitt, I, Brostoff, J, and Male, D: Immunology, ed 2. CV Mosby, St Louis, 1989, p 9.8.
17. Oppenheim, JJ, Ruscetti, FW, and Faltynek, C: Cytokines. In Stites, DP and Terr, AI: Basic and Clinical Immunology, ed 7. Appleton & Lange, Norwalk, CT, 1991, p 86.
18. Bryant, NJ: Laboratory Immunology and Serology, ed 3. WB Saunders, Philadelphia, 1992, pp 68–69.
19. Owen, M: Major histocompatibility complex. In Roitt, I, Brostoff, J, and Male, D: Immunology, ed 2. CV Mosby, St Louis, 1989, p 4.1.
20. Swartz, BD: The human major histocompatibility human leukocyte antigen (HLA) complex. In Stites, DP and Terr, AI: Basic and Clinical Immunology, ed 7. Appleton & Lange, Norwalk, CT, 1991, p 49.
21. Goodman, JW: Immunoglobulin structure and function. In Stites, DP and Terr, AI: Basic and Clinical Immunology, ed 7. Appleton & Lange, Norwalk, CT, 1991, p 109.
22. Bryant, NJ: Laboratory Immunology and Serology, ed 3. WB Saunders, Philadelphia, 1992, p 72.
23. Goodman, JW: Immunoglobulin structure and function. In Stites, DP and Terr, AI: Basic and Clinical Immunology, ed 7. Appleton & Lange, Norwalk, CT, 1991, pp 109–118.

24. Nance, SJ, Arndt, PA, and Garratty, G: Correlation of IgG subclass with the severity of hemolytic disease of the newborn. Transfusion 30:381, 1990.
25. Goodman, JW: Immunoglobulin structure and function. In Stites, DP and Terr, AI: Basic and Clinical Immunology, ed 7. Appleton & Lange, Norwalk, CT, 1991, p 117.
26. Rieben, R, et al: Antibodies to histo-blood group substances A and B: Agglutination titers, Ig class, and IgG subclasses in healthy persons of different age categories. Transfusion 31: 607, 1991.
27. Sokol, RJ, et al: Red cell autoantibodies, multiple immunoglobulin classes, and autoimmune hemolysis. Transfusion 30:714, 1990.
28. Walker, RH: AABB Technical Manual, ed 10. American Association of Blood Banks, Arlington, VA, 1990, p 422.
29. Kerr, WG, Hendershot, LM, and Burrows, PD: Regulation of IgM and IgD expression in human B-lineage cells. J Immunol 146:3314, 1991.
30. Hay, F: The generation of diversity. In Roitt, I, Brostoff, J, and Male, D: Immunology, ed 2. CV Mosby, St Louis, 1989, p 6.2.
31. Walker, RH: AABB Technical Manual, ed 10. American Association of Blood Banks, Arlington, VA, 1990, p 128.
32. Zaleski, MB, et al: Allotopy of Immunoglobulins, Immunogenetics. Pitman Publishing, Marshfield, MA, 1983, p 171.
33. Goodman, JW: Immunoglobulin structure and function. In Stites, DP and Terr, AI: Basic and Clinical Immunology, ed 7. Appleton & Lange, Norwalk, CT, 1991, p 115..
34. Mollison, PL: Red cell antigens and antibodies and their interactions. In Blood Transfusion in Clinical Medicine, ed 8. Blackwell Scientific Publications, Oxford, 1987, pp 254–255.
35. Frank, MM: Complement and kinin. In Stites, DP and Terr, AI: Basic and Clinical Immunology, ed 7. Appleton & Lange, Norwalk, CT, 1991, p 161.
36. Walport, M: Complement. In Roitt, I, Brostoff, J, and Male, D: Immunology, ed 2. CV Mosby, St Louis, 1989, p 13.11.
37. Bryant, NJ: Laboratory Immunology and Serology, ed 3. WB Saunders, Philadelphia, 1992, p 47.
38. Frank, MM: Complement and kinin. In Stites, DP and Terr, AI: Basic and Clinical Immunology, ed 7. Appleton & Lange, Norwalk, CT, 1991, pp 167–169.
39. Frank, MM: Complement and kinin. In Stites, DP and Terr, AI: Basic and Clinical Immunology, ed 7. Appleton & Lange, Norwalk, CT, 1991, p 166.
40. O'Connor, KL: The Rh blood group system. In Harmening, D: Modern Blood Banking and Transfusion Practices, ed 2. FA Davis, Philadelphia, 1989, p 112.
41. Mollison, PL: ABO, Lewis, Ii, and P groups. In Blood Transfusion in Clinical Medicine, ed 8. Blackwell Scientific Publications, Oxford, 1987, pp 307–308.
42. Widmann, FK: Adverse effects of blood transfusion. In Harmening, D: Modern Blood Banking and Transfusion Practices, ed 2. FA Davis, Philadelphia, 1989, p 124.
43. Moulds, JM, et al: The C3b/C4b receptor is recognized by the Knops, McCoy, Swain-Langley, and York blood group antisera. J Exp Med 173:1159, 1991.
44. Rao, N, et al: Identification of human erythrocyte blood group antigens on the C3b/C4b receptor. J Immunol 146:3502, 1991.
45. Bryant, NJ: Laboratory Immunology and Serology, ed 3. WB Saunders, Philadelphia, 1992, p 55.
46. Schleuning, M, et al: Complement activation during storage of blood under normal blood bank conditions. Effects of proteinase inhibitors and leukocyte depletion. Blood 79:3071, 1992.
47. Goodman, JW: Immunogenicity and antigenic specificity. In Stites, DP and Terr, AI: Basic and Clinical Immunology, ed 7. Appleton & Lange, Norwalk, CT, 1991, p 101.
48. Issitt, PD: Applied Blood Group Serology, ed 3. Montgomery Scientific Publications, Miami, 1985, p 224.
49. Roitt, I: Essential Immunology, ed 7. Blackwell Scientific Publications, Oxford, 1991, pp 68–74.
50. Turgeon, ML: Fundamentals of Immunohematology. Lea & Febiger, Philadelphia, 1989, pp 158, 187.
51. Roitt, I: Essential Immunology, ed 7. Blackwell Scientific Publications, Oxford, 1991, pp 169–170.
52. Walker, RH: AABB Technical Manual, ed 10. American Association of Blood Banks, Arlington, VA, 1990, pp 182–183.
53. Howard, J and Male, D: Immunological tolerance. In Roitt, I, Brostoff, J, and Male, D: Immunology, ed 2. CV Mosby, St Louis, 1989, p 12.1.
54. Oppenheim, JJ, Ruscetti, FW, and Faltynek, C: Cytokines. In Stites, DP and Terr, AI: Basic and Clinical Immunology, ed 7. Appleton & Lange, Norwalk, CT, 1991, p 84.
55. Issitt, PD: Applied Blood Group Serology, ed 3. Montgomery Scientific Publications, Miami, 1985, p 11.
56. Oppenheim, JJ, Ruscetti, FW, and Faltynek, C: Cytokines. In Stites, DP and Terr, AI: Basic and Clinical Immunology, ed 7. Appleton & Lange, Norwalk, CT, 1991, p 99.
57. Elliott, MJ, et al: Inhibition of human monocyte adhesion by interleukin 4. Blood 77:2739, 1991.
58. Roitt, I: Essential Immunology, ed 7. Blackwell Scientific Publications, Oxford, 1991, pp 155–157.
59. Goodman, JW: The immune response. In Stites, DP and Terr, AI: Basic and Clinical Immunology, ed 7. Appleton & Lange, Norwalk, CT, 1991, pp 40–41.
60. Walker, RH: AABB Technical Manual, ed 10. American Association of Blood Banks, Arlington, VA, 1990, pp 139–141.
61. Walker, RH: AABB Technical Manual, ed 10. American Association of Blood Banks, Arlington, VA, 1990, p 137.
62. Issitt, PD: Applied Blood Group Serology, ed 3. Montgomery Scientific Publications, Miami, 1985, pp 34–35.
63. Issitt, PD: Applied Blood Group Serology, ed 3. Montgomery Scientific Publications, Miami, 1985, p 37.
64. Kutt, SM, et al: Rh Blood Group System Antigens, Antibodies, Nomenclature, and Testing. Ortho Diagnostic Systems, Raritan, NJ, 1990, pp 13–14.
65. Stites, DP and Rodgers, RP: Clinical laboratory methods for detection of antigens and antibodies. In Stites, DP and Terr, AI: Basic and Clinical Immunology, ed 7. Appleton & Lange, Norwalk, CT, 1991, p 253.
66. Turgeon, ML: Fundamentals of Immunohematology. Lea & Febiger, Philadelphia, 1989, p 77.
67. Issitt, PD: Applied Blood Group Serology, ed 3. Montgomery Scientific Publications, Miami, 1985, p 64.
68. Kutt, SM, Larison, PJ, and Kessler, LA: Solving Antibody Problems, Special Techniques. Ortho Diagnostic Systems, Raritan, NJ, 1992, pp 11–12.
69. Walker, RH: AABB Technical Manual, ed 10. American Association of Blood Banks, Arlington, VA, 1990, p 584.
70. Issitt, PD: Applied Blood Group Serology, ed 3. Montgomery Scientific Publications, Miami, 1985, p 68.
71. Hybridomas and Monoclonal Antibodies. Bioeducational Publications, Rochester, NY, 1982, p 19.
72. Lau, P, et al: Group A variants defined with a monoclonal anti-A reagent. Transfusion 30:142, 1990.
73. Turgeon, ML: Fundamentals of Immunohematology. Lea & Febiger, Philadelphia, 1989, pp 72, 158.
74. Walker, RH: AABB Technical Manual, ed 10. American Association of Blood Banks, Arlington, VA, 1990, p 144.
75. Ammann, AJ: Mechanisms of immunodeficiency. In Stites, DP and Terr, AI: Basic and Clinical Immunology, ed 7. Appleton & Lange, Norwalk, CT, 1991, p 319.
76. Walker, RH: AABB Technical Manual, ed 10. American Association of Blood Banks, Arlington, VA, 1990, p 183.
77. Terr, AI: Mechanisms of hypersensitivity. In Stites, DP and Terr, AI: Basic and Clinical Immunology, ed 7. Appleton & Lange, Norwalk, CT, 1991, p 367.
78. Walker, RH: AABB Technical Manual, ed 10. American Association of Blood Banks, Arlington, VA, 1990, p 422.
79. Turgeon, ML: Fundamentals of Immunohematology. Lea & Febiger, Philadelphia, 1989, pp 158, 353.
80. Roitt, I: Essential Immunology, ed 7. Blackwell Scientific Publications, Oxford, 1991, p 269.
81. Bryant, NJ: Laboratory Immunology and Serology, ed 3. WB Saunders, Philadelphia, 1992, p 78.
82. Parker, JW and Lukes, RJ: Neoplasms of the immune system. In Stites, DP and Terr, AI: Basic and Clinical Immunology, ed 7. Appleton & Lange, Norwalk, CT, 1991, p 617.

83. Walker, RH: AABB Technical Manual, ed 10. American Association of Blood Banks, Arlington, VA, 1990, p 187.
84. Steinberg, AD: Mechanisms of disordered immune regulation. In Stites, DP and Terr, AI: Basic and Clinical Immunology, ed 7. Appleton & Lange, Norwalk, CT, 1991, pp 432–437.
85. Goodman, JW: Immunoglobulin structure and function. In Stites, DP and Terr, AI: Basic and Clinical Immunology, ed 7. Appleton & Lange, Norwalk, CT, 1991, p 117.

Bibliography

Bryant, NJ: Laboratory Immunology and Serology, ed 3. WB Saunders, Philadelphia, 1992.

Elliott, MJ, et al: Inhibition of human monocyte adhesion by interleukin 4. Blood 77:2739, 1991.

Hybridomas and Monoclonal Antibodies, Bioeducational Publications, Rochester, NY, 1982.

Issitt, PD: Applied Blood Group Serology, ed 3. Montgomery Scientific Publications, Miami, 1985.

Kerr, WG, Hendershot, LM, and Burrows, PD: Regulation of IgM and IgD expression in human B-lineage cells. J Immunol 146:3314, 1991.

Kutt, SM, et al: Rh Blood Group System Antigens, Antibodies, Nomenclature and Testing. Ortho Diagnostic Systems, Raritan, NJ, 1990.

Kutt, SM, Larison, PJ, and Kessler, LA: Solving Antibody Problems, Special Techniques. Ortho Diagnostic Systems, Raritan, NJ, 1992.

Lau, P, et al: Group A variants defined with a monoclonal anti-A reagent. Transfusion 30:142, 1990.

Miller, LE, et al: Manual of Laboratory Immunology, ed 2. Lea & Febiger, Philadelphia, 1991.

Moulds, JM, et al: The C3b/C4b receptor is recognized by the Knops, McCoy, Swain-Langley, and York blood group antisera. J Exp Med 173:1159, 1991.

Nance, SJ, Arndt, PA, Garratty, G: Correlation of IgG subclass with the severity of hemolytic disease of the newborn. Transfusion 30:381, 1990.

Rao, N, et al: Identification of human erythrocyte blood group antigens on the C3b/C4b receptor. J Immunol 146:3502, 1991.

Rieben, R, et al: Antibodies to histo-blood group substances A and B: Agglutination titers, Ig class, and IgG subclasses in healthy persons of different age categories. Transfusion 31:607, 1991.

Roitt, I: Essential Immunology, ed 7. Blackwell Scientific Publications, Oxford, 1991.

Roitt, I, Brostoff, J, and Male, D: Immunology, ed 2. CV Mosby, St Louis, 1989.

Schleuning, M, et al: Complement activation during storage of blood under normal blood bank conditions. Effects of proteinase inhibitors and leukocyte depletion. Blood 79:3071, 1992.

Sokol, RJ, et al: Red cell autoantibodies, multiple immunoglobulin classes, and autoimmune hemolysis. Transfusion 30:714, 1990.

Stites, DP and Terr, AI: Basic and Clinical Immunology, ed 7. Appleton & Lange, Norwalk, CT, 1991.

Turgeon, ML: Fundamentals of Immunohematology. Lea & Febiger, Philadelphia, 1989.

Walker, RH: AABB Technical Manual, ed 10. American Association of Blood Banks, Arlington, VA, 1990.

Waytes, AT, Malbran, A, Bobak, DA, and Fries, LF: Preligation of CR1 enhances IgG-dependent phagocytosis by cultured human monocytes. J Immunol 146:2694, 1991.

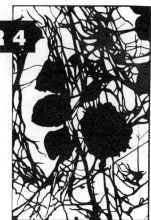

CHAPTER 4

The Antihuman Globulin Test

Ralph E. B. Green, BAppSci, FAIMS, MACE
Peggy Perkins Simpson, MT(ASCP)

OBJECTIVES

Upon completion of this chapter, the learner should be able to:

1 Name the proteins present in polyspecific antihuman globulin.

2 Discuss the advantages and disadvantages of anticomplement activity in polyspecific antihuman globulin.

3 Name a clinically significant antibody whose detection is enhanced by anticomplement activity in polyspecific antihuman globulin.

4 Describe the preparation of antihuman globulin reagents.

5   State the advantages of a low ionic strength solution indirect antiglobulin test using monospecific anti-IgG.

6   Define the applications and limitations of different antihuman globulin reagents for direct antiglobulin testing and indirect antiglobulin testing.

7   Compare and contrast the indirect antiglobulin test and the direct antiglobulin test. Include an explanation of (1) principle, (2) applications, and (3) red cell sensitization.

8   List the reasons for the procedural steps in the direct antiglobulin test and in the indirect antiglobulin test.

9   List the sources of error associated with the performance of the antiglobulin test.

10 List the factors affecting the antiglobulin test that may result in increased sensitivity.

11 Interpret the results of a direct antiglobulin test panel correctly.

History of the Antihuman Globulin Test

With Landsteiner's discovery in 1901 of the ABO blood group system, the first steps toward a rational approach to blood transfusion became possible. Nearly a half century later, the next advance occurred: the introduction of serologic techniques permitting the detection of "incomplete" antibodies, which are nonagglutinating immunoglobulin G (IgG) antibodies that sensitize (coat) red blood cells (RBCs). During the 1940s albumin,[1] enzymes,[2] and the antihuman globulin[3,4] techniques were introduced.

In 1945, Coombs et al.[3] described the use of the antihuman globulin test for the detection of weak and nonagglutinating Rh antibodies in serum. In 1946, Coombs et al.[4] described the use of antihuman globulin to detect in vivo sensitization of the red cells of babies suffering from hemolytic disease of the newborn. Although the test initially was of great value in the investigation of Rh hemolytic disease of the newborn, it was not long before its versatility for the detection of other IgG blood group antibodies became evident. The first of the Kell blood group system antibodies[5] and its associated antigen were reported only weeks after Coombs had described the test.

Although Coombs and his coworkers were instrumental in introducing the antihuman globulin test to blood group serology, the principle of the test had in fact been described by Moreschi in 1908.[6] Moreschi's studies involved the use of rabbit antigoat serum to agglutinate rabbit red cells, which were sensitized with low nonagglutinating doses of goat antirabbit red cell serum.

Coombs' procedure involved the injection of human serum into rabbits to produce antihuman serum. After absorption to remove heterospecific antibodies, the antiserum was diluted to an appropriate concentration such that prozone was avoided, while still retaining sufficient antibody activity to permit cross-linking of adjacent RBCs sensitized with IgG antibodies. The cross-linking of sensitized RBCs by the antihuman

globulin produced hemagglutination, indicating that the RBCs had been sensitized by an antibody that had reacted with an antigen present on the cell surface. The use of antihuman globulin to detect in vitro sensitization of RBCs is referred to as the *indirect test*, whereas its use to detect in vivo sensitization is called the *direct test* (Fig. 4–1).

Basic Concepts of Antiglobulin Testing

Two major classes of antibodies react with RBC antigens. "Complete" or saline agglutinins will agglutinate RBCs suspended in saline; these are usually IgM. "Incomplete" agglutinins do not react in saline and require special techniques to agglutinate RBCs; these

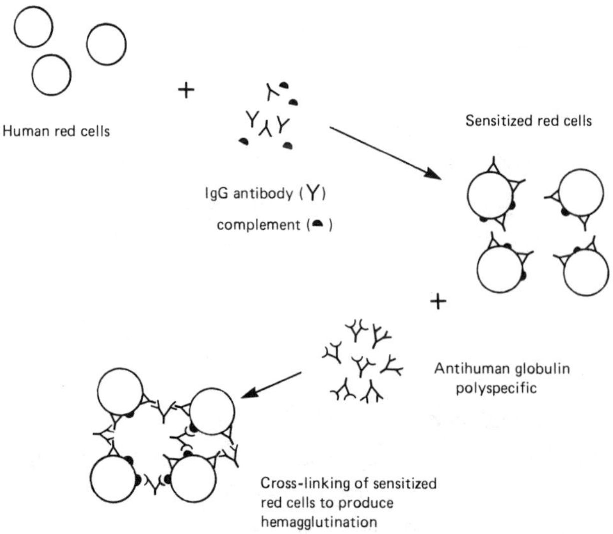

FIGURE 4–1 Antihuman globulin test. The indirect test is employed to determine in vitro sensitization of red cells whereas the direct test is used to detect in vivo sensitization. Polyspecific antihuman globulin contains anti-IgG and anticomplement activity.

are IgG. After combining to their corresponding antigen, some blood group antibodies have the ability to activate and bind complement to the RBC membrane. Antiglobulin tests are used to detect IgG or complement-sensitized RBCs. Sensitization can occur either in vivo or in vitro. The presence of alloantibodies, autoantibodies, and complement components can be detected by antihuman globulin serum in the antiglobulin test (AGT).

Antiglobulin sera are made by injecting human serum or purified globulin into rabbits. The human globulin behaves as a foreign antigen, the rabbit's immune response is triggered, and an antibody to human globulin is produced. For example, human IgG is injected; anti-IgG is produced. The antibodies produced react with their antigen immediately at room temperature.

For in vitro antigen-antibody reactions, the indirect antiglobulin test tasks are listed and explained:

Task	Why
1. Incubate RBCs with antisera.	1. Allows time for antibody molecule attachment to RBC antigen
2. Perform three saline washings.	2. Removes free globulin molecules
3. Add antiglobulin reagent.	3. Forms RBC agglutinates (RBC antigen + antibody + anti-IgG + antibody + RBC antigen)
4. Centrifuge.	4. Accelerates agglutination by bringing cells closer together
5. Examine for agglutination.	5. Interprets test as positive or negative
6. Grade agglutination reactions	6. Determines the strength of reaction
7. Add antibody-coated RBCs to those with negative reactions.	7. Checks for neutralization of antihuman sera by free globulin molecules (the Coombs control cells are D-positive RBCs that are coated with anti-D)

The direct antiglobulin test does not require the incubation phase because the antigen-antibody complexes have formed in vivo.

Antibodies Required in Antihuman Globulin for Indirect and Direct Test Procedures

ANTI-GAMMA GLOBULIN ACTIVITY

Antihuman globulin must contain antibody activity to nonagglutinating blood group antibodies. The vast majority of these antibodies are IgG, mainly IgG_1 or IgG_3, or both subclasses. Very occasionally these antibodies may be IgG_2 or IgG_4. Rarely, nonagglutinating IgM antibodies may be found; however, they have been shown always to fix complement and may be detected by anticomplement.[7] IgA antibodies with Rh specificity have been reported; however, IgG antibody

activity has always been present as well. The only blood group alloantibodies that have been reported as being solely IgA have been examples of anti-Pr,[8] and those antibodies were agglutinating. IgA autoantibodies have been reported, albeit very rarely.[9] Therefore, anti-IgG activity must be present. Anti-IgM and anti-IgA activity may be present, but neither is essential. The presence of anti–light chain activity will allow the detection of all immunoglobulin classes.

ANTICOMPLEMENT ACTIVITY

Early antihuman globulin reagents were prepared using a crude globulin fraction as the immunogen. In 1947, Coombs and Mourant showed that the antibody activity that detected Rh antibodies was associated with the anti–gamma-globulin fraction in the reagent. The first indication that another antibody activity might be present that had an influence on the final reaction was presented by Dacie in 1951.[10] He observed that different reaction patterns were obtained when dilutions of antihuman globulin were used to test cells sensitized with "warm" versus "cold" antibodies. In 1957, Dacie et al.[11] published data showing that the reactivity of antihuman globulin to cells sensitized with "warm" antibodies was due to anti–gamma-globulin activity, whereas anti–nongamma-globulin activity was responsible for the activity of cells sensitized by "cold" antibodies. The nongamma-globulin component was shown to be beta globulin and had specificity for complement. Later studies[12,13] revealed that the complement activity was due to C3 and C4.

During the 1960s many reports were published indicating the need for anticomplement activity in antihuman globulin to allow the detection of antibodies by the indirect test.[14–17] Many of the specificities mentioned in these reports were ones that are now generally considered to be of little clinical significance (e.g., anti-Le^a, anti-P, and anti-O[H]). However, one specificity that was consistently mentioned is considered to be clinically significant: anti-Jk^a. It was also shown that the presence of anticomplement activity would enhance the reactions of some antibodies (e.g., anti-Fy^a and anti-K).[14]

In a 3-year study, Howard et al.[18] found eight patients whose antibodies were detected primarily or solely by antihuman globulin containing anticomplement activity. Seven of these antibodies had anti-Jk^a or anti-Jk^b specificity. Some of them could be detected using homozygous Jk^a or Jk^b cells and an antihuman globulin containing only anti-IgG activity. Two of the anti-Jk^a antibodies were associated with delayed hemolytic transfusion reactions. The complement-only Kidd antibodies represented 23 percent of all Kidd antibodies detected during the study. The authors concluded that they would continue to use polyspecific antihuman globulin reagent for routine compatibility testing (Table 4–1).

TABLE 4-1 **DEVELOPMENT OF ANTIHUMAN GLOBULIN REAGENT**

1945 Coombs and Mourant	Discovered anti–gamma globulin for detecting nonagglutinating antibodies
1951, 1957 Dacie et al.	Discovered anticomplement activity Differentiated between anti–gamma globulin activity to detect "warm" antibody sensitization and anti–non–gamma globulin activity to detect cold antibody sensitization
1976 Garratty and Petz	Confirmed need for anti-C3d activity in antihuman globulin Concluded anti-C4 activity in broad-spectrum antihuman globulin should be excluded
1982 Howard et al.	Found proof that some antibodies were detected primarily by anticomplement activity in antihuman globulin reagent

Mechanism of Complement Component Degradation

By the late 1960s the mechanism of complement activation was becoming better understood, and it was known that both C3 and C4 were split into two components as part of the activation process. C3b and C4b were bound to the cell membrane, whereas C3a and C4a passed into the fluid phase. Further degradation of C3b and C4b could then occur by removal of C3c and C4c, to leave C3d and C4d firmly attached to the cell membrane.[19-21]

C3d SENSITIZATION

The final degradation step was shown to occur in vivo[22] and, in fact, was a common occurrence in both warm and cold types of autoimmune hemolytic anemia. In the latter type of autoimmune hemolytic anemia, C3d is invariably the only material detected on the cell. Engelfriet et al.[23] also have shown that, provided a long enough incubation period, degradation to C3d could occur in vitro.

C3d ACTIVITY IN ANTIGLOBULIN TESTING

In 1976, Garratty and Petz[24] reported on the significance of red cell–bound complement components. Using in-house antisera, they confirmed the need for anti-C3d activity in antihuman globulin for use in the direct test. They also confirmed Engelfriet's observation that, given sufficient incubation time, cell-bound C3b could be degraded to C3d in vitro.

Consequently, the anti-C3d activity in antihuman globulin could be used for the indirect test as well as the direct test. However, the level of anti-C3d activity in the antihuman globulin was shown to be critical. If the activity was too high, many weakly positive results could be obtained, owing to the presence of comple-

ment fixing clinically insignificant cold antibodies in the serum under investigation. This was particularly a problem whenever a room temperature incubation phase was followed by incubation at 37°C before performance of the antihuman globulin test. Attachment of C3d to RBCs has also been shown to occur naturally by incubation of normal RBCs and serum at 37°C.[25]

Thus the anti-C3d activity needed to be carefully standardized to minimize the occurrence of insignificant weak positive reactions in the indirect test. Garratty and Petz[24] did point out that commercial broad-spectrum reagents available then did not have excess anti-C3d activity and consequently were not prone to giving unwanted positive reactions.

C4d SENSITIZATION

Another important observation from Garratty and Petz[24] was that RBCs stored as clots at 4°C and then used in direct antihuman globulin tests produced a very high incidence of positive results. These results were due to the presence of C4d, and to a lesser extent of C3d, on the cells. When anticoagulated donor segment cells were tested, positive reactions were obtained only for C4d and then only on *some* of the cell samples. It was concluded that attachment of complement to the cells was most probably facilitated by the presence of cold antibodies and "normal incomplete cold antibody." Commercial reagents were shown to be nonreactive with both clots and donor segment cells.

The authors concluded that anti-C4 activity in broad-spectrum antihuman globulin was undesirable and that its exclusion would not decrease the efficiency of the reagent for use in the indirect test.

ANTIGLOBULIN TESTING WITH LOW IONIC STRENGTH SOLUTION

During the 1970s the low ionic strength solution (LISS) antihuman globulin technique came into vogue.[26-30] The advantage of this technique was the significantly shortened incubation times that could be used to achieve sensitization of the red cells being tested. However, even though the ionic strength is adjusted to minimize the nonspecific uptake of complement,[26] many laboratories that used the technique began to find a high level of "grainy" or weakly positive results when using polyspecific antihuman globulin, especially when reading the results microscopically. Petz et al.[31] examined 39,436 fresh or freshly frozen sera using the LISS technique and polyspecific antihuman globulin. They found that the LISS technique detected all potentially clinically significant antibodies. However, it also detected many clinically insignificant antibodies, especially when the technique used a room temperature incubation that was then carried through to 37°C. If anti-IgG was used in place of the polyspecific reagent, the detection of clinically insignificant antibodies was markedly reduced; however, at the same time, five clinically significant antibodies (anti-Jk[a]) were missed. Ninety-three percent of the unwanted positive reactions detected by the polyspecific reagent were shown to be due to C3 on the cells.

Current licensing requirements for polyspecific antihuman globulin require the presence of both anti-IgG and anti-C3d activity, with the presence of other antibody specificities being optional. A decision on the use of the reagent for indirect tests is the prerogative of the individual blood bank. The decision on whether to use polyspecific or IgG antihuman globulin depends heavily on the technique used for the indirect test.[32]

Preparation of Antihuman Globulin Reagents

POLYSPECIFIC REAGENT

Antihuman globulin is usually prepared in rabbits, although when large volumes of antibody are required, sheep or goats may be used. In contrast with the early production methods, in which a crude globulin fraction of serum was used as the immunogen, modern production commences with the purification of the immunogen from a large pool of normal sera. IgG is prepared and its purity determined before immunization of the animals. The monoclonal antibody technique devised by Kohler and Milstein[33] has been used and proven particularly useful in producing high-titer antibodies with well-defined specificities to the fragments of C3.[34-36] In fact, the C3g fragment of C3 was first defined using a monoclonal antibody.[37] Figure 4–2 summarizes the manufacture of polyspecific antihuman globulin.

In the production of polyclonal antisera, the animals are hyperimmunized to produce high-titer, high-avidity IgG antibodies. With monoclonal antibodies, the hybrid clones are screened for antibodies with the required specificity and affinity. The antibody-secreting clones may then be propagated in culture or by inoculation into mice, in which case the antibody is collected as ascites. Monoclonal anticomplement antibodies may be either IgM or IgG.

In polyclonal antisera production, blood specimens are drawn from the immunized animals, and the antibody titer and specificity are then determined. Assuming that the specificity of the antibodies is as required and that the titer has reached a sufficient level, the

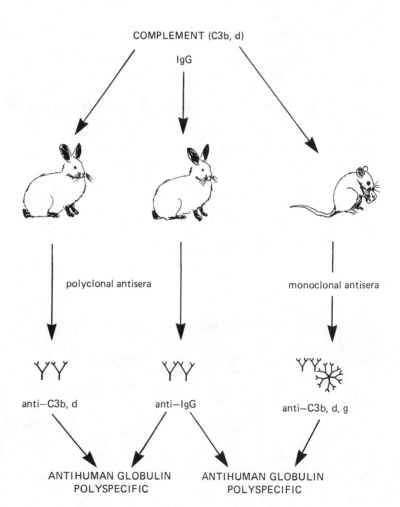

FIGURE 4–2 Antihuman globulin manufacture. Polyspecific antihuman globulin may be manufactured by combining polyclonal anti-IgG with either polyclonal or monoclonal anticomplement components. Antisera to the "g" portion of C3 have been made using only monoclonal technology.

animals are then bled for a production batch of reagent. Separate blends of the anti-IgG and anticomplement antibodies are made, and each pool is then absorbed with A_1, B, and O cells to remove heterospecific antibodies. The total antibody content of each pool is determined, and the pools are then analyzed by block titration to calculate the optimum antibody dilution for use. Block titrations are performed by reacting dilutions of each antibody against cells sensitized with different amounts of IgG and complement. This is a critical step in the manufacturing process because excess antibody, especially with anti-IgG, may lead to prozoning and hence false-negative test results. Once the required performance characteristics of the trial blend are obtained, a production blend of the separate anti-IgG and anticomplement pools is made.

The final product is one that contains both anti-IgG and anticomplement activity at the correct dilution for immediate use. The reagent also contains buffers, stabilizers, and bacteriostatic agents and may be dyed green for identification purposes.

MONOSPECIFIC REAGENTS

Monospecific reagents for use in the direct antihuman globulin test are prepared by a similar production process; however, they contain only one antibody specificity. The one exception, is anti-IgG. If not gamma-chain specific, anti-IgG may contain anti–light chain activity and therefore will react with cells sensitized with IgM and IgA antibodies as well as with IgG.

Before the antihuman globulin is available for purchase, manufacturers must subject their reagents to an evaluation procedure, the results of which must be submitted to the Food and Drug Administration (FDA) for approval. The evaluation procedure involves parallel testing of the manufacturer's reagents and a reference standard supplied by the Office of Biologics Research and Review (OBRR). In addition to supplying the reference standard, the OBRR stipulates recommended methods that must be used in the evaluation process. The procedure for evaluation has been reviewed by Case.[38] Table 4–2 summarizes the procedure for the preparation of antihuman serum.

Principles of the Antiglobulin Test

According to the American Association of Blood Banks (AABB) Technical Manual, the antiglobulin test is based on the following simple principles:[39]

1. Antibody molecules and complement components are globulins.
2. Injecting an animal with human globulin stimulates the animal to produce antibody to the foreign protein (i.e., antihuman globulin [AHG]). Serologic tests employ a variety of AHG reagents reactive with various human globulins including anti-IgG, antibody to the C3d component of human complement, and polyspecific reagents that contain both anti-IgG and anti-C3d activity.
3. AHG will react with human globulin molecules either bound to RBCs or free in serum.
4. Washed RBCs coated with human globulin are agglutinated by AHG.

Direct Antihuman Globulin Test

PRINCIPLE AND APPLICATION OF THE DIRECT ANTIGLOBULIN TEST

The direct antiglobulin test is used to detect in vivo sensitization of RBCs. Clinical conditions that can result in in vivo coating of RBCs with antibody or complement or both are (1) hemolytic disease of the newborn (HDN), (2) hemolytic transfusion reaction (HTR), and (3) autoimmune and drug-induced hemolytic anemias (AIHA). Table 4–3 lists the clinical application and in vivo sensitization detected for each situation.

DIRECT ANTIGLOBULIN TESTING PANEL

Initial direct antiglobulin testing (DAT) should include both anti-IgG and anti-C3d reagents or polyspecific (anti–IgG-C3d) reagent. Subsequent testing using monospecific reagents determines the type of protein sensitizing the cell. Table 4–4 defines the application and limitations of polyspecific reagents (anti–IgG-C3d) and monospecific reagents (e.g., anti-IgG or anti-C3d). A DAT panel using polyspecific and monospecific reagents characterizes the type of protein sensitization that has occurred in vivo. A DAT

TABLE 4–2 PREPARATION OF ANTIHUMAN SERUM

Immunization of animal	Injection of purified immunoglobulin into rabbit; either C3 or IgG
Harvest antisera	Animal bled to make pool of anti-C3 and anti-IgG
Purify pool of antisera	Pool absorbed with A_1, B, and O cells to remove heterospecific antibodies
Adjust antibody titer	Remove excess antibody by block titration
Validate performance	Antibody titer and specificity verified by evaluation

TABLE 4–3 DIRECT ANTIGLOBULIN TEST

Principle: Detects In Vivo Red Cell Sensitization	
Application	**In Vivo Sensitization**
HDN	Maternal antibody coating fetal RBCs
HTR	Recipient antibody coating donor RBCs
AIHA	Autoantibody coating individual's RBCs

TABLE 4–4 APPLICATIONS AND LIMITATIONS OF DIFFERENT ANTIHUMAN GLOBULIN REAGENTS

Direct Antiglobulin Tests	ANTI-Ig, -C3d (POLYSPECIFIC)		ANTI-IgG		ANTI-C3b, -C3d (ANTI-C3)	
	Rabbit	Mono-clonal	Rabbit	Mono-clonal	Rabbit	Mono-clonal
Diagnosis of HDN	Yes	Yes	Yes	Yes	NA	NA
Investigation of transfusion reactions	Yes	Yes	Yes*	Yes*	Yes*	Yes*
Investigation of drug-induced red cell sensitization	Yes	Yes	Yes*	Yes*	Yes*	Yes*
Investigation of autoimmune hemolytic anemia	Yes	Yes	Yes*	Yes*	Yes*	Yes*
General identification of cell surface coat (e.g., complement or immunoglobulin)	NA	NA	Yes	NA	NA	NA
Specific identification of cell surface coat (e.g., C3, IgG, IgM, IgA)	NA	NA	NA	Yes	Yes	Yes
Compatibility testing	Yes	Yes	†	†	NA	NA
Screening for unexpected antibodies in donors	Yes	Yes	Yes†	Yes†	NA	NA
Screening for unexpected antibodies in patients	Yes	Yes	†	†	NA	NA
Identification of antibodies	Yes	Yes	Yes	Yes	Yes	Yes
Detection of antigens	Yes	Yes	Yes	Yes	NA	NA

*The cells should be tested for the presence of both IgG and C3d, using either anti-IgG/C3d (polyspecific) or antihuman globulin reagents that contain these components separately (e.g., anti-IgG and anti-C3d).

†Some literature indicates that anti-IgG occasionally fails to detect antibodies that are demonstrable by means of an antihuman globulin reagent containing an anti-C3 component. In some cases, antibodies not detected by anti-IgG may be clinically significant. Anti-IgG may be used for antibody screening and for compatibility testing, but the worker should be aware that current scientific data do not wholly support the exclusive use of anti-IgG for these purposes.

panel is useful in determining whether the patient's RBCs are coated with antibody, complement, or both. Patterns of reactivity and the type of protein sensitization in AIHA are summarized in Table 4–5.

Significance of a Positive DAT Result

The AABB Technical Manual[39] states that clinical consideration should dictate the extent to which a positive DAT result is evaluated. Interpreting the significance of a positive DAT result requires knowledge of the patient's diagnosis, drug therapy, and recent transfusion history. Table 4–6 describes the in vivo phenomena that may be associated with transfusion, drug-induced hemolytic anemia, warm and cold AIHA, hypergammaglobulinemia, and hemolytic disease of the newborn. A positive DAT may occur without clinical manifestations of immune-mediated hemolysis.

EVALUATION OF A POSITIVE DAT RESULT

The AABB Technical Manual states that "results of serological tests are not diagnostic; their significance can only be assessed in relationship to the patient's clinical condition."[39] Answering the following questions before investigating a positive DAT result for patients other than neonates will help determine what further testing is appropriate:

1. Is there evidence of in vivo hemolysis?
2. Has the patient been transfused recently?
3. Does the patient's serum contain unexpected antibodies?
4. Is the patient receiving any drugs?
5. Has the patient received blood products or components containing ABO-incompatible plasma?
6. Is the patient receiving antilymphocyte globulin (ALG) or antithymocyte globulin (ATG)?

Indirect Antihuman Globulin Test Applications

This test determines in vitro sensitization of red cells and is used in the following situations:

1. Detection of incomplete antibodies to potential donor red cells (compatibility testing) or to screening cells (antibody screen) in serum
2. Identification of antibody specificity using a panel of red cells with known antigen profiles

TABLE 4–5 DAT PANEL PATTERNS OF REACTIVITY IN AIHA*

Anti IgG	Anti C3d	Type of AIHA
+	+	Warm (67%)
+	−	Warm (20%)
−	+	CHD, PCH, Warm (13%)

Modified from the AABB Technical Manual.[39]

*The direct antiglobulin test with monospecific antiglobulin reagents is helpful in classifying AIHAs. Other procedures and studies are necessary to diagnose and characterize which form of autoimmune disease is present (see Chapter 20).

AIHA = autoimmune hemolytic anemia; CHD = cold hemagglutinin disease; PCH = paroxysmal cold hemoglobinuria.

TABLE 4-6 IN VIVO PHENOMENA ASSOCIATED WITH A POSITIVE DAT RESULT

Transfusion	1. Recipient alloantibody and donor antigen	Alloantibodies in the recipient of a recent transfusion that react with antigen on donor RBCs
	2. Donor antibody and recipient antigen	Antibodies present in donor plasma that react with antigens on a transfusion recipient's RBCs
Drug-induced	1. Drug absorption	Penicillin absorbed to RBCs in vivo; antipenicillin will react with the penicillin bound to the RBCs; penicillin-coated RBCs become coated with IgG
	2. Immune complex absorption	Drug and specific antibody form complexes that attach nonspecifically to RBCs and initiate complement activation on the RBC surface
	3. Membrane modification	RBCs coated with cephalothin (Keflin) will absorb albumin, IgA, IgG, IgM, and α and β (is complement) globulins
	4. Autoimmunity	Following α-methyldopa therapy, autoantibodies are formed that react with intrinsic RBC antigens
AIHA	1. Warm AIHA IgG and/or C3	Autoantibody reacts with patient's RBCs in vivo
	2. CHD C3	Cold-reactive IgM autoagglutinin binds to RBCs in peripheral circulation (temperature 32°C); IgM binds complement; as RBCs return to warmer parts of circulation, IgM dissociates, leaving RBCs coated only with complement
	3. PCH IgG	IgG autoantibody reacts with RBCs in colder parts of body, causes complement to be bound irreversibly to RBCs, and then elutes at warmer temperature
HDN	1. Maternal alloantibody crosses placenta	Maternal alloantibody, specific for fetal antigen, coats fetal RBCs
Miscellaneous	1. Administration of equine preparations of antilymphocyte globulin and antithymocyte globulin	Heterophile antibodies that are present in ALG or ATG coat recipient's RBCs
	2. Administration of high dose intravenous gamma globulin	Non–antibody-mediated binding of immunoglobulin to RBCs in patients with hypergammaglobulinemia

Modified from the AABB Technical Manual.[39]
AIHA = autoimmune hemolytic anemia; CHD = cold hemagglutinin disease; PCH = paroxysmal cold hemoglobinuria.

3. Determination of red cell phenotype using known antisera (e.g., Kell typing, D^u testing)
4. Titration of incomplete antibodies

Table 4-7 lists the indirect antiglobulin tests and the in vitro sensitization detected for each application.

The complete procedures for the direct and indirect antihuman globulin tests can be found in the procedural appendix at the end of this chapter. **Color Plate 1** summarizes the methodology of both tests.

Factors Affecting the Antihuman Globulin Test

The antihuman globulin test may be able to detect between 150 and 500 IgG molecules per red cell.[40,41] In the study performed by Merry et al.,[40] complete agglutination occurred once a cell had been sensitized with approximately 1000 molecules of IgG. Similar results were obtained for both direct and indirect antihuman globulin tests. The test, therefore, is a poor indicator of the amount of antibody actually sensitizing red cells, inasmuch as there is a very narrow dose-response curve between the number of antibody molecules on the cells and the degree of hemagglutination. In a study employing monoclonal antibodies to C3 fragments, Merry et al.[42] found that the antihuman globulin test had sensitivity for C3 similar to that for IgG.

For the indirect antihuman globulin test, therefore, there must be between 100 and 200 IgG or C3 molecules on the cell to obtain a positive reaction. The number of IgG molecules that will sensitize a red cell and the rate at which sensitization occurs can be influenced by several factors, outlined here:

1. **Ratio of serum to cells.** Increasing the ratio of serum to cells will increase the sensitivity of the test system. Generally, a minimum ratio of 40:1

TABLE 4-7 INDIRECT ANTIGLOBULIN TEST

Principle: Detects In Vitro Sensitization		
Application	**Tests**	**In Vitro Sensitization**
Antibody detection	Compatibility testing, antibody screening	Recipient antibody reacting with donor cells Antibody reacting with screening cells
Antibody identification	Antibody panel	Antibody reacting with panel cells
Antibody titration	Rh antibody titer	Antibody and selected Rh cells
Red cell phenotype	D^u test	Anti-D and Rh_o-negative RBCs to detect weak antigen

should be aimed for, and this can be achieved by using 2 drops of serum and 1 drop of a 5-percent volume of solute per volume of solution (v/v) suspension of cells.[43] When using cells suspended in saline, it is often advantageous to increase the ratio of serum to cells in an effort to detect weak antibodies (e.g., 4 drops of serum with 1 drop of a 3-percent v/v cell suspension will give a ratio of 133:1).

2. **Temperature.** The rate of reaction for the vast majority of IgG antibodies is optimal at 37°C; hence this is the usual incubation temperature for the indirect antihuman globulin test. This is also the optimum temperature for complement activation.

3. **Incubation time.** For cells suspended in saline, incubation times may vary between 30 and 120 minutes. The vast majority of clinically significant antibodies can be detected after 30 minutes of incubation, and extended incubation times are usually not necessary. If using a LISS technique,[26,27] incubation times may be shortened to 10 to 15 minutes. With these shortened incubation times, it is essential that tubes be incubated at a temperature of 37°C. Extended incubation (i.e., up to 40 minutes) in the LISS technique has been shown to cause antibody to elute from the red cells, causing a decrease in the sensitivity of the test.[44] However, this could not be confirmed by Voak et al.[45]

4. **Reaction medium.** In 1965, Stroup and Mac-Ilroy[46] reported on the increased sensitivity of the indirect antihuman globulin if albumin was incorporated into the reaction medium. Their reaction mixture, consisting of 2 drops of serum, 2 drops of 22 percent weight per volume (w/v) bovine albumin, and 1 drop of 3 to 5 percent v/v cells, was shown to provide the same sensitivity at 30 minutes of incubation as a 60-minute saline test. The proposed function of albumin was to reduce the ionic strength and at the same time to raise the dielectric constant of the reaction mixture. The reduction in ionic strength would increase the rate of antibody uptake on the cell. However, many workers were not able to show this increase, probably because they were not using salt-poor albumin. The use of albumin does not seem to provide any advantage over LISS techniques and does add to the cost of the test.[47] Petz et al.[31] also showed that use of an albumin technique may miss a number of clinically significant antibodies.

The LISS technique introduced by Low and Messeter[26] has critical requirements with respect to the serum-to-cell ratio. Moore and Mollison[27] showed that optimum reaction conditions were obtained using 2 drops of serum and 2 drops of a 3 percent v/v suspension of cells in LISS. Increasing the serum-to-cell ratio increased the ionic strength of the reaction mixture, leading to

a decrease in sensitivity, thus counteracting the shortened incubation time of the test.

5. **Washing of cells.** After either in vivo or in vitro sensitization, RBCs must be washed before adding antihuman globulin reagent. This represents another critical stage in the technique.

Cells should be saline washed three or four times to remove all free protein. The washing should be performed in as short a time as possible to minimize the elution of low-affinity antibodies. The cell pellet should be completely resuspended before adding the next saline wash. All saline should be discarded completely following the final wash, because residual saline will dilute the antihuman globulin reagent and therefore will decrease the sensitivity of the test.

Centrifugation at each wash should be sufficient to provide a firm cell pellet and therefore to minimize the possible loss of cells with each discard of saline. Washing may be performed using an automatic cell washer.[48]

6. **Saline for washing.** Ideally the saline used for washing should be fresh or alternatively buffered to a pH of 7.2 to 7.4. Saline stored for periods of time in plastic containers has been shown to decrease in pH, which may increase the rate of antibody elution during the washing process.[49] These pH changes may have important implications when monoclonal antihuman globulin is used, inasmuch as monoclonal antibodies have been shown sometimes to have very narrow pH ranges for optimum reactivity. Significant levels of bacterial contamination in saline has been reported,[50] and this can contribute to false-positive results.

7. **Addition of antihuman globulin.** Antihuman globulin should be added to the washed cells immediately after washing to minimize the chance of antibody eluting from the cell and subsequently neutralizing the antihuman globulin reagent. The volume of antihuman globulin added should be as indicated by the manufacturers. However, Voak et al.[51] have shown that adding two volumes of antihuman globulin may overcome washing problems when low levels of serum contamination remain. They point out that the neutralization of antihuman globulin is only a problem with IgG and not with the anti-complement activity, inasmuch as the complement fragments against which antibody activity is directed are not normally present in serum.

8. **Centrifugation for reading.** Centrifugation of the cell pellet for reading of hemagglutination, along with the method used for resuspending the cells, is a crucial step in the technique. The OBRR-recommended method for the evaluation of antihuman globulin employs 1000 relative centrifugal force (RCF) for 20 seconds, although the technique described in this chapter suggests 500 RCF for 15 to 20 seconds. The use of higher

RCFs will yield more sensitive results; however, depending on how the pellet is resuspended, it may produce weak false-positive results owing to inadequate resuspension or alternatively may give a negative result if resuspension is too vigorous. The optimum centrifugation conditions should be determined for each centrifuge.

Sources of Error

Some of the more common sources of error associated with the performance of the antihuman globulin test have been outlined in the previous section. Table 4–8 lists those, along with some other, less frequently occurring problems. Additional information on problems associated with the performance of antihuman globulin tests may be found in the excellent article by Voak et al.[48] and in the AABB Technical Manual.[52]

The daily quality control on polyspecific antihuman globulin reagents is best performed by adding weakly sensitized cells to all negative test result specimens. Any negative antiglobulin test result must be confirmed by adding Coombs' control cells. Adding IgG-coated RBCs to nonreactive test result specimens will demonstrate impaired AHG activity.

Modified and Automated Antihuman Globulin Techniques

Modifications to the antihuman globulin technique have been mentioned (LISS, LISS additive, and albumin); however, some other modifications may be used in special circumstances. Unger[53] reported on the use

TABLE 4–8   **SOURCES OF ERROR IN THE ANTIHUMAN GLOBULIN TECHNIQUE**

False-Positive Results

1. Autoagglutinable cells
2. Bacterial contamination of cells or saline used in washing
3. Cells with a positive DAT used for the indirect antiglobulin test
4. Saline contaminated by heavy metals or colloidal silica
5. Dirty glassware
6. Overcentrifugation and overreading
7. Polyagglutinable cells
8. Preservative-dependent antibody in LISS reagents[62]
9. Contaminating antibodies in the antihuman globulin reagent

False-Negative Results

1. Inadequate or improper washing of cells
2. Antihuman globulin reagent nonreactive owing to deterioration or neutralization
3. Antihuman globulin reagent not added
4. Serum not added in the indirect test
5. Serum nonreactive owing to deterioration of complement
6. Inadequate incubation conditions in the indirect test
7. Cell suspension either too weak or too heavy
8. Undercentrifuged or overcentrifuged
9. Poor reading technique

of enzymes to pretreat cells prior to performing the indirect antihuman globulin test. With this technique he was able to detect very low titers of Rh_o antibodies. The technique was also shown to be useful in detecting anti-Jk[a].[54]

In their 1961 paper, Polley and Mollison[14] reported on the use of a two-stage ethylenediaminetetraacetic acid (EDTA) technique to detect complement-fixing antibodies. This technique is particularly suitable for the detection of many Jk[a] and Le[a] antibodies, especially when investigating "aged" serum samples.

In 1980, Lalezari and Jiang[55] reported on the adaption of the automated low-ionic polybrene (LIP) technique for use as a manual procedure. The technique relies on low-ionic conditions rapidly to sensitize cells with antibody. Polybrene, a potent rouleaux-forming reagent, is added to allow the sensitized cells to approach each other to permit cross-linking by the attached antibody. A high-ionic strength solution is then added to reverse the rouleaux; however, if agglutination is present, it will remain. The test can be carried through to an antihuman globulin technique if required. If this is performed, a monospecific anti-IgG reagent must be used, as the low-ionic conditions cause considerable amounts of C4 and C3 to coat the cells and would give false-positive reactions if a polyspecific reagent were used.

Antihuman globulin tests may be performed in reaction vessels other than test tubes. The capillary tube technique, originally introduced by Chown and Lewis[56] for Rh blood grouping, was adapted by them in 1957[57] for the antihuman globulin test. Postoway and Garratty[58] have reported on the use of the capillary tube technique in the determination of IgG subclasses using specific subclass-typing antisera.

The antihuman globulin test also has been performed using microplates. Crawford et al.[59] used microplates for a number of different grouping procedures, including the indirect antihuman globulin test. Microplate technology is increasingly used in blood group serology, and many techniques are being adapted for it. Redman et al.[60] have adapted the LIP technique for use in microplates. Although their report does not include the use of an antihuman globulin phase, this additional step could easily be included.

One modification that is attracting considerable attention is the use of solid-phase serology for the performance of antihuman globulin tests. A number of different techniques have been reported using either test tubes[61] or microplates.[62,63] With the availability of microplate readers, this modification lends itself to the introduction of partial automation.

Solid phase involves the addition of sensitized red cells to a well coated with antihuman globulin. Following centrifugation, the cells will adhere to the walls of the well as a monolayer, if they are sensitized by antibody, or will pellet to the bottom of the well, if they are not sensitized. Plapp et al.[64] have provided an excellent review on solid-phase assays and their use in blood bank serology.

Immucor Incorporated manufactures a solid-phase

system for the detection and identification of alloantibodies. Group O reagent RBC membranes are bound to the surfaces of polystyrene microtitration strip wells. IgG antibodies from patient or donor sera are bound to the membrane antigens. After incubation, unbound immunoglobulins are rinsed from the wells; then a suspension of anti-IgG–coated indicator RBCs is added to the wells. Centrifugation brings the indicator RBCs in contact with antibodies bound to the reagent RBC membranes. If the test result is negative, a pellet of indicator RBCs will form in the bottom of the wells. A positive test result will cause adherence of the indicator RBCs forming anti-IgG–IgG complexes and a second immobilized RBC layer.

One form of automation for the performance of antihuman globulin tests has been introduced by Gamma Biologics, Incorporated. The Gamma STS-A (Standardised Test System–Antiglobulin) performs the antihuman globulin test in a specially designed cuvette that allows for the automated addition of cells and serum, washing of sensitized cells, addition of antihuman globulin, centrifugation, and finally analysis of the cell suspension for the presence of agglutinates.

The changes in blood bank technology being introduced, along with changes in emphasis on the importance of crossmatching versus antibody screening, will likely further modify the role of the antihuman globulin test over the coming years. At the moment, however, it still remains the most important test in the blood bank for the detection of clinically significant antibodies to red cells and for the detection of immune hemolysis.

Basic Case Studies

Case 1

A 50-year-old woman is admitted to the hospital for cardiac surgery. Six units of blood are ordered. The patient is blood type O Rh$_o$ positive. The pretransfusion antibody screen is negative and the abbreviated immediate spin crossmatch is compatible. The patient is transfused 4 units of type O Rh$_o$-positive blood. Ten days after transfusion the patient is slightly jaundiced, develops malaise and weakness, and voids dark urine. The results of a transfusion-reaction investigation, before and after laboratory testing, are as follows:

Test	Pretransfusion Sample	Posttransfusion Sample
Serum haptoglobin	—	Decreased
Urine hemoglobin	Negative	4+
Hematocrit	35%	30%
Antibody screen	Negative	Negative
DAT	—	2+
Reticulocyte count	—	7.2%
Indirect bilirubin	0.7 mg/dl	3.0 mg/dl

No clerical errors are detected.

Questions

1. Explain the positive DAT result on the posttransfusion sample.
2. What antiglobulin testing is indicated on the posttransfusion sample?

Answers

1. The positive DAT result on the posttransfusion sample is due to an alloantibody present in the patient's serum reacting with recently transfused donor RBC antigen. It was not detected in the pretransfusion sample because of a low titer. The titer increased when the corresponding donor antigen caused an anamnestic response and an increase in antibody.
2. An antibody identification performed on the RBC eluate should be done to confirm the possibility of a delayed hemolytic transfusion reaction. Because the DAT result is positive and the antibody screen is negative, this confirms the presence of antibody-coated transfused cells. After primary immunization some alloantibodies may diminish to undetectable levels in the serum. A secondary response to recently transfused red cell antigens leads to an increased level of IgG antibodies that react with transfused cells.

Case 2

During preadmission testing on a 45-year-old man, a positive DAT result is demonstrated. A DAT panel is performed to characterize the type of protein sensitizing the red blood cells.

DAT Panel		
Polyspecific Anti-Human Serum	Anti-IgG	Anti-C3d
Patients' RBCs +	−	+

Questions

1. Interpret the DAT panel by indicating what type of protein is sensitizing the RBCs.
2. Name two reasons for this type of protein sensitization.
3. What questions answered before investigating a positive DAT result will help determine what further testing is appropriate?

Answers

1. Complement is sensitizing the RBCs.

2. Cold agglutinins and drugs associated with the immune complex mechanism activate complement.

3. See p 75, questions 1 through 6.

Advanced Case Study

An obstetric patient, 32 years of age, was referred to the Laboratory Blood Bank at the Regional Medical Center. Blood bank records from 1983 indicated that this patient's red cells were found to have a weak D antigen detectable only by the antihuman globulin test (AGT). In December 1991 the woman was again typed as having a weak D antigen. Because of anemia, she was given 2 units of D-positive blood. During prenatal testing in June 1992, she was discovered to have a positive DAT result and an anti-D titer of 8. The patient has never received Rh immunoglobulin and has had multiple pregnancies.

A reference laboratory was consulted for further investigative studies. The patient's red cells typed as group A_2 and C−E+c+e+ and were nonreactive after incubation at 37°C, with a commercial anti-D reagent (a blend of monoclonal and polyclonal anti-D). Because of the positive DAT result, before the AGT to detect weak D antigens was performed, the patient's RBCs were treated with EDTA–glycine acid to remove the IgG coating them. The EDTA–glycine acid–treated red cells were tested with five different examples of anti-D by the AGT using polyethylene glycol additive (PEG) for antibody enhancement. All five reagents were reactive with the patient's RBCs, although reactivity was weaker than that of control cells and varied from $2+^s$ microscopic to 2+ macroscopic. The 6-percent albumin control was nonreactive by the same method (AGT using PEG), indicating that no detectable IgG coating remained on the patient's treated cells and that the results with the anti-D may therefore be considered valid. These results indicate that the patient's red cells are weakly D positive.

The patient's serum was tested against a panel with LISS and ficin techniques. Anti-D was detected by AGT with LISS; reactivity with the ficin-pretreated panel was stronger. All panel cells, regardless of D status, were reactive on immediate spin; after incubation at 37°C, reactivity with D-positive RBCs was greatest. By ficin AGT only, D-positive RBCs were reactive.

Reactivity with untreated D-negative RBCs was enhanced when PEG was used for the AGT (strongest reactivity 2+ microscopic). By this method, the patient's red cells treated with EDTA–glycine acid were 2+ microscopic, suggesting that, in addition to a probable alloanti-D, the patient's serum contains warm reactive autoantibody.

An acid eluate prepared from the patient's cells was tested against the following: (1) first six cells of the panel, (2) the patient's EDTA–glycine acid–treated cells, (3) two examples of D—cells, (4) two examples of Rh_{null} cells, and (5) a D-positive LW-negative sample. The only nonreactive cells were the Rh_{null} cells. All D-positive cells reacted 3+ macroscopic; D-negative cells and the autocontrol reacted $1+^w$ to $1+^s$ macroscopic. These results further indicate that autoantibody is present in the patient's serum.

An aliquot of the patient's RBCs was ficin treated and used to autoabsorb her serum. After four absorptions, only anti-D remained; D-negative cells and the patient's own cells were nonreactive.

Questions

1. What is the patient's most probable Rh genotype?
2. Explain the presence of anti-D coexisting with weakly D-positive cells.
3. What technique was used to remove the IgG from the patient's RBCs before performing an AGT for the presence of the antigen?
4. What type of blood should be transfused to a recipient with weakly D-positive cells?
5. Based on the investigative studies, what can be concluded?
6. What further studies are indicated or would be helpful?

Answers

1. The patient's most probable genotype is *C(D)E/cde (R₂r)*. The *(D)* denotes a weak D antigen.
2. The patient's RBCs may express a partial D antigen. A partial D antigen may give the reactivity of a normal-strength D antigen or may appear as a weak D. The existence of rare D-positive people, who have made alloanti-D, is well documented. These people are thought to lack one or more epitopes of the D antigen. If exposed to the missing epitopes by transfusion or pregnancy, these individuals may make alloanti-D, reactive with all cells and having a normal expression of D.
3. Because cells coated with IgG may yield a positive result regardless of D status, IgG was removed from the patient's RBCs by the EDTA–glycine acid method to avoid nonspecific positive reactions with anti-D used by AGT.
4. It is common practice to transfuse patients with weakened expression of D, who have not made anti-D, with D-positive blood.
5. This patient may represent a rare or unusual blood type. Although her red cells type as D positive, a portion or epitope of the D antigen is lacking, allowing the development of alloanti-D. The positive DAT result is due to an autoantibody. When people with partial D antigens first make alloanti-D, autoantibody may also be detected. This autoanti-D does not usually react with D-negative cells, although occasionally it may resemble anti-LW.
6. A study of the patient's family, particularly her parents, siblings, children, and their respective fathers, may give insight into her true Rh genotype. Also, when the patient's cells are negative in the DAT repeat testing should be done.

Review Questions

1. The direct antihuman globulin test is used to detect _____ sensitization of red cells.
   A. In viva
   B. In vivo
   C. In vitra
   D. In vitro

2. After adding control cells to a negative antiglobulin test result specimen, a positive result was obtained. Which of the following could be a reason?
   A. Reagent had deteriorated.
   B. Reagent was contaminated.
   C. Reagent was neutralized.
   D. The control cells were properly coated with IgG.

3. To determine a red cell phenotype, such as a Jk^a typing, a technologist would employ:
   A. A direct antiglobulin test
   B. An indirect antiglobulin test
   C. Both a direct antiglobulin test and an indirect antiglobulin test
   D. Neither

4. What is the ideal pH range for saline washing?
   A. 6.8 to 7.0
   B. 7.0 to 7.2
   C. 7.2 to 7.4
   D. 7.4 to 7.6
   E. 7.6 to 7.8

5. DAT panel results on three patients follow:

	Polyspecific AHG	Anti-IgG	Anti-C3d
Patient No. 1	+	+	+
Patient No. 2	+	−	+
Patient No. 3	+	+	−

A correct interpretation of the type of protein coating each patient's RBCs corresponds to:

	Patient 1	Patient 2	Patient 3
A.	IgG only	C3d only	IgG only
B.	Both IgG and C3d	C3d only	IgG only
C.	Both IgG and C3d	IgG only	C3d only
D.	Both IgG and C3d	IgG only	IgG only

6. False-positive DAT results are most often associated with:
   A. Use of refrigerated, clotted blood sample in which complement components coat RBCs in vitro
   B. A recipient of a recent transfusion manifesting an immune response to recently transfused RBCs
   C. Presence of heterophile antibodies from administration of globulin
   D. A positive autocontrol caused by polyagglutination

7. Which of the following is a clinically significant antibody whose detection is enhanced by anticomplement activity in polyspecific antihuman globulin reagent?
   A. Anti-Jk^a
   B. Anti-Le^a

C. Anti-P
D. Anti-H

8. Block titrations are performed when preparing antihuman globulin reagents to avoid prozone caused by:
   A. Antibody excess, which could cause a false-positive result
   B. Antigen excess, which could cause a false-negative result
   C. Antibody excess, which could cause a false-negative result
   D. Antigen excess, which could cause a false-positive result

9. Cold hemagglutinin disease is associated with which DAT pattern of reactivity?

	Anti-IgG	Anti-C3d	Anti-IgG-C3d
A.	−	−	+
B.	+	+	+
C.	−	+	+
D.	+	−	+

10. An in vivo phenomenon associated with a positive DAT result is:
    A. Detection of incomplete antibodies to potential donor red cells
    B. Identification of antibody specificity using a panel of red cells
    C. Determination of red cell phenotype using known antisera
    D. Titration of incomplete antibodies
    E. Attachment of immune complexes nonspecifically to RBCs and fixation of complement

11. A principle of the antiglobulin test is:
    A. IgG and C3d are required for red cell sensitization.
    B. Human globulin is eluted from RBCs during red cell washings.
    C. Injection of an animal with human globulin engenders passive immunity.
    D. Antihuman globulin will react with human globulin molecules either bound to RBCs or all in serum.

12. A patient whose blood type is O Rh_o negative is transfused 3 units of O Rh_o-negative blood on June 1, 1993. Two more units of blood are ordered on June 10, 1993. During pretransfusion testing for the additional units a weakly positive autocontrol is demonstrated, and the antibody screen is negative. The results on a DAT panel on the pretransfusion (6/1/93) and posttransfusion (6/10/93) specimens are as indicated:

	Polyspecific Antihuman Serum	Anti-IgG	Anti-C3d	Control
Pretransfusion	−	−	−	−
Posttransfusion	+	+	−	−

The most likely explanation for the posttransfusion positive DAT result and negative antibody screen is the presence of:

A. An alloantibody formed in response to recently transfused donor RBC antigens not detected because of in vivo attachment to the patient's RBCs

B. An autoantibody attached to recently transfused donor RBCs

C. An autoantibody attached to patient's RBCs

D. An amnestic response that stimulated alloantibody formation not detectable in the indirect antiglobulin test because of in vivo attachment to recently transfused donor RBCs

Answers to Review Questions

1. B (p 70)
2. D (p 76)
3. B (p 74)
4. C (p 77)
5. B (p 74)
6. A (Table 4–7)
7. A (p 71)
8. C (p 73)
9. C (Table 4–5)
10. E (Table 4–6)
11. D (p 70)
12. D (Table 4–4)

References

1. Diamond, LK and Denton, RL: Rh agglutination in various media with particular reference to the values of albumin. J Lab Clin Med 30:821, 1945.
2. Morton, JA and Pickles, MM: Use of trypsin in the detection of incomplete and anti-Rh antibodies. Nature 159:779, 1947.
3. Coombs, RAA, Mourant, AE, and Race, RR: A new test for the detection of weak and "incomplete" Rh agglutinins. Br J Exp Pathol 26:255, 1945.
4. Coombs, RRA, Mourant, AE, and Race, RR: In vivo isosentisation of red cells in babies with haemolytic disease. Lancet i:264, 1946.
5. Race, RR and Sanger, R: Blood Groups in Man, ed 6. Blackwell Scientific Publications, Oxford, 1975, p 283.
6. Moreschi, C: Neue Tatsachen uber die Blutkorperchen Agglutinationen. Zentralbl Bakteriol 46:49, 1908. Cited by Mollison, PL: Blood Transfusion in Clinical Medicine, ed 7. Blackwell Scientific Publications, Oxford, 1983, p 502.
7. Mollison, PL: Blood Transfusion in Clinical Medicine, ed 7. Blackwell Scientific Publications, Oxford, 1983, p 502.
8. Garratty, G, et al: An IgA high titre cold agglutinin with an unusual blood group specificity within the Pr complex. Vox Sang 25:32, 1973.
9. Petz, LD and Garratty, G: Acquired immune hemolytic anemias. Churchill Livingstone, New York, 1980, p 193.
10. Dacie, JV: Differences in the behavior of sensitized red cells to agglutination by antiglobulin sera. Lancet ii:954, 1951.
11. Dacie, JV, Crookston, JH, and Christensen, WM: "Incomplete" cold antibodies: Role of complement in sensitization to antiglobulin serum by potentially haemolytic antibodies. Br J Haematol 3:77, 1957.
12. Harboe, M, et al: Identification of the component of complement participating in the antiglobulin reaction. Immunology 6:412, 1963.
13. Jenkins, GC, Polley, MJ, and Mollison, PL: Role of C4 in the antiglobulin reaction. Nature 186:482, 1960.
14. Polley, MJ and Mollison, PL: The role of complement in the detection of blood group antibodies. Special reference to the antiglobulin test. Transfusion 1:9, 1961.
15. Polley, MJ, Mollison, PL, and Soothill, JK: The role of 19S gamma-globulin blood group antibodies in the antiglobulin reaction. Br J Haematol 8:149, 1962.
16. Stratton, F, Gunson, HH, and Rawlinson, VI: The preparation and uses of antiglobulin reagents with special reference to complement fixing blood group antibodies. Transfusion 2:135, 1962.
17. Stratton, F, Smith, DS, and Rawlinson, VI: Value of gel fixation on Sephadex G-200 in the analysis of blood group antibodies. J Clin Pathol 21:708, 1968.
18. Howard, JE, et al: Clinical significance of the anti-complement component of antiglobulin antisera. Transfusion 22:269, 1982.
19. Lachman, PJ and Muller-Eberhard, HJ: The demonstration in human serum of "conglutinogen-activating-factor" and its effect on the third component of complement. J Immunol 100:691, 1968.
20. Muller-Eberhard, HJ: Chemistry and reaction mechanisms of complement. Adv Immunol 8:1, 1968.
21. Cooper, NR: Isolation and analysis of mechanisms of action of an inactivator of C4b in normal human serum. J Exp Med 141:890, 1975.
22. Brown, DL, Lachman, PJ, and Dacie, JV: The in vivo behaviour of complement-coated red cells: Studies in C6-deficient, C3-depleted and normal rabbits. Clin Exp Immunol 7:401, 1970.
23. Engelfriet, CPKW, et al: Autoimmune haemolytic anemias. 111 preparation and examination of specific antisera against complement components and products, and their use in serological studies. Clin Exp Immunol 6:721, 1970.
24. Garratty, G and Petz, LD: The significance of red cell bound complement components in development of standards and quality assurance for the anti-complement components of antiglobulin sera. Transfusion 16:297, 1976.
25. Stratton, F and Rawlinson, VI: C3 components on red cells under various conditions. In International Symposium on the Nature and Significance of Complement Activation, Ortho Research Institute of Medical Science, Raritan, NJ, 1976, p 113.
26. Low, B and Messeter, L: Antiglobulin test in low-ionic strength salt solution for rapid antibody screening and cross-matching. Vox Sang 26:53, 1974.
27. Moore, HC and Mollison, PL: Use of a low-ionic strength medium in manual tests for antibody detection. Transfusion 16:291, 1976.
28. Wicker, B and Wallas, CH: A comparison of a low ionic strength saline medium with routine methods for antibody detection. Transfusion 16:469, 1976.
29. Rock, G, et al: LISS—An effective to increase blood utilisation. Transfusion 18:228, 1978.
30. Lown, JAG, Barr, AL, and Davis, RE: Use of low ionic strength saline for crossmatching and antibody screening. J Clin Pathol 32:1019, 1979.
31. Petz, LD, et al: Compatibility testing. Transfusion 21:633, 1981.
32. Garratty, G: Problems in standardizing antiglobulin reagents in the USA. Biotest Bull 3:23, 1986.
33. Kohler, G and Milstein, C: Continuous cultures of fused cells secreting antibody of predefined specificity. Nature 256:495, 1975.
34. Lachman, PJ, et al: Use of monoclonal antibodies to character-

ize the fragments of C3 that are found on erythrocytes. Vox Sang 45:367, 1983.

35. Holt, PDJ, et al: NBTS/BRIC 8. A monoclonal anti-C3d antibody. Transfusion 25:267, 1985.

36. Voak, D, et al: Monoclonal antibodies—C3 serology. Biotest Bull 1:339, 1983.

37. Lachman, PJ, Pangburn, MK, and Oldroyd, RG: Breakdown of C3 after complement activation: Identification of a new fragment, C3g, using monoclonal antibodies. J Exp Med 156:205, 1982.

38. Case, J: Quality control of anti-human globulin. Biotest Bull 3:33, 1986.

39. Walker, RH (ed): Technical Manual, ed 10. American Association of Blood Banks, Arlington, VA, 1990.

40. Merry, AH, et al: Quantitation of IgG on erythrocytes: Correlation of numbers of IgG molecules per cell with the strength of the direct and indirect antiglobulin tests. Vox Sang 47:73, 1984.

41. Petz, LD and Garratty, G: Acquired immune hemolytic anemias. Churchill Livingstone, New York, 1980, p 307.

42. Merry, AH, et al: The quantification of C3 fragments on erythrocytes: Estimation of C3 fragments on normal cells, acquired haemolytic anaemia cases and correlation with agglutination of sensitized cells. Clin Lab Haematol 5:387, 1983.

43. Voak, D, et al: Improved antiglobulin tests to detect different antibodies: Detection of anti-Kell by LISS. Med Lab Sci 39:363, 1982.

44. Jorgensen, J, et al: The influence of ionic strength, albumin and incubation time on the sensitivity of indirect Coombs' test. Vox Sang 36:186, 1980.

45. Voak, D, et al: Low-ionic strength media for rapid antibody detection: Optimum conditions and quality control. Med Lab Sci 37:107, 1980.

46. Stroup, MA and MacIlroy, M: Evaluation of the albumin antiglobulin technic in antibody detection. Transfusion 5:184, 1965.

47. Mollison, PL: Blood Transfusion in Clinical Medicine, ed 7. Blackwell Scientific Press, Oxford, 1983, p 519.

48. Voak, D, et al: Quality control of antihuman globulin tests: Use of replicate tests to improve performance. Biotest Bull 3:41, 1986.

49. Bruce, M, et al: A serious source of error in antiglobulin testing. Transfusion 26:177, 1986.

50. Green, C, et al: Quality assurance of physiological saline used for blood grouping. Med Lab Sci 43:364, 1968.

51. Voak, D, et al: Antihuman globulin reagent specification. The European and ISBT/ICSH view. Biotest Bull 3:7, 1986.

52. Widman, FK (ed): Technical Manual of the American Association of Blood Banks, ed 9. American Association of Blood Banks, Arlington, VA, 1985, p 95.

53. Unger, LJ: A method for detecting Rh₀ antibodies in extremely low titre. J Lab Clin Med 37:825, 1951.

54. Lown, JA, Holland, PA, and Barr, AL: Inhibition of serological reactions with enzyme treated red cells by complement binding alloantibodies. Vox Sang 46:300, 1984.

55. Lalezari, P and Jiang, RF: The manual polybrene test: A simple and rapid procedure for detection of red cell antibodies. Transfusion 20:206, 1980.

56. Chown, B and Lewis, M: The slanted capillary method of rhesus blood grouping. J Clin Pathol 4:464, 1951.

57. Chown, B and Lewis, M: The Kell antigen in American Indians, with a note about anti-Kell sera. Am J Phys Anthropol 15:149, 1957.

58. Postoway, N and Garratty, G: Standardization of IgG subclass antiserums for use with sensitized red cells. Transfusion 23:398, 1983.

59. Crawford, MN, Gottman, FE, and Gottman, CA: Microplate system for routine use in blood bank laboratories. Transfusion 10:258, 1970.

60. Redman, M, Malde, R, and Knight, RC: Typing of red cells on microplates by low-ionic polybrene technique. Med Lab Sci 43:393, 1986.

61. Rosenfield, RE, Kochwa, S, and Kaczera, Z: Solid phase serology for the study of human erythrocytic antigen-antibody reactions. Proc 15th Congr Int Soc Blood Trans, Paris, 1976, p 27.

62. Moore, HH: Automated reading of red cell antibody identification tests by a solid phase antiglobulin technique. Transfusion 24:218, 1984.

63. Plapp, FV, et al: A solid phase antibody screen. Am J Clin Pathol 82:719, 1984.

64. Plapp, FV, et al: Solid phase red cell adherence tests in blood banking. In Smit Sibinga, C Th, Das, PC, and Greenwalt, TJ: Future Development in Blood Banking. Martinus Nijhoff, Boston, 1986, p 177.

Bibliography

Beck, ML and Marsh, WL: Letter to the editor: Complement and the antiglobulin test. Transfusion 17:529, 1977.

Black, D and Kay, J: Influence of tube type on the antiglobulin test. Med Lab Sci 43:169, 1986.

Freedman, J, Chaplin, H, and Mollison, PL: Further observations on the preparation of antiglobulin reagents reacting with C3d and C4d on red cells. Vox Sang 33:21, 1977.

Freedman, J and Mollison, PL: Preparation of red cells coated with C4 and C3 subcomponents and production of anti-C4d and anti-C3d. Vox Sang 31:241, 1976.

Federal Register 42:41920, 1977.

Federal Register 50:5579, 1985.

Garratty, G and Petz, LD: An evaluation of commercial antiglobulin sera with particular reference to their anticomplement properties. Transfusion 11:79, 1971.

Giles, C and Engelfriet, P: Working party on the standardization of antiglobulin reagents of the expert panel of serology. Vox Sang 38:178, 1980.

Graham, HA, et al: A new approach to prepare cells for the Coombs test. Transfusion 22:408, 1982.

Issitt, PD, Issitt, CH, and Wilkinson, SL: Evaluation of commercial antiglobulin sera over a two-year period. Part 1. Anti-beta 1A, anti-alpha 2D, and anti-beta 1E levels. Transfusion 14:93, 1974.

Judd, WJ, Steiner, EA, and Cochran, RK: Paraben-associated autoanti-Jkᵃ antibodies. Three examples detected using commercially prepared low-ionic strength saline containing parabens. Transfusion 22:31, 1982.

Petz, LD: Complement in immunohaematology and in neurologic disorders. In International Symposium on the Nature and Significance of Complement Activation. Ortho Research Institute of Medical Science, Raritan, NJ, 1976, p 87.

PROCEDURAL APPENDIX

Manual Antihuman Globulin Techniques

I. Direct antihuman globulin test

A. Procedure

1. Label two 10 or 12 × 75 mm glass test tubes. Test and control, respectively, and add 1 drop of a 3-percent v/v suspension of test cells to each.
2. Wash the cells a minimum of three times with saline and *ensure that all saline is completely decanted after the last wash.*
3. To the tube labeled "test," add 1 to 2 drops of antihuman globulin as recommended by the manufacturer, and mix.
4. To the control tube, add 1 to 2 drops of 3 percent w/v bovine albumin in saline, and mix.
5. Centrifuge both tubes at 500 RCF for 15 to 20 seconds.
6. Following centrifugation, completely resuspend the cell pellet by gently tipping and rolling the tube. Read and score agglutination macroscopically with the aid of a background light source and low-power magnification.
7. Incubate the tubes for another 5 minutes at room temperature, and repeat steps 5 and 6. Most manufacturers now recommend this additional step inasmuch as it has been shown that some negative or even weak reactions may increase in strength. These reactions have been attributed to the presence of C3d and, to a lesser extent, IgA on the cell surface. Conversely, the reaction with some cells may weaken after the extra incubation; this has been attributed to either detachment of IgG antibody or, alternatively, prozoning when excess anti-IgG has been added.

B. Controls

To all negative tubes, add 1 drop of control cells weakly sensitized with IgG, mix the cells, and repeat steps 5 and 6. A mixed-field weakly positive reaction should now be obtained, indicating the antihuman globulin had been added to the tube and that it was still reactive. All negative results could therefore be considered valid. If, after addition of the control cells, a negative result was obtained, it would indicate the antihuman globulin had not been added or that, if added, it was nonreactive. This could occur if:

1. The reagent had deteriorated on storage.
2. The reagent had been contaminated by serum and the antibody activity neutralized.
3. The cells had been insufficiently washed and residual serum or plasma had neutralized the antihuman globulin reagent when added to the tube.

Control cells weakly sensitized with complement should be used with monopecific anti-C3d reagent to validate negative results.

The control tube containing cells and 3-percent w/v bovine albumin should give a negative result. If positive, it indicates that the cells are autoagglutinable and that the test cannot be properly interpreted.

For reasons previously outlined, the cells used for direct antihuman globulin tests should be collected into either EDTA or citrates containing anticoagulant to minimize the possibility of the in vitro attachment of complement components.

II. Indirect antihuman globulin test

A. Procedure

1. Into a labeled glass 10 or 12 × 75 mm test tube, place 2 to 4 drops of test serum and 1 drop of a washed 3-percent v/v suspension if red cells.

2. Mix the cell suspension and incubate for 30 minutes in a 37°C water bath.
3. Centrifuge the tube at 500 RCF for 15 to 20 seconds.
4. Following centrifugation, completely resuspend the cell pellet by gently tapping and rolling the tube. Read and score agglutination macroscopically with the aid of a background light source and low-power magnification.
5. Wash the cells a minimum of three times with saline and *ensure that all saline is completely decanted following the final wash.*
6. Add 1 to 3 drops of antihuman globulin as recommended by the manufacturer and mix.
7. Repeat steps 3 and 4.

B. Controls

To all negative tubes, add 1 drop of control cells weakly sensitized with IgG, mix the cells, and repeat steps 3 and 4. Negative results can be considered valid if a weakly positive mixed-field reaction is obtained, following addition of the control cells. If this reaction is not obtained, the test should be repeated.

When phenotyping red cells using an antihuman globulin reactive typing serum, it is important to follow the antisera manufacturer's recommendations for the use of the reagent.

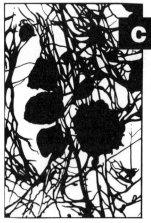

CHAPTER 5

The ABO Blood Group System

Denise M. Harmening, PhD, MT(ASCP), CLS(NCA)
Deborah Firestone, MA, MT(ASCP)SBB

OBJECTIVES

Upon completion of this chapter, the learner should be able to:

1 Describe the reciprocal relationship between ABO antigens and antibodies for
  blood types O, A, B, and AB.

2 Identify the frequencies of the four major blood types in the white, black,
  Mexican, and Asian populations.

3 Explain the effect of age on the production of ABO agglutinins.

4 Describe the immunoglobulin classes of ABO antibodies in group O, A, and B individuals.

5 Predict the ABO phenotypes and genotypes of offspring from various ABO matings.

6 Explain the formation of H, A, and B antigens on the red cells from precursor substance to immunodominant sugars.

7 Discuss the formation of H, A, and B antigens in secretory cells.

8 Explain the principle of the hemagglutination inhibition assay for the determination of secretor status.

9 Describe the qualitative and quantitative differences between the A_1 and A_2 phenotypes.

10 Describe the reactivity of *Ulex europaeus* with the various ABO groups.

11 Describe the characteristics of the weak subgroups of A (A_3, A_x, A_{end}, A_m, A_y, A_{el}).

12 Describe the characteristics of the Bombay phenotype.

13 Explain the effects of disease on the expression of ABH antigens and antibodies.

14 Interpret the results from an ABO typing and resolve any discrepancies if present.

Historic Perspective

Karl Landsteiner truly opened the doors of blood banking with his discovery of the first human blood group system, ABO. This marked the beginning of the concept of individual uniqueness defined by the red cell antigens present on the red cell membrane. The ABO system still remains the most important of all blood groups in transfusion practice. Transfusion of an incorrect ABO type can result in death of the patient.

In 1901, Landsteiner drew blood from himself and five associates, separated the cells and the serum, and then mixed each cell sample with each serum. He was inadvertently the first individual to perform forward and reverse groupings. Forward grouping is defined as using known sources of reagent antisera (antibodies) to detect antigens on an individual's red cells (Table 5–1). Reverse grouping is defined as using reagent cells with known ABO antigens and testing the serum of the patient for ABO group antibodies (Table 5–2).

Groups A, B, and O were the first blood groups described by Landsteiner. He found that serum from group B individuals agglutinated group A red blood cells and, therefore, that an antibody to A antigens was present in group B serum. Conversely, serum from

TABLE 5–1 ABO FORWARD GROUPING

Patient's Red Cells	Reaction with Anti-A	Reaction with Anti-B	Interpretation of Blood Group
1	Negative	Negative	O
2	+	Negative	A
3	Negative	+	B
4	+	+	AB

+ = visual agglutination.

TABLE 5–2 ABO REVERSE GROUPING

Patient's Serum	Reaction with Reagent A_1 Cells	Reaction with Reagent B Cells	Interpretation of Blood Group
1	+	+	O
2	Negative	+	A
3	+	Negative	B
4	Negative	Negative	AB

+ = visual agglutination.

group A individuals agglutinated group B red cells and, therefore, an antibody to B antigens was present in group A serum. Serum from group O individuals agglutinated both A and B cells, indicating the presence of antibodies to both A and B in group O serum (Table 5–2).

In 1902, Landsteiner's associates, Sturle and von Descatello, discovered the fourth ABO blood group, AB. As can be seen from Table 5–2, serum from group AB individuals does not agglutinate group A or group B cells, indicating the absence of antibodies to both A and B.

The frequency of these blood groups in the white population is as follows: group O, 45 percent; group A, 41 percent; group B, 10 percent; and group AB, 4 percent.[1] Therefore, O and A are the most common blood group types and blood group AB the rarest. However, frequencies of ABO groups differ in a few selected populations and ethnic groups (Table 5–3).[1-4] For example, group B is found twice as frequently in blacks and Asians as in whites; subgroup A_2 is rarely found in Asians.

Landsteiner concluded from the reactions he observed that in the ABO blood group system, individuals have naturally occurring antibodies in their serum directed against the missing ABO antigen on the sur-

TABLE 5–3 **ABO PHENOTYPE FREQUENCIES IN US POPULATIONS**

Phenotype	Whites (%)	Blacks (%)	Mexican (%)	Asian (%)
O	45	49	56	43
A₁	33	19	22	27
A₂	8	8	6	Rare
B	10	19	13	25
A₁B	3	3	4	5
A₂B	1	1	Rare	Rare

face of their red blood cell. This term "naturally occurring" is really a misnomer, inasmuch as substantial evidence suggests that anti-A and anti-B are stimulated by substances that are ubiquitous in nature. Bacteria have been shown to be chemically similar to human ABO antigens and may serve as a source of stimulation of antibody formation. Springer et al.[5] have demonstrated that Leghorn chickens kept in a germ-free environment from birth lacked ABO antibodies, compared with control chickens raised under normal conditions, who had ABO antibodies. Various seeds from pollinating plants are also chemically similar to human ABO antigens, so much so that they can be used as a source of antisera (e.g., the reagent anti-A₁ lectin; see ABO Subgroups, later in this chapter).

Whether the source of stimulation to ABO antigens the individual lacks is pollen particles, bacteria, or other natural substances, there is a general processing of that particular antigen. This results in a consistent immune response reflected in antibody production. These antibodies are always present in normal, healthy individuals. ABO antibodies are a result of a cross-reactivity and are initiated at birth upon exposure to foreign substances ubiquitous in nature. Titers are usually too low for detection until the individual is 3 to 6 months old. As a result, it is logical to perform only forward grouping on cord blood from newborn infants. The antibody production peaks when the individual is 5 to 10 years old and then declines progressively with advanced age. Patients older than age 65 usually have low titers, so that antibodies may be undetectable in the reverse grouping. The ABO blood group system is unique in that all normal, healthy individuals consistently have present in their serum antibodies to antigens they lack on their red cells. The other defined blood group systems do not have persistently present in their serum "naturally occurring"

antibodies to antigens they lack. Most other blood group systems require the introduction of foreign red cells by transfusion or pregnancy. Some blood groups, however, can occasionally have antibodies present that are not related to the introduction of foreign red cells. These antibodies are usually the IgM type and are not consistently present in everyone's serum. Performance of a reverse grouping is, therefore, unique to the ABO blood group system.

Testing of ABO is relatively easy; therefore, the regular occurrence of anti-A or anti-B, or both, in persons lacking the corresponding antigens serves as a confirmation of results in the forward grouping. Complete absence of anti-A and anti-B is very rare in healthy individuals (except in AB subjects), occurring at less than 0.01 percent in a random population.[6]

The consistently present ABO antibodies, however, create a treacherous situation as far as blood transfusion is concerned. If group B (or A) red cells are given to a patient whose serum contains anti-B (or anti-A), the donor's red cells will be destroyed almost immediately, being lysed at a rate of approximately 1 ml of red cells per minute. This produces a very severe, if not fatal, transfusion reaction in the patient. Therefore, both forward and reverse groupings must be performed on all patient samples, noting the correct reciprocal relationship of antigens and antibodies in a given blood group type (Table 5–4).

ABO Antibodies

ABO antibodies are usually IgM. Characteristically, IgM antibodies are cold-reacting antibodies that do not cross the placenta and can bind complement. (For a review of other characteristic properties of IgM antibodies, see Chapter 3.)

In a given serum sample from a group A and/or B individual, anti-B or anti-A or both may be IgM entirely, a mixture of IgM and IgG, a mixture of IgM and IgA, or a mixture of all three immunoglobulins.[7] However, the majority of anti-A from a group B individual and anti-B from a group A individual contains IgM antibody predominantly, with minor amounts of IgG or IgA present, if detectable at all. The "immune" form of anti-A or anti-B can be produced by individuals exposed to foreign red cell stimulation, either by transfusion or pregnancy.

Serum from group O individuals contains not only

TABLE 5–4 **SUMMARY OF FORWARD AND REVERSE GROUPINGS**

Patient	PATIENT CELLS TESTED WITH		Interpretation: Forward Group	PATIENT SERUM TESTED WITH		Interpretation: Reverse Group
	Anti-A	Anti-B		A₁ Cells	B Cells	
1	Negative	Negative	O	+	+	O
2	+	Negative	A	Negative	+	A
3	Negative	+	B	+	Negative	B
4	+	+	AB	Negative	Negative	AB

anti-A and anti-B but also anti-A,B. Anti-A,B antibody activity, originally thought to be just a mixture of anti-A and anti-B, cannot be separated into a pure specificity when absorbed with either A or B cells. Activity toward both A and B cells still remains with anti-A,B, even after repeated absorptions with A or B cells.[8,9] Anti-A,B, therefore, possesses serologic activity not found in mixtures of anti-A plus anti-B.

Anti-A,B from group O individuals has been reported to be a mixture of IgG and IgM or of IgG, IgM, and IgA. Anti-A,B will cross the placenta more frequently than anti-A or anti-B, confirming the presence of IgG. The "immune" form of anti-A,B can be produced by O individuals exposed to A or B red cells by either transfusion or pregnancy. These anti-A,B "immune" antibodies are predominantly IgG. IgG anti-A and anti-B antibodies develop far more commonly in group O individuals than in A or B individuals. Knowledge of the amount of IgG anti-A, anti-B, or anti-A,B in a woman's serum sometimes allows prediction or diagnosis of hemolytic disease of the newborn caused by ABO incompatibility (see Chapter 20).

There is a wide variation in the titers of ABO isoagglutinins in a random population. Generally, anti-A from a group O individual has a higher titer than that from a group B individual, and anti-A from a group B individual usually has a higher titer than anti-B from a group A individual. Anti-A,B from group O individuals is a higher titer of anti-A and anti-B than that found in group A and B individuals. This makes A,B antiserum a convenient reagent to use to detect weak ABO antigens; therefore, this serum from group O individuals is routinely used in the forward grouping.

Inheritance of the ABO Blood Groups

The theory for the inheritance of the ABO blood groups was first described by Bernstein in 1924. He demonstrated that each individual inherits one ABO gene from each parent and that these two genes determine which ABO antigens are present on the red cell membrane. One position, or locus, on each chromosome number nine is occupied by an A, a B, or an O gene. The O gene is considered an amorph (a silent allele), inasmuch as no detectable antigen is produced in response to the inheritance of this gene. The designations A or B refer to phenotypes, whereas *AA*, *BO*, and *OO* denote genotypes. In the case of an O individual, both phenotype and genotype are the same, because that individual would have to be homozygous for the O gene. Table 5–5 lists possible ABO phenotypes and genotypes from various matings. The inheritance of ABO antigens, therefore, follows simple mendelian genetics. ABO, like most other blood group systems, is codominant in expression. (For a review of genetics, refer to Chapter 2.)

FORMATION OF A, B, AND H ANTIGENS

The ABO genes do not actually code for the production of ABO antigens, but rather produce specific glycosyltransferases that add sugars to a basic precursor substance. Figure 5–1 illustrates the red blood cell precursor structure. A "donor" nucleotide derivative supplies the sugar that confers ABO specificity (Table 5–6). Also, ABO genes genetically interact with sev-

TABLE 5–5 ABO GROUPS OF THE OFFSPRING FROM THE VARIOUS POSSIBLE ABO MATINGS

Mating Phenotypes	Mating Genotypes	Offspring Possible Phenotypes (and Genotypes)
A × A	AA × AA	A (AA)
	AA × AO	A (AA or AO)
	AO × AO	A (AA or AO) or O (OO)
B × B	BB × BB	B (BB)
	BB × BO	B (BB or BO)
	BO × BO	B (BB or BO) or O (OO)
AB × AB	AB × AB	AB (AB) or A (AA) or B (BB)
O × O	OO × OO	O (OO)
A × B	AA × BB	AB (AB)
	AO × BB	AB (AB) or B (BO)
	AA × BO	AB (AB) or A (AO)
	AO × BO	AB (AB) or A (AO) or B (BO) or O (OO)
A × O	AA × OO	A (AO)
	AO × OO	A (AO) or O (OO)
A × AB	AA × AB	AB (AB) or A (AA)
	AO × AB	AB (AB) or A (AA or AO) or B (BO)
B × O	BB × OO	B (BO)
	BO × OO	B (BO) or O (OO)
B × AB	BB × AB	AB (AB) or B (BB)
	BO × AB	AB (AB) or B (BB or BO) or A (AO)
AB × O	AB × OO	A (AO) or B (BO)

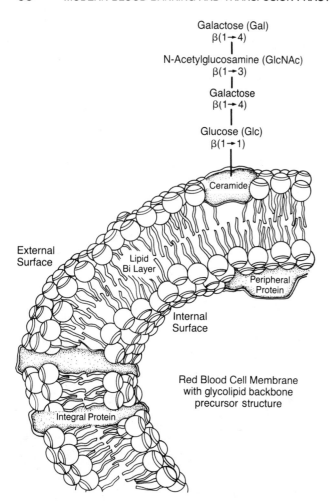

Galactose (Gal)
β(1→4)
|
N-Acetylglucosamine (GlcNAc)
β(1→3)
|
Galactose
β(1→4)
|
Glucose (Glc)
β(1→1)
|
Ceramide

External Surface

Lipid Bi Layer

Peripheral Protein

Internal Surface

Red Blood Cell Membrane with glycolipid backbone precursor structure

Integral Protein

FIGURE 5-1 Red blood cell precursor structure: lacto-N-neotetraosylceramide (a type-2 chain paragloboside). (Adapted from Harmening-Pittiglio[27].)

eral other separate, independent blood group systems, resulting in addition of sugar residues to a common precursor substance. The action of the H gene is intimately related to the formation of the ABO antigens. The inheritance of the H gene is independent of the inheritance of the ABO genes, but A, B, and H antigens are all formed from the same basic precursor material, which is itself a genetic product. The basic material has a glycoprotein or glycolipid backbone (depending on whether an ABH red cell antigen or soluble substance is being produced) to which sugars are attached in response to specific enzyme transferases elicited by an inherited gene. The ABH glycolipid antigens are built on a common carbohydrate residue, which represents a paragloboside (**see Color Plate 3**).

The precursor substance on erythrocytes is referred to as type 2. This means that the terminal galactose on the precursor substance is attached to the N-acetylglucosamine in a beta-1→4 linkage (**see Color Plate 4**). A type-1 precursor substance, which will be discussed later, refers to beta-1→3 linkage between galactose and N-acetylglucosamine.

TABLE 5-6 **DONOR NUCLEOTIDES AND IMMUNODOMINANT SUGARS RESPONSIBLE FOR H, A, AND B ANTIGEN SPECIFICITIES**

Gene	Glycosyltransferase	Nucleotide (Sugar Donor)	Immunodominant Sugar	Antigen
H	α-2-L-fucosyltransferase	GDP-Fuc	L-fucose	H
A	α-3-N-acetylgalactosaminyltransferase	UDP-GalNAc	N-acetyl-D-galactosamine	A
B	α-3-D-galactosyltransferase	UDP-Gal	D-galactose	B

Adapted from Harmening-Pittiglio,[27] p 3.
GDP-Fuc = guanosine-diphosphate L-fucose; UDP-GalNAc = uridine diphosphate-N-acetyl-D-galactose; UDP-Gal = uridine diphosphate galactose.

INTERACTION OF Hh AND ABO GENES

Inheritance of the H gene elicits an enzyme, L-fucosyltransferase, which transfers the sugar L-fucose from the guanosine-diphosphate-L-fucose (GDP-Fuc) donor nucleotide to the terminal galactose of the precursor chain. The H gene is very common in the random population, with greater than 99.99 percent inheriting the H gene. The allele of H, h, is quite rare, and the genotype, *hh*, is extremely rare. This *hh* genotype is called the Bombay phenotype and lacks normal expression of the ABO genes. Even though Bombay (*hh*) individuals may inherit ABO genes, normal expression reflected in the formation of A, B, or H antigens does not occur. (A discussion of the Bombay phenotype can be found later in this chapter.)

The H substance must be formed first by the inheritance of at least one H gene (genotype *HH* or *Hh*) in order for the other sugars to be attached in response to an inherited A gene or B gene or both. Therefore, the Bombay phenotype is devoid of all antigens of the ABO system. Remember, however, that for all practical purposes all individuals possess the H gene, in which H substance is formed first, and then other sugars attach to this, depending on the ABO genes inherited. The sugars that occupy the terminal positions of this precursor chain and confer blood group specificity are called the immunodominant sugars. Therefore, L-fucose is the sugar responsible for H specificity (**see Color Plate 5**).

The A gene codes for the production of *N*-acetylgalactosaminyltransferase, which transfers an *N*-acetylgalactosamine (GalNAc) sugar from the uridine-diphosphate-*N*-acetyl-D-galactose (UDPGalNAc) donor nucleotide to the H structure. This sugar is responsible for A specificity (**see Color Plate 6**). The A-specific immunodominant sugar is linked to a type 2 chain glycolipid precursor that now contains H substance through the action of the H gene. Only type 2 paragloboside chains are found in the erythrocyte membrane being synthesized by the red cell precursors.

The A gene tends to elicit higher concentrations of glycosyltransferase than the B gene. This leads to the conversion of practically all the H antigen on the red cell to A antigen sites. As many as 810,000 to 1,170,000 antigen sites exist on an A adult red cell in response to inherited genes.

The B gene codes for the production of D-galactosyltransferase, which transfers a D-galactose (Gal) sugar from the uridine-diphosphate-galactose (UDP-Gal) donor nucleotide to the H substance. This sugar is responsible for B specificity (**see Color Plate 7**). From 600,000 to 830,000 B antigen sites exist on a B adult red cell in response to the conversion of the H antigen by the glycosyltransferase elicited by the B gene.

When A and B genes are both inherited, the B enzyme (D-galactosyltransferase) seems to compete more efficiently for the H structure and the A enzyme (*N*-acetylgalactosaminyltransferase) is not as successful. Therefore, the average number of A antigens on an AB adult cell is approximately 600,000 sites, compared with an average of 720,000 B antigen sites.

The O gene is an amorph that does not elicit a transferase and, therefore, adds no additional sugar to the H structure. As a result, the O blood group has the highest concentration of H antigen. Interaction of the Hh and ABO genes is reviewed in Figure 5–2.

Studies at the molecular level using complementary DNA clones have revealed that the difference in the specificities of the A and B transferases may be caused by a difference in four amino acids between the A and B genes. In addition, O genes were identified as having a single base deletion near the N terminus when compared with A genes. This deletion of a single DNA base pair creates a premature stop codon resulting in an *O*-transferase, which is functionally inactive and incapable of modifying the H antigen. It is unlikely, therefore, that O individuals would express a protein that is immunologically related to that produced by either A or B transferases.[10]

All the ABH antigens develop as early as day 37 of fetal life but do not increase very much in strength during the gestational period. Typically, ABH reactivity of the newborn erythrocyte is not as strong as that of the adult cell. The red cells of the newborn infant have been estimated to carry between 25 and 50 percent of the number of antigenic sites found on the adult red cell. In addition to age, the phenotypic expression of ABH antigens may vary with race, genetic interaction, and disease states. The genetic interaction of the ABO blood group system with the Lewis, Ii, and P blood groups is reflected in the synthesis of all these antigens by the sequential addition of sugar residues to a common precursor substance previously described for ABO (Fig. 5–3).

FORMATION OF A-, B-, AND H-SOLUBLE ANTIGENS

In addition to red cells, ABH antigens can be found in epithelium tissues, organs such as bone marrow and kidneys, lymphocytes, and platelets. It has recently been reported that ABH antigens are not present on granulocytes.[11] In fact, ABH-soluble antigens can be synthesized and secreted by tissue cells. Therefore, ABH blood group specific substances can be found in all the body secretions, depending on the ABO genes inherited as well as on the inheritance of another set of genes (secretor genes) that regulates their formation.

INTERACTIONS OF THE Sese, Zz, AND ABH GENES

It is believed that two other genetic systems control the expression of ABH genes. More specifically, they control the H gene, which, in turn, influences the A and B genes. The systems are the Sese and the Zz. Both systems are inherited independently of the ABO and H genes. Approximately 78 percent of the random US population has inherited the Se gene possess-

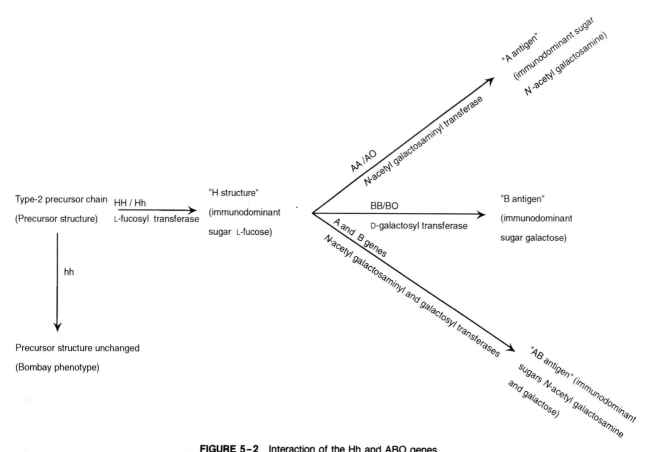

FIGURE 5-2   Interaction of the Hh and ABO genes.

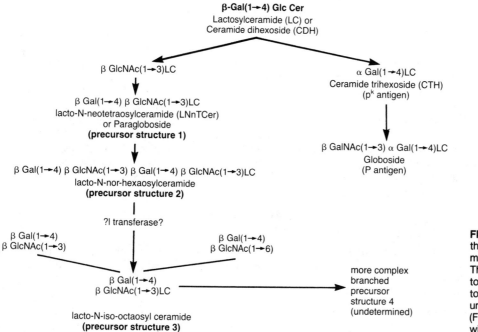

FIGURE 5-3 Possible biosynthetic pathway leading to the formation of precursor structures. The blood group I activity is likely to be associated with the galactose - *N* - acetylglucosamine-lined units of the precursor structure. (From Harmening-Pittiglio,[27] p 15, with permission.)

ing the genotype *SeSe* or *Sese*, given the name secretor. The Sese system regulates the formation of H antigen and, subsequently, of A and B antigens in secretory cells. The secreted A, B, and/or H antigens are glycoproteins, as opposed to glycolipids on red blood cell surfaces. People who inherit sese genes are termed nonsecretors. The exact mechanism of how the Se gene functions to regulate tissue secretory cells is not known. However, the H-specific transferase (L-fucosyltransferase) is found only in the secretions of secretors, indicating that the secretor gene controls the expression of the H gene in the secretory cells. The Se gene does not, however, affect the formation of A, B, or H antigens on the red cell and does not control the presence of A, B, or H transferases in hemopoietic tissue. In fact, A or B transferase enzymes, unlike A or B glycoprotein substances or antigens, are found in the secretions of A_1 or B individuals regardless of their secretor status. However, it is the presence of the H gene–specified L-fucosyltransferase (which depends on the inheritance of the Se gene) that determines whether ABH-soluble substances will be secreted, inasmuch as H substances must be synthesized before the formation of A or B substances (**see Color Plate 8**).

The Zz system regulates production of H antigen on erythrocytes. If a person inherited zz genes, a very rare occurrence, then no H antigen would be formed regardless of the presence of the H gene (Fig. 5–4). As with the Sese system, the exact mechanism involved in control of the Hh genes by the Zz system is unknown.

DISTINCTION OF A, B, AND H ANTIGENS AND A-, B-, AND H-SOLUBLE SUBSTANCES

The formation of soluble A, B, and H substances is the same as described for the formation of A, B, and H antigens on the red cells except for a few minor distinctions:

1. The secreted substances are glycoproteins; the red cell antigens are glycolipids.
2. The first sugar in the common carbohydrate residue of the precursor substance is *N*-acetylgalactosamine for the glycoprotein secretions, and glucose for the red cell antigens (**review Color Plates 3, 4, and 8**).
3. In the biosynthesis of the glycoprotein secretions, both type 1 and type 2 linkages occur in the precursor structures. In the case of the red cell ABH glycolipid antigens, only type 2 precursor chains are involved. Note that type 1 chain refers to a beta-1→3 linkage in which the number one carbon of the galactose is attached to the number three carbon of the *N*-acetylglucosamine sugar of the precursor substance, as opposed to a beta-1→4 linkage previously described for a type 2 chain.
4. Inasmuch as the H structure or substance is the precursor or acceptor substrate for sugars transferred by the A or B gene-specified enzymes, the Sese system regulates the H-gene activity in secretions but not in the red cell. The Zz system regulates the H-gene activity in the red cell.

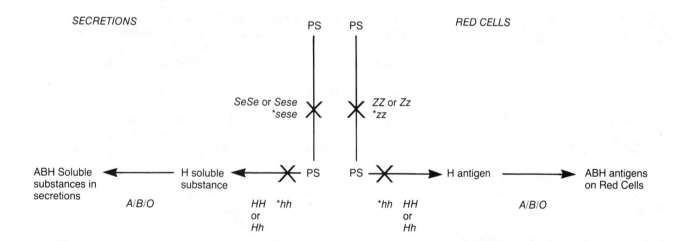

*inherited recessive genes block pathway at the indicated points (X) resulting in either no production of A, B, H soluble substances in secretions or no A, B, H red cell antigens.

FIGURE 5–4 Proposed pathway for genetic control of formation of A, B, and H antigens. (From Harmening-Pittiglio,[27] p 10, with permission.)

TABLE 5-7 **ABH SUBSTANCES IN THE SALIVA OF SECRETORS (SeSe OR Sese)***

ABO Group	SUBSTANCES IN SALIVA		
	A	B	H
O	None	None	↑↑
A	↑↑	None	↑
B	None	↑↑	↑
AB	↑↑	↑↑	↑

*Nonsecretors (sese) have no ABH substances in saliva.

↑↑ and ↑ respectively represent high and some concentration of ABH substances in saliva.

Tests for ABH secretion may establish the true ABO group of an individual whose red cell antigens are poorly developed. The demonstration of the A, B, and H substances in saliva is evidence for the inheritance of an A gene, a B gene, an H gene, and an Se gene. The term "secretor" refers only to secretion of A-, B-, or H-soluble antigens in body fluids. The glycoprotein-soluble substances (or antigens) normally found in the saliva of secretors are listed in Table 5-7. The procedure for determination of secretor status can be found in the Procedural Appendix at the end of this chapter. Table 5-8 summarizes the body fluids in which ABH-soluble substances can be found.

ABO Subgroups

A SUBGROUPS

Basic Concepts

In 1911 von Dungern described two different A antigens based on reactions with anti-A and anti-A_1 antisera. Serum from group B individuals contains a mixture of two antibodies, anti-A and anti-A_1, which can be separated by absorption techniques using appropriate red cells. Group A red cells that react with anti-A only and not with anti-A_1 are classified as A_2 subgroup. When anti-A is purposely absorbed from the serum of a group B individual using A_2 red cells, the serum left after the cells and attached anti-A are removed by centrifugation is referred to as absorbed serum (anti-A_1). Group A red cells that react with both anti-A and anti-A_1 are classified as A_1 (Table 5-9).

TABLE 5-8 **FLUIDS IN WHICH A, B, AND H SUBSTANCES CAN BE DETECTED IN SECRETORS**

Saliva	Milk
Tears	Amniotic fluid
Urine	Pathologic fluids: pleural, peritoneal,
Digestive juices	pericardial, ovarian cyst
Bile	

From Harmening-Pittiglio,[27] p 30, with permission.

TABLE 5-9 **A_1 VERSUS A_2 PHENOTYPES**

Blood Group	REACTIONS OF PATIENT'S RED CELLS WITH	
	Anti-A (from B Sera)	Anti-A_1 Lectin
A_1	+	+
A_2	+	Negative

Another source of anti-A_1, besides absorbed serum, is anti-A_1 lectin. Lectins are seed extracts that agglutinate human cells with some degree of specificity. The seeds of the plant *Dolichos biflorus* serve as the source of the anti-A_1 lectin. This reagent agglutinates A_1 or A_1B cells but does not agglutinate A_2 or A_2B cells.

Classification into A_1 and A_2 phenotypes accounts for 99 percent of all group A individuals. The cells of approximately 80 percent of the group A population are A_1, and the remaining 20 percent are A_2 or weaker subgroups. The difference between A_1 and A_2 is both quantitative and qualitative, and the production of both types of antigens is still a result of an inherited gene at the ABO locus (Table 5-10). Inheritance of an A_1 gene converts almost all of the H precursor structure to A_1 antigens on the red cells, because this gene elicits high concentrations of the enzyme N-acetylgalactosaminyltransferase. Remember, this enzyme transfers the immunodominant sugar N-acetylgalactosamine to the H antigen conferring A specificity to these red cells. A_1 is a very potent gene that creates from 810,000 to 1,170,000 A_1 antigen sites on the adult A_1 red cell. Inheritance of an A_2 gene results in the production of only 240,000 to 290,000 A_2 antigen sites on the adult A_2 red cell. These quantitative differences have been reflected not only in the number of antigen sites but also in the concentration of N-acetylgalactosaminyltransferase. Studies on the transferases from A_1 and A_2 individuals have demonstrated greater activity in the sera of A_1 individuals than in A_2 individuals by their ability to convert group O cells to A cells.[12,13] Qualitative differences also exist, inasmuch as 1 to 8 percent of A_2 individuals produce anti-A_1 in their serum and 22 to 35 percent of A_2B individuals produce anti-A_1. In fact, some investigators have dem-

TABLE 5-10 **ADDITIONAL ABO GENOTYPES, PHENOTYPES, AND FREQUENCIES**

Genotype	Phenotype	US FREQUENCIES	
		Whites	Blacks
A_1A_1 A_1A_2 A_1O	A_1	33%	19%
A_2A_2 A_2O	A_2	7%	5%
A_1B	A_1B	2%	2%
A_2B	A_2B	1%	2%

onstrated that anti-A$_1$ can be found in the sera of all A$_2$B individuals if sensitive techniques are used. Therefore, some subtle qualitative differences between A$_1$ and A$_2$ antigens must exist, even though the same immunodominant sugar is attached by the same transferase in each case. There must be some change in the antigenic structure, because the A$_2$ and A$_2$B individuals cannot recognize the A$_1$ antigen as being part of their own red cell makeup and are immunologically stimulated to produce a specific A$_1$ antibody that does not cross-react with A$_2$ red cells.

It is generally presented, however, that A$_1$ has two antigens, A and A$_1$, whereas A$_2$ has only one, A antigen (**see Color Plate 9**A). However, to simplify the concept, one can think of A$_1$ as having only A$_1$ antigen sites and A$_2$ as having only A antigen sites. Anti-A serum (from group B donors) contains two antibodies, anti-A plus anti-A$_1$; therefore, this antibody mixture will react with both A$_1$ and A$_2$ red cells. Pure anti-A$_1$ antibody will react only with A$_1$ antigen sites (**see Color Plate 9**B). Regardless of which conceptual presentation is used, the fact remains that group A red cells can be subdivided by the results of tests with anti-A (from B donor sera), anti-A,B (from O donor sera), and anti-A$_1$ (from absorbed serum or lectin). The characteristics of the A$_1$ and A$_2$ phenotypes are presented in Table 5–11.

Most group A infants appear to be A$_2$ at birth, inasmuch as ABO antigens are not fully developed on the red cells at this time. However, no difficulty is usually encountered in grouping cord red cells because most reagents contain potent anti-A and anti-A,B. Most cord A$_2$ cells will eventually group as A$_1$ individuals after a given amount of time for development (usually a few months).

Group AB red cells can also be similarly classified into subgroups. To include these subgroups in the genetic pathways of the biosynthesis of ABH antigens, we must again start with the basic precursor substance. In the diagram in Figure 5–5, one can see that the H gene appears to be necessary for the formation of the A, B, and H antigens. H antigen is found in greatest concentration on the red cells of group O individuals. Group A$_1$ individuals will not possess a great deal of H antigen. In the presence of the A$_1$ gene, almost all of the H antigen is converted to the A$_1$ antigen by placing that large N-acetylgalactosamine sugar on the H substance. Because so many A$_1$ antigens exist, the H antigen may be so hidden that A$_1$ and A$_1$B red cells may

not react with anti-H antisera. In the presence of an A$_2$ gene, only some of the H antigen is converted to A antigens and the remaining H antigen is expressed on the cell. Therefore, weak subgroups of the A antigen will often have large amounts of H antigen exposed and a lower number of A antigens formed. The H antigen in A$_1$ and A$_1$B red cells is so well hidden by the addition of that large immunodominant sugar that anti-H is occasionally found in their serum. This anti-H is a "naturally occurring" IgM cold agglutinin that reacts best below room temperature. As can be expected, this antibody is formed in response to a natural substance and reacts most strongly with cells of group O individuals. It is an insignificant antibody in terms of transfusion purposes, inasmuch as it has no reactivity at 37°C, body temperature. However, high-titered anti-H may react at room temperature and may be a problem in compatibility testing (see Chapter 12). It can be detectable during antibody screening procedures, inasmuch as the reagent cells used are all group O red cells (see Chapter 11). However, because 80 percent of the A and AB donors are A$_1$ and A$_1$B, these would probably be selected for the appropriate patient and would be compatible with anti-H in the patient's serum.

Anti-H lectin from the extract of *Ulex europaeus* closely parallels the reactions of human anti-H. Both agglutinate cells of group O and A$_2$ and react very weakly or not at all with A$_1$ and A$_1$B. Group B cells give reactions of variable strength (Fig. 5–6). Apparently the difference in the accessibility of the fucose sugar that determines H specificity contributes to the reactivity of anti-H among the various red cell ABO groups (for review, **refer to Color Plates 5 through 7**).

Advanced Concepts

The discussion thus far has presented a basic overview of the two major ABO subgroups, A$_1$ and A$_2$. A more plausible, yet more detailed theory of ABO subgroups has been proposed by the identification of four different forms of H antigens, two of which are unbranched chains and two of which are branched chains. H$_1$ and H$_2$ are unbranched straight chains, and H$_3$ and H$_4$ are more complex branched chains (**see Color Plate 10**). H$_1$ through H$_4$ correspond to the precursor structures upon which the A$_1$ enzyme can act to convert H antigen to blood group A active glycolipids. Although the chains differ in length and

TABLE 5–11 **CHARACTERISTICS OF A$_1$ AND A$_2$ PHENOTYPES**

| Pheno-types | TESTING OF RED CELLS | | | | | "NATURALLY OCCURRING" ANTIBODIES IN SERUM | | Substances Present in Saliva of Secretors | Presence of a Transferase in Serum | Number of Antigen Sites per Red Cell × 10^3 |
	Anti-A	Anti-B	Anti-A,B	Anti-H	Anti-A$_1$	Common	Unexpected			
A$_1$	++++	0	++++	0	++++	Anti-B	None	A, H	Pos (pH = 6)	810–1170
A$_2$	+++	0	+++	+++	0	Anti-B	Anti-A$_1$ (1–8% of cases)	A, H	Pos (pH = 7)	240–290

From Harmening-Pittiglio,[27] p 19, with permission.

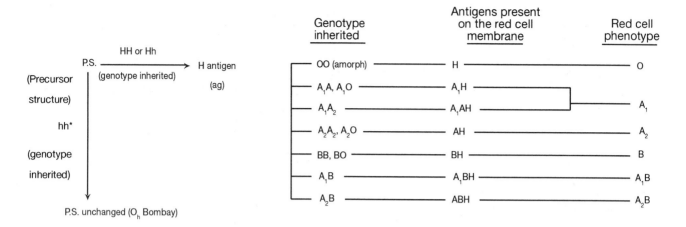

* Bombay individuals may inherit ABO genes (e.g., genotype OO, A_1O, A_1A_2, A_1B) but red blood cells are devoid of ABO antigen.

FIGURE 5–5 Summary of the genetic pathway for the biosynthesis of ABH antigens.

$$O > A_2 > B > A_2B > A_1 > A_1B$$

greatest	least
amount of	amount of
H	H

FIGURE 5–6 Reactivity of anti-H antisera or anti-H lectin with ABO blood groups.

TABLE 5–12 STRUCTURAL CHARACTERISTICS OF A_1 AND A_2 RED CELLS

A_2 red cells: A^a and A^b predominantly and unconverted H_3 and H_4 antigen sites

A_1 red cells: A^a, A^b, A^c, and A^d determinant and no unconverted H_3 and H_4 antigen sites

complexity of branching, the terminal sugars giving rise to their antigenic specificity are identical. Studies on the chemical and physical characteristics of the A_1 and A_2 enzyme transferases have demonstrated that these two enzymes are different qualitatively.[13,14] Straight chain H_1 and H_2 glycolipids can be converted to A^a and A^b antigens, respectively, by both A_1 and A_2 enzymes, with the A_2 enzyme being less efficient. The more complex branched H_3 and H_4 structures can be converted to A^c and A^d antigens by A_1 enzyme and only very poorly by A_2 enzyme. As a result, more unconverted H antigens (specifically H_3 and H_4) are available on group A_2 red cells, and only A^a and A^b A determinants are formed from H_1 and H_2 structures. In the red cells of some A_2 individuals, A^c is extremely low and A^d is completely lacking (Table 5–12). It is feasible to expect that these are the individuals in whom one would find an anti-A_1 in the serum. This anti-A_1 antibody could really be an antibody to A^c and A^d A determinants, which these A_2 individuals lack. Also, in 22 to 35 percent of A_2B individuals, anti-A_1 can be found in the serum. Inasmuch as the B enzyme transferase is usually more efficient than the A enzyme in converting H structures to the appropriate antigen,

A_2 enzymes would probably fail completely when paired with a B enzyme. As a result, A_2B individuals would be far more likely to lack A^c and A^d components, with subsequent production of anti-A^c and anti-A^d (anti-A_1).

Most group A infants appear to be A_2 at birth, with subsequent development of A_1 a few months later. Newborn infants, however, have been found to have a deficiency of the branched H_3 and H_4 antigens and, therefore, also the A^c and A^d antigens, possibly accounting for the A_2 phenotype. Adult cells contain a higher concentration of branched H_3 and H_4 structures and, therefore, A^c and A^d variants of the A antigen of A_1 individuals.

WEAK A SUBGROUPS

Basic Concepts

Inasmuch as 99 percent of the subgroups encountered in the laboratory are A_2, subgroups are mainly of academic interest. Group A phenotypes demonstrating weaker serologic reactivity than A_2 are designated

TABLE 5–13 **CHARACTERISTICS OF WEAK ABO PHENOTYPES**

Phenotypes	TESTING OF RED CELLS				"NATURALLY OCCURRING" ANTIBODIES IN SERUM		Substances Present in Saliva of Secretors	Presence of a Transferase in Serum	Number of Antigen Sites per Red Cell 10^3
	Anti-A	Anti-B	Anti-A,B	Anti-H	Common	Unexpected			
A_3	++mf	0	++mf	+++	Anti-B	Sometimes anti-A_1	A, H	Weak pos	30
A_x	wk/0	0	++	++++	Anti-B	Almost always anti-A_1	H	Very weak pos	4
A_{end}	wk mf	0	wk mf	++++	Anti-B	Sometimes anti-A_1	H	Neg	See text
A_m*	0	0	0	++++	Anti-B	No anti-A_1	A, H	Pos (two types)	0.2–1.9
A_y*	0	0	0	++++	Anti-B	No anti-A_1	A, H	Weak pos	—
A_{el}*	0	0	0	++++	Anti-B	Usually anti-A_1; sometimes anti-A also	H	Neg	0.1–1.4

From Harmening-Pittiglio,[27] p 19, with permission.
*A specificity demonstrated only by adsorption/elution procedures.
mf = mixed field agglutination; wk = weak; 0 = negative.

weak subgroups. Reactivity with anti-H may be used to classify the weaker subgroups of A along with the reactions using anti-A and anti-A,B. Also, the presence or absence of anti-A_1 in the serum as well as secretor studies and adsorption-elution tests can all be used to subdivide A individuals into A_3, A_x, A_{end}, and so on (Table 5–13).

Occasionally weak subgroups of A may present practical problems if, for example, an A_x donor is mistyped as group O. This is potentially dangerous because the group O patient possesses anti-A,B, which will agglutinate and lyse A_x red cells. Occasional problems also arise when A_2 or A_2B individuals demonstrate anti-A_1 in their serum. Because anti-A_1 is a "naturally occurring" IgM cold antibody, it is unlikely to cause a transfusion reaction, but it will be detected in the compatibility testing as well as in reverse grouping.

Advanced Concepts

Most of these weak A phenotypes may result from expression of an alternate weak allele present at the ABO locus. Some very rare subgroups may result from modifying genes that regulate expression of ABO genes. Weak subgroup A alleles, when paired with an O gene, exhibit a dominant mode of inheritance, except in subgroup A_y, which is inherited in a recessive manner.[15] The rare phenotype A_y apparently does not represent an alternate allele because it is inherited in a recessive fashion and can be observed only in siblings. This observation suggests inheritance of a double dose of a recessive regulatory gene segregating independently of the ABO locus, which modifies expression of the inherited A gene.[14] Glycosyltransferase studies of gene products of these alternate alleles at the A locus have demonstrated evidence of heterogeneous en-

zymes in A_3 and A_m subgroups and absence of transferase activity in the A_{end} and A_{el} subgroups.[16] It should be noted that there are still some reported A variants that do not fit into any of the weak subgroups described, alluding to existence of new alternate alleles or regulation by modifier genes.[14]

Weak A phenotypes can be serologically differentiated using the following techniques:

1. Forward agglutination with anti-A, anti-A,B, and anti-H
2. Serum grouping of ABO antibodies and the presence of anti-A_1
3. Adsorption-elution tests with anti-A
4. Saliva studies for presence of A and H substances

Additional special procedures such as serum glycosyltransferase studies for detection of A enzyme can be performed for differentiation of weak subgroups. Absence of a disease process should be confirmed before subgroup investigation, because ABH antigens are altered in various malignancies and other hematologic disorders (see ABH Antigens-Antibodies in Disease, later in this chapter).

Weak A subgroups can be distinguished as A_3, A_x, A_{end}, A_m, A_y, and A_{el} using the serologic techniques mentioned earlier (see Table 5–13). The characteristics of each weak A subgroup are now presented.

A_3 A_3 red cells characteristically demonstrate a mixed-field (mf) pattern of agglutination with anti-A and anti-A,B reagents.[17] The estimated number of A antigen sites is approximately 30,000 per red cell.[14] Weak N-acetylgalactosaminyltransferase activity is detectable in the serum. However, there appears to be a heterogeneity in the A_3 glycosyltransferases isolated from various A_3 phenotypes. Individuals tested were divided into three groups.[16] Group 1 consisted of A_3

phenotypes with low levels of detectable serum A enzyme, which had an optimal pH of approximately 7.0. Group 2 consisted of A_3 individuals with no detectable A enzyme. Group 3 consisted of an A_3 phenotype demonstrating a serum A enzyme level at 50 percent of the control level and an optimal pH activity of 6.0. Additionally, serum from this A_3 individual in group 3 was capable of converting O red cells into A red cells.[16] A_3 enzyme is a product of an allele at the ABO locus inherited in a dominant manner. Anti-A_1 may be present in serum of A_3 individuals, and A substance is detected in saliva of A_3 secretors.

A_x A_x red cells characteristically are not agglutinated by anti-A reagent but demonstrate weak agglutination with anti-A,B.[17] The estimated number of A antigen sites is approximately 4000 per red cell.[15] A very weak A enzyme has been detected in the serum of this subgroup, which represents the gene product of an alternate allele inherited in a dominant mode at the ABO locus.[16] In some rare exceptions, this mode of inheritance has been questioned. A_x individuals almost always produce anti-A_1 in their serum. Routine secretor studies detect the presence of only H substance in A_x secretors. However, A_x secretors contain A substance detectable only by agglutination-inhibition studies using A_x red cells as indicators.[15] Caution should be used in interpreting results of secretor studies using A_x indicator cells and anti-A, inasmuch as not all A_x cells are agglutinated by anti-A.

A_{end} A_{end} red cells characteristically demonstrate weak mf agglutination with anti-A and anti-A,B, but only a very small percentage (no greater than 10 percent) of the red cells agglutinate.[17] The estimated number of A antigen sites on the few agglutinable red cells is approximately 200,000, whereas no detectable A antigens are demonstrated on red cells that do not agglutinate.[15] No A glycosyltransferase is detectable in the serum of A_{end} individuals.[16] The A_{end} phenotype is the expression of an A allele inherited in a dominant mode at the ABO locus. Secretor studies detect the presence of only H substance in saliva of A_{end} secretors. Some investigators consider the phenotypes of A_{finn} and A_{bantu} as variants of the A_{end} subgroup.[15]

A_m A_m red cells are characteristically unagglutinated by anti-A or anti-A,B. A strongly positive adsorption-elution of anti-A confirms the presence of A antigenic sites. The estimated number of A antigen sites varies from 200 to 1900 per red cell in A_m individuals.[15] An A enzyme of either the A_1 or the A_2 type previously described is detectable in the serum of A_m subgroups.[18] This A_m enzyme is a product of an alternate allele at the ABO locus that is inherited in a dominant manner and results in the A_m phenotype. These individuals usually do not produce anti-A_1 in their sera. A substance in normal quantities is easily detected in saliva of A_m secretors.

A_y A_y red cells are unagglutinated by anti-A or anti-A,B. Adsorption-elution of anti-A is the method used to confirm the presence of A antigens. Activity of eluates from A_y red cells is characteristically weaker than that of eluates from A_m red cells. Weak A glycosyltransferase is detectable in the serum of A_y individuals, and saliva secretor studies demonstrate H and A substance, with A substance below normal quantities.[16] A_y individuals usually do not produce anti-A_1. The A_y phenotype can be observed in siblings, implicating a recessive mode of inheritance. This phenotype does not represent expression of an alternate allele at the ABO locus but suggests the action of a separate independent genetic system, designated Yy, regulating expression of the A gene. It is hypothesized that inheritance of a double dose of the recessive regulatory gene (yy) results in suppression of the A gene, leading to formation of the A_y phenotype.[15]

A_{el} A_{el} red cells typically are unagglutinated by anti-A or anti-A,B. Often, adsorption and elution of anti-A is positive when monospecific anti-IgG antisera is used in indirect antiglobulin testing. No detectable A enzyme activity can be demonstrated in the serum of A_{el} individuals by glycosyltransferase studies.[16] The A_{el} phenotype is an expression of an alternate A allele at the ABO locus inherited in a dominant manner when paired with an O gene. A_{el} individuals usually produce an anti-A_1 that is reactive with A_1 cells and sometimes produce an anti-A that agglutinates A_2 red cells.[15] Secretor studies demonstrate the presence of only H substance in the saliva of A_{el} secretors.

A general flow chart for the process of elimination and identification of various subgroups is presented in Figure 5–7, with the assumption that the patient's medical history (e.g., recent transfusion, disease states) has been investigated and excluded as a source of discrepancy.

FORMATION OF B ANTIGEN

Advanced Concepts

The B gene codes for a D-galactosyltransferase, which transfers a galactose sugar to the H antigen previously formed. Isoelectric focusing of group B serum has demonstrated two B enzyme activities, one with an isoelectric point (pI) equal to 4.8 to 5.2 and the other with a pI of 8.2 to 8.8.[19] Activity of both enzymes in serum is optimum at pH 6.5 and requires the presence of the metallic cofactor Mn^{++}. Both B glycosyltransferases are specific for the same nucleotide sugar donor (UDP-Gal) and transfer the same immunodominant sugar, D-galactose, to confer B specificity. As a result of the four types of H substrate available to B glycosyltransferases, four types of B antigenic structures are possible, as previously described for the A blood groups. These B antigens are designated B_I, B_{II}, B_{III}, and B_{IV}, with the addition of D-galactose to the respective H glycolipid variant.[20] Only B_I and B_{II} glycolipid variants have been isolated and characterized. B_{III} and B_{IV} structures remain to be isolated and characterized from red blood cells but are

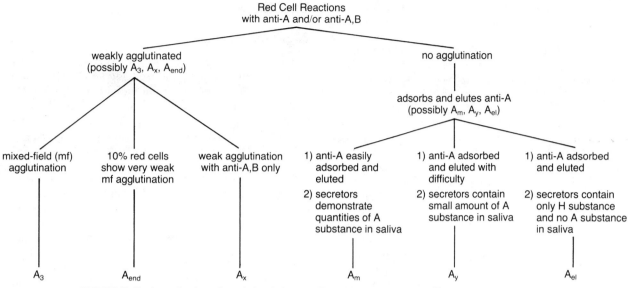

FIGURE 5-7   Investigation of weak A subgroups. (From Harmening-Pittiglio,[27] p 22, with permission.)

considered to be branched structures inasmuch as they are built upon H_3 and H_4 glycolipids.[20]

B SUBGROUPS

Basic Concepts

Subgroups of B are very rare and occur less frequently than do subgroups of A. Red cells demonstrating serologic activity weaker than normal are designated weak B phenotypes or B subgroups and include B_3, B_x, B_m, and B_{el} phenotypes[15] (Table 5-14). There are no B subgroups reported that are equivalent to A_{end} or A_y. A classification similar to A subgroups has been used because of common serologic characteristics. Subgroups of B are usually recognized by variations in the strength of the reaction using anti-B and anti-A,B. In addition, an anti-B lectin, *Bandeiraea simplicifolia* (modified BS-1 lectin), has been prepared for differentiating group B variants. The most important finding of this new lectin, however, is its ability to differentiate true B antigens from "acquired B–like" antigens on red blood cells. Modified BS-1 lectin does not agglutinate acquired B antigens, only true B antigens (see ABH Antigens-Antibodies in Disease, later in this chapter). This lectin is not widely available yet (as is the anti-A_1 lectin) and, therefore, is not routinely used in the laboratory.

Advanced Concepts

Inheritance of B subgroups, similar to that of most A subgroups, is considered to be due to alternate alleles at the B locus. Criteria used for differentiation of weak B phenotypes include (1) type of agglutination with anti-B, anti-A,B, and anti-H, (2) presence or absence of antibodies in the serum, (3) adsorption-elution studies with anti-B, and (4) presence of B substance in saliva. These serologic techniques can be used to characterize B subgroups in the following manner.

TABLE 5-14   **CHARACTERISTICS OF B PHENOTYPES**

Phenotypes	TESTING OF RED CELLS				"NATURALLY OCCURRING" ANTIBODIES IN SERUM		Substances Present in Saliva of Secretors	Presence of B Transferase in Serum
	Anti-A	Anti-B	Anti-A,B	Anti-H	Common	Unexpected		
B	0	++++	++++	++	Anti-A	None	B, H	Pos (normal amount)
B_3	0	mf ++	++ mf	+++	Anti-A	None	B, H	Wk pos
B_x	0	wk/0	+	+++	Anti-A	Weak anti-B	H	Neg
B_m*	0	0	0	+++	Anti-A	None	B, H	Wk pos
B_{el}*	0	0	0	+++	Anti-A	Sometimes a weak anti-B	H	Neg

From Harmening-Pittiglio,[25] p 26, with permission.
*B specificity demonstrated only by adsorption/elution procedures.
mf = mixed field; wk = weak; 0 = negative.

B$_3$ An mf pattern and rapid agglutination is the typical reaction of the B$_3$ phenotype with anti-B reagent.[17] B glycosyltransferase is present in the serum of these individuals, but enzyme activity varies from 10 to 100 percent of control levels.[15] This variability suggests heterogeneity of B enzyme in B$_3$ individuals, which is characteristic also for the subgroup A$_3$. Anti-B is absent in the serum of B$_3$ phenotypes, but B substance is present in normal amounts in the saliva of secretors. The B$_3$ subgroup is the most frequently occurring weak B phenotype.[15]

B$_x$ B$_x$ red cells typically demonstrate weak agglutination with anti-B antisera without mf agglutination, although some examples of red cells may not agglutinate at all.[14] Similar to the A$_x$ phenotype, B$_x$ erythrocytes agglutinate stronger with anti-A,B than with anti-B.[17] B glycosyltransferase has not been detected in the serum of B$_x$ phenotypes, but a weakly reactive anti-B usually is produced.[15] B$_x$ red cells readily adsorb and elute anti-B. Secretor studies demonstrate large amounts of H substance, but B substance is undetectable using group B indicator red cells. When B$_x$ indicator red cells are used, a weak B substance can be detected in secretor studies.[15]

B$_m$ B$_m$ red cells characteristically are unagglutinated by anti-B or anti-A,B. The B$_m$ red cells easily adsorb and elute anti-B. B glycosyltransferase is present in the serum of B$_m$ phenotypes but is usually lower in activity and varies from individual to individual.[21]

Reduced activity of B enzyme in hemopoietic tissue is clearly the defect causing the formation of the B$_m$ subgroup, inasmuch as normal B plasma incubated with B$_m$ red cells and UDP-Gal transforms them into a normal group B phenotype. Anti-B is not characteristically present in the serum of B$_m$ individuals. Normal quantities of H and B substance are found in the saliva of B$_m$ secretors.

The B$_m$ phenotype is usually the result of inheritance of a rare allele at the ABO locus, although the subgroup B$_m$ may be the product of an interacting modifying gene linked closely to the ABO locus.[21] This modifier gene may depress expression of the B gene, resulting in decreased B enzyme activity.[21] The B$_m$ subgroup is reported to occur more frequently in Japan.[15]

B$_{el}$ B$_{el}$ red cells are unagglutinated by anti-B or anti-A,B. This extremely rare phenotype must be determined by adsorption and elution of anti-B. No B glycosyltransferase has been identified in the serum of B individuals. A weak anti-B may be present in the serum of this subgroup. Only H substance is demonstrated in saliva of B$_{el}$ secretors.

Other weak B phenotypes have been reported that do not possess the appropriate characteristics for classification into one of the groups previously discussed.[22] These may represent new classifications and new representations of ABO polymorphism.

The Bombay Phenotypes (O$_h$)

BASIC CONCEPTS

The H gene appears to be necessary for the formation of A and B antigens (see Fig. 5–5). It is very common; 99.99 percent of all individuals have an *HH* or *Hh* genotype. The allele h is very rare and does not produce the L-fucose transferase necessary for formation of the H structure. The genotype *hh* or *H$_{null}$* is extremely rare and is known as the Bombay phenotype, or O$_h$.

Bombay cells cannot be converted to group A or B by the specific transferases. This supports the concept that the H structure serves as the acceptor molecule or precursor substance for the product of the A or B gene-specified transferases. Bombay individuals lack all normal expression of the A, B, or O genes they inherited (see Fig. 5–5). The Bombay phenotype was first reported by Bhende in 1952 in Bombay, India. More than 130 Bombay phenotypes have now been reported in various parts of the world. These red cells are devoid of normal ABH antigens. The Bombay red cells fail to react with anti-A, anti-B, and anti-H. Bombay serum contains anti-A, anti-B, anti-A,B, and anti-H. Unlike the anti-H found occasionally in the serum of A$_1$ and A$_1$B individuals, the Bombay anti-H is active over a wide thermal range. It is an IgM antibody that can bind complement and cause red cell lysis. Because the H antigen is common to all ABO blood groups, Bombay blood is incompatible with all ABO donors. In routine forward grouping, using anti-A, anti-B and anti-A,B, the Bombay would phenotype as an O blood group. However, transfusing normal group O (with the highest concentration of H antigen) would cause immediate cell lysis by the potent anti-H of the Bombay individual. Therefore, only blood from another Bombay individual can be transfused to a Bombay recipient. Table 5–15 lists the general characteristics of Bombay phenotypes.

TABLE 5–15 GENERAL CHARACTERISTICS OF BOMBAY O$_H$ (H$_{null}$) PHENOTYPES

1. Absence of H, A, and B antigens; no agglutination with anti-A, anti-B, anti-A,B, or anti-H
2. Presence of anti-A, anti-B, anti-A,B, and a potent wide thermal range anti-H in the serum
3. A, B, H nonsecretor (no A, B, or H substances present in saliva)
4. Absence of α-2-L-fucosyltransferase (H enzyme) in serum and red cells
5. Presence of A or B enzymes in serum and red cells
6. Strong reactivity with anti-I reagents (possibly owing to an increase in number of I receptors)
7. A recessive mode of inheritance (identical phenotypes in children but not in parents)

From Harmening-Pittiglio,[27] p 45, with permission.

Inheritance of the genotype *hh* usually occurs in the children of consanguineous marriages. When family studies demonstrate which ABO genes are inherited in the Bombay phenotype, then the genes are written as superscripts (O_h^A, O_h^B, O_h^{AB}).

The serum of Bombay individuals who are genetically A or B contains the specific A or B transferases, demonstrated by the ability of the Bombay serum to convert group O cells to A or B. O_h (hh) individuals are all nonsecretors of ABH substances, because both the H gene and the Se gene must be inherited for the ABH antigens to be found in secretions.

ADVANCED CONCEPTS

The Bombay phenotype has now been divided into four different categories that depend on the inheritance of the alleles of H (hh) or modifying genes (zz) that are responsible for the variable expression of H and, in turn, A and B antigens.

Category 1: Classic Bombay

As discussed earlier, this group arises from the inheritance of the *hh* genotypes. These cells lack all H antigen and react stronger with examples of anti-I. This phenomenon gives credence to the theory that I antigen is a precursor to H antigen and A and B antigens. If a person inherited the normal A or B gene, or both, the respective enzymes could be detected, and the person would be designated O_h^A, O_h^B, O_h^{AB}.

Category 2: Deficient Bombay Nonsecretors

Red cells of these persons have a slight amount of ABH antigens that are primarily detected by adsorption and elution studies. If a person is genetically A or B, the respective enzymes can be detected, but no H enzyme is detectable even though it has been shown that there is some slight H antigen production.[23] It is postulated that rather than hh being inherited, alternate genes are present at the H loci that give rise to a small amount of H antigen. The persons are designated A_h, B_h, or AB_h.[24] These designations are also referred to as para-Bombay.

Category 3: H-Deficient Bombay Secretors: Recessive Inheritance

These Bombay secretors arise out of the inheritance of a double dose of the recessive gene z. As discussed earlier, the Z gene is a regulator gene that is needed in conjunction with an H gene to produce normal ABO antigen on red blood cells. In zz persons, ABO determinants cannot be expressed, but what is unique is that normal ABH substances are present in secretions, provided that the person has at least one Se gene (remember that there is a normal H gene present).

The description for these persons is H_z, H_z^A, H_z^B, or H_z^{AB}.[24]

Category 4: H-Deficient Bombay Secretors: Dominant Inheritance

This is the most recently discovered Bombay category.[24] These persons inherit H-deficient red cells via a dominant gene; however, they contain normal ABH substances if they are secretors. Weak expressions of A, B, and H antigens can be detected along with their corresponding enzymes. The theory contends that an alternate gene is present at the Zz loci, resulting in the particular Bombay type. However, only one family has been identified with this characteristic.

Table 5–16 summarizes the various Bombay classifications.

ABH Antigens-Antibodies in Disease

Associations among ABH antigens and practically any known disorder can be found throughout medical literature. Even more profound are the associations of blood group specificity and such things as a more pronounced "hangover" in A blood group individuals, criminality in group B, and good teeth in group O. There are also several papers correlating blood groups with personality traits. It is no surprise that many scientists refer to these associations as a part of blood group mythology. However, more relevant associations between blood groups and disease are important to the blood banker in terms of blood group serology.

Various disease states seem to alter red cell antigens and result in progressively weaker reactions or additional acquired "pseudoantigens" during forward grouping. Leukemia, for example, has been shown to depress antigen strength. Often the cells will appear to be an mf agglutination (tiny agglutinates in a sea of unagglutinated cells). These weakened A or B antigens may demonstrate the type of serologic reactions shown in Table 5–17.

The weakening of the antigen tends to follow the course of the disease. The antigen strength will increase again as the patient enters into remission. The isoagglutinins (anti-A, anti-B, or anti-A,B) also may be weak or absent in those leukemias demonstrating hypogammaglobulinemia, such as chronic lymphocytic leukemia (CLL). Various lymphomas, such as the malignant (non-Hodgkin's) variety, may yield weak isoagglutinins owing to moderate decreases in the gamma globulin fraction. Also, immunodeficiency diseases, such as congenital agammaglobulinemia, will also yield weak or absent isoagglutinins. If this problem is suspected, a simple serum protein electrophoresis will confirm or deny this condition. Hodgkin's disease also has been reported to weaken or to depress

TABLE 5–16 CHARACTERISTICS REPORTED OR POSTULATED FOR THE CATEGORIES OF H-DEFICIENT PHENOTYPES (BOMBAYS)

Classification	Proposed Genes Inherited	¶Glycosyltransferases	Red Cell Antigens: A, B, and H Detected and Lewis Phenotype	A, B, and H Soluble Substances in Secretions	Antibodies In Serum	Mode of Inheritance
1. Classical Bombay O_h, O_h^B, O_h^A, O_h^{AB}	Z hh sese	None or A and/or B† in serum or red cell stoma	None detectable Le(a + b −)‡ or Le(a − b −)	None detectable	Anti-A, anti-B, anti-H	Recessive
2. Para-Bombay A_h, B_h, AB_h	A hh* sese	A and/or B† in serum and red cell stoma	Weak A/B† Residual H when A or B immunodominant sugar is removed with appropriate enzymes Le(a + b −)† or Le(a − b −)	None detectable	Anti-A/anti-B† Weak anti-IH or anti-H	Recessive
3. H_z Bombay (formerly O_m^h or O_{Hm}) Group 1: H_z, H_z^A, H_z^B, H_z^{AB} Group 2: AH_z, BH_z, ABH_z	zz HSe zz HSe	A and/or B† in serum/red cells	None Le(a − b −) Weak A or B† Le(a − b −)	H substance (normal amounts) H substance A/B† (all normal amounts)	Weak IH or anti-H‡ Weak anti-IH	Recessive Recessive
4. H_m Bombay§ H_m, A_{Hm}, B_{Hm}, AB_{Hm}	zz HSe	H in serum and red cell stroma (normal activity); A and/or B† in serum and red cell stroma (normal activity)	Weak A/B† and H Le(a − b −)	H substance A/B† (all normal amounts)	Anti-A/anti-B† Anti-A/anti-B†	Dominant

From Harmening-Pitiglio,[27] p 49, with permission.

* = Weak variant present at the Hh locus.
† = Dependent on ABO genotype.
‡ = Majority of cases.
§ = One family reported.
¶ = Refer to Figure 5–3.

TABLE 5-17 **SEROLOGIC REACTIONS TYPICAL OF LEUKEMIA**

Patient Phenotype	FORWARD GROUPING REACTION OF PATIENT CELLS WITH			REVERSE GROUPING REACTION OF PATIENT SERUM WITH	
	Anti-A	Anti-B	Anti-A,B	A₁ Cells	B Cells
A	+ mf	Neg	++ mf	Neg	+++
B	Neg	±/+	+	++++	Neg
Patient Diagnosis: Leukemia					

mf = mixed field.

ABH red cell antigens, resulting in variable reactions during forward grouping similar to those found during leukemia.

The very young and the elderly populations also have weak expression of the ABO isoagglutinins. In the elderly patient, immunoglobulin production is depressed. In infants, ABO isoagglutinin production is undetectable until 3 to 6 months of age. Also, A antigen production is not fully complete at birth, and newborn cells will appear as the subgroup A_2. Discrepancies in the reverse grouping are thus observed even in the absence of disease.

Individuals with intestinal obstruction, carcinoma of the colon or rectum, or other disorders of the lower intestinal tract will have increased permeability of the intestinal wall, which allows passage of the bacterial polysaccharides from *Escherichia coli* serotype O86 into the patient's circulation. This results in the "acquired B" phenomenon in group A individuals. The patient's group A red cells absorb the B-like polysaccharide, which reacts with anti-B. This reaction is always weaker than the reaction of the true A antigen with anti-A. The acquired B phenomenon has also been associated with septicemic infections from *Proteus vulgaris*. An acquired A phenomenon has been associated with asepticemic infections from *P. mirabilis*.

A lack of detectable ABO antigens can occur in patients with carcinoma of the stomach or pancreas. The patient's red cell antigens have not been changed, but the serum contains excessive amounts of blood group–specific soluble substances (BGSS) that neutralize the antisera used in the forward grouping. The individual's red cells can be grouped correctly when they are washed three times with saline to remove any residual patient serum.

All these disease states previously mentioned result in discrepancies between the forward and reverse groupings, indicating that the patient's red cell group is not what it seems. All ABO discrepancies must be resolved before blood is released for that patient. In some cases saliva studies may help confirm the patient's true ABO group.

ABO Discrepancies

ABO discrepancies are usually technical in nature and can be simply resolved by correctly repeating the

TABLE 5-18 **COMMON SOURCES OF TECHNICAL ERRORS RESULTING IN ABO DISCREPANCIES**

1. Inadequate identification of blood specimens, test tubes, or slides
2. Cell suspension either too heavy or too light
3. Clerical errors
4. A mix-up in samples
5. Missed observation of hemolysis
6. Failure to add reagents
7. Failure to follow manufacturer's instructions
8. Uncalibrated centrifuge
9. Contaminated reagents
10. Warming during centrifugation

testing and carefully checking reagents with meticulous reading and recording of results. Some of the more common causes of technical errors leading to ABO discrepancies in the forward and reverse groupings are listed in Table 5–18. Occasionally, however, the discrepancy may be due to a real problem with the patient's ABO group. Before trying to resolve the discrepancy, it helps to acquire essential information regarding the patient's age, diagnosis, transfusion history, medications, immunoglobulin levels (if determined), and history of pregnancy.

ABO discrepancies may be arbitrarily divided into four major categories, which will be considered separately.

GROUP I DISCREPANCIES

These discrepancies are between forward and reverse groupings owing to weak-reacting or missing antibodies. Discrepancies in group I are more common than those in the other groups listed. When a reaction in the reverse grouping is weak or missing, weak or missing antibodies should be suspected because, normally, forward and reverse grouping reactions are very strong (4+). The reason for the missing or weak isoagglutinins is that the patient has depressed antibody production or cannot produce the ABO antibodies. Some of the more common populations with discrepancies in this group are:

1. Newborn infants
2. Elderly patients
3. Patients with leukemias demonstrating hypogammaglobulinemia (e.g., CLL)

4. Patients with lymphomas demonstrating hypogammaglobulinemia (e.g., malignant lymphomas)
5. Patients using immunosuppressive drugs that yield hypogammaglobulinemia
6. Patients with congenital agammaglobulinemia
7. Patients with immunodeficiency diseases
8. Patients with bone marrow transplantations (patients develop hypogammaglobulinemia from therapy and start producing another different red cell population from the transplanted bone marrow)

The best way to resolve this discrepancy is by enhancing this reaction in the reverse group. This, of course, is done after technical errors, as outlined in Table 5–18, have been accounted for. To enhance the reverse group reaction, incubate the patient serum with the reagent cells at room temperature for approximately 15 minutes. If there is still no reaction, incubate the serum-cell mixtures at 4°C for 15 to 30 minutes. (Some blood banks have a 16°C incubator; this can be tried before 4°C.) An autocontrol and an O cell control must always be tested concurrently with the reverse typing when trying to solve the discrepancy because the lower temperature (4°C) of testing will enhance the reactivity of other naturally occurring cold autoagglutinins present in everyone's serum. Table 5–19 shows a type of discrepancy that may be seen with weak or missing antibodies.

One of the rare causes of a weak or missing ABO isoagglutinin is chimerism. Figure 5–8 illustrates an example of chimera twins. Chimerism is defined as the presence of two cell populations in a single individual. Detecting a separate cell population may be easy or difficult, depending on what percentage of cells of the minor population is present. Reactions from chimerism will typically be mf agglutination. More commonly, artificial chimeras occur, yielding mixed cell populations that are due to (1) blood transfusions (e.g., group O cells given to a group A or B patient); (2) transplanted bone marrows; (3) exchange transfusions; and (4) fetal-maternal bleeding. True chimerism is rarely found and occurs in twins in which two cell populations will exist through the life of the individual. In utero exchange of blood occurs because of vascular anastomosis. As a result, two cell populations emerge that are both recognized as self, and the individuals do not produce anti-A or anti-B. Therefore, no detectable isoagglutinins are present in the reverse grouping. If the patient or donor has no history of a twin, then the chimera may be due to dispermy (two sperm fertilizing one egg) and indicates mosaicism.

GROUP II DISCREPANCIES

These discrepancies are between forward and reverse groupings owing to weak-reacting or missing antigens. This group is probably the least frequently encountered. Some of the causes of discrepancies in this group include the following:

1. Subgroups of A or subgroups of B, or both, may be present (see ABO Subgroups).
2. Leukemias may yield weakened A or B antigens (see Table 5–17).
3. Hodgkin's disease has been reported sometimes to mimic the depression of antigens found in leukemia.
4. Excess amounts of BGSS present in the plasma in association with certain diseases, such as carcinoma of the stomach and pancreas, will neutralize the reagent anti-A or anti-B, leaving no unbound antibody to react with the patient cells. This yields a false-negative or weak reaction in the forward grouping. Washing the patient cells free of the BGSS with saline should alleviate the problem, resulting in correlating forward and reverse groupings.
5. Acquired B phenomenon results from intestinal obstruction, carcinoma of the colon or rectum, and other disorders associated with the lower intestinal tract. Two modes of acquisition have been recognized; the most common seems to be a bacterial enzymatic effect on the A receptors in group A_1 individuals suffering from organic bowel disorders or infection. The other acquired B phenomenon results from increased permeability of the intestinal wall and subsequent adsorption of the bacterial polysaccharide onto the red cells yielding B specificity in group A or O patients with infections of *P. vulgaris* and *E. coli* O_{86}. The acquired B antigen has also been reported with septicemic infections from *P. vulgaris*. An acquired A antigen has been reported in association with an infection caused by *P. mirabilis*. The reaction of the appropriate antiserum with these acquired antigens demonstrates a weak reaction, often yielding an mf appearance.

TABLE 5–19 **EXAMPLE OF ABO DISCREPANCY SEEN WITH WEAK OR MISSING ANTIBODIES**

	FORWARD GROUPING REACTION OF PATIENT CELLS WITH			REVERSE GROUPING REACTION OF PATIENT SERUM WITH	
	Anti-A	**Anti-B**	**Anti-A,B**	**A₁ Cells**	**B Cells**
Patient	Neg	+++	++++	Neg	Neg
	Patient's Probable Group: B (Elderly Patient)				

	αA	αB	αA,B	A₁	B		
Pt. 1	0	2+MF	2+MF	4+	0	Twin 1	70% B
							30% 0
Pt. 2	0	+Wk	+Wk	4+	0	Twin 2	30% B
							70% 0

FIGURE 5-8 Patients 1 and 2 are examples of chimera twins.

Table 5–20 shows the type of discrepancy in the forward and reverse groupings that one may recognize owing to an acquired B antigen. It has been reported that acidifying the anti-B typing reagent to pH 6.0 would differentiate between true and acquired B antigens, inasmuch as the acidified anti-B antisera will agglutinate only true B antigens.[25] In addition to acidifying the anti-B reagent, secretor studies could be performed. If the patient is in fact a secretor, only A substance will be secreted in the acquired B phenomenon. The discovery of the molecular genetics of glycosyltransferases provides an additional approach to the diagnosis of acquired B status. Because these individuals are genetically blood group B, the B transferase activity will be absent.[26]

6. Antibodies to low incidence antigens may be present in the reagent anti-A or anti-B. It is impossible for manufacturers to screen reagent antisera against all known red cell antigens. It has been reported (although rarely) that this additional antibody in the reagent antisera has reacted with the corresponding low-incidence antigen present on the patient's red cell. This gives an unexpected reaction of the patient cells with anti-A, anti-B, or both, mimicking the presence of a weak antigen (Table 5–21).

In this example, once acquired B antigen is ruled out, the best way to resolve this discrepancy is by using anti-B with a different lot number. If the cause of the discrepancy is a low-incidence antibody in the reagent antisera reacting with a low-incidence antigen on the patient's cells, then the chances are that the antibody will not be present in a different lot number of anti-B. The same solution could also be used for a weak-reacting A typing.

GROUP III DISCREPANCIES

These discrepancies are between forward and reverse groupings owing to protein or plasma abnormalities and have the following causes:

1. Elevated levels of globulin from certain disease states, such as multiple myeloma, Waldenström's macroglobulinemia, and other plasma cell dyscrasias, as well as certain moderately advanced cases of Hodgkin's lymphomas, result in rouleaux formation. Also, increased levels of fibrinogen can enhance rouleaux formation. Rouleaux of red cells result from a stacking of erythrocytes that adhere in a coinlike fashion, giving the appearance of agglutination (**see Color Plate 2J**). Washing the patient's red cells with saline or adding a drop or two of saline to the test tube will free the cells in the case of rouleaux formation. In the case of true agglutination, red cell clumping will still remain after the addition of saline.

2. Plasma expanders, such as dextran and polyvinylpyrrolidone (PVP), also will cause rouleaux formation as previously described. Washing the red cells with saline will alleviate this problem. The type of discrepancy in the forward and reverse groupings caused by rouleaux formation is shown in Table 5–22.

3. Wharton's jelly is a viscous mucopolysaccharide material present on cord bloods that causes spontaneous rouleaux, resembling agglutination. Washing the cord cells six to eight times should alleviate this problem. Even though it is rather illogical to perform reverse groupings on cord samples, a few hospitals still routinely carry out this procedure. Therefore, the student should be aware that washing the cord cells with saline will result in an accurate forward grouping. However, the reverse grouping may still not correlate with the forward grouping because the antibodies detected are usually of maternal origin.

GROUP IV DISCREPANCIES

These discrepancies are between forward and reverse groupings owing to miscellaneous problems and have the following causes:

1. Polyagglutination (spontaneous red cell aggluti-

TABLE 5-20 EXAMPLE OF ABO DISCREPANCY CAUSED BY AN ACQUIRED B ANTIGEN

	FORWARD GROUPING REACTION OF PATIENT CELLS WITH			REVERSE GROUPING REACTION OF PATIENT SERUM WITH	
	Anti-A	Anti-B	Anti-A,B	A₁ Cells	B Cells
Patient	++++	+	++++	Neg	++++
Patient's Probable Group: A					

TABLE 5–21 **EXAMPLE OF ABO DISCREPANCY CAUSED BY LOW-INCIDENCE ANTIBODIES IN THE REAGENT ANTISERA**

	FORWARD GROUPING REACTION OF PATIENT CELLS WITH			REVERSE GROUPING REACTION OF PATIENT SERUM WITH	
	Anti-A	Anti-B	Anti-A,B	A₁ Cells	B Cells
Patient	++++	+	++++	Neg	++++
	Patient's Probable Group: A				

TABLE 5–22 **EXAMPLE OF ABO DISCREPANCY CAUSED BY ROULEAUX FORMATION**

	FORWARD GROUPING REACTION OF PATIENT CELLS WITH			REVERSE GROUPING REACTION OF PATIENT SERUM WITH	
	Anti-A	Anti-B	Anti-A,B	A₁ Cells	B Cells
Patient	++++	++	++++	++	++++
	Patient's Probable Group: A				

nation by most normal human serum) can occur owing to exposure of a hidden erythrocyte antigen (T antigen) in patients with bacterial or viral infections. Bacterial contamination in vitro or in vivo produces an enzyme that alters and exposes the hidden antigen on red blood cells, leading to T activation. All normal human serum contains anti-T, which reacts with this now-exposed hidden T antigen. The strength of the reaction depends on how much anti-T antibody is in the serum. An example of the type of discrepancy in the forward and reverse groupings caused by T activation is shown in Table 5–23.

If polyagglutination is suspected, then lectin studies should be performed. This consists of testing the patient cells with a series of lectins. Commercial lectin kits are available. Based on the reactions obtained, the type of polyagglutination can be determined (see Chapter 22). "Tn activation," although rarely encountered, is another type of polyagglutinability. This condition is permanent, not transient, and is not associated with bacterial or viral infections. Acquired A antigen phenomenon has been reported in Tn activation (see Chapter 22).

2. Potent cold autoantibodies can cause spontaneous agglutination of the patient's cells. These cells will often yield a positive direct Coombs' test result (see Chapter 21). If the antibody in the serum reacts with all adult cells (e.g., anti-I [see Ii Blood Group System, in Chapter 8]), then the reagent A and B cells used in the reverse grouping will also agglutinate. The type of discrepancy in the forward and reverse groupings caused by cold autoantibodies is shown in Table 5–24.

To resolve this discrepancy, the patient cells could be washed with 37°C saline three times, and then retyped. As for the serum, an autoabsorption could be performed to remove the autoantibody from the serum and then a panel could be performed to identify the cold antibody.

Patients with warm autoimmune hemolytic anemia or those taking drugs such as methyldopa may have red cells coated with sufficient antibody to promote spontaneous agglutination that will react more weakly at room temperature than at 37°C. Also, transfusion reactions resulting in antibody production owing to transfused foreign red cell antigens can result in antibody-coated

TABLE 5–23 **EXAMPLE OF ABO DISCREPANCY CAUSED BY T ACTIVATION**

	FORWARD GROUPING REACTION OF PATIENT CELLS WITH			REVERSE GROUPING REACTION OF PATIENT SERUM WITH	
	Anti-A	Anti-B	Anti-A,B	A₁ Cells	B Cells
Patient	++	+	++++	++++	++++
	Patient's Probable Group: O				

TABLE 5–24 **EXAMPLE OF ABO DISCREPANCY CAUSED BY COLD AUTOANTIBODIES**

	FORWARD GROUPING REACTION OF PATIENT CELLS WITH			REVERSE GROUPING REACTION OF PATIENT SERUM WITH	
	Anti-A	Anti-B	Anti-A,B	A₁ Cells	B Cells
Patient	++	++++	++++	++++	+++
	Patient's Probable Group: B				

red cells that produce a positive direct Coombs' test result. This may promote an mf or weak agglutination in the forward grouping, resulting in an ABO discrepancy. These warm-reacting antibodies, which are coating the patient's red cells, will yield weaker reactions at room temperature than at 37°C during ABO testing. The type of discrepancy in the forward and reverse groupings caused by warm autoantibodies or transfusion reactions yielding antibody-coated red cells is shown in Table 5–25.

When a technologist suspects that warm autoantibodies are causing false-positive reactions in the forward grouping, he or she can treat the cells in a manner that removes the bound immunoglobulin. Treating the cells with chloroquine diphosphate is one such way. Chloroquine diphosphate removes the bound immunoglobulins, and the cells can then be retested.

3. Unexpected ABO isoagglutinins in the patient's serum react at room temperature with the corresponding antigen present on the reagent cells. Examples of this type of ABO discrepancy include A₂ and A₂B individuals who can produce "naturally occurring" anti-A₁, or A₁ and A₁B individuals who may produce "naturally occurring" anti-H. (For review, refer to previous sections on ABO subgroups.)

4. Unexpected alloantibodies in the patient's serum other than ABO isoagglutinins may cause a discrepancy in the reverse grouping. Reverse grouping cells possess other antigens in addition to A and B, and it is possible that other unexpected antibodies present in the patient's serum will react with these cells (Table 5–26). In this situation, a panel should be performed with the patient's serum. Once the unexpected alloantibodies are identified, then A and B cells negative for the corresponding antigen can be used in the reverse typing.

5. Antibodies other than anti-A and anti-B may react to form antigen-antibody complexes that may then adsorb to the patient's red cells. For example, acriflavine is the yellow dye used in some commercial anti-B reagents. Some individuals have antibodies against acriflavine in their

TABLE 5–25 **EXAMPLE OF ABO DISCREPANCY CAUSED BY WARM AUTOANTIBODIES OR TRANSFUSION REACTIONS YIELDING ANTIBODY-COATED RED CELLS**

	FORWARD GROUPING REACTION OF PATIENT CELLS WITH			REVERSE GROUPING REACTION OF PATIENT SERUM WITH	
	Anti-A	Anti-B	Anti-A,B	A₁ Cells	B Cells
Patient	+	+	+	++++	++++
	Patient's Probable Group: O				

TABLE 5–26 **EXAMPLE OF ABO DISCREPANCY CAUSED BY UNEXPECTED ALLOANTIBODIES IN PATIENT'S SERUM**

	FORWARD GROUPING REACTION OF PATIENT CELLS WITH			REVERSE GROUPING REACTION OF PATIENT SERUM WITH	
	Anti-A	Anti-B	Anti-A,B	A₁ Cells	B Cells
Patient	++++	++++	++++	+	+
	Patient's Probable Group: AB				

TABLE 5-27 **EXAMPLE OF ABO DISCREPANCY CAUSED BY A RED CELL–ABSORBED, SOLUBLE, ANTIGEN-ANTIBODY COMPLEX**

	FORWARD GROUPING REACTION OF PATIENT CELLS WITH			REVERSE GROUPING REACTION OF PATIENT SERUM WITH	
	Anti-A	**Anti-B**	**Anti-A,B**	**A₁ Cells**	**B Cells**
Patient	Neg	+++	Neg	++++	++++
	Patient's Probable Group: O				

serum, which combine with the dye and attach to the patient's red cells, resulting in agglutination in the forward grouping. The type of discrepancy in the forward grouping caused by this red cell–adsorbed, soluble, antigen-antibody complex is shown in Table 5–27. Washing the patient's cells three times with saline and then retyping them should resolve this discrepancy.

6. The serum of most "cis-AB" individuals (a rare occurrence) contains a weak anti-B, which leads to an ABO discrepancy in the reverse grouping. Cis-AB refers to the inheritance of both AB genes from one parent carried on one chromosome and an O gene inherited from the other parent. This results in the offspring inheriting three ABO genes instead of two (Fig. 5–9). The designation cis-AB is used to distinguish this mode of inheritance from the more usual AB

phenotype in which the alleles are located on different chromosomes. Usually the B antigen yields a weaker reaction with the anti-B from random donors, with mf agglutination typical of subgroup B_3 reported in several cases. The serum of most cis-AB individuals contains a weak anti-B, which reacts with all ordinary B red cells, yet not with cis-AB red cells. Some investigators have suggested that the B antigen in the cis-AB represents only a piece of the normal B antigen. Cis-AB blood can be divided into four categories: A_2B_3, A_1B_3, A_2B, and A_2B_x. Various hypotheses have been offered to explain the cis-AB phenotype. Many favor a crossing-over of a portion of a gene resulting in unequal expression by the recombinant. However, the banding pattern of the distal end of the long arm of chromosome 9 representing the ABO locus is normal. There

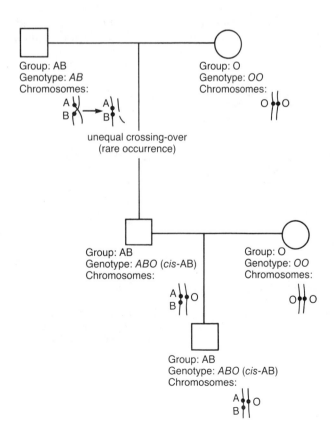

FIGURE 5-9 Example of cis-AB inheritance to unequal crossing-over. □ = male; ○ = female. (From Harmening-Pittiglio,[27] p 7, with permission.)

TABLE 5–28 ABO DISCREPANCIES BETWEEN FORWARD AND REVERSE GROUPING*

Patient	FORWARD GROUPING			REVERSE GROUPING			Auto Control	Possible Causes	Resolution Steps
	Anti-A	Anti-B	Anti-A,B	A₁ Cells	B Cells	O Cells			
1	Neg	Neg	Neg	Neg	Neg	Neg	Neg	Group O newborn or elderly patient; patient may have hypogammaglobulinemia or agammaglobulinemia, or may be taking immunosuppressive drugs	Check age of patient and immunoglobulin levels if possible; incubate at RT for 30 min or at 4°C for 15 min
2	4+	Neg	4+	1+	4+	Neg	Neg	Subgroup of A; probable A_2 with anti-A_1	Use anti-A_1 lectin
3	4+	4+	4+	2+	2+	2+	2+	1. Rouleaux (multiple myeloma patient; any patient with reversed albumin-to-globulin ratio or patients given plasma expanders)	(1) Wash red cells; use saline replacement
								2. Cold autoantibody (probable group AB with an auto anti-I)	(2) Perform cold panel and autoabsorb or rabbit erythrocyte stroma (REST) absorb (see Chapter 11)
								3. Cold autoantibody with underlying cold or RT reacting alloantibody (probable group AB with an auto anti-I and a high-frequency cold antibody (e.g., anti-P_1, anti-M, anti-Le^b)	(3) Perform cold panel, autoabsorb or REST, and run panel on absorbed serum; select reverse cells lacking antigen for identified alloantibody; repeat reverse group on absorbed serum to determine true ABO group
4	3+	4+	4+	1+	Neg	Neg	Neg	Subgroup of AB; probable A_2B with anti-A_1	Use anti-A_1 lectin
5	4+	Neg	4+	Neg	4+	3+	Neg	A_1 with potent anti-H	Confirm A_1 group with anti-A_1 lectin; test additional A_2, O, and A_1 cells and an O_h if available
6	Neg	Neg	Neg	4+	4+	4+	Neg	O_h Bombay	Test with anti-H lectin; test O_h cell if available; send to reference laboratory for confirmation
7	Neg	Neg	2+	2+	4+	Neg	Neg	Subgroup of A; probable A_x with anti-A_1	Perform saliva studies or absorption/elution
8	4+	2+	4+	Neg	4+	Neg	Neg	Group A with an "acquired B" antigen	Check history of patient for lower gastrointestinal problem or septicemia; use modified BS-1 lectin if available, or acidify anti-B typing reagent to pH 6.0 by adding 1 or 2 drops of 1N HCl to 1 ml of anti-B antisera, and measure with a pH meter (this acidified anti-B antisera would agglutinate only true B antigens, *not* acquired B antigens)
9	4+	4+	4+	2+	Neg	2+	Neg	Alloantibody	Perform antibody screen and panel
10	Neg	4+	4+	4+	1+	1+	1+	Group B with cold autoantibody	Enzyme treat red cells and perform autoabsorption or REST absorption at 4°C or perform prewarmed testing

*Absorptions should not be performed on patient cells that have been transfused within the last 3 months.
REST = rabbit erythrocyte system; RT = room temperature.

have been other examples of cis-ABs that do not fit this scenario. In these examples, there was a mutation at the ABO locus, and an enzyme was produced that was capable of transferring both A- and B-specific sugars to the precursor molecule.

RESOLUTION OF ABO DISCREPANCIES

Most ABO discrepancies are detected because forward and reverse groupings do not agree. Therefore, the first step in problem solving is to repeat all tests to be sure that the cell suspension is not too heavy or too light; that the red cells, reagents, and equipment are free of contamination; and that there is no sample mix-up. If repeat testing confirms the original results, then a complete work-up should be performed. This should include:

1. A direct antihuman globulin test (DAT) (see Chapter 4)
2. Performance of the forward grouping using red cells that have been washed three times with saline and resuspended in saline (reagents anti-A, anti-B, anti-A,B, and anti-A_1 should all be used)
3. Performance of reverse grouping with three examples of A_1, A_2, and B cells, as well as group O cord cells, O screening cells, and an autologous control (patient's serum mixed with patient's red cells)
4. Incubation of all tests at room temperature for 15 to 30 minutes and, if necessary, at 4°C for 5 to 15 minutes before reading and recording results to resolve the discrepancy

Some examples of serologic reactions involving ABO discrepancies have been provided with answers for review and self-evaluation at the end of this chapter (Table 5–28). Also, the procedure for determination of secretor status is provided in the procedural appendix at the end of this chapter. Finally, you have been briefly introduced to ABO, the first and simplest blood group system known.

Review Questions

1. An ABO type on a patient gives the following reactions:

REACTION OF PATIENT CELLS WITH			REACTION OF PATIENT SERUM WITH	
Anti-A	Anti-B	Anti-A,B	A_1 Cells	B Cells
+	+	+	Neg	Neg

What is the patient's blood type?
A. O
B. A
C. B
D. AB

2. The major immunoglobulin class of anti-B in a group A individual is:
A. IgM
B. IgG
C. IgA
D. All of the above

3. What are the possible ABO phenotypes of the offspring from the mating of a group A to a group B individual?
A. O, A, B
B. A, B
C. A, B, AB
D. O, A, B, AB

4. The immunodominant sugar responsible for blood group A specificity is:
A. L-fucose
B. N-acetyl-D-galactosamine
C. D-galactose
D. Uridine diphosphate-N-acetyl-D-galactose

5. What ABH substances would be found in the saliva of a group B secretor?
A. H
B. H and A
C. H and B
D. H, A, and B

6. An ABO type on a patient gives the following reactions:

REACTION OF PATIENT CELLS WITH				REACTION OF PATIENT SERUM WITH	
Anti-A	Anti-B	Anti-A,B	Anti-A_1	A_1 Cells	B Cells
+	+	+	Neg	+	Neg

The reactions above may be due to:
A. Patient is A_1 with acquired B
B. Patient is A_1B with anti-A_1
C. Patient is A_2B with anti-A_1
D. Patient has increased concentrations of protein in the serum

7. Which of the following ABO blood groups contains the least amount of H substance?
A. A_1B
B. A_2
C. B
D. O

8. You are working on a laboratory specimen that you believe to be a "Bombay phenotype." Which of the following reactions would you *not* expect to see?
A. Patient cells + *U. europaeus* = No agglutination
B. Patient cells + *U. europaeus* = Agglutination

C. Patient serum + Group O donors = Agglutination

D. Patient serum + A_1 and B cells = Agglutination

9. An example of a technical error that can result in an ABO discrepancy is:
   A. Acquired B phenomenon
   B. Missing isoagglutinins
   C. Clerical error
   D. Acriflavin antibodies

10. An ABO type on a patient gives the following reactions:

REACTION OF PATIENT CELLS WITH			REACTION OF PATIENT SERUM WITH			
Anti-A	Anti-B	Anti-A,B	A_1 Cells	B Cells	O Cells	Auto Control
+	Neg	+	+	+	+	Neg

To resolve this discrepancy, you would:
A. Check the age and immunoglobulin levels of the patient
B. Perform antibody screen and panel
C. Perform cold panel and autoabsorption of serum
D. Wash red cells and use saline replacement

Answers to Review Questions

1. D (p 88)
2. A (p 89)
3. D (p 89)
4. B (p 91)
5. C (p 94)
6. C (p 94)
7. A (p 95)
8. B (p 100)
9. C (p 103)
10. B (p 107)

References

1. Mourant, AE, et al: The Distribution of the Human Blood Groups and Other Biochemical Polymorphisms, ed 2. Oxford University Press, Oxford, 1976.
2. Reed, TE: Distributions and tests of independence of seven blood group systems in a large multiracial sample from California. Am J Hum Genet 20:142, 1968.
3. Wiener, AS: Problems and pitfalls in blood grouping tests for non-parentage: Distribution of the blood groups. Am J Clin Pathol 51:9, 1969.
4. Schreffler, DC, et al: Studies on genetic selection in a completely ascertained US Caucasian population. I. Frequencies, age, and sex effects and phenotype associations for 12 blood group systems. Tecumseh, Michigan: Population 10,000 West European ancestry. American Society of Human Genetics, Bethesda, MD, 1971.
5. Springer, GF, et al: Origin of anti-human blood group B agglutinins in white leghorn chicks. J Exp Med 110:221, 1959.
6. Dobson, A and Ikin, E: The ABO blood groups in the United Kingdom: Frequencies based on a very large sample. J Pathol Bacteriol 58:221, 1946.
7. Kunkel, HG and Rockey, JH: B2$_A$ and other immunoglobulins in isolated anti-A antibodies. Proc Soc Exp Biol Med 113:278, 1963.
8. Landsteiner, K and Witt, DH: Observations on the human blood groups. Irregular reactions. Isoagglutinin in sera of group 4. The factor A_1. J Immunol 2:221, 1926.
9. Dodd, BE, Lincoln, PJ, and Boorman, KE: The cross-reacting antibodies of group O sera: Immunological studies and a possible explanation of the observed facts. Immunology 12:39, 1967.
10. Yamamoto, F, Clausen, H, and White, T: Molecular genetic basis of the histo-blood group ABO system. Nature 345:229, 1990.
11. Kelton, JG and Bebenek, G: Granulocytes do not have surface ABO antigens. Transfusion 25:567, 1985.
12. Schachter, H, et al: A quantitative difference in the activity of blood group A specific N-acetylgalactosaminyl-transferase in serum from A_1 and A_2 human subjects. Biochem Biophys Res Commun 45:1011, 1971.
13. Schachter, H, et al: Qualitative differences in the alpha-N-acetyl-galactosaminyl transferases produced by human A_1 and A_2 genes. Proc Natl Acad Sci USA 7:220, 1973.
14. Tilley, CA, et al: Human blood group A- and H-specified glycosyltransferase levels in the sera of newborn infants and their mothers. Vox Sang 34:8, 1978.
15. Salmon, C, Cartron, JP, and Rouger, P: The Human Blood Groups. Masson Publishing, New York, 1984, p 420.
16. Cartron, JP, et al: Study of the α-N-acetyl-galactosaminyltransferase of sera and red cell membranes of human A subgroups. J Immunogenet 5:107, 1978.
17. Lopez, M, et al: Activity of IgG and IgM ABO antibodies against some weak A (A_3, A_x, A_{end}) and weak B (B_3, B_x) red cells. Vox Sang 37:281, 1979.
18. Cartron, JP, et al: Assay of α-N-acetylgalactosaminyltransferase in human sera. Further evidence for several types of A_m individuals. Vox Sang 28:347, 1975.
19. Topping, MD, and Watkins, WM: Isoelectric points of the human blood group A_1, A_2 and B gene-associated glycosyltransferases in ovarian cysts fluids and serum. Biochem Biophys Res Commun 6:89, 1975.
20. Hakomori, SI: Blood group ABH and Ii antigens of human erythrocytes: Chemistry, polymorphism and their developmental change. Semin Hematol 18:39, 1981.
21. Koscielak, J, Pacuszka, T, and Dzierzkowa-Borodej, W: Activity of B-gene-specified galactosyltransferase in individuals with Bm phenotypes. Vox Sang 30:58, 1976.
22. Boose, GM, Issitt, C, and Issitt, PD: Weak B antigen in family. Transfusion 18:570, 1978.
23. Watkins, WM: Changes in the specificity of blood-group mucopolysaccharides induced by enzymes from Trichomonas foetus. Immunology 5:245, 1962.
24. Salmon, C, et al: H deficient phenotypes. A proposed practical classification Bombay A_h, H_2, H_m. Blood Transfus Immunohaematol 23:233, 1980.
25. Cheng, MS: Two similar cases of weak agglutination with anti-B reagent. Lab Med 12:506, 1981.
26. Fischer, GF, Fae, I, and Dub, E: Analysis of the gene polymorphism of ABO blood group specific transferases helps diagnosis of acquired B status. Vox Sang 62:113, 1992.
27. Harmening-Pittiglio, D: Genetics and biochemistry of A, B, H and Lewis antigens. In Wallace, ME and Gibbs, FL (eds): Blood Group Systems: ABH and Lewis. American Association of Blood Banks, Arlington, VA, 1986, pp 1–56.

Bibliography

Abe, K, Levery, SB, and Hakomori, S: The antibody specific to type 1 chain blood group A determinant. J Immunol 132:1951, 1984.
Adatia, A, et al: Comparison of the absorption of allo-anti-B by red cells and by a synthetic immunoabsorbent using the autoanalyzer. Rev Fr Transfus Immunohematol 26:585, 1983.

Anderson, DE and Haas, C: Blood type A and familial breast cancer. Cancer 54:1845, 1984.

Atichartakarn, V, et al: Autoimmune hemolytic anemia due to anti B autoantibody. Vox Sang 49:301, 1985.

Baechtel, FS: Secreted blood group substances: Distributions in semen and stabilities in dried semen stains. J Foren Sci 30:1119, 1985.

Bakacs, T, Ringwald, G, and Jokuti, I: Direct ADCC lysis of O, Rh-positive (R 1 R2) erythrocytes by lymphocytes of individuals sensitized against antigen D. Immunol Lett 4:53, 1982.

Beattie, KM, et al: Two chimeras detected during routine grouping test by Autoanalyzer. Transfusion 17:681, 1977.

Beattie, KM, et al: Blood group chimerism as a clue to generalized tissue mosaicism. Transfusion 4:77, 1964.

Bensinger, WI, Buckner, CD, and Clift, RA: Whole blood immunoadsorption of anti-A or anti-B antibodies. Vox Sang 48:357, 1985.

Bensinger, WI, et al: Immune adsorption of anti-A and anti-B antibodies. Prog Clin Biol Res 88:295, 1982.

Bernoco, M, et al: Detection of combined ABH and Lewis glycosphingolipids in sera of H-deficient donors. Vox Sang 49:58, 1985.

Bolton, S and Thorpe, JW: Enzyme-linked immunoabsorbent assay for A and B water soluble blood group substances. J Forensic Sci 31:27, 1986.

Boose, GM, Issitt, C, and Issitt, P: Weak B antigen in a family. Transfusion 18:570, 1978.

Bracey, AW and Van-Buren, C: Immune anti-A1 in A2 recipients of kidneys from group O donors. Transfusion 26:282, 1986.

Brand, A, et al: ABH antibodies causing platelet transfusion refractoriness. Transfusion 26:463, 1986.

Breimer, ME and Karlsson, KA: Chemical and immunological identification of glycolipid-based blood group ABH and Lewis antigens in human and kidney. Biochim Biophys Acta 755:170, 1983.

Brouwers, HA, et al: Sensitive methods for determining subclasses of IgG anti-A and anti-B in sera of blood-group O women with a blood-group-A or B child. Br J Haematol 66:267, 1987.

Cartron, J, et al: Study of the alpha-N-acetylgalactosaminyltransferase in sera and red cell membranes of human A subgroups. J Immunogenet 5:107, 1978.

Cartron, J, et al: Assay of alpha-N-acetylgalactosaminyltransferases in human sera. Further evidence for several types of Am individuals. Vox Sang 28:347, 1975.

Cartron, J, et al: "Weak A" phenotypes. Relationship between red cell agglutinability and antigen site density. Immunology 27:723, 1974.

Cheng, MS: Two similar cases of weak agglutination with anti-B reagent. Lab Med 12:506, 1981.

Clausen, H, Holmes, E, and Hakomori, S: Novel blood group H glycolipid antigens exclusively expressed in blood group A and AB erythrocytes (type 3 chain H). II. Differential conversion of different H substrates by A1 and A2 enzymes, and type 3 chain H expression in relation to secretor status. J Biol Chem 261:1388, 1986.

Clausen, H, Levery, SB, Nudelman, E, et al: Further characterization of type 2 and type 3 chain blood group A glycosphingolipids from human erythrocyte membranes. Biochemistry 25:7075, 1986.

Clausen, H, Watanabe, K, Kannagi, R, et al: Blood group A glycolipid (Ax) with globo-series structure which is specific for blood group A1 erythrocytes: One of chemical bases for A1 and A2 distinction. Biochem Biophys Res Commun 124:523, 1984.

Cohen, F and Zuelzer, WW: Interrelationship of the various subgroups of the blood group A: Study with immunofluorescence. Transfusion 5:223, 1965.

Dodd, BE and Wood, NJ: Elution of group-specific substance A from RBC of various subgroups of A and its effect on the agglutination of AX RBC. Vox Sang 43:248, 1982.

Dodd, BE and Lincoln, PJ: Serological studies of the H activity of Oh red cells with various anti-H reagents. Vox Sang 35:168, 1978.

Dunstan, RA: Status of major red cell blood group antigens on neutrophils, lymphocytes and monocytes. Br J Haematol 62(2):301, 1986.

Economidou, J, Hughes-Jones, N, and Gardner, B: Quantitative measurements concerning A and B antigen sites. Vox Sang 12:321, 1967.

Feng, CS, et al: Variant of type B blood in an El Salvador family. Expression of a variant B gene enhanced by the presence of an A2 gene. Transfusion 24:264, 1984.

Finne, J: Identification of the blood group ABH-active glycoprotein components of human erythrocyte membrane. Eur J Biochem 104:181, 1980.

Fukuda, MN and Hakomori, S: Structures of branched blood group A-active glycosphingolipids in human erythrocytes and polymorphism of A- and H-glycolipids in A1 and A2 subgroups. J Biol Chem 257:446, 1982.

Furukawa, K, Mattes, MJ and Lloyd, KO: A1 and A2 erythrocytes can be distinguished by reagents that do not detect structural differences between the two cell types. J Immunol 135:4090, 1985.

Gardas, A and Koscielak, J: A, B and H blood group specificities in glycoprotein and glycolipid fractions of human erythrocyte membrane. Absence of blood group active glyco-proteins in the membrane of non-secretors. Vox Sang 20:137, 1971.

Gart, JJ and Nam, JM: A score test for the possible presence of recessive alleles in generalized ABO-like genetic systems. Biometrics 40:887, 1984.

Gemke, RJ, Kanhai, HH, Overbeeke, MA, et al: ABO and Rhesus phenotyping of fetal erythrocytes in the first trimester of pregnancy. Br J Haematol 64:689, 1986.

Greenwell, P, Ball, MG, and Watkins, WM: Fucosyltransferase activities in human lymphocytes and granulocytes. Blood group H-gene-specified alpha-2-L-fucosyltransferase is a discriminatory marker of peripheral blood lymphocytes. FEBS Lett 164:314, 1983.

Hakomori, S, Stellner, K, and Watanabe, K: Four antigen variants of blood group A glycolipid: Examples of highly complex, branched chain glycolipid of animal cell membrane. Biochem Biophys Res Commun 49:1061, 1972.

Handa, V, Oza, RM, Patel, RZ, et al: The Oh (Bombay group) phenotype. J Indian Med Assoc 82:446, 1984.

Hanfland, P: Characterization of B and H blood group active glycosphingolipids from human B erythrocyte membranes. Chem Phys Lipids 15:105, 1975.

Herron, R, et al: A specific antibody for cells with acquired B antigen. Transfusion 22:525, 1982.

Hirschfeld, J: Conceptual framework shifts in immunogenetics. I. A new look at cis AB antigens in the ABO system. Vox Sang 33:286, 1977.

Hummel, K, et al: Inheritance of cis-AB in three generations (Family Lam). Vox Sang 33:290, 1977.

Kannagi, R, Levery, SB, and Hakomori, S: Blood group H antigen with globo-series structure. Isolation and characterization from human blood group O erythrocytes. FEBS Lett 175:397, 1984.

Knowles, RW, et al: Monoclonal anti-type 2 H: An antibody detecting a precursor of the A and B blood group antigens. J Immunogenet 9:69, 1982.

Kogure, T and Furukawa, K: Enzymatic conversion of human group O red cells into group B-active cells by alpha-N-galactosyltransferase of sera and salivas from group B and its variant types. J Immunogenet 3:147, 1976.

Koscielak, J, et al: Structures of fucose containing glycolipids with H and B blood group activity and of sialic acid and glucosamine containing glycolipid of human erythrocyte membrane. Eur J Biochem 37:214, 1973.

Koscielak, J, et al: Weak A phenotypes possibly caused by mutation. Vox Sang 50:187, 1986.

Le-Pendu, J, et al: Alpha-2-L-fucosyltransferase activity in sera of individuals with H-deficient red cells and normal H antigen in secretions. Vox Sang 44:360, 1983.

Levine, P, Uhlir, M, and White, J: Ah, an incomplete suppression of A resembling Oh. Vox Sang 6:561, 1961.

Lin-Chu, M, et al: The para-Bombay phenotype in Chinese persons. Transfusion 27:388, 1987.

Lopez, M, et al: Activity of IgG and IgM ABO antibodies against some weak A (A3, Ax, Aend) and weak B (B3, Bx) red cells. Vox Sang 37:281, 1979.

Madsen, G and Heisto, H: A Korean family showing inheritance of A and B on the same chromosome. Vox Sang 14:211, 1968.

Makela, O, Ruoslahti, E, and Ehnholm, C: Subtypes of human ABO blood groups and subtype-specific antibodies. J Immunol 3:763, 1969.

Marsh, WL, et al: Inherited mosaicism affecting the blood groups. Transfusion 15:589, 1975.

Mohn, JF, et al: An inherited blood group A variant in the Finnish population. I. Basic characteristics. Vox Sang 25:193, 1973.

Moores, PP, et al: Some observations on "Bombay" bloods, with comments on evidence for the existence of two different O$_h$ phenotypes. Transfusion 15:237, 1975.

Oriol, R, Le-Pendu, J, and Mollicone, R: Genetics of ABO, H, Lewis, X and related antigens (Review). Vox Sang 51:161, 1986.

Pacuszka, T, et al: Biochemical serological and family studies in individuals with cis AB phenotypes. Vox Sang 29:292, 1975.

Poretz, RD and Watkins, WM: Galactosyltransferases in human submaxillary glands and stomach mucosa associated with the biosynthesis of blood group specific glycoproteins. Eur J Biochem 25:455, 1972.

Race, C and Watkins, WM: The action of the blood group B gene-specified alpha-galactosyltransferase from human serum and stomach mucosal extracts on group O and "Bombay" O$_h$ erythrocytes. Vox Sang 23:385, 1972.

Race, RR and Sanger, R: Blood Groups in Man, ed 6. Blackwell Scientific Publications, Oxford, 1975, pp 522–524, 531–535.

Rawson, AJ and Abelson, N: Studies in blood group antibodies. III. Observations on the physiochemical properties of isohemagglutinins and isohemolysins. J Immunol 85:636, 1960.

Reed, TE and Moore, BPL: A new variant of blood group A. Vox Sang 9:363, 1964.

Renkonen, KO: Blood-group-specific haemagglutinins in seed extracts. Vox Sang 45:397, 1983.

Roath, S, Todd, CE, and Shavv, D: Transient acquired blood group B antigen associated with diverticular bowel disease. Acta Haematol (Basel) 77:188, 1987.

Romano, EL, Mollison, PL, and Linares, J: Number of B sites generated on group O red cells from adults and newborn infants. Vox Sang 34:14, 1978.

Romans, DG, Tilley, CA, and Dorrington, KJ: Monogamous bivalency of IgG antibodies. I. Deficiency of branched ABHI-active oligosaccharide chains on red cells of infants causes the weak antiglobulin reactions in hemolytic disease of the newborn due to ABO incompatibility. J Immunol 124:2807, 1980.

Rubinstein, P, Allen, F, and Rosenfield, RE: A dominant suppressor of A and B. Vox Sang 25:377, 1973.

Sabo, B, et al: The cis AB phenotype in three generations of one family. Serological enzymatic and cytogenetic studies. J Immunogenet 5:87, 1978.

Salmon, C, et al: Quantitative and thermodynamic studies of erythrocytic ABO antigens. Transfusion 16:580, 1976.

Sathe, MS, Gorakshakar, AC, and Bhatia, HM: Blood group specific transferases in Bombay (O$_h$) Para-Bombay and weaker A and B variants. Indian J Med Res 81:53, 1985.

Schenkel-Brunner, H: Blood-group-ABH antigens of human erythrocytes. Eur J Biochem 104:529, 1980.

Schenkel-Brunner, H, Chester, MA, and Watkins, WM: Alpha-L-fucosyl-transferases in human serum from donors of different ABO, secretor and Lewis blood group phenotypes. Eur J Biochem 30:269, 1972.

Schenkel-Brunner, H, Prohaska, R, and Tuppy, H: Action of glycosyltranferases upon "Bombay" (O$_h$) erythrocytes. Conversion to cells showing blood group H and A specificities. Eur J Biochem 56:591, 1975.

Schenkel-Brunner, H and Tuppy, H: Enzymatic conversion of human O into A erythrocytes and of B into AB erythrocytes. Nature 223:1272, 1969.

Schenkel-Brunner, H and Tuppy, H: Enzymatic conversion of human blood group O erythrocytes into A$_2$ and A$_1$ cells by alpha-N-acetyl-D-galacto-saminyltransferases of blood group A individuals. Eur J Biochem 34:125, 1973.

Schmidt, P, et al: A hemolytic transfusion reaction due to the transfusion of A$_x$ blood. J Lab Clin Med 54:38, 1959.

Seyfried, H, Waleska, I and Werblinska, B: Unusual inheritance of ABO group in a family with weak B antigens. Vox Sang 3:268, 1964.

Smalley, CE and Tucker, EM: Blood group A antigen site distribution and immunoglobulin binding in relation to red cell age. Br J Haematol 54:209, 1983.

Solomon, J, Waggoner, R, and Leyshon, CW: A quantitative immunogenetic study of gene suppression involving A$_1$ and H antigens of the erythrocyte without affecting secreted blood group substances. The ABH phenotypes A^h and O^h. Blood 25:470, 1965.

Stayboldt, C, Rearden, A, and Lane, TA: B antigen acquired by normal A1 red cells exposed to a patient's serum. Transfusion 27:41, 1987.

Sturgeon, P, Moore, BPL, and Weiner, W: Notations for two weak A variants: A$_{end}$ and A$_{el}$. Vox Sang 9:214, 1964.

Takasaki, S and Kobata, A: Chemical characterization and distribution of ABO blood group active glycoprotein in human erythrocyte membrane. J Biol Chem 251:3610, 1976.

Takasaki, S, Yamashita, K, and Kobata, A: The sugar chain structures of ABO blood group active glycoproteins obtained from human erythrocyte membrane. J Biol Chem 253:6086, 1978.

Topping, MD and Watkins, WM: Isoelectric points of the human blood group A$_1$, A$_2$ and B gene-associated glycosyltransferases in ovarian cyst fluids and serum. Biochem Biophys Res Commun 34:89, 1975.

Tuppy, H and Schenkel-Brunner, H: Occurrence and assay of alpha-N-acetyl-galactosaminyltransferase in the gastric mucosa of humans belonging to blood group A. Vox Sang 17:139, 1969.

Viitala, J, Finne, J, and Krusius, T: Blood group A and H determinants in polyglycosyl peptides of A1 and A2 erythrocytes. Eur J Biochem 126:401, 1982.

Watanabe, K, Laine, RA, and Hakomori, S: On neutral fucoglycolipids having long branched carbohydrate chains: H-active I-active glycosphingolipids of human erythrocyte membranes. Biochemistry 14:2725, 1975.

Watkins, WM: Glycoproteins: Their composition, structure and function. In Gottschalk, A (ed): Glycoproteins, ed 2. Elsevier, Amsterdam, 1972, pp 830–891.

Watkins, WM: Blood group substances: Their nature and genetics. In Surgenor, D (ed): The Red Blood Cell. Academic Press, New York, 1974, p 303.

Westerveld, A, et al: Assignment of the AK$_1$: Np: ABO linkage group to human chromosome 9. Proc Natl Acad Sci 73:895, 1976.

Wiener, AS and Cioffi, AF: A group B analogue of subgroup A3. Am J Clin Pathol 58:693, 1972.

Wiener, AS and Socha, WW: Macro and microdifferences in blood group antigens and antibodies. Int Arch Allergy Appl Immunol 47:946, 1974.

Wittemore, NB, et al: Solubilized glycoprotein from human erythrocyte membranes possessing blood group A, B and H activity. Vox Sang 17:289, 1969.

Wrobel, DM, et al: "True" genotypes of chimeric twins revealed by blood group gene products in plasma. Vox Sang 27:395, 1974.

Wu, AM, et al: Immunochemical studies on blood groups: The internal structure and immunological properties of water-soluble human blood group A substance studied by Smith degradation, liberation, and fractionation of oligosaccharides and reaction with lectins. Arch Biochem Biophys 215:390, 1982.

Yamaguchi, H: A review of cis AB blood. Jinrui Idengaku Zasshi 18:1, 1973.

Yamaguchi, H, Okubo, Y, and Hazama, F: Another Japanese A$_2$B$_3$ blood group family with the propositus having O group father. Proc Jpn Acad 42:517, 1966.

Yamaguchi, H, Okubo, Y, and Tanaka, M: Cis AB bloods found in Japanese families. Jinrui Idengaku Zasshi 15:198, 1970.

Yokoyama, M, Stacey, SM, and Dunsford, I: B$_x$ A new subgroup of the blood group B. Vox Sang 2:348, 1957.

Yoshida, A, et al: An enzyme basis for blood type A intermediate status. Am J Hum Genet 34:919, 1982.

Yoshida, A, et al: A case of weak blood group B expression (Bm) associated with abnormal blood group galactosyltransferase. Blood 59:323, 1982.

Yoshida, A, Yamaguchi, YF, and Dave, V: Immunologic homology of human blood group glycosyltransferase and genetic background of blood group (ABO) determination. Blood 54:344, 1979.

PROCEDURAL APPENDIX

Determination of the Secretor Property

PRINCIPLE

Certain blood group substances occur in soluble form in secretions, such as saliva and gastric juice (see Table 5–8), in a large proportion (78 percent) of individuals. Such individuals are termed "secretors" (they possess the Se gene) and secrete A-, B-, or H-soluble antigens. These water-soluble blood group substances are readily detected in very minute quantities because they have the property of reacting with their corresponding antibodies, thereby neutralizing or inhibiting the capacity of the antibody to agglutinate erythrocytes possessing the corresponding antigen. The reaction is termed hemagglutination inhibition and provides a means of assaying the relative activity or potency of these water-soluble blood group substances.

MATERIALS

1. Paraffin wax
2. Saliva
3. Anti-A serum
4. Anti-B serum
5. Test tubes
6. 2 to 5 percent washed group A cells
7. 2 to 5 percent washed group B cells
8. 2 to 5 percent washed group O cells

PROCEDURE

1. Chew a piece of paraffin wax to stimulate secretion of saliva.
2. Collect about 2 to 3 ml of saliva in a test tube.
3. Place stoppered tube of saliva in a boiling water bath for 10 minutes. This inactivates enzymes that might otherwise destroy blood group substances.
4. Centrifuge hard for 10 minutes.
5. Collect clear supernatant into a clean tube.
6. Add 1 drop of diluted antiserum to an appropriately labeled tube (anti-A, anti-B, anti-H). For dilution, titrate anti-H, anti-A, and anti-B, testing against appropriate cells at immediate spin. Select the dilution giving 2+ agglutination and prepare a sufficient quantity to complete the test.
7. Add 1 drop of supernatant saliva to each tube. Incubate at room temperature for 10 minutes.
8. Add 1 drop of the 2 to 5 percent saline suspension of washed A, B, or O cells to the appropriate tube.
9. Allow serum-saliva-cell mixture to stand at room temperature for 30 to 60 minutes.
10. Centrifuge.
11. Observe for macroscopic agglutination.

CONTROL

1. Add 1 drop diluted antiserum; no saliva is added.
2. Add 1 drop of a 2 to 5 percent saline cell suspension of appropriate blood group.
3. Incubate 30 to 60 minutes (in parallel with tests), then centrifuge and read for agglutination.

INTERPRETATIONS

1. Nonsecretor: Agglutination of red cells by antiserum-saliva mixture; control tube positive.
2. Secretor: No agglutination of red cells by antiserum and saliva mixture; control tube positive. The antiserum has been neutralized by the soluble blood group substances or antigens in the saliva, which react with their corresponding antibody. Therefore, no antibody sites in the antisera are free to react with the antigens on the reagent red cells used in the testing. This negative reaction is a positive test result for the presence of ABH-soluble antigens and indicates the individual is a secretor.

ABH Substances in Saliva

ABO GROUP	ABH SUBSTANCES IN SALIVA		
	A	B	H
Secretors			
A	Much	None	Some
B	None	Much	Some
O	None	None	Much
AB	Much	Much	Some
Nonsecretors			
A, B, O, and AB	None	None	None

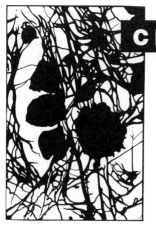

CHAPTER 6

The Rh Blood Group System

Merilyn Wiler, MA Ed, MT(ASCP)SBB

OBJECTIVES

Upon completion of this chapter, the learner should be able to:

1 Explain the derivation of the term Rh.
2 Differentiate Rh from LW.
3 Compare and contrast the Fisher-Race, Wiener, and Tippett theories of Rh inheritance.
4 Translate the five major Rh antigens, genotypes, and haplotypes from one nomenclature to another, including Fisher-Race, Wiener, Rosenfield, and ISBT nomenclatures.

  5 Define the basic biochemical structure of Rh.

  6 Compare and contrast the genetic pathways for the inherited Rh_{null} and the amorphic Rh_{null}.

  7 Describe and differentiate three mechanisms that result in weak D expression on red blood cells.

  8 List three instances when the Du status of an individual must be determined.

  9 List and differentiate four types of Rh typing reagents and give two advantages for each.

  10 Define three characteristics of Rh antibodies.

  11 Describe three symptoms associated with an Rh hemolytic transfusion reaction.

  12 Compare and contrast Rh_{null} and Rh_{mod}.

  13 List four Rh antigens (excluding DCcEe) and give two classic characteristics of each.

The term Rh refers not only to a specific red cell antigen but also to a complex blood group system that is currently comprised of nearly 50 different antigenic specificities. Although the Rh antibodies were some of the first to be described and scientists have spent years unraveling the complexities of the Rh system and its mode of inheritance, the genetic control of the Rh system and the biochemical structure of the Rh antigens still elude scientists.

History of the Rh System

Before 1939 the only significant blood group antigens recognized were those of the ABO system. Transfusion medicine was thus based on the matching of ABO groups. In spite of ABO matching, blood transfusions continued to result in morbidity and mortality.

As the decade of the 1930s ended, two significant discoveries were made that would further the safety of blood transfusion and eventually result in defining the most extensive blood group system known. It began when Levine and Stetson[1] described a hemolytic transfusion reaction in an obstetric patient. Following delivery of a stillborn infant, the woman required transfusions. Her husband, who had the same ABO type, was selected as her donor. After transfusion, the recipient demonstrated the classic symptoms of an acute hemolytic transfusion reaction. Subsequently an antibody was isolated from the mother's serum that reacted both at 37°C and 20°C with the father's red blood cells. It was postulated that the fetus and the father possessed a common factor that the mother lacked. While the mother carried the fetus, the mother was exposed to this factor and subsequently built up an antibody that reacted against the transfused red cells from the father and resulted in the hemolytic transfusion reaction.

A year later, Landsteiner and Wiener[2] reported on an antibody made by guinea pigs and rabbits when they were transfused with rhesus monkey red cells.

This antibody, which agglutinated 85 percent of human red cells, was named "Rh." Another investigation by Levine et al.[3] demonstrated that the agglutinin that had caused the hemolytic transfusion reaction and the antibody described by Landsteiner and Wiener appeared to define the same blood group. Many years later it was recognized that the two antibodies were different. However, the name Rh was retained for the human-produced antibody, and the antirhesus formed by the animals was renamed anti-LW in honor of those first reporting it (Landsteiner and Wiener).

Further research resulted in defining the cause of hemolytic disease of the newborn (erythroblastosis fetalis) and a significant cause of hemolytic transfusion reactions. Continued investigation[4-7] showed additional blood group factors associated with the original agglutinin. By the mid-1940s five antigens made up the Rh blood group system. Today the Rh blood group system is composed of nearly 50 different specificities.

Nomenclature of the Rh System

The terminology used to describe the Rh system is derived from four sets of investigators. Two of the terminologies are based on the postulated genetic mechanisms of the Rh system. The third terminology describes only the presence or absence of a given antigen. The fourth is the result of the efforts of the International Society of Blood Transfusion (ISBT) Working Party on Terminology for Red Cell Surface Antigens. The genetic pathways are described in detail after the discussion of the nomenclatures, although reference to the former may be included here.

FISHER-RACE: THE DCE TERMINOLOGY

In the early 1940s Fisher and Race[8] were investigating the antigens found on human red blood cells, including the newly defined Rh antigen. They postu-

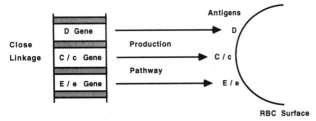

FIGURE 6-1 Fisher-Race concept of Rh (simplified). Each gene produces one product.

lated that the antigens of the system were produced by three closely linked sets of alleles. This is illustrated in Figure 6-1. Each gene was responsible for producing a product (or antigen) on the red cell surface. Each antigen and corresponding gene were given the same letter designation; however, when referring to the gene, the letter is italicized.

Fisher and Race named the antigens of the system D, d, C, c, E, and e. To date, no d antigen has been found, and it is considered an amorph (silent allele) or the absence of D antigen. The phenotype (blood type observed during testing) of a given red cell is defined by the presence or absence of *D, C, c, E,* and *e.* The gene frequency for each Rh antigen is given in Table 6-1 and the Rh haplotype (the complement of genes inherited from either parent) frequencies are given in Table 6-2. Notice how the frequencies vary with race.

According to the Fisher-Race proposal, each person inherits a set of *Rh* genes from each parent (i.e., one *D* or *d,* one *C* or *c,* and one *E* or *e*). This is detailed in Figure 6-1. Because *Rh* genes are codominant, each inherited gene expresses its corresponding antigen on the red cell. The combination of maternal and paternal haplotypes determines one's genotype (the Rh genes inherited from each parent) and dictates one's phenotype (the antigens expressed on the red cell that can be detected serologically). An individual's Rh phenotype is reported as DCE rather than CDE because Fisher postulated that the C/c locus lies between D/d and E/e loci. This information is based on frequencies of the various gene combinations.

It is essential to remember that d does not represent an antigen but simply the absence of the D antigen. C, c, E, and e represent actual antigens recognized by specific antibodies. For many students the Fisher-Race nomenclature represents the easiest way to think

about the five major Rh system antigens, but it has shortcomings in that many of the newer Rh antigens are not assigned names using the Fisher-Race nomenclature.

WIENER: THE Rh-Hr TERMINOLOGY

In his early work defining the Rh antigens, Wiener[10] believed that the gene responsible for defining Rh actually produced an agglutinogen that contained a series of blood factors. According to Rh-Hr terminology, this *Rh* gene produces at least three factors within an agglutinogen (Fig. 6-2). The agglutinogen may be considered the phenotypic expression of the haplotype. Each factor is an antigen recognized by an antibody. Antibodies can recognize single or multiple factors (antigens).

Table 6-3 lists the major agglutinogens and their respective factors, along with the shorthand term that has come to represent each agglutinogen. The Wiener terminology is complex and unwieldy; nevertheless, it is used by many blood bankers interchangeably with the other nomenclatures.

Fisher-Race nomenclature may be converted to Wiener nomenclature and vice versa. It is important to remember that an agglutinogen in the Wiener nomenclature actually represents the presence of a single haplotype composed of three different antigens (Table 6-3). When describing an agglutinogen, the uppercase R denotes the presence of the original factor, the

TABLE 6-2 FISHER-RACE PHENOTYPES OF THE Rh SYSTEM: FREQUENCIES IN THE UNITED STATES

Gene Combination	FREQUENCY (%)			
	White	Black	Native American	Asian
DCe	42	17	44	70
dce	37	26	11	3
DcE	14	11	34	21
Dce	4	44	2	3
dCe	2	2	2	2
dcE	1	0	6	0
DCE	0	0	6	1
dCE*	0	0	0	0

From Widmann,[9] p 130, with permission.
*Frequency less than 1%, but phenotype has been found.

TABLE 6-1 GENE FREQUENCY OF Rh ANTIGENS

Gene	Frequency (%)
D	85
d (absence of D)	15
C	70
E	30
c	80
e	98

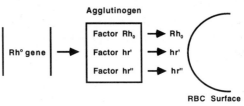

FIGURE 6-2 Wiener's agglutinogen theory. Antibody will recognize each factor within the agglutinogen.

TABLE 6–3 **Rh-Hr TERMINOLOGY OF WIENER**

Gene	Agglutinogen	Blood Factors	Shorthand Designation	Fisher-Race Antigens
Rh^o	Rh_o	$Rh_o hr'hr''$	R_o	Dce
Rh^1	Rh_1	$Rh_o rh'hr''$	R_1	DCe
Rh^2	Rh_2	$Rh_o hr'rh''$	R_2	DcE
Rh^z	Rh_z	$Rh_o rh'rh''$	R_z	DCE
rh	rh	$hr'hr''$	r	dce
rh'	rh'	$rh'hr''$	r'	dCe
rh''	rh''	$hr'rh''$	r''	dcE
rh^y	rh_y	$rh'rh''$	r^y	dCE

D antigen. The lowercase r indicates the absence of the D antigen. The presence of uppercase C is indicated by a one (1) or single prime ('). Lowercase c is implied when there is no 1 or ' indicated; that is, R_1 is the same as DCe, r' denotes dCe, and R_o is equivalent to Dce. The presence of E is indicated by the Arabic numeral two (2) or double prime ("). Lowercase e is implied when there is no 2 or " indicated; that is, R_2 is the same as DcE, r'' denotes dcE, and r is equivalent to dce. When both C and E are uppercase, the letter z or y is used. R_z denotes CDE, and r^y is CdE. Italics and superscripts are used when describing the Rh genes in the Wiener nomenclature. Standard type is used to describe the gene product or agglutinogen. Subscripts are used with the uppercase R and superscripts with the lowercase r.

When referring to the Rh antigens (or factors) in Wiener nomenclature, the single prime (') refers to either C or c and the double prime (") to either E or e. If the r precedes the h (i.e., rh' or rh"), we are referring to C or E antigens, respectively. When the h precedes the r, we are referring to either c (hr') or e (hr") antigen. Rh_o is equivalent to D. In the Wiener nomenclature, there is no designation for the absence of D antigen. By using these designations, the worker should be able to recognize immediately which factors are present on the red cells described. However, it is difficult to use the Wiener nomenclature to describe adequately additional alleles within an agglutinogen. Because of this, many of the more recently described antigens of the Rh system have not been given Rh-Hr designations.

ROSENFIELD AND COWORKERS: ALPHANUMERIC TERMINOLOGY

As the Rh blood group system expanded, it became more difficult to assign names to new antigens using existing terminologies. In the early 1960s Rosenfield et al.[11] proposed a system that assigns a number to each antigen of the Rh system in order of its discovery or recognized relationship to the Rh system (Table 6–4). This system has no genetic basis but simply demonstrates the presence or absence of the antigen on the red cell. A minus sign preceding a number designates the absence of the antigen. If an antigen has not been typed for, its number will not appear in the sequence. An advantage of this nomenclature is that the red cell phenotype is thus succinctly described.

For the five major antigens, D is assigned Rh1, C is Rh2, E is Rh3, c is Rh4, and e is Rh5. For red cells that type D + C + E + c negative e negative, the Rosenfield designation is Rh:1,2,3,−4,−5. If the sample was not tested for e, the designation would be Rh:1, 2, 3, −4. All Rh system antigens have been assigned a number.

The numeric system is well suited to electronic data processing. Its use expedites data entry and retrieval. Its primary limiting factor is that there is a similar nomenclature for numerous other blood groups such as Kell, Duffy, Kidd, Lutheran, Scianna, and more. K:1,2 refers to the K and k antigens of the Kell blood group system. Therefore, when using the Rosenfield nomenclature in the computer, one must use both the

TABLE 6–4 **COMMON Rh TYPES BY THREE NOMENCLATURES**

	GENOTYPE			Frequency (%) (approximate, whites)
	Wiener	Fisher-Race	Rosenfield	
Common genotypes	R^1r	DCe/dce	$Rh:1,2,-3,4,5$	33
	R^1R^1	DCe/DCe	$Rh:1,2,-3,-4,5$	18
	rr	dce/dce	$Rh:-1,-2,-3,4,5$	15
	R^1R^2	DCe/DcE	$Rh:1,2,3,4,5$	11
	R^2r	DcE/dce	$Rh:1,-2,3,4,5$	9
	R^2R^2	DcE/DcE	$Rh:1,-2,3,4,-5$	2
Rarer genotypes	$r'r$	dCe/dce	$Rh:-1,2,-3,4,5$	1
	$r'r'$	dCe/dCe	$Rh:-1,2,-3,-4,5$	0.01
	$r''r$	dcE/dce	$Rh:-1,-2,3,4,5$	1
	$r''r''$	dcE/dcE	$Rh:-1,-2,3,4,-5$	0.03
	R^0r	Dce/dce	$Rh:1,-2,-3,4,5$	2
	R^0R^0	Dce/Dce	$Rh:1,-2,-3,4,5$	0.1
	r^yr	dCE/dce	$Rh:-1,2,3,4,5$	Rare

From Geenwalt, TJ and Steane, EA (eds): Handbook of Clinical Laboratory Science. CRC Press, Boca Raton, FL, 1977, p 342, with permission.

alpha (Rh:, K:) and the numeric (1, 2, −3, etc.) to denote a phenotype.

INTERNATIONAL SOCIETY OF BLOOD TRANSFUSION: NUMERIC TERMINOLOGY

As the world of blood transfusion began to cooperate and share data, it became apparent that there was a need for a universal language. The ISBT formed the Working Party on Terminology for Red Cell Surface Antigens. Its mandate was to establish a uniform nomenclature that is both eye and machine readable, and in keeping with the genetic basis of blood groups.[12] They adopted a six-digit number for each authenticated blood group specificity. The first three numbers represent the system and the remaining three the antigenic specificity. The number 004 was assigned to the Rh blood group system, then each antigen assigned to the Rh system was given a unique number to complete the six-digit computer number. Table 6–5 provides a complete listing of these numbers.

When referring to individual antigens, an alphanumeric designation similar to the Rosenfield nomenclature may be used. The alphabetic names formerly

TABLE 6–5 ANTIGENS OF Rh BLOOD GROUP SYSTEM IN FOUR NOMENCLATURES

Numeric	Fisher-Race	Weiner	ISBT Number	Other Names or Comments
Rh1	D	Rh_o	004001	
Rh2	C	rh′	004002	
Rh3	E	rh″	004003	
Rh4	c	hr′	004004	
Rh5	e	hr″	004005	
Rh6	ce	hr	004006	f
Rh7	Ce	rh_i	004007	
Rh8	C^W	rh^{W1}	004008	
Rh9	C^X	rh^X	004009	
Rh10	ce^S	hr^V	004010	V
Rh11	E^W	rh^{W2}	004011	
Rh12	G	rh^G	004012	
Rh13		Rh^A	004013	
Rh14		Rh^B	004014	
Rh15		Rh^C	004015	
Rh16		Rh^D	004016	
Rh17		Hr_o	004017	
Rh18		Hr	004018	
Rh19		hr^S	004019	
Rh20	e^S		004020	VS
Rh21	C^G		004021	
Rh22	CE	rh	004022	Jarvis
Rh23	D^W		004023	Wiel
Rh24	E^T		004024	
Rh25*†			004025	
Rh26	c-like		004026	Deal
Rh27	cE	rh_{ii}	004027	
Rh28		hr^H	004028	Hernandez
Rh29			004029	total Rh
Rh30	D^{cor}		004030	Go^a
Rh31		hr^B	004031	
Rh32		$\bar{\bar{R}}^N$	004032	Troll
Rh33		R_o^{Har}	004033	Hill
Rh34		Hr^B	004034	Bastiaan
Rh35			004035	1114
Rh36			004036	Be^a (Berrens)
Rh37			004037	Evans
Rh38†			004038	Duclos
Rh39	C-like		004039	
Rh40	Tar		004040	Targett
Rh41	Ce-like		004041	
Rh42	Ce^S	rh_i^S	004042	Thornton
Rh43			004043	Crawford
Rh44			004044	Nou
Rh45			004045	Riv
Rh46	"Allelic" to $\bar{\bar{R}}^N$		004046	Sec
Rh47			004047	Dav
Rh48			004048	JAL
Rh49			004049	Stem
Rh50			004050	FPTT

*Rh25 was formerly assigned to the LW antigen. LW is now known as LW^a and is no longer considered a member of the Rh system.
†Obsolete names: Rh25, formerly LW; Rh38, formerly Duclos.

used (e.g., Rh, Kell) were left unchanged but were converted to all uppercase letters (e.g., RH, KELL). Therefore, D is RH1, C is RH2, etc. (Note: There is no space between the RH and the assigned number.)

The phenotype designation includes the alphabetical symbol that denotes the blood group, followed by a colon and then the specificity numbers of the antigens defined. A minus sign preceding the number indicates the antigen was tested for but is not present. The phenotype D+ C− E+ c+ e+ or DccEe or R_2r would be written RH:1,−2,3,4,5.

When referring to a gene, an allele, or a haplotype, the symbols are italicized, followed by a space or asterisk, and then the numbers of the specificities are separated by commas. R^1 or *DCe* would be *RH 1, 2, 5.*

SUMMARY: Rh TERMINOLOGIES

Blood bankers must be familiar with the Fisher-Race, Wiener, Rosenfield, and ISBT nomenclatures and must be able to translate among them when reading about, writing about, or discussing the Rh system.

Tables 6–4 and 6–6 summarize the data presented in this section. These tables also include probable genotypes based on the antigens found in selected red blood cell populations.

Table 6–6 correlates Rh phenotypes with the most probable genotype in a designated population. It is important to remember that results of typing do not define genotype, only phenotype. Other genotypes that can occur with the given test results are also listed, but they are not commonly seen.

Determining probable genotypes is useful for percentage studies as well as for population studies. Probable genotypes also may be useful in predicting the potential for hemolytic disease of the newborn (HDN) in offspring of an Rh-negative woman with an Rh antibody.

There are substantial differences in the probable genotypes of various populations. These differences must be remembered when trying to locate compatible blood for recipients with unusual or multiple Rh antibodies.

To further emphasize the interchangeable use of the terminologies for the basic antigens, Table 6–4 defines common genotypes using the Fisher-Race, Wiener, and Rosenfield nomenclatures. The frequencies listed are for those found in the white population.

Proposed Genetic Pathways

BIOCHEMISTRY OF THE Rh ANTIGENS

Before discussing the genetic pathways, it is necessary to understand the result of gene action. The final result of gene action in red blood cell groups is the production of a biochemical structure; in the Rh system it is a nonglycosylated protein. This means that there are no carbohydrates attached to the protein.

TABLE 6–6 18 POSSIBLE REACTION PATTERNS WITH FIVE ANTISERA

TEST RESULTS WITH Rh ANTISERA							PROBABLE GENOTYPES		
D	C	E	c	e	Whites (%)*	Blacks (%)*	Whites	Blacks	Other Possibilities (Both Groups)
+	+	−	+	+	35	26	DCe/dce	DCe/Dce	dCe/Dce
+	+	−	−	+	19	3	DCe/DCe	DCe/DCe	DCe/dCe
+	+	+	+	+	13	4	DCe/DcE	DCe/DcE	DCe/dcE dCe/DcE, DCE/dce DCE/Dce or dCE/Dce
+	−	+	+	+	12	16	DcE/dce	DcE/Dce	dcE/Dce
+	−	+	+	−	2	1	DcE/DcE	DcE/DcE	DcE/dcE
+	−	−	+	+	2	42	Dce/dce	Dce/Dce or Dce/dce	—
−	−	−	+	+	15	7	dce/dce	dce/dce	—
−	+	−	+	+	1	1	dCe/dce	dCe/dce	—
−	−	+	+	+	1	Rare	dcE/dce	dcE/dce	—
−	+	+	+	+	Each of these phenotypes occurs with a frequency of < 0.2% in both racial groups.			dCe/dcE	dCE/dce
−	+	−	−	+				dCe/dCe	—
−	−	+	+	−				dcE/dcE	—
+	+	+	−	+				DCE/DCe	DCE/dCe
+	+	+	+	−				DCE/DcE	DCE/dcE
+	+	+	−	−				DCE/DCE	DCE/dCE
−	+	+	−	+				dCE/dCe	—
−	+	+	+	−				dCE/dcE	—
−	+	+	−	−				dCE/dCE	—

*Percentages are rounded off.

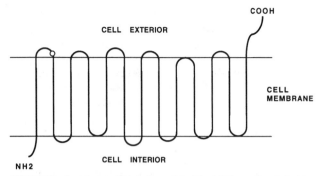

FIGURE 6-3 Model of Rh polypeptide. The NH2 terminus is inside the cell and the COOH terminus is outside the cell membrane. "O" denotes where the sequence of D diverges from C/c or E/e. (From Agre,[14] p 556, with permission.)

The Rh antigen is a transmembrane polypeptide and is an integral part of the red cell membrane.[13] Agre and Cartron[14] have shown that the D-associated protein is linked to the membrane skeleton (Fig. 6-3). The antigen specificity appears to depend on cofactors or specific conformational requirements that are achieved only if the protein is embedded in the cell membrane bilayer in a very specific configuration.

Because Rh antigens are found only on red blood cells and lose their specificity when removed from the membrane, it is difficult to harvest sufficient material to characterize the protein structure fully. It is known, however, that the protein is one of low molecular weight. The reader is referred to other references for an in-depth analysis of the biochemical research on the Rh antigen.

As part of the research on the biochemistry of the Rh antigens, investigations have been performed to determine the quantity of antigen sites on red blood cells of various Rh blood group phenotypes. In comparison with ABO and Kell (K) blood groups, A_1 cells possess approximately 1.0×10^6 A antigens, whereas homozygous Kell cells have 6000 K sites. The number of D antigen sites, measured on a variety of Rh phenotypes by Hughes-Jones and coworkers, are summarized in Table 6-7.[15] The greatest number of D antigen sites are on cells of the rare Rh phenotype D--.

(D-- cells carry only D antigen and completely lack Cc and Ee.) However, of the commonly encountered Rh phenotypes, R2R2 cells possess the largest number of D antigen sites.

MECHANISMS OF ANTIGEN PRODUCTION

Many theories have been proposed to explain genetically the results of serologic and biochemical studies in the Rh system. Two theories of Rh genetic control were initially postulated. Wiener postulated that a single gene produced a single product that contained separately recognizable factors (see Fig. 6-2). In contrast, Fisher and Race proposed that the Rh locus contains three distinct genes that control the production of their respective antigens (see Fig. 6-1).

It is currently accepted that there are only two closely linked genes that control the expression of Rh: the first gene codes for *D* and the second gene for *CcEe*[15,16] (Fig. 6-4). Locus one contains one of two alleles, *D* or *d*. The *d* may result from the absence of the *D* allele or may be an allele that is an inactive gene. The second locus contains one of four alleles: *Ce*, *cE*, *ce*, or *CE*.

It has been demonstrated through linkage studies that the Rh locus is located on chromosome 1, along with the genes for elliptocytosis, 6-phosphogluconate dehydrogenase (PGD), phosphoglucomutase (PGM), and phosphopyruvate hydratase (PPH).[17]

The Rh antigens are inherited as codominant alleles. Offspring inherit one Rh haplotype from each parent. Figure 6-5 illustrates an example of a normal Rh inheritance pattern.

It has been postulated that the genes contained at the Rh locus are very closely linked, so much so that crossing over is extremely rare. The frequencies of the various Rh gene complexes strongly support this theory. If the genes were not closely linked, all of the gene complex frequencies would be similar.

One mechanism of Rh antigen production, first proposed by Race, uses the concept of precursor substances as the building blocks for Rh antigens. Different sets of genes sequentially affect the final expression of the Rh antigens in a given individual. This concept has been used to describe the formation of

TABLE 6-7 NUMBER OF D ANTIGEN SITES OF CELLS WITH VARIOUS PHENOTYPES

Rh Phenotype	Number of D Antigen Sites
R_1r	9,900-14,600
R_0r	12,000-20,000
R_2r	14,000-16,600
R_1R_1	14,500-19,300
R_1R_2	23,000-31,000
R_2R_2	15,800-33,300
D--	110,000-202,000

From Stroup, M: Complexities of the D Antigen. Ortho Diagnostic Systems, Raritan, NJ, 1988, p 5, with permission.

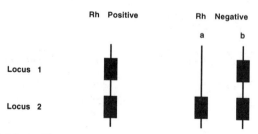

FIGURE 6-4 Rh inheritance: the two-loci theory. Locus 1 codes for the presence of D/d. (*A*) Illustrates the absence of the D gene, (*B*) illustrates the presence of an amorphic (dd) gene. Locus 2 codes for the presence of Ce, cE, ce, or CE.

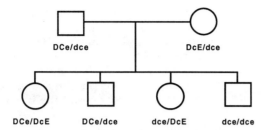

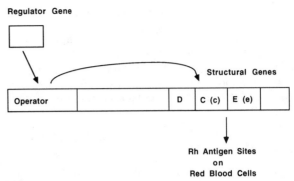

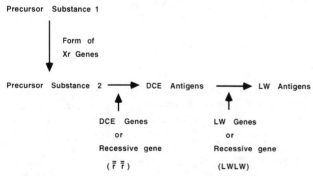

FIGURE 6-5 Example of a normal pattern of Rh inheritance.

FIGURE 6-7 Operon model of Rh antigen production (simple operon).

many other common blood group antigens. When only a few alleles exist, it appears to be an adequate explanation. With the complexity of the Rh system, modification of this proposal is required.

The modification illustrated in Figure 6–6 is based on serologic data gathered during the 1960s.[18] Variation within the Rh_{null} phenotype (phenotype that demonstrates no Rh antigens on the red cell surface) and the discovery that the Rh genes are not linked to the LW genes are better explained by Giblett's interpretation. According to Giblett,[19] precursor substance 1 is acted upon by one of several genes at the Xr locus. Under normal circumstances precursor 1 is converted to precursor 2 in the presence of the X^1r gene. (The X^1r may be either homozygous or heterozygous.) In the presence of *DCE* genes, precursor 2 is converted to DCE antigens. The LW gene(s) then act to express the LW antigens. When the *LW/LW* genotype (the amorphic genotype) is present, the cells express no LW antigens and type as LW^{a-b-}.

When homozygous $X^\circ r/X^\circ r$ genes are inherited at the Xr loci, precursor 1 is not converted to precursor 2. Even though the individual has normal *CDE* and *LW^a* or *LW^b* genes and can transfer these genes to offspring, neither the CDE nor LW antigens will be expressed on this individual's red blood cells. When no Rh antigens are expressed on the red cell, the cells are said to be Rh_{null}. Because the $X^\circ r/X^\circ r$ genes are inherited independently from the Rh genes, this type of Rh_{null} is called the regulator or inhibitor type Rh_{null}.

Because these individuals carry no Rh antigens on their red cells, they are capable of making antibody to any or all of the Rh antigens.

When homozygous X^Qr/X^Qr genes are inherited at the Xr loci, only a limited amount of precursor 1 is converted to precursor 2. This results in a weakened expression of all Rh antigens on the red cell. People with the Rh_{mod} phenotype do not produce antibody to the Rh antigens that they possess.

When the X^1r gene is inherited in combination with the $\bar{r}\bar{r}$ genes, the individual is said to have the amorphic Rh_{null} phenotype. Precursor 1 is converted to precursor 2; however, the $\bar{r}\bar{r}$ genes at the DCE loci do not alter precursor 2. This results in no DCE antigens or LW antigens being produced.

As the understanding of genetics grew, the way of looking at blood group inheritance also changed. The 1973 paper by Rosenfield et al.[20] is a comprehensive description of the operon model. This model postulates that an operator gene directs production of a messenger, that in turn directs a structural gene to produce a polypeptide chain (the antigen itself). Furthermore, there may be a regulator gene at another locus that can influence the sequence described. This may result in either altered genetic products or in no production of genetic products. Compatible with this model is the occurrence of mutations that can result in varied expression of products from the Rh locus. The model is diagrammatically interpreted in Figure 6–7. Rosenfield defines a conjugated operon that further explains the unique gene products associated with the Rh system.

As work in the fields of genetics and blood groups advances, it may be possible to define the actual pathway of antigen production. As new data become available, new concepts and hypotheses may evolve from current theories and proposals.

Variations of the Rh_o(D) Antigen

WEAK D OVERVIEW

When Rh-positive red cell samples are typed for the D antigen, it is expected that they will react strongly

FIGURE 6-6 Giblett's modification of Race's Rh genetic pathway. Alternative forms of Xr gene: X^{1}r, X$^\circ$r, or X^{Q}r. Inheriting X^{1}r in either the homozygous or heterozygous form results in expected conversion of precursor 1 to precursor 2. Inheriting homozygous X$^\circ$rX$^\circ$r results in the regulator or inhibitor Rh_{null}. Inheriting homozygous X^{Q}rX^{Q}r results in Rh_{mod} expression.

(macroscopically) with anti-D reagents. However, with certain red cells the testing must be carried through the antiglobulin phase of testing to demonstrate the presence of the D antigen. Red cells carrying the weaker D antigen have historically been referred to as having the Du type. Three different mechanisms have been described that can explain the weakened expression of the D antigen.

GENETIC WEAK D

The first mechanism results from inheritance of *D* genes that code for a weakened expression of the D antigen.[21] The D antigens expressed appear to be complete but few in number. Inheritance of these genes can be tracked vertically from one generation to the next and are seen most frequently in blacks. The "genetic Du" is rarely found in whites.

C TRANS

The second mechanism that may result in weakened expression of the D antigen is described as a position effect or gene interaction effect.[22] In individuals showing the gene interaction Du, the allele carrying *D* is trans (or in the opposite haplotype) to the allele carrying *C*—for example, *Dce/dCe*. The Rh antigen on the red cell is normal, but the steric arrangement of the C antigen in relationship to the D antigen appears to interfere with the expression of the D antigen. This interference with D expression does not occur when the *C* gene is inherited in the cis position to *D*, such as *DCe/dce*. It is not possible to distinguish the genetic weak D from the position-effect weak D serologically. Family studies are necessary to distinguish which type of weakened D antigen is being demonstrated. Practically speaking, this is unnecessary because the D antigen is structurally complete. These individuals can receive D-positive red cells with no adverse effects.

D MOSAIC

The third mechanism by which the D antigen expression can be weakened is the D mosaic. In this mechanism, one or more parts of the D antigen are missing. Cells with a mosaic D antigen usually type weaker than expected with most commercial anti-D reagents.

In the early 1950s several reports[23,24] described individuals who typed D-positive but made an anti-D that reacted with all D-positive samples except their own. The formation of alloanti-D by D-positive individuals required explanation.

Wiener and Unger[25] postulated that the D antigen is made of antigenic subparts, genetically determined, that could be absent in rare instances. If an individual lacks one (or more) pieces or epitopes of the total D antigen, alloantibody can be made to the missing fraction(s), if exposed to red cells that possess the complete D antigen. This theory has become well accepted.

Two additional theories were proposed to further delineate what is called the D-antigen mosaic. Wiener and Unger postulated that the complete D (Rh$_o$) antigen has four parts, designated Rh^A, Rh^B, Rh^C, and Rh^D. A lowercase superscript of a, b, c, and d is used to indicate when the corresponding portion(s) of the mosaic is missing; for example, Rh^b means the B portion is absent.

Tippett and Sanger[26] continued to work with red blood cells and sera of D-mosaic individuals to classify these antigens further. Their work, which was based on the reactivity of anti-D sera from D-positive people, with red cells from D-positive people who also make anti-D, has led to a second method of categorizing the D mosaic. Seven categories were recognized, designated by Roman numerals I through VII. Category I is now obsolete and a few of the categories have been subdivided further. Table 6–8 presents a summary of the partial D categories.

Although the nomenclature for D-mosaic red cells can be confusing, it is important to remember that the anti-D made by D-mosaic individuals can cause HDN or transfusion reactions, or both. Once anti-D is identified, Rh-negative blood should be used for transfusion. It would be ideal to differentiate weak D antigens resulting from inheritance of a weak *D* gene or the *D/C* trans effect from those caused by the *D*-mosaic before transfusion. However, this cannot be done by routine testing. The identification of a person with a *D*-mosaic gene routinely occurs after the person begins producing anti-D. This discovery should prompt collection of additional samples to be sent to a reference laboratory for *Rh$_o$(D)* classification.

Determination of Du Status

Determining the D status of a red cell sample is essential when testing donor blood samples. Blood for transfusion is considered Rh positive if either the D or the Du test result is positive. Any donor blood sample that types Rh$_o$(D) negative by the slide or rapid tube method must be tested further by an indirect antihuman globulin technique (**see Color Plate 11**). If both test results are negative, the donor sample is considered Rh negative. If the D slide type, the rapid tube test, or Du test is reactive, the donor sample is considered Rh positive.

For transfusion recipients, the application of the Du test remains controversial. Because the Du position effect and the genetic Du recipients clearly have the complete D antigen and cannot make alloanti-D, Rh-positive blood may be transfused. The very rare D-mosaic individuals can form alloanti-D when exposed to D-positive red cells. However, many workers believe that the number of individuals homozygous for the D-mosaic gene is so rare, the risk of sensitizing a D-mosaic individual is so small, and the supply of Rh-negative blood so precious that an intended blood recipient that types Du positive should be given Rh-

TABLE 6-8 CLASSIFICATION OF PEOPLE WITH D ON THEIR CELLS AND ALLOANTI-D IN THEIR SERA

Cells	II	III a	III b	III c	IV a	IV a	IV b	V a	V b	V c	VI i	VI ii	VII	G	Anti-Goᵃ	Dᵂ	Tar
II	−	+	+	+	+	+	w	+	+	w	+	+	nt	+	−	−	−
IIIa*	+	−	+	−	+	+	+	+	+	+	+	+	w	+	−	−	−
b	+	−	−	−	+	+	+	w	+	+	+	+	nt	−	−	−	−
c	+	−	+	−	+	+	+	+	+	+	+	+	+	+	−	−	−
IVa	−	w	+	−	−	−	−	+	+	−	+	+	+	+	+	−	−
b	−	w	+	w	−	−	−	−	+	w	+	−	nt	+	−*	−	−
Va	+	−	+	−	+	w	+	−	w	−	+	−	−	+	−	+	−
b	+	−	+	−	+	−	−	−	−	−	−	−	nt	+	−	−	−
c	+	−	+	−	w	−	w	−	−	−	+	−	nt	+	−	−	−
VI	−	−	+	−	+	−	+	−	−	−	−	−	−	+	−	−	−
VII	+	±	+	±	+	+	+	±	+	+	+	+	−	+	−	−	+

Category I	Obsolete. In retrospect, some of these may have been due to presence of a transient anti-D.
Category II	Primary classification: failure to react with serum from founder member Mcl. None of the original three propositi (all white) is still available for cross-testing. The partial D was traveling with *Ce* in two of the families tested.
Category III	Primary classification: failure to react with serum from immunized IIIa individuals. The founder member was Mrs. DS, who made the original anti-Rhᴰ of Sachs and associates.[28]
Categories IIIa and IIIb	Phenotype is C negative E negative; some have an aberrant V − VS + phenotype. Most propositi are black.
Category IIIb	G negative and sometimes also hrˢ negative. The immune response of this subdivision is very complex: the IIIb serum used also contains anti-G.
Category IIIc	Not yet shown to be inherited. Phenotype is C + G + V − VS −. All propositi are white.
Category IV	Primary classification: failure to react with serum from immunized IVa individuals and selected anti-D made by D-negative people; weak reaction with IIIa serum.
Category IVa	Positive reaction with anti-Goᵃ, an antibody defining a low-frequency Rh antigen.[29] Partial D travels with *ce* in several families (mostly black).
Category IVb*	No positive reaction with anti-Goᵃ in direct testing, but possible weak expression detectable by adsorption-elution tests (Giles, CM, Personal communication, Tippett, P and Lomas, CG, Unpublished observations). Although lacking part of the D mosaic, the remaining D antigen appears to be elevated as judged by a few incomplete anti-D that agglutinate saline suspensions of Dᴵⱽ cells. The very rare gene complex (C)Dᴵⱽ− also lacks some public Rh antigens but expresses three private Rh antigens.
Category V	Primary classification: failure to react with immune sera from category Va individuals and from IIIa and selected VI individuals. Selected anti-D from D-negative people fail to react with category V cells.
Category Va	Positive reaction with anti-Dᵂ, an antibody defining a low-frequency Rh antigen.[30] The partial D is traveling with *ce* in some families (mostly black) and *Ce* in other families (mostly white); it has been found with *cE*.
Category Vb	Dᵂ negative and negative with all VI sera. One family only, white.
Category Vc	Dᵂ negative.
Category VI	Primary classification: characteristic pattern of reactions with selected anti-D from D-negative people and failure to react with anti-D from D-positive people except those from IVb and some IVa people. However, cells of different members react with different percentages of anti-D made by D-negative people; this appears to be a quantitative difference. Partial D travels with *Ce* in most families, only rarely with *ce* or *cE*. Majority of propositi are white. The anti-D made by some members reacts with Dᴵⱽᵃ and Dⱽ cells, but that of others does not. The possibility that members of category VI have an unusual G antigen must be borne in mind.[26,27]
Category VII	Primary classification: positive reaction with anti-Tar, a low-frequency Rh antigen,[31] and characteristic pattern of reactions with selected anti-D from D-negative people. Partial D travels with *Ce* in one family tested; this had been shown to be the common phenotype for Tar+ people who had not made anti-D.[31] Lomas and coworkers[32] found only weak anti-D but strong anti-E in the sera of the two propositi. The checkerboard of cross-reactions is incomplete because cells from some categories are no longer available.

*Notes on D categories from Tippett and Sanger[27] and Lomas, C and Tippett, PA (unpublished observations), with permission. From Tippett, PA: Rh blood group system: The D antigen and high- and low-frequency Rh antigens. In Vengelen-Tyler, V and Pierce, S (eds): Blood Group Systems: Rh. American Association of Blood Banks, Arlington, VA, 1987, p 32, with permission.

+ = positive; − = negative; w = weak; nt = not tested; ± = positive with some sera and negative with others.

positive blood. Policy regarding transfusion of weak D recipients is established individually within each transfusion service. Regulatory agencies do not require routine Du testing of blood recipients unless the intended recipient has, or in the past has had, anti-D in his or her serum.

Determining the Rh₀(D) status (including Du status) of obstetric patients is critical. All Rh-negative, Du-negative obstetric patients are candidates for Rh immune globulin (RhIg) (a drug injected to prevent Rh-negative individuals who are exposed to Rh-positive red cells from developing anti-D). Likewise, when the mother is Rh negative and the newborn types Rh negative by slide or rapid tube test, the Du status of the newborn must be determined to assess the likelihood of maternal sensitization and the need for Rh immune globulin prophylaxis for the mother.

There are instances when an accurate Rh type cannot be determined through routine testing. If a newborn's cells are coated with maternal IgG anti-D in utero, very few D antigen sites will be available to react with reagent anti-D. Elution of the sensitizing antibody (removing the antibody) and identifying it as anti-D will verify that the infant's red cells are D positive. Other complex Rh typing difficulties arise in persons suffering from warm autoimmune hemolytic anemia. Many of the antibodies produced in this disorder are directed against the patient's own red cells and react as though they are Rh specific. Resolution of these anomalies is beyond the scope of this chapter and frequently require referral to reference laboratories for resolution or confirmation.

Detection of Rh Antibodies and Antigens

Rh ANTIBODIES

Although the Rh system was first recognized by saline tests used to detect IgM antibodies, most Rh antibodies are IgG and react optimally at 37°C or following the addition of antiglobulin reagent. Rh antibodies are usually produced after exposure of the individual's immune system to foreign red cells, either through transfusion or pregnancy. Rh antigens are highly immunogenic; the D antigen is the most potent.[33] A comparison of the immunogenicity of the common Rh antigens is presented in Figure 6–8. Exposure to less than 1 ml of Rh-positive red cells can stimulate antibody production in an Rh-negative person.

IgG_1, IgG_2, IgG_3, and IgG_4 subclasses of Rh antibodies have been reported. IgG_1 and IgG_3 are of the greatest clinical significance because the reticuloendothelial system rapidly clears IgG_1 and IgG_3 coated red cells from the circulation. IgA Rh antibodies have also been reported but are not routinely tested for in the blood bank.[26]

As with most blood group antigen sensitization, IgM Rh antibodies are formed initially, followed by a transition to IgG. Rh antibodies often persist in the circulation for years. An individual with low-titer Rh antibody may experience an anamnestic (secondary) antibody response if exposed to the same sensitizing

D > c > E > C > e

Highly Immunogenic   Rarely Immunogenic

FIGURE 6–8 Immunogenicity of common Rh antigens. Fifty to seventy-five percent of D-negative people exposed to D-positive red cells will form anti-D. (For a detailed discussion, refer to Mollison.[33])

antigen. Therefore, in the clinical setting, accuracy of D typing is essential, as is the careful checking of patient history to determine whether an Rh antibody has been identified previously. Most commonly found Rh antibodies are considered clinically significant. Therefore, antigen negative blood must be provided to any patient with a history of Rh antibody sensitization, whether the antibody is currently demonstrable or not.

Rh antibodies do not bind complement. For complement to be fixed (or the complement cascade activated), two IgG molecules must attach in close proximity on the red cell surface. Rh antigens (to which the antibody would attach) are not situated on the red cell surface this closely. Therefore, when an Rh antibody coats the red cells intravascularly, complement-mediated hemolysis cannot occur. Red cell destruction due to Rh antibodies is primarily extravascular. This type of hemolysis classically characterizes a delayed hemolytic transfusion reaction.

Because Rh antibodies are primarily IgG and can traverse the placenta, and because Rh antigens are well developed early in fetal life, Rh antibodies formed by Rh-negative pregnant women do cross the placenta and may coat fetal red cells that carry the corresponding antigen. This results in the fetal cells testing positive by the direct antiglobulin test and in what is known as hemolytic disease of the newborn (HDN), if the coated fetal cells are removed prematurely from the fetal circulation (see Chapter 20). Until the discovery of Rh immune globulin, anti-D was the most frequent cause of HDN.

Rh ANTIGEN TYPING REAGENTS

The reagents used to type for D and for the other Rh antigens may be derived from a variety of sources. The reagents may be high or low protein based, saline based, chemically modified, or monoclonal.

Saline reactive reagents, which contain IgM, were the first typing reagents available to test for the D antigen. Saline anti-D has the advantage of being low protein based and can be used to test cells that are coated with IgG antibody. The primary disadvantages of saline typing reagents are their limited availability, cost of production, and lengthy incubation time. Because saline anti-D is IgM, it cannot be used for Du typing.

In the 1940s high-protein anti-D reagents were developed. Human plasma containing high-titer D-specific antibody is used as the raw material. Potentiators of bovine albumin and macromolecular additives such as dextran or polyvinylpyrrolidone are added to the source material to optimize reactivity in the standard slide and rapid tube tests.[34] These reagents are commonly referred to as high protein reagents. The presence of potentiators and the higher protein concentration, however, increase the likelihood of false positive reactions. To assess the validity of the high protein Rh typing results, a control reagent was manufactured and had to be tested in parallel with each Rh test. If the control reacted, the test result was invalid and had to be repeated using a different technique or reagent anti-D. The major advantages of high protein anti-D reagents are reduced incubation time and the ability to perform Du testing and slide typing with the same reagent.

In the late 1970s, scientists chemically modified the IgG anti-D molecule by breaking the disulfide bonds, which maintain the antibody's rigid shape.[35] This allows the antibody to relax and span the distance between red cells in a low protein medium. The chemically modified reagents can be used for both slide and tube testing and do not require a separate, manufactured Rh control as long as the samples type as A, B, or O. When samples test AB Rh positive or when performing the Rh test by itself, a separate saline control must be used to ensure the observed reactions are true agglutination and not due to spontaneous agglutination. Fewer false positive test reactions are obtained because of the lower protein suspending medium. Because of its lower protein base and ready availability, the chemically modified anti-D replaced the need for saline anti-D reagents.

Monoclonal antibody reagents have become available recently. These reagents are derived from single clones of antibody producing cells. The antibody producing cells are hybridized with myeloma cells to increase their reproduction rate and, thereby, maximize their antibody producing capabilities. Because the D antigen appears to be a mosaic and the monoclonal Rh antibodies have a narrow specificity, monoclonal anti-D reagents are usually a combination of monoclonal anti-Ds from several different clones to ensure reactivity with a broad spectrum of Rh positive red cells. Some companies also blend monoclonal anti-IgM and anti-IgG anti-D to maximize visualization of reactions at immediate spin testing and to allow indirect antiglobulin testing for Du with the same reagent. The monoclonal blends can be used for slide, tube, microwell, and most automated Rh testing. Because these reagents are not human derived, they lack all potential for transmitting infectious disease.

As with all commercial typing reagents, Rh antigen typing must be performed with strict adherence to manufacturer's directions, use of proper controls, and accurate interpretation of test and control results. Table 6–9 summarizes several common causes of false Rh typing results and suggested corrective actions that may be taken to obtain an accurate Rh type.

Clinical Considerations

TRANSFUSION REACTIONS

Rh antigens are highly immunogenic. The D antigen is the most immunogenic antigen outside the ABO system. When anti-D is detected, a careful medical history will reveal red cell exposure through pregnancy or transfusion of red cell containing products. Circulating antibody appears within 120 days after a primary exposure and within 2 to 7 days after a secondary exposure.

TABLE 6–9 FALSE REACTIONS WITH Rh TYPING REAGENTS

FALSE POSITIVES		FALSE NEGATIVES	
Likely Cause	Corrective Action	Likely Cause	Corrective Action
1. Cold agglutinins	1. Wash with warm saline, retype	1. Cell suspension too heavy	1. Adjust suspension, retype
2. Test incubated too long or drying (slide)	2. Follow manufacturer's instructions precisely	2. Immunoglobulin-coated cells (in vivo)	2. Use saline-active typing reagent
3. Rouleaux	3. Use saline-washed cells, retype	3. Saline-suspended cells (slide)	3. Use unwashed cells
4. Fibrin interference	4. Use saline-washed cells, retype	4. Failure to follow manufacturer's directions precisely	4. Review directions, repeat test
5. Contaminating low-incidence antibody in reagent	5. Try another manufacturer's reagent or use a known serum antibody	5. Omission of reagent	5. Always add reagent first and check before adding cells
6. Polyagglutination	6. See Chapter 22, on polyagglutination	6. Resuspension too vigorous	6. Resuspend all tube tests gently
7. Bacterial contamination of reagent vial	7. Open new vial of reagent, retype	7. Incorrect reagent selected	7. Read vial label carefully, repeat test
8. Incorrect reagent selected	8. Read vial label, repeat test	8. Variant antigen	8. Refer sample for further investigation
		9. Reagent deterioration	9. Open new vial

Rh-mediated hemolytic transfusion reactions, whether due to primary sensitization or secondary immunization, usually result in extravascular destruction of immunoglobulin coated red cells. The transfusion recipient may have an unexplained fever, a mild bilirubin elevation, and decrease in hemoglobin and haptoglobin. The direct antihuman globulin test result is usually positive, and the antibody screen may or may not demonstrate circulating antibody. When the direct antiglobulin test indicates that the recipient's red cells are coated with IgG, elution studies may be helpful in defining the offending antibody specificity. If antibody is detected in either the serum or eluate, subsequent transfusions should lack the implicated antigen. It is not unusual for a person with a single Rh antibody to produce additional Rh antibodies if further stimulated.[33]

HEMOLYTIC DISEASE OF THE NEWBORN

Hemolytic disease of the newborn, or erythroblastosis fetalis, is briefly described here because of the historic significance of the discovery of the Rh system in elucidating its cause. Anti-D was discovered in a woman following delivery of a stillborn fetus. The mother required transfusion. The father's blood was transfused and the mother subsequently experienced a severe hemolytic transfusion reaction. Levine and Stetson[1] postulated that the antibody causing the transfusion reaction also crossed the placenta and destroyed the red blood cells of the fetus, causing its death. The offending antibody was subsequently identified as anti-D.[3]

Hemolytic disease of the newborn caused by Rh antibodies is often severe because the antigens are well developed on fetal cells, and Rh antibodies are primarily IgG, which readily cross the placenta.

After years of research, a method was developed to prevent susceptible (Rh$_o$D negative) mothers from forming anti-D, thus preventing Rh$_o$(D) HDN. Rh immune globulin, a purified preparation of anti-D, is given to D negative women during pregnancy and following delivery of a D positive fetus.[36] Rh immune globulin is effective only in preventing anti-D HDN. No effort is being made at this time to develop immunoglobulin products for other Rh antigens (C, c, E, e, etc.). When present, Rh HDN may be severe and may require aggressive treatment. Refer to Chapter 20 for a more detailed discussion of HDN—its etiology, serology, and treatment.

Rh$_{null}$ SYNDROME; Rh$_{mod}$

The rare individual who lacks all Rh antigens is said to have the Rh$_{null}$ syndrome and demonstrates a mild compensated hemolytic anemia,[37] reticulocytosis, stomatocytosis, a slight to moderate decrease in hemoglobin and hematocrit, an increase in hemoglobin F, a decrease in serum haptoglobin, and possibly an elevated bilirubin. The severity of the syndrome is highly variable from individual to individual even within one family. When transfusion of individuals with Rh$_{null}$ syndrome is necessary, only Rh$_{null}$ blood can be given.

Individuals of the Rh$_{mod}$ phenotype exhibit features similar to those with the Rh$_{null}$ syndrome; however, the clinical symptoms of these individuals are usually less severe and rarely clinically remarkable.[38] Rh$_{null}$ and Rh$_{mod}$ red cells exhibit other blood group antigens; however, S, s, and U antigen expression may be depressed.[39] Rh$_{null}$ red cells are negative for FY5.

Unusual Phenotypes and Rare Alleles

A brief discussion follows of some of the less frequently encountered Rh antigens. Refer to other references for in-depth discussions.[13,17]

C^w

The C^w antigen was originally considered an allele at the C/c locus.[40] Later studies showed that it can be expressed in combination with both C and c and in the absence of either allele. Although C^w is usually found in combination with C, its exact origin is not clear. C^w is found in about 2 percent of whites and is very rare in blacks. Anti-C^w has been identified in individuals without known exposure to foreign red cells as well as after transfusion or pregnancy. Anti-C^w may show dosage (i.e., reacting more strongly with cells from individuals who are homozygous for C^w). Because of the low incidence of the C^w, C^w antigen negative blood is readily available.

f (ce)

The f antigen is expressed on the red cell when both c and e are present on the same haplotype or are in the cis position and has been called a "compound" antigen.[41] However, f is a single entity. Phenotypically the following samples appear the same when tested with the five major Rh antisera: *Dce/DCE* and *DcE/DCe*. However, when tested with anti-f, only the former will react. Anti-f has been reported to cause HDN and transfusion reactions.

rh$_i$ (Ce)

Like anti-f, anti-rh$_i$ is present when C and e are in the cis configuration, has been called a "compound" antigen, and is a single entity.[41] A sample with the phenotype D+C+E+c+e+ can be either *DcE/DCe* or *Dce/DCE*. Anti-rh$_i$ will react only with *Dce/DCE* red cells.

G

G is an antigen that is present on most D-positive and all C-positive red blood cells. In the test tube anti-G reacts as though it is a combination of anti-C plus anti-D.[42] G was originally described in an *rr* person who received Dccee red blood cells. Subsequently the recipient produced an antibody that appeared to be anti-D+C, which should be impossible because the C antigen was not on the transfused red cells. Further investigation showed that the antibody was directed toward D+G.

Rh:13, Rh:14, Rh:15, Rh:16

Rh:13,14,15,16 define four different parts of the D mosaic, as it was originally described. Although these parts are included in the D mosaic categories II through VII as defined by Tippett and Sanger,[26,27,43] they are not directly comparable.

Hr$_o$

Hr$_o$ is an antigen present on all red blood cells with the "common" Rh phenotypes (i.e., R_1R_1, R_2R_2, rr, etc.)[44] When red cells phenotype as D--, the most potent antibody they make is often one directed against Hr$_o$.

Rh:23, Rh:30, Rh:40

Rh:23, Rh:30, and Rh:40 are all low frequency antigens associated with a specific category of D mosaic. Rh:23 (also known as Wiel and D^w) is an antigenic marker for category Va D mosaic,[30] Rh:30 (also known as Go^a or D^{cor}) is a marker for category IVa D mosaic,[29] and Rh:40 (also known as Tar or Targett) is a marker for category VII.[31]

Rh:33

The low incidence antigen Rh:33 is associated with a rare variant of the R^o *(Dce)* gene called $R_o{}^{Har}$.[45] $R_o{}^{Har}$ gene codes for normal amounts of c, reduced amounts of e, reduced f, reduced Hr$_o$, and reduced amounts of D antigen. The D reactions are frequently so weak that the cells are frequently mistakenly typed as Rh negative. To denote the weakened expression of an antigen in Fisher-Race nomenclature, the letter is placed in parentheses. The $R_o{}^{Har}$ gene expresses (D)c(e) and has been found in whites.

Rh:32

Rh:32 is a low frequency antigen associated with a variant of the R^1 *[D(C)(e)]* gene, which is called $\overline{\overline{R}}{}^N$.[46] The C and e antigen are expressed weakly. The D antigen expression is exaggerated or exalted. This gene has been found primarily in blacks.

e VARIANTS

It appears, especially in the black population, that the e antigen may exhibit the same mosaic quality described for D. Because of these variations, e typings can be unreliable.[17,47]

Among the variants at the e locus are hr^S, hr^B, and $VS(e^S)$, with a variant R^O or r gene making e plus one or the other of these pieces. Such variants are usually recognized when they make antibodies that behave as anti-e yet their red cells type as e positive with routine Rh typing reagents.

V, VS

The V(ce^S) antigen is found in about 30 percent of randomly selected American blacks. In selected individuals it serologically appears to be the counterpart of *f* because it is present when c is cis with e^S.[48] The VS(e^S) antigen is also relatively common in blacks, reacting with all V-positive red cells and additionally with $r's$ red cells.[49] Although the relationship of *V* to *VS* remains somewhat less than clear, both are markers associated with the black population.

DELETIONS

Some very uncommon phenotypes demonstrate no Cc and/or Ee reactivity. Many examples lacking all *Cc* or *Ee* often have an unusually strong D antigen expression, frequently called an exalted D. The deletion phenotype is indicated by the use of a dash (-), as in the following examples: DC-, Dc-, D-E, D--. The antibody made by D-- people is called anti-Rh 17 or anti-Hr$_o$.

A variation has been recognized within the deletion D--, called D··. The D antigen in the D·· is stronger than that in DC-, D-E, Dc-, or D-e samples, but weaker than that of D-- samples. A low incidence antigen called Evans (Rh:37) accompanies the Rh structure of D·· cells.[50]

Deleted complexes are of particular interest and concern in parentage testing. The absence of antigens can make interpretation of parentage testing results difficult. Transfusion of individuals with a deletion or D·· phenotype is difficult if multiple antibodies are present; blood of a similar phenotype would be required.

The LW Antigen

A discussion of the LW antigen begins at the time Rh antigens were first recognized. The antibody produced by injecting rhesus monkey red cells into guinea pigs and rabbits was identified as having the same specificity as the antibody Levine and Stetson[1] described earlier. The antibody was given the name anti-Rh, for anti-rhesus, and the blood group system was established. Many years later it was recognized that the two antibodies were not identical, and the anti-rhesus described by Landsteiner and Wiener[2] was renamed anti-LW in their honor.

Phenotypically there is a similarity between the Rh and LW systems. Anti-LW reacts strongly with most D positive red cells, weakly (sometimes not at all) with Rh negative red cells, and never reacts with Rh$_{null}$ cells. The independent segregation of *LW* from the *Rh*

TABLE 6–10 **LW PHENOTYPES AND GENOTYPES***

Phenotype	Genotype
LW(a+b−)	LW^aLW^a or LW^aLW
LW(a+b+)	LW^aLW^b
LW(a−b+)	LW^bLW^b or LW^bLW
LW(a−b−)	$LWLW$

From Sistonen and Tippett,[52] p 252, with permission.

*Rh_null individuals are phenotypically LW(a−b−) because of the genetic mechanism causing the Rh_null status. The *LW* genotype of Rh_null may be determined by family studies.

blood group genes was established by a family study on a D-positive, LW-negative woman; other family studies support this point.[46,51]

The nomenclature describing the various expressions of the LW antigen has evolved over time.[52] An excellent description of this is found in other reference texts.[47]

There are three alleles at the LW locus: LW^a, LW^b, and *LW* (a silent allele). Persons lacking LW antigen altogether are *LW/LW* and express no LW on the red cells. Refer to Table 6–10 for a summary of LW phenotypes and genotypes. LW^a is very common, and LW^b somewhat less common. The relationship of LW antigen production to the Rh antigens is summarized in Figure 6–9. Under normal circumstances precursor substance is acted on by the *Rh* genes to produce normal Rh antigens. The *LW* genes then exert their influence to express LW antigen on the red cell surface.

When the Rh_null suppressor genes (X^orX^or) are present, the *Rh* and *LW* genes are not expressed on the red cell; however, the *Rh* and *LW* genes are normal and, when passed to offspring with the X^Ir gene, are expressed normally. The amorphic Rh_null individual inherits the $\overline{\overline{rr}}$ genes, which do not express Rh antigens; therefore, *LW* genes cannot be expressed.

Anti-LW usually reacts more strongly with D positive red cells than with D negative adult red cells. A weak anti-LW may react only with D positive red cells, and enhancement techniques may be required to demonstrate its reactivity with D negative cells. Anti-LW reacts equally well with cord cells, regardless of D typing.[17] This is an important characteristic to remember when trying to differentiate anti-LW from anti-D. Also, anti-LW more frequently appears as an auto-antibody, which does not present clinical problems. Autoanti-LW is occasionally seen in autoimmune hemolytic anemia.

Because of the complexity of the Rh blood group system, a tremendous amount of literature exists. The inquisitive reader can continue to piece together the puzzle by consulting the sources included in the references.

Review Questions

1. The Rh system was first recognized in a case report about:
   - A. A hemolytic transfusion reaction
   - B. HDN
   - C. Circulatory overload
   - D. Autoimmune hemolytic anemia

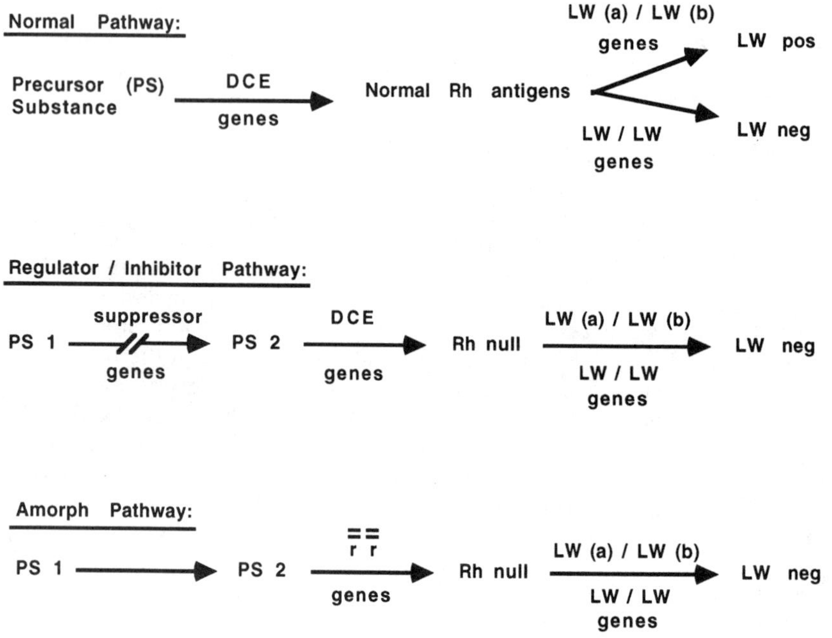

FIGURE 6–9 Genetic pathways relating Rh and LW antigens. Rh antigen precursor substance must be available for LW to be made.

2. The _____ antigen is found in 85 percent of whites and is always significant for transfusion purposes.
   A. d
   B. c
   C. D
   D. E
   E. e

3. Weaker than expected reactions with anti-D typing reagents are expected with _____.
   A. Rh$_{null}$
   B. Du
   C. DAT positive
   D. D^w

4. Cells carrying a weak D antigen require the use of the _____ to demonstrate its presence.
   A. Indirect antiglobulin test
   B. Direct antiglobulin test
   C. Microplate test
   D. Warm auto absorption test

5. Rh antigens are inherited as _____.
   A. Autosomal recessive alleles
   B. Sex-linked genes
   C. Codominant alleles
   D. X-linked

6. Rh antigens are _____.
   A. Glycophorins
   B. Simple sugars
   C. Proteins
   D. Lipids

7. Rh antibodies react best at _____ °C.
   A. 22
   B. 18
   C. 15
   D. 37

8. Rh antibodies are primarily of the _____ class.
   A. IgA
   B. IgM
   C. IgG
   D. IgD
   E. IgE

9. Rh antibodies have been associated with which of the following clinical conditions?
   A. Erythroblastosis fetalis
   B. Thrombocytopenia
   C. Hemolytic transfusion reactions
   D. Hemophilia A
   E. More than one above

10. Rh$_{null}$ cells lack:
    A. Lewis antigens
    B. Normal oxygen-carrying capacity
    C. Rh antigens
    D. MNSs antigens

11. The antigen system closely associated phenotypically with Rh is known as:
    A. McCoy
    B. Lutheran
    C. Duffy
    D. LW

12. Anti-LW will not react with which of the following?
    A. Rh-positive red cells
    B. Rh-negative red cells
    C. Rh$_{null}$ red cells
    D. Rh:33 red cells

13. Convert the following genotypes from Wiener nomenclature to Fisher-Race and Rosenfield nomenclatures and list the antigens present in each haplotype.
    A. R_1r
    B. R_2R_o
    C. R_zR_1
    D. r^yr

14. The Rh phenotype that has the strongest expression of D is _____.
    A. R_1r
    B. R_1R_2
    C. R_2r
    D. R_2R_2
    E. D--

Answers to Review Questions

1. A (p 117)
2. C (Table 6–1)
3. B (p 124)
4. A (p 124)
5. C (p 122)
6. C (p 121)
7. D (p 126)
8. C (p 126)
9. E (p 127–128)
10. C (p 128)
11. D (p 129)
12. C (p 130)

13. R_1r DCe/cde   Rh:1,2,−3,4,5
    R_2R_o DcE/cDe   Rh:1,−2,3,4,5
    R_zR_1 DCE/DCe   Rh:1,2,3,−4,5
    r^yr CE/cde   Rh:−1,2,3,4,5
    (see Table 6–3)
14. E (p 122)

References

1. Levine, P and Stetson, RE: An unusual case of intragroup agglutination. JAMA 113:126, 1939.
2. Landsteiner, K and Wiener, AS: An agglutinable factor in human blood recognized by immune sera for rhesus blood. Proc Soc Exp Biol (NY) 43:223, 1940.
3. Levine, P, et al: The role of isoimmunization in the pathogenesis of erythroblastosis fetalis. Am J Obstet Gynecol 42:925, 1941.
4. Race, RR, et al: Recognition of a further common Rh genotype in man. Nature 153:52, 1944.
5. Mourant, AE: A new rhesus antibody. Nature 155:542, 1945.
6. Stratton, F: A new Rh allelomorph. Nature 158:25, 1946.
7. Levin, P: On Hr factor and Rh genetic theory. Science 102:1, 1945.
8. Race, RR: The Rh genotypes and Fisher's theory. Blood 3(suppl 2):27, 1948.
9. Widmann, FK (ed): Technical Manual of the American Association of Blood Banks, ed 9. American Association of Blood Banks, Arlington, VA, 1985.
10. Wiener, AS: Genetic theory of the Rh blood types. Proc Soc Exp Biol (NY) 54:316, 1943.
11. Rosenfeld, RE, et al: A review of Rh serology and presentation of a new terminology.
12. Lewis, M (Chair): Blood group terminology 1990. Vox Sang 58:152, 1990.
13. Issitt, PD: Serology and Genetics of the Rh Blood Group System. Montgomery Scientific Publications, Cincinnati, 1985.
14. Agre, P and Cartron, J: Molecular biology of the Rh antigen. Blood 78:551, 1991.
15. Hughes-Jones, NC, Gardner, B, and Lincoln, PJ: Observations of the number of available c, D, and E antigen sites on red cells. Vox Sang 21:210, 1971.
16. Tippett, PA: A speculative model for the Rh blood groups. Ann Hum Genet 50:241, 1986.
17. Race, RR and Sanger, R: Blood Groups in Man, ed 6. Blackwell Scientific Publications, Oxford, 1975.
18. Race, RR: Modern concepts of the blood group systems. Ann NY Acad Sci 127:844, 1965.
19. Giblett, ER: Genetic Markers in Human Blood. Blackwell Scientific Publications, Oxford, 1969.
20. Rosenfield, RE, Allen, FH, Jr, and Rubinstein, P: Genetic model for the Rh blood group system. Proc Natl Acad Sci 70:1303, 1973.
21. Race, RR, Sanger, R, and Lawler, SD: The Rh antigen Dᵘ. Ann Eugen Lond 14:171, 1948.
22. Capellini, R, Dunn, LC, and Turri, M: An interaction between alleles at the Rh locus in man which weakens the reactivity of the Rh₀ factor (Dᵘ). Proc Natl Acad Sci 41:283, 1955.
23. Shapiro, M: The ABO, MN, P and Rh blood group systems in South African Bantu: A genetic study. South Afr Med J 25:187, 1951.
24. Argall, CI, Ball, JM, and Trentelman, E: Presence of anti-D antibody in the serum of Dᵘ patient. J Clin Lab Med 41:895, 1953.
25. Wiener, AS and Unger, LJ: Rh factors related to the Rh₀ factor as a source of clinical problems. JAMA 169:696, 1959.
26. Tippett, P and Sanger, R: Observations on subdivisions of the Rh antigen D. Vox Sang 7:9, 1962.
27. Tippett, PA and Sanger, R: Further observations on subdivisions of the Rh antigen. Arztl Lab 23:476, 1977.
28. Sachs, MS, et al: Isosensitization to a new blood group factor Rhᴰ with special reference to its clinical importance. Ann Intern Med 51:740, 1959.
29. Lewis, M, et al: Blood group antigen Goᵃ and the Rh system. Transfusion 7:440, 1967.
30. Chown, B, et al: The Rh antigen Dʷ (Wiel). Transfusion 4:169, 1964.
31. Lewis, M, et al: Assignment of the red cell antigen Targett (Rh 40) to the Rh blood group systems. Am J Hum Genet 31:630, 1979.
32. Lomas, C, et al: Tar + individuals with anti-D, a new category Dᵛᴵᴵ (abstract). Transfusion 26:560, 1986.
33. Mollison, PL: Blood Transfusion in Clinical Medicine, ed 6. Blackwell Scientific Publications, Oxford, 1988.
34. Diamond, LK and Denton, RC: Rh agglutination in various media with particular reference to the value of albumin. J Clin Lab Med 30:821, 1945.
35. Romans, DG, et al: Conversion of incomplete antibodies to direct agglutinins by mild reduction. Proc Natl Acad Sci USA 74:2531, 1977.
36. Queenan, JT: Modern Management of the Rh Problem, ed 2. Harper & Row, New York, 1977.
37. Schmidt, PJ and Vos, GH: Multiple phenotypic abnormalities associated with Rh_null (---/---). Vox Sang 13:18, 1967.
38. Chown, B, et al: An unlinked modifier of Rh blood groups: Effects when heterozygous and when homozygous. Am J Hum Genet 24:623, 1972.
39. Schmidt, PJ, et al: Aberrant U blood group accompanying Rh_null. Transfusion 7:33, 1967.
40. Callendar, ST and Race, RR: A serological and genetic study of multiple antibodies formed in response to blood transfusion by a patient with lupus erythematosus diffusus. Ann Eugen Lond 13:102, 1946.
41. Rosenfield, RE and Haber, GV: An Rh blood factor, rh_i (Ce) and its relationship to hr (ce). Am J Hum Genet 10:474, 1958.
42. Allen, FH and Tippett, PA: A new Rh blood type which reveals the Rh antigen G. Vox Sang 3:321, 1958.
43. Wiener, AS and Unger, LJ: Further observations on the blood factors Rhᴬ, Rhᴮ, Rhᶜ, Rhᴰ. Transfusion 2:230, 1962.
44. Allen, FH, Jr and Corcoran, PA: Evidence for "New" blood-group antigen of nearly universal occurrence. Proc 11th Annual Meeting, AABB, Cincinnati, Abstract, 1958.
45. Giles, CM, et al: An Rh gene complex which results in a 'new' antigen detectable by a specific antibody, anti-Rh 33. Vox Sang 21:289-301, 1971.
46. Rosenfield, RE, et al: Problems in Rh typing as revealed by a single Negro family. Am J Hum Genet 12:147, 1960.
47. Issitt, PD: Applied Blood Group Serology, ed 3. Montgomery Scientific Publications, Miami, 1985.
48. DeNatale, A, et al: A "new" Rh antigen, common in Negroes, rare in white people. JAMA 159:247, 1955.
49. Sanger, R, et al: An Rh antibody specific for V and Rˢ. Nature (Lond) 186:171, 1960.
50. Contreras, M, et al: The Rh antigen Evans. Vox Sang 34:208, 1978.
51. Vos, GH, et al: A sample of blood with no detectable Rh antigens. Lancet i:14, 1961.
52. Sistonen, P and Tippett, P: A "new" allele giving further insight into the LW blood group system. Vox Sang 42:252, 1982.

CHAPTER 7

The Lewis System

Denise M. Harmening, PhD, MT(ASCP), CLS(NCA)
Mitra Taghizadeh, MS, MT(ASCP)

OBJECTIVES

Upon completion of this chapter, the learner should be able to:

1 Describe the formation and secretion of Lewis antigens and their adsorption onto the red cells.

2 Discuss the inheritance of the Lewis genes and their interactions with the other blood group genes.

3 List substances present in secretions and the Lewis phenotypes based on a given genotype.

4 Define the role of secretor genes in formation of Lewis antigens.

5 Diagram the proposed genetic pathway for formation of Lewis antigens.

6 List the Lewis phenotypes and their frequencies in the white and black populations.

7 Indicate the process of development of the Lewis antigens after birth.

8 Describe the changes in the Lewis phenotypes during pregnancy.

9 List the characteristics of the Lewis antigens.
10 List the characteristics of the Lewis antibodies.
11 Discuss the significance of Lewis antibodies.

The Lewis blood group system is unique in that it is believed to be the only system that is not manufactured by the red blood cell. Lewis antigens are not synthesized by the red cell and incorporated into the red cell membrane structure. Instead, these antigens are manufactured by tissue cells and secreted into body fluids. Therefore, the Lewis system is referred to as a system rather than a blood group because Lewis antigens are primarily found in the secretions and the plasma. These antigens are then adsorbed onto the red cell membrane from plasma, but they are not really an integral part of the membrane structure. Because Lewis-soluble antigens are manufactured by tissue cells, antigen production depends not only on the inheritance of Lewis genes but also on the inheritance of the secretor and *Hh* genes. Genetic interaction exists also between the Lewis and ABO genes, because the amount of Lewis antigen detectable on the red cell is influenced by the ABO genes inherited.

Inheritance

Similar to ABO genes, the Lewis gene (*Le*) does not actually code for the production of Lewis antigens but, rather, produces a specific glycosyl transferase, L-fucosyltransferase. This enzyme adds L-fucose to the basic precursor substance. The Le gene is thought to be located on chromosome 19 linked to the C3 complement locus.[1] In whites, 90 percent of the population possesses *Le* gene. This gene codes for a specific glycosyltransferase, α-4-L-fucosyltransferase, which transfers L-fucose to type 1 chain oligosaccharide on glycoprotein or glycolipid structures. Type 1 chain refers to the beta linkage of the number 1 carbon of galactose to the number 3 carbon of *N*-acetylglucosamine (GlcNAc) residue of the precursor structure (Fig. 7–1). The inheritance of *Le* acts in competition with ABO genes, adding L-fucose to the GlcNAc sugar of the common precursor structure manufactured by tissue cells (Fig. 7–2 and **Color Plate 12**). The structure formed is known as Le^a-soluble antigen. It is then secreted and adsorbed onto the red cell membrane from plasma. In the addition of L-fucose to type 1 chain catalyzed by Lewis enzyme, the number 1 carbon of L-fucose is attached to the number 4 carbon of GlcNAc. This transfer reaction can occur in type 1 precursor structures only. Addition of L-fucose cannot occur with type 2 precursor structures, inasmuch as in type 2 structures, number 4 carbon of GlcNAc is already linked to galactose (Fig. 7–1).

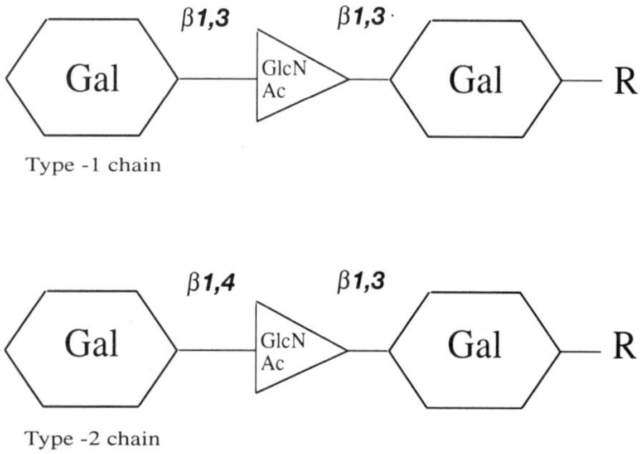

FIGURE 7–1 Structure of type 1 and type 2 chains. Gal = D-galactose; GlcNAc = *N*-acetyl-D-glucosamine; R = other biochemical residues.

Basic Concepts: The Lewis Phenotypes

THE LEWIS (a+b−) PHENOTYPE NONSECRETORS

Le^a substance is secreted regardless of the secretor status. The term "secretor" refers only to the presence of water-soluble ABH antigen substances in the body fluids and is influenced by the independently inherited secretor genes *Se* and *se*. (For a review of secretors, refer to Chapter 5.) Therefore, an individual can be a nonsecretor (*sese*) of ABH and still secrete Le^a into the body fluids, producing the phenotype Lewis a-positive b-negative [Le(a+b−)] on the red blood cells. All Le(a+b−) individuals are nonsecretors of ABH substances. Lewis enzyme has been detected in saliva, milk, submaxillary glands, gastric mucosa, kidney, and cyst fluids.[2] Lewis fucosyltransferase has not been detected in plasma or in red cell stroma. Lewis antigens produced in saliva and other secretions are glycoproteins, but Lewis cell-bound antigens absorbed from plasma onto the red cell membranes are glycolipids. Formation of Le^a from type 1 precursor structure is depicted in Figures 7–3 and 7–4.

THE LEWIS (a−b+) PHENOTYPE SECRETORS

The genetically independent *Sese*, ABO, *Hh*, and Lewis genes are intimately associated in the formation of the Le^b antigen. Le^a and Le^b are not alleles. The phenotype Le(a−b+) is the result of the genetic interaction of *Hh*, *Lele*, and *Sese* genes. Le^b antigen repre-

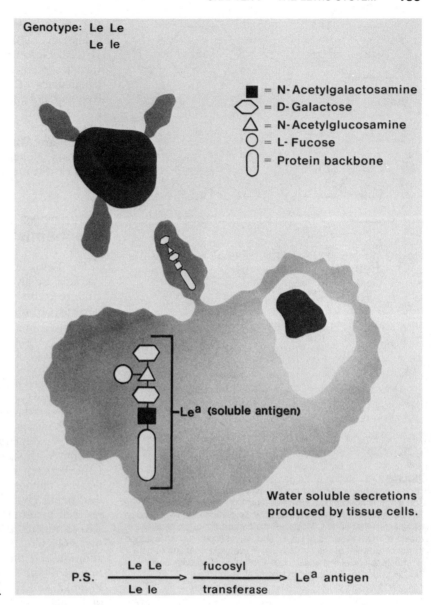

Genotype: Le Le
         Le le

■ = N-Acetylgalactosamine
⬡ = D-Galactose
△ = N-Acetylglucosamine
○ = L-Fucose
▯ = Protein backbone

—Le^a (soluble antigen)

**Water soluble secretions
produced by tissue cells.**

$$\text{P.S.} \xrightarrow[\text{Le le}]{\text{Le Le}} \xrightarrow[\text{transferase}]{\text{fucosyl}} \text{Le}^a \text{ antigen}$$

FIGURE 7-2 Formation of Le^a substance.

sents the product of genetic interaction among *Le, Se,* and *H* genes. In secretions, *Se* gene regulates expression of *H* gene, resulting in production of the H enzyme α-2-L-fucosyltransferase, which adds L-fucose to the D-galactose of the type 1 precursor resulting in H-soluble antigen (Figs. 7–3 and 7–4). The inheritance of the *Le* gene codes for the addition of another L-fucose that is added to the subterminal *N*-acetylglucosamine forming Le^b antigen (Figs. 7–3 and 7–4). Some precursor chains are not acted on by the H fucosyltransferase but may accept L-fucose from the Lewis fucosyltransferase forming Le^a (Fig. 7–5 and **Color Plate 13**). Therefore, both Le^a- and Le^b-soluble antigens can be found in the secretions. However, only Le^b adsorbs onto the red cell from plasma. This is probably because of the fact that higher concentrations of Le^b in plasma allow Le^b-soluble antigen to compete more successfully for sites of adsorption onto

the red cell membrane. As a result, the red cells of these individuals always phenotype as Le(a−b+), even though both Le^a and Le^b soluble antigens are present in the secretions and plasma. In secretors, biochemical studies indicate that Le and H fucosyltransferases compete for type 1 chain precursor.[3] H glycosyltransferase catalyzes synthesis of H on type 1 chain precursor structures. The respective amounts of Le^a and type 1 H substances formed in secretions are determined by the ratio of these two fucosyltransferases. In nonsecretors (*sese*), only Le^a antigens are formed in secretions, inasmuch as no H enzyme is present in secretory cells, even though the *H* gene is inherited. As a result, all type 1 chain precursor glycoproteins are available for the Le enzyme α-4-L-fucosyltransferase. The *H* gene does, however, function in adding L-fucose to D-galactose of type 2 chain on the red cell membrane paragloboside structure, forming the H antigen as de-

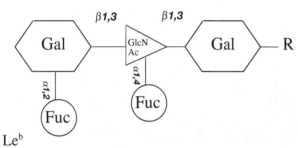

Le^a

Type-1 H substance

Le^b

FIGURE 7-3 Action of Le gene transferase enzyme. Le^a = gene codes for L-fucosyltransferase that add L-fucose (FUC) to the carbon #4 of *N*-acetylglucosamine of type 1 precursor structure. Type 1 H substance = *H* gene activated by *Se* gene codes for L-fucosyl transferase that adds L-fucose to the carbon #2 of terminal galactose. Le^b = in presence of Le, H, and Se, a second fucose is added to the carbon #4 of the subterminal *N*-acetylglucosamine of type 1 H substance. Gal = D-galactose; GlcNAc = *N*-acetylglucosamine; FUC = L-fucose; R = other biochemical residues.

scribed for formation of ABH antigens (see Chapter 5). Therefore, only Le^a antigen will be secreted by the tissue cells and subsequently adsorbed onto the erythrocyte from plasma yielding the phenotype Le(a+b−). Lewis antigens have been also detected on the surface of platelets and lymphocytes, regardless of the secretor status, but not on the surface of granulocytes or monocytes.[4,5]

THE LEWIS (a−b−): *lele* INDIVIDUALS

Lack of inheritance of the Le gene (*lele*) leads to a third type of red cell phenotype, Lewis a-negative b-negative [Le(a−b−)] (Figs. 7−6 and 7−7). The *lele* genotype is much more common in blacks than in whites. The frequencies of the Lewis red cell phenotypes in the white population are as follows: Le(a−b+), 72 percent; Le(a+b−), 22 percent; Le(a−b−), 6 percent. In the black population the frequencies are Le(a−b+), 55 percent; Le(a+b−), 23 percent;

Le(a−b−), 22 percent (Table 7−1). All Le(a−b+) individuals are ABH secretors and also secrete Le^a and Le^b. All Le(a+b−) individuals are ABH nonsecretors, yet all secrete Le^a. It is no surprise, then, that the frequencies of these Lewis phenotypes parallel the frequency of the secretor gene. Approximately 78 to 80 percent of whites are secretors and 20 percent nonsecretors. In terms of Le(a−b−) individuals, 80 percent are ABH secretors and 20 percent ABH nonsecretors. Neither Le^a nor Le^b is found in the secretions of this phenotype (Figs. 7−6 and 7−7).

Advanced Concepts: Biochemistry of Lewis Antigens

The Lewis antigens or substances found in the secretions are glycoproteins, as are the ABH substances from secretors. The glycoproteins are composed of 80 percent carbohydrates and 15 percent amino acids.[6] In plasma, Lewis antigens are glycolipids (glycosphingolipids). These antigens are carried by lipoproteins present in plasma that adhere to red cell membranes, forming glycosylceramides. All of the Lewis antigens found on red cells have been absorbed from plasma. Using plasma as a source of Lewis glycosphingolipids, Le(a−b−) red cells incubated with Le^a-positive or Le^b-positive plasma can be converted to Le(a+b−) or Le(a−b+), depending on the substance present in the plasma. With saliva as a source of Lewis substances, Le(a−b−) red cells cannot be converted into Lewis-positive phenotypes because Lewis substances in saliva, being glycoproteins, are not adsorbed onto the red cell membranes. The Lewis specificity similar to ABH antigens resides in the carbohydrate portion of the molecule. Both Le^a and Le^b are formed by the addition of a fucose molecule to the precursor structure of a type 1 chain in secretions (Fig. 7−2, **Color Plate 12**; and Fig. 7−5, **Color Plate 13**). In addition, A or B enzymes in secretor individuals can form A or B antigens in secretions by adding the appropriate sugar residue to type 1 or type 2 H substances. The substances present in secretions and antigens present on red cells, depending on *Lele*, *Hh*, and ABO genes inherited, are listed in Table 7−2. The Le^a gene-specified fucosyltransferase competes with A and B gene-specified enzymes for the same type 1 H substrate. As a result, those individuals who inherit *Le* and *Se* genes have more Lewis and fewer A or B plasma glycolipids than *Se lele* individuals. Le^a and Le^b antigens, once formed in secretions, can no longer be used as substrates for H and A or B enzymes, owing to chain termination signaled by the Lewis transferase. As a result, presence or absence of *Le* gene affects the concentration of H, A, and B type 1 chain substances found in secretions. *Le* gene does not affect synthesis of type 2 chain H, A, and B-soluble antigens found in secretions. Antigens of all other blood group systems are built on type 2 precursor chains found on the red cell membrane because these determinants are manufactured by the red cell. Characteristics of Lewis and

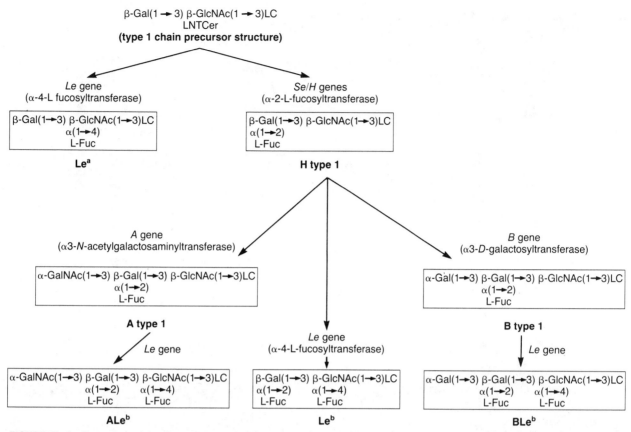

β-Gal(1 → 3) β-GlcNAc(1 → 3)LC
LNTCer
(type 1 chain precursor structure)

Le gene
(α-4-L fucosyltransferase)

β-Gal(1→3) β-GlcNAc(1→3)LC
α(1→4)
L-Fuc

Le^a

Se/H genes
(α-2-L-fucosyltransferase)

β-Gal(1→3) β-GlcNAc(1→3)LC
α(1→2)
L-Fuc

H type 1

A gene
(α3-*N*-acetylgalactosaminyltransferase)

α-GalNAc(1→3) β-Gal(1→3) β-GlcNAc(1→3)LC
α(1→2)
L-Fuc

A type 1

Le gene

α-GalNAc(1→3) β-Gal(1→3) β-GlcNAc(1→3)LC
α(1→2)   α(1→4)
L-Fuc   L-Fuc

ALe^b

Le gene
(α-4-L-fucosyltransferase)

β-Gal(1→3) β-GlcNAc(1→3)LC
α(1→2)   α(1→4)
L-Fuc   L-Fuc

Le^b

B gene
(α3-*D*-galactosyltransferase)

α-Gal(1→3) β-Gal(1→3) β-GlcNAc(1→3)LC
α(1→2)
L-Fuc

B type 1

Le gene

α-Gal(1→3) β-Gal(1→3) β-GlcNAc(1→3)LC
α(1→2)   α(1→4)
L-Fuc   L-Fuc

BLe^b

FIGURE 7-4 Formation of Lewis antigens (le^a, le^b, Ale^b, Ble^b) absorbed from plasma. Note: LC (lactosylceramide) = β-Gal(1→4) β-Glc(→1)Cer; LNTCer = lacto-*N*-tetraosylceramide; Gal = D-galactose; GlcNAc = *N*-acetylglucosamine; Fuc = L-fucose; GalNAc = *N*-acetylgalactosamine. (From Harmening-Pittiglio,[25] p 33, with permission.)

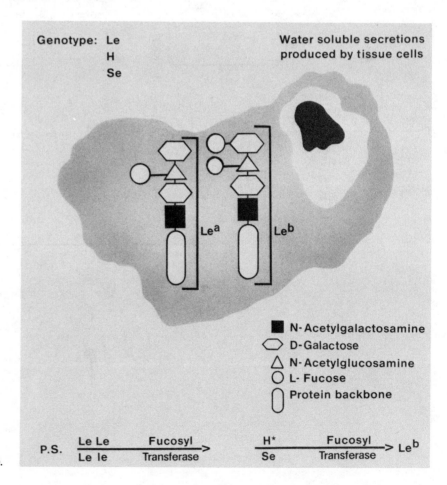

FIGURE 7-5 Formation of Le^b substance.

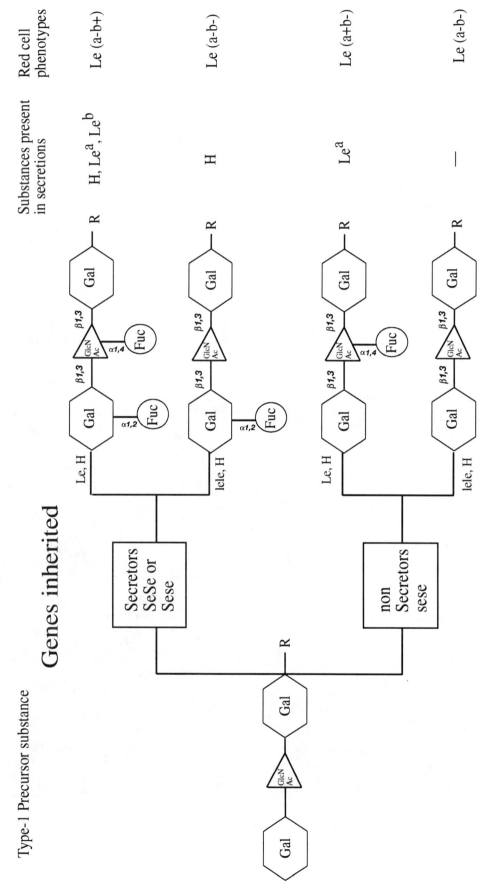

FIGURE 7-6 Formation of Lewis antigens in secretors and nonsecretors. Gal = *D*-galactose; GlcNAc = *N*-acetyl-*D*-glucosamine; FUC = L-fucose; R = other biochemical residues.

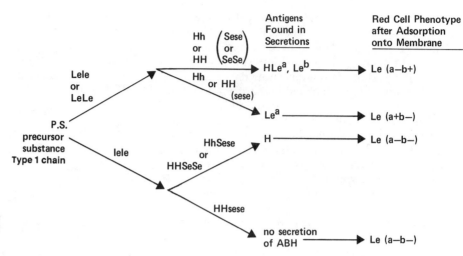

FIGURE 7-7 Proposed genetic pathway for formation of Lewis antigens.

TABLE 7-1 PHENOTYPES AND FREQUENCIES IN THE LEWIS SYSTEM

| Phenotype | ADULT PHENOTYPE FREQUENCY (%) | |
	Whites	Blacks
Le(a+b−)	22	23
Le(a−b+)	72	55
Le(a−b−)	6	22

ABH substances found in secretions are compared in Table 7-3.

Development and Changes of Lewis Antigens After Birth

Depending on the genes inherited, Le^a and Le^b glycoproteins as well as ABH substances will be present in the saliva of newborn infants. In plasma there are no

TABLE 7-2 SUBSTANCES PRESENT ON SECRETIONS AND ANTIGENS PRESENT ON RED CELLS, DEPENDING ON THE LEWIS, *Hh*, AND ABO GENES INHERITED

Genes Inherited	Substances Present in Secretions	Red Cell Phenotype
Le, Se, H, A/B/O	Le^a, Le^b, H, A, B	ABH, Le(a−b+)
lele, Se, H, A/B/O	H, A, B	ABH, Le(a−b−)
Le, sese, H, A/B/O	Le^a	ABH, Le(a+b−)
lele, sese, H, A/B/O	—	ABH, Le(a−b−)
Le, Se, hh, A/B/O	Le^a	(O$_h$), Le(a+b−)

From Harmening-Pittiglio,[25] p 34, with permission.

detectable Lewis glycosphingolipids at birth.[7] Therefore, cord blood and red cells from newborn infants phenotype as Le(a−b−). It is the low level of plasma Lewis antigens that accounts for this fact, because the plasma of newborn infants has been demonstrated

TABLE 7-3 CHARACTERISTICS OF LEWIS, A, B, AND H SUBSTANCES FOUND IN SECRETIONS

	Lewis Substances in Secretion	ABH Substances in Secretion
Genetic control	*Le* gene (Le^a formation is not dependent or controlled by *Se* gene)	*Se* gene
Glycosyltransferase	α-4-L-fucosyltransferase (Le)	α-2-L-fucosyltransferase (H) α-3-*N*-acetylgalactosaminyltransferase (A) α-3-D-galactosyltransferase (B)
Substrate precursor structure	Type 1 chains	Type 1 or type 2 chains
Factors affecting formation	1. Once forced, Le^a and Le^b are no longer substrates for H or AB enzymes, respectively. 2. Lewis and H fucosyltransferases compete for type 1 chain precursor structure. 3. Lewis and AB enzymes compete for type 1 H substance.	1. Type 2 chain, A, B, and H substance formation is unaffected by the presence of the Lewis enzyme. 2. A or B type 1 substances can act as substrates for Lewis enzyme forming ALe^b or BLe^b "compound" antigenic glycoproteins. 3. Formation of type 1 chain, A, B, and H substances is competitively inhibited by the presence of Lewis enzyme.

From Harmening-Pittiglio,[25] p 36, with permission.

to be incapable of transforming Le(a−b−) adult cells into Lewis-positive phenotype. However, Le(a−b−) erythrocytes from infants can be transformed into Le(a+b−) phenotype by incubation with plasma from an Le(a+b−) adult.[8] When inheriting the genotype *Le, sese, H,* Lewis antigens (Le[a] and Le[b]) are not detectable on cord red cells, but these infants do secrete Le[a] substance in their saliva. Lewis glycosphingolipids become detectable in plasma after approximately 10 days of life. In those individuals who inherit *Le* and *Se/H* genes, a transformation can be followed from Le(a−b−) phenotype at birth to Le(a+b+) after 10 days, and finally to Le(a−b+), the true Lewis phenotype. The Le(a−b+) phenotype can be acquired as early as 2 years of age. In contrast, those individuals who inherit *Le* and *sese/H* genes will phenotype as Le(a−b−) at birth and transform to Le(a+b−) after 10 days. The Le(a+b−) phenotype persists throughout life. Individuals with *lele* genes phenotype as Le(a−b−) at birth and for the rest of their lives.

Changes in Lewis Phenotype

A decrease in expression of Lewis antigens has been demonstrated on red cells from many pregnant women, resulting in Le(a−b−) phenotypes during gestation.[9] The mechanism causing production of this phenotype during pregnancy is uncertain. It has been suggested that physiologic changes in the composition of blood, which affects distribution of Lewis glycolipid between plasma and red cells, is responsible for this phenomenon. Of the total Lewis glycolipids in whole blood, approximately one third of Le[b] is associated with red cells, and the rest is bound to plasma lipoproteins.[9] Other investigators have proposed that the large increase in the ratio of plasma lipoproteins to red cell mass that occurs during pregnancy is responsible for Le(a−b−) phenotypes.[10] In this instance, a greater amount of Le[b] glycolipids would be bound to plasma lipoproteins instead of adsorbing onto red cells. Lack of expression of Lewis antigens (Le[a] and Le[b]) has been demonstrated on red cells of patients with cancer. This transformation of Lewis-positive phenotypes to Lewis-negative phenotypes is due to neoplastic changes occurring in cancer patients.[11,12] A summary of Lewis antigens can be found in Table 7–4.

Lewis Antibodies

BASIC CONCEPTS

Antibodies to the Lewis blood group antigen (anti-Le[a] and anti-Le[b]) are frequently detected in antibody screening procedures. Lewis antibodies are generally produced by Le(a−b−) persons. Lewis antibodies are

TABLE 7–4 LEWIS ANTIGENS

Poorly developed at birth
Reversibly adsorbed to red cells from plasma
Not found on cord blood or newborn red cells Le(a−b−)
Lewis glycosphingolipids detectable in plasma after approximately 10 days of life
Transformation of Lewis phenotype after birth seen in individuals who inherit *Le, Se,* and *H* genes: Le(a−b−) to Le(a+b−) to Le(a+b+) to Le(a−b+) (the true phenotype)
Decrease in expression demonstrated in red cells from many pregnant women, resulting in Le(a−b−) phenotypes during gestation

considered naturally occurring because they are present without prior exposure to the antigen positive red cells. They are generally immunoglobulin M (IgM) in nature and do not cross the placenta to cause hemolytic disease of the newborn (HDN). However, because they are IgM antibodies these hemolysins can activate complement and, therefore, occasionally can cause in vivo and in vitro hemolysis. An interesting aspect of Lewis antibodies is that they occur quite frequently in the sera of pregnant women.[13] Lewis antibodies are more reactive with enzyme-treated cells than with untreated cells and more reactive with group O cells than with group A or B cells. Anti-Le[a] and anti-Le[b] may occur together.

Anti-Le[a]

Anti-Le[a] is the most commonly encountered antibody of the Lewis system produced in individuals of Le(a−b−) phenotypes. The antibody is often of IgM class; however, some may have IgG components or may be entirely IgG.[14] The IgG form of anti-Le[a] does not bind to the red cells as efficiently as the IgM form does and thereby is not generally detected in routine blood bank procedures. However, IgG anti-Le[a] has been detected on red cells using enzyme-linked immunosorbent assay (ELISA).[14] The IgG Lewis antibodies can be formed following massive transfusions of Lewis-positive antigens in individuals whose serum lacks Lewis antibodies prior to Lewis-positive red cell transfusion.[13,15] The IgM form of Le[a] antibody binds complement and, therefore, can cause in vivo and in vitro hemolysis. The antibody reactivity is enhanced by enzyme-treated red cells. The Le[a] antibody is frequently detected with saline-suspended cells at room temperature. However, it sometimes reacts at 37°C and Coombs phase and therefore can cause hemolytic transfusion reactions. Anti-Le[a] is easily neutralized with plasma or saliva that contains Le[a] substance. Persons who are Le(a−b+) do not make anti-Le[a] because the Le[a] antigen structure is contained within Le[b] antigen epitope. Additionally, Le(a−b+) persons have Le[a] substance present in their plasma and saliva. Caution must be used, however, because the agglutinates can be dispersed easily if the red blood cells are not resuspended gently.

TABLE 7-5 LEWIS ANTIBODIES

Usually naturally occurring
Predominantly IgM
May cause in vivo hemolysis of red cells
Sometimes reacts at 37°C and Coombs phase more weakly than at
 room temperature
Enhanced by enzymes
Readily neutralized by Lewis blood group substances
Rarely causes in vitro hemolysis; however, in vitro posttransfusion
 hemolysis reported in cases in which Lewis Ab strongly reacted
 in Coombs phase

Anti-Le^b

Anti-Le^b is not as common nor generally as strong as anti-Le^a. Although it is usually an IgM agglutinin, it does not fix complement as readily as anti-Le^a. Anti-Le^b is usually produced by an Le(a−b−) individual; only occasionally will an Le(a+b−) individual produce an anti-Le^b. Like anti-Le^a, anti-Le^b is neutralized by plasma or saliva containing Le^b substance. A summary of Lewis antibodies can be found in Table 7–5.

ADVANCED CONCEPTS

Anti-Le^b

An interesting aspect of anti-Le^b is that it can be classified into two categories: anti-Le^{bH} and anti-Le^{bL}. Anti-Le^{bH} reacts best when the Le^b and the H antigens are both present on the red cell such as group O and A$_2$ cells. Anti-Le^{bH} is probably an antibody to a compound antigen. One must be cautioned that when phenotyping red cells, especially A$_1$ and A$_1$B cells, the antisera being used is not anti-Le^{bH}. Anti-Le^{bL} is the Le^b antibody that recognizes any Le^b antigen regardless of the ABO type. Anti-Le^{bH} can be neutralized by either H or combined H and Le^b substance, whereas anti-Le^{bL} is inhibited only by Le^b substance. Anti-Le^{bL} is the antibody of choice for phenotyping red cells.

Neither anti-Le^{bH} nor anti-Le^{bL} is frequently implicated in hemolytic transfusion reaction, and the lack of reports in the literature suggests that anti-Le^b in general has no clinical significance.[13] Formation of possible Lewis antibodies in different red cell phenotypes is summarized in Table 7–6.

Anti-Le^x

Anti-Le^x agglutinates all Le(a+b−) and Le(a−b+) red cells and is formed by all individuals lacking *Le*

gene. Anti-Le^x also agglutinates approximately 90 percent of all white cord blood initially phenotyping as Le(a−b−). In 1981, Schenkel-Brunner and Hanfland[16] defined the binding site of Le^x antibodies by immunoadsorption studies. The binding site of Le^x antibodies was found to be the smaller disaccharide structure of fucose-$\alpha(1{\rightarrow}4)$GlcNAc-R[7,16] (Fig. 7–8). The reactivity of Le^x determinant as defined by these authors is inhibited by the Le^a glycolipid similar to the inhibition of normal anti-Le^a because the specificities of both antibodies are determined by a fucose-$\alpha(1{\rightarrow}4)$GlcNAc linkage, which is present in both Le^x and Le^a antigens as a product of the Lewis α-4-L-fucosyltransferase.

Le(a−b−x+) cord cells do not react with anti-Le^a or anti-Le^b. This may be due to the hidden nature of the Le^x determinant, which is covered by the addition of many more carbohydrates to the disaccharide chain. A somewhat similar analogy can be made with the A, B, and H antibodies and antigens, in that H-positive O cells, analogous to Lewis (a−b−x+) cells, do not react with anti-A or anti-B, but anti-H (analogous to anti-Le^x) does agglutinate selected B and A cells. The fact that the reactivity of anti-Le^x cannot be separated using Le(a+b−) or cord red cells indicates that this antibody is detecting a Lewis precursor antigen present in the biochemical structure of Le^a and Le^b.

Clinical Significance of Lewis Antibodies

Although some cases of hemolytic transfusion reactions caused by anti-Le^a have been reported and there have been cases of in vivo red cell destruction due to anti-Le^b, Lewis antibodies are generally considered insignificant in blood transfusion practices. This is because

1. Lewis antibodies can be neutralized by the Lewis substances present in the plasma and can thereby be decreased in quantity.
2. The Lewis antigens dissociate from the red cells as readily as they bind to the red cells. In other words, the Lewis-positive donor red cells can become Lewis-negative red cells following transfusion into an individual with a Lewis-negative phenotype. These antigens released into the plasma can further neutralize any Lewis antibodies present in the recipient plasma.
3. Lewis antibodies are generally IgM and therefore cannot cross the placenta and cause HDN. In addition, Lewis antigens are not fully developed at birth (Table 7–7).

For these reasons the presence of Lewis antibodies in a patient's serum does *not* require transfusion of Lewis-negative red cells, as long as pretransfusion tests performed at 37°C and Coombs phase are compatible and there is no evidence of in vitro hemolysis. The Lewis antibodies reactive at 37°C and antihuman

TABLE 7-6 LEWIS ANTIGEN ON THE RED CELLS AND POSSIBLE ANTIBODIES PRODUCED IN THE PLASMA

Red Cell Phenotype	Possible Antibodies Produced
Le(a+b−)	Anti-Le^b
Le(a−b+)	—
Le(a−b−)	Anti-Le^a, Anti-Le^b
Le^x	—

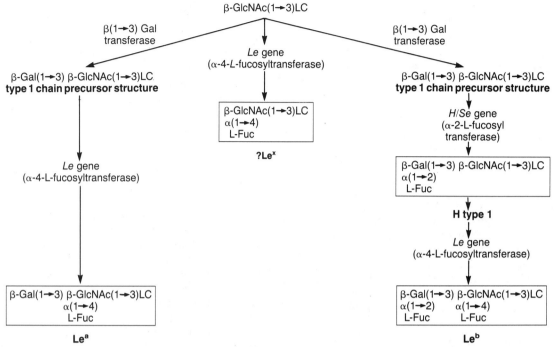

FIGURE 7–8 A hypothetical pathway: formation of Le^a, Le^b, and Le^x substance absorbed from plasma. (From Harmening-Pittiglio,[25] p 40, with permission.)

TABLE 7–7 FACTORS CONTRIBUTING TO CLINICAL INSIGNIFICANCE OF LEWIS ANTIBODIES

Neutralization of Lewis antibodies by Lewis substances present in the plasma
Loss of red cell Lewis antigen(s) into the plasma
Lack of reactivity at 37°C and antihuman globulin phase
Generally IgM in nature and incapable of crossing placenta
Lewis antigens poorly developed in newborn infants

globulin phase, however, should not be ignored because these antibodies can cause in vivo red cell destructions.

Other Lewis Antigens

Le^c AND Le^d

Le^d antigen was first described by Potapov,[17] who reported an antibody in the serum that reacted with red cells from Le(a–b–) ABH-secretor individuals. In his report, he predicted another hypothetical antibody, anti-Le^c, which would detect the Lewis antigen on red cells of Lewis (a–b–) ABH nonsecretors. In 1972, Gunson and Latham reported such an antibody that defined the Le^c antigen.[18]

Le^c and Le^d type 1 chain structures have been proposed by Graham[19] and Hanfland et al.,[20] who obtained anti-Le^c and anti-Le^d antibodies following immunization of goats with human saliva. In their

investigation, anti-Le^d was strongly inhibited by a fucose containing saccharide of the type 1 H chain structure. These investigators suggest that no Le^c and Le^d antigens are associated with the Lewis system. Le^c represents type 1 precursor structure, and Le^d is type 1 H structure (Fig. 7–9). More recent findings suggest that Le^c antigen is not only a type 1 precursor. Study of purified fractions of human sphingolipids from *lele* nonsecretors demonstrated a more complex structure for Le^c antigen. This Le^c antigen is a branched structure with a combination of type 1 and type 2 chains,[21,22] depicted here:

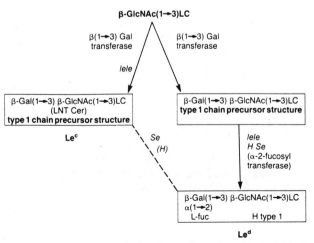

FIGURE 7–9 A hypothetical pathway: formation of Le^c and Le^d. Based on the work of Graham et al.[19] and Hanfland et al.[20] (From Harmening-Pittiglio,[25] p 39, with permission.)

TABLE 7–8 REVIEW OF THE GENETIC INTERACTION AMONG LEWIS, _Hh_, SECRETOR, AND ABO GENES

Hypothetic Genotype	Substances Present in Saliva	Red Cell Phenotype
LeLe HH SeSe AA	A, H, Le^a, Le^b	A Le(a−b+)
lele Hh Sese AO	A, H	A Le(a−b−)
Lele Hh sese AO	Le^a	A Le(a+b−)
lele HH sese AO	None	A le (a−b−)
lele HH sese AB	None	AB Le(a−b−)
LeLe HH Sese AB	A, B, H, Le^a, Le^b	AB Le(a−b+)
lele Hh SeSe AB	A, B, H	AB Le(a−b−)
Lele Hh sese AB	Le^a	AB Le(a+b−)
Lele HH SeSe OO	H, Le^a, Le^b	O Le(a−b+)
lele Hh SeSe OO	H	O Le(a−b−)
LeLe HH sese OO	Le^a	O le(a+b−)
lele Hh sese OO	None	O Le(a−b−)
lele hh Sese (any ABO genotype)	None	O$_h$ Le(a−b−)
LeLe hh SeSe (any ABO genotype)	Le^a	O$_h$ Le(a+b−)
Lele hh sese (any ABO genotype)	Le^a	O$_h$ Le(a+b−)
lele hh sese (any ABO genotype)	None	O$_h$ Le(a−b−)

β-Gal (1→3) β-GlcNAc 1

$$>3,6\ \beta\text{-Gal (1}\rightarrow\text{3) }\beta\text{-GlcNAc}$$

(1→3) β-Gal (1→4) β-Glc (1→1) Cer

β-Gal (1→4) β-GlcNAc 1

α (1→3)

Fuc

Formation of Lewis antigens in secretions and through their adsorption onto red cells depends on the genetic makeup of the individual (Table 7–8).

The Le^c and Le^d antigens are found in individuals who lack the Le gene (_lele_) and have a phenotype of Le(a−b−). Le^c antigen is found only in Le(a−b−) individuals who are ABH nonsecretors. Le^d antigen is found only in Le(a−b−) individuals who are ABH secretors. In view of these findings, perhaps Lewis phenotype would be more correctly written as Le(a−b−c+d−) and Le(a−b−c−d+), similar to the two new phenotypes previously described. Le^c is analogous to Le^a; they are biochemically very similar and secreted only by ABH nonsecretors (_sese_). Similarly Le^c is adsorbed onto the red cell only after exposure to the plasma or secretion containing the soluble antigen. This close similarity between Le^a and Le^c accounts for the observation that the Le(a−b−) individuals who produced anti-Le^a were all ABH secretors with an Le(a−b−c−d+) phenotype.

The presence of Le^c in Le(a−b−) ABH nonsecretors probably prevents the formation of anti-Le^a, inasmuch as Le^c and Le^a are biochemically very similar. Saliva from these Le(a−b−c+d−) ABH nonsecretors has been found to contain Le^c-soluble antigens.

Le^d antigen is analogous to the Le^d antigen and is found only in Le(a−b−) secretors; its correct phenotype is Le(a−b−c−d+). Le^d is also thought to be biochemically similar to Le^b. The Le^c- and Le^d-soluble antigens subsequently adsorb (as all Lewis antigens do) to the red cell membrane after exposure to the plasma containing the soluble antigen.

In the rare Bombay phenotype, O$_h$ (see Chapter 5), the individuals cannot synthesize the H, A, B, or Le^b antigens because the H structure as well as the genetic interaction of these various blood groups is necessary for their formation (see Fig. 7–2, **Color Plate 12**; and Fig. 7–5, **Color Plate 13**). As a result, all O$_h$ individuals will have a phenotype of either Le(a+b−), if the Lewis gene (_Le_) is inherited, or Le(a−b−), if the Lewis genotype is _lele_ (Fig. 7–10). A more specific phenotype for the O$_h$ individual of the Lewis genetic makeup (_lele_) would be Le(a−b−c+d−), inasmuch as all O$_h$ individuals are nonsecretors of all ABH substances yet are capable of secreting Le^c substances in the saliva.

To make the Lewis system even more complicated and intriguing, interaction among ABO, H, _Se_, and _Le_ genes results not only in the formation of the Le^a and Le^b substances but also in the compound antigen products ALe^b and BLe^b. This has been confirmed because an anti-A^1 Le^b antibody has been described in the Lewis system. The compound antibody reacts only with red cells that possess both the A$_1$ and Le^b antigenic determinants and is felt to be the result of genetic interaction among the A$_1$, _Le_, H, and _Se_ genes.[23] For a review of the genetic interaction that occurs between the _Le_, H, _Se_, and ABO genes, which results in the various substances found in secretions as well as red cell phenotypes, the reader should study Table 7–8, which gives various hypothetical genotypes.

Le^x AND Le^y

Le^x reactive with anti-Le^x previously discussed is present in every individual who inherits the _Le_ gene, Le(a+b−) or Le(a+b−). This structure is made by addition of an L-fucose to the GlcNAc of the precursor substance before addition of _N_-galactose and formation of the type 1 chain[7,16] (see Fig. 7–8). It is postulated that Le^x (fucose-α (1→4)GlcNAc-R) may represent a hidden determinant of the biochemical structure of both Le^a and Le^b antigens. The use of

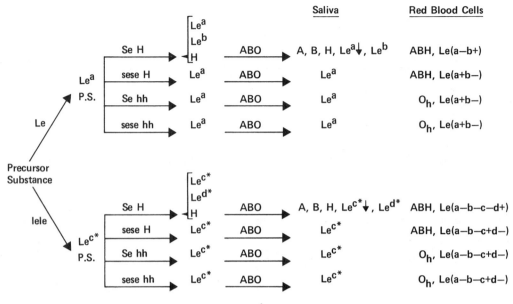

*Provisional place for Le^c and Le^d antigens

FIGURE 7-10 Genetic pathway for the production of the A, B, H, Le^a, and Le^b blood group substances.

protease-treated red cells to enhance reactivity of anti-Le^x antibodies confirms the hidden nature of the Le^x antigen. Some investigators have suggested that Le^x determinant does not represent a separate Lewis antigen. This conclusion was based on studies using hemagglutination inhibition and quantitative passive hemagglutination, which demonstrated the ability of anti-Le^x antibodies to react with traces of Le^b substance present on fetal red cells that were not detectable by anti-Le^a.[16] These techniques demonstrated that the reactivity of anti-Le^x when compared with anti-Le^a shared equal affinity for Le^a determinant.[16] However, according to Watkins et al.[3] and Mollison et al.,[13] Le^x is referred to as a type 2 isomer of Le^a, which is formed by addition of fucose-α (1→3) GlcNAc linkage on type 2 chain (Fig. 7-11). This Le^x is the same antigenic structure called stage-specific embryonic antigen-1 (SSEA-1),[1] which is different from Le^x as a binding site for the anti-Le^x discussed previously. In recent studies three types of α-3-L-fucose transferases have been demonstrated that transfer L-fucose to the three carbon of GlcNAc of type 2 chains. These α-3-L-fucose transferases—myeloid fucosyltransferase, serum α-3-fucosyltransferase, and α-3/4-fucosyltransferase—transfer L-fucose to type 1 and type 2 precursor chains.[22] The fucose transferase that adds L-fucose to type 2 precursor chain is controlled either by *Le* gene or by another gene, possibly called *X*.[22,24] The *X* gene fucose transferase is demonstrated in serum, whereas the *Le* gene fucose transferase is not.

It has been postulated that the expression of α-3-fucosyltransferase is independent of *Le* gene and this enzyme is demonstrated in serum of almost every individual.[3] However, it is worth noting that lack of the

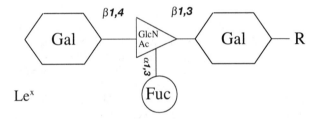

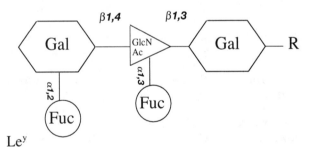

FIGURE 7-11 Structure of Le^x and Le^y from type 2 chains. Gal = D-galactose; GlcNAc = N-acetylglucosamine; R = other biochemical residues.

enzyme α-3-fucosyltransferase has been found in a few nonsecretor individuals who also lack the *Le* gene, and their phenotype was Le(a−b−). This indicates that the *Le* gene and the gene for α-3-fucosyltransferase might be closely linked.

Le^y is defined as a type 2 isomer of Le^b and is made by addition of fucose-α (1→3) GlcNAc linkage on type 2 H substance (Fig. 7-11). Further studies are needed to clarify the discrepancies between type 1 and type 2 Le^x antigenic structures.

Summary

Traditionally, six antigens have been associated with the Lewis system: Le^a, Le^b, Le^c, Le^d, Le^x, and Le^y. All these antigens can be detected in secretions and on red cell (after absorption from plasma). The Lewis system represents a tissue group, inasmuch as Lewis antigens are not synthesized by red cells but rather are adsorbed from plasma. In secretions, these antigens exist as glycoproteins. In plasma and on red cells, they are glycolipids. The structure of the Le^a and Le^b glycosphingolipids from human plasma and red cells has been defined biochemically. Le^a represents a lacto-*N*-fucopentaosyl (II) ceramide, depicted here:

β-Gal(1→3) β-GlcNAc(1→3) β-Gal(1→4)

β-Glc(1→1)Cer

α(1→4)
Fuc

Type 1 chain

Le^b represents a lacto-*N*-difucohexaosyl (1) ceramide, depicted here:

β-Gal(1→3) β-GlcNAC(1→3) β-Gal(1→4)

β-Glc(1→1)Cer

α(1→2) α(1→4)
Fuc   Fuc

Type 1 chain

Le^c is found in *lele* nonsecretors, Le^d in *lele* secretors. The biochemical structure of Le^c and Le^d are type 1 precursor and type 1 H substance, respectively (see Fig. 7–9). Le^c as a compound structure (type 1 and type 2) has also been demonstrated. Le^x as a separate and distinct structure, α-3-fucosyltransferase on type 2 chain, has been detected and is present in the serum

of almost all individuals. The exact gene responsible for expression of Le^x antigen is not fully understood. It is postulated that Le^x antigen might be controlled by a gene other than the *Le* gene. Le^y antigen is defined as type 2 isomer of Le^b. The formation of Lewis antigens adsorbed from plasma is summarized in Figure 7–12.

Case Study

A 35-year-old woman is seen by her obstetrician for prenatal care examination. A blood test for prenatal type and screen showed the following:

ABO-Rh Typing					
Anti-A	Anti-B	Anti-D	Rh Control	A$_1$ Cell	B Cell
O	4+	4+	O	4+	O
Antibody Screen					
		IS	37°C	Antihuman Globulin	
I	R$_1$R$_1$	1+	1+	1+	
II	R$_2$R$_2$	1+	1+	O	

The results of a 10–red cell panel indicate that anti-Le^a and anti-Le^b are present in the patient's serum. The anti-Le^b reactivity is seen only to IS and 37°C, with the 37°C reactivity most likely a carryover from the IS reading. Therefore, anti-Le^b is not clinically significant because it does not react to antihuman globulin.

The anti-Le^a reactivity is present to all phases—IS, 37°C, and antihuman globulin. A prewarmed antibody screen should be performed before considering the anti-Le^a to be clinically significant. The majority of the anti-Le^a antibodies are nonreactive to antihuman globulin using the prewarmed technique.

The results in this case illustrate that:

1. Lewis antibodies are present in the serum of the pregnant woman.

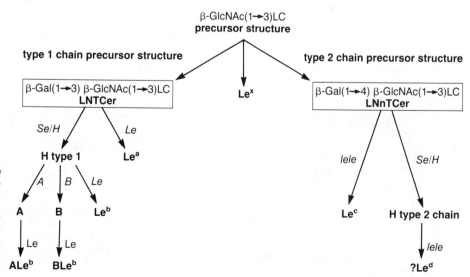

FIGURE 7–12 Summary of the formation of Lewis antigens absorbed from plasma. Le^a, Le^b, Le^c, Le^d, Le^x, ALe^b, and BLe^b. LC = lactosylceramide; LNnTCer = lacto - *N* - neotetraosylceramide; LNTCer = lacto - *N* - tetraosylceramide. (From Harmening-Pittiglio,[25] p 43, with permission.)

2. The antibodies are insignificant or are not associated with HDN, or both, as newborn infants lack the Lewis antigens and IgM antibodies do not cross the placenta.

Review Questions

1. Where are the Lewis antigens produced?
   A. Platelets
   B. Red blood cells
   C. White blood cells
   D. Tissue cells

2. Biochemically, Lewis antigens are classified as _____ in secretions.
   A. Glycoproteins
   B. Glycolipids
   C. Polyproteins
   D. Glycophorins

3. Biochemically, Lewis antigens are classified as _____ in plasma and on red cells. (Use answer choices for question 2.)

4. Which of the following characteristics best describes Lewis antibodies?
   A. IgM, naturally occurring, causes HDN.
   B. IgM, naturally occurring, does not cause HDN.
   C. IgG, in in vitro hemolysis, causes hemolytic transfusion reactions.
   D. IgG, in in vitro hemolysis, does not cause hemolytic transfusion reactions.

5. The *Le* gene codes for a specific glycosyltransferase that transfers an L-fucose to the *N*-acetylglucosamine on:
   A. A type 1 precursor chain
   B. A type 2 precursor chain
   C. Type 1 and 2 precursor chains
   D. Either type 1 or type 2 in any one individual but not in both

6. Secretions of a person with the genes *B, H, Se,* and *Le* will contain the following:
   A. B substance, H substance, Le^a and Le^b substances
   B. B substance, Le^a substance
   C. H substance, Le^a and Le^b substances
   D. H substance, Le^a substance

7. Secretions of a person with the genes *B, H, sese,* and *Le* will contain the following:
   A. B substance, Le^a substance
   B. H substance, Le^a substance
   C. H substance, Le^a and Le^b substance
   D. Le^a substance

8. An individual with genes *A, H, Se,* and *lele* will have the following phenotypes:

A. ABH, Le(a−b−)
B. ABH, Le(a+b−)
C. AH, Le(a−b−)
D. AH, Le(a+b−)

9. Transformation to Le^b phenotype after birth is as follows:
   A. Le(a−b−) to Le(a+b+) to Le(a−b+)
   B. Le(a+b−) to Le(a−b−) to Le(a−b+)
   C. Le(a−b+) to Le(a+b−) to Le(a−b+)
   D. Le(a+b+) to Le(a+b−) to Le(a−b+)

10. In what way do the Lewis antigens change during pregnancy?
    A. Le^a antigen increases only.
    B. Le^b antigen increases only.
    C. Le^a and Le^b both increase.
    D. Le^a and Le^b both decrease.

11. Le^c and Le^d antigens are found in individuals with the phenotype of:
    A. Le(a−b−)
    B. Le(a+b−)
    C. Le(a−b+)
    D. Le(a+b+)

12. Anti-Le^x agglutinates which of the following antigens?
    A. All Le(a+b−) red cells
    B. All Le(a−b+) red cells
    C. All Le(a−b−) red cells
    D. Two of the above

Answers to Review Questions

1. D (p 134)
2. A (p 134)
3. B (p 134)
4. B (p 140)
5. A (p 134)
6. A (p 136)
7. D (p 136)
8. C (p 136)
9. A (p 140)
10. D (p 140)
11. A (p 142)
12. D (p 141)

References

1. Oriol, R, LePendu, J, and Mollicone, R: Genetics of ABO, H, Lewis, X and related antigens. Vox Sang 51:161, 1986.
2. Salmon, C, Cartron, JP, and Rouger, P: The human blood groups. Masson Publishing, New York, 1984, p 162.
3. Watkins, WM, et al: Regulation of expression of carbohydrate blood group antigens. Biochimie 70:1597, 1988.
4. Dunstan, RA: Status of major red cell blood group antigens on neutrophils, lymphocytes, and monocytes. Br J Haematol 62:301, 1986.

5. Dunstan, RA: The expression of ABH antigens during in vitro megakaryocyte maturation: Origin of heterogeneity of antigen density. Br J Haematol 62:587, 1986.

6. Watkins, WM: Blood group substances. In the ABO system the genes control the arrangement of sugar residues that determines blood group specificity. Science 152:172, 1966.

7. Wendell, RF: Clinical Immunohematology: Basic Concept and Clinical Applications. Blackwell Scientific Publications, Oxford, 1990, pp 187–199.

8. Hanfland, P, and Graham, HA: Immunochemistry of the Lewis blood-group system: Partial characterization of Le^a, Le^b, and H-type 1 (Le^{dH}) blood group active glycosphingolipids from human plasma. Arch Biochem Biophys 210:383, 1981.

9. Churchill, WH and Kutz, SR: Transfusion Medicine. Blackwell Scientific Publications, Oxford, 1988, p 57.

10. Hammar, L, et al: Lewis phenotype of erythrocytes and Le^b active glycolipid in serum of pregnant women. Vox Sang 40:27, 1981.

11. Langkilde, NC, Wolf, H, and Orntoft, TF: Letter to the Editor. Lancet 1:926, 1990.

12. Idikio, HA and Manickavel V: Lewis blood group antigens (a and b) in human breast tissues. Loss of Lewis-b in breast cancer cells and correlation with tumor grade. Cancer 68:1303, 1991.

13. Mollison, PL, Engelfriet, CP, and Contreras, M: Blood Transfusion in Clinical Medicine, ed 9. Blackwell Scientific Publications, Oxford, 1993, pp 175–198.

14. Cowles, JW, Spitalnik, SL, and Blumberg, N: The fine specificity of Lewis blood group antibodies. Evidence for maturation of immune response.[1] Vox Sang 56:107, 1989.

15. Cheng, MS, and Lukomskyj, L: Lewis antibody following a massive blood transfusion. Vox Sang 57:155, 1989.

16. Schenkel-Brunner, H, and Hanfland, P: Immunochemistry of the Lewis blood group system. III. Studies on the molecular basis of the Le^x property. Vox Sang 40:358, 1981.

17. Potapov, MI: Detection of the antigen of the Lewis system, characteristic of the erythrocytes of the secretor group Le(a−b−). Probl Hematol Blood Transfus (USSR) 11:45, 1970.

18. Gunson, HH, and Latham, V: An agglutinin in human serum reacting with cells from Le(a−b−) non-secretor individuals. Vox Sang 22:344–353, 1972.

19. Graham, HA, Hirsch, HF, and Davies, DM, Jr: Genetic and immunochemical relationships between soluble and cell-bound antigens of the Lewis system. In Mohn, JF, et al (eds): Human Blood Groups. Proceedings of the Fifth International Convocation on Immunology. Karger, Basel 1977, pp 257–267.

20. Hanfland, P, et al: Immunochemistry of the Lewis blood-group system. FEBS Lett 142:77, 1982.

21. Hanfland, P, et al: Immunochemistry of the Lewis blood-group system: Isolation and structures of Lewis-c active and related glycosphingolipids from the plasma of blood-group O Le(a−b−) nonsecretors.[1] Arch Biochem Biophys 246:655, 1986.

22. Oriol, R: Genetic control of the fucosylation of ABH precursor chains. Evidence for new epstatic interactions in different cells and tissues. J Immunogenet 17:235, 1990.

23. Seaman, MJ, Chalmers, DJ, and Franks, D: Siedler. An antibody which reacts with A, (Le(a−b−) red cells. Vox Sang 15:25, 1968.

24. Watkins, WM: Monoclonal antibodies as tools in genetic studies on carbohydrate blood group antigens. J Immunogenet 17:259, 1990.

25. Harmening-Pittiglio, D: Genetic and biochemistry of A, B, H and Lewis antigens. In Wallace, ME and Gibbs, FL (eds): Blood Group Systems: ABH and Lewis. American Association of Blood Banks, Arlington, VA, 1986, pp 31–43.

Bibliography

Abhyankar, S, et al: Positive cord blood "DAT" due to anti-Le^a: Absence of hemolytic disease of the newborn. Am J Pediatr Hematol Oncol 11:185, 1989.

Bernoco, M, et al: Detection of combined ABH and Lewis glycosphingolipids in sera of deficient donors. Vox Sang 49:58, 1985.

Boorman, KE, Dodd, BE, and Lincoln, PJ: Blood Group Serology, ed 6. Churchill Livingstone, New York, 1988, pp 69–80.

Caillard, T, et al: Failure of expression of alpha-3-fucosyltransferase in human serum is coincident with the absence of the X (or Le(x)) antigen in the kidney but not on leukocytes, Exp Clin Immunogenet 5:15, 1988.

Clausen, H, and Hakomori, S: ABH and related histo-blood group antigens; immunochemical differences in carrier isotypes and their distribution. Vox Sang 56:1, 1989.

Cowles, JW, et al: Comparison of monoclonal antisera with conventional antisera for Lewis blood group antigen determination. Vox Sang 52(1–2):83, 1987.

Hanfland, P, et al: Immunochemistry of the Lewis blood group system: Isolation and structures of Lewis-c active and related glycosphingolipids from the plasma of blood group Le(a−b−) nonsecretors. Arch Biochem Biophys 246:655, 1986.

Issitt, PD: Applied Blood Group Serology, ed 3. Montgomery Scientific Publications, Miami, 1985, pp 169–187.

Le-Pendu, J, et al: Expression of ABH and X (Le^x) antigens in various cells. Biochimie 70:1613, 1988.

Mollicone, R: Expression of ABH and X (Le^x) on platelets and lymphocytes. Blood 71(4):1113, 1988.

Mollicone, R, et al: Acceptor specificity and tissue distribution of three human alpha-3-fucosyltransferase. Eur J Biochem 191:169, 1990.

Mollison, PL, Engelfriet, CP, and Contreras, M: Blood Transfusion in Clinical Medicine, ed 9. Blackwell Scientific Publications, Oxford, 1993, pp 175–198.

Oriol, R: Genetic regulation of the expression of ABH and Lewis antigens in tissues. Apmis (suppl) 27:28, 1992.

Rossi, EC, Simon, TL, and Moss, GS: Principles of Transfusion Medicine. Williams & Wilkins, Baltimore, 1992, p 70.

Shulman, IA: Problem Solving in Immunohematology, ed 4. ASCP Press, Chicago, 1992, pp 62–64.

Turgeon, ML: Fundamentals of Immunohematology: Theory and Technique. Lea & Febiger, Philadelphia, 1989, pp 137–159.

Ura, Y, et al: Quantitative dot blot analyses of blood group related antigens in paired normal and malignant human breast tissues. Int J Cancer 50:57, 1992.

Watkins, WM, et al: Regulation of expression of carbohydrate blood group antigens. Biochimie 70:1597, 1988.

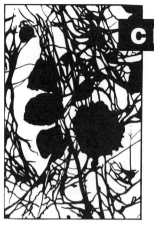

CHAPTER 8

Other Major Blood Group Systems

Loni Calhoun, MT(ASCP)SBB

OBJECTIVES

Upon completion of this chapter, the learner should be able to:

Antigen Characteristics

1 List the antigen frequencies for the common antigens K, M, S, s, Fy^a, Fy^b, Jk^a, Jk^b, and P_1.

2 Define Kp^a, Js^a, and Lu^a as low-frequency antigens and Kp^b, Js^b, Lu^b, and I as high-frequency antigens.

3 Associate the antigen phenotypes S-s-U-, Js(a+), and Fy(a—b—) with blacks.

4 Define the null phenotypes En(a—), U—, M^k, p, K_o, Fy(a—b—), Jk(a—b—), Lu(a—b—) and describe their role in problem solving.

5 Compare both dominant and recessive forms of the Lu(a—b—) and Jk(a—b—) phenotypes.

6 Describe the reciprocal relationship of I antigen to i.

7 Associate I, P_1, and Lutheran antigens as being poorly expressed on cord cells.

8 Define the association of MN with glycophorin A and Ss with glycophorin B.

Antibody Characteristics

9 Define M, N, I, and P_1 antibodies as naturally occurring, room temperature agglutinins that are usually clinically insignificant.

10 Describe K, k, S, s, Fy^a, Fy^b, Jk^a, and Jk^b antibodies as immune, antiglobulin reactive antibodies that are clinically significant.

11 Differentiate the antibody specificities that commonly show dosage (M/N, S/s, K/k, Jk^a/Jk^b) from those that show dosage less easily (Fy^a/Fy^b and Lu^a/Lu^b).

12 Differentiate those antibodies whose reactivity is destroyed by routine blood bank enzymes (M, N, S, s, Fy^a, Fy^b) from those whose reactivity is enhanced (Ii, P_1, Jk^a, Jk^b).

13 List the antibodies in the Kell and Lutheran blood group systems that do not react with 2-aminoethylisothiouronium–treated red cells and those antibodies in the Kell, MNSs, and Duffy systems that do not react with ZZAP-treated red cells.

Clinical Significance and Disease Association

14 Identify or correlate the common 37°C–antihuman globulin–reactive antibodies K, k, S, s, Fy^a, Fy^b, Jk^a, and Jk^b with transfusion reactions and hemolytic disease of the newborn.

15 Describe why Kidd antibodies are a common cause of delayed hemolytic transfusion reactions.

16 Describe the association of autoanti-I with *Mycoplasma pneumoniae* infections and autoanti-i with infectious mononucleosis.

17 Describe the common characteristics of the McLeod phenotype, including very weak Kell antigen expression, acanthocytosis, and late onset of muscular dystrophy – like syndrome.

18 Describe the association of the Fy(a−b−) phenotype with *Plasmodium vivax* resistance.

19 Identify Jk(a−b−) red cells with an inability to lyse normally in 2M urea, a common diluting fluid used for automated platelet counters.

20 Define those autoantibodies that sometimes have specificity to antigens in certain blood group systems and describe why the strength of the corresponding antigen sometimes weakens during this time.

This chapter contains more information than blood bank technologists or technicians need to work capably at the bench. It is hoped that the extra details will challenge them to learn more and serve as a good reference when the antigens and antibodies are encountered in real-life situations.

Students need information "in a nutshell," however, summarized for easy review. This has been provided on the front and back inside covers of this book. Students should review the objectives, read the material, then refer to the antigen-antibody characteristic chart to see how much they really know.

Terminology

A blood group system is a group of antigens produced by alleles at a single gene locus or at loci so closely linked that crossing over does not occur or is very rare.[1] With a few notable exceptions, most blood group genes are located on the autosomal chromosomes and are inherited in straightforward mendelian fashion.

Most blood group alleles are codominant and express a corresponding antigen. For example, a person who inherits alleles *K* and *k* carries both K and k antigens on his or her red cells. Some genes code for complex structures that carry more than one antigen (e.g., the glycophorin B structure that carries S or s antigen also carries 'N' and U specificity).

Silent or amorphic alleles that produce no antigen are rare. When paired chromosomes carry the same silent allele, a null phenotype results. Red cells with null phenotypes can be very helpful when evaluating antibodies to unknown high-frequency antigens. For example, an antibody reacting with all test cells except those with the phenotype Lu(a−b−) is directed against the antigens in the Lutheran system or an antigen phenotypically related to the Lutheran system.

Some blood group systems have regulator or modifying genes that alter antigen expression. These are not necessarily located at the same locus as the blood group genes they affect and may segregate independently. One such modifying gene is *In(Lu)*, which inhibits or suppresses the expression of all the antigens in the Lutheran blood group system as well as many other antigens including P_1 and i. It is a rare dominant gene inherited independently of Lutheran, P, and Ii.

Although gene and antigen names seem confusing at first, certain conventions are followed when writing alleles, antigens, and phenotypes.[1] Some examples are given in Table 8–1. Genes are underlined or written in italics and their allele number or letter is usually superscript. Antigen names are not italicized and are most easily learned by everyday use. Phenotype designation depends on the antigen nomenclature and whether letters or numbers are used. These are also best learned through use. It is not appropriate to refer to an antigen by its system or historic name (e.g., the antigens Fy[a] and K are called "Fya" and "Big K," not "Duffy A" and "Kell"). Antibodies are described by their antigen notation with the prefix "anti-".

TABLE 8–1 **EXAMPLES OF CORRECT BLOOD GROUP TERMINOLOGY**

| Gene | Antigen | PHENOTYPE | | BLOOD GROUP | |
		Antigen Positive	Antigen Negative	Antibody	System
K	K	K+	K−	Anti-K	Kell
Jk[a]	Jk[a]	Jk(a+)	Jk(a−)	Anti-Jk[a]	Kidd
P[1k]	P_1	P_1+	P_1−	Anti-P_1	P
Fy[4]	Fy4	Fy:4	Fy:−4	Anti-Fy4	Duffy

To help standardize blood group system and antigen names, the International Society of Blood Transfusion (ISBT) Working Party of Terminology for Red Cell Surface Antigens has devised a numeric system based on nomenclature first proposed by Rosenfield and colleagues.[2] Each known system is given a number and letter designation, and each antigen within the system is numbered sequentially in order of discovery. For example, the Kell blood group system is 006 or KEL; the K antigen is 006001 or KEL1.

One must remember that serologic tests determine only red cell phenotype, not genotype. Genotype is determined usually by family studies. Genetic studies and statistic analyses of inheritance data are required before an antigen is assigned to a blood group system.

Evaluating Antigen Biochemistry

Although blood bank personnel use routine serologic methods to detect red cell antigens, researchers use new technical advances to analyze their biochemistry. Because these methods contribute so greatly to our knowledge of antigen biochemistry, inheritance, and function, students should understand the principles behind some of the basic research tools.[3]

To prepare red cell membranes for antigen analysis, a large volume of cells is lysed osmotically to produce ghost cells. Intact ghost cell membranes can be stained or labeled for proteins, but more often they are dissociated first into lipid and protein components. Lipids are separated with organic solvents; loosely bound proteins are solubilized by changing pH or ionic strength or by using chelating agents; and tightly bound proteins are solubilized with detergents. Sodium dodecyl sulfate (SDS), an anionic detergent that also dissociates complex proteins into smaller polypeptides, is most commonly used.

Solubilized membrane proteins are separated from one another using polyacrylamide gel electrophoresis (PAGE). The porous gel allows small molecules to move freely but retards the movement of larger ones. Protein migration depends on molecular size and charge. When SDS and PAGE are used together, the negative charge of the detergent overpowers the charge of the protein and separation occurs by size alone. By comparing relative electrophoresis mobilities with SDS-PAGE, protein molecular weights can be determined. SDS-PAGE analysis has become a basic tool for studying solubilized membrane protein.

After proteins are separated, the electrophoretic bands are stained by one of several methods: Coomassie blue R 250, which stains protein; or periodic acid–Schiff (PAS), which stains carbohydrates. Bands detected with PAS represent glycoprotein. The common membrane proteins identified with SDS-PAGE and Coomassie blue/PAS stains are summarized elsewhere.[1,4,5] Some help maintain red cell shape and structure; others are associated with glycophorin structures, which carry MNSs and other antigens.

Membrane proteins can also be separated according to their biologic activity by passing them through affinity chromatography columns. The support media in a column can be coupled with specific antibodies, lectins, membrane receptors, or special enzymes. Only high-affinity proteins will bind; others can be washed away. Once isolated, the bound protein can be eluted and its amino acid sequence determined.

The carbohydrates attached to glycoproteins and glycolipids also can be studied. Glycopeptide linkages (i.e., where sugars attach to protein) have been found to be either N-glycosidic (N-acetylglucosamine [GlcNAc] attached to asparagine [Asn]) or O-glycosidic (sugars, usually N-acetylgalactosamine [GalNAc] or galactose [Gal], attached to serine [Ser] or threonine [Thr]). The sugars within a carbohydrate chain itself are sequenced by systematically degrading or removing them with specific glycosidase enzymes.

The MNSs Blood Group System

Following the discovery of the ABO blood group system, Landsteiner and Levine began immunizing rabbits with human red cells, hoping to find new antigen specificities. Among the antibodies recovered from these rabbit sera were anti-M and anti-N, both of which were reported in 1927.[6,7] Data from family studies suggested that the genes coding for M and N were alleles to one another. Thus, MN became a blood group system.

In 1947, after the implementation of the antiglobulin test, Walsh and Montgomery[8] discovered S, a distinct antigen genetically linked to MN. Its antithetical partner, s, was found in 1951,[9] and the MN system became MNSs, a two-loci system.

In 1953, an antibody to a high-frequency antigen, U, was reported by Wiener et al.[10] The observation by Greenwalt et al.[11] that all U− red cells were also S−s− resulted in the inclusion of U in the system. The phenotypic frequencies of MN and Ss are listed in Table 8–2, along with some key facts.

TABLE 8–2 FREQUENCY OF MNSs PHENOTYPES AND KEY FACTS*

Phenotype	Whites (%)	Blacks (%)
M+N−	28	26
M+N+	50	44
M−N+	22	30
S+s−	11	3
S+s+	44	28
S−s+	45	69
S−s−U−	0	<1

*Antigens: Well developed at birth.
Antibodies: Anti-MN: Clinically insignificant; some examples are pH/glucose dependent.
Anti-Ss: Clinically significant.
Reactivity is destroyed by enzymes; S reactivity is also destroyed by bleach.
Usually show dosage.

Since these initial discoveries, many other antigens have been described, making the MNSs system equal to Rh in size and complexity (Table 8–3). Many of these represent low-frequency variants of the structures associated with MNSs activity. Some behave as antithetical antigens to MNSs; others as extra antigens inherited along with MNSs. Some are high-frequency antigens, representing epitopes on the basic protein carrying MN or Ss activity.

To recognize its early discovery, the MNSs system is assigned the ISBT numeric designation 002, second after ABO.

TABLE 8–3 **SUMMARY OF MNSs ANTIGENS**

Number	Common Name	Alternate Name	Frequency (%)	Year Discovered	Comments
			I. Common Antigens Encoded by MNSs Loci		
1	M	—	78	1927	GPA aa1-5:Ser-Ser-Thr-Thr-Gly
2	N	—	72	1927	GPA aa1-5:Leu-Ser-Thr-Thr-Glu
3	S	—	55	1947	GPB aa29:Met
4	s	—	89	1951	GPB aa29:Thr
			II. Low-Frequency Antigens Encoded by MNSs Loci		
6	He	Henshaw	0.8	1951	Variant GPB
(7)	Mi^a	Miltenberger	<1	1951	See Miltenberger subsystem
8	M^c	—	<0.1	1953	GPA aa1-5:Ser-Ser-Thr-Thr-Glu
9	Vw	Verweyst	<1	1954	See Miltenberger subsystem
10	Mur	Murrell	<0.1	1961	See Miltenberger subsystem
11	M^g	Gilfeather	<0.01	1958	GPA aa1-5:Leu-Ser-Thr-Asn-Glu
12	V^r	Verdegaal	<0.1	1958	—
13	M^e	—	<1	1961	Factor common to M and He
14	Mt^a	—	0.25	1962	—
15	St^a	Stones	<0.1	1962	—
16	Ri^a	Ridley	<0.1	1962	—
17	Cl^a	Caldwell	<0.1	1963	—
18	Ny^a	Nyberg	<0.1	1964	—
19	Hut	Hutchinson	<0.1	1966	See Miltenberger subsystem
20	Hil	Hill	<0.1	1966	See Miltenberger subsystem
21	M^v	Armstrong	<0.6	1966/1980	Variant GPB
22	Far	Kamhuber	<0.1	1977	—
23	s^D	Dreyer	<0.01	1981	Variant s-SGP?
24	Mit	Mitchell	0.12	1980	—
25	Dantu	—	<0.1	1981/1984	GPB-GPA hybrid
26	Hop	—	<0.1	1982	See Miltenberger subsystem
27	Nob	—	<0.1	1982	See Miltenberger subsystem
29	En^{a}KT	—	<0.1	1985	GPA-GPB hybrid
31	Or	Orrill	(Low)	1987	Variant GPB
32	DANE	—	(Low)	1991	See Miltenberger subsystem
33	TSEN	—	(Low)	1992	GPA-GPB^S hybrid junction
34	MINY	—	(Low)	1992	GPA-GPB hybrid junction
			III. High-Frequency Antigens Encoded by MNSs Loci		
5	U	—	>99.9	1953	Common Ss-SGP
28	En^a	—	>99.9	1969	Common MN-SGP
30	'N'	—	>99.9	1978	Common Ss-SGP
			IV. Antigens Associated With MNSs but Biochemistry/Genetics Uncertain		
	Hu	Hunter	<1W/7B	1934	Altered MN-SGP?; 53% are Tm+
	M$_1$	—	<1W/16B	1960	M1:M as A1:A; altered CHO
	Sul	Sullivan	<0.1	1967	—
	Sj	Stenbar-James	2W/4B	1968	All Sj+ are N+
	Can	Canner	27W/60B	1979	M with NeuNAc
	Tm	Sheerin	25W/31B	1965	Altered N-SGP; O-CHO
	Shier	—	Rare	1969	Many Shier+ are N+Tm+
	M^A	—	78	1966	Subfactor of M?
	N^A	—	72	1971	Subfactor of N?
	U^x	—	>99.9	1978	Associated with MN/Ss-SGP
	U^z	—	>99.9	1972	Associated with Ss-SGP

B = blacks; W = whites.

BASIC CONCEPTS

MN Antigens

The M and N antigens are found on a well-characterized glycoprotein called MN-sialoglycoprotein (MN-SGP), α-sialoglycoprotein (α-SGP), or glycophorin A (GPA). The antigens are defined by the first and fifth amino acid (aa) on this structure (see Biochemistry subsection farther on, and Figure 8–1), but antibody reactivity may also encompass nearby carbohydrate chains that are rich in sialic acid.

There are about 10^6 copies of MN-SGP/red cell.[12] The antigens exhibit dosage. For example, red cells from people who are homozygous *MM* carry a double dose of the M antigen and react more strongly with anti-M than do red cells from heterozygous *MN* individuals who carry only a single dose of M.

The antigens can be detected as early as 9 weeks' gestational age and they are well developed at birth. This makes them very useful in paternity exclusion cases involving newborn infants or the very young (when only well-developed antigens can be reliably typed).

Because MN antigens are at the outer end of GPA, they are easily destroyed or removed by the routine blood bank enzymes ficin, papain, and bromelin, and by less common enzymes trypsin and pronase. The antigens are also destroyed by ZZAP, a solution of dithiothreitol (DTT) and papain, but they are not affected by DTT alone or by 2-aminoethylisothiouronium bromide (AET). They are slightly depressed with chymotrypsin. Treating red cells with neuraminidase, which cleaves sialic acid (also known as neuraminic acid [NeuNAc]) abolishes reactivity with only some examples of antibody. MN antibodies can be heterogeneous: some may recognize only specific amino acids, whereas others recognize both amino acids and carbohydrate chains.

M and N are primarily red cell antigens. Although older data suggested that M antigen may be present on lymphocytes,[13] M and N were not detected on lymphocytes, monocytes, or granulocytes by immunofluorescence flow cytometry;[14] nor have they been detected on platelets. MN antigens have been detected on renal capillary endothelium.[15] This is especially interesting because a strain of *Escherichia coli* associated with urinary tract infection has been identified as having recognition sites for the NH_2 terminal end of M-SGP.[16]

Ss Antigens

Ss antigens are located on a glycoprotein very similar to MN called Ss-sialoglycoprotein (Ss-SGP), δ-SGP, or glycophorin B (GPB) (see Biochemistry and Figure 8–1). The aa at position 29 on GPB is critical to antigen expression—S has methionine, whereas s has threonine—but the epitope may also include the glutamic acid residue at position 28 and the glycosidic chain attached to threonine at position 25.[17] Ss-SGP complexes with Rh protein, which helps Ss-SGP stabilize or incorporate into the red cell membrane.[5] Rh_{null} red cells have greatly reduced Ss expression.

There are about 2.5×10^5 copies of Ss-SGP/red cell,[12] but not all of these may be available for antibody attachment. Masouredis et al.[18] found only 12,000 available s sites on *ss* red cells. Data also suggest that red cells from *SS* people carry more copies of GPB than those from *ss* people.[17] Like MN, Ss antigens exhibit dosage. They also are well developed at birth and appear on red cells at an early gestational age (12 weeks).

The Ss antigens are less easily degraded by enzymes because the antigens are located farther down the glycoprotein, and enzyme-sensitive sites are less accessible. Ficin, papain, bromelin, propase, and chymotrypsin can destroy Ss activity, but the amount of degradation may depend on the strength of the enzyme solution, length of treatment, and enzyme-to-cell ratio. Trypsin does not destroy Ss activity; neither does AET. Weak concentrations (0.0005 to 0.005 percent) of sodium hypochlorite, or common household bleach, selectively destroy S reactivity by oxidizing the methionine amino acid at position 29. Such bleach-treated cells can be useful in identifying antibodies found in combination with anti-S.[19] Like MN, Ss are considered red cell antigens. They are not found on platelets, lymphocytes, monocytes, and granulocytes.[14]

Anti-M

Most examples of anti-M are naturally occurring, cold-reactive saline agglutinins. Although we may think of them as IgM, 50 to 80 percent are IgG or have an IgG component.[1] They usually do not bind complement, regardless of their immunoglobulin class, and they do not react with enzyme-treated red cells. The frequency of finding saline reactive anti-M in routine blood donors is 1 in 2500 to 5000.[14] It appears to be more common in infants than in adults.

Because of antigen dosage, M antibodies react better with M+N− red cells (genotype *MM*) than with M+N+ red cells (genotype *MN*). Very weak anti-M may not react with M+N+ red cells at all, making panel identification difficult. Antibody reactivity can be enhanced by increasing the serum-to-cell ratio or incubation time, or both, by decreasing incubation temperature or by adding potentiating medias such as albumin or low-ionic strength solution (LISS).

Some examples of anti-M are pH dependent, reacting best at pH 6.5. These may be detected in plasma, which is slightly acidic from the anticoagulant, but not in unacidified serum. It is suggested that their antibody-binding site includes the histidine residue at position 9 on M-SGP, because its steric orientation is known to vary with pH.[1]

Other examples of anti-M react only with red cells exposed to glucose solutions. Such antibodies react with M+ reagent red cells or donor cells stored in preservative solutions containing glucose but not with freshly collected M+ cells. The significance of both

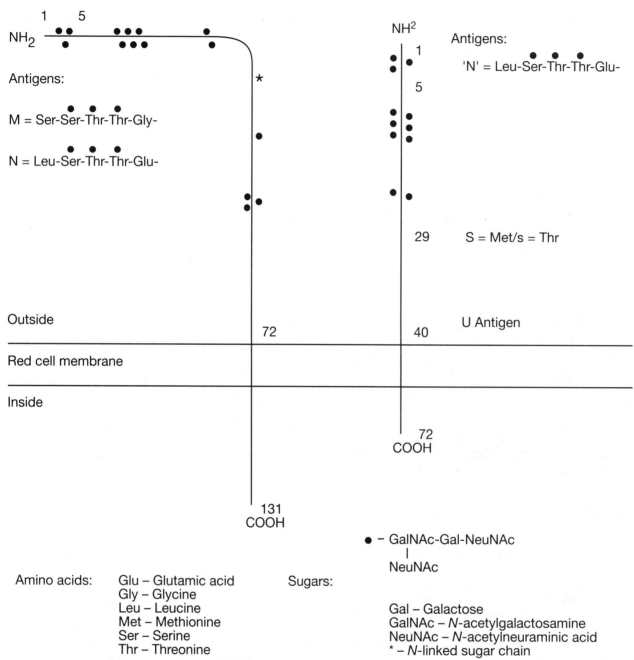

FIGURE 8-1 Comparison of MN and Ss-SGP.

pH and glucose-dependent antibodies in transfusion is questionable.

As long as anti-M does not react at 37°C, it is not clinically significant in transfusion. It is sufficient to provide units that are crossmatch compatible at 37°C and in the antiglobulin phase without typing for M antigen. Sometimes compatible units carry the M antigen (e.g., M+N+ red cells, which do not react with weak anti-M). Only rarely do such units stimulate a change in the antibody's thermal range.

Anti-M rarely causes hemolytic transfusion reactions, decreased cell survival, or hemolytic disease of the newborn (HDN). However, when 37°C-reactive IgG anti-M is found in a pregnant woman, her physician should be forewarned; some HDN cases have been severe.[1]

Anti-N

The serologic characteristics of anti-N are similar to those of anti-M: it is a cold-reactive IgM or IgG saline agglutinin that does not bind complement or react with enzyme-treated red cells. It demonstrates dosage, reacting better with M−N+ (*NN*) red cells than with M+N+ (*MN*) ones. Rare examples are glucose dependent, as are some anti-M.[20]

Also like anti-M, anti-N is not clinically significant unless it reacts at 37°C. It has only been implicated with rare cases of HDN.

Anti-N is more rare than anti-M because the terminal end of Ss-SGP carries the same amino acid sequence and sugars as the N antigen on GPA. This N-like structure, called 'N', may prevent N− individuals from recognizing N as a foreign antigen. In a series of 86,000 patients, only two examples of anti-N were seen.[14] The most potent antibodies are found in rare individuals who type M+N−S−s− and lack N and 'N'.

Anti-N is also seen in renal patients, regardless of their MN type, who are dialyzed on equipment sterilized by formaldehyde. Dialysis-associated anti-N reacts with any N+ or N− red cell treated with formaldehyde and is called anti-N^f. Formaldehyde may alter the MN antigen so that it is recognized as foreign. The antibody titer decreases when dialysis treatment and exposure to formaldehyde stops. Because anti-N^f does not react at 37°C, it is clinically insignificant in transfusion. However, it has been associated with the rejection of a chilled transplanted kidney.[21]

Anti-S and Anti-s

Most examples of anti-S and anti-s are IgG, reactive at 37°C in the antiglobulin phase. A few express optimal reactivity at colder temperatures. If S or s specificity is suspected, incubating tests at room temperature or colder and performing a "cold" antiglobulin test may help in its identification.

The antibodies may or may not react with enzyme-treated red cells, depending on the degree of treatment. Treated red cells should be tested for Ss reactivity with known antisera before enzyme reactions are interpreted. As discussed earlier, anti-S will not react with bleach-treated cells.

Although seen less often than anti-M, Ss antibodies are more likely to be clinically significant. They may bind complement, and they have been implicated with severe hemolytic transfusion reaction with hemoglobinuria. They have also caused HDN.

Units selected for transfusion must be antigen negative and crossmatch compatible. Because only 11 percent of whites and 3 percent of blacks are s−, providing blood for a patient with anti-s can be difficult. S− units are much easier to find (45 percent of whites and 69 percent of blacks are S−), but antibodies to low-frequency antigens are commonly found in sera containing anti-S,[14] and these can cause unexplained incompatible crossmatches.

ADVANCED CONCEPTS

Biochemistry

MN-SGP or GPA has a molecular weight of 36 kD and contains 131 aa.[22] The hydrophilic NH$_2$ terminal end, which lies outside the red cell membrane, has 71 aa residues, 15 O-glycosidically linked oligosaccharide chains (GalNAc-Ser/Thr), and 1 N-glycosidic chain (sugar-Asn). The portion that traverses the membrane is hydrophobic and contains 29 aa. The hydrophilic COOH end of the peptide chain, which contains 21 aa and no carbohydrates, lies inside the membrane and interacts weakly with the membrane cytoskeleton. MN antigens differ in their aa residue at positions 1 and 5 (Fig. 8−1): M has serine and glycine at these positions, whereas N has leucine and glutamic acid.

The Ss-SGP or GPB has a molecular weight of 20 kD and contains 72 aa and 11 O-linked oligosaccharide chains.[22] It has an outer glycosylated portion of 39 aa and a hydrophobic portion of about 31 aa that traverses the red cell membrane. The small remaining "tail" may imbed in the lipid layer or may rest at the surface of the cytoplasmic compartment.

Because the first 26 aa on GPA are identical to those on GPB, cells truly negative for N were not found and researchers thought perhaps N was a precursor to M. We now call the N-like structure on GPB 'N' and recognize that it can react with some anti-N. Other similarities between GPA and GPB exist: GPB residues 27 to 35 and 46 to 71 are almost identical to GPA residues 59 to 67 and 75 to 100, respectively. However, the middle portion of GPB has no counterpart on GPA, and GPB carries no N-linked carbohydrate chain on aa 26.

Most O-linked carbohydrate structures on GPA and GPB are branched tetrasaccharides containing one GalNAc, one Gal, and two NeuNAc (sialic acid). Heterogeneity does occur within these chains — they can lack a sugar or have sugar substitutions[5,17] — but their significant feature is NeuNAc, which helps give the red cell its negative charge. About 70 percent of a red cell's NeuNAc is carried by GPA; about 16 percent by GPB.[17]

Other antigens within the MNSs system have been evaluated biochemically (Table 8−3). Some have altered GPA because of aa substitutions or changes in carbohydrate chains, or both. Others appear to be variants of GPB. Still others are hybrids of both GPA and GPB, probably arising from gene crossover during meiosis. Such hybrid structures can have the outer NH$_2$ portion of GPA attached to the inner COOH end of GPB, or vice versa. This results in changes in glycosylation, changes in molecular weight, loss of high-frequency antigens, appearance of novel low-frequency antigens, and alterations in the expression of MNSs antigens.[17,23]

Both GPA and GPB can exist in dimeric form in the red cell membrane. Whereas GPB appears to complex with Rh protein, GPA most likely associates with Protein Band 3. The area of association between GPA or

GPB with these other structures may give rise to additional antigen specificities.[12]

The heterogeneity of GPA and GPB leads to speculation about their physiologic function. Red cells that lack GPA or GPB are not associated with disease or decreased survival. Perhaps these glycoproteins and their negative charge prevent red cells from adhering to each other or to vessel walls. Perhaps the water attracted to their carbohydrates helps protect red cells from damage during circulation.[1]

Genetics

The genes that code for GPA and GPB represent two closely linked loci on the long arm of chromosome 4. The known alleles for *GPA* (i.e., *M/N*) and *GPB* (i.e., *S/s*) are codominant. Because of their many similarities and primate antigen studies, it is thought that *GPB* arose from a duplication of an ancestral *GPA* gene and that the other alleles arose by further point mutations.[1,22] The most common gene complex is *Ns*, followed by *Ms*, *MS*, then *NS*.

GPA is organized into seven exons (portions that are translated into functional protein—the unused portions or introns are spliced out): A1 encodes for a leader protein, which helps insert the structure into the membrane during formation; A2 encodes the first 26 aa; A3 has inverted repeat sequences known to be sites for DNA recombination; A4, the remaining extracellular portion; A5, the transmembrane protein; A6 and A7, the cytoplasmic portion.[22] A7 also contains the stop code.

In size and arrangement *GPB* is similar to *GPA* but has only five exons: B1 and B2, which are nearly identical to A1 and A2, encode a leader protein and aa 1 through 26; B3 is analogous to A4, encoding the portion of the molecule that carries Ss; B4 is similar to A5, encoding a larger transmembrane portion because of a mutation that affects a messenger RNA splice site; B5 encodes the cytoplasmic portion and final stop code. There is no A3 counterpart because of another splice site mutation, nor is there an A6 or an A7 counterpart.

Now that the genetic complexity of GPA and GPB is understood, it is easy to account for the variant alleles. There may be point mutations, deletions, and unequal pairing with subsequent recombination (Fig. 8–2), resulting in hybrids. A *GPA-GPB* hybrid (called Lepore type for a similar hemoglobin hybrid) encodes only altered structures that contain the beginning NH$_2$ end of GPA and the COOH end of GPB. A *GPB-GPA* hybrid (called anti-Lepore type) encodes normal GPA, normal GPB, as well as a hybrid structure that contains the NH$_2$ end of GPA and the COOH end of GPA.[22,23]

M and N Lectins

A number of plant lectins have proved useful in studying MN-SGP biochemistry, some with a practical application.[1,24] Those having N reactivity include *Bau-*

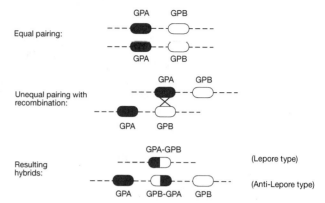

FIGURE 8-2 How unequal pairing and recombination during meiosis can lead to *GPA-GPB* hybrids.

hinia variegata, B. candicans, B. bonatiana, B. purpura, and *Vicia graminea. V. graminea* lectin is most commonly used. It reacts with the *O*-linked tetrasaccharides near the NH$_2$ end of M- and N-SGP, but when properly diluted it will appear to react only with N-SGP and so makes an appropriate typing reagent.[1]

Anti-M reactivity has been found in seeds from the plants *Iberis amara, I. umbellata, I. semperivens,* and the Japanese turnip. *Maclura aurantiaca,* made from the Osage orange, reacts with the tetrasaccharides on both M-SGP and N-SGP and has been used to screen for rare red cells lacking MN-SGP.[24]

When antigen typing red cells with lectins, one must keep in mind that only specific carbohydrate structures are recognized by these reagents. Results may not parallel those obtained with human antibody or other lectins, especially when altered or variant SGPs are tested.

Null Phenotypes

U Negative Phenotype The U (for "universal") antigen is located on Ss-SGP very close to the red cell membrane, and its steric presentation may be influenced by nearby protein and lipid structures.[17] This high-frequency antigen is found in all individuals except about 1 percent of American blacks (and 1 to 35 percent of African blacks[22]), who lack Ss-SGP because of a partial or complete deletion of *GPB*. They usually type S—s—U— and make anti-U in response to transfusion or pregnancy.

Not all examples of anti-U react the same with U— red cells.[24] Some cells absorb and elute anti-U and are referred to as U variants. It may be that "true" U— individuals lack Ss-SGP, whereas those having U variants have lost only part, or had aa substitutions or changes in surrounding lipids so that expression is altered. Because U antibodies are individualistic, U— units selected for transfusion must be crossmatched. Simply knowing the unit types U— does not guarantee it will be compatible. To complicate matters, even an antihuman globulin (AHG) crossmatch may not detect a U-variant cell. Some patients may tolerate a U-variant unit; others may not. Additionally, when the antibody producer is also N−, the antibody may actually have N, 'N', and U specificity. These units are even more difficult to find.

As mentioned earlier, Rh$_{null}$ and Rh$_{mod}$ individuals have less Ss-SGP and may appear U−. However, U is present and can be confirmed by absorption-elution.

The antigens U^x and U^z are not U variants, but rather distinct antigens in the MNSs system. They were given a U designation because some examples of anti-U block the site with which their antibody reacts. U^x appears to involve NeuNAc containing receptors within the outer portions of MN and Ss-SGP. U^z may be located between aa residue 29 to 40 on Ss-SGP.[17]

En^a Negative Phenotype In 1969, Darnborough et al.[25] and Furuhjelm et al.[26] described an antibody to a high-frequency antigen, called En^a (for "envelope"), which reacted with all cells except those of the propositi. Both En(a−) individuals appeared to be M−N− with reduced NeuNAc on their red cells, but had normal Ss expression.

Although the gene responsible for this phenotype has been termed *En*, it is now known that Finnish En(a−) individuals lack MN-SGP because of a complete or nearly complete deletion of *GPA*. English En(a−) individuals have a Lepore type *GPA-GPB* hybrid gene that encodes a small amount of M (designated 'M') and S.

Most En(a−) adults produce anti-En^a, which defines portions of GPA unrelated to M or N, and not all antibodies detect the same portion. For example, anti-En^{a}TS recognizes a trypsin-sensitive (TS) area on GPA between residues 20 and 39. Anti-En^{a}FS reacts with a ficin-sensitive (FS) area between residues 46 and 56, and anti-En^{a}FR reacts with a ficin-resistant (FR) area around residues 62 to 70.[17]

Wr(a−b−) Phenotype In 1975, Issitt et al.[27] discovered that En(a−) red cells were Wr(a−b−), which led to much speculation about the association of Wr^b with MN-SGP. Wr^b was described 4 years earlier as the high-frequency antithetic antigen to Wr^a.[28] Red cells of the original Wr(a+b−) propositus had normal En^a antigen and MN-SGP, so there was no previous association of Wr^b with MN. In fact, Wr and MN appear to be genetically independent. The ISBT has placed Wr^a and Wr^b in the antigen collection 211 and designated them 211001 and 211002, respectively.

Wr^b, like En^{a}FR, is protease-resistant and thought to be associated with MN-SGP near the red cell membrane. Recent studies suggest that antigen activity lies between residues 65 and 70 and results from interaction of this region with another membrane component; the primary candidate is protein band 3.[12]

M^k Phenotype The rare silent gene *M^k* was identified in 1964 by Metaxas and Metaxas-Buhler[29] in the heterozygous state when they studied an M−N+ (*NM^k*) mother who had an M+N− (*MM^k*) child. The red cells of these rare individuals expressed half the amount of normal MN and Ss on SDS-PAGE analysis. In 1979,

Tokunaga et al.[30] reported finding two related homozygous *M^{k}M^k* blood donors in Japan. These null individuals typed M−N−S−s−U− but had a normal hematologic picture. Three more have been identified since, and it is now known that the *M^k* gene represents a single, near-complete deletion of both *GPA* and *GPB*.[22]

The Miltenberger Subsystem

The Miltenberger subsystem was developed to explain the relationship of several very low–frequency antigens in the MNSs blood group system. They appeared to be related to one another because red cells containing one of these antigens often had more than one, which would be statistically unlikely if they were genetically independent.

After the first five antigens were defined, Cleghorn performed a series of cross tests with their respective antibodies and separated the red cells into five classes or phenotypes: Mi^I, Mi^{II}, Mi^{III}, Mi^{IV}, and Mi^V.[31] These classes have been redefined and expanded to nine with the discovery of additional antigens (Table 8–4).[32,33] Reactions with the original Miltenberger serum (anti-Mi^a) have been included for historic reasons, but Mi^a is no longer thought to be an antigenic determinant as the serum was later found to contain anti-V^w plus anti-MUT.[33]

Biochemical and molecular studies have simplified our understanding of the Miltenberger classes. Each class represents a distinct variant GPA or hybrid molecule; these are summarized in Table 8–4. Tippett et al.[33] proposed that the Miltenberger terminology be dropped in favor of one that recognizes the glycoprotein and the name of the first propositus. Many other variant MN glycoproteins associated with the Miltenberger phenotypes are described in the article by Tippett et al.[33]

Other Antibodies in the MNSs System

Antibodies to antigens other than M, N, S, and s are rarely encountered and can usually be grouped into two categories: those directed against low-frequency antigens and those directed against higher-frequency antigens.

Antibodies to higher-frequency antigens are easily detected with antibody screening cells. Antibodies to low-frequency antigens are rarely detected by the antibody screen but are seen as an unexpected incompatible crossmatch or an unexplained case of HDN. Few hospital blood banks have the test cells available to identify the specificity, but enzyme reactivity and MNSs antigen typings may offer clues.

It is common practice with these antibodies to transfuse units that are crossmatch compatible at 37°C and in the antiglobulin phase—an easy task if the antigen frequency is low but quite a difficult one if it is high. Typing sera for other MNSs specificities are

TABLE 8–4 **THE MILTENBERGER SUBSYSTEM**[32,33]

Current Class	Proposed[33] Terminology	(Mi^a)*	Vw	Mur	Hil	Hut	Hop	Nob	DANE	MUT	TSEN	MINY	Biochemistry
Mi.I	GP.Vw	+	+	0	0	0	0	0	0	0	0	0	GPA: aa28 Thr→Met
Mi.II	GP.Hut	+	0	0	0	+	0	0	0	+	0	0	GPA: aa28 Thr→Lys
Mi.III	GP.Mur	+	0	+	+	0	0	0	0	+	0	+	GPB-GPA-GPB: aa29 Thr †
Mi.IV	GP.Hop	+	0	+	0	0	+	0	0	+	+	+	GPB-GPA-GPB: aa29 Thr †
Mi.V	GP.Hil	0	0	0	+	0	0	0	0	0	0	+	GPA-GPB: aa29 Thr
Mi.VI	GP.Bun	+	0	+	+	0	+	0	0	+	0	+	GPB-GPA-GPB: aa29 Thr †
Mi.VII	GP.Nob	0	0	0	0	0	0	+	0	0	0	0	GPA: aa49 Arg→Thr aa52 Thr→Ser
Mi.VIII	GP.Joh	0	0	0	0	0	+	+	0	0	NT	0	GPA: aa 48 Arg→Thr
Mi.IX	GP.Dane	0	0	+	0	0	0	0	+	0	0	0	Variant GPA— molecular structure not known

*Mi^a is no longer considered an antigen (see text).
†Double crossover; associated with normal GPA and a GP(B-A-B) hybrid.
NT = not tested.

not generally available, so the antigen status of compatible units seldom can be confirmed.

Autoantibodies

Autoantibodies to M, N, and S have been reported but are very rare. Autoantibodies to U, En^a, and Wr^b are more common and may be associated with warm-type autoimmune hemolytic anemia.

Not all examples of anti-M in M+ individuals or anti-N in N+ individuals are autoantibodies. Many fail to react with the patient's own cells. It may be that these individuals have altered MN-SGP and that their antibody is specific for a portion of the common SGP that they lack.

Disease Associations

As already mentioned, M-SGP may serve as the receptor by which certain pyelonephritogenic strains of *E. coli* gain entry to the urinary tract.

The malaria parasite *Plasmodium falciparum* may use sites associated with the glycophorins or the NeuNAc attached to glycophorins, or both, for cell invasion. In an attempt to identify the receptor, its invasion rate into cells with normal and rare phenotypes has been studied. Reduced invasion is seen with En(a−) cells, U− cells, M^kM^k cells, Tn and Cad cells (which have altered oligosaccharides on their SGP), and normal cells treated with neuraminidase and trypsin.[34] The extent to which MN and Ss-SGP is involved is unclear. Hadley et al.[34] suggested that *P. falciparum* merozoites may use several receptors: a NeuNAc-dependent site (perhaps on MN-SGP) and a NeuNAc-independent site.

The P Blood Group System

The P blood group system was introduced in 1927 by Landsteiner and Levine.[7] In their search for new antigens, they injected rabbits with human red cells and produced an antibody, initially called anti-P, that divided human red cells into two groups: P+ and P−.

In 1959, Levine et al.[35] described anti-Tj^a (now known as anti-PP$_1$P^k), an antibody to a high-frequency antigen that Sanger[36] later related to the P system. Because it defined an antigen common to P+ and P− cells and was made by an apparent P-null individual, the original antigen and phenotypes were renamed. Anti-P became anti-P$_1$; the P+ phenotype became P$_1$; the P− phenotype became P$_2$; and the rare P-null individuals became known as p individuals.

The P blood group became more complex in 1959, when Matson et al.[37] described the P^k phenotype. These rare individuals lack an antigen, P, which is common to all red cells except those with the phenotype p or P^k. In its place is another high-frequency antigen, P^k, one not commonly seen on red cells but one that is well expressed on all fibroblasts except those from p individuals. The puzzling association of P and P^k was not truly understood until the biosynthetic pathway became known.

This knowledge has prompted the ISBT to divide the antigens into both a blood group system and an associated antigen "collection." The antigen P$_1$ is assigned to the P blood group system (designated P1 or 003) and given the number 003001. The antigens P, P^k, and Luke are assigned to the globoside collection of antigens (209) and are given the numbers 209001, 209002, and 209003, respectively; p antigen has not yet been assigned. To simplify things for the reader, this section will refer to all the antigens as part of a loosely termed "P system."

TABLE 8-5   **P SYSTEM PHENOTYPES, ANTIGENS, AND ANTIBODIES**

Phenotype	Detectable Antigens*	Possible Antibodies†	FREQUENCY Whites	FREQUENCY Blacks
P_1	P_1,P	—	79%	94%
P_2	P	Anti-P_1	21%	6%
p	—	Anti-PP$_1$P^k	Rare	Rare
$P_1{}^k$	P_1,P^k	Anti-P	Very rare	Very rare
$P_2{}^k$	P^k	Anti-P, Anti-P_1	Most rare	Most rare

*Antigens: P_1 poorly developed at birth; combined frequency of rare phenotypes 10:1,000,000.

†Antibodies: Anti-P_1: Usually clinically insignificant. Anti-PP$_1$P^k: Hemolytic; associated with early abortion. Anti-P: Hemolytic; associated with Donath-Landsteiner antibody and early abortion. Reactivity enhanced by enzymes.

The antigens and phenotypes associated with the P system are summarized in Table 8–5. The P_1 and P_2 phenotypes are analogous to A_1 and A_2 in the ABO system. The antibodies generally fall into two categories: clinically insignificant or potently hemolytic.

BASIC CONCEPTS

The P system antigens are biochemically related to the carbohydrate chains that make up the ABH and I antigens. P_1, P, and P^k are found on red cells, platelets, leukocytes, tissue fibroblasts, and uroepithelial cells; P and P^k have also been found in plasma as glycosphingolipids. The antigens have not been identified in secretions.[14]

The P_1 Antigen

The expression of P_1 changes during fetal development. The antigen has been found on fetal red cells as early as 12 weeks but it weakens with gestational age.[38] Ikin et al.[39] found that young fetuses were more frequently and more strongly P_1+ than were older fetuses. The antigen is poorly expressed at birth and may take up to 7 years to be fully expressed.[40]

Antigen strength in adults varies from one individual to another, a fact first noted by Landsteiner and Levine,[7] who found that some P_1+ people were P_1 strong and others were P_1 weak. These differences appear to be quantitative, not qualitative, and may either be genetically controlled or represent homozygous versus heterozygous inheritance of the gene making P_1. The strength of P_1 also varies with race. Blacks have a stronger expression of P_1 than whites. The rare dominant gene *In(Lu)* (discussed in The Lutheran Blood Group System) inhibits the expression of P_1 so that P_1 individuals who inherit it may serologically type P_2.

The P_1 antigen deteriorates rapidly on storage. When old cells are typed or used as controls for typing reagents, or when older cells are used to detect anti-P_1 in serum, false-negative reactions may result.

Anti-P_1

Anti-P_1 is a common, naturally occurring IgG antibody in the sera of P_2 individuals. It is usually a weak, cold-reactive saline agglutinin not seen in routine testing. Stronger examples react at room temperature or bind complement, which is detected in the antiglobulin test when polyspecific reagents are used. Antibody activity can be neutralized or inhibited with soluble P_1 substance.

Because P_1 antigen expression on red cells varies and deteriorates during storage, antibodies may react only with cells having the strongest expression and may produce inconclusive patterns of reactivity when panel identification is performed. Laboratory staff can incubate tests in the cold or pretreat test cells with enzymes to enhance reactions and confirm specificity, but most will repeat the tests using prewarmed methods instead. If activity is no longer seen, the antibody may be considered clinically insignificant and specificity need not be identified.

Providing units that are crossmatch compatible at 37°C and in the antiglobulin phase, regardless of their P_1 status, is an acceptable approach to transfusion. Giving P_1+ units under these circumstances does not cause a rise in antibody titer or a change in its thermal range of reactivity.[14]

When P_1 antibodies truly do react at 37°C, they must be evaluated very carefully because they can cause in vivo red cell destruction; both immediate and delayed hemolytic transfusion reactions have been reported.[41,42] These rare antibodies react well in the antiglobulin phase, bind complement, and may lyse enzyme-treated test cells. Although it is tempting to assume that such antibodies are IgG, many have been identified as IgM; IgG forms actually are rare. HDN is not associated with anti-P_1, presumably because the antigen is so poorly developed on fetal cells.

ADVANCED CONCEPTS

Biochemistry

The antigens of the P system exist as glycosphingolipids and glycoproteins. Like ABO, the antigens are

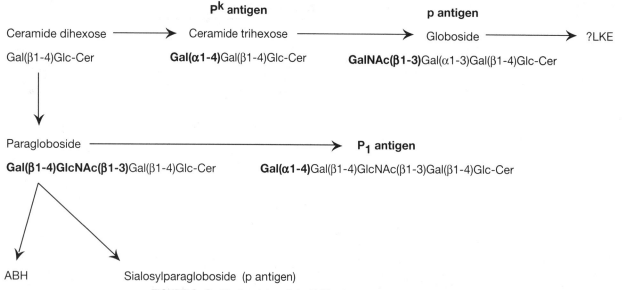

FIGURE 8–3 Biochemistry of the P blood group glycosphingolipids.

immunodominant sugars added sequentially to a precursor structure. Biochemical analyses have shown that the structures carrying P determinants also carry I and ABH antigens. However, the genes of the P system act first; hence, their antigens are closer to the membrane than A, B, H, or I.

The biosynthetic pathway of the P^k, P, and Luke antigens is shown in Figure 8–3.[14] Ceramide dihexose (CDH), also called lactosylceramide, is a glycolipid precursor that can be acted on by several different sugar transferases. The addition of galactose in an $\alpha 1 - 4$ linkage makes ceramide trihexose (CTH), or the P^k antigen. With another sugar addition, the P^k structure becomes globoside, or the P antigen. This explains why the high-frequency antigen P^k is not readily apparent on red cells; the P sugar makes P^k less accessible to its antibody. In sheep, globoside is the precursor for the Forssman antigen; in humans, it may be the precursor for the LKE or Luke antigen.

In an alternate biosynthetic pathway, CDH can acquire two more sugars and become paragloboside, a precursor for the P_1 antigen, the p antigen (discussed later), or the ABH antigens.

Genetics

The problem with the biosynthetic pathway is finding a genetic model that fits serologic data. Several have been suggested, but the two-loci model proposed by Graham and Williams[43] is most simple. Its genes and gene products are given in Table 8–6. The first locus is thought to contain three alleles. Two, P^{1k} and P^k, are common and make a galactosyl transferase that adds the same sugar to one or two precursors. The third allele, P, is very rare and makes no transferase. The second locus contains two alleles: P^2 has a very high frequency and makes a transferase that converts CTH to globoside; $P^{2.0}$ has a very low frequency and is silent like p.

The P phenotype of an individual depends on the alleles inherited at both loci (Fig. 8–4). When p is inherited in the homozygous state, antigens cannot form even with a p^2 gene because the precursor is not made. Such individuals are very rare, 5.8 of 1 million. The p gene is slightly more common in Japan, in northern Sweden, and in an Amish group in Ohio.[1] Individuals homozygous for $P^{2.0}$ have the P^k phenotype. Whether or not they express P_1 antigen will depend on their alleles at locus 1. Data suggest that the gene coding for P_1 is located on chromosome 22.[14]

Other Sources of P_1 Antigen and Antibody

The discovery of strong anti-P_1 in two P_2 individuals infected with *Echinococcus granulosus* tapeworms led to the identification of P_1 and P^k substance in hydatid

TABLE 8–6 **PROPOSED GENES AND GENE PRODUCTS FOR THE P SYSTEM[1,43]**

Gene	Alleles	Frequency	Gene Product	Substrate or Precursor	Action
Locus 1	P^k	0.5	α-galactosyl transferase	CDH	Converts CHD→Pk
	P^{1k}	0.5	α-galactosyl transferase	CDH and paragloboside	Converts CDH→Pk and paragloboside→P_1
	P	<0.001	(none)	—	—
Locus 2	P^2	>0.999	β-galactosyl transferase	CTH	Converts Pk→P
	$P^{2.0}$	<0.001	(none)	—	—

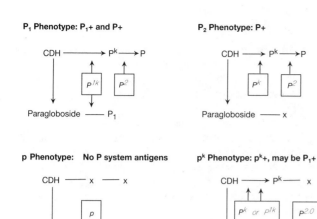

FIGURE 8-4 Proposed inheritance of P blood group antigens. Inherited gene alleles are indicated by boxes.

cyst fluid.[44] This fluid was used in many of the investigations that elucidated the biochemical structure of P system antigens.

A P_1–like antigen has also been found in the red cells, plasma, and droppings of pigeons and turtledoves as well as the egg white of turtledoves. Exposure to these birds may place P_2 bird handlers at risk of making strong, clinically significant anti-P_1. The P_1 antigen in bird droppings may be attributed to certain gram-negative avian bacteria rather than to the birds themselves.[45]

Strong antibodies to P_1 also have been associated with fascioliasis (bovine liver fluke disease), *Clonorchis sinensis*, and *Opisthorchis viverrini* infections.[46] P_1 substance has been identified in extracts of *Lumbricus terrestris* (the common earthworm) and *Ascaris suum*.[47]

Soluble P_1 substances have potential use in the blood bank and are commercially available. When it is necessary to confirm antibody specificity or to identify underlying antibodies, these substances can be used to neutralize anti-P_1 if prewarmed methods do not eliminate reactivity.

Antibodylike substances, similar to plant lectins, also have been reported. Extracts of salmon and trout roe contain activity for P_1, P^k, and B antigen. Serum from the snake *Python sebae* contains an anti-P activity detected with enzyme-treated red cells.

Anti-PP₁Pᵏ

Originally called Tj[a], this antibody was first described in the serum of Mrs. Jay, a p individual with adenocarcinoma of the stomach.[35] Her tumor cells carried P system antigens, and the antibody was credited as having cytotoxic properties that may have helped prevent metastatic growth postsurgery (the T of Tj[a] refers to *tumor*).

Anti-PP₁Pᵏ is produced by all p individuals early in life without red cell sensitization and reacts with all red cells except those of other P-null individuals. Unlike the system-reactive antibodies made by other blood group–null individuals, most examples are a mixture of separable anti-P, anti-P_1, and anti-P^k. The antibodies are predominantly IgM, sometimes IgG. They react over a wide thermal range and efficiently bind complement, which makes them potent hemolysins. Anti-PP₁Pᵏ has the potential to cause severe hemolytic transfusion reactions and HDN.[14]

The antibody is also associated with spontaneous abortions in early pregnancy. Although the reason for this is not fully known, it has been suggested that having an IgG anti-P component is an important factor.[48] Women with such antibodies and a history of multiple abortions have successfully delivered infants after being plasmapheresed to reduce their antibody level during pregnancy.[49]

Vos et al.[50] described an unusual Tj[a]–like autoantibody in the serum of habitual aborters found transiently only during pregnancy and only in Australia. The antibody did not agglutinate cells or react in an antiglobulin test; it was only detected by its hemolysis. This activity was not complement dependent, although it was destroyed by heat, and may reflect some Australian environmental factor.

Anti-P

In addition to being an antibody component in p individuals (see earlier), anti-P is found as a naturally occurring alloantibody in the sera of all P^k individuals. Its reactivity is similar to anti-PP₁Pᵏ in that it is usually a potent hemolysin reacting with all cells except the autocontrol and those with a P-null phenotype. However, it also does not react with cells having the extremely rare P^k phenotype, and the individual making the antibody may type P_1+.

Alloanti-P is rarely seen in the blood bank, but because it is hemolytic with a wide thermal range of reactivity, it is very significant in transfusion. IgG fractions may occur and have been associated with habitual early abortion.

Anti-P specificity is also associated with the cold-reactive IgG autoantibody in patients with paroxysmal cold hemoglobinuria (PCH). This autoimmune disorder is seen transiently in children following viral infections and in tertiary syphilis. Antibody activity is biphasic. It attaches to red cells in the cold and lyses them as they warm. The autoantibody reacts only weakly or not at all with routine test methods. Its true hemolytic nature is best demonstrated by the Donath-Landsteiner test. The etiology and diagnosis of PCH are more fully discussed in Chapter 21.

Anti-Pᵏ

This antibody has been isolated from some examples of anti-PP₁Pᵏ by selective absorption with P_1 cells. Its activity has also been reported in the serum of P_1 individuals with biliary cirrhosis and autoimmune hemolytic anemia.[38] Anti-P^k activity can be inhibited with hydatid cyst fluid.

Antibodies to Compound Antigens

Considering the biochemical relationship of the P system antigens to ABH and I, it is not surprising that antibodies requiring more than one antigenic determinant have been described, including IP_1, iP_1, I^TP_1, and IP. Most examples are cold-reactive agglutinins.

Luke (LKE) Antigen and Antibody

In 1965, Tippett et al.[51] described an antibody in the serum of a patient with Hodgkin's lymphoma that divided the population into three phenotypes: 84 percent tested Luke+, 14 percent were weakly positive or Luke(w), and 2 percent were Luke−. Although this mendelian-dominant gene segregated independently of the P system, it was thought to be phenotypically related because the antibody reacted with all cells except those having the rare p and P^k phenotypes, and 2 percent of P_1+. All individuals with the p and P^k phenotype are Luke−, and more P_2 individuals have Luke−/Luke(w) phenotypes than do P_1 individuals. Also, the Luke−/Luke(w) phenotypes are associated more with the A_1 blood group than with A_2, B, or O.

Luke's association with the ABO and P systems has become more understandable, thanks to a murine monoclonal antibody with Luke specificity. Its antigen is called LKE for Luke erythrocyte antigen.[52] Anti-LKE is inhibited by NeuNAc(a2−3)Gal(B1−3)GalNAc−, the structural equivalent of globoside (P antigen) with galactose and neuraminic acid attached. Although no such structure has yet been isolated from the red cell membrane, LKE− people may lack the terminal neuraminic acid, possibly the galactose, on globoside.[52]

Only four human antibodies have been described. The original was a saline agglutinin that reacted best at 4°C. Using enzyme methods and additional complement, it became a potent hemolysin. The other examples were much weaker and clinically insignificant. The rarity of human antibody makes monoclonal anti-LKE a truly important tool.

The p Antigen and Antibody

In 1972, Englefriet et al.[53] described a transient antibody in the serum of a P_1 individual that reacted best with p red cells, less well with P_2 cells, and weakest with P_1 cells. Because of this pattern of reactivity, it was called anti-p. The antigen it detects is sialosylparagloboside; that is, paragloboside with NeuNAc (sialic acid) attached. This oligosaccharide is present in great quantity on p cells but is neither a precursor to P system antigens nor genotypically related.

Only a few examples of anti-p have been reported. They react preferentially with p red cells either at 4°C or in the antiglobulin phase. Reactions can be inhibited with sialosylparagloboside. Anti-p reactivity is destroyed with neuraminidase but enhanced with papain.

Disease Associations

A number of diseases and pathologic conditions associated with the P system have been described here: parasitic infections are associated with anti-P_1; early abortions with anti-PP_1P^k or anti-P; and PCH with anti-P.

The antigens may also be associated with urinary tract infections. Some pyelonephritogenic strains of *E. coli* may ascend the urinary tract in a ladderlike fashion by adhering to P_1 or P^k glycolipids on uroepithelial cells. The fimbriae or pili of such organisms have receptor sites for structures involving a Gal(α1−4)Gal(β1−4) moiety, which represent the terminal sugars for P_1 and P^k.[54−56]

Lomberg et al.[57] reported more urinary infections in young girls who are P_1+ than in those who are P_1−, and it has been shown that persons with the p phenotype are not susceptible to acute pyelonephritis related to significant strains of *E. coli*. However, specific receptor molecules may vary or be influenced by other factors because Mullholland et al.[58] found more infections in a P_1− postmenopausal group.

The I Blood Group Collection

The existence of cold agglutinins in the serum of people with acquired hemolytic anemia has long been recognized. In 1956, Wiener et al.[59] gave a name to one such agglutinin, calling its antigen "I" for "individuality." The antibody reacted with all but 5 of 22,000 blood specimens tested (i.e., most were I+). The nonreactive, or I−, specimens were thought to be homozygous for a rare gene producing the "i" antigen. Many cold autoagglutinins were found to have I specificity. In 1960, Marsh and Jenkins[60] reported finding anti-i, and the unique relationship between I and i began to unfold.

Because I and i are not discrete antithetical antigens produced by allelic genes, they are classified not as a system but rather as a "collection" of blood group antigens that has been given the numeric designation 207 by the ISBT.[2] They represent common related structures defined by a heterogeneous collection of autoantibodies. Individuality and heterogeneity are indeed a hallmark.

BASIC CONCEPTS

The Ii Antigens

The antigens are best introduced by classic serologic facts. Both I and i are high-frequency antigens expressed in a wide range of strengths that are inversely proportional to one another. At birth, infant red cells are rich in i; I is almost undetectable. During the first 18 months of life, the quantity of i slowly decreases as that of I increases, until adult proportions are reached. Most adult red cells are rich in I and have little i expression.

TABLE 8-7   **Ii PHENOTYPES AND KEY FACTS***

Phenotype	I Antigen Content	i Antigen Content	Frequency
I	Strong	Weakest	Common in adults
I_{int}	Intermediate	Intermediate	Rare in adults (?heterozygote)
i Cord	Weak	Strong	Common in newborn infants
i_2	Weaker	Stronger	1:10,000 black adults
i_1	Weakest	Strongest	<1:10,000 white adults

*Antigens: Infants are born with i antigen.
        I normally developing by 18 months of age.
        I activity based on ABH precursor branching.
Antibodies: Anti-I: Common cold reactive autoantibody; associated with *M. pneumoniae.*
        Anti-i: Rare autoantibody; associated with infectious mononucleosis.
        Reactivity enhanced by enzymes.

Among adults, there is a wide normal range of reactivity with both anti-I and anti-i.[14] Data suggest that a red cell's i reactivity is inversely proportional to marrow transit time as well as age in circulation. The number of I sites on adult cells has been found to vary from 0.3 to 5×10^5; i sites on cord cells from 0.2 to 0.65×10^5.

Some people appear not to change their i status after birth: they become the rare "adult i" individuals. Two adult i phenotypes have been reported:[60,61] i_1 has the least amount of I antigen and is found in whites; i_2 has a little more I antigen and is associated with blacks. Ii phenotypes and their characteristics are listed in Table 8-7.

Anti-I

Anti-I is a common autoantibody that can be benign or pathologic.[1,62] Consistently strong reactions with adult cells and weak reactions with cord cells define its classic activity but are no guarantee of its specificity. Cord cells have weak expression of other antigens and additional testing may be needed to confirm or rule out these specificities. Those of high frequency, such as Yt[a], may mimic anti-I but should not cause a positive autocontrol result as anti-I typically does. Table 8-8 gives common reactivity patterns.

Benign anti-I, found in the serum of many normal healthy individuals, is not associated with in vivo red cell destruction. It is usually a weak, naturally occurring, saline-reactive, IgM agglutinin that goes undetected in routine testing because it reacts best at 4°C. Stronger examples agglutinate test cells at room temperature or bind complement, which can be detected in the antiglobulin test if polyspecific reagents are used. Some may react only with the strongest I+ cells and give inconsistent panel reactions.

Although incubating tests in the cold enhance anti-I reactivity and help confirm its identity, many blood bankers prefer to repeat tests using prewarmed methods. If the weak reactions disappear, they are clinically insignificant and can be ignored. If identification is necessary, albumin and enzyme methods also enhance I reactivity. Using enzymes with slightly acidified serum may even promote hemolysis. Examples of thimerosol-dependent autoanti-I have also been reported. They are seen only when thimerosol is present in the test system.[63]

Pathologic antibodies are more potent IgM agglutinins with higher titers and a broader thermal range of activity (i.e., reacting up to 32°C or warmer). When peripheral circulation cools in response to low ambient temperatures, these antibodies attach in vivo and cause autoagglutination and vascular occlusion (Raynaud's phenomenon) or intravascular hemolysis (see Chapter 21).

Such strong examples of anti-I can react with adult and cord cells equally well, and antibody specificity may not be apparent unless the serum is diluted or warmed to 37°C. Potent cold autoantibodies can also mask clinically significant underlying alloantibodies and complicate transfusions. Procedures to deal with

TABLE 8-8   **TYPICAL REACTIONS OF SOME COLD AUTOANTIBODIES***

Antibody	A_1 Adult	A_2 Adult	B Adult	O Adult	O Cord	A Cord	O_h Adult	O_i Adult
Anti-I	++++	++++	++++	++++	0/+	0/+	++++	(0)
Anti-i	0/+	0/+	0/+	0/+	++++	++++	0/+	++++
Anti-H	0/+	++	+++	++++	+++	0/+	(0)	+++
Anti-IH	0/+	++	+++	++++	0/+	0/+	(0)	(0)
Anti-IA	++++	+++	0/+	0/+	0/+	0/+	(0)	(0)

*Reactions vary with antibody strength; very potent examples may need to be diluted before specificity can be determined.
0 = negative; + = positive.

these problems are discussed in other chapters. When a patient with pathologic autoanti-I must be transfused, use of a blood warmer is advised, especially when fast infusion rates are required. Blood warmers are not needed with weaker benign examples of anti-I or with slow infusion rates.

The production of autoanti-I may be stimulated by microorganisms carrying I-like antigen on their surface. Patients with *Mycoplasma pneumoniae* infections often develop strong cold agglutinins with I specificity as a cross-reactive response to the mycoplasma antigen.[64] They may experience a transient episode of acute abrupt hemolysis just as the infection begins to resolve. A *Listeria monocytogenes* organism from a patient with cold autoimmune hemolytic anemia has been reported to absorb anti-I and stimulate its production in rabbits.[65]

Anti-I also exists as an IgM or IgG alloantibody in the serum of the rare i adult. It has been traditional to transfuse compatible i units to these people, although such a practice may be unnecessary.[1] Whether or not the antibody is clinically significant depends on its reactivity: does it react at 37°C? Technologists must be aware that strong autoanti-I can mimic alloanti-I; if enough autoantibody attaches to a patient's red cells, they may falsely type I—.

Anti-I is not associated with HDN because the antigen is poorly expressed on infant red cells.

Anti-i

Most examples of anti-i are IgM and react best with saline-suspended cells at 4°C. Only very strong antibodies are detected in routine testing because standard test cells (except cord cells) have poor i expression (see Table 8–7).

Unlike anti-I, anti-i is not seen as a common benign antibody in healthy individuals. Potent examples are associated with infectious mononucleosis (Epstein-Barr virus infections) and diseases of the reticuloendothelial system (i.e., reticuloses, myeloid leukemias, and alcoholic cirrhosis). High-titered antibodies with a wide thermal range may contribute to hemolysis but because of the generally weak antigen expression, they seldom cause significant hemolysis. IgG anti-i has also been described and has been associated with HDN.[66]

ADVANCED CONCEPTS

Biochemistry and Genetics

An early association of Ii to ABH was demonstrated by complex antibodies involving both ABH and Ii specificity (see Antibodies to Compound Antigens, farther on). It was also known that I activity increased when ABH sugars were removed with specific enzymes and that adults with the Bombay phenotype (O_h) had the greatest amount of I antigen on their cells.[67] Thanks to these observations and works by Feizi, Hakomori, Watanabe, and Kabat (reviewed elsewhere[62,68,69]), we now know that Ii antigens are defined by a series of carbohydrates on the inner portion of ABH oligosaccharide chains.

ABH determinants on the red cell membrane are carried on four H-active precursor structures (H_1, H_2, H_3, and H_4), which attach to either proteins or lipids (Fig. 8–5). Little i activity is defined by at least two repeating N-acetyllactosamine (Galβ[1–4]GlcNAc) units on a linear structure. Branched carbohydrates containing repeating N-acetyllactosamine units are associated with I activity. Consequently, H_2 has i activity; H_3 has I activity; and H_1 carries no Ii activity because it is too short. H_4 is heterogeneous and not well characterized but contains both branched and linear regions. Studies on rabbit cells suggest that the linear regions on H_4 may contribute to the expression of i on adult red cells.[62]

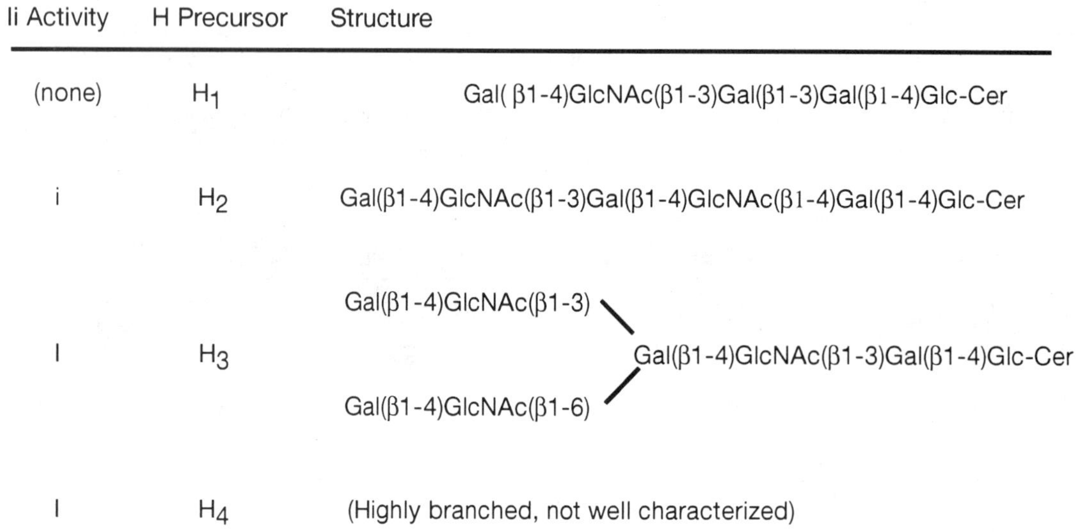

Ii Activity	H Precursor	Structure
(none)	H_1	Gal(β1-4)GlcNAc(β1-3)Gal(β1-3)Gal(β1-4)Glc-Cer
i	H_2	Gal(β1-4)GlcNAc(β1-3)Gal(β1-4)GlcNAc(β1-4)Gal(β1-4)Glc-Cer
I	H_3	Gal(β1-4)GlcNAc(β1-3) ＼ ⟩ Gal(β1-4)GlcNAc(β1-3)Gal(β1-4)Glc-Cer Gal(β1-4)GlcNAc(β1-6) ／
I	H_4	(Highly branched, not well characterized)

FIGURE 8–5 ABO precursor structures having Ii activity.

In summary, fetal, cord, and adult i red cells predominantly carry unbranched H_1 and H_2 chains and have an i phenotype.[69] Normal adult cells have the more branched structures H_3 and H_4 and express the I antigen. Although it has yet to be proven, the I gene most likely codes for the enzyme responsible for branching, $\alpha(1-6)$glucosaminyltransferase.

Family studies show that the adult i phenotype is recessive. Heterozygous children having one I parent and one i parent have intermediate I expression. One family in India has a reported I—i— phenotype: 15 of 93 family members had greatly reduced I and i, and six had partial depression of both. Perhaps their Ii antigens have a variant spatial relationship preventing them from reacting with common forms of both anti-I and anti-i.[1]

Other Sources of Ii Antigen

Ii antigens are found on the membranes of leukocytes and platelets in addition to red cells. Indeed, some potent Ii antibodies have been shown to be lymphocytotoxic. It is quite likely that the antigens exist on other tissue cells, much like ABH, but this is not confirmed.

I and i have also been found in the plasma and serum of adults and newborn infants, in saliva, and in human milk. The antigens in secretions do not correlate with red cell expression and are thought to develop under separate genetic control. For example, the quantity of I antigen in the saliva of adult i individuals and newborn infants is quite high.

Technologists occasionally attempt to neutralize potent examples of anti-I with human milk or saliva in order to identify underlying alloantibodies. Because so few antibodies will neutralize, this technique is not as helpful as it might appear.

The I antigen has been found on the red cells of other animal species including rabbit, sheep, cattle, and kangaroo.[14]

The I^T Antigen and Antibody

In 1965, Curtain et al.[70] reported in Melanesians a cold agglutinin that did not demonstrate classic I or i specificity. In 1966, Booth et al.[71] confirmed the antibody's high incidence and carefully described its reactivity. It reacted strongly with cord cells, weaker with normal adult cells, and weakest with adult i cells. These investigators concluded that the antibody might represent a transitional state of i into I, and designated the specificity I^T. Although the association of this antibody to transitional I (hence its name) has since been questioned, its serologic pattern of reactivity is not in dispute.

Anti-I^T is a common, naturally occurring antibody in several populations: the Melanesians, coastal residents of Paupa and New Guinea, and the Yanomama Indians in Venezuela. Whether or not it is associated with an organism or parasite indigenous to these regions is unknown.

The antibody has also been associated with Hodgkin's disease. Garratty et al.[72] investigated more than 50 patients with Hodgkin's disease: three of the four patients in this group with evidence of warm autoimmune-mediated hemolysis demonstrated IgG autoanti-I^T. The antibody has also been reported in a patient with non-Hodgkin's lymphoma, in patients with hemolytic anemia, and in a few patients with no evidence of hemolysis.[1]

The Specificities I^D, I^F, and I^S

In 1971, Marsh et al.,[73] thinking that the I antigen might be a mosaic, proposed two subdeterminants that could be serologically distinguished. I^F (for "fetal") described the I antigen that was detected on cord cells and that remained constant on all cells, including i adults throughout life. I^D (for "developed") referred to the I antigen that was not detected on cord cells but that developed later at the expense of i antigen. Anti-I^D appeared as a common benign example of antibody and could be inhibited with human milk. In contrast, anti-I^F was not inhibited and was seen as the pathologic component in hemolytic antibodies.

I^S described the soluble I antigen in secretions (human milk and saliva). The rare anti-I^S reported in 1975 by Dzierzkowski-Borodej et al.[74] was completely inhibited by saline and IgA colostrum and appears to parallel the inhibitable I^D antibodies of Marsh et al.[73]

Understanding these specificities (I^T, I^F, I^D, and I^S) is difficult until one considers the complex biochemistry of Ii. These specificities will represent different heterogeneous portions of ABH oligosaccharides.

Antibodies to Compound Antigens

Many other I-related antibodies have been described: IA, IB, IAB, IH, iH, IP_1, I^TP_1, ILe^{bH}, and $iHLe^b$. Bearing in mind the close relationship of I to the biochemical structures of ABH, Lewis, and P, one should not be surprised to find antibodies that recognize compound antigens. Such antibodies require both antigens in order to react best. Table 8–8 summarizes some common specificities with this collection.

Disease Associations

Well-known associations between strong autoantibodies and disease or microorganisms have already been discussed: anti-I and *M. pneumoniae*; anti-i and infectious mononucleosis; and anti-I^T and Hodgkin's disease. Cold autoantibodies have also been reported in influenza infections, but other associations are rare. Isolated cases include *Coxsackievirus* type A infection, acute cytomegalovirus infection, relapsing fever, malaria, trypanosomiasis, and bacterial infections.[62]

Diseases can also alter the expression of Ii antigen on red cells. Conditions associated with increased i antigen include those that stress the bone marrow or shorten the marrow maturation time of red cells: acute leukemias, hypoplastic anemias, megaloblastic anemias, sideroblastic anemias, hemoglobinopathies, chronic hemolytic anemias, and even patients phlebotomized too much and too often. Except in some cases of leukemia, this increase in i is not usually associated with a decrease in I antigen. The expression of I antigen can appear normal or sometimes enhanced.

Chronic dyserythropoietic anemia type II or hereditary erythroblastic multinuclearity with a positive acidified serum (HEMPAS) test result is associated with having much greater i activity on red cells than control cord cells. HEMPAS cells are very susceptible to lysis with both anti-i and anti-I; lysis by anti-I appears to be due to increased antibody uptake and increased sensitivity to complement.[14]

Reactive lymphocytes in infectious mononucleosis are reported to have increased i antigen. Those from patients with chronic lymphocytic leukemia have less i antigen than normal control subjects. In the Japanese population, the gene coding for i is linked to an autosomal recessive gene for congenital cataracts.[14]

The Kell Blood Group System

The Kell blood group system is an interesting mix of high- and low-frequency antigens. The first one was discovered in 1946 shortly after the introduction of antiglobulin testing.[75] It was defined by an antibody in the serum of Mrs. Kellacher, which reacted with the red cells of her newborn infant, her older daughter, her husband, and about 9 percent of the random population. The antigen was called K (Kell). In 1949, Levine et al.[76] reported its high-frequency antithetical partner k (Cellano).

Kell remained a two-antigen system until Allen et al.[77,78] described the antithetical antigens Kpª and Kpᵇ in 1957 and 1958. Inheritance patterns and statistics confirmed their relation to the Kell system. Likewise, Jsª, described in 1958 by Giblett,[79] and Jsᵇ, described in 1963 by Walker et al.,[80] were found to be antithetical and related to the Kell system.

The discovery of the null phenotype in 1957,[81] designated K$_o$, has helped associate many other antigens with the Kell system. Antibodies that react with all red cells except those with the K$_o$ phenotype recognize high-frequency antigens that are phenotypically related. Some of these are made by closely linked loci to K/k; for others the genetic status is not clear. These are called para-Kell or Kell-like antigens.

The description of the McLeod phenotype by Allen et al.[82] in 1961, with its weakened expression of Kell antigens and associated pathologic syndrome, has brought into focus another antigen, Kx, made by a gene on the X chromosome. Research aimed at understanding the association of Kell and Kx has expanded our knowledge of the system's inheritance and biochemistry.

The 21 antigens now included in the Kell blood group system, designated KEL or 006 by the ISBT, are listed in Table 8–9. The associated antigen Kx is part of the XK system, which carries the numeric designation 19.

BASIC CONCEPTS

Kell blood group antigens are found only on red cells. They have been found neither on platelets nor on lymphocytes, granulocytes, and monocytes using immunofluorescent flow cytometry.[14]

The K antigen can be detected on fetal cells as early as 10 weeks (k at 7 weeks) and is well developed at birth. The total number of K antigen sites and red cells is quite low and shows dosage: Hughes-Jones and Gardner[83] found about 6000 sites on K+k− red cells and only 3500 sites on K+k+ red cells. Despite this low number, K is very immunogenic and reacts well with its antibody.

The antigens are not denatured by routine blood bank enzymes ficin and papain but are destroyed by trypsin and chymotrypsin used in combination with one another.[84] Solutions of DTT and ZZAP (which contains DTT) denature all Kell antigens except Kx and Km; AET destroys all Kell antigens except Kx. β-mercaptoethylamine (MEA) and 2-mercaptoethanol (2ME) are known to denature the Kell antigens K, k, Kpª, Kpᵇ, Jsª, Jsᵇ, and Ku. The frequencies of common Kell phenotypes and key facts are listed in Table 8–10.

K and k Antigens

These antithetical antigens warrant special attention because they are so immunogenic. K is rated second only to D in immunogenicity. When K− people are transfused with 1 unit of K+ blood, the probability of their developing anti-K may be as high as 10 percent.[85] Fortunately, the frequency of K is low and the chance of receiving a K+ unit small. If anti-K develops, compatible units are easy to find.

Blood banks are seldom involved with the k antigen. Only 2 in 1000 individuals lack k and are capable of developing the antibody. The likelihood that these few individuals have been transfused and become sensitized is even more rare.

Kpª, Kpᵇ, and Kpᶜ Antigens

Alleles Kpª and Kpᶜ are low-frequency mutations of their high-frequency partner Kpᵇ. The Kpª antigen is found in about 2 percent of whites. Its gene is unique because it suppresses the expression of other Kell genes in cis position, including k, Jsᵇ, K11, K14, and K18.[86]

The Kpᶜ antigen is even more rare. In 1979, Yamaguchi et al.[87] discovered several siblings from a consanguineous marriage in Japan who typed Kp(a−b−) but otherwise had normal Kell antigens. They concluded that both parents carried a new allele, Kpᶜ, that the children inherited in a homozygous state. Gavin et al.[88] then showed that Kpᶜ and Levay,[89] the first low-

TABLE 8-9 **SUMMARY OF KELL ANTIGENS**

Number	Common Name	Alternate Name	Frequency (%)	Year Discovered	Comments
			I. Antigens Known to Be Encoded by the Kell Gene		
K1	K	Kell	9	1946	Antithetical to k
K2	k	Cellano	99.8	1949	Antithetical to K
K3	Kpª	Penney	2W	1957	Antithetical to Kpᵇ
K4	Kpᵇ	Rautenberg	>99.9	1958	Antithetical to Kpª
K6	Jsª	Sutter	<0.1W/20B	1958	Antithetical to Jsᵇ
K7	Jsᵇ	Matthews	>99.9W/99B	1963	Antithetical to Jsª
K10	Ulª	—	<3 Finns	1968	
K11	—	Cote	>99.9	1976	Antithetical to K17
K17	Wkª	Weeks	0.3	1974	Antithetical to K11
K21	Kpᶜ	Levay	<0.1	1945/1979	Antithetical to Kpª/Kpᵇ
			II. Para-Kell Antigens (Phenotypically Related/Genetics Uncertain)		
K5	Ku	—	>99.9	1961	
K12	—	Boc	>99.9	1973	
K13	—	Sgro	>99.9	1974	
K14	—	Santini	>99.9	1973	Antithetical to K24
K16	—	(k-like)	99.8	1976	
K18	—	V.M.	>99.9	1975	
K19	—	Sub	>99.9	1979	
K20	Km	—	>99.9	1979	
K22	—	N.I.	>99.9	1982	
K23	—	—	<0.5	1987	
K24	—	Cls	<2.0	1985	Antithetical to K14
			III. Associated Antigen Encoded by the XK Gene		
Xk1	—	Kx	>99.9	1975	

Note: ISBT considers K8 (for Kw), K9 (for KL), and K15 (for Kx) obsolete.
B = blacks; W = whites.

TABLE 8-10 **FREQUENCIES OF COMMON KELL PHENOTYPES AND KEY FACTS***

Phenotype	Whites (%)	Blacks (%)
K−k+	91.0	96.5
K+k+	8.8	3.5
K+k−	0.2	<0.1
Kp(a+b−)	<0.1	0
Kp(a+b+)	2.3	Rare
Kp(a−b+)	97.7	100
Js(a+b−)	0	1
Js(a+b+)	Rare	19
Js(a−b+)	100	80

*Antigens: Well developed at birth.
Expression very weak on McLeod phenotype cells.
Antibodies: Anti-K: Most common antibody after anti-D; reacts less well in low-ionic media.
Clinically significant.
Reactivity destroyed by AET and DTT.
May show dosage.

frequency antigen ever described, were identical. Levay was not placed into the system when it was first reported because Kell had not yet been discovered.

Jsª and Jsᵇ Antigens

The Jsª antigen, antithetical to the high-frequency antigen Jsᵇ, is found in about 20 percent of blacks but in less than 0.1 percent of whites. It is interesting that the frequency of Jsª in blacks is almost six times greater than that of the K antigen in blacks. Jsª and Jsᵇ were linked to the Kell system when it was discovered that K₀ red cells were Js(a−b−).

Anti-K

Besides ABO and Rh antibodies, anti-K is the most common antibody seen in the blood bank.[14] It is usually an IgG (often IgG1) antibody reactive in the antiglobulin phase, but some examples agglutinate saline-suspended cells. About 20 percent bind complement up to C3, but they are seldom lytic. The antibody is made in response to antigen exposure through pregnancy and transfusion and can persist for many years.

Naturally occurring IgM examples of anti-K are more rare and have been associated with bacterial infections. Marsh et al.[90] studied anti-K in an untransfused 20-day-old infant with an *E. coli* 0125:B15 infection; the infant's mother did not make anti-K. The organism was shown to have a somatic K-like antigen that reacted with the infant's antibody, which was thought to have been the stimulus. The antibody disappeared after recovery. Other organisms implicated with naturally occurring anti-K or known to react with anti-K include mycobacterium, *Streptococcus faecium,*

Morganella morganii, Campylobacter fetus subsp *jejuni,* and *Campylobacter coli.*[14,91]

Some examples of anti-K react poorly in low ionic medias such as LISS and LISS-polybrene (LIP), and in some automated systems.[91] The most reliable method of detection is the indirect antiglobulin test, but even this is no guarantee, especially when LIP is used. Routine blood bank albumin or enzyme methods do not affect antibody reactivity, but using DTT, ZZAP, 2ME, MEA, or AET does because these solutions destroy most Kell antigens. The potentiating medium polyethylene glycol (PEG) may increase reactivity.

Anti-K shows a dosage effect, as do many other Kell antibodies; however, dosage may not always be evident. Many factors other than gene zygosity can weaken or affect antigen expression (see farther on).

The K antibody has been implicated in severe hemolytic transfusion reactions. Although some antibodies bind complement, in vivo red cell destruction is usually extravascular via the macrophages in the spleen. Some reactions have been due to interdonor incompatibility—that is, when a K− patient is unknowingly given a unit of K+ blood and a unit of blood containing anti-K. This situation would occur only if the units were not screened (and most are) and if the anti-K titer were very high.

Anti-K is also associated with severe HDN. Titer does not always accurately predict the severity of disease, as stillbirth has been seen with an antihuman globulin (AHG) titer as low as 1:64. When a pregnant woman is identified as making anti-K, it is prudent to type the father for the K antigen and, if he is K+, to monitor the fetus carefully for signs of HDN.[91]

Antibodies to Kpᵃ, Jsᵃ, and Other Low-Frequency Kell Antigens

These antibodies are rare because so few people are exposed to the antigen. Because routine antibody screening cells do not carry low-frequency antigens, the antibodies are most often detected through unexpected incompatible crossmatches or cases of HDN. Not all blood banks have the antigen-positive cells needed to confirm the specificity, but everyone should be able to provide compatible units for transfusion.

The serologic characteristics and clinical significance of these antibodies parallel those of anti-K except that HDN has been mild. The original anti-Kpᵃ was naturally occurring, but most antibodies are immune.

Antibodies to k, Kpᵇ, Jsᵇ, and Other High-Frequency Kell Antigens

Antibodies to high-frequency Kell antigens are rare, because so few people lack the antigen. They also parallel anti-K in serologic characteristics and clinical significance but have only been associated with mild cases of HDN.

The antibodies are easy to detect but difficult to work with because most blood banks have neither the antigen-negative panel cells needed to rule out other alloantibodies nor typing reagents to phenotype the patient's red cells. However, if the antibody does not react with AET-treated red cells, this is a good clue that it may be related to Kell, and it provides the technologist with more "rule-outs" for other specificities.

Finding compatible units for transfusion can be difficult; siblings and rare donor inventories are the most likely sources. Patients with these kinds of antibody should be encouraged to donate autologous units.

ADVANCED CONCEPTS

Biochemistry

Kell and Para-Kell Antigens Early evidence suggested that Kell antigens involved both protein and carbohydrates. They were destroyed by 56°C heat, formaldehyde, and sulfhydral compounds, all of which denature protein. The K-related antigen on *E. coli* 0125:B15 that stimulated production of anti-K was dialyzable and thermostable like a sugar.[92]

The glycoprotein was finally isolated by sensitizing red cells with Kell antibody, solubilizing the membranes, separating the antibody-antigen complexes, and analyzing them with SDS-PAGE. The same 93-kD protein has been isolated using antibodies to K, k, Kpᵇ, Ku, Jsᵇ, K12, K13, K14, K19, K22, and K23, indicating all these specificities rest on the same structure. Periodic acid–Schiff (PAS) staining shows it to be a glycoprotein, and enzyme studies suggest that it carries five to six *N*-linked oligosaccharide chains. Under nonreducing conditions, the protein is complexed with other membrane proteins, including band 4.1, spectrin, and a protein similar to actin.

The *Kell* gene was recently cloned and, from its complementary DNA, the Kell protein is deduced to be a unique transmembrane glycoprotein with 732 aa.[22] About 47 aa at the *N*-terminus reside in the cell cytoplasm and probably complex with the cell cytoskeleton.[92] A 655-aa segment on the extracellular surface of the cell has six *N*-glycosylation sites, which concurs with biochemical data, and 15 cysteines, which suggests protein folding and disulfide bonds. Antigen activity probably depends on the folded configuration of the protein, and surrounding lipids may be important in maintaining its conformation.

Kx Antigen Because the expression of Kell antigens depends on another antigen, Kx (also called XK1), Kx was believed to be a precursor or backbone for Kell, but this is no longer thought to be true. Kx activity has been isolated on a 37-kD protein that is not a part of the Kell glycoprotein. Perhaps Kx helps to stabilize the red cell membrane and cytoskeleton. When Kell antigens are denatured with AET or DTT, Kx expression increases.[93,94]

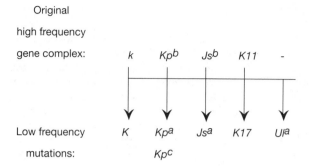

FIGURE 8-6 The Kell autosomal gene complex.

Genetics

***Kell* Gene** The Kell antigens are encoded by a gene complex that has at least five subloci (Fig. 8–6). The alleles within each subloci are expressed as mendelian codominants. A rare silent gene called *K^O* has also been identified. When inherited in a homozygous *K^O K^O* state, no Kell antigens are expressed.

Given all the subloci and alleles, many gene complexes are possible, but only a few have been found (Fig. 8–6). The most common combination, *kKp^b Js^b K11*, is thought to be the primary complex in humans, with the other alleles arising by simple mutation within this complex.[95] However, 29 examples of chimpanzee red cells tested K−k+, Kp(a−b+), Js(a+b−), K:11, so *kKp^b Js^a K^{11}* may be the ancestral gene, with *Js^b* arising by mutation after the human and chimp evolutionary lines separated.[86,92]

A gene complex codes for only one low-frequency antigen — never two or more — because this would require two or more mutations within one complex or recombination between two complexes. People who test positive for two low-frequency Kell antigens have always been found to carry them on different chromosomes. For example, someone who tests Kp(a+) and Js(a+) is genetically *kKp^a Js^b* on one chromosome and *kKp^b Js^a* on the other.

The *Kell* gene is linked with the Yt blood group and the gene that enables us to taste phenylthiocarbamide (PTC). Data suggested possible assignment of *Kell* to chromosome 5 and then to chromosome 6. Most recently, DNA marker and linkage studies show that *Kell* resides on the long arm of chromosome 7, between positions 7q32 and qter.[14]

***XK* Gene** The Kx antigen is encoded by the gene *XK* on the X chromosome, possibly near position Xp21.1.[86] Two alleles are proposed: *XK1*, which codes for Kx antigen; and *XKO*, which does not produce Kx and results in the McLeod phenotype. However, *XKO* may actually represent a small or partial deletion of the X chromosome in this area.

The K_O Phenotype

K^O is a silent *Kell* allele or some closely linked gene regulator. Inheriting two *K^O* genes results in a recessive null phenotype that expresses no Kell or para-Kell antigens, although Kx antigen expression is enhanced. K_O cells have no membrane abnormality and survive normally in circulation. The phenotype is rare, occurring in 1 in 25,000 whites.[86]

When K_O individuals are immunized, they can make antibodies to any or all Kell antigens they lack, including Ku (K5), a "universal" Kell antigen present on all cells except K_O. The true nature of Ku is not known. Its antibody is clearly different from anti-Js^b, but sufficient studies have not been done to prove it is not a complex mixture of Kell antibodies.[1]

Because K_O red cells are negative for k, Kp^b, Js^b, etc., they are very useful in investigating complex antibody problems. They can help confirm Kell specificity or rule out other underlying specificities. When K_O cells are not available, they can be made by treating normal cells with AET. Caution is needed when interpreting results with AET-made K_O cells because AET also denatures other high-frequency antigens including JMH, Yk^a, Hy, Kn^a, McC^a, and Vel.[1] DTT-treated cells must be used with similar cautions.

Other Kell Antigens

K11 and K17 In 1971, Guevin et al.[96] described anti-Cote (K11), which reacted with all red cells tested except those of the propositus, two of her eight siblings, and Kell null cells. Its antigen appeared to be phenotypically related to the Kell system. Three years later, Strange et al.[97] discovered that the low-frequency antigen Wk^a (Weeks) was strongly expressed on K:−11 red cells and definitely traveled with the Kell gene complex. Once this antithetical relationship was confirmed, Wk^a was given the name K17 to indicate its placement into the Kell system. *K^{11}/K^{17}* represents the fourth sublocus of the *KEL* gene.

Ul^a Ul^a describes a low-frequency antigen found in about 3 percent of randomly tested Finns, 0.46 percent of Japanese, and one of 12 Chinese. Three informative families helped place Ul^a (K10) into the Kell system. A high-frequency antithetical antigen has not yet been described.

Para-Kell Antigens

K12, K13, K18, K19, and K22 These discrete, very high–frequency antigens are phenotypically related to the Kell system because they are not present on K_O red cells and they are only weakly expressed on McLeod phenotype red cells. Although most have been found on the same glycoprotein as the Kell antigens, they are not controlled by the *Kell* gene. In fact, there is only one identified K:−18 individual, so K18 is not yet known to be inherited.

K14 and K24 K14, like the para-Kell antigens already described, is a high-frequency antigen. In 1985, its antithetical low-frequency antigen, K24, was described.[98] Anti-K24 reacts best with rare K:−14,24 red cells, moderately well with K:14,24 cells, and not at all with common K:14,−24 or AET-treated K:24 red cells. *K14/K24* may represent a sixth sublocus within the Kell system.

K23 K23 was described by Marsh et al.[99] in 1987 as a low-frequency antigen in one family. Because of its rarity, conventional genetic analyses could not be used to place it within a blood group system. However, using protein isolation techniques, it was found to be an epitope on the 93-kD Kell protein and therefore related to the Kell system.

Miscellaneous Kell Antigens The antigens K8 (also called K^w) and K9 (KL) are now obsolete and no longer used. K15 is also obsolete: its antigen Kx has been moved to the XK system and given the designation XK1. The specificities KL, Kx, and Km (K20) are related: A young boy named Claas with both the McLeod phenotype and probable chronic granulomatous disease made an antibody called anti-KL, which was found to be two separable antibodies to Kx and Km.[100] Kx and Km are high-frequency antigens present on all red cells, with two exceptions: cells with the McLeod phenotype are Kx−,Km−; and K$_O$ cells are Kx+,Km−. The expression of Kell antigens on red cells with common, McLeod, and K$_O$ phenotypes is summarized in Figure 8–7.

K16 refers to a high-frequency k-like antigen seen on k+ red cells, but which is expressed differently on McLeod red cells.

The McLeod Phenotype

In 1961, Allen et al.[82] described a young male blood donor who initially appeared to be Kell null but who demonstrated weak expression of k, Kp^b, and Js^b with absorption-elution methods. This unusual phenotype was called McLeod after the donor.

More than 60 examples of this rare phenotype have now been identified. All are male, all lack Kx (XK1) and Km (K20) on their red cells, and all have poor expression of Kell and para-Kell antigens. These individuals demonstrate a variety of associated clinical

anomalies collectively called the McLeod syndrome.[92,101]

Red cells lacking Kx have abnormal morphology. Many are acanthocytic (having irregular shapes and protrusions) and are removed from circulation in the spleen. As a result, people with the McLeod phenotype have a chronic, but often well-compensated, hemolytic anemia with reticulocytosis, bilirubinemia, splenomegaly, and reduced serum haptoglobin levels.

The red cells have normal enzymes, sodium-potassium-phosphorus transport, intracellular adenosine triphosphate (ATP), membrane microviscosity, and phospholipid ratios. However, some have a reduction in total lipid content, and abnormal shape may be due to a lipid deficiency on the inner membrane bilayer.[102] McLeod red cells have enhanced transbilayer mobility of phosphatidylcholine and show increased phosphorylation of protein band 3 and the B band of spectrin. Whether or not these changes are due to the lack of Kx is unknown.

Individuals having McLeod syndrome develop a slow, progressive form of muscular dystrophy between the ages of 40 and 50 associated with areflexia (a lack of deep tendon reflexes); choreiform movements (well-coordinated, involuntary movements); and cardiomegaly leading to cardiomyopathy. These individuals have elevated serum creatinine phosphokinase (CPK) levels of the MM type (cardiac-skeletal muscle) and elevated carbonic anhydrase III levels.

An association between the McLeod phenotype and X-linked chronic granulomatous disease (CGD) was made in 1971, when Giblett et al.[103] reported that the rare McLeod phenotype was common among young boys suffering the equally rare disorder CGD. CGD is characterized by the inability of phagocytes to make nicotinamide-adenine dinucleotide (NADH)–oxidase, an enzyme important in generating H_2O_2, which is used to kill ingested bacteria.[104] Children with CGD die at an early age of overwhelming infections.

At one time CGD was believed to be caused by a lack of Kx on white cells, and several alleles at the *XK* locus were proposed to explain Kx expression on McLeod red cells and CGD white cells. More recent data have disproved this theory. The *Xk* gene appears to reside

			Red cell antigen expression			
X-linked gene	+ Autosomal Kell gene	=	Kell antigens	Km	Kx	Phenotype
Xk1	+ kKp^{b}Js^b K11 ⟶		k, Kp^b, Js^b, K11 ...	Strong	Weak	Common
Xk1	+ K$_O$	⟶	None	None	Strong	Ko
Xk0	+ kKp^{b}Js^b K11 ⟶		k, Kp^b, Js^b, K11 ... trace only	None	None	McLeod

FIGURE 8–7 Summary of Kell antigens on red cells having normal, K$_O$, and McLeod phenotypes.

on the X chromosome near position Xp21, and near deletions associated with CGD, Duchenne's dystrophy, and even retinitis pigmentosa.[102]

The expression of Kx in women who are carriers of the McLeod phenotype (*XK1,XK0*) follows the Lyon hypothesis, which states that in early embryo development, one of the two X chromosomes in female cells randomly shuts down. All cells descending from the resulting cell line express only the allele on the active chromosome. Hence, McLeod carriers exhibit two red cell populations: one having Kx and normal Kell antigens, the other having the McLeod phenotype and atypical morphology.

Altered Expressions of Kell Antigens

Weaker than normal Kell antigen expression is associated with the McLeod phenotype, the suppression by *Kp^a* on *cis* Kell antigens, and the dosage effect seen when *Kp^a* is paired with *K^O*.

Depressed Kell and para-Kell antigens are also seen on red cells with the K:−13 phenotype and the Gerbich-negative phenotypes Ge:−1,−2,−3 and Ge:−2,−3. These Gerbich-negative cells lack normal β- and γ-sialoglycoproteins, which may influence the configuration of Kell antigens.[86]

Marsh and Redman[105] propose the umbrella term "K$_{mod}$" to describe other phenotypes with weak Kell expression, including those called Day and Mullins. As a group, these phenotypes have very weak Kell antigens and enhanced Kx expression, and some make nonidentical Ku-like antibodies.

Patients with autoimmune hemolytic anemia, in which the autoantibody is directed against a Kell antigen, may have depressed expression of that antigen. Antigen strength returns to normal when the anemia resolves. This phenomenon appears more common in the Kell system than in other systems.[1]

Finally, red cells may appear to acquire Kell antigens. McGinnis et al.[106] described a K− patient who acquired a K-like antigen during a *Streptococcus faecium* infection. Cultures containing the disputed organism converted K− cells to K+ cells, but bacteria-free filtrates did not.

Autoantibodies

Marsh et al.[107] reported that 1 in 250 autoantibodies do not react with K$_O$ red cells and are therefore related to the Kell system. The actual frequency of these antibodies could be much higher because their study detected autoantibody with pure Kell specificity, not with mixtures of Kell with other autoantibodies.[1] These antibodies may be benign or hemolytic.

Most Kell autoantibodies are directed against undefined, high-frequency Kell antigens, but identifiable autoantibodies to K, Kp^b, and K13 have also been reported. Issitt[1] has noted a possible association between autoanti-K and head injuries or brain tumors.

Mimicking specificities have been reported, such as when an autoanti-K is eluted from K− red cells. Not all

of these antibodies may have true mimicking specificity, however. It may be that the patient is truly K+ and has concurrent weakened K expression.

The Duffy Blood Group System

The Duffy blood group system was named for Mr. Duffy, a multiply transfused hemophiliac who, in 1950, was found to have the first described example of anti-Fy^a.[108] One year later the antibody defining its antithetical antigen Fy^b was described by Ikin et al.[109] in the serum of a woman who had had three pregnancies.

In 1955, Sanger et al.[110] reported that the majority of blacks tested were Fy(a−b−). The gene responsible for this null condition was called *Fy*. Although *FyFy* appeared to be a common genotype in blacks, especially in Africa, the gene was exceedingly rare in whites. In 1975, Miller et al.[111] provided an explanation for this observation: Fy(a−b−) red cells were shown to resist infection by the malaria organism *P. knowlesi* and, as we now know, by *P. vivax*—an example of natural selection in human beings.

Additional Duffy antibodies have since been recognized. Although rarely seen in the blood bank, their antigens—Fy3, Fy4, Fy5, and Fy6—have contributed to our understanding of the blood group system, which is designated FY or 008 by the ISBT.

BASIC CONCEPTS

Fy^a and Fy^b Antigens

The Duffy antigens most important in routine blood bank serology are Fy^a and Fy^b. They can be identified on fetal red cells as early as 6 to 7 weeks' gestational age and are well developed at birth. Masouredis et al.[18] estimated the number of Fy^a sites on Fy(a+b−) red cells to be 13,300 per cell; a Fy(a+b+) cell carries only 6900 sites. The antigens have not been found on platelets, lymphocytes, monocytes, or granulocytes.[14]

The frequencies of the common phenotypes in the Fy system are given in Table 8–11. The disparity in distribution in different races is quite notable.

TABLE 8–11 **FREQUENCY OF DUFFY PHENOTYPES AND KEY FACTS***

Phenotype	Whites (%)	American Blacks (%)	Chinese (%)[117]
Fy(a+b−)	17	9	90.8
Fy(a+b+)	49	1	8.9
Fy(a−b+)	34	22	0.3
Fy(a−b−)	Very rare	68	0

*Antigens: Well developed at birth.
　　　　　Moderately immunogenic.
　　　　　Fy(a−b−): Resistant to malaria infection.
Antibodies: Clinically significant.
　　　　　Reactivity destroyed by enzymes.
　　　　　Dosage not obvious.

Fy antigens do not store well, even frozen. They tend to elute from red cells stored in a media with low pH or low ionic strength. This can lead to inhibitory substances in the supernatant fluid, which can weaken the reactivity of an anti-Fy[a] or anti-Fy[b].[14] They also elute from red cells stored in saline for 2 weeks at pH 7.0. These changes are not seen in red cells stored in licensed anticoagulants or the reagent solutions used by commercial manufacturers.[1]

Fy[a] and Fy[b] antigens are destroyed by common proteolytic enzymes such as ficin, papain, bromelin, and chymotrypsin, and the IgG cleaving reagent ZZAP. They are also denatured by formaldehyde or by 56°C heat applied for 30 minutes. They are not affected by the reagent AET, but prolonged exposure to chloroquine diphosphate can weaken Fy[b]. Neuraminidase may reduce the molecular weight of Fy[a] and Fy[b], but it does not destroy antigenic activity; neither does purified trypsin.

The ability of bromelin to denature Fy[a] and Fy[b] antigen puzzled those who detected their antibodies using autoanalyzer methods and bromelin. Rosenfield et al.[112] suggested that in such systems, the antibody may bind first and protect the antigen from enzyme degradation.

Anti-Fy[a] and Anti-Fy[b]

Because Duffy antigens are only moderate immunogens, anti-Fy[a] occurs three times less frequently than anti-K. Anti-Fy[b] is more rare and often occurs in combination with other antibodies. Fy[a] appears to be more immunogenic in Fy(a−b+) whites than in Fy(a−b−) blacks: in two series, only 25 of 130 patients with anti-Fy[a] were Fy(a−b−) blacks.[14]

The antibodies are usually IgG (IgG1) and react best in the antiglobulin phase. About half bind complement up to C3. A few examples are saline agglutinins; these are sometimes seen following a second stimulation. Antibody activity is enhanced in a low ionic strength medium. Anti-Fy[a] and anti-Fy[b] do not react with enzyme-treated red cells, a helpful characteristic to know when identifying multiple antibodies in a serum containing anti-Fy[a] or −Fy[b].

The antibodies may or may not show dosage. This discrepancy occurs because it is difficult to differentiate the genotype of some cells. For example, an Fy(a+b−) red cell may have a double or single dose of Fy[a] antigen, depending on whether the donor's genotype is *Fy[a]Fy[a]* or *Fy[a]Fy*. Other antigen typings may offer important clues: cells testing R[O], S−s−, V+VS+, Js(a+), or Le(a−b−) are more likely to be from black donors and to be heterozygous. Dosage is also more likely to be seen with saline agglutinating antibodies and with more sensitive techniques.

Anti-Fy[a] and anti-Fy[b] have been associated with hemolytic transfusion reactions, although hemolysis is seldom severe. Once the antibody is identified, antigen-negative blood must be given and finding such units in a random population is not difficult. Duffy antibodies have been implicated in delayed hemolytic transfusion reactions, especially in Fy(a−b−) patients with sickle cell disease having multiple antibodies. Duffy specificity should be looked for or carefully ruled out in such situations.

Anti-Fy[a] is associated with mild to severe HDN.[113] Anti-Fy[b] has the same potential.

Rare autoantibodies with mimicking Fy[a] and Fy[b] specificity have been reported (e.g., anti-Fy[b] that can be adsorbed onto and eluted from Fy[a+b−] red cells). Issitt[1] suggests that these may represent alloantibodies with "sloppy" specificity made early in an immune response.

ADVANCED CONCEPTS

Biochemistry

Enzymes, membrane solubilization methods, SDS-PAGE analysis, immunoblotting, and radiolabeling have all been used to study the biochemistry of the Duffy antigens.[114] It appears that Fy[a] activity resides on a heavily glycosylated protein that has a molecular weight of at least 35 kD with a trailing end extending to 66 kD. This trailing edge may be due to variable glycosylation. Tanner et al.[115] suggest that 40 to 50 percent of its mass consists of *N*-glycosidically linked oligosaccharides. Its mobility characteristics are similar to MN-SGP and protein band 3, but it is not associated with the red cell skeleton and is most likely on a structure not yet described.

The Fy[x] Gene

The gene *Fy[x]* was described in 1965 by Chown et al.[116] as a new allele at the *Duffy* locus. It does not produce a distinct antigen but rather an inherited weak form of Fy[b] that reacts with some but not all examples of anti-Fy[b]. Fy(x+) individuals may type Fy(b−), but their red cells absorb and elute anti-Fy[b]. They also have depressed expression of their Fy3 antigen. The red cells from *Fy[x]Fy[x]* people also react weakly with anti-Fy5 and anti-Fy6.[117]

Presence of the gene can cause confusion in paternity studies if the gene is not detected. *Fy[x]* and the silent allele *Fy* or *Fy4* can initially mimic one another, as illustrated by the family study in Figure 8–8. *Fy[x]* is probably more common than *Fy* in whites, but both are rare.

Anti-Fy[x] has never been described.

Fy3 Antigen and Antibody

In 1971, Albrey et al.[118] reported finding anti-Fy3 in the serum of an Fy(a−b−) white Australian female. It reacted with all red cells tested except those of the Fy(a−b−) phenotype. Because it was an inseparable anti-Fy[a]Fy[b], it was thought to react with an antigenic determinant or precursor common to both Fy[a] and

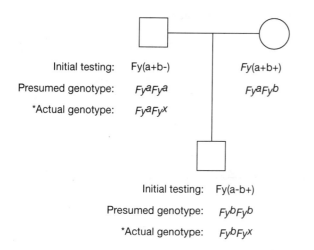

Initial testing: Fy(a+b−)   Fy(a+b+)

Presumed genotype: *Fy^aFy^a*   *Fy^aFy^b*

*Actual genotype: *Fy^aFy^x*

Initial testing: Fy(a-b+)

Presumed genotype: *Fy^bFy^b*

*Actual genotype: *Fy^bFy^x*

*After father's weak Fy^b is confirmed by absorption-elution.

FIGURE 8–8 How inheriting the *Fy^x* gene can confuse genotype determinations in a white family.

Fy^b, and was called Fy3. Unlike Fy^a and Fy^b, the Fy3 antigen is not destroyed by enzymes.

Other examples of anti-Fy3 have been reported, but considering the great number of Fy(a−b−) individuals transfused annually, the antibody is very rare. It is now thought that people making anti-Fy3 are "special" Fy(a−b−) nulls who also lack a common Duffy precursor or determinant (see Genetic Summary, farther on).

Anti-Fy3 producing nulls have been found in white, black, and Cree Native American families.[1] Examples of anti-Fy3 produced by nonblacks appear to react with all Duffy-positive cells equally well. Those made by blacks are similar but react weakly or not at all with Duffy-positive cord cells.

Fy4 Antigen and Antibody

For many years, Fy(a−b−) individuals were thought to be homozygous for a silent allele *Fy*. That concept changed when, in 1973, Behzad et al.[119] discovered anti-Fy4 in the serum of a young Fy(a+b+) black female with sickle cell anemia. The antibody reacted with red cells from all Fy(a−b−) blacks, with those from many Fy(a+b−) and Fy(a−b+) blacks, but not with those from Fy(a+b+) blacks nor from whites of any Duffy type. It was concluded that most Fy(a−b−) blacks carried an antigen called Fy4, perhaps in place of Fy^a and Fy^b, and were genetically *Fy^4Fy^4*. The *Fy^4* gene is very common in blacks; its frequency in whites is low. The Fy4 antigen, like Fy3, is not destroyed by enzymes.

It has been suggested that Fy4 offers protection from immunization to Fy^a and Fy^b because so many transfused Fy(a−b−) blacks do not produce corresponding antibodies. This may lead a technologist to think falsely that immunization cannot occur, when in reality it does occur.[120,121]

Fy5 Antigen and Antibody

Anti-Fy5 was discovered by Colledge et al.[122] in 1973 in the serum of an Fy(a−b−) black child who later died of leukemia. Initially it was thought to be anti-Fy3 because it reacted with all Fy(a+) or Fy(b+) red cells but not with Fy(a−b−) cells. His antibody differed in that it reacted with the cells from an Fy(a−b−)Fy:−3 white female; but it did not react with Fy(a+) or Fy(b+) Rh_null red cells and only reacted weakly with Fy(a+) or Fy(b+) D-- red cells.

The Fy5 antigen appears to be the result of an interaction between Rh and Duffy genes. People who are *Fy^4Fy^4* or Rh_null, or both, who do not make Fy5 are at risk of making the antibody, although few do so. The antigen is common in whites, but much less common in blacks. Like Fy3 and Fy4, it is not destroyed by enzymes. Its existence provides even more evidence that the genetic background of the common Fy(a−b−) black is very different from the rare Fy(a−b−) person making anti-Fy3.

Fy3, Fy4, and Fy5 Antibody Characteristics

As a group, the antibodies to Fy3, Fy4, and Fy5 are immune, IgG, and antiglobulin reactive. They react with enzyme-treated red cells, sometimes with enhanced reactivity. Although not all have been so implicated, they have the potential to cause transfusion reactions and HDN.

These antibodies are rarely seen in routine blood banking, and their special patterns of reactivity may not be immediately recognized on standard antibody panels. A summary of Duffy antibody reactivity with common and rare cells is given in Table 8–12. Anti-Fy3 and anti-Fy5 initially appear to be a mixture of anti-Fy^a plus anti-Fy^b, but the reactivity is not destroyed by enzymes. The identification of anti-Fy4 takes a bit more thinking; the antibody will react with all Fy(a−b−) panel cells, perhaps with some Fy(a+b−) and Fy(a−b+) cells, but with no Fy(a+b+) cells. Typing the patient's red cells for Duffy and Rh antigens can provide helpful clues.

Fy6 Antigen and Antibody

In 1987, Nichols et al.[123] described a murine monoclonal antibody they had prepared that reacted much like anti-Fy3 except that its reactivity was destroyed by ficin, papain, and chymotrypsin. Trypsin enhanced its reactivity.

The antibody appears to define the Duffy receptor that *P. vivax* uses to penetrate red cells. This antigen is a protein with a molecular mass of 46 kD, similar to Fy^a. Approximately 12,200 determinant sites have been quantitated on Fy:6 red cells.

Anti-Fs

This weak antiglobulin reactive antibody was discovered in the serum of a black Brazilian female whose

TABLE 8–12 **REACTIVITIES OF ANTI-Fy3, ANTI-Fy4, ANTI-Fy5, AND ANTI-Fy6**[117]

Red Cell Phenotype	Anti-Fy3	Anti-Fy4	Anti-Fy5	Anti-Fy6
White Fy(a+b−)	+	0	+	+
White Fy(a−b−)	+	0	+	+
White Fy(a−b+)	+	0	+	+
Black Fy(a+b−)	+	Most +	+	+
Black Fy (a+b+)	+	0	+	+
Black Fy(a−b+)	+	Most +	+	+
Black Fy(a−b−)	0	Most +	0	0
White Fy(a−b−)*	0	+w	+	0
White Fy(a+b+), Rh$_{null}$	+	0	0	+
White Fy(a−b+w), *Fy^{x}Fy^x*	+w	NT	+w	+w

*Producer of anti-Fy3.
NT = not tested; w = weak reactivity.

red cells typed Fy(a−b−)Fy:3,5.[124] It reacted with 79 percent of Fy(a−b−) red cell samples and 14 percent of Fy(a+) or Fy(b+) samples, or both, from blacks and whites. Its reactivity preference for Fy(a−b−) cells associates it with the Duffy blood group system, but the nature of the association is not clear. Limited family studies showed that Fs+ children may be born to Fs− parents. The authors concluded that if Fs was inherited as a simple mendelian characteristic, the controlling gene must segregate independent of the *Fy* gene.

Genetic Summary

In 1968, the *Duffy* gene was linked to a visible inherited abnormality of chromosome 1,[125] thus becoming the first human gene to be assigned to a specific chromosome. It appears to be located near the centromere in the p21 to q23 area, but whether it is on the short (p) arm or the long (q) arm of the chromosome is unclear.[117] The *Fy* locus is syntenic to *Rh*, which is located near the tip of the short arm; that is, they are on the same chromosome but segregate independently.

Speculation arises when trying to fit the antigens Fy3 and Fy4 into a genetic model. The genes coding for Fy^a, Fy^b, and Fy^x may also produce Fy3, or Fy3 may be some interaction product. It has also been suggested that the Duffy system is coded for by two closely linked loci with alleles *Fy^a*, *Fy^b*, *Fy^x*, and *Fy* at one locus and alleles *Fy^3* and *Fy^4* at the other.[126] Figure 8–9 summarizes possible gene complexes.

The alleles are inherited in straightforward mendelian fashion: *Fy^a/Fy^b/Fy^x* are considered codominant, as are *Fy^3/Fy^4*, whereas *Fy* is silent. The Fy^x phenotype could also be caused by a rare mutant operator gene that suppresses or weakens the expression of Fy^b and Fy3.

How Fy5 and Fy6 fit also is not known. One gene may be responsible for related antigens; certainly the antibodies to Fy3, Fy5, and Fy6 are similar in their reactivity. Perhaps the Fy3 protein consists of an enzyme-resistant area (Fy3) and an enzyme-sensitive area (Fy6), and Fy5 expression may depend on the interaction of normal Rh genes with *Fy^3*.[117]

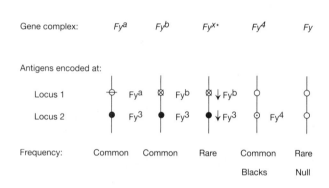

*Antigen expression may be depressed by a variant operator.

⅄ = depressed antigen expression.

FIGURE 8–9 Model proposed by Salmon et al.[126] for the inheritance and expression of Duffy antigens.

Duffy antigen typings have been performed using the red cells of chimpanzees, gorillas, and Old and New World monkeys. The results suggest that Fy3 developed first, followed by Fy^b, but that Fy^a arose during human evolution.[117]

The Duffy-Malaria Association

A correlation between the Duffy antigens and malaria infection has long been suspected. Since 1955, it was known that African and American blacks were resistant to infection by *P. vivax* and that these same populations were Fy(a−b−).

Because *P. vivax* could not be grown in culture at that time, Miller et al.[111] conducted in vitro studies with the simian parasite *P. knowlesi*, which could be cultured and would invade human red cells. They confirmed that malaria merozoites invaded only red cells carrying normal Fy^a and Fy^b antigen. When antigen sites were blocked by antibody or denatured with certain enzymes, the cells became resistant to invasion. Because the resistance factors for *P. knowlesi* and for *P. vivax* were parallel in West African populations, it was suggested that Fy[a] and Fy[b] might also be the invasion receptor for *P. vivax*.

In vivo data support this hypothesis. During a malarial vaccine study[127] in which 16 people were exposed to *P. vivax*, all five Fy(a−b−) blacks were resistant, but all six blacks and five whites who were Fy(a+) or Fy(b+) became infected. In another study of 13 black servicemen who contracted *P. vivax* in Vietnam, all typed Fy(a+) or Fy(b+)—a highly significant finding considering the antigen frequency in black servicemen.[128] Finally, a study in Honduras that tested 420 people for Duffy antigens, malarial infection, and parasite antibody supported the conclusion that either the Fy(a−b−) phenotype was the basis for resistance or Fy[a] or Fy[b] acted as receptors for invasion.[129]

Close evaluation of the invasion process of *P. knowlesi* suggests that two receptor sites are involved: one for attachment and one for junction.[34,114] Initial attachment occurs regardless of Duffy type and is characterized by the formation of thin filaments between the merozoite and the red cell surface. Junction, the point where the merozoite and red cell membranes actually join, which leads to invagination of the red cell membrane and formation of a parasitophorous vacuole (i.e., invasion), is Duffy antigen dependent.

Analyses of the Duffy antigens on human and Old and New World monkey red cells, and their resistance to invasion before and after treatment with various enzymes, has led researchers to conclude that Fy6 is the receptor for invasion for *P. vivax* without exception, but that Fy3 is a more probable receptor for *P. knowlesi*.[117]

The Kidd Blood Group System

The Kidd blood group is the simplest and most straightforward system to be discussed. In 1951, Allen et al.[130] reported finding anti-Jk[a] in the serum of Mrs. Kidd, whose infant had HDN. Its antithetical antigen, Jk[b], was found 2 years later by Plaut et al.[131] The null phenotype, Jk(a−b−), was described by Pinkerton et al.[132] in 1959. The propositus made an antibody to a high-frequency antigen called Jk3, which was present on any red cell positive for Jk[a] or Jk[b]. No other antigens have been described.

The Kidd system, designated JK or 009 by the ISBT, is especially significant to routine blood banking because of its antibodies, which can be difficult to detect and are a common cause of hemolytic transfusion reactions.

BASIC CONCEPTS

Jk[a] and Jk[b] Antigens

Jk[a] and Jk[b] are common red cell antigens. Table 8–13 summarizes the frequencies of the four known phenotypes. There are notable racial differences in antigen frequency: 91 percent of blacks and 77 percent of whites but only 50 percent of Chinese are

TABLE 8–13 FREQUENCIES OF KIDD PHENOTYPES AND KEY FACTS*

Phenotype	Whites (%)	Blacks (%)	Asians (%)
Jk(a+b−)	28	57	23
Jk(a+b+)	49	34	50
Jk(a−b+)	23	9	27
Jk(a−b−)	Exceedingly rare	Exceedingly rare	0.9–<0.1

*Antigens: Well developed at birth.
       Not very immunogenic.
       Jk(a−b−): Resistant to urea lysis.
Antibodies: Clinically significant; associated with delayed hemolytic transfusion reactions.
       Bind complement well.
       Fade quickly from circulation.
       Reactivity is enhanced by enzymes.
       Demonstrate dosage well.

Jk(a+); 57 percent of blacks and only 28 percent of whites are Jk(b−).

Jk[a] antigens are detected on fetal red cells as early as 11 weeks' gestation, Jk[b] at 7 weeks' gestation. These antigens are well developed at birth, which contributes to the potential for HDN. Red cells from homozygous *Jk[a]Jk[a]* individuals express the antigen more strongly than heterozygous *Jk[a]Jk[b]* individuals; *Jk[a]Jk[a]* red cells carry 14,000 antigen sites per cell.[18]

Kidd antigens are not altered by enzymes, ZZAP, chloroquine diphosphate, or AET, reagents that readily affect many other blood group antigens. They are probably not very accessible on the red cell surface and may well be clustered.[133] Both could explain why they do not always react well with their antibody, but antibody that is bound activates complement. They are also not strong immunogens: the risk of making anti-Jk[a] after one exposure to Jk(a+) blood appears to be 7 of 1000.[133]

The antigens are not found on platelets, lymphocytes, monocytes, or granulocytes using sensitive radioimmunoassay or immunofluorescent techniques.[14]

Anti-Jk[a] and Anti-Jk[b]

Kidd antibodies have a notorious reputation in the blood bank. They show dosage, are often weak, and are found in combination with other antibodies, all of which make them difficult to detect. Their reactivity is not proportional to their clinical significance in transfusion.

Anti-Jk[a] is more common than anti-Jk[b]. Both are IgG (primarily IgG3) and antiglobulin reactive, although IgM examples have been reported.[14] Antibodies are made in response to pregnancy or transfusion; naturally occurring examples have not been reported.

Kidd antibodies bind complement very well. This can be detected in the antiglobulin test using polyspecific reagents; it may also cause in vitro hemolysis. Rare examples are detected only by the complement they bind (i.e., they are nonreactive in antiglobulin tests using anti-IgG reagents. Using polyspecific reagents with both anti-IgG and anticomplement can be helpful in these situations.[1]

Antibody reactivity can also be enhanced by using LISS or PEG methods (to promote IgG attachment), by using four drops of serum instead of two (to increase the antibody-antigen ratio), or by using enzymes such as ficin or papain. Enzymes may cleave surrounding proteolytic structures and make the antigen more accessible to react with its antibody; this also promotes hemolysis. Hemolysis may be influenced by antigen dose. Haber and Rosenfield[134] described one anti-Jk[a] that lysed 100 percent of ficin-treated Jk(a+b−) red cells but only 25 percent of Jk(a+b+) cells.

The ability of Jk antibodies to show dosage can confound inexperienced blood bank technologists. An anti-Jk[a] that reacts only with Jk(a+b−) red cells (which carry a double dose of the antigen) can give inconclusive panel results and appear compatible with Jk(a+b+) cells (which carry only a single dose). Readers are urged to rule out Kidd antibodies only with homozygous *Jk[a]Jk[a]* panel cells and type all cross-match-compatible units with commercial antisera to make sure they are antigen negative. To ensure that these stored reagents can indeed detect weak expressions of the antigen, Jk(a+b+) positive control cells should be tested in parallel.

Kidd antibodies do not store well. When Jk[a] or Jk[b] specificity cannot be confirmed in a serum, which can happen when reference laboratories test samples sent from hospitals, sample freshness and complement activity must be considered. To boost complement levels and enhance Jk reactivity with polyspecific antiglobulin reagents, some add fresh serum,[1] whereas others use a two-stage ethylenediaminetetra-acetic acid (EDTA) method.[135] Identification is easiest when the freshest possible sample is used.

Unlike most blood group antibodies, anti-Jk[a] and anti-Jk[b] fade quickly from circulation. A strong antibody identified today may be undetectable in a few months. This confirms the need to check blood bank records for previously identified antibodies before a patient is transfused. It is equally important to inform the patient that he or she has such an antibody and to provide a wallet card that notes the specificity in case the patient is transfused elsewhere.

Jk antibodies are a common cause of hemolytic transfusion reactions, especially of the delayed type. Although intravascular hemolysis has been noted in severe reactions, coated red cells more often are removed extravascularly in the liver. The rate of clearance of incompatible red cells can vary, so that once a delayed reaction is suspected the patient should be carefully monitored for hemolysis.

Contrary to their hemolytic reputation in transfusion, most Kidd antibodies are associated with relatively infrequent and mild cases of HDN. In a review of 14 cases, only two infants required exchange transfusion and both of these occurred before 1969.[136] Perhaps the facts that Jk antibodies have lower titers

and that an affected fetus carries only a single dose of the antigen help protect an infant at risk.

ADVANCED CONCEPTS

Biochemistry

For many years, all that was known about the biochemistry of Kidd antigens was that they were protein: they were inactivated by heating to 56°C for 5 minutes but not by sulfhydral compounds. Using newer methods of immunoblotting and electrophoresis, Sinor et al.[137] identified the Jk[a] protein as a single protein band with a molecular weight of 45,000 kD. It is not affected by reduction or alkylation and appears not to be glycosylated.

The Kidd protein may be associated with the urea-water transport system of the red cell. Heaton and McLoughlin[138] reported in 1982 that Jk(a−b−) red cells resist lysis in 2M urea, a solution commonly used to lyse red cells in a sample before it is used in some automated platelet counting instruments. Urea crosses the red cell membrane and causes an osmotic imbalance and an influx of water, which rapidly lyses normal cells. With Jk(a−b−) cells, lysis is delayed 15 to 30 minutes.

Because both urea and water enter the red cell through transport systems, these have become primary areas of research. Whether the anomaly lies in the movement of urea, water, or both is not clear. Water movement across the membrane of Jk(a−b−) red cells may be restricted in the presence of urea.[139,140]

Urea uptake is influenced by pH, leading some to hypothesize that a critical protein might be different on Jk(a−b−) red cells, a variant with a different net charge. SDS-PAGE analysis, which separates proteins only by weight, shows normal membrane proteins on these rare cells; however, PAGE without SDS, which separates protein by both weight and charge, reveals an unique protein with a molecular weight of 67 kD.[141]

No clinical abnormalities have been associated with the Jk(a−b−) phenotype to date, but kidney function studies are in progress. Although urea transport has no apparent function in red cell physiology, it may be important in renal circulation, where red cells are exposed to high concentrations of urea.[140]

Genetics

The alleles *Jk[a]* and *Jk[b]* are mendelian codominant. Although *Jk* is called a silent allele (because null cells carry no Kidd antigens), it most likely makes a protein, albeit abnormal, given the results of PAGE with and without SDS as discussed earlier.

Early evidence based on Kidd and Colton inheritance in people with deletions of the long arm of chromosome 7 or monosomy of chromosome 7 suggested the *Kidd* and *Colton* genes were synthesized on that chromosome. Later analyses[142] suggested linkage between *Jk* and *Km*, which was assigned to chromosome 2 by in situ hybridization studies. Most recently, Geitvik et al.[143] linked *Jk* to chromosome 18 using a restriction fragment polymorphism. Studies indicate it may be near the centromere, between 18q11 and p21.

Jk(a–b–) Phenotype

People with the null phenotype lack Jk[a], Jk[b], and the common antigen Jk3. Although very rare, most of these individuals have been identified in the Far East and the Pacific Ocean area (Hawaii, New Zealand, Samoa, Tonga, and Polynesia).[1] The null phenotype has also been reported in several white families and in the Mato Grosso Indians of Brazil. The delayed lysis of Jk(a–b–) red cells in 2M urea has proved an easy way to screen families or populations (or both) for this rare phenotype.

Family studies show that most Jk(a–b–) nulls are homozygous for the rare silent allele *Jk*. Parents of *JkJk* offspring and children of *JkJk* parents type Jk(a+b–) or Jk(a–b+) but never Jk(a+b+), because they are genetically *Jk[a]Jk* or *Jk[b]Jk*. These individuals also demonstrate a single dose of Jk[a] or Jk[b] antigen in titration studies. Serologists must consider the presence of the *Jk* allele whenever Kidd discrepancies are encountered in paternity studies.

Another genetic explanation for the Jk(a–b–) phenotype was reported by Okubo et al.[141] They discovered a dominant pattern of inheritance within a Japanese family and proposed the existence of a dominant inhibitor to the Kidd system, *In(Jk)*, analogous to *In(Lu)* in the Lutheran blood group system. Dominant type Jk(a–b–) red cells absorb and elute anti-Jk[a] and anti-Jk3, indicating that the antigens are expressed but only very weakly.

Other evidence for suppression or heterogeneity in the Kidd blood group system has been offered. Arcara et al.[144] described a Jk(a–b–) mother who had seven Jk(a+b–) children, five with a double dose of Jk[a] on their red cells and two with a single dose. She never made anti-Jk[a] or anti-Jk3, although her Jk(a–b–) brother did. They suggested the brother was truly *JkJk*, whereas she carried a *Jk[a]* gene she could not express. Humphrey and Morel[145] also encountered unexpected titration and dose results when testing *Jk[a]Jk* and *Jk[b]Jk* individuals. Their red cells appeared to carry single doses of Jk[a] and Jk[b], but double doses of Jk3 except for an Asian who demonstrated a single dose of both Jk[a] and Jk3. How these data fit into a genetic picture is still not clear.

Anti-Jk3

Alloanti-Jk3 is an IgG, antiglobulin-reactive antibody that looks like an inseparable anti-Jk[a]Jk[b]. Because panel cells are Jk(a+) or Jk(b+), or both, anti-Jk3 reacts with all cells tested except the autocontrol. Most blood banks do not have the rare cells needed to confirm the identity of anti-Jk3; however, they can

easily determine its most probable specificity through antigen typings. The individual making the antibody will type Jk(a–b–). As with other Kidd antibodies, enzymes enhance the reactivity.

Anti-Jk3 is associated with mild HDN and delayed hemolytic transfusion reactions. Compatible units are best found by typing siblings or searching the rare donor files. One example of the antibody has been found in an untransfused male.

Autoantibodies

Autoantibodies with Kidd specificity (Jk[a], Jk[b], and Jk3) are rare, but they have been associated with autoimmune hemolytic anemia.[133] Some examples are drug related: One was found in a patient taking alphamethyldopa (Aldomet)[146]; another was chlorpropamide dependent[147] (i.e., it reacted with Jk(a+) red cells only when the drug was present). Because the patient was Jk(a+) and being treated with the drug, a hemolytic anemia developed. This antibody crossreacted with three other drugs, all containing a urea group: acetohexamide, tolbutamide, and tolazamide.

Examples of benign autoanti-Jk[a] have been associated with butyl, ethyl, methyl, and propyl esters of parahydroxybenzoate or paraben.[148] These chemicals are used in some commercially prepared LISS, cosmetics, food preservatives, and pharmaceuticals. The antibodies are seen when paraben-containing LISS is used in antibody detection tests with Jk(a+) cells. These antibodies may arise from viral or bacterial stimulation.

As with other blood groups, Kidd autoantibodies may have mimicking specificity or be associated with depressed antigen expression. One pregnant woman with an apparent compensated anemia was found to have mimicking autoanti-Jk[b] and -Jk3; the antibodies could be absorbed by Jk(a+b–) and Jk(a–b–) red cells.[149] In another report, a woman who was Jk(a+b–) transiently typed as Jk(a–b–) and had anti-Jk3.[150]

Disease Associations

Although Jk[a] and Jk[b] are thought to be human red cell antigens, three organisms have been associated with Jk[b]-like specificity. Two, *Streptococcus faecium* and *Micrococcus*, were able to convert Jk(b–) cells to Jk(b+); and one, *Proteus mirabilis*, may have been the stimulus for an autoanti-Jk[b].[151]

The Lutheran Blood Group System

Lutheran antigens have been recognized since 1945, when the first example of anti-Lu[a] was discovered in the serum of a patient with lupus erythematosus diffuses, following the transfusion of a unit of blood carrying the corresponding low-frequency antigen.[89] (Interestingly, this patient also made anti-c, anti-N, the first example of anti-C[w], and anti-Levay,

TABLE 8-14 **SUMMARY OF THE LUTHERAN ANTIGENS**

Number	Common Name	Frequency (%)	Year Discovered	Comments
I. Antigens Known to be Encoded by the Lutheran Gene				
Lu1	Lu^a	8.0	1945	Antithetical to Lu^b
Lu2	Lu^b	99.8	1956	Antithetical to Lu^a
Lu3	—	>99.9	1963	—
Lu6	—	>99.9	1972	Antithetical to Lu9
Lu8	—	>99.9	1972	Antithetical to Lu14
Lu9	—	2.0	1973	Antithetical to Lu6
Lu14	—	2.4	1977	Antithetical to Lu8
Lu18	Au^a	80.0	1961	Antithetical to Au^b
Lu19	Au^b	50.0	1989	Antithetical to Au^a
II. Para-Lutheran Antigens (Phenotypically Related; Genetics Uncertain)				
Lu4	—	>99.9	1971	
Lu5	—	>99.9	1972	
Lu7	—	>99.9	1972	
Lu11	—	>99.9	1974	
Lu16	—	>99.9	1980	
Lu17	—	>99.9	1979	
III. Phenotypically Related Antigens Probably not Produced by Lutheran				
(Lu12)	Much	>99.9	1973	
(Lu13)	Hughes	>99.9	1983	

Note: ISBT considers Lu10 (for singleton) and Lu15 (for An/Wj) obsolete.

now known as Kp^c.) The new antibody was named Lutheran, a misinterpretation of the donor's name Luteran.[152] In 1956, Cutbush and Chanarin[153] described anti-Lu^b, which defined the antithetical partner to Lu^a.

The blood group system appeared complete until 1961, when Crawford and coworkers[154] described the first Lu(a−b−) phenotype. Unlike most null phenotypes at the time, this one was inherited in a dominant fashion. In 1963, Darnborough et al.[155] found a more traditional Lu(a−b−) phenotype inherited as a recessive silent allele.

With rare Lu(a−b−) red cells to test antibodies to unknown high-frequency antigens, some sera showed a phenotypic relationship to Lutheran. That is, they reacted with all red cells tested except those having the Lu(a−b−) phenotype, even though the antibody producers appeared to have normal Lutheran antigens. These specificities were not identical to one another and were given numeric designations Lu4, Lu5, Lu6, and so on, to represent their association to the system. Some of these antigens have been found to be products of allelic genes at the *Lutheran* locus; others may be independent and are referred to as para-Lutheran antigens. All are summarized in Table 8-14.

The ISBT designation of the Lutheran blood group system is LU or 005.

BASIC CONCEPTS

Blood bankers seldom deal with the serology of Lutheran blood group system because the antigens have either very high or very low frequency. Either so many people have the antigen that only a few are capable of making alloantibody, or the antigens are so rare that only a few people are ever exposed. Consequently, the antibodies are infrequently seen. The antigens also have questionable immunogenicity.[14]

Lu^a and Lu^b Antigens

Lu^a and Lu^b are antigens produced by allelic codominant genes. Common phenotypes are listed in Table 8-15. Most individuals are Lu(b+); only a few are Lu(a+).

Although the antigens have been detected on fetal red cells as early as 10 to 12 weeks' gestation, they are poorly developed at birth and do not reach adult levels for many years. Using a murine monoclonal antibody

TABLE 8-15 **FREQUENCIES OF LUTHERAN PHENOTYPES AND KEY FACTS***

Phenotypes	Whites (%)	Blacks (%)
Lu(a+b−)	0.15	0.1
Lu(a+b+)	7.5	5.2
Lu(a−b+)	92.35	94.7
Lu(a−b−)	Very rare	Very rare

*Antigens: Poorly developed at birth.
       Lu(a−b−): Dominant, recessive, and X-linked types.
Antibodies: Questionable clinical significance.
       May be IgM, IgG, or IgA.
       Dosage not obvious.
       Reactivity possibly destroyed by AET.

with anti-Lu[b] activity, the number of Lu[b] sites per red cell is estimated to be 1630 to 4070 on Lu(a−b+) cells and 845 to 1820 on Lu(a+b+) cells.[156]

The antigens show dosage, with clear differences noted between homozygous and heterozygous members within the same family. However, antigen expression varies greatly from one family to another[38] and is more pronounced with Lu[a] than with Lu[b].

Lutheran antigens are thought to be red cell antigens, but Lu[b]-like glycoproteins have been recently found on kidney endothelial cells and liver hepatocytes (especially in fetal livers) using the monoclonal antibody BRIC 108.[157] Lutheran antigens have not been detected on platelets, lymphocytes, monocytes, or granulocytes using sensitive radioimmunoassay or immunofluorescent techniques.[14]

Anti-Lu[a]

Most examples are naturally occurring saline agglutinins that react better at room temperatures than 37°C. A few react at 37°C by indirect antiglobulin test. Some are capable of binding complement, but no in vitro hemolysis has been reported. Lutheran antibodies are unusual in that they may be IgA as well as IgM and IgG.[14]

Anti-Lu[a] often goes undetected in routine testing because most reagent cells are Lu(a−). They are more likely encountered as an incompatible crossmatch or during an antibody workup for another specificity. Experienced technologists recognize Lutheran antibodies by their characteristic loose, mixed-field reactivity in a test tube. In capillary testing, their agglutination resembles a pine tree.[158]

Antibody reactivity is not profoundly altered with the common blood bank enzymes ficin and papain, but it can be destroyed with trypsin, chymotrypsin, pronase, and AET.[14] Although anti-Lu[a] can show dosage, this may not be apparent because antigen expression is so variable.

Most Lu[a] antibodies are clinically insignificant in transfusion. Lu(a+) red cells have been reported to have normal or near-normal survival in a patient making anti-Lu[a].[159] Such transfusions do not appear to increase antibody production or change its thermal range of reactivity. In fact, some antibodies have been observed to disappear several months after detection.[158]

Because Lutheran antigens are poorly expressed on cord cells, most cases of HDN associated with anti-Lu[a] are mild. Infants may exhibit weakly positive or negative Direct Antiglobulin Test (DATs) and mild to moderate elevations in bilirubin. Many require no treatment, whereas others respond to simple phototherapy. In one report of mild HDN, the mother's antibody titer rose to 1:4096.[160]

Anti-Lu[b]

Although the first example of anti-Lu[b] was a room temperature agglutinin and although IgM and IgA antibodies have been noted, most anti-Lu[b] are IgG (often IgG4) and reactive at 37°C and in the antiglobulin phase. They are made in response to pregnancy or transfusion.

Alloanti-Lu[b] reacts with all cells tested except the autocontrol, and reactions are often weaker with Lu(a+b+) red cells and cord cells. Ficin or papain does not significantly alter reactivity, although AET may. Autologous red cells will test Lu(a+) if typing sera are available.

Anti-Lu[b] has been implicated in shortened survival of transfused cells and posttransfusion jaundice, but severe or acute hemolysis has not been reported. Chromium survival studies demonstrate a rapid initial clearance of some Lu(b+) red cells, but much slower removal of those remaining.[14] Anti-Lu[b] may be regarded as clinically significant, but blood should not be withheld in emergency situations just because compatible units cannot be found. Like anti-Lu[a], Lu[b] antibodies are associated with only mild HDN.

ADVANCED CONCEPTS

Biochemistry

In 1981, Marcus et al.[161] found Lu[b] activity on red cell gangliosides, most of which contain paragloboside as found in P$_1$ and Ii. They proposed that Lutheran determinants contained this glycolipid or a homologous structure.

Lutheran antigens also may reside on a glycoprotein: early work showed that the antigens are thermolabile and, in cold butanol extractions, are found in the aqueous phase.[156] Dahr and Kruger[162] found they were solubilized from the red cell membrane using Triton X-100, a detergent that makes integral membrane proteins soluble.

Using immunoblot methods and a new monoclonal antibody BRIC 108 that has Lu[b]-like activity, Parsons et al.[163] identified two proteins with molecular weights of 85 and 78 kD. The Lu[b] activity of these two glycoproteins depends on at least one N-glycosidically linked oligosaccharide and intrachain disulfide bonds.

Daniels and Khalid,[164] using human antibodies to Lu[a], Lu[b], Lu3, Lu4, Lu6, Lu8, and Lu12, showed that probably all are located on the same membrane components and that these appear identical to those defined by BRIC 108. Studies with anti-Lu17 identified structures with a mobility similar to that of Lutheran glycoproteins but having different blot characteristics.

All Lutheran and para-Lutheran antigens are destroyed by trypsin, chymotrypsin, and pronase. Papain has little effect except on Lu8 and Lu14, which it destroys.[156] Ficin destroys Lu8, Lu14, and Lu12, and may partially alter Lu[a], Lu[b], and Lu3.[14] Red cells treated with 6 percent AET or 200 mM DTT, which break disulfide bonds, also fail to react with Lutheran antibodies, although some researchers report otherwise.[156] Perhaps minor variations in treatment resulted in the discrepant findings, or perhaps there are different specificities of anti-Lu[b], some affected by AET and some not. Some examples of anti-Lu[b] may recognize a relevant carbohydrate only on a particular peptide structure.[14]

Genetics

The *Lu* gene is located on chromosome 19, along with *H, Se, Le, LW, C3,* and genes coding for Ok[a], apolipoprotein C-II (APO), and myotonic dystrophy. Gene order on the chromosome may be *Ok-Le-C3-LW-APO-Lu-Se-H*,[156,158] with *Lu* residing at position 19q13.2.[14] *Lu* is closely linked to *Se* and was the first example of autosomal linkage described in humans.[1]

Because *H, Se,* and *Le* all encode or control fucosyltransferases and Lutheran antigens are associated with glycosylated structures, Daniels[156] suggests that chromosome 19 carries a whole family of glycosyltransferase genes that glycosylate polypeptides or lipids.

The *Lutheran* gene is probably a complex of at least four closely linked loci, each having two known codominant alleles: *Lu[a]/Lu[b], Lu[6]/Lu[9], Lu[8]/Lu[14],* and *Au[a]/Au[b]*. Like the *Kell* gene model, the original *Lu* complex may have coded for the high-frequency antigens Lu[b], Lu6, Lu8, and Au[a], and point mutations may explain their lower-frequency antithetical antigens Lu[a], Lu9, Lu14, and Au[b].

Several genetic explanations for the Lu(a−b−) phenotype have been described. These are summarized in Figure 8−10 and explained in the next section.

Lu(a−b−) Phenotypes

Dominant *In(Lu)* Type The first Lu(a−b−) family study was reported by the propositus herself.[154] Because the phenotype was seen in successive generations in 50 percent of her family members and others, and because null individuals passed normal Lutheran genes to their offspring, the expression of *Lutheran* was thought to be suppressed by a rare dominant

regulator gene later called *In(Lu)* for "inhibitor of Lutheran." *In(Lu)* segregates independently from *Lutheran.* Blood donor screenings have shown the frequency of this type of Lutheran null to be 1:3000 to 1:5000.[165]

Dominant type Lu(a−b−) red cells carry trace amounts of Lutheran and para-Lutheran antigens, as shown by absorption-elution studies. For example, a person who inherits two normal *Lu[b]* genes plus *In(Lu)* will type Lu(a−b−) using routine typing methods but will absorb and elute anti-Lu[b]. This trace amount may protect individuals from making alloanti-Lu[b].

Inheriting just one *In(Lu)* gene prevents normal expression of all Lutheran antigens, as well as P[1], i, and An/Wj, which are genetically independent. The I antigen appears unaffected. Other unrelated antigens that are suppressed include Cs[a], Yk[a], Kn[a], Sl[a], In[a] and In[b], MER2, epitopes on the common glycoprotein CDw44, concanavalin A receptor, and the receptor for horse antilymphocyte globulin.[156]

Because *In(Lu)* affects the synthesis or expression of so many antigens outside the Lutheran system, Marsh et al.[166] have proposed changing its name to *SYN-1* (for "synthesis"), with *SYN-1A* representing the common allele and *SYN-1B* representing *In(Lu)*. Although many agree that the name *In(Lu)* is outmoded, they prefer not to change it until the mechanism of the action is better understood. Some propose that *In(Lu)* causes abnormal glycosylation of a common carbohydrate sequence present in many glycoproteins and some glycolipids. It may also alter membrane conformation and affect antigen quantity or its ability to bind with antibody.[156]

In(Lu) may also affect red cell shape and metabolism. Udden et al.[167] observed abnormal poikilocytosis and acanthocytosis in some *In(Lu)* individuals, although this was variable within families. Red cells from the original *In(Lu)* propositus appear morphologically normal when first collected but become abnormal

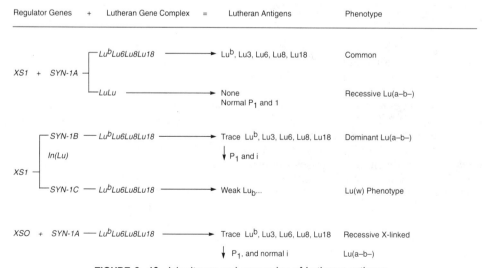

FIGURE 8-10 Inheritance and expression of Lutheran antigens.

during storage more quickly than those with normal typings. These red cells also hemolyze more during 4°C storage in modified Alsever's solution.[156] The osmotic fragility of *In(Lu)* red cells is normal, but these cells significantly resist lysis when incubated in plasma at 37°C for 24 hours. *In(Lu)* red cells have been shown to lose more K+ than they acquire in Na+ under these conditions.[156]

Recessive *LuLu* Type In some families, the Lu(a−b−) phenotype is inherited in a recessive fashion, the result of having two rare silent alleles *LuLu* at the *Lutheran* locus.[155] The parents and offspring of these nulls may type Lu(a−b+), but dosage studies and titers show them to carry a single dose of Lu[b].

Unlike *In(Lu)* null individuals, recessive Lu(a−b−) people lack all Lutheran and para-Lutheran antigens and can make an inseparable anti-Lu[ab] called anti-Lu3. They also have normal antigen expression of P1, i, and the many other antigens *In(Lu)* affects. This distinction emphasizes the importance of testing an antibody against recessive Lu(a−b−) red cells before calling its antigen phenotypically related.

Recessive Sex-linked Inhibitor Type In 1986, Norman et al.[168] described a Lu(a−b−) phenotype that fit neither an *In(Lu)* nor a *LuLu* pattern. All Lu(a−b−) family members were male and carried trace amounts of Lu[b] detected by absorption-elution. Although P1 expression was weak, i was well expressed but I was depressed. The pattern of inheritance suggested an X-borne inhibitor to *Lutheran*. They proposed calling the locus *XS*, with *XS1* being the common allele and *XS2*, the rare inhibitor that suppresses in a hemizygous state.

Lu(w) Phenotype A number of Lu(a−b+[w]) and Lu(a+[w]b+[w]) individuals with weakened Lutheran antigens have been described. Although not proved, this phenotype, also known as Lu(w), may result from *In(Lu)* with a lesser degree of penetrance or an allele to *In(Lu)* that causes less suppression (*SYN-1C*).

Anti-Lu3

Anti-Lu3 is a rare antibody that reacts with all red cells except those testing Lu(a−b−). The antibody looks like inseparable anti-Lu[ab] and recognizes a common antigen, Lu3, that is present whenever Lu[a] or Lu[b] are present (much like Jk3's association with Jk[a] and Jk[b]). It is usually antiglobulin reactive.

This antibody is made only by *LuLu* individuals. Perhaps the very weak expression of Lu3 found on dominant *In(Lu)* and sex-linked *XS2* type nulls protects them from making this antibody. Red cells from dominant and sex-linked type Lutheran nulls can be safely transfused to patients with anti-Lu3.

Lu6/Lu9 and Lu8/Lu14

In 1972, Lu6[169] and Lu8[170] designations were given to two nonidentical antibodies directed against high-frequency antigens related to the Lutheran system.

The antibodies reacted with all red cells except autologous and Lu(a−b−) cells, but they were made by Lu(a−b+) individuals.

In 1973, Molthan et al.[171] described anti-Lu9, an antibody that reacted with 2 percent of random donors and that gave very strong reactions with Lu:−6 red cells. In 1976, Judd et al.[172] reported on anti-Lu14, another antibody to a low-frequency antigen that was strongly expressed on Lu:−8 red cells.

It is now known that these antigens are made by two pairs of closely linked alleles at the Lutheran locus, *Lu6/Lu9* and *Lu8/Lu14*, which are related to *Lu[a]/Lu[b]* the way *Kp[a]/Kp[b]* and *Js[a]/Js[b]* are related to *K/k*.

Au[a] (Lu18) and Au[b] (Lu19)

Au[a] (for Auberger) was described in 1961 by Salmon et al.[173] as an antigen found in 80 percent of whites. In 1989, its antithetical antigen, Au[b], was reported by Frandson et al.[174] Because the antigens were suppressed by *In(Lu)* and *XS2*, and destroyed by trypsin, chymotrypsin, and pronase, they were closely associated with the Lutheran system except that in one family study, they were inherited independently. Serologists considered them just another set of antigens suppressed by Lutheran inhibitors, and assigned them to an antigen collection (204) with the designations 204001 and 204002.

This has all recently changed.[175,176] Au[a] and Au[b] are found on the same glycoprotein expressing Lu[a], Lu[b], Lu3, Lu4, Lu6, and Lu12 activity and are known to be absent on *LuLu* red cells. The Au(a−) family members associated with the earlier genetic exclusion were retested and found to test Au(a+), so this exclusion is not invalid. Finally, through DNA linkage studies, they were shown to reside on chromosome 19 at position 19q13.2, the *Lutheran* locus. Au[a] and Au[b] are now considered a fourth closely linked pair of alleles at the *Lutheran* locus and have been redesignated *Lu18* and *Lu19*, respectively.

Lu4, Lu5, Lu7, Lu11, Lu16, and Lu17

These antigens represent discrete, high-frequency antigens phenotypically related to Lutheran. Their antibodies parallel the characteristics of anti-Lu6 and anti-Lu8: they do not react with Lu(a−b−) red cells or autologous cells that carry otherwise normal Lutheran antigens. However, there is no conclusive evidence that their genes are part of the *Lutheran* locus.

Anti-Lu4 is known to detect Lutheran glycoproteins (GPs) in immunoblotting studies. Anti-Lu17 reacts with two GPs different from Lutheran GPs, which have the same mobility.[164]

Lu12, Lu13, An/Wj, and Singleton

These antigens have been associated with, but are probably independent of, the Lutheran system.

Lu12 describes the discrete high-frequency antigen

"Much," which is not present on *In(Lu)* and *LuLu* red cells. Its antiglobulin reactive antibody was found in the serum of a woman who tested weakly positive for Lu^b, Lu5, Lu7, Lu8, and Lu11. Family studies showed that the *Much* gene segregates independently from *Se*.[158] Because *Lutheran* and *Se* are linked, *Much* must also segregate independent of *Lutheran*. However, it has been found on the Lu glycoprotein and is still considered a para-Lutheran antigen.

Lu13 is reserved for another high-frequency antigen (called MEH or Hughes) present on all samples except Lu(a—b—) and the patient's own red cells. The antibody may be associated with anti-An/Wj.[1]

An/Wj is an interesting high-frequency antigen defined by alloantibodies (anti-Anton) and autoantibodies (anti-Wj), which were found to recognize the same specificity. Infants are born An/Wj— but become An/Wj+ almost overnight within 2 months of birth.[156]

The antigen is acquired, not inherited, by all individuals except those with the rare *In(Lu)* Lu(a—b—) and An/Wj— phenotypes. Some strains of *Haemophilus influenzae* bind to red cells by the An/Wj antigen, although this does not appear to be the organism's receptor on epithelial cells.[156] Lu15 was originally reserved for the antigen when it was first associated with *In(Lu)* red cells, but because it is present on *LuLu* cells the designation is no longer appropriate. The ISBT has given An/Wj the high-frequency antigen designation 900030.

Lu10 is another designation that is no longer used. It was at one time reserved for the Singleton antigen that was thought to be the allele of Lu5. The antibody reacted strongly with red cells from a Lu:—5 individual. However, five other examples or Lu:—5 cells were later tested and found to be negative with the Singleton serum.[1]

TABLE 8–16 **SUMMARY OF ANTIBODY CHARACTERISTICS**

Antibody	REACTIVITY ≤RT	37	AHG	Enzymes	Bind Complement	In Vitro Hemolysis	HTR	HDN	Compatible in U.S. Population (%)	Comments
M	Most	Few	Few	Destroy	(Rare)*	No	Few	Mild–severe	22	Usually clinically insignificant
N	Most	Few	Few	Destroy	(Rare)	No	Rare	Moderate	28	
S	Some	Some	Most	Variable effect	Some	No	Yes	Mild	45 W 69 B	
s	Few	Few	Most	Variable effect	Few	No	Yes	Mild–severe	11 W 3 B	
U	Rare	Some	Most	No change	(Rare)	No	Yes	Mild–severe	<1 B	
P₁	Most	Some	Rare	Enhance	Rare	Rare	Rare	(No)	21	Usually clinically insignificant
PP₁Pᵏ	Most	Some	Some	Enhance	Most	Most	(Yes)	Mild	<0.1	Potent hemolysins
P	Most	Some	Some	Enhance	Most	Some	(Yes)	Mild–severe	<0.1	May be associated with early abortions
I	Most	Few	Few	Enhance	Most	Few	Rare	(No)	See text	Usually autoantibodies clinically insignificant
i	Most	Few	Few	Enhance	Most	Few	(?)	Mild	See text	
K	Some	Some	Most	No change	Some	No	Yes	Mild–severe	91	
k	Few	Few	Most	No change	(Some)	No	Yes	Mild	0.2	
Kpᵃ	Some	Some	Most	No change	(Some)	No	Yes	Mild	99.7	
Kpᵇ	Few	Few	Most	No change	(Some)	No	Yes	Mild	<0.1	
Jsᵃ	Few	Few	Most	No change	(Some)	No	Yes	Moderate	100 W 80 B	
Jsᵇ	(No)	(No)	Most	No change	(Some)	No	Yes	Mild–moderate	1 B	
Fyᵃ	Rare	Rare	Most	Destroy	Some	No	Yes	Mild–severe	34 W	
Fyᵇ	Rare	Rare	Most	Destroy	Some	No	Yes	(Yes)	17 W 77 B	
Jkᵃ	Few	Few	Most	Enhance	All	Some	Yes	Mild	23	Associated with severe delayed HTR
Jkᵇ	Few	Few	Most	Enhance	All	Some	Yes	Mild	28 W 57 B	
Luᵃ	Most	Few	Few	Variable effect	Some	No	(?)	Mild	92	IgG₄ and IgA antibody classes seen
Luᵇ	Few	Few	Most	Variable effect	Some	No	Yes	Mild	0.15	

*Comments in parentheses are postulated and not based on reported cases.
B = blacks; HDN = hemolytic disease of the newborn; HTR = hemolytic transfusion reactions; ≤ RT = room temperature or colder; W = whites.

Applications to Routine Blood Banking

The major blood group systems outside of ABO and Rh become important only after patients develop unexpected antibodies. Then a fundamental knowledge of antibody characteristics, clinical significance, and antigen frequency is needed to help confirm antibody specificity and select appropriate units for transfusion.

Only a few antibody specificities are commonly seen: M, P_1, and I react at room temperature and are considered clinically insignificant; K, S, s, Fy^a, Fy^b, Jk^a, and Jk^b react in the antiglobulin phase and are clinically significant. These and selected others are summarized in Table 8–16.

Not all antibody problems are easily solved, however; panel reactions are sometimes inconclusive. This is when all the esoteric information about the blood groups should be searched for clues. What other antibodies should be considered? What other special techniques or special cells might be used? What information will be gained by antigen typing the patient's cells? If antigen typings are weaker than normal, what is the reason? A systematic review of the blood groups may provide the answer.

Laboratory staff performing paternity tests need to be aware of inheritance patterns and the existence of silent genes, regulators, inhibitors, and modifying situations. Knowing the genetics and biochemistry of the blood group antigens can provide insight into their red cell function and observed disease associations. Perhaps this esoterica will stimulate readers to learn more.

Review Questions

1. Which of the following best describes MN antigens and antibodies?
   A. Well developed at birth, susceptible to enzymes, generally saline reactive
   B. Not well developed at birth, susceptible to enzymes, generally saline reactive
   C. Well developed at birth, not susceptible to enzymes, generally saline reactive
   D. Well developed at birth, susceptible to enzymes, generally antiglobulin reactive

2. Evidence suggests that the Ii antigens are associated with which blood group system?
   A. ABH
   B. Kell
   C. Duffy
   D. Lutheran

3. The antigens Js^b and K^b belong to which system?
   A. MNSs
   B. Kell
   C. Duffy
   D. Lutheran

4. Which blood group system is associated with resistance to malaria?
   A. P
   B. Kell
   C. Duffy
   D. Kidd

5. Which antibody does *not* fit with the others with respect to optimum temperature of reactivity?
   A. Anti-S
   B. Anti-P_1
   C. Anti-Fy^a
   D. Anti-Jk^b

6. An antibody reacts with 1 in 10 random test cells in the antiglobulin phase. Reactivity is not effected by enzymes, but is destroyed by AET. The antibody is most likely:
   A. Anti-i
   B. Anti-K
   C. Anti-P_1
   D. Anti-Jk^a

7. Antibody screening cells will *not* routinely detect:
   A. Anti-M
   B. Anti-Kp^a
   C. Anti-Fy^a
   D. Anti-Lu^b

8. About how many donors will need to be antigen typed to find three Fy(a−) units for crossmatch?
   A. 3
   B. 5
   C. 10
   D. 12

9. Which blood group system is known for showing dosage?
   A. I
   B. P
   C. Kidd
   D. Lutheran

10. Which antibody is most commonly associated with delayed hemolytic transfusion reactions?
    A. Anti-s
    B. Anti-k
    C. Anti-Lu^a
    D. Anti-Jk^a

11. A patient with an infection from *Mycoplasma pneumoniae* will most likely develop a cold autoantibody with specificity to:
    A. I
    B. i
    C. P
    D. P_1

12. Which antigen is routinely destroyed by enzymes?
    A. P_1
    B. Js^a
    C. Fy^a
    D. Jk^a

Answers to Review Questions

1. A (p 153)
2. A (p 164)
3. B (p 166)
4. C (pp 171 and 174)
5. B (p 159)
6. B (p 166)
7. B (p 168)
8. C (Table 8–16)
9. C (p 175)
10. D (p 176)
11. A (p 164)
12. C (p 172)

References

1. Issitt, PD: Applied Blood Group Serology. Montgomery Scientific Publications, Miami, 1985.
2. Lewis, M, et al: Blood group terminology 1990. Vox Sang 58:152, 1990.
3. Plapp, FV: How to dissect membrane structure. In Vengelen-Tyler, V and Judd, WJ (eds): Recent Advances in Blood Group Biochemistry. American Association of Blood Banks, Arlington, VA, 1986.
4. Brown, PJ: Basic red cell membrane structure. In Pierce, SR and Steane, S (eds): Biochemistry for Blood Bankers. American Association of Blood Banks, Arlington, VA, 1983.
5. Dahr, W: Immunochemistry of sialoglycoproteins in human red blood cell membranes. In Vengelen-Tyler, V and Judd, WJ (eds): Recent Advances in Blood Group Biochemistry. American Association of Blood Banks, Arlington, VA, 1986.
6. Landsteiner, K, and Levine, P: A new agglutinable factor differentiating individual human bloods. Proc Soc Exp Biol 24:600, 1927.
7. Landsteiner, K, and Levine, P: Further observations on individual differences of human blood. Proc Soc Exp Biol 24:941, 1927.
8. Walsh, RJ, and Montgomery, C: A new human isoagglutinin subdividing the MN blood groups. Nature 160:504, 1947.
9. Levine, P, et al: A new blood group factor, s, allelic to S. Proc Soc Exp Biol 78:218, 1951.
10. Wiener, AS, Unger, LJ, and Gordon, EB: Fatal hemolytic transfusion reaction caused by sensitization to a new blood group factor U. JAMA 153:1444, 1953.
11. Greenwalt, TJ, et al: An allele of the S(s) blood group genes. Proc Natl Acad Sci USA 40:1126, 1954.
12. Anstee, DJ: Blood group-active surface molecules of the human red blood cell. Vox Sang 58:1, 1990.
13. Stoltz, JF, Strieff, F, and Genetet, B: Demonstration of M antigen on human lymphocytes by liquid phase electrophoresis. Vox Sang 26:467, 1974.
14. Mollison, PL, Engelfriet, CP, and Contreras, M: Blood Transfusion in Clinical Medicine, ed 9. Blackwell Scientific Publications, Oxford, 1993.
15. Hawkins, P, et al: Localization of MN blood group antigens in kidney. Transplant Proc 17:1697, 1985.
16. Vaisanen, V, et al: Blood group M specific haemagglutinin in pyelonephritogenic Escherichia coli. Lancet ii:1192, 1982.
17. Rolih, S: Biochemistry of MN Antigens. In Unger, PJ and Laird-Fryer, B (eds): Blood Group Systems: MN and Gerbich. American Association of Blood Banks, Arlington, VA, 1989.
18. Masouredis, SP, et al: Quantitative immunoferritin microassay of Fy^a, Fy^b, Jk^a, U and Di^b antigen site numbers on human red cells. Blood 56:969, 1980.
19. Rygiel, SA, Issitt, CH, and Fruitstone, MJ: Destruction of the S antigen by sodium hypochlorite. Transfusion 25:274, 1985.
20. Morel, P, et al: Sera exhibiting hemagglutination of N red blood cells stored in media containing glucose (abstr). Transfusion 15:522, 1975.
21. Belzer, FO, Kountz, SL, and Perkins, HA: Red cell cold autoagglutinins as a cause of failure of renal transplantation. Transplantation 11:422, 1971.
22. Lutz, P, and Dzik, WH: Molecular biology of red cell blood group genes. Transfusion 32:467, 1992.
23. Reid, ME: Hybrid sialoglycoproteins, Gerbich, Webb and Cad blood group determinants. In Vengelen-Tyler, V and Judd, WJ (eds): Recent Advances in Blood Group Biochemistry. American Association of Blood Banks, Arlington, VA, 1986.
24. Holliman, SM: The MN blood group system: Distribution, serology and genetics. In Unger, PJ and Laird-Fryer, B (eds): Blood Group Systems: MN and Gerbich. American Association of Blood Banks, Arlington, VA, 1989.
25. Darnborough, J, Dunsford, I, and Wallace, JA: The En^a antigen and antibody: A genetical modification of human red cells affecting their blood grouping reactions. Vox Sang 17:241, 1969.
26. Furuhjelm, V, et al: The red cell phenotype En(a−) and anti-En^a: serological and physicochemical aspects. Vox Sang 17:256, 1969.
27. Issitt, PD, et al: An En(a−) sample that types as Wr(a−b−). Transfusion 15:353, 1975.
28. Adams, J, et al: An antibody in the serum of a Wr(a−) individual, reacting with an antigen of very high frequency. Transfusion 11:290, 1971.
29. Metaxas, MN, and Metaxas-Buhler, M: M^k: An apparently silent allele at the MN locus. Nature 202:1123, 1964.
30. Tokunaga, E, et al: Two apparently healthy Japanese individuals of type M^kM^b have erythrocytes which lack both the blood group MN and Ss-active sialoglycoproteins. J Immunogenet 6:383, 1979.
31. Cleghorn, TE: A memorandum on the Miltenberger blood groups. Vox Sang 11:219, 1966.
32. Dahr, W: Miltenberger subsystem of the MNSs blood group system: Review and outlook. Vox Sang 62:129, 1992.
33. Tippett, P, et al: The Miltenberger subsystem: Is it obsolescent? Transfus Med Rev 4:170, 1992.
34. Hadley, TJ, McGinniss, MH, and Miller, LH: Blood group antigens and invasion of erythrocytes by malarial parasites. In Garratty, G (ed): Red Cell Antigens and Antibodies. American Association of Blood Banks, Arlington, VA, 1986.
35. Levine, P, et al: Isoimmunization by a new blood factor in tumor cells. Proc Soc Exp Biol 77:403, 1951.
36. Sanger, R: An association between the P and Jay systems of blood groups. Nature 176, 1163, 1955.
37. Matson, GA, et al: A "new" antigen and antibody belonging to the P blood group system. Am J Hum Genet 11:26, 1959.
38. Race, RR, and Sanger, R: Blood Groups in Man, ed 6. Blackwell Scientific Publications, Oxford, 1975.
39. Ikin, EW, et al: P_1 antigen in the human foetus. Nature 192:883, 1961.
40. Heiken, A: Observations on the blood group receptor P_1 and its development in children. Hereditas 56:83, 1966.
41. Moureau, P: Les reactions post-transfusionnelles. Rev Bel Sci Med 16:258, 1945.
42. Dinapoli, JB, et al: Hemolytic transfusion reaction caused by IgG anti-P_1 (abstr). Transfusion 18:383, 1978.
43. Graham, H: An overview of the biochemistry of the Lewis, ABH and P systems. In Bell, CA (ed): A Seminar on Antigens on Blood Cells and Body Fluids. American Association of Blood Banks, Washington, DC, 1980.
44. Cameron, GL, and Staveley, JM: Blood group P substance in hydatid cyst fluids. Nature 179:147, 1957.

45. Roland, FP: P₁ blood group and urinary tract infection. Lancet i:946, 1981.
46. Ben-Ishmail, R, et al: Anti-P₁, allohemagglutinins associated with Clonorchis sinensis and Opisthorchis viverrini infections in patients from Southeast Asia. Southeast Asian J Trop Med Public Health 13:86, 1982.
47. Prokop, I, and Schlesinger, D: Über das Vorkommen von P₁-Blutgruppensubstanz bei einigen Metazoen, insbesondere Ascaris suum und Lumbricus terrestris. Z Immun Forsch 129:344, 1965.
48. Cantin, G, and Lyonnais, J: Anti-PP₁Pᵏ and early abortion. Transfusion 23:350, 1983.
49. Shirey, RS, et al: Plasmapheresis and successful pregnancy after fourteen miscarriages in the P₁ᵏ with anti-P (abstr). Transfusion 24:427, 1984.
50. Vos, GH, et al: Relationship of a hemolysin resembling anti-Tjᵃ to threatened abortion in western Australia. Transfusion 4:87, 1964.
51. Tippett, P, et al: An agglutinin associated with the P and the ABO blood group systems. Vox Sang 10:269, 1965.
52. Tippett, P: Contributions of monoclonal antibodies to understanding one new and some old blood group systems. In Garratty, G (ed): Red Cell Antigens and Antibodies. American Association of Blood Banks, Arlington, VA, 1986.
53. Englefriet, CP, et al: Haemolysins probably recognizing the antigen p. Vox Sang 23:176, 1972.
54. Källenius, G, et al: Occurrence of P-fimbriated Escherichia coli in urinary tract infection. Lancet 2:1369, 1981.
55. Källenius, G, et al: Structure of carbohydrate part of receptor on human uroepithelial cells for pyelonephritogenic Escherichia coli. Lancet 2:604, 1981.
56. Anstall, HB, and Blaylock, RC: The P blood group system: Biochemistry, genetics and clinical significance. In Moulds, JM and Woods, LL (eds): Blood Groups: P, I, Sdᵃ and Pr. American Association of Blood Banks, Arlington, VA, 1991.
57. Lomberg, H, et al: P₁ blood group and urinary tract infection. Lancet 1:551, 1981.
58. Mulholland, SG, Mooreville, M, and Parson, CL: Urinary tract infections and P blood group antigens. Urology 24:232, 1984.
59. Wiener, AS, et al: Type-specific cold autoantibodies as a cause of acquired hemolytic anemia and hemolytic transfusion reactions, biologic test with bovine red cells. Ann Intern Med 44:221, 1956.
60. Marsh, WL, and Jenkins, WJ: Anti-i: A new cold antibody. Nature 188:753, 1960.
61. Marsh, WL: Anti-i: A cold antibody defining the Ii relationship in human red cells. Br J Haematol 7:200, 1961.
62. Beck, ML: The I blood group collection. In Moulds, JM and Woods, LL (eds): Blood Groups: P, I, Sdᵃ and Pr. American Association of Blood Banks, Arlington, VA, 1991.
63. Shirey, S, Harris, J, and Moore, L: An autoanti-I greatly enhanced in the presence of Thimerosol (abstr). Transfusion 19:642, 1979.
64. Taney, FA, Lee, LT, and Howe, C: Cold hemagglutinin crossreactivity with Mycoplasma pneumoniae. Infect Immun 22:29, 1978.
65. Costea, N, Yakulis, V, and Heller, P: Experimental production of cold agglutinins in rabbits. Blood 26:323, 1965.
66. Gerbal, A, et al: Sensibilisation des hematies d'un nouveauné par un auto-anticorps anti-i d'origine maternelle nature IgG. Nouv Rev Hematol 11:689, 1971.
67. Moores, PP, et al: Some observations on "Bombay" bloods with comments on evidence for the existence of two different Oₕ phenotypes. Transfusion 15:237, 1975.
68. Feizi, T: The blood group Ii system: A carbohydrate antigen system defined by naturally monoclonal or oligoclonal autoantibodies of man. Immunol Commun 10:127, 1981.
69. Hakomori, S: Blood group ABH and Ii antigens on human erythrocytes: Chemistry, polymorphism and their developmental change. Semin Hematol 18:39, 1981.
70. Curtain, DD, et al: Cold haemagglutinins: Unusual incidence in Melanesian populations. Br J Haematol 11:247, 1965.
71. Booth, PB, Jenkins, WL, and Marsh WL: Anti-Iᵀ: A new antibody of the I blood group system occurring in certain Melanesian sera. Br J Haematol 12:341, 1966.
72. Garratty, G, et al: Autoimmune hemolytic anemia in Hodgkins desease associated with anti-Iᵀ. Transfusion 14:226, 1974.
73. Marsh, WL, Nichols, ME, and Reid, ME: The definition of two I antigen components. Vox Sang 20:209, 1971.
74. Dzierzkowski-Borodej, W, Seyfried, H, and Lisowka, E: Serological classification of anti-I sera. Vox Sang 28:110, 1975.
75. Coombs, RR, Mourant, AE, and Race, RR: In-vivo isosensitization of red cells in babies with hemolytic disease. Lancet i:264, 1946.
76. Levine, P, et al: A new human hereditary blood property (Cellano) present in 99.8 percent of all bloods. Science 109:464, 1949.
77. Allen, FH, and Lewis, SJ: Kpᵃ (Penney), a new antigen in the Kell blood group system. Vox Sang 2:81, 1957.
78. Allen, FH, Lewis, SJ, and Fudenberg, HH: Studies of anti-Kpᵇ, a new alloantibody in the Kell blood group system. Vox Sang 3:1, 1958.
79. Giblett, ER: Js, a "new" blood group antigen found in negroes. Nature 181:1221, 1958.
80. Walker, RH, et al: Anti-Jsᵇ, the expected antithetical antibody of the Sutter blood group system. Nature 197:295, 1963.
81. Chown, F, Lewis, M, and Kaita, H: A "new" Kell blood group phenotype. Nature 180:711, 1957.
82. Allen, FH, Krabbe, SM, and Corcoran, PA: A new phenotype (McLeod) in the Kell blood group system. Vox Sang 6:555, 1961.
83. Hughes-Jones, NC, and Gardner, B: The Kell system: Studies with radioactively labelled anti-K. Vox Sang 21:154, 1971.
84. Judson, PA, and Anstee, DJ: Comparative effect of trypsin and chymotrypsin on blood group antigens. Med Lab Sci 34:1, 1977.
85. Kornstad, L and Heisto, H: The frequency of formation of Kell antibodies in recipient of Kell-positive blood. Proc 6th Congr Europ Soc Haematol, Copenhagen, 1957.
86. Daniels, G: The Kell blood group system: Genetics. In Laird-Fryer, B, et al. (eds): Blood Group Systems: Kell. American Association of Blood Banks, 1990.
87. Yamaguchi, H, et al: A "new" allele, Kpᶜ, at the Kell complex locus. Vox Sang 36:29, 1979.
88. Gavin, J, et al: The red cell antigen once called Levay is the antigen Kpᶜ of the Kell system. Vox Sang 36:31, 1979.
89. Callender, ST, Race, RR, and Paykos, ZV: Hypersensitivity to transfused blood. Br Med J 2:83, 1945.
90. Marsh, WL, et al: Naturally occurring anti-Kell stimulated by E. coli entercolitis in a 20-day old child. Transfusion 18:149, 1978.
91. Schultz, MH: Serology and clinical significance of Kell blood group system antibodies. In Laird-Fryer, B, et al. (eds): Blood Group System: Kell. American Association of Blood Banks, Arlington, VA, 1990.
92. Marsh, WL, and Redman, CM: The Kell blood group system: A review. Transfusion 30:158, 1990.
93. Advani, H, et al: Inactivation of Kell blood group antigens by 2-aminoethylisothiouronium bromide. Br J Haematol 51:107, 1982.
94. Branch, DR, Sy Siak Hian, AL, and Petz, LD: Unmasking of Kx antigen by reduction of disulfide bonds on normal McLeod red cells. Br J Haematol 59:505, 1985.
95. Chown, B: XIIIth John G. Gibson II Lecture. Columbia Presbyterian Medical Center College of Physicians and Surgeons, New York, 1964.
96. Guevin, RM, Taliano, V, and Waldmann, O: The Cote serum, an antibody defining a new variant in the kell system (abstr). 24th Annual Meeting Abstract Booklet, American Association of Blood Banks, 1971.
97. Strange, JJ, et al: Wkᵃ (Weeks), a new antigen in the Kell blood group system. Vox Sang 27:81, 1974.
98. Eicher, C, et al: A new low frequency antigen in the Kell system: K24 (Cls) (abstr). Transfusion 25:448, 1985.
99. Marsh, WL, et al: K23: A low-incidence antigen in the Kell blood group system identified by biochemical characterization. Transfusion 27:36, 1987.

100. Van der Hart, M, Szaloky, A, and Van Loghem, JJ: A "new" antibody associated with the Kell blood group system. Vox Sang 15:456, 1968.

101. Marsh, WL: Deleted antigens of the rhesus and Kell blood groups: Association with cell membrane defects. In Garratty, G (ed): Blood Group Antigens and Disease. American Association of Blood Banks, Arlington, VA, 1983.

102. Rouger, P: Defects of McLeod red blood cells and association with disease. In Laird-Fryer, B, Levitt, J and Daniels, G (eds): Blood Groups Systems: Kell. American Association of Blood Banks, Arlington, VA, 1990.

103. Giblett, ER, et al: Kell phenotypes in chronic granulomatous disease: A potential transfusion hazard. Lancet 1:1235, 1971.

104. Marsh, WL, Uretsky, SC, and Douglas, SD: Antigens of the Kell blood group system on neutrophils and monocytes: Their relation to chronic granulomatous disease. J Pediatr 87:1117, 1975.

105. Marsh, WL, and Redman, CM: Recent developments in the Kell blood group system. Transfus Med Rev 1:4, 1987.

106. McGinnis, MH, Maclowry, JD, and Holland, PV: Acquisition of K:1-like antigen during terminal sepsis. Transfusion 24:28, 1984.

107. Marsh, WL, Dinapoli, J, and Øyen, R: Autoimmune hemolytic anemia caused by anti-K13. Vox Sang 36:174, 1979.

108. Cutbush, M, Mollison, PL, and Parkin, DM: A new human blood group. Nature 165:188, 1950.

109. Ikin, EW, et al: Discovery of the expected hemagglutinin, anti-Fy^b. Nature 168:1077, 1951.

110. Sanger, R, Race, RR, and Jack, J: The Duffy blood groups of New York Negroes: The phenotype Fy(a−b−). Br J Haematol 1:370, 1955.

111. Miller, LH, et al: Erythrocyte receptors for (Plasmodium knowlesi) malaria: Duffy blood group determinants. Science 189:561, 1975.

112. Rosenfield, RE, Szymanski, O, and Kochwa, S: Immunochemical studies of the Rh system: III. Quantitative hemagglutination that is relatively independent of source of Rh antigens and antibodies. Cold Spring Harbor Symp Quant Biol 29:427, 1964.

113. Greenwalt, TJ, Saski, T, and Gajewski, M: Further examples of hemolytic disease of the newborn due to anti-Duffy (anti-Fy^a). Vox Sang 4:138, 1959.

114. Valko, DA: The Duffy blood group system: Biochemistry and role in malaria. In Pierce, SR and Macpherson, CR (eds): Blood Group System: Duffy, Kidd and Lutheran. American Association of Blood Banks, Arlington, VA, 1988.

115. Tanner, MJA, et al: Effect of endoglycosidase F preparations on the surface components of the human erythrocyte. Carbohydr Res 178:203, 1988.

116. Chown, B, Lewis, M, and Kaita, H: The Duffy blood group system in Caucasians: Evidence for a new allele. Am J Hum Genet 17:384, 1965.

117. Beattie, KM: The Duffy blood group system: Distribution, serology and genetics. In Pierce, SR and Macpherson, CR (eds): Blood Group Systems: Duffy, Kidd and Lutheran. American Association of Blood Banks, Arlington, VA, 1988.

118. Albrey, JA, et al: A new antibody, anti-Fy3, in the Duffy blood group system. Vox Sang 20:29, 1971.

119. Behzad, O, et al: A new anti-erythrocyte antibody in the Duffy system: Anti-FY4. Vox Sang 24:337, 1973.

120. Sosler, SD, et al: The relative prevalence of Duffy antibodies in a population of known racial make-up (abstr). Transfusion 26:546, 1986.

121. Baldwin, M, et al: The incidence of anti-Fy^a and anti-Fy^b antibodies in Black and White patients (abstr). Transfusion 26:546, 1986.

122. Colledge, KI, Pezzulich, M, and Marsh, WL: Anti-Fy5, an antibody disclosing a probable association between the Rhesus and Duffy blood group genes. Vox Sang 24:193, 1973.

123. Nichols, ME, et al: A new Duffy blood group specificity defined by a murine monoclonal antibody. J Exp Med 166:776, 1987.

124. Palanik, M, Junqueira, PC, and Alves, ZMS: Fs: An antigenic determinant possibly related to the Duffy blood group. Rev Fr Transfus Immunohematol 6:629, 1982.

125. Donahue, RP, et al: Probable assignment of the Duffy blood group locus to chromosome 1 in man. Proc Natl Acad Sci USA 61:949, 1968.

126. Salmon, C, Cartron, JP, and Rouger, P: The Human Blood Groups. Masson Publishing, New York, 1984.

127. Mason, SJ, et al: The Duffy blood group determinants: Their role in susceptibility of human and animal erythrocytes to Plasmodium knowlesi malaria. Br J Haematol 36:327, 1977.

128. Miller, LH, et al: The Duffy blood group phenotype in American blacks infected with Plasmodium vivax in Vietnam. Am J Trop Med 27:1069, 1978.

129. Spencer, HC, et al: The Duffy blood group and resistance to Plasmodium vivax in Honduras. Am J Trop Med 27:664, 1978.

130. Allen, FH, Diamond, LK, and Niedziela, B: A new blood group antigen. Nature 167:482, 1951.

131. Plaut, G, et al: A new blood group antibody, anti-Jk^b. Nature 171:431, 1953.

132. Pinkerton, FJ, et al: The phenotype Jk(a−b−) in the Kidd blood group system. Vox Sang 4:155, 1959.

133. Mougey, R: The Kidd blood group system: Serology and genetics. In Pierce, SR and Macpherson, CR (eds): Blood Group Systems: Duffy, Kidd and Lutheran. American Association of Blood Banks, Arlington, VA, 1988.

134. Haber, G, and Rosenfield, RE: Ficin treated red cells for hemagglutination studies. In Andresen PH: Papers in Dedication of His 60th Birthday. Munksgaard, Copenhagen, 1957.

135. Polley, MT, and Mollison, PL: The role of complement in the detection of blood group antibodies. Special reference to the antiglobulin test. Transfusion 1:9, 1961.

136. Dorner, I, Moore, JA, and Chaplin, H: Combined maternal erythrocyte autosensitization and materno-fetal Jk^a incompatibility. Transfusion 14:211, 1974.

137. Sinor, LT, et al: Dot-blot purification of the Kidd blood group antigen (abstr). Transfusion 26:561, 1986.

138. Heaton, DC, and McLoughlin, K: Jk(a−b−) red blood cells resist urea lysis. Transfusion 22:70, 1982.

139. Edwards-Moulds, J, and Kasschau, MR: The effect of 2 molar urea on Jk(a−b−) red cells. Vox Sang 55:181, 1988.

140. Edwards-Moulds, J: The Kidd blood group system: Drug-related antibodies and biochemistry. In Pierce, SR and Macpherson, CR (eds): Blood Group System: Duffy, Kidd and Lutheran. American Association of Blood Banks, Arlington, VA, 1988.

141. Okubo, Y, et al: Heterogeneity of the phenotype Jk(a−b−) found in Japanese. Transfusion 26:237, 1986.

142. Lewis, M, et al: Analysis of linkage relationship of Co, Jk and K with each other and with chromosome 2 loci ACP1 and Km. Ann Hum Genet 46:349, 1982.

143. Geitvik, GA, et al: The Kidd (Jk) blood group locus assigned to chromosome 18 by close linkage to a DNA-RFLP. Hum Genet 77:205, 1987.

144. Arcara, PC, O'Conner, MA, and Dimmette, RM: A family with three Jk(a−b−) members (abstr). Transfusion 9:282, 1969.

145. Humphrey, AJ and Morel, PA: Heterogeneity within the Kidd system. Transfusion 16:242, 1976.

146. Patten, E, et al: Autoimmune hemolytic anemia with anti-Jk^a specificity in a patient taking Aldomet. Transfusion 17:517, 1977.

147. Sosler, SD, et al: Acute hemolytic anemia due to a chloropropamide-dependent autoanti-Jk^a (abstr). Transfusion 19:641, 1979.

148. Judd, WJ, Steiner, EA, and Cochrane, RK: Paraben-associated autoanti-Jk^a antibodies. Transfusion 22:31, 1982.

149. Ellisor, SS, et al: Autoantibodies mimicking anti-Jk^b plus anti-Jk3 associated with autoimmune hemolytic anemia in a primipara who delivered an unaffected infant. Vox Sang 45:53, 1983.

150. Obarski, G, et al: The Jk(a−b−) phenotype, probably occurring as a transient phenomenon (abstr). Transfusion 27:548, 1987.

151. McGinnis, MH: The ubiquitous nature of human blood group antigens as evidenced by bacterial, viral and parasitic infections. In Garratty, G (ed): Blood Groups Antigens and Disease. American Association of Blood Banks, Arlington, VA, 1983.

152. Marsh, WL: Recent advances relating to the Duffy and Lutheran blood groups. In Walker, RH, et al. (eds): A Seminar on Recent Advances in Immunohematology. American Association of Blood Banks, Washington, DC, 1973.

153. Cutbush, M, and Chanarin, I: The expected blood group antibody, anti-Lu^b. Nature 178:855, 1956.

154. Crawford, MN, et al: The phenotype Lu(a–b–) together with unconventional Kidd groups in one family. Transfusion 1:228, 1967.

155. Darnborough, J, et al: A "new" antibody anti-Lu^{a}Lu^b and two further examples of the genotype Lu(a–b–). Nature 198:796, 1963.

156. Daniels, G: The Lutheran blood group system: Monoclonal antibodies, biochemistry and the effect of In(Lu). In Pierce, SR and Macpherson, CR (eds): Blood Group System: Duffy, Kidd and Lutheran. American Association of Blood Banks, Arlington, VA, 1988.

157. Anstee, DJ, et al: Evidence for the Occurrence of Lu^b-Active Glycoproteins in Human Erythrocytes, Kidney and Liver (abstr). International Congress ISBT-BBTS Book of Abstracts, Les Ulis, France, 1988, p 263.

158. Crawford, M: The Lutheran blood group system: Serology and genetics. In Pierce, SR and Macpherson, CR (eds): Blood Group System: Duffy, Kidd and Lutheran. American Association of Blood Banks, Arlington, VA, 1988.

159. Greendyke, RM, and Chorpenning, FW: Normal survival of incompatible red cells in the presence of anti-Lu^a. Transfusion 2:52, 1960.

160. Francis, BJ, and Hatcher, DE: Hemolytic disease of the newborn apparently caused by anti-Lu^a. Transfusion 1:248, 1961.

161. Marcus, DM, Kunku, SK, and Suzuki, A: The P blood group system: Recent progress in immunochemistry and genetics. Semin Hematol 18:63, 1981.

162. Dahr, W, and Kruger, J: Solubilization of various blood group antigens by Triton X-100. Proceedings of the 10th Congress of the Society for Forensic Haemogenetics. Munich, 1983, p 141.

163. Parsons, SF, et al: Evidence that the Lu^b blood group antigen is located on red cell membrane glycoproteins of 85 and 78 kd. Transfusion 27:61, 1987.

164. Daniels, G, and Khalid, G: Identification, by immunblotting, of the structures carrying Lutheran and Para-Lutheran blood group antigens. Vox Sang 57:137, 1989.

165. Poole, J: Review: The Lutheran blood group system—1991. Immunohematology 8:1, 1992.

166. Marsh, WL, Johnson, CL, and Mueller, KA: Proposed new notation for the In(Lu) modifying gene. Transfusion 24:371, 1984.

167. Udden, MM, et al: New abnormalities in the morphology, cell surface receptors, and electrolyte metabolism in In(Lu) erythrocytes. Blood 69:52, 1987.

168. Norman, PC, Tippett, P, and Beal, RW: A Lu(a–b–) phenotype caused by an X-linked recessive gene. Vox Sang 51:49, 1986.

169. Marsh, WL: Anti-Lu5, anti-Lu6 and anti-Lu7. Three antibodies defining high frequency antigens related to the Lutheran blood group system. Transfusion 12:27, 1972.

170. MacIlroy, M, McCreary, J, and Stroup, M: Anti-Lu8, an antibody recognizing another Lutheran-related antigen. Vox Sang 23:455, 1972.

171. Molthan, L, et al: Lu9, another new antigen of the Lutheran blood group system. Vox Sang 24:468, 1973.

172. Judd, WJ, et al: Anti-Lu14: A Lutheran antibody defining the product of an allele at the Lu8 blood group locus. Vox Sang 32:214, 1977.

173. Salmon, C, et al: Un nouvel antigene de groupe sanguin erythrocytaire present chez 80% des sujets du race blanche. Nouv Rev Fr Hematol 1:649, 1961.

174. Frandson, S, et al: Anti-Au^b: The antithetical antibody to anti-Au^a. Vox Sang 56:54, 1989.

175. Daniels, GL, et al: The red cell antigens Au^a and Au^b belong to the Lutheran system. Vox Sang 60:191, 1991.

176. Zelinski, T, et al: Assignment of the Auberger red cell antigen polymorphism to the Lutheran blood group system: Genetic justification. Vox Sang 61:275, 1991.

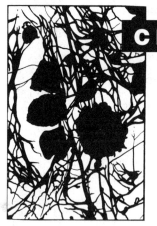

CHAPTER 9

Miscellaneous Blood Group Systems

Denise M. Harmening, PhD, MT(ASCP), CLS(NCA)
Felicia E. Dawson-Batcha, MT(ASCP)BB, CLS(NCA)

OBJECTIVES

Upon completion of this chapter, the learner should be able to:

1 Discuss the significant characteristics of antigens in the following blood group systems.

   a sex-linked (Xg) blood group system
   b Wright (Wr) blood group system
   c Cartwright (Yt) blood group system
   d Diego (Di) blood group system
   e Scianna (Sc) blood group system
   f Dombrock (Do) blood group system
   g Colton (Co) blood group system
   h Auberger (Au) blood group system

2 Discuss the significant characteristics of the following unrelated red cell antigens.

   a Antigens Cost (Csᵃ), York (Ykᵃ), Knops (Knᵃ), and McCoy (McCᵃ and McCᵇ)
   b Antigen Chido (Chᵃ)

   c Antigen Rodgers (Rg[a])
   d Antigen John Milton Hagen (JMH)
   e Bg Antigens
3 Have a general understanding of antigens of high incidence and antigens of low
   incidence and examples of these antigens on the red cells.

In the category of miscellaneous blood groups, approximately 300 blood group antigens have been described that may or may not represent independent blood group systems. In light of this, it would be difficult to try to present all these miscellaneous antigens. As a result, only the more commonly studied blood group systems are presented here briefly, depending on the information currently available. All the other antigens will be grouped into various categories or under certain headings for simplicity.

The Sex-Linked Blood Group System: Xg[a]

The Xg[a] blood group was discovered in 1962,[1] and other examples soon followed (Cook et al.[2] and Sausais et al.[3]). This blood group is unique in that it is believed to be the only one produced under the control of a gene located on the X chromosome. Many family studies have confirmed the inheritance of Xg[a] on an X-linked basis; therefore, a difference in the frequency of the Xg[a] antigen is noted between the sexes. Approximately 89 percent of the female population is Xg(a+), whereas 67 percent of the male population is Xg(a+).[4]

Men can be of genotype *Xg[a]* or *Xg*, whereas women can be *Xg[a]Xg[a]*, *Xg[a] Xg*, or *XgXg*. Thus the mating of an Xg(a+) man with an Xg(a−) woman would produce all Xg(a+) daughters and Xg(a−) sons.

Several examples of anti-Xg[a] have been described. Most of these antibodies are IgG immunoglobulins reactive only in the antihuman globulin phase of in vitro testing and are destroyed by enzymes (bromelyn, ficin, papain, trypsin, and pronase) but not by neuraminidase.

The majority of Xg[a] antibodies can bind complement but have not been demonstrated to produce in vitro hemolysis. Most Xg[a] antibodies are the result of red cell stimulation but have not been implicated in transfusion reactions or hemolytic disease of the newborn (HDN). Therefore, Xg[a] antigen does not appear to be an efficient immunogen. One example of autoanti-Xg[a] has been reported (Yokoyama et al.[5]).

The Wright Blood Group System: Wr[a] and Wr[b]

The Wright blood group system, discovered in 1953,[6] is composed of two allelic antigens: Wr[a], a low-frequency antigen occurring in less than 0.1 per-

cent of the random population; and Wr[b], a high-frequency antigen occurring in 99.9 percent of the random population.

Although the antigen Wr[a] is extremely rare, the antibody anti-Wr[a] has been reported quite frequently. Two types of Wr[a] exist. The first is an IgM antibody that is naturally occurring, usually agglutinates Wr(a+) red cells in saline, and reacts better at 20°C than at 37°C. It is frequently found in the serum of individuals who have never been pregnant or transfused. The second type is an IgG antibody that is reactive only in the antihuman globulin phase of in vitro testing. The IgG anti-Wr[a] is a red cell–stimulated antibody that has been reported to cause moderately severe HDN as well as severe transfusion reactions. Anti-Wr[a] is also commonly found in the sera of patients suffering from warm autoimmune hemolytic anemia.

The Wr[a] antigen, which is rare, has been detected only in whites. Only one example of an antibody that appeared to have anti-Wr[b] specificity has been described.[7] Anti-Wr[b] may be found as a warm autoantibody in patients with autoimmune hemolytic anemia.

The Cartwright Blood Group System: Yt[a] and Yt[b]

The Cartwright blood group system, discovered in 1956,[8] is probably composed of two antigens: Yt[a], a high-frequency antigen occurring in 99.7 percent of random whites; and Yt[b], a low-frequency antigen occurring in 8 percent of random whites. Three phenotypes have been described, virtually with the same frequencies in both the white and black populations: Yt(a+b−) occurs at 91.9 percent; Yt(a+b+) at 7.8 percent; and Yt(a−b+) at 0.3 percent. The phenotype Yt(a−b−) has not been reported.[9]

The Yt[a] antigen is poorly developed at birth; therefore, cord bloods are usually Yt[a] negative. However, the Yt[a] antigen is an efficient immunogen, and consequently, the antibody anti-Yt[a] is not that uncommon in spite of the rare Yt(a−b+) phenotype.[10]

The Yt[b] antigen appears to be a poor immunogen. Therefore, anti-Yt[b] is rare and has been reported only in patients who have been transfused a great deal and who have produced multiple antibodies.[11]

Both anti-Yt[a] and anti-Yt[b] are reactive only in the antihuman globulin phase of in vitro testing and appear to be IgG. These antibodies are considered clinically significant, are usually red cell stimulated, but have not been implicated in HDN. Studies by Eaton et al.[8] and by Giles et al.[12] have shown both Yt[a] and Yt[b] to be inherited as dominant characters.

The Diego Blood Group System: Di[a] and Di[b]

The Diego blood group system was discovered in 1955 when the antibody to the Di[a] antigen was described. Di[b] was described in 1967 when the antibody anti-Di[b] was reported. The Di[a] antigen appears to be inherited as a dominant character, extremely rare in whites but more frequent in individuals of Mongolian background. The Di[a] antigen is therefore useful as a genetic marker for Mongolian derivation and is significant in anthropologic studies. South American, Central American, and North American Indians have been shown to have a high incidence of Di[a]. Di[a] is found in 3 to 5 percent of Chinese people and in 8 to 12 percent of Japanese people. Di[b] is a high-frequency antigen in whites. Both anti-Di[a] and anti-Di[b] are reactive only in the antihuman globulin phase of in vitro testing and appear to be IgG and not to be enhanced by complement. Although both antibodies have been implicated in causing HDN, anti-Di[b] causes only mild forms of the disease. Both anti-Di[a] and anti-Di[b] are usually red cell stimulated.

The Scianna Blood Group System: Sm (Sc1) and Bu[a] (Sc2)

In 1962 the antibody to the Sm antigen was reported. In 1963 an antibody to the Bu[a] antigen was described; however, the investigators were not aware that this was an allele to Sm. A new terminology for the Scianna blood group system was devised in 1974.[13] Antigen Sm became Sc1, and Bu[a] antigen Sc2. Sc1 is a high-frequency antigen in whites, occurring in approximately 100 percent of the population. Sc2 is a low-frequency antigen, occurring in less than 1 percent of the random population, and not at all in blacks.[9] Sc1 and Sc2 are inherited as codominant characters (Anderson et al.[14]; Lewis et al.[13]). Both anti-Sc1 and anti-Sc2 are rare antibodies. Most anti-Sc1 antibodies are red cell stimulated and react only in the antihuman globulin phase of in vitro testing. Some anti-Sc2 antibodies react in the saline phase and are naturally occurring, whereas others react only in the antihuman globulin phase and are red cell stimulated. Neither anti-Sc1 nor anti-Sc2 has been implicated in HDN or in transfusion reactions.

The phenotype Sc:−1,−2 was found by McCreary et al.[15] in two members of a highly inbred population living on Likiep Atoll in the Marshall Islands. Furthermore, an antibody reacting with all red cells except those of Sc:−1,−2 was reported by Nason et al.[16] The antibody called anti-Sc3 did not contain separate specificities in absorption studies. Thus, Sc1 and Sc2 red

cells appear also to be Sc3, whereas Sc:−1,−2 red cells are Sc:−3.

In 1982 Skradski et al.[17] discovered a patient who had made antibodies against C, e, Jk[b], and an antigen of very high frequency. When the last antibody was adsorbed onto and eluted from C−, e−, Jk(b−) red cells, it was shown to be nonreactive with the red cells of the antibody maker, his brother, and two Sc:−1,−2 red cells. The red cells of the antibody maker and his brother that lacked the common antigen were found to be Sc:1,−2. Thus, we do not know if the newly defined antigen is part of the Scianna system or whether it is simply absent from Sc:−1,−2 red cells.

Devine et al.[18] described antibodies directed against high-frequency red blood cell antigens in sera of three persons whose red blood cells contained the common phenotype Sc:1,−2. Sera or eluates or both from these persons did not react with Sc:1,−2 red blood cells. The samples were not mutually compatible. Sc:−1,−2 cells may lack multiple high-frequency antigens.

The Dombrock Blood Group System: Do[a] and Do[b]

The Dombrock blood group system was discovered in 1965 when the antibody to the Do[a] antigen was described.[19] Do[b] was defined in 1973 when the antibody anti-Do[b] was reported.[20] The Do[a] antigen can be found in 67 percent of whites; however, it appears to have a lower frequency in black as well as in Native Americans. Do[b] antigen can be found in approximately 83 percent of whites. Three phenotypes have been described in the Dombrock system with the following approximate frequencies: Do(a+b−) occurs at 17.2 percent; Do(a+b+) at 49.5 percent; and Do(a−b+) at 33.3 percent. The phenotype Do(a−b−) has not been reported.

Both anti-Do[a] and anti-Do[b], which react only in the antihuman globulin phase of in vitro testing, appear to be IgG. These antibodies showed marked preferences to some anti-IgG reagents and were not detectable with others. These antibodies occur infrequently, they are usually red cell stimulated, and their reactivity appears to be enhanced when enzyme-treated red cells are used. Anti-Do[a] has been implicated in a mild case of HDN, but neither anti-Do[a] nor anti-Do[b] has been implicated in transfusion reactions. Both anti-Do[a] and anti-Do[b] have been shown to demonstrate dosage.

The Colton Blood Group System: Co[a] and Co[b]

The Colton blood group system was discovered in 1967 when the antibody to the Co[a] antigen was described.[21] Co[b] was defined in 1970 when the antibody anti-Co[b] was reported.[22] Co[a], a high-frequency antigen, occurs in 99.7 percent of the random white population. Co[b] can be found in 9.7 percent of the random white population. Three phenotypes have been described in the Colton system with the following approximate frequencies: Co(a+b−), 90.3 percent; Co(a+b+), 9.4 percent; Co(a−b+), 0.3 percent; and Co(a−b−), less than 0.01 percent. The phenotype Co(a−b−) has been described in two patients with monosomy −7.[23] Although they are rarely found, both anti-Co[a] and anti-Co[b] are usually red cell stimulated. Some of these antibodies are reactive only in the antihuman globulin phase of in vitro testing, and others react only with enzyme-treated red cells. Both anti-Co[a] and anti-Co[b] appear to be IgG. Anti-Co[a] has been implicated in a mild case of HDN and has been suspected to cause transfusion reactions.

The Auberger Blood Group System: Au[a]

In 1961 the Au[a] antigen was described.[24] Approximately 90.5 percent of all whites are Au(a+). The Auberger antigen is well developed at birth, and its expression depends not only on the *Au[a]* gene but also on the inheritance of the *Lutheran* genes (see Chapter 8). The inheritance of the *In(Lu)* gene may be responsible for the dominant Lu(a−b−) phenotype and also may suppress the expression of the Au[a] antigen. The rare anti-Au[a] antibodies appear to react only in the antihuman globulin phase of in vitro testing.

Miscellaneous Antigens

For simplicity some of the other miscellaneous antigens are listed in Tables 9−1 and 9−2. Numerous other antigens have been described in the category of high-frequency antigens found in Table 9−2. Refer to other texts, such as *Applied Blood Group Serology* (third edition) by Issitt,[9] and *Blood Groups in Man* by Race and Sanger,[4] for further discussion of other antigens.

High Titer, Low Avidity

High titer and low avidity (HTLA) is used to describe a group of antibodies that demonstrate high-titered (greater than 64) reactivity but low avidity (1+ or less) for the corresponding antigen, usually in the antihuman globulin phase of testing (Tables 9−1 and 9−3). Titer is the reciprocal number of the highest serial dilution of serum that still causes visible agglutination of red cells containing the appropriate antigen. Avidity is the strength of agglutination (size of clumping) of the antigen-antibody reaction during a particular phase of testing.

High-titer, low-avidity antibodies may cause difficulty in routine antibody screening, identification, and compatibility testing. Table 9−4 lists the "classic" antibodies included in this group. The majority of these antibodies define antigens that are considered to be high-frequency red cell antigens (found in greater than 98 percent of the population). In addition, these antigens are not stable during storage and frequently show variable strength of reactivity from individual to individual.

Characteristically, HTLA antibodies are IgG that do not bind complement, react poorly in routine LISS procedures, and are considered clinically insignificant antibodies. They have not been implicated in causing hemolytic transfusion reactions or HDN. Generally,

TABLE 9−1 **HTLA ANTIBODIES* AND HLA-RELATED SYSTEMS**

Antigen	Blood Group System or Nomenclature		Approximate Percentage of Population Positive	General Characteristics
Yk[a]†	York	} White cell determinants expressed on RBCs and in plasma	92 (W); 98 (B)	
Cs[a]†	Cost-Sterling		98 (W)	
Kn[a]†	Knops	} White cell determinants expressed on RBCs and in plasma	99 (W)	Antibody found more often in whites
McC[a]†	McCoy		99 (W); 98 (B)	Antibody found more often in blacks
Ch[a]	Chido	} Determinants on the C4d fragment present in plasma that is coded for by the HLA locus	98 (W)	Demonstrated to be HTLA antibodies; Ch[a] and Rg[a] (C4) absorb onto red cell membrane
Rg[a]	Rodgers		97 (W)	
JMH	John Milton Hagen		98 (W); 98 (B)	
Bg[a]	} Originally called the Donna, Bennett, Goodspeed (DBG) antigen	Correlation with HLA has been demonstrated		HLA-B7 = Bg[a] HLA-Bw17 = Bg[b] HLA-A28 = Bg[c]
Bg[b]	Ho antigen			These anti-HLA and anti-Bg antibodies are therefore synonymous
Bg[c]	Ot antigen Also grouped together as the Bg antigens			

*Holley (Hy) and Gregory (Gy[a]) have been placed in the HTLA category by some immunohematologists.
†Demonstrated to be HTLA antibodies.
B = black; RBC = red blood cell; W = white.

TABLE 9-2 **HIGH-FREQUENCY ANTIGENS**

Antigen	Blood Group System or Nomenclature	General Characteristics	Approximate Percentage of Population Positive
Vel 1 Vel 2	Vel	Antibodies are usually IgM, complement binding, some IgG, usually red cell stimulated, HDN not reported, Vel antigens not well developed at birth	100
Gy^a Hy	Gregory Holley	Antibody usually IgG, AHG reactive only, red cell stimulated, implicated in transfusion reactions, antigens not well developed at birth, HDN not reported	100
Sd^a	Sid	Soluble antigen found in saliva and urine of Sd(a+) individuals; the amount of Sd^a present on red cells varies greatly from person to person; rare "super-Sid" or Sd(a++) red cells exist, which possess a high concentration of Sd^a antigen and have been termed "Cad" (the Cad, or super-Sid, red cell characteristic is the only known form of inherited polyagglutination [see Chapter 22]); antibody is usually IgM, complement binding, few are IgG; most antibodies are "naturally occurring"; almost all adult serum contains anti-Cad or anti-Sd(a++); rarely implicated in transfusion reactions; HDN not reported; agglutination pattern is unique and shows a very refractile mixed-field clumping with tight agglutinates in a sea of free cells; antibody neutralizable with fresh urine	96
Ge:1 Ge:2 Ge:3	Gerbich	Most antibodies are IgG, a few are IgM, some are red cell stimulated, others are "naturally occurring"; antibodies have been implicated in causing a mild HDN	100
En^a	En^a antigen	Antibody is usually IgG reacting in all phases of in vitro testing, most are red-cell stimulated; antibody has been implicated in transfusion reactions, suspected in causing HDN; En^a-negative individual's red cells have reduced sialic acid as well as reduced or depressed M and N antigens	100
Lan	Langereis	Antibody is usually IgG, most reactive in only AHG phase, some reactive in both albumin and AHG phases; most are red-cell stimulated and have been implicated in causing a mild HDN	100
Pr(Sp)	Pr(Sp) antigen	Antibodies are usually IgM, some are IgA, some are IgG; most are "naturally occurring." Pr(Sp) antigens are destroyed by enzyme treatment, most antibodies present as high-titered cold autoagglutinins (see Chapter 21)	100

AHG = antihuman globulin.

TABLE 9-3 **TYPICAL PATTERN OF AN HTLA ANTIBODY DURING ANTIBODY IDENTIFICATION**

Panel Number	PHASE OF REACTIVITY			
	35°C	AHG	Prewarm	Monospecific IgG
1	0	±	±	±
2	0	±	±	±
3	0	±	±	±
4	0	±	±	±
5	0	±	±	±
6	0	±	±	±
7	0	±	±	±
8	0	±	±	±
9	0	±	±	±
10	0	±	±	±

AHG = antihuman globulin.

TABLE 9-4 **THE MOST COMMON HTLA ANTIBODIES**

Anti-Ch^a	(Chido)
Anti-Rg^a	(Rodgers)
Anti-Cs^a	(Cost-Sterling)
Anti-Yk^a	(York)
Anti-Kn^a	(Knops)
Anti-Kn^b	(Knops)
Anti-McC^a	(McCoy)
Anti-McC^b	(McCoy)

HTLA antibodies have been found in patients with a history of multiple transfusions or in transfused multiparous women. Difficulty, however, arises when the reaction patterns of these antibodies do not fit a specific pattern during antibody identification, and the technologist may confuse this with a combination of specificities (e.g., anti-Jk^a and anti-K) to explain the results. This requires the patient to receive antigen-negative blood unnecessarily, thereby delaying transfusion therapy.

A few special techniques can be employed to determine the presence of HTLA antibodies. It is important to identify their presence, because these antibodies can mask other clinically significant antibodies directed against such systems such as Kidd, Kell, Duffy, and Rh. Underlying alloantibodies have been reported in approximately 25 percent of samples being investigated for HTLA antibodies. In addition, potentially serious antibodies such as anti-Vel, anti-Di^b, or anti-Cr^a, which cause rapid red cell hemolysis, could mimic HTLA antibodies.

If an HTLA antibody is suspected and a titration study is performed, one should be aware that the stan-

TABLE 9-5 **TITRATION OF AN HTLA ANTIBODY COMPARED WITH OTHER COMMON ANTIBODIES DETECTED**

Titer	Avidity		1	2	4	8	16	32	64	128	256	512
High	Low	(HTLA)	1+	1+	1+	1+	1+	1−	1+	+w	+w	+w
High	High	(K)	4+	4+	4+	4+	3+	3−	3+	2+	2+	1+
Low	High	(Jkª)	3+	2+	1+	0	0	0	0	0	0	0
High	Low	(Lu6)	1+	1+	1+	1+	1+	1−	1+	+w	+w	+w

dard method for performing the indirect antihuman globulin test (2 drops of serum and 1 drop of a 3 to 4 percent cell suspension incubated at 37°C for 15 minutes) may not be sensitive enough to detect a weak HTLA antibody. Many immunohematologists recommend using 6 to 8 drops of serum with 1 drop of cells and an incubation of 60 minutes. An HTLA antibody can be suspected if results demonstrate the same weakly positive reactions in virtually all dilutions (Table 9–5). It should be noted that other antibodies also can demonstrate HTLA reactions with most of the panel cells tested, such as those in the Lutheran or Cartwright systems. Therefore, additional testing should be performed before one concludes that the antibody is clinically insignificant inasmuch as it gave HTLA reactions. Other antibodies, such as those in the Bg system, also can mimic HTLA antibodies by yielding HTLA reactions. However, the Bg system contrasts with the HTLA group by detecting low-frequency antigens, thereby reacting with only a few of the panel cells tested.

The use of enzymes can greatly facilitate the differentiation of the HTLA antibodies. Generally, the HTLA antibodies react with the same degree of strength or weaker with enzyme-treated red cells, with the exception of anti-Chido (Chª), anti-Rodgers (Rgª), and anti–John Milton Hagen (JMH), which are usually nonreactive. In addition, anti-Chª and anti-Rgª are the only two HTLA antibodies that can be neutralized or inhibited by plasma that is positive for these antigens. The plasma inhibition study has been provided in the procedural appendix following this chapter. It has been discovered that Chido and Rodgers are part of the C4 component complement. As a result, the use of C4d in plasma or serum absorbs anti-Chido and anti-Rodgers, thereby facilitating the screening for other underlying alloantibodies. This makes these two HTLA antibodies the easiest of this group to identify. Chido and Rodgers are only two IgG HTLA antibodies that will react at room temperature with C4d-coated red cells suspended in saline.

Cord cells also may assist in determining the HTLA specificity of the antibody. The majority of the HTLA antibodies react the same or less well with cord red cells than with red cells of an adult. However, Chido and Rodgers antibodies react weakly or not at all with cord cells. Other antibodies of clinical significance, such as anti-Ytª, anti-Vel, or anti-Luᵇ, also share this characteristic.

Of interest, anti-JMH is the only reported "naturally occurring" HTLA antibody. Because anti-JMH is not found in plasma, it is not neutralizable with antigen-positive plasma. It is the only nonneutralizable HTLA antibody that does not react with enzyme-treated red cells. Again, other clinically significant antibodies directed against high-frequency antigens in the Lutheran and Cartwright systems are not neutralizable with antigen-positive plasma and react weakly or not at all with enzyme-treated red cells.

SUMMARY

High-titer, low-avidity antibodies do not represent a separate blood group system. HTLA is a general description of the classic serologic reactions demonstrated by a variety of different antibodies. HTLA antibodies are generally IgG and display weakly variable reactions in the antihuman globulin phase of testing. They can be divided into neutralizable (Chido and Rodgers) and nonneutralizable (other) antibodies. The nonneutralizable HTLA antibodies are exclusively red cell antigens, not found on platelets or leukocytes. The majority of these antibodies are clinically insignificant and do not cause transfusion reactions or HDN. The HTLA antibodies may be troublesome during routine compatibility testing, creating a delay in the transfusion. Any incompatibility problem must be investigated, and the presence or absence of other underlying alloantibodies must be thoroughly confirmed prior to transfusion. All variable or weakly positive reactions in the antihuman globulin phase of testing cannot be assumed to be due to an HTLA antibody. Other serologic problems can mimic an HTLA antibody, yielding similar results in initial panel studies. Some of these problems include the presence of multiple weak alloantibodies, warm or cold autoagglutinins, or weak examples of antibodies directed against high-frequency antigens. Table 9–6 compares some of the serologic patterns that may be confused with the reactivity of HTLA antibodies. Each laboratory should develop a standard approach toward resolution of an incompatibility suspected to be caused by an HTLA antibody.

Bg Antibodies

Bg antibodies are primarily directed toward and define white blood cell antigens. Antigenic expression of variable strength is present on some red cells, and correlation with human leukocyte antigen (HLA) has been demonstrated. The Bgª antigen can be demon-

TABLE 9-6 **CHARACTERISTICS OF SOME ASSORTED ANTIBODIES**

Antibody Specificity	Opt Rxn In Vitro Sal/AHG/Enz	IgG/IgM	Binds Compl Yes/No	In Vitro Lysis Yes/No	Implicated in Trans Rxn HDN	W Pos (%)
Anti-Xg^a	x	x	Most/some	x		87F;64M
Anti-Do^a	x x	x		x	Mild	67
Anti-Do^b	x x			x		83
Anti-Yt^a	x	Most		x		99.8
Anti-Yt^b	x			x		8
Anti-Di^a	Some/x	x		x	x	Rare
Anti-Di^b	x x	x		x	Mild	100
Anti-Sc1	x			x		100
Anti-Sc2	Some/x			x		Rare
Anti-Wr^a	Some/some	x		x	x/x	Rare
Anti-Wr^b	x		x	x	Prob	100
Anti-Co^a	Some/x	x		x	Prob/mild	99.7
Anti-Co^b	Some/x	x		x		9.7
Vel system	Some/some/x	Few/many	x	x	x	100
Gerbich system	Most	Most/few		x	Mild	100
Anti-Lan	Most	x		x	x/mild	100
Anti-Gn^a	x			x		100
Anti-Gy^a and Anti-Hy	x	x		x	x	100
Anti-Kn^a	x			x	Mild	99.8
Anti-Sd^a	Some/some/x	Few/most	Most	x	Rare	96.1
Anti-En^a	x/ x/x	x		x	x/poss	100
Pr(Sp) system	Most/ few/none	Some/some		x	DAT+	100

AHG = antihuman globulin; F = female; M = male; W = white.

TABLE 9-7 **GENERAL CHARACTERISTICS OF HTLA ANTIBODIES**[1,4]

1. Produce weak reactions with red blood cells in the antihuman globulin phase.
2. Rarely react at room temperature or 37°C.
3. Often display inconsistent or nonreproducible results.
4. Demonstrate variable reaction strengths with different red blood cells.
5. Possible difficulty in distinguishing between weakly reactive and negative reactions.
6. Possibly decreased reactions with storage of red cells.
7. Antibodies IgG and noncomplement binding.
8. Antibodies negative with patient's own cells.
9. Possibly weaker or negative reactions with cord red cells.
10. Difficulty in absorption and elution.
11. Easily washed off (therefore, use handwashing, not machine washing).
12. Difficult to reproduce the serologic reactions.

strated on the red cells of 93 percent of HLA-B7 donors, and Bg^b on those of 80 percent of HLA-B17 donors using manual capillary tube testing.[22] However, the Bg antigens are present only on the red cells of a very few individuals in the random population (Table 9-1).

Bg antibodies also fit into the serologic criteria of HTLA but, unlike the HTLA group, these antibodies typically do *not* react with all panel cells tested. Bg antibodies classically differ from HTLA antibodies by reacting with only a few panel cells (Table 9-7).

Review Questions

1. Which blood group antigen is under control of a gene located on the X chromosome?
   A. Bg^a
   B. Di^a
   C. Do^a
   D. Xg^a
   E. Yt^a

2. Which of the following are high-frequency antigens?
   A. Co^a Wr^a Yt^a
   B. Co^a Wr^a Yt^b
   C. Co^a Wr^b Yt^a
   D. Co^b Wr^b Yt^b
   E. Co^b Wr^b Yt^a

3. Which of the following best describes HTLA antigens?
   A. Frequency greater than 98 percent of the population, instability during storage, variable strength of reactivity from individual to individual
   B. Frequency less than 2 percent, instability during storage, variable strength of reactivity from individual to individual
   C. Frequency greater than 98 percent, instability during storage, variable strength of reactivity from individual to individual
   D. Frequency greater than 98 percent, instability during storage, constant strength of reactivity from individual to individual
   E. Frequency greater than 98 percent, instability during storage, constant strength of reactivity from individual to individual

4. Which of the following are neutralizable HTLA antibodies?
   A. John Milton Hagen and Chido
   B. York and Chido
   C. Knops and McCoy
   D. McCoy and Rodgers
   E. Chido and Rodgers

5. The antibody to this antigen is easily neutralized with fresh urine:
   A. En^a
   B. Ge:1
   C. Lan
   D. Pr
   E. Sd^a

6. Proteolytic enzymes can be of value in enhancing the reactions of antibodies in which blood group system?
   A. Xg
   B. Do
   C. Lewis
   D. Co
   E. Duffy

7. Antigens in which of the following blood group systems commonly bind complement?
   A. The Kidd blood group system
   B. HTLA
   C. The sex-linked (Xg) blood group system
   D. The Rh/Hr blood group system
   E. The ABO blood group system

8. The first example of autosomal linkage in humans was found between which of the following gene complexes?
   A. Rh and Duffy
   B. Lutheran and Lewis
   C. Lutheran and Auberger
   D. Lutheran and secretor

9. Match the system name from column II with the correct antibody in column I.

Column I	Column II
A. Anti-Do^a	1. ABO
B. Anti-Yt^b	2. Auberger
C. Anti-Di^a	3. Xg
D. Anti-Xg^a	4. Lewis
E. Anti-Wr^b	5. Cartwright
F. Anti-Sc2	6. Wright
G. Anti-Co^b	7. Duffy
H. Anti-Au^a	8. Dombrock
	9. Vel
	10. Diego
	11. Colton
	12. Kidd
	13. Scianna

10. **True or False:** Studies have shown that Yt^a and Yt^b are inherited as a dominant character.

Answers to Review Questions

1. D (p 189)
2. C (pp 189–190)
3. A (p 191)
4. E (p 193)
5. E (Table 9–2)
6. B (p 190)
7. A, C, E (p 189)
8. C (p 191)
9. A = 8 (p 190)
   B = 5 (p 189)
   C = 10 (p 190)
   D = 3 (p 189)
   E = 6 (p 189)
   F = 13 (p 190)
   G = 11 (pp 190–191)
   H = 2 (p 191)
10. True

References

1. Mann, J, et al: A sex-linked blood group. Lancet i:8, 1962.
2. Cook, IA, et al: A second example of anti-Xg^a. Lancet i:857, 1963.
3. Sausais, L, et al: Characteristics of a third example of Anti-Xg^a (abstract). Transfusion 4:312, 1964.
4. Race, RR, and Sanger, R: Blood Groups in Man, ed 5. FA Davis, Philadelphia, 1968.
5. Yokoyama, M, et al: The first example of autoanti Xg^a. Vox Sang 12:138, 1967.
6. Holman, C: A new rare human blood group antigen (Wr^a). Lancet ii:119, 1953.
7. Adams, J, et al: An antibody in the serum of a Wr(a$^-$) individual, reacting with an antigen of very high frequency. Transfusion 11:290, 1971.
8. Eaton, BR, et al: A new antibody, anti-Yt^a, characterizing a blood group antigen of high incidence. Br J Haematol 2:333, 1956.
9. Issitt, PD: Applied Blood Group Serology, ed 3. Montgomery Scientific Publications, Miami, 1985.
10. Giles, CM, et al : A family showing independent segregation of Bu^a and Yt^b. Vox Sang 18:265, 1970.
11. Bettigole, R, et al: Rapid in vivo destruction of Yt(a+) red cells in a patient with anti-Yt^a. Vox Sang 14:143, 1968.
12. Giles, CM, et al: Studies in the Yt blood group system. Vox Sang, 13:171, 1967.
13. Lewis, M, et al: Scianna blood group system. Vox Sang 27:261, 1974.
14. Anderson, C, et al: An antibody defining a new blood group antigen, Bu^a. Transfusion 3:30, 1963.
15. McCreary, J, et al: Another minus-minus phenotype: Bu(a−) two examples in one family (abstract). Transfusion 13:350, 1973.
16. Nason, SG, et al: A high incidence antibody (anti-Sc3) in the serum of a SC:−1,−2 patient. Transfusion 20:531–535, 1980.
17. Skradski, KJ, et al: An antibody against a high frequency antigen absent on red cells of the Scianna:−1, −2 phenotype (abstract). Transfusion 22:406, 1982.
18. Devine, P, et al: Serologic evidence that Scianna null (SC:−1,−2) red cells lack multiple high-frequency antigens. Transfusion 28:4, 1988.

19. Swanson, JL, et al: A "new" blood group antigen, Do^a. Nature 206:313, 1965.
20. Molthan, L, et al: Enlargement of the Dombrock blood group system: The finding of anti-Do^b. Vox Sang 24:382, 1973.
21. Heisto, H, et al: Three examples of a red cell antibody, anti-Co^a. Vox Sang 12:18, 1967.
22. Giles, CM, et al: Identification of the first example of anti-Co^b. Br J Haematol 19:267, 1970.
23. De la Chapelle, A, et al: Monosomy-7 and the Colton blood groups. Lancet ii:817, 1975.
24. Salmon, C, et al: Un nouvel antigene de group sanguine erythrocytaire present chez 80% des sujets de race blanch. Nouv Rev Franc Haematol 1:649, 1961.
25. Moulds, MK: Serological investigation and clinical significance of high-titered, low-avidity (HTLA) antibodies. Am J Med Tech 10:794, 1981.

PROCEDURAL APPENDIX

Plasma Inhibition Studies*

MATERIALS AND METHODS

Sera (plasmas) and cells: unknown patient serum, indicator cells (screening cells) Chido-Rodgers positive plasma: Ch(a+) Rg(a+) plasma, Ch(a+) Rg(a−) plasma

1. Set up two sets of each of the following mixtures and incubate at room temperature for 15 minutes:
    A. 2 drops unknown serum, 1 drop Ch(a+) Rg(a−) plasma
    B. 2 drops unknown serum, 1 drop Ch(a−) Rg(a+) plasma
    C. 2 drops unknown serum, 1 drop Ch(a+) Rg(a+) plasma
2. Incubate a set of selected screening cells with the foregoing three mixtures for 60 minutes at 37°C. Wash three times with saline and convert to the antihuman globulin test.
3. If multiple alloantibodies are suspected after the previous results are obtained, test a complete genotyped panel of donors with the appropriate mixture.

INTERPRETATION OF RESULTS

1. If mixture A is reactive with both screening cells and mixtures B and C are nonreactive, the antibody is anti-Rg^a and no other alloantibodies are detected in the unknown serum.
2. If mixture B is reactive and mixtures A and C are nonreactive with the screening cells, the antibody is anti-Ch^a and no other alloantibodies are detected in the unknown serum.
3. If mixture C is reactive and either mixture A or mixture B is nonreactive, it could mean that there is not sufficient quantity of Ch^a or Rg^a substance in the Ch^a- or Rg^a-positive plasma to inhibit the antibody but that there is enough in mixture A or mixture B plasma to inhibit the antibody.
4. If all three mixtures are nonreactive, the serum antibody is too weak to allow dilution studies.
5. If one screening cell is negative and the other positive with any of the mixtures, then anti-Ch^a and anti-Rg^a and a second or third antibody may be present in the serum. The appropriate mixtures should then be incubated with a panel of selected genotyped cells.

*From Moulds,[25] p 794, with permission.

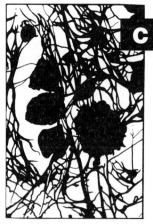

CHAPTER 10

Donor Selection and Component Preparation

Patricia A. Wright, BA, MT(ASCP)SBB

OBJECTIVES

Upon completion of this chapter, the learner should be able to:

1 Identify the demographic information required from every prospective blood donor to ensure adequate identification and, if necessary, recall (six items).

2 Give the minimum acceptable levels for the following tests, for both allogenic and autologous donors:
   a Weight
   b Temperature
   c Pulse
   d Blood pressure
   e Hemoglobin
   f Hematocrit

3 Select an acceptable allogenic blood donor when given the results of the physical examination and medical history.

4 State the medical history information that would be cause for permanent, indefinite deferral.

5 Identify information that would be cause for temporary deferral, and state the length of time for the deferral.

6 List the special medical history and physical examination information required of a pheresis donor.

7 Explain the four major types of autologous blood donation procedures.

8 State the procedure for performing a whole blood donor phlebotomy including arm preparation, blood collection, and postphlebotomy care instructions for the donor.

9 Recognize a donor reaction; identify the difference between mild, moderate, and severe reactions; and state the recommended treatments for each.

10 List the 10 tests that are required to be performed on all allogenic blood donor units.

11 List the information that is required to be on the blood unit label.

12 Identify the primary ingredient, storage conditions, shelf life, quality control requirements, and indications for use for each of the following blood components:
   a Red blood cells
   b Leukocyte-reduced red blood cells
   c Washed red blood cells
   d Frozen, deglycerolized red blood cells
   e Platelet concentrates (random, single donor)
   f Single-donor plasma (fresh frozen, frozen within 24 hours, liquid, frozen)
   g Cryoprecipitate concentrate
   h Granulocyte concentrate
   i Factor VIII concentrates
   j Factor IX concentrates
   k Rh immunoglobulin
   l Plasma derivatives (immune serum globulin, plasma protein fraction, normal serum albumin, volume expanders)

Donor Selection

The process of blood donor selection is designed to provide the blood bank with the answers to two major questions: (1) Will a donation of approximately 450 ml of whole blood at this time be harmful to the donor? and (2) Could blood drawn from this donor at this time potentially transmit a disease to the recipient? If the answer to each of these questions is no, then the donation can proceed. If the answer to either question is yes, the donor must be deferred either temporarily or indefinitely, depending on the circumstances.

The following are the guidelines established by the blood banking community, which are considered to be the minimum acceptable standards. They are designed to protect both the donor and the public.

REGISTRATION INFORMATION AND GENERAL REQUIREMENTS

Each donor must be clearly and uniquely identified so that a specific donor can be traced through the entire process and, if necessary, recalled.[1] Please note the top section of the donor card (Fig. 10–1). This demographics section of the donor card is designed to fulfill the identification and recall requirements. The following data are required:

1. **Donor's name.** First name, last name, and middle initial are needed.
2. **Donor's address and phone number.** If the donor works outside the home, it is helpful to have the business address and phone number also.
3. **Gender.**
4. **Date of birth and age.** Prospective donors must be at least 17 years of age. The minimum age limit may be exempted for autologous blood donors. This exception should be determined by the blood bank medical director and then stated in writing in the facility's procedure manual. In some states donors between 17 and 21 years of age may, by law, be considered minors, and therefore require parental permission before donation. Check individual state laws. There is no longer an upper age limit for blood donors. Any individual who is in good health and meets all the other donor requirements may donate.
5. **Date of donation.**
6. **Donor's consent.** The donor must provide written, informed consent for the blood bank to take and use his or her blood; the consent must be obtained before the donation. All aspects of the donation procedure must be explained in terms that the donor can understand, including information on significant risks in the procedure and any tests that will be performed on the donated unit. The donor should be given the opportunity to ask questions about the procedure and to refuse consent. Informed consent for a minor must be in accordance with applicable state laws.[2]

Although not required by the American Association of Blood Banks (AABB) standards, the following information may be useful to have as part of the donor record:

7. **Additional identification.** Social security or driver's license number is good because these are unique numbers and most donors will have one or the other.
8. **Donor's occupation.** Donors with hazardous jobs or activities (e.g., police, fire fighters, pilots, heavy machinery operators, runners) will need to be informed and cautioned concerning safe return to their full range of job activities.
9. **Time of last meal.** It is better that a donor not be fasting at the time of donation. If it has been longer than 4 hours since the last meal, the donor should be given something to eat and drink before the donation.
10. **Race.** It may prove useful later to know the racial origin of the donor when screening for some phenotypes (e.g., Lewis or Duffy negatives).
11. **Intended recipient, replacement credit, donor group.** Many blood donations are designated by the donor for a specific donor group or patient. When this occurs, it is important to obtain the patient or credit information to ensure proper crediting. Even if the donor is rejected or deferred, the information may still be useful or necessary. Any of the following information may be needed: (1) patient name and hospital, (2) patient identification or hospital number, or (3) donor group name.

PHYSICAL EXAMINATION

A brief physical examination is required and is primarily designed to ensure the donor's safety. The elements of the examination should rule out or defer any donor whose physical condition is such that a blood donation at this time could be detrimental. It must be done on the day of donation and generally is performed at the time of donation along with the medical history.

1. **General appearance.** The donor should appear to be in good health. If there are signs of alcohol or drug intoxication or obvious symptoms of a cold or other infection or disease, the donor should be deferred.
2. **Weight: 110 lb (50 kg).** The donation of a unit of blood should not exceed approximately 10 percent of the donor's blood volume. This means that for the standard donation of 525 ml including pilot tubes, the donor should weigh at least 110 lb (50 kg). Blood can be drawn from donors who weigh less than 110 lb, provided the amount of blood collected is proportionately reduced. If less than 300 ml is to be drawn, the amount of anticoagulant in the bag must be reduced accordingly. The following formulas can be used to calculate the amount of anticoagulant to be removed from the primary bag.

    a. Amount of blood to be drawn

    $$\frac{\text{Donor's weight (lb)}}{110 \text{ lb}} \times 450 \text{ ml} = \text{Allowable amount (ml)}$$

    b. Amount of anticoagulant needed

    $$\frac{\text{Allowable amount}}{100} \times 14 = \text{Anticoagulant needed (ml)}$$

    c. Amount of anticoagulant to remove

    $$63 \text{ ml} - \text{anticoagulant (ml)} = \text{Anticoagulant to remove (ml)}$$

DONOR CARD **MARYLAND GENERAL HOSPITAL—BLOOD BANK** BLOOD TYPE

NAME LAST FIRST M.I.	AGE	DATE OF BIRTH	SEX	DATE TODAY (MDY)	WHOLE BLOOD NUMBER	
STREET ADDRESS	HOME PHONE		DIRECTED DONOR ONLY ☐			
CITY STATE ZIP CODE	BUSINESS PHONE		PERSONAL PHYSICIAN		DEFERRED UNTIL (MDY)	INDEFINITE DEFERRAL ☐
IDENTIFICATION SS#			HOSPITAL		NO. PREVIOUS DONATIONS	DATE LAST DONATION

WEIGHT	TEMP.	PULSE	B.P.	Hgb	ARMS S U	PD FILE CK:		LOT NUMBER	SIGNATURE

		YES	NO
1	EVER HAD YELLOW JAUNDICE, LIVER DISEASE, HEPATITIS OR A POSITIVE BLOOD TEST FOR HEPATITIS?	☐	☐
2	EVER TAKEN SELF-INJECTED DRUGS?	☐	☐
3	IN THE PAST 12 MONTHS RECEIVED BLOOD TRANSFUSIONS, BLOOD INJECTIONS OR TATTOOS?	☐	☐
4	IN THE PAST 12 MONTHS BEEN EXPOSED TO ANYONE WITH YELLOW JAUNDICE, HEPATITIS, OR ON A KIDNEY MACHINE?	☐	☐
5	EVER HAD MALARIA OR ANTI-MARLARIAL DRUGS IN 3 YEARS?	☐	☐
6	IN THE PAST THREE YEARS BEEN OUTSIDE THE UNITED STATES?	☐	☐
7	EVER HAD ANY SERIOUS ILLNESS?	☐	☐
8	IN THE PAST 12 MONTHS BEEN HOSPITALIZED?	☐	☐
9	ARE YOU FEELING WELL TODAY?	☐	☐
10	IN THE PAST MONTH TAKEN ANY MEDICATIONS?	☐	☐
11	EVER BEEN DEFERRED AS A BLOOD DONOR OR HAD PROBLEMS DONATING?	☐	☐
12	EVER HAD HEART DISEASE, CHEST PAIN OR SHORTNESS OF BREATH?	☐	☐
13	BLOOD DISEASE AND PROLONGED BLEEDING?	☐	☐
14	EVER HAD CONVULSIONS, SEIZURES, OR FAINTING SPELLS?	☐	☐
15	EVER HAD CANCER?	☐	☐
16	IN THE PAST YEAR HAD ANY VACCINATIONS OR IMMUNIZATIONS?	☐	☐
17	HAVE YOU EVER HAD CHAGAS DISEASE OR BABESIOSIS?	☐	☐
18	IN THE PAST THREE DAYS HAD ANY DENTAL WORK OR MINOR SURGERY?	☐	☐
19	DO YOU HAVE POLYCYTHEMIA?	☐	☐
20	HAVE YOU EVER RECEIVED PITUITARY GROWTH HORMONE?	☐	☐
21	HAVE YOU READ THE AIDS INFORMATION?	☐	☐
22	BEEN PREGNANT IN THE PAST SIX MONTHS?	☐	☐
23	HAVE YOU - EVER TAKEN STREET DRUGS BY NEEDLE, EVEN ONCE? - BEEN A SEX PARTNER OF AN IV DRUG ABUSER SINCE 1977?	☐	☐
24	SINCE 1977 HAVE YOU - TO YOUR KNOWLEDGE, HAD A POSITIVE TEST FOR HIV (AIDS)? - BEEN EXPOSED TO ANYONE WITH AIDS OR WITH A POSITIVE TEST FOR AIDS? - EXCHANGED SEX FOR DRUGS OR MONEY? - TAKEN CLOTTING FACTOR CONCENTRATES FOR A BLEEDING DISORDER SUCH AS HEMOPHILIA OR HAD SEX WITH SOMEONE WHO HAS?	☐	☐
25	FOR MEN, HAVE YOU - HAD SEX, EVEN ONCE, WITH ANOTHER MAN SINCE 1977? - HAD SEX WITH A FEMALE PROSTITUTE IN THE LAST 12 MONTHS?	☐	☐
26	FOR WOMEN, HAVE YOU - HAD SEX, EVEN ONCE, WITH A MAN WHO HAD SEX WITH ANOTHER MAN SINCE 1977? - HAD SEX WITH A MALE PROSTITUTE IN THE LAST 12 MONTHS?	☐	☐
27	HAD NIGHT SWEATS, UNEXPLAINED FEVER OR WEIGHT LOSS, LUMPS IN NECK, ARM PITS OR GROIN, DISCOLORED AREAS OF SKIN OR MOUTH, PERSISTENT COUGH OR PERSISTENT DIARRHEA?	☐	☐
28	HISTORY OF GONORRHEA OR SYPHILLIS OR TREATMENT FOR EITHER IN THE PAST 12 MONTHS?	☐	☐
29	ANY HISTORY OF LUNG DISEASE, TROUBLE BREATHING NOW?	☐	☐

THE INFORMATION I HAVE GIVEN FOR THIS FORM IS CORRECT. I DONATE MY BLOOD OR PLASMA FOR USE AS NEEDED. I UNDERSTAND THE INFORMATION THAT HAS BEEN GIVEN TO ME TODAY ABOUT THE SPREAD OF THE AIDS VIRUS THROUGH DONATED BLOOD AND PLASMA. IF I AM AT RISK FOR SPREADING THE AIDS VIRUS, I AGREE NOT TO DONATE BLOOD OR PLASMA FOR TRANSFUSION TO ANOTHER PERSON. ☐ ☐

DONOR SIGNATURE

X

REMARKS LISTED ON BACK OF CARD L-19-2

FIGURE 10–1 Front of the donor history card for allogenic donation. (Courtesy Maryland General Hospital, Baltimore, Maryland.)

For institutions that routinely want or need to draw blood from donors weighing less than 110 lb and that have a need for low-volume units of blood, donor bags are available that are designed to draw 150 ml or 250 ml rather than 450 ml.

3. **Temperature: Orally should not exceed 99.6°F (37.5°C).** The purpose of determining the donor's temperature is to eliminate any donor who may have an infection or disease that may be transmissible through the donated blood. Fever is a symptom of infection. There is no low-temperature limit because a low temperature is most frequently caused by cold environmental temperatures and is rarely associated with disease.[3]

   Care should be taken to ensure that sufficient time has elapsed since eating, drinking, or smoking so that the temperature reading will not be affected.

4. **Pulse: 50 to 100 beats per minute.** The pulse should be checked for at least 30 seconds, and if there is any doubt about the rate or rhythm, assessment should be extended to a full minute. Pulse rates greater than 100 beats per minute must be further evaluated. Increased pulse rates may be caused by physiologic factors such as anxiety, fear, or recent physical exercise. Allow the donor to relax for 10 to 15 minutes, then check the pulse again for a full minute. If it is still elevated, consult the blood bank medical director, or defer the donor, or both.

   Pulse rates of less than 50 beats per minute may frequently occur in athletes who have a high tolerance to exercise (e.g., marathon runners, professional ball players). A statement indicating the athletic activity and its frequency should be made a part of the permanent donor record. Any irregularities in heart rhythm should be cause for deferral.

5. **Blood pressure: Systolic no greater than 180 mm Hg, diastolic no greater than 100 mm Hg.** Donors with pressure readings higher than these limits must be evaluated by the blood bank medical director before being accepted.

6. **Hematocrit and hemoglobin: 38 percent (12.5 g/dl), venipuncture or fingerstick.** Although determination of either hemoglobin (Hb) or hematocrit (Hct) is acceptable, large donor collection sites will probably prefer the hemoglobin determination using a copper sulfate ($CuSO_4$) method. This method uses the principle that a drop of whole blood when dropped into a solution of $CuSO_4$, which has a given specific gravity, will maintain its own density for approximately 15 seconds. The density of the drop is directly proportional to the amount of hemoglobin in that drop. If the drop is denser than the specific gravity of the solution, the drop sinks to the bottom; if not, it will float on top. The test solution should have a specific gravity of 1.053. This is not a quantitative test, but it is quick, easy, and

quite accurate for screening donors. If a donor fails this procedure or there is a question concerning the results, it is advisable to confirm the results with a microhematocrit. Hemoglobin levels can also be determined using spectrophotometric methods, which are very accurate but more expensive. Several small, portable, easy-to-use hemoglobinometers are available that are well suited for mobile operation use. Smaller donor operations—fewer than 10 to 20 donors per day—may still elect to use a microhematocrit method because at that level it is the cheapest method.

7. **Skin lesions, arm check.** The antecubital area of both arms must be inspected for evidence of habitual drug use or the presence of skin eruptions such as poison ivy, rash, or psoriasis. If there is evidence of self-injected drug use that the donor does not adequately explain, the donor must be indefinitely deferred. There is an extremely high risk of hepatitis and human immunodeficiency virus (HIV) infection in abusers of self-injected drugs. If there is evidence of a rash or infection at the phlebotomy site, the donor must be deferred until the problem has cleared up. This is to help protect both the donor and the donated unit from contamination.

8. **Review of permanent deferral file.** All donors must be checked against a file of indefinitely deferred donors. This check must be performed at some time before the release of the unit from quarantine to distribution.

MEDICAL HISTORY

The medical history is both fact finding and diagnostic. Its purpose is to obtain a profile of the prospective donor's health status in order to determine his or her suitability for donating blood.[4] The questions are designed to determine whether the donation might be harmful to the donor or whether the blood obtained might transmit disease. The questions should be phrased so that the donor can answer with a simple "yes" or "no" that can be elaborated on if necessary.

The interviewer should be familiar with the questions so that he or she can observe the donor during the interview, be aware of the donor's body postures and facial expressions, and be ready to elaborate on any question if the donor seems not to understand it.

The medical history must be performed on the day of donation and is usually performed at the same time as the physical examination. The interview must be conducted in a somewhat secluded place that has few distractions and permits privacy.

It is recognized that the safety of the country's blood supply is critically tied to the quality and effectiveness of the predonation donor medical history. In response to this, the AABB Ad Hoc Committee on Donor History/Interview Process has developed a uniform set of questions that everyone can use and that ensures adherence to both the AABB standards and the Food and Drug Administration (FDA) regulations and recommendations. It is hoped that the use of these questions will help ensure that the donor history is comprehensive, understandable, and dependable to the degree that that is possible.[5]

1. Have you ever had yellow jaundice, liver disease, hepatitis, or a positive test result for hepatitis? In the past 12 months, have you received blood or had an organ or tissue transplant? In the past 12 months, have you had a tattoo, ear or skin piercing, acupuncture, or an accidental needlestick? In the past 12 months, have you had close contact with a person with yellow jaundice or hepatitis, or have you been given hepatitis B immunoglobulin (HBIg)? Have you ever used a needle, even once, to take any drug (including steroids)?

All of these questions are considered "hepatitis questions." Laboratory tests are not 100 percent effective in eliminating units of blood that are capable of transmitting viral hepatitis. The medical history cannot completely eliminate the hazard either, but in combination with sensitive testing methods and an emphasis on volunteer donors, the risk has been significantly reduced. (Donors with a history of abuse of self-injected drugs also are at high risk for HIV infection.)

A donor must be indefinitely or permanently deferred if he or she:

1. Gives a history of viral hepatitis after the age of 10
2. Currently has or previously has had a confirmed positive test result for hepatitis B surface antigen (HBsAg)
3. Has had more than one reactive test result for hepatitis B core antibody (anti-HBc)
4. Has present or past evidence (either clinical or laboratory) of hepatitis C infection
5. Presents with an elevated alanine aminotransferase (ALT) level, more than twice the highest acceptable level on any one occasion or above the acceptable high level on two occasions
6. Indicates past or present abuse of self-injected drugs
7. Was the donor of the only unit involved in a documented case of posttransfusion hepatitis

A 12-month deferral is given to a potential donor who has had close contact with someone who has hepatitis. "Close contact" is defined as sharing the same household, kitchen, or bathroom facilities. This may include a student living in a dormitory where several cases of hepatitis have occurred or any person who is institutionalized in a prison, psychiatric hospital, or institution for the retarded. It does *not* routinely apply to hospital personnel performing normal duties, but care should be taken to ensure that hospital workers are aware of and follow infection and body fluid precaution protocols (gloves, gowns, and masks as appropriate). Guidelines for the selection or deferment of

personnel working in dialysis centers or units must be defined by the blood bank medical director.

Donors who have received blood transfusions or injections of blood or blood products, an organ or tissue transplant (including skin allografts), a tattoo, ear or other skin piercing, acupuncture, or an accidental needlestick injury should also be deferred from allogeneic donation for 12 months.

There is a 12-month deferral also for any donor who has received HBIg because HBIg is given for exposure to possible infection and it may delay the onset of symptoms of disease. Receipt of hepatitis B vaccine is, however, *not* a cause for deferral. The vaccine is now generally made from recombinant material and is given prophylactically, not as a result of exposure.

2. In the past 3 years, have you had malaria or taken antimalarial drugs? In the past 3 years, have you been outside the United States or Canada?

Malaria parasites reproduce in the red blood cells (RBCs) and can remain in the blood and tissues for years. After the initial infection, some people develop a chronic infection, characterized by periodic relapses.[6] Prospective donors who have had malaria or have been treated for malaria must be deferred for 3 years following therapy, or departure from the endemic area, or both. They must remain asymptomatic and not take antimalarial drugs during the 3-year period.

Visitors, immigrants, or refugees from an area considered to be endemic for malaria by the Centers for Disease Control (CDC) Malaria Programs must be deferred for 3 years after departure from the area and must remain asymptomatic and not take antimalarial drugs for that period.

Donors who have traveled to areas considered endemic for malaria are deferred for 6 months after departure from the area, provided they remain asymptomatic and have not taken antimalarial drugs. It is not necessary to defer a donor who has started antimalarial therapy in preparation for travel but who has not yet been to the endemic area.[7]

3. In the past 12 months, have you been under a doctor's care or had a major illness or surgery?

A "yes" answer here requires the interviewer to investigate further. Prospective donors who have recently undergone surgical procedures need to be evaluated to identify those who received blood or blood product (except Rh immune globulin) transfusions at the time. A blood transfusion requires a 12-month deferral owing to the risk of exposure to hepatitis, HIV, or other viral disease. Surgical procedures that are uncomplicated and do not require any blood transfusions are cause for deferral only until healing is complete and the donor has resumed his or her full range of activity. It is not necessary to distinguish between major and minor surgery as long as blood transfusions are not involved and the donor has returned to normal activities.[8]

Any indication that a biopsy was performed should be evaluated further, inasmuch as a large number of patients with acquired immunodeficiency syndrome (AIDS) or AIDS-related complex (ARC) have had lymph node biopsies.[9] If the biopsy findings indicate or suggest either of these diagnoses, the donor must be deferred indefinitely. A person who has been hospitalized for AIDS or AIDS-related diseases must be deferred permanently.

4. Are you feeling well and healthy today?

The prospective donor should be in general good health and free from any acute upper respiratory infection or disease. Donors who have active cold or flu symptoms must be deferred until the symptoms are gone. Be aware that many people take over-the-counter medications that mask or eliminate the signs and symptoms of colds and flu. Remember also that some sore throats and nasal stuffiness may be caused by smoking, shouting, environmental pollution, allergies, low humidity, or air conditioning.

This question is the only one that requires a "yes" answer. It can be used as a general lead-off question to help relax the donor and to begin the questioning process, or it can be used in the middle of the interview to help ensure that both the donor and the interviewer are alert and listening to the questions and answers.

5. Have you ever taken Tegison for psoriasis? In the past 4 weeks, have you taken any pills, medications, or Accutane? In the past 3 days, have you taken aspirin or anything that has aspirin in it?

This question is designed to help identify those donors who are being treated for a serious illness or condition that could defer him or her as a blood donor. In most cases it is not the medication itself that is a cause for deferral but rather the underlying condition for which it is prescribed.[10] The blood bank should maintain a list of drugs and medications (generic and brand names) that cause temporary or indefinite deferral.

Although there is no specific requirement concerning Tegison, the Food and Drug Administration's (FDA) Inspection Checklist and Report recommends that donors taking Tegison be deferred for 3 years following the final dose.[11] This drug is potentially teratogenic and may remain in the donor for up to 3 years following the last dose. Accutane (isotretinoin, for acne therapy) is also a potent teratogen that can remain in the blood for several weeks and therefore carries a recommended 4-week deferral. Teratogens in the donor unit could be harmful to an embryo or fetus of a pregnant recipient.[12]

The following common medications generally *do not* disqualify a donor: oral contraceptives, mild analgesics, minor tranquilizers, psychic energizers, vitamins, diet pills, hormones, and marijuana (if not currently under the influence). Aspirin and aspirin-containing medications are acceptable provided the donor is not being evaluated for a platelet pheresis procedure.

Aspirin causes a significant decrease in platelet function for up to 3 days.

6. In the past 8 weeks have you given blood, plasma, or platelets? Have you ever been refused as a blood donor or told not to donate blood? Have you ever given blood under a different name?

The time interval between whole blood donations is 8 weeks (56 days). If a donor has been participating in a pheresis program (plasma, platelets, leukocytes), there must be a 48-hour interval between the last pheresis donation and the anticipated whole blood donation. Pheresis donors will need to wait 8 weeks after a whole blood donation before returning to the pheresis program.

The second part of this question is a leading one. If the answer is "yes," further investigation as to why the donor was deferred or told not to donate is required.

Regarding the last part of this question, the FDA now requires that donors be asked if they have ever donated under a different name so that a more accurate check of a Donor Deferral Register can be made. It is thought that this will help increase the probability that unsuitable donors will be identified and that units or products from these persons will be removed from the transfusable blood supply.

7. Have you ever had chest pain, heart disease, or lung disease?

A history of cardiovascular, coronary, or rheumatic heart disease is usually cause for deferral. In cases in which there is no disability, no limitations of activity, or restrictions imposed by the primary physician, the donor may be acceptable upon approval of the blood bank medical director.

Active pulmonary tuberculosis (TB) or other active pulmonary disease is cause for deferral. Donors who have had TB that has been successfully treated and that is now nonactive are acceptable, as are donors who have a positive skin test (Purified Protein Derivative [PPD]) result but no other signs (on x-ray examination) or symptoms of the disease.

8. Have you ever had cancer, a blood disease, or a bleeding problem? Have you ever taken clotting factor concentrates for a bleeding problem such as hemophilia?

A history of cancer, leukemia, or lymphoma is generally a cause for indefinite deferral. Exceptions can be made for some cases such as basal or squamous cell (skin) cancer, carcinoma in situ of the cervix, and papillary thyroid carcinoma that have been surgically removed and cured. Any donor presenting with a history of any type of cancer should be reviewed by the blood bank medical director before being accepted. A history of leukemia, lymphoma, Kaposi's sarcoma, aplastic anemia, granulocytopenia, sickle cell anemia, thalassemia, any of the hemoglobinopathies or polycythemia is cause for indefinite deferral.

Any history of prolonged or abnormal bleeding following surgery, childbirth, tooth extraction, or cuts and abrasions must also be further evaluated. Persons with a history of abnormal bleeding should be deferred because they may experience excessive bleeding from the venipuncture and because their plasma may lack significant levels of some clotting factors. Persons with a history of hemophilia A or B, von Willebrand's disease, or severe thrombocytopenia, and a history of having ever received clotting factor concentrates, must be permanently deferred from donating blood or blood products.

9. Have you had convulsions, seizures, or fainting spells?

A donor with a history of epilepsy or frequent convulsions, other than febrile convulsions in early childhood, is usually deferred because of the possibility of a serious donor reaction. Donors whose seizures are well controlled with or without medication may be accepted. Final decision of acceptability of these donors lies with the blood bank medical director. It should be noted that this question is no longer required by either the AABB or the FDA but is still included on many donor history cards.

10. In the past 4 weeks, have you had any shots or vaccinations? In the past 12 months, have you been given rabies shots?

Killed viral, bacterial, rickettsial vaccines or toxoids are acceptable if the donor is afebrile and symptom free. These include diphtheria, pertussis, typhoid, tetanus, paratyphoid, cholera, hepatitis B, typhus, Rocky Mountain spotted fever, influenza (killed virus), plague, Salk (polio), and rabies (duck embryo or human diploid). Attenuated virus vaccines such as smallpox, Sabin (oral) polio, measles (rubeola), mumps, yellow fever, and influenza (live virus) carry a 2-week deferral. German measles (rubella) vaccine carries a 4-week deferral. Rabies vaccine, if given after the bite of a rabid animal, requires a 12-month deferral, as does HBIg. If a prospective donor has received IV immune serum globulin (IVIg), he or she must be evaluated and deferred, if necessary, based on the underlying reason for the immunization.[13]

11. Have you had a tooth extraction or dental work in the past 3 days? (not a required question)

Although not required, this question may still be used by many blood banks or blood centers. There may be some risk of bacterial infection following oral surgery, and some procedures require the prophylactic use of antibiotics, which may be cause for a temporary deferral. The final ruling on this question rests with the blood bank medical director.

12. In the past 6 weeks have you been pregnant, or are you pregnant now?

A prospective donor should be deferred during pregnancy and for 6 weeks following a third-trimester delivery. Exceptions can be made by the blood bank medical director for autologous donation or if the woman's blood is needed for the exchange transfusion of her infant.

A first- or second-trimester abortion or miscarriage need not be a cause for deferral. If however, blood is transfused during or following an abortion or delivery, the donor must be deferred for 12 months.

13. Have you ever been given growth hormone?

Because of the risk of transmission of Creutzfeldt-Jacob disease (CJD) through infected blood transfusions, a prospective donor who has ever received pituitary growth hormone of human origin must be permanently deferred. Recombinant growth hormones (Protropin, Humatrope) do not require deferral, but it must be clear that the donor had received *only* recombinant hormones.[14]

14. Have you ever had Chagas' disease or babesiosis?

Any history of Chagas' disease or babesiosis is cause for permanent deferral.

15. In the past 12 months, have you had a positive test result for syphilis? In the past 12 months, have you had or been treated for syphilis or gonorrhea?

Prospective donors who have had or been treated for syphilis or gonorrhea are to be deferred for at least 12 months following completion of treatment. Any person with a positive result to a serologic test for syphilis (STS) must be deferred for 12 months. The reason for deferral is not so much a fear of transmission of either syphilis or gonorrhea but that, as they are sexually transmitted diseases, the donor has a higher than normal risk of exposure to HIV and hepatitis infections.

16. Have you ever had night sweats; unexplained fever or weight loss; lumps in the neck, armpits, or groin; discolored areas of the skin or mouth; persistent cough; or persistent diarrhea?

A donor who has any of the foregoing symptoms must be further evaluated to determine whether or not these symptoms are consistent with AIDS or ARC. Any donor whose symptoms are consistent with the diagnosis of AIDS or ARC (briefly described here) must be indefinitely deferred.

1. Persistent night sweats (repeated sweating at night so that the sheets are wet)
2. Fever of greater than 99°F for more than 10 days
3. Unexplained weight loss of 10 lb or more in less than 2 months
4. Lymphadenopathy (swollen lymph nodes in the neck, armpits, or groin)
5. Discolored areas of the skin (bluish purple areas under the skin typical of Kaposi's sarcoma) or white spots in the mouth or mucous membranes

(typical of opportunistic thrush infection), or both

6. Persistent diarrhea that lasts for several days or weeks and returns frequently

7. Persistent cough or shortness of breath

8. Malaise (fatigue, loss of energy)

17. Do you have AIDS or have you had a positive test result for the AIDS virus? In the past 12 months, have you had sex, even once, with anyone who has AIDS or tested positive for the AIDS virus?

Donors who have tested positive for the HIV antibody must be indefinitely deferred. Donors who have had sexual contact with a person who had AIDS, ARC, or tested positive for the HIV antibody must also be indefinitely deferred.

18. In the past 12 months, have you had sex with anyone who has ever used a needle, even once, to take any drug (including steroids)? In the past 12 months, have you ever had sex, even once, with anyone who has ever taken clotting factor concentrates for a bleeding problem such as hemophilia?

Sexual contact with any person who is at high risk of exposure to HIV infection must be deferred for 12 months from the date of last high-risk sexual contact. The 12-month deferral should provide adequate time for seroconversion to occur if the sexual contact has resulted in the donor's infection with the HIV virus.

19. At any time since 1977, have you taken money or drugs for sex? In the past 12 months, have you had sex, even once, with anyone who has done so? In the past 12 months, have you given money or drugs to anyone to have sex with you?

Prostitution is a high-risk behavior. Many drug abusers use prostitution to support their drug habit, and frequent, casual sexual contact with many different partners dramatically increases a person's risk of becoming infected with HIV or the hepatitis virus, or both.

Permanent deferral is required for anyone who, since 1977, has traded sex for drugs or money. A 12-month deferral must be given to anyone who, even once, has given someone money or drugs in payment for sex or who has ever had sex with someone they know to have exchanged money or drugs for sex.

20. *Male donors:* Have you had sex with another male, even once, since 1977?
Female donors: In the past 12 months, have you had sex with a male who has had sex, even once since 1977, with another male?

These too are questions that inquire about a donor's possible participation in high-risk behavior. HIV is very prevalent in the male homosexual population and sexual contact by men or women with a homosexual or bisexual man is cause for deferral.

Permanent deferral is required for any male donor who, since 1977, has had *any* homosexual episode with another male. A 12-month deferral is required of any female donor who has had sex with a bisexual male. As in the previous questions, this 12-month deferral should provide time for seroconversion to take place and be detectable upon routine donor testing.

21. Are you giving blood in order to be tested for AIDS?

There are no specific requirements by either the AABB or the FDA to ask this question, but it is a good question to evaluate further a donor's motivation for donating at this time. It is well known publicly that donors' blood is tested for the HIV antibody and that if the result is positive the donor will be notified. It is also known that this test is completely free of charge to the donor. If performed by a private physician, the test is quite expensive. Although many clinics, health departments, and blood centers provide free and anonymous testing, many people still feel threatened by going to such a place for the testing.

22. Do you understand that if you have the AIDS virus, you can give it to someone else even though you may feel well and test negative for HIV?

The FDA recommends that, as part of an effort to educate the general public more fully about AIDS and HIV infection, blood donors need to be informed about the time ("window period") between early infection when a person is able to transmit the virus and the development of the HIV antibody that is detectable in the screening test.[15]

23. Have you read and understood all the donor information presented to you, and have all your questions been answered?

The FDA requires that donors be provided with written information about high-risk behaviors, signs and symptoms of disease, the risk of transmitting HIV through blood transfusion, and the importance of self-exclusion. It requires that this information be written in language that the donor can understand and that the interviewer provide an opportunity for the donor to ask questions about anything that he or she does not understand. Figure 10–2 is an example of an information sheet that should be given to every donor each time they present for donation. This example also includes information on other transfusion-transmitted diseases and the tests that will be performed on the donated unit of blood.

24. The information I have given for this form is correct. I donate my blood or plasma for use as needed. If I am at risk for spreading the AIDS virus, I agree not to donate blood or plasma for transfusion to another person.

This is the informed consent statement that the donor must read and sign at the completion of the medical history screening. Figure 10–3 is an example of an additional self-exclusion form that every donor should be asked to complete. It is designed to be a confidential form that the donor can complete in private, seal, and return before the donation. The form should *not* be reviewed until later, usually at the time of donor processing. Many large donor centers use a machine-readable (bar code) sticker that the donor selects and places on the donor card. It provides a mechanism for donors who are at risk but afraid to be deferred at the donor site, to ensure that their donation is not used for transfusion purposes.

PHERESIS DONOR SELECTION

The donor selection requirements for a pheresis donor are generally the same as those for a whole blood (WB) donor. Under normal conditions, a pheresis donor must meet all the criteria for a whole blood donor. In addition, the following criteria are specific for the potential pheresis donor and need to be investigated before proceeding with the donation.

Medical History

1. **A history of donor reactions, particularly to previous pheresis procedures.** Possible adverse reactions to hydroxyethyl starch (HES), steroids, or heparin must be determined and carefully evaluated.
2. **A history of bleeding problems or thrombocytopenia, or both.** This may be critical if a procedure using heparin is to be performed. It is best to defer female donors from heparin procedures during menses.
3. **Allergies to beef or pork.** They are generally a source of heparin.
4. **An indication or history of fluid retention problems.** This may be a significant problem if using HES or steroids or both in the pheresis procedure.
5. **An underlying medical condition that may be aggravated by steroids.** These include hypertension, tuberculosis, and diabetes mellitus.
6. **The donor weight.** The size of the bowl used in the procedure (225 ml or 375 ml) will alter the volume of blood that is outside the body (extracorporeal) and therefore will change the donor's weight requirements. No more than 15 percent of the donor's total blood volume can be extracorporeal. The small bowl requires 110 lb; the large about 150 lb.
7. **Medications.** Use of any medication that might increase the donor's risk or decrease the effectiveness of the product, most particularly aspirin (or aspirin-containing substances), must be evaluated. The donor should be free of aspirin ingestion for 3 to 5 days before platelet pheresis or leukopheresis.

Physical Examination and Laboratory Tests

As with the medical history, the pheresis donor must meet all the minimum physical examination require-

ments of a WB donor. Depending on which pheresis procedure is being performed, the following additional laboratory tests must be performed before each donation:

1. Hemoglobin and hematocrit
2. Serum protein
3. Platelet count (not less than 50,000/ml)
4. White blood cell (WBC) count and differential
5. Partial thromboplastin time (PTT), if using heparin

Perform the following tests after the donation:

1. Hemoglobin and hematocrit
2. Platelet count
3. WBC count

Protein electropheresis should be performed every 4 months if the donor is a regular, biweekly plasma donor.

AUTOLOGOUS DONOR SELECTION

An autologous donor is one who is donating blood for his or her own future use. Autologous blood is the safest transfusion possible. There is no risk of disease transmission; alloimmunization to RBCs, platelets, WBCs, or plasma proteins; or transfusion reactions, and the phlebotomy process stimulates the bone marrow to increase cell production. The use of autologous blood decreases the need for allogeneic blood, frequently decreases the total amount of blood needed, and may actually increase the supply of allogeneic blood if the unused autologous units are "crossed over" into the general inventory.[16] All of this adds up to a big advantage to the donor recipient and a strong reason for blood banks and physicians to encourage its use.

There are four types of autologous donations-transfusions. Predeposit donation refers to blood that is drawn sometime before the anticipated transfusion and stored, usually liquid but occasionally frozen, in the blood bank. Intraoperative autologous transfusion occurs when blood is collected during a surgical procedure and usually reinfused immediately. A third type of autologous donation is the immediate preoperative hemodilution. In this procedure, once the patient is in the operating room 1 to 3 units of WB are collected and the volume is replaced with colloid or crystalloid, or both, thus reducing the patient's hemoglobin level by about 1 to 3 g/dl. The blood remains in the operating room and is used for transfusion during the surgical procedure. The fourth type of autologous donation is postoperative "salvage," in which a drainage tube is placed in the surgical site and postoperative bleeding is salvaged, cleaned, and reinfused.

Predeposit Donation

Predeposit autologous donation is usually performed for a scheduled elective surgical procedure in

MARYLAND GENERAL HOSPITAL

827 Linden Avenue
Baltimore, Maryland 21201
301 225-8000

<u>AN IMPORTANT MESSAGE TO ALL BLOOD DONORS</u>

 Please read this information sheet carefully before you agree to donate blood today. At the completion of the medical history review you will be asked to sign a statement that says you have read this information today, that you understand it and that if you are at risk for spreading the AIDS virus you will not donate blood or plasma for transfusion to another person. If any of the information below applies to you, **DO NOT DONATE BLOOD, BECAUSE IT MIGHT HARM THE PATIENT WHO RECEIVES IT.**

AQUIRED IMMUNE DEFICIENCY SYNDROME (AIDS)

AIDS is a disease in which the body's normal defense mechanisms against certain diseases and infections has been broken down. AIDS can be spread through donated blood and plasma. AIDS is associated with the HIV (HTLV-I) virus. Blood tests to detect antibody to the AIDS virus are very good, but they are not perfect. It is possible for a person in the early stage of infection to have a negative test result. Therefore, <u>people who are at risk for getting AIDS must not donate blood or plasma.</u>

You are at risk of getting AIDS and spreading the AIDS virus if:

- You are a man who has had sex with another man since 1977, **even one time!**
- You have ever taken ("shot up") illegal drugs by needle.
- You have AIDS or one of its signs or symptoms which include:
    *Unexplained weight loss (10 pounds or more in less than 2 months)
    *Night sweats (reoccurring sweating at night which wets the sheets)
    *Blue/purple spots on or under the skin or in the mouth (Kaposi Sarcoma)
    *Long lasting white spots in the mouth (Thrush infection)
    *Swollen lymphnodes (lumps in the neck, arm pits or groin) lasting more
     than a month.
    *Fever of greater than 99 degrees lasting for several days or weeks and/or
     reoccurring frequently
    *Persistant diarrhea (lasting more than a month)
- You have ever had a positive test for AIDS or the AIDS virus (Anti-HIV)
- You are a hemophiliac who has taken clotting factor concentrates since 1977
- You have, since 1977, had sex with any person described above.
- You are a woman or a man who has been a prostitute at any time since 1977.
- You are a man who has had sex with a female prostitute or a woman who has
  had sex with a male prostitute in the past 12 months.

HEPATITIS

If you have ever had hepatitis (a liver disease that can be caused by a virus), **DO NOT DONATE BLOOD OR PLASMA.**

If you have ever had a positive test for hepatitis (HBsAg, Anti-HCV, Anti-HBc), **DO NOT DONATE BLOOD OR PLASMA**

SYPHILIS and/or GONORRHEA

If you have or have been treated for syphilis or gonorrhea, in the past 12 months, **DO NOT DONATE BLOOD OR PLASMA**

(OVER)

FIGURE 10-2 Donor information sheet for viral marker testing. (Courtesy Maryland General Hospital, Baltimore, Maryland.)

MALARIA

If you have visited or lived in a country where malaria exists, DO NOT DONATE BLOOD FOR 6 MONTHS AFTER YOU LEAVE THAT COUNTRY.

If you are a native of a country where malaria exists, DO NOT DONATE BLOOD FOR 3 YEARS after you have left the area and entered the United States.

If you have had malaria or have taken anti-malarial drugs, DO NOT DONATE BLOOD FOR 3 YEARS after your last attack of malaria and/or after stopping your anti-malarial drug therapy.

IF ANY OF THE ABOVE INFORMATION APPLIES TO YOU, DO NOT DONATE BLOOD OR PLASMA, **EVEN IF YOU FEEL HEALTHY.** YOU MAY LEAVE NOW WITHOUT PROVIDING AN EXPLANATION. IF YOU ARE NOT SURE YOU SHOULD DONATE, PLEASE TALK PRIVATELY WITH THE DONOR ROOM PHLEBOTOMIST.

Your blood will be tested for hepatitis viruses, syphilis, the AIDS virus (HIV)

and certain other viruses.

If the tests for hepatitis show that you probably are a carrier of hepatitis, or if the HIV antibody test shows that you probably have been exposed to the AIDS virus, we will not use your blood or plasma. You will be notified confidentially of the test results and we will put your name and other identifying information on a confidential list of persons who should not donate blood or plasma.

If the results of your hepatitis tests or HIV antibody test are unclear, we will not use your blood or plasma even though you are probably healthy. Your name will be put on a confidential list for special testing the next time you donate blood. You will not however, be informed of these unclear results unless the blood bank medical director decides that the special test results mean that your health might be affected.

We report positive test results to applicable health departments as required by federal, state and local law.

WE APPRECIATE THE TIME AND EFFORT INVOLVED IN MAKING A TRIP TO THE BLOOD BANK AND HOPE THAT ALL DONORS WILL RECOGNIZE THE NECESSITY OF THE VOLUNTARY SCREENING PROCEDURES WHICH HAVE BEEN INSTITUTED.

FIGURE 10–2 *Continued.*

which there is a reasonable chance that transfusion will be required. Because the donor will also be the recipient, the donor requirements can be significantly different from those required of an allogeneic, WB donor (Fig. 10–4).

General Requirements

1. The donor-patient must have a signed written statement from his or her physician requesting the procedure (Fig. 10–5).
2. The physician's request must be reviewed and approved by the blood bank medical director (Fig. 10–6).
3. The donor-patient must give signed, informed consent (Fig. 10–7).

Donor Criteria

1. **Age.** Generally no age limits exist, although a child should be old enough to understand what is happening and be cooperative. Almost any person who is a good candidate for elective surgery can be an autologous donor. The final decision rests with the donor-patient's physician and the blood bank medical director.
2. **Weight.** No strict weight requirements exist. If the donor weighs less than 110 lb (50 kg), a proportionately smaller volume of blood must be drawn. (See the guidelines provided in the discussion of the physical examination, earlier in this chapter, for calculations necessary.) As a rule

MARYLAND GENERAL HOSPITAL

827 Linden Avenue
Baltimore, Maryland 21201
301 225-8000

DONOR SELF-EXCLUSION FORM

PLEASE READ AND COMPLETE THIS FORM BEFORE YOU LEAVE THE DONOR ROOM

AIDS can be spread through blood and plasma. Therefore, blood or plasma from people at risk for getting AIDS and spreading the AIDS virus must not be transfused to another person.

YOU ARE AT RISK FOR GETTING AIDS AND SPREADING IT THROUGH YOUR BLOOD AND PLASMA IF:

- You are a man who has had sex with another man since 1977, <u>even one time.</u>
- You have ever taken illegal drugs by needle.
- You are a native of Haiti, Burundi, Kenya, Rwanda, Tanzania, Uganda or Zaire who has entered the United States since 1977.
- You have AIDS or one of the signs or symptoms of AIDS. (listed on the "An Important Message To All Blood Donors" sheet)
- You have ever had a positive test for HIV (HTLV-III) antibody, showing past exposure to the AIDS virus.
- You have hemophilia.
- You are or have been the sex partner of any person described above.
- You are a woman or man who is now or has been a prostitute since 1977.
- You have been the heterosexual partner of a male or female prostitute within the last twelve (12) months.

If any of the above information applies to you, your blood or plasma <u>MUST NOT BE TRANSFUSED</u> TO ANOTHER PERSON. Please take time to think about this important issue and then mark the correct box below.

SYPHILIS OR GONORRHEA: <u>DO NOT</u> donate blood for transfusion to another person if:

- You have or have been treated for syphilis in the last twelve (12) months.
- You have or have been treated for gonorrhea in the last twelve (12) months.

YOU MUST MARK ON OF THE BOXES BELOW IN ORDER FOR YOUR BLOOD TO BE USED. FAILURE TO MARK ONE OF THE BOXES WILL REQUIRE THAT YOUR BLOOD BE DISCARDED.

MARK ONLY ONE BOX! YOUR RESPONSE IS STRICTLY CONFIDENTIAL!

I believe my blood is <u>SAFE FOR TRANS-FUSION</u> to another person.

My blood should <u>NOT BE TRANSFUSED</u> to another person.

After marking the correct box, fold and seal the form so that nobody can see your answer. Do not put your name on the form. Give the sealed form to the Donor Room nurse.

THANK YOU FOR YOUR INTEREST IN DONATING BLOOD AND FOR HELPING US MAINTAIN A SAFE BLOOD SUPPLY.

FIGURE 10-3 Donor self-exclusion form. (Courtesy Maryland General Hospital, Baltimore, Maryland.)

DONOR CARD   **MARYLAND GENERAL HOSPITAL—BLOOD BANK**   BLOOD TYPE

| NAME LAST | FIRST | M.I. | AGE | DATE OF BIRTH | SEX | DATE TODAY (MDY) | **WHOLE BLOOD NUMBER** |

| STREET ADDRESS | | HOME PHONE | AUTOLOGOUS USE ONLY ☐ | |

| CITY | STATE | ZIP CODE | BUSINESS PHONE | PERSONAL PHYSICIAN | DEFERRED UNTIL (MDY) | INDEFINITE DEFERRAL ☐ |

| IDENTIFICATION SS# | | HOSPITAL | NO. PREVIOUS DONATIONS | DATE LAST DONATION |

| WEIGHT | TEMP. | PULSE | B.P. | Hgb | ARMS S U | TIME START | TIME COMPLETED | LOT NUMBER | SIGNATURE |

					YES	NO
1	HAVE YOU BEEN PREVIOUSLY REJECTED/IF SO WHY?				☐	☐
2	ILLNESS, INFECTIOUS DISEASE RECENTLY (SPECIFICALLY DIARRHEA, NAUSEA, VOMITING, OR ABDOMINAL PAIN WITHIN THE LAST 7 DAYS?)				☐	☐
3	CONVULSIONS/FAINTING SPELLS/ABNORMAL BLEEDING?				☐	☐
4	MINOR OR DENTAL SURGERY WITHIN THE LAST 3 DAYS?				☐	☐
5	MAJOR SURGERY IN THE LAST 12 MONTHS?				☐	☐
6	FEELING WELL TODAY?				☐	☐
7	RECEIVED BLOOD/BLOOD PRODUCTS IN THE LAST 12 MONTHS?				☐	☐
8	HAVE YOU EVER HAD CHEST PAIN, HEART, KIDNEY, LIVER, OR LUNG DISEASE?				☐	☐
9	DO YOU HAVE DIABETES?				☐	☐
10	ARE YOU ON ANY DRUG THERAPY INCLUDING ANTIBIOTICS?				☐	☐
11	HAVE YOU HAD ANY UNEXPLAINED WEIGHT LOSS?				☐	☐
12	ARE YOU PREGNANT OR BEEN PREGNANT WITHIN THE LAST 6 MONTHS?				☐	☐

DATE | DONOR NUMBER | Anti A | Anti B | Cells A₁ B | Anti D | Rh Cont | Du | Check Cell | Du Cont | Check Cell | Interp. | Tech.

LABELING INFO: I   II   III

Date Drawn: RT 37°C   RT 37°C   RT 37°C

| DATE | I.S. Sal | 10' LISS | AHG | Check Cell | I.S. Sal | 10' LISS | AHG | Check Cell | I.S. Sal | 10' LISS | AHG | Check Cell |

Date Expires:

Labeled By:

Label Checked By: REMARKS:

THE INFORMATION I HAVE GIVEN FOR THIS FORM IS CORRECT. I DONATE MY BLOOD OR PLASMA FOR USE AS NEEDED. IF I AM AT RISK FOR SPREADING THE AIDS VIRUS, I AGREE NOT TO DONATE BLOOD OR PLASMA FOR TRANSFUSION TO ANOTHER PERSON.   YES ☐ NO ☐   DONOR SIGNATURE X

L-19 (Rev. 9-92)

FIGURE 10-4 Donor history card for autologous donation. (Courtesy Maryland General Hospital, Baltimore, Maryland.)

of thumb, reduce the volume to be drawn by 4 ml for each pound under 110.

3. **Hemoglobin and hematocrit.** The hemoglobin should not be less than 11 g/dl; the hematocrit, not less than 34 percent.

4. **Frequency.** Donations should not be more frequent than every 3 days, and the final donation must be completed at least 3 days before the scheduled surgical procedure. This allows the donor's plasma volume to return to normal before surgery. It is recommended that donors be placed on oral iron therapy if several units are to be drawn or the units are to be drawn very frequently.

5. **Medical history.** Because the donor will also be the recipient, most medical history questions need not be cause for deferral. Any medical condition that could make the phlebotomy dangerous to the donor-patient must be evaluated by the patient's physician and the blood bank medical director (see Fig. 10–4).

Intraoperative Blood Collection

During a surgical procedure blood is collected, by aspiration, from the surgical site. It is then processed by centrifugation, washing, and filtering, and is reinfused to the patient during or immediately after surgery.

The procedure can be used in most procedures as long as there is no contamination (sepsis or penetrating bowel wound) of the surgical site or contamination with malignant tumor cells. It has frequently been used in orthopedic, vascular, cardiac, obstetric and gynecologic, and neurosurgical procedures.[17] The procedure tends to be somewhat expensive so it is advisable to limit the use of this method to those situations in which multiple (three or more) units of blood may be needed.

Blood collected by this method is not suitable for transfusion to any other patient. It can be stored at room temperature for up to 4 hours and generally does not leave the operating or recovery room. If longer storage is desired, harvested units can be sent to the blood bank to store at 1°C to 6°C for up to 24 hours. If this is done, there must be a system in place to identify the unit positively before leaving the operating room and a mechanism, in the blood bank, to prevent accidental release of the blood to the general inventory or the wrong patient. There must be a written protocol for the intraoperative procedure, the blood bank medical director should be involved in establishing the protocol, and the hospital's transfusion committee must approve it.[18]

827 Linden Avenue
Baltimore, Maryland 21201   **PHYSICIAN ORDER FORM FOR PREDEPOSIT AUTOLOGOUS TRANSFUSION**
410 225-8000

PATIENT NAME: _____

ADDRESS: _____

TELEPHONE: _____ BIRTHDATE: _____ HOSP. # _____

I request that the above-named patient donate_____units of autologous blood in

advance of his/her surgical procedure_____scheduled
                                        (PROCEDURE)

for _____.
          (DATE)

I have explained this procedure to my patient, including the advantages and disadvantages. In view of my patient's current medical status, I do not foresee any
contraindications to this procedure. I have advised my patient to begin a high
iron diet or prescribed oral iron with the instructions to begin the recommended
iron regime one (1) week prior to the first phlebotomy.

I authorize the release of all unused autologous blood components from this patient
after the post-operative interval specified below. They may be used for transfusion
to other patients or any other use deemed appropriate by the blood bank medical
director. I may extend the holding period by contacting the blood bank at any time
through the end of the originally designated interval. If only autologous red
blood cells are requested, I authorize release of other components immediately
following donation.

_____   _____, M.D.
    (Date)   (Requesting Physician's Signature)

- -
UNLESS OTHERWISE SPECIFIED, THE FOLLOWING CONDITIONS ARE UNDERSTOOD:

Components reserved for autologous use:	Red Cells (only)	_____ (specify FFP if desired)
Minimum donor hematocrit:	34%	
Minimum interval between donations:	7 days	_____ (specify other)
		_____ (specify other)
Minimum interval between last donation & date of surgery:	72 hours	
		_____ (specify other)
Blood held after surgery:	72 hours	
		_____ (specify other)
Oral iron therapy begun: _____ (date)	Dose: _____	

FIGURE 10-5 Front of the physician's order form for autologous donation. (Courtesy Maryland General Hospital, Baltimore, Maryland.)

BLOOD BANK USE ONLY
_____

Medical Director's review and approval   APPROVED: YES_____ NO_____

COMMENTS: _____

_____

_____

_____

_____

_____   _____
(Signature)   (Date)

FIGURE 10-6 Back of the physician's order form for autologous donation; the blood bank medical director's review and approval. (Courtesy Maryland General Hospital, Baltimore, Maryland.)

Immediate Preoperative Hemodilution

This procedure is used particularly with heart surgery (cardiopulmonary bypass [CPB]) procedures. After the patient is under anesthesia and before the bypass surgery begins, 1 to 3 units of blood are removed and the blood volume is restored using volume expanders (colloid or crystalloid or both). The patient's hematocrit is typically lowered to about 20 percent.

The advantages of this procedure include:

1. Surgical bleeding occurs at a lower hematocrit, and therefore the amount of RBC mass that is lost is less.
2. The donated blood that can be reinfused during or immediately after surgery is very fresh and contains viable platelets, adequate protein levels, and good levels of all the plasma clotting factors.[19]
3. The blood flow through the microcirculation is improved because of the greatly reduced hematocrit.[20]

The collected blood usually does not leave the operating room. It can be stored at room temperature for up to 4 hours, or in the refrigerator (1°C to 6°C) for up to 24 hours. As with the intraoperative collection, longer storage should be handled by the blood bank, and all procedures and policies must be in place to ensure proper collection, handling, storage, identification, distribution, and disposition of the blood.

Postoperative "Shed" Blood Collection

This procedure collects blood from a drainage tube placed in the surgical site. It is particularly useful in collecting "shed" blood from a chest tube following CPB surgery and is frequently used following total knee surgery. The procedure can be used alone or in conjunction with other autologous blood collection procedures. The blood collected by this method must be used within 6 hours of collection.

WHOLE BLOOD COLLECTION AND PHLEBOTOMY

Once the donor has been registered and has successfully passed the physical examination and medical history requirements, the next step is the actual collection of the donor unit.

1. The personnel performing the phlebotomy procedure must be well trained and under the supervision of a qualified, licensed physician.
2. The blood must be drawn in an aseptic manner, using a sterile, closed system and a single venipuncture.
   a. The phlebotomy site on the donor's arm(s), usually the antecubital area, must be free of any skin lesions or rash, or both, which could cause contamination of the unit or infection to the donor.
   b. The venipuncture site must be thoroughly cleaned and disinfected. A surgical preparation is used to provide maximum protection. Table 10-1 lists two acceptable methods used by most blood banks.
3. A system must be established that will uniquely and positively identify each donor unit, subsequent product prepared, the medical history form, and all pilot tubes. The system may use numbers, letters, or other symbols, or various combinations thereof. It must, however, provide positive donor identification that is traceable. The numbers (or other identification system) must be applied to the bags, medical history form, and pilot tubes before proceeding with the phlebotomy.
4. Any of the following anticoagulants and additive solutions are considered acceptable by the FDA. Additive solutions (AS) are added to the RBCs after the plasma has been removed:
   a. Acid-citrate-dextrose (ACD)
   b. Heparin
   c. Citrate-phosphate-dextrose (CPD)
   d. Citrate-phosphate-dextrose-adenine (CPDA-1)
   e. CPD plus AS-1 or AS-2, consisting of saline, dextrose, mannitol, and adenine
   f. Citrate-phosphate-double dextrose (CP2D) plus AS, consisting of saline, dextrose, and adenine
5. The pilot samples to be used for donor processing should be attached firmly to the container before the phlebotomy. They must be filled at the time the donor unit is being drawn, usually immediately following the collection of the unit, by the same individual who drew the unit.

   Samples (segments) to be used for subsequent compatibility testing must be prepared from the integral tubing (the tubing that runs from the needle to the primary bag) in a manner that allows each segment to be separated without contamination of the unit.
6. Phlebotomy procedure and pilot tube collection. DO NOT LEAVE THE DONOR UNATTENDED AT ANY TIME DURING THE PHLEBOTOMY PROCEDURE.
   a. Make the donor comfortable. Confirm the donor's identification.

MARYLAND GENERAL HOSPITAL

827 Linden Avenue
Baltimore, Maryland 21201
301 225-8000

PRE-DEPOSIT AUTOLOGOUS DONOR PROGRAM

STATEMENT OF CONSENT FOR AUTOLOGOUS DONATION AND TRANSFUSION

A. The advantages, nature and purpose of autologous donation/transfusion, the risks involved and the possibility of complications have been explained to me by _____, M.D. I acknowledge such counseling.

I understand that:

1. The blood drawn from me for later transfusion to me is the safest blood for me to receive and that there is virtually no risk of my aquiring hepatitis or AIDS from the transfusion of such blood.

2. The procedure for donating my own blood is identical to routine blood donation. Each unit (approximately 1 pint) is collected by placing a needle into a vein in my arm; blood flows into a sterile plastic bag containing an anticoagulant. After the procedure, the needle is removed and pressure and a bandage are applied to my arm to prevent bleeding. Each unit is labeled and stored for my own use during my subsequent hospitalization.

3. A mild anemia and/or decrease in my blood volume may temporarily result from frequent blood donations for autologous transfusion. Because of these possible changes, I should refrain from strenuous athletic events and hazardous occupations or endeavors between the time the first unit is drawn and the scheduled use of predeposit units.

4. I may be asked to take oral iron supplements to replenish the iron lost with each donated unit.

5. I should contact my personal physician or the blood bank if I feel faint, weak, lightheaded, dizzy or otherwise ill. The blood bank is open Monday-Friday from 8:00am - 5:00pm for any questions I may have about symptoms related to autologous donation. The Blood Bank phone # is 225-8462.

6. The blood which I am donating for autologous purposes may not be used to transfuse me if my physician determines that autologous transfusion is not medically appropriate. I also understand that there may be situations where additional blood products are required. In any event, I agree to accept homologous (other donor's) blood if my physician determines that such transfusion(s) is(are) appropriate.

7. If I am physically and mentally able, I must identify my signature on the autologous transfusion tag prior to the administration of each unit of autologous blood.

8. If the scheduled procedure is delayed for any reason, it may be necessary to transfuse an older unit back to me and withdraw a fresh unit to prevent expiration and discarding of the older unit.

9. If the blood is to be transfused at Maryland General Hospital, no infectious disease testing will be performed on the donated unit.

(OVER)

FIGURE 10-7 Predeposit consent form for autologous donation. (Courtesy Maryland General Hospital, Baltimore, Maryland.)

10. If I or my physician request that the donated blood be transfered to another facility or hospital, all infectious disease testing required by state and federal law will be performed. These include tests for Hepatitis B surface Antigen (HBsAg), Hepatitis C Virus Antibody (Anti-HCV), Aminoalanine transaminase (ALT), Antibody to the Hepatitis B core antigen (Anti-HBc), Human Immunodeficiency Virus Antibody (Anti-HIV), Human T-lymphotropic Virus Type I Antibody (Anti-HTLV-I).

11. If the tests for infectious deseases show that I am a carrier of hepatitis or have been exposed to the AIDS virus, I will be notified confidentially of the test results and my name and other identifying information will be placed on a confidential list of persons who should not donate blood or plasma for transfusion to other people.

12. If Maryland state laws or federal laws require that these positive test results be reported to state or federal health authorities, this will be done in accordance with such laws.

B. I consent to the withdrawl of blood, by authorized members of the staff of the Maryland General Hospital Blood Bank, for autologous transfusion purposes and further consent to such additional procedures pursuant to autologous transfusion as may be necessary or desirable. Should I not require transfusion of the blood withdrawn for autologous transfusion, during the time frame specified by my physician/surgeon, I further consent to the disposal of my blood in any manner deemed appropriate by the blood bank medical director.

(Date)	Donor/Patient Signature or Authority to Consent if not the Patient's own signature
(Date)	Witness

DR-1 rev. 9/90

FIGURE 10-7 _Continued._

TABLE 10–1 ARM PREPARATION METHODS

Method I

1. Scrub the site (2 × 2 inches) for 30 seconds using an aqueous iodophor scrub solution (0.7 percent). Iodophor is a polyvinylpyrrolidone-iodine or poloxamer iodine complex. Remove excess foam. Area need not be dry before proceeding.
2. Apply iodophor complex and let stand for 30 seconds. Use a concentric spiral motion, starting in the center and moving outward. Do not go back toward the center. Removal of the iodophor solution is not necessary. The iodine is complexed and will not usually cause skin irritation.
3. Site is now ready for venipuncture. Cover with a sterile gauze until ready for needle insertion.

Method II

1. Scrub vigorously for 30 seconds using a 15-percent aqueous solution of soap ("green soap"). Scrub area should be at least 2 × 2 inches around the intended venipuncture site. The scrub is designed to remove dirt, oils, and loose skin cells.
2. Remove the soap using an alcohol (70 percent) and acetone (10 percent) solution (9 : 1 ratio). Apply solution in the aforementioned concentric, spiral motion. Allow to dry.
3. Apply a tincture of iodine solution (3 percent iodine in 70 percent alcohol). Use the same concentric motion as with the alcohol. Allow to dry.
4. Remove the iodine with the alcohol and acetone solution as in step 2. The iodine should be removed; it is no longer needed in order to maintain the cleanliness of the area and, if left on, may cause skin irritation.
5. Site is now ready for venipuncture. Cover with a sterile gauze until ready for needle insertion.

b. Select and locate the desired vein. Marking may be necessary if the vein is deep and does not distend visually.

c. Prepare the site and cover.

d. Set up and check the bag and scale unless previously completed.

e. Place a clamp on the tubing between the needle and the primary bag.

f. Give the donor something to squeeze. Instruct the donor to clench the fist a couple of times and then hold it tight.

g. Use a tourniquet or blood pressure cuff (maximum 60 mm Hg) to increase the distention of the vein.

h. Perform the venipuncture. Place the thumb of your free hand below the prepared site and pull the skin taut. With the needle at a 45-degree angle to the skin, make a quick clean puncture. Once in the skin, reduce the angle of the needle to about 10 to 20 degrees, orient the line of the vein, and make a second push through the vein wall; thread the needle up the vein about one-half inch to aid in securing the needle.

i. Release the clamp on the tubing, and check to make sure the flow is fairly rapid and steady.

j. Tape the needle and tubing lightly to the arm. This will help prevent accidentally pulling the needle out. Cover with a sterile gauze.

k. Reduce the tourniquet or blood pressure cuff to approximately 40 mm Hg.

l. Continue to monitor the donor for signs of a reaction. Continue to observe the flow rate and periodically mix the blood to insure contact with the anticoagulant. Mixing is not required if vacuum equipment is being used.

m. When the primary unit has tripped the preset scale, instruct the donor to stop squeezing and clamp off (or tie a knot in) the tubing. The volume-weight conversion for whole blood is 1.06 g/ml. A unit of WB should weigh between 430 and 525 g plus the weight of the bag, anticoagulant, and the empty pilot tubes.

n. Collect the pilot tubes before removing the needle from the donor's arm. The most convenient system is one with an in-line needle or in-line pouch; however, this is not mandatory.

o. Release the tourniquet or blood pressure cuff.

p. Permanently clamp or seal the donor tubing close to the needle.

q. Remove the needle from the donor's arm, apply pressure to the site (over the gauze), and instruct the donor to raise his or her arm with the elbow straight, and continue pressure to the site. Once the bleeding has stopped (approximately 2 minutes), have the donor lower his or her arm. Check for bleeding and place a bandage over the site.

r. Strip the tubing to ensure that the blood is completely mixed with the anticoagulant. Allow the tubing to refill, being careful to avoid any bubbles. Seal the tubing in segments at approximately 3-inch intervals, making sure that the lot number is present on each segment. The seal between each segment should be clean and should allow for easy separation. These segments will be used for compatibility testing (see step 5).

s. Place the units in storage. All units except those that will be used for platelet production are to be stored at 1°C to 6°C or placed into a container for transportation, which will gradually reduce the temperature to 4°C. Those units destined for platelet production are to be stored at 20°C to 24°C until the platelets have been removed.

7. Before allowing the donor to leave the area, instruct him or her in postphlebotomy care. The following are some examples of instructions that should be given:

a. Increase fluid intake for the next few hours (may be up to 24 hours). Have something to eat or drink, or both, before leaving the donor area. Remain in the area for at least 10 minutes.

b. Do not drink alcoholic beverages before the next meal.

c. Do not smoke for the next half hour.

d. Leave the bandage on for a few hours.

e. Do not put strong pressure on or try to lift or carry heavy objects with the donating arm for the next few hours.

f. If bleeding occurs from the phlebotomy site, reapply direct pressure until it stops.

g. If you feel dizzy or faint, sit down with your head lowered between your knees or lie down with your feet elevated. If the symptoms continue, return to the blood bank or see your doctor.

h. Refrain from very strenuous activity or hazardous work for a few hours.

DONOR REACTIONS

Although the majority of donations proceed without any complications, occasionally a donor will have an adverse reaction to the donation. Most reactions are vasovagal reactions. The reactions may result from psychologic influences, such as the sight of blood, excitement, fear, or apprehension or may be a neurophysiologic response to the actual donation. The reactions can be roughly grouped into three categories based on the degree of severity.

Mild Reactions

Mild reactions are the most frequently encountered type of reaction, in which the donor exhibits signs of shock but does not lose consciousness. The signs and symptoms of mild reactions include one or more of the following:

1. Nervousness, anxiety
2. Complaints of feeling warm
3. Pallor, sweating
4. Increased or thready pulse (lacking a complete vibration in the beat)
5. Increased respirations leading to hyperventilation
6. Decreased blood pressure
7. Nausea and possibly vomiting

In general, treatment for mild reactions include:

1. Stop the donation; remove the tourniquet and needle from the donor's arm.
2. Have the donor breathe into a paper bag, which will counteract the effects of hyperventilation by increasing the amount of carbon dioxide (CO_2) in the air the donor is breathing.
3. Loosen any tight clothing, particularly a necktie or shirt buttoned around the neck.
4. Ensure that the donor has a clear airway.
5. Have the donor pull his or her knees up (with feet on the donor bed) or raise his or her feet (approximately 45 degrees) for a while. The feet may be lowered as the donor recovers.
6. Apply a cold towel to the forehead and neck and use aromatic spirits of ammonia if necessary.

7. Talk to the donor as the treatment is being given to reassure the donor and to reduce his or her stress or anxiety or both, which may have been the primary causes of the reaction.
8. If the donor does not quickly respond and recover, additional medical help should be summoned.
9. DO NOT LEAVE THE DONOR.

Moderate Reactions

Moderate reactions are characterized by signs and symptoms similar to those found in mild reactions, plus the fact that the donor loses consciousness. In moderate reactions, the following signs and symptoms, in addition to those listed for mild reactions, may occur:

1. Periods of unconsciousness (which may be repetitive)
2. Decreased pulse rate
3. Rapid, shallow respirations and hyperventilation
4. Continued decrease in blood pressure (hypotension; systolic pressure may drop as low as 60 mm Hg)

The recommended countermeasures for moderate reactions include the following:

1. Proceed with the appropriate measures listed for treatment of mild reactions.
2. Check blood pressure, pulse, and respirations frequently until they return to normal.
3. Administer 95 percent oxygen (O_2); 5 percent CO_2.
4. Separate the donor from the general donor area by use of screens or move the donor to another room. Sight of a reaction in one donor may trigger reactions in others.

Severe Reactions

To classify a severe reaction, add convulsions to the previously listed symptoms. Convulsions or seizures can be caused by cerebral ischemia associated with vasovagal syncope (reduced blood flow to the brain owing to the deepening shock symptoms); by marked hyperventilation (severe CO_2 depletion can cause convulsions or tetany); or by epilepsy. These severe reactions can be further categorized by the symptoms they produce.

1. Hyperventilation tetany (the earliest stage of convulsions caused by hyperventilation)
   a. The donor has not lost consciousness and may complain of stiffness or tingling in the fingers.
   b. The fingers and thumb may spasm and assume an unnatural position.
   c. The symptoms will progress to deeper, more pronounced convulsions if CO_2 intake is not increased.

The recommended countermeasures include:
a. Remain calm; do not alarm other donors if possible.
b. Have the donor rebreathe air from a paper bag.
c. DO NOT LEAVE THE DONOR. However, help should be summoned inasmuch as the reaction may progress to a more severe state.
2. Mild convulsions
a. Short lapse of consciousness
b. Voice fadeout
c. Slight involuntary movement of the arms and legs
3. Severe convulsions
a. Rigid body and tightly clenched teeth
b. Temporary loss of breathing, followed by a rasping or stertorous type breathing
c. Slight involuntary movement of the arms and legs

The recommended countermeasures for both moderate and severe convulsions include:
a. Gently restrain to prevent the donor from injuring himself or herself. It may be necessary to move the donor from the donor couch to the floor.
b. Summon help immediately. Remain calm and with the donor.
c. Ensure an adequate airway.
d. 95 percent O_2; 5 percent CO_2 may be administered.
e. Maintain observation of donor until fully recovered and released by the blood bank physician.

Cardiac and/or Respiratory Problems

If the donor develops respiratory difficulties or appears to be having cardiac problems, call for medical assistance immediately. If the donor goes into cardiac arrest, administer cardiopulmonary resuscitation (CPR) until medical help arrives.

Hematomas

Hematomas are not an uncommon complication of the phlebotomy process. They can occur if the needle is not seated properly and there is leakage of blood around the needle entry site into the tissue or if the needle went through the vein and punctured the back wall. If a hematoma develops, remove the tourniquet and the needle. Apply pressure to the venipuncture site and raise the arm for 5 to 10 minutes. Make sure the bleeding has completely stopped, then apply a bandage. If the arm is stiff or sore, a cold (ice) pack can be used over the dressing. Caution the donor that a "black-and-blue" area will develop and, if it is sore or uncomfortable, that ice packs can be applied. If the arm becomes painful, the donor should see a doctor or return to the donor center. The discoloration will last awhile and will gradually change colors from blue-black to purple to red-brown to yellow.

A report of any adverse reaction should be kept on file in the blood bank as a part of the donor record.

DONOR PROCESSING

All donor units must be processed to some degree before being released for compatibility testing and transfusion. Although there are some minor differences between the AABB standards and the FDA regulations as to which tests are needed, the following criteria will satisfy both organizations' minimum requirements.

All reagents used in donor blood testing and screening must meet or exceed the minimum standards for reactivity established by the FDA. The commercially prepared reagents that are licensed by the FDA must meet these standards, so the blood bank need not be concerned with reagent testing other than routine quality control procedures (see Chapter 13). Each major step of the testing and processing system must be documented and the records maintained so that any unit or component or both can be traced. The example given in Figure 10–8 uses a system in which the processing test results are kept as part of the donor record (on the back of the medical history card).

ABO Grouping

Regulations require that two different tests be used to determine the ABO type of each donor unit. The detection of the antigens present on the red cells is commonly called a "forward or front" type and requires the use of anti-A and anti-B sera. The use of anti-A,B is optional, although still in some use, particularly to confirm the forward type of group O units. The detection of the antibodies present in the plasma or serum is commonly called the "reverse or back" type. Reagent A_1 cells and B cells are required; A_2 cells are optional.

The results of both tests must be recorded, compared, and found in agreement before the unit can be released. Any discrepancies must be investigated and resolved before releasing the unit, and the results of the investigation must be kept as part of the processing record.

Rh Typing

The Rh type is determined by the use of anti-Rh_o (D) serum. If the test result is positive after the immediate spin phase (D-positive), the unit is labeled "Rh-positive." If the immediate spin phase is negative, an anti-human globulin (AHG) or Coombs phase to detect the D variant (D^u) antigen is performed.

Large automated blood typing machines are now being used (mostly in large blood centers) that are so sensitive that the Rh type can be accurately determined without the need for the AHG phase.

DATE	DONOR NUMBER	Anti A	Anti B	Cells A₁	Cells B	Anti D	Rh Cont	Du	Check Cell	Du Cont	Check Cell	Interp.	Tech.		TEST	RESULT	DATE	TECH
															HBsAg			
															ALT			
LABELING INFO:		I				II				III					Anti-HBc			
Date Drawn:		RT	37°C			RT	37°C			RT	37°C				Anti-HIV			
Date Expires:		I.S. Sal	10' LISS	AHG	Check Cell	I.S. Sal	10' LISS	AHG	Check Cell	I.S. Sal	10' LISS	AHG	Check Cell		STS/RPR			
Labeled By:															HTLV-I/II			
Label Checked By:															HCV			

PHLEB S U	REACTION SL M SEV.	TIME STARTED	TIME COMPLETED	WEIGHT GMS

REMARKS:

FIGURE 10-8 Form for blood testing for allogenic donation (back of the donor history card; see Fig. 10-1). (Courtesy Maryland General Hospital, Baltimore, Maryland.)

Antibody Screen

Although an antibody screen is required only on those donors who give a history of previous pregnancy or transfusion or both,[21] it is standard practice to perform an antibody screen on all donor units. The procedure must be designed so that the presence of clinically significant antibodies will be detected. Most antibody screening procedures consist of an incubation at 37°C in saline, low-ionic-strength solution, or albumin (a new enhancement media, polyethylene glycol, is becoming widely used also) and an AHG phase. Because it is widely agreed that antibodies that react only in the cold (less than 37°C) have little or no clinical significance, the use of the immediate spin or a 22°C (room temperature) incubation phase, or both, has generally been dropped. It is acceptable practice to use serum pooled from several donors or pooled screening cells or both when performing the antibody screening test on donor units. Donor units in which clinically significant antibodies have been detected should be used for transfusion as RBCs. The plasma must not be used for the preparation of single-donor plasma liquid or fresh frozen and should not be used for the production of platelet concentrates or cryoprecipitate.

Serologic Test for Syphilis

The serologic test for syphilis (STS) is a test that detects previous exposure to syphilis. The rapid plasma reagent (RPR) test is quick, easy to perform, and inexpensive, which makes it good for mass screening of blood donors. However, the test is also prone to false-positive results. Consequently, any positive RPR test result must be confirmed with the more specific but far more expensive and complicated, fluorescent treponemal antibody absorption (FTA-ABS) test.

Over the years there has been much debate as to the need for an STS. Most have believed that the test is unnecessary because the *Treponema pallidum* spirochete does not survive in citrated blood, stored at 1°C to 6°C, for more than 72 hours, meaning platelet concentrates are about the only products at risk of transmitting the disease and there have been no documented cases of transfusion-transmitted syphilis. At the time the previous edition of this book was written, the AABB had dropped their requirement for performing the STS, but the FDA and many state and municipal laws still required it. Then in 1991, in the 14th edition of the AABB Standards, the STS was reinstated as a required test.

Today the return of the STS as a universally required donor screening test is not because there is a concern with transfusion-transmitted syphilis but rather because syphilis is, like hepatitis B, hepatitis C, and HIV, a sexually transmitted disease. A donor who proves to be syphilis positive is probably at higher risk for exposure to hepatitis and HIV because it implies that "safe" sexual practices have not been followed.[22]

If the RPR test result is positive, the donor unit is not to be used for transfusion purposes. If the FTA-

ABS test result also is positive, the donor needs to be notified.

Hepatitis B Surface Antigen

The test procedure used must be one approved by the FDA or a documented equivalent method. The methods currently approved are radioimmunoassay (RIA), enzyme-linked immunosorbent assay (ELISA), and reverse passive hemagglutination (RPHA). Of these approved methods the ELISA is by far the most common procedure in use. All of the newer viral marker tests use the ELISA method and many facilities perform all of the tests on a single instrument.

Any unit found to be positive for HBsAg must not be used for transfusion. (Units drawn for autologous transfusion only can be accepted.)

In an emergency, blood and blood products can be released before HBsAg testing is completed, provided the test is performed, the results are transmitted to the transfusion service as soon as possible, and the unit is conspicuously labeled or tagged to indicate that testing is not complete. Record of the early release and the subsequent test results must be maintained. If the test result should be positive, the recipient's physician must be notified and a record of that notification must be maintained.[23]

Hepatitis C Antibody

The hepatitis C virus (HCV) was identified in 1988 and accounts for most, but not all, of what we used to call "non-A, non-B hepatitis." The test is an ELISA procedure that detects the presence of antibody formed against the hepatitis C virus (anti-HCV). Any donor unit that tests positive for anti-HCV must not be used for transfusion except, as with HBsAg testing, as an autologous transfusion.

The rules for emergency release of a unit, before testing for anti-HCV, are the same as for HBsAg testing.

Hepatitis Surrogate Testing

In late 1986, surrogate testing for non-A, non-B hepatitis was instituted based on the results of two major studies: one by the National Institutes of Health (NIH) and the other by a multi-institutional cooperative study (Transfusion-Transmitted Virus Study [TTVS]). These studies indicated a significant incidence of elevated ALT levels or anti-HBc or both present in donor units implicated in posttransfusion non-A, non-B hepatitis infection.[24] Even with the identification of HCV and the presence of a direct test for anti-HCV, both ALT and anti-HBc testing methods are still in use.

ALT: This enzyme is found in large amounts in the liver. Normally, serum levels are very low, but liver damage, particularly hepatitis, can cause very high serum elevations.[25] According to AABB guidelines, units that have an ALT level 2.25 standard deviations above the log mean normal value, as determined by the individual blood bank, should not be used for transfusion. In blood banks where ALT testing is already established, or where a particular reagent manufacturer's normal range is used, the acceptable cutoff level is 1.5 times the upper limit of normal. Units with levels between 1.5 and 3.0 times the upper limit must be discarded. Permanent deferral and donor notification are required if the level is more than three times the upper limit or if levels between 1.5 and 3.0 occur on at least two consecutive donations.

Anti-HBc: This antibody is directed against a "core" or interior protein on the hepatitis B virus. It usually develops before general symptoms of disease are apparent and has been found in donor units that have been implicated in non-A, non-B transfusion-transmitted hepatitis (TTH). Any unit that is repeatedly reactive for anti-HBc should not be used for transfusion.

Human Immunodeficiency Virus Antibody

All donor units must be screened for the presence of the HIV-1/2 antibody using an ELISA procedure approved by the FDA. If the ELISA screening test result is positive, the test is repeated. If the repeat test result is negative, the unit can be used for transfusion. If the repeat screening test result is positive, the unit is discarded and a confirmation Western blot test performed. If the Western blot test result is negative or inconclusive, the donor's name is placed in a temporary holding file. The donor need not be notified or deferred from future donations. If the Western blot test result is positive, the donor must be notified, preferably in person, and counseled on what the test results mean. The donor is indefinitely deferred.

HIV-2 has been isolated from several patients with frank AIDS. Although common in West Africa, this virus is quite rare in the United States.[26] In 1992, in an effort to ensure the safest blood supply possible, all donor blood was required to be tested for the presence of both HIV-1 and HIV-2 antibodies (anti-HIV 1/2). In most centers this is done by the use of a new, combined test.

Human T-Cell Lymphotropic Virus Type I Antibody

This virus is believed to cause adult T-cell leukemia (ATL) and has been associated with a neurologic disorder called tropical spastic paraparesis (TSP). Because the incubation period for the diseases associated with HTLV-1 infection may be very long and because the results of an American Red Cross study in 1986–1987 indicated a possible transfusion-transmitted infection rate of 2800 recipients per year, this virus has been added to the growing list of viral markers that must be screened for in all donor blood.[27]

As with the other viral marker tests, this is an ELISA procedure to detect the presence of the HTLV-1 antibody. Any unit that tests positive must not be used for transfusion purposes except as an autologous transfusion.

Testing Requirements for Autologous Donors

Units that are donated exclusively for autologous transfusion must be tested for ABO and Rh only if the unit is to be transfused at the same facility that collected it. However, if the unit is to be shipped from the collecting facility to a transfusing facility, the first unit from a specific donor within a 30-day period must be tested for HBsAg, anti-HIV 1/2, anti-HCV, anti-HBc, STS, and any other test that is required or recommended by the FDA.[28]

If any of the disease marker test results are found to be positive, a "biohazard" label must be attached to the unit. If either the HBsAg or the anti-HIV 1/2 tests are confirmed to be reactive, the unit must not be shipped unless *written* request and consent is obtained from the patient's physician. The patient's physician must also be notified if the anti-HBc, anti-HCV, or STS is found to be repeatedly reactive.

If an autologous donor has met all of the standard requirements for an allogeneic blood donor and the blood bank wishes to use the unit for allogeneic (cross-over) transfusion, should it not be needed by the donor, all of the standard tests identified in this section must be performed.

Labeling

Once all testing is completed, the WB or component(s) must be labeled. The label shall include the following information (Fig. 10–9):

1. Classification of the donor (volunteer or paid)
2. Name of the component and any modifier(s), if applicable
3. Name of the anticoagulant used (not required for components prepared by hemapheresis or for frozen, deglycerolized, rejuvenated, or washed RBCs)
4. Amount of blood collected or, for platelets, fresh frozen plasma, or low-volume red blood cells, volume in the container
5. Donor or WB number (the alphanumeric identification system)
6. Name, address, and registration or license number of the collecting facility
7. Required storage temperature for the specific component
8. ABO group and Rh type of the donor
9. Expiration date (month, day, and year) and, if appropriate, time
10. "See circular of information for indications, contraindications, cautions, and methods of infusion"
11. "Caution: Federal law prohibits dispensing without prescription"
12. "Properly identify intended recipient"
13. "This product may transmit infectious agents"

Repeat Testing

If the blood-collecting facility is separate from the transfusion facility, the latter is required to perform some repeat testing before issuing the blood or component for transfusion. The tests that must be repeated are:

1. ABO group on all WB and RBC units
2. Rh type on all Rh-negative WB and RBC units (immediate spin phase is required, but D^u testing is *not* required)

These tests are to be performed on a segment sample from the attached integral tubing.

Component Preparation

Today effective transfusion therapy depends on the availability of many different blood components. These components, used separately or in various combinations, can adequately meet most patient transfusion needs while keeping the risk of transfusion to a minimum.

Component transfusion therapy has the added benefit of using a limited natural resource more effectively by providing needed therapeutic material to several patients from a single donation.

The following section reviews each of the major components in terms of their preparation and general use. Table 10–2 outlines the various components.

RED BLOOD CELLS

Red blood cells are prepared by removing approximately 80 percent of the plasma from a unit of WB. Regulations require that the final hematocrit of an RBC unit not exceed 80%. The average hematocrit is between 65 percent and 80 percent.

Red blood cells contain the same RBC mass and therefore the same O_2-carrying capacity as WB, but with approximately one-half the volume (average volume is 250 to 300 ml). They can be used in any situation that requires increased O_2-carrying capacity. RBCs are particularly useful in patients who require the increased RBC mass but may be at risk of circulatory overload (e.g., patients with chronic severe anemia with a compensated [normal] blood volume or those with anemia along with cardiac failure). The advantages of using RBCs rather than WB include:

1. Equal O_2 capacity in half the volume
2. Significant reduction in the level of isoagglutinins (anti-A and anti-B), thus facilitating the safe transfusion of group O cells to non–group O recipients

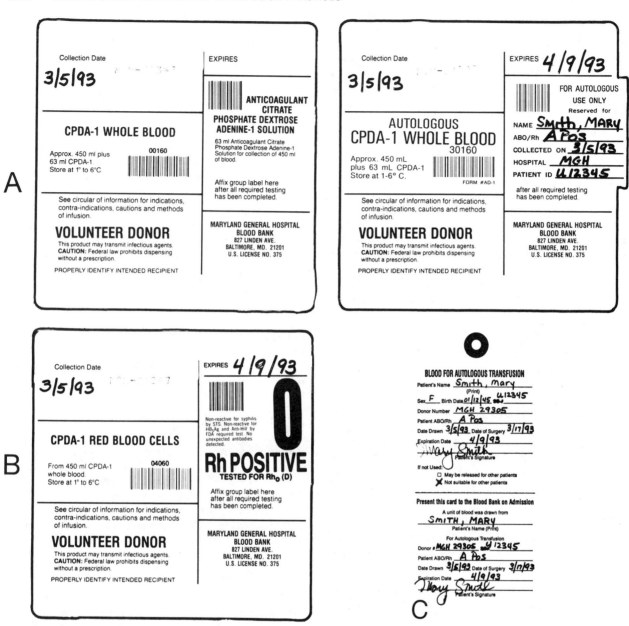

FIGURE 10-9   Donor base labels: (*A*) at time of collection, (*B*) after completion of all testing, and (*C*) for an autologous donor's unit.

3. Significant reduction in the levels of acid, citrate, and potassium in units prepared just before transfusion. This reduces the risk of acid level, citrate toxicity, and potassium load in patients with cardiac, renal, or liver disease. Units that are prepared at the time of collection have reduced levels of acid and citrate (most of the anticoagulant is removed with the plasma), but potassium, which is released as the RBCs age, will remain a problem.

Red blood cells can be prepared anytime during the normal dating period by centrifugation or sedimentation. Between 200 and 250 ml of plasma are usually removed from units collected in CPDA-1. An extra 50 ml of plasma can be removed from units drawn in CPD plus adenine-saline because 150 ml of adenine-saline preservative solution will be added to the cells, returning the hematocrit to about 80 percent. The expiration date of RBCs prepared in a closed system will not change from that of the WB (35 days for CPDA-1 and 42 for CPD plus adenine-saline). Should the unit have to be entered, the expiration date is reduced to 24 hours from the time the unit was entered. Sterile docking-connecting devices are now available that allow entrance to a unit without altering the original expiration date.

The following is a general procedure for RBC production using centrifugation:

1. Weigh and balance each unit.

TABLE 10–2 SUMMARY OF BLOOD COMPONENTS

Component	Shelf Life	Storage Temperature	Quality Control Requirements	Volume	Indications for Use	Content	Dosage Effect	Transfusion Criteria
RBCs	CPD = 21 days CPDA-1 = 35 days CPD-AS = 42 days Heparin = 2 days	1°C–6°C	Hematocrit must be 80% or less (usually 65–80%)	250–300 ml	Restore O_2-carrying capacity in symptomatic anemia (acute or chronic)	RBCs (65–80%) Plasma (20–35%) Some: Platelets WBCs Storage lesion by products	1 unit RBC ↑ Hct 3% ↑ Hb 1 g	ABO and Rh specific X-match compatible
Leukocyte-reduced RBCs	Closed system: same as for RBCs Open system: 24 hours	1°C–6°C	5×10^6 residual WBC 80% recovery of RBC 80% Hct if unit is to be stored	250–300 ml	Patients who require replacement of RBC mass and reduced exposure to WBC: febrile reactions, BMT, etc (see text)	RBCs (80–95%) Plasma (5–20%) Residual WBCs ($<5 \times 10^6$)	Same as for RBC	ABO and Rh specific X-match compatible
Washed RBCs	24 hours (open system)	1°C–6°C	Plasma removal If procedure is being used to prepare leukocyte-reduced RBCs, all criteria for leukocyte-reduced RBCs must also be met	250–350 ml	Patients who require replacement of red cell mass and have a history of plasma protein antibodies, diagnosis of PNH, history of febrile reactions	RBCs (60–80%) Saline (20–40%)	Same as for RBC	ABO and Rh specific X-match compatible
Frozen, thawed, deglycerolized RBCs	Frozen: (−65°C or −150°C) Deglycerolized = 24 hours (open system) Frozen = 10 years	Frozen: (−65°C or −150°C) Deglycerolized: 1°C–6°C	80% recovery RBC mass <1% residual glycerol (420 mOsm) <300 mg residual-free hemoglobin	200–300 ml	Long-term storage of "rare" units and/or autologous units	RBCs (60–80%) Saline with dextrose (20–40%) <1–2% residual WBCs, platelets	Same as for RBC	ABO and Rh specific X-match compatible Frequently typed for other RBC antigens
Platelets Random-donor (prepared from WB)	5 days 2 days	20°C–24°C (room temp) 1°C–6°C	5.5×10^{10} platelets pH = 6.0 or greater at end of storage time Prepared within 6 hours of WB collection	50–65 ml 30–40 ml	To correct thrombocytopenia due to decreased platelet function, or production; increased platelet consumption (bleeding, platelet disorders, DIC, massive transfusion)	Platelets: 5.5×10^{10} Plasma: 50–65 ml Residual WBCs	↑ platelet count: 5,000–10,000 per unit	ABO and Rh compatible (if possible)

Continued

TABLE 10–2 SUMMARY OF BLOOD COMPONENTS (Continued)

Component	Shelf Life	Storage Temperature	Quality Control Requirements	Volume	Indications for Use	Content	Dosage Effect	Transfusion Criteria
Platelets Single-donor (prepared by pheresis)	5 days (closed system) 24 hours (open system)	20°C–24°C	3.0×10^{11} platelets pH = 6.0 or greater at the end of the storage time	300 ml	To correct thrombocytopenia in patients who demonstrate refractoriness to random-donor platelets (platelet antibodies)	Platelets: 3.0×10^{11} Plasma: 300 ml approx. May have significant RBC and WBC	↑ platelet count: 30–60.000 per unit	ABO and Rh compatible HLA typed (sometimes) X-match compatible (may be required)
Single-donor plasma FFP or SDP-24	Frozen = 1 year Thawed = 24 hours	−18°C 1°C–6°C	FFP: Prepare within 6 hours of whole blood collection SDP-24: Prepare within 24 hours of whole blood collection	150–250 ml	Treatment of multiple coagulation factor deficiencies (massive transfusion, trauma, liver disease, DIC, unidentified deficiency)	Plasma, all coagulation factors except platelets 400 mg fibrinogen 1 unit/ml all other factors	Increase factor levels 20–30% per dose of 10–15 ml/kg of body weight	ABO compatible
Single-donor plasma (SDP) Liquid/frozen	Liquid: up to 5 days beyond whole blood expiration date (26–40 days) Frozen: 5 years	1°C–6°C −18°C or colder	Must be frozen within 6 hours of transfer to final container	150–250 ml	Treatment of stable clotting factor deficiencies Source plasma for manufacture into NSA, PPF, ISG	Plasma stable clotting factors only		ABO compatible
Cryoprecipitated antihemophilic factor (Cryo)	Frozen: 1 year Thawed: 6 hours Pooled: 4 hours	−18°C or colder 20°C–24°C	Factor VIII:C (80 IU) Thaw at 37°C	10–25 ml	Correction of F VIII deficiency (hemophilia A, von Willebrand's) F XIII deficiency Fibrinogen deficiency owing to congenital hypofibrinogenemia Some fibrinogen consumption problems Source of "fibrin glue"	Factor VIII:C (80–150 IU) Fibrinogen: (150–250 mg) Factor XIII (20–30% of WB level) vWF (40–70% of WB level)	Plasma volume × % factor level needed = No. units needed ÷ 80–100 = No. cryoprecipitate bags needed	ABO compatible
Granulocyte concentrate	24 hours	20°C–24°C	1.0×10^{10} granulocytes Total WBC count with differential	200–600 ml	Correct severe neutropenia (<500 polymorpho-nuclear neutrophils/ml)	Granulocytes: 1.0×10^{10} WBCs Platelets Plasma RBCs (15% Hct)		ABO and Rh specific HLA matched (usually) X-match compatible

Component	Shelf Life	Storage Temperature	Volume		Indications	Composition	Dosage	Special Instructions
					Fever unresponsive to antibiotic therapy for 24–48 hours Myeloid hypoplasia of bone marrow with reasonable chance of survival			
Factor VIII concentrate (AHF)	Varies (expiration date listed on each vial)	1°C–6°C (lyophilized)	10–30 ml	—	Treatment of moderate to severe factor VIII deficiencies (hemophilia A)	Factor VIII:C (level stated on label of each vial) Some fibrinogen	See cryoprecipitate for dosage calculations 1 U factor VIII per kilogram body weight should ↑ factor VIII level by 2%	Reconstitute before infusion
Factor IX concentrate (prothrombin complex)	Varies (expiration date listed on each vial)	1°C–6°C (lyophilized)	20–30 ml	—	Treatment of factor IX deficiency (hemophilia B, Christmas disease) Treatment of some factor II, VII, X deficiencies	Factors II, VII, IX, X (levels stated on each vial)	See cryoprecipitate for dosage calculations 1 U factor IX per kilogram body weight should ↑ factor IX level by 1.5%	Reconstitute before infusion
ISG	3 years: Intramuscular injection 1 year: Intravenous solution		Varies according to patient size and indications for use	—	Prophylactic treatment for exposure to certain diseases such as hepatitis, chickenpox	Gamma globulins (intramuscular = 16.5 g/dl) (intravenous = 5 g/dl) Primarily IgG, some IgA, IgM		Intramuscular or intravenous, depending on product used
NSA 5 or 25%	3 years 5 years	20°C–24°C 1°C–6°C	50 ml or 250 ml	—	Plasma volume expansion: surgery, trauma, burns, etc.	96% Albumin 4% Globulin		
PPF 5%	3 years 5 years	20°C–24°C 1°C–6°C	250 ml	—	Plasma volume expansion	Albumin (80–85%) Globulin (15–20%)		

Continued

TABLE 10-2 SUMMARY OF BLOOD COMPONENTS (Continued)

Component	Shelf Life	Storage Temperature	Quality Control Requirements	Volume	Indications for Use	Content	Dosage Effect	Transfusion Criteria
Synthetic volume expanders	Varies	—	—	Varies	Plasma volume expansion (colloid or crystalloid)	Normal saline Ringer's Electrolyte solution Dextran HES	—	—
$Rh_o(D)$ immunoglobulin	3 years	1°C–6°C	—	1 ml	Prevention of $Rh_o(D)$ immunization	Full dose = 300 μg anti-D Mini dose = 150 μg anti-D	Full dose: term delivery, termination at 12 weeks or more, antipartum, transfusion exposure Mini dose: bleeding or termination at <12 weeks (1st trimester)	Injection given within 12 hours of delivery, abortion, or miscarriage Rh-negative recipient No evidence of serum anti-$Rh_o(D)$

2. Place the balanced units into the centrifuge. The centrifuge of choice is a swinging bucket type. It produces a better pack and a better plasma-cell interface. The refrigerated centrifuges should be checked on each day of use for correct speed and temperature (calibration should be performed every 6 months), and quality-control documents should be maintained.
3. Centrifuge for the specified time and speed. Although the average speed is approximately 3600 rpm for about 5 minutes, each centrifuge must be calibrated individually to ensure a quality product. The speed and time will change, depending on the plasma product(s) prepared. The AABB *Technical Manual* contains some centrifuge calculation data and procedures.[29]
4. When the centrifuge has come to a complete stop, remove the unit carefully and place on an expressor.
5. Express the plasma into the attached satellite bag. The hematocrit can be estimated by expressing enough plasma to bring the plasma-cell interface to the top corner (shoulder) of the bag or by removing a specified weight of plasma. The AABB *Technical Manual* suggests 232 to 258 g.
6. When the desired amount of plasma has been removed, seal the tubing using a dielectric heat sealer or metal clips.
7. Separate the plasma and the RBCs. Store the RBCs at 4°C. The plasma can be stored at 4°C, 22°C, or −30°C, depending on the product desired.

As part of the quality control program, each month hematocrit values must be calculated on a representative number of units (usually 1 to 4 units, depending on the total number prepared). Seventy-five percent of samples tested must meet the approved criteria (80 percent or less).

Irradiation

In the past several years the use of irradiated blood products (primarily RBCs and platelets) has risen dramatically. It has long been known that gamma irradiation of blood products would reduce the risk of transfusion-associated graft versus host (TA-GVH) disease in patients receiving allogeneic bone marrow transplants (BMT), and for such patients it is standard practice to irradiate any blood product that is contaminated with donor lymphocytes. More recently it has become clear that other patients are also at risk for TA-GVH disease. The risk appears to be well defined in BMT patients, patients with congenital immunodeficiency syndrome, or Hodgkin's disease; for intrauterine transfusions; and for blood transfusions from first-degree family members. Still under investigation, but also felt to carry some degree of risk, are premature newborn infants, solid organ transplant patients, patients with non-Hodgkin's malignancies, and those with solid tumors. It is interesting that to date there

has been no reported incidence of TA-GVH disease in AIDS patients.[30]

Most blood product irradiation uses either cesium-137 (^{137}Cs) or cobalt-60 (^{60}Co) as the source of gamma rays. AABB requires that products be given a minimum of 25 Gy, and the range can run as high as 35 Gy.

The shelf life of irradiated RBCs has been under much discussion. Studies have shown that there is an increase in extracellular potassium after irradiation,[38] and it has been suggested that blood should be used within 2 weeks of irradiation, but as yet no change in the original expiration date of the product is required.

LEUKOCYTE-REDUCED RED BLOOD CELLS

Leukocyte-reduced RBCs are products in which the absolute WBC count in the unit is less than 5×10^6 (5×10^8 is acceptable for the prevention of febrile transfusion reactions). The method used must also ensure that at least 80 percent of the original RBC mass is retained. It has been thought for some time that donor leukocytes in blood transfusions are responsible for febrile nonhemolytic (FNH) transfusion reactions and transfusion-related acute lung injury (TRALI). More recently there have been concerns about transfusion-transmitted infectious agents such as cytomegalovirus (CMV), Epstein-Barr virus (EBV), and HTLV-1, all known to be carried primarily in the leukocytes, as well as TA-GVH disease.[31] Many patients, including multiply transfused, leukemia, aplastic anemia, immunosuppressed, and immunodeficient patients, and multiparous women, are potential candidates for leukocyte-reduced blood products.

Several techniques exist for preparing leukocyte-reduced RBCs. Which technique is used may depend on the patient's particular need, the equipment available in the blood bank, whether the method can be done in a closed system, and the cost. The following is a brief summary of the acceptable techniques.

Centrifugation

This is one of the easiest and least costly of the methods and it can be done in a closed system, but it is also the least efficient. It reduces the WBC level only by 70 to 80 percent (less than 1 log reduction) and sacrifices as much as 20 percent of the RBC volume.[32] In some instances this technique may not produce a finished product that meets minimum standards for WBC reduction. Today, this method has largely been replaced by other, more effective techniques.

Filtration

There are many types of filters available today that can produce an acceptable leukocyte-reduced product depending on the purpose for the WBC reduction and the intended recipient.

Microaggregate filters are typically polyester or plastic screen filters with a pore size of 20 to 40 μm.[33] The unit is generally centrifuged before filtration. This will increase the size of the microaggregates (e.g., platelets, WBCs), which are then filtered out during the administration of the unit. The effectiveness of the leukocyte reduction can be increased by cooling the unit at 4°C for 3 hours after centrifugation and before filtering. Filters of this type usually give a 1- to 2-log reduction (90 to 99 percent) of leukocytes in the unit and recover most of the original RBC volume.[34] The procedure is easy, quick, and relatively inexpensive. RBC units prepared by this method are quite suitable for patients who have experienced FNH transfusion reactions or for those who are receiving transfusions outside the hospital (e.g., home transfusions), where FNH reactions should be avoided.

Newer leukocyte-reducing filters use selective adsorption of leukocytes or leukocytes and platelets. They are made of polyester or cellulose acetate and will produce a 2- to 4-log (more than 99.9 percent) reduction of the WBCs or platelets or both.[35] As with the microaggregate filters, there is very little loss of RBC volume and the procedure is quite easy. With the use of a sterile connecting device, the closed system can be maintained and these filters can be used either in the blood bank or at the patient's bedside. Because these filters are so effective in eliminating the leukocytes or platelets or both, they can be used to help prevent alloimmunization to HLA antigens, CMV transmission-reactivation, and FNH reactions. They are suitable for use with BMT patients, patients receiving intrauterine transfusions, and chemotherapy patients.[36] The drawbacks to these filters are that (1) they are expensive; (2) they reduce the flow rate of blood if using the bedside filtering procedure and if the filtering is done in the blood bank without an expensive sterile connecting device; (3) the system is open; and (4) there is a 24-hour expiration date on the final product.

Freezing, Deglycerolizing, and Saline Washing

All of these techniques can produce a leukocyte-reduced product. They are not as efficient at removing WBCs as the newer filters (95 to 99 percent reduction), but because they all have a saline-washing step, they remove all of the donor plasma. This makes these products particularly good for patients with plasma protein problems such as paroxysmal nocturnal hemoglobinuria (PNH) or immunoglobulin A (IgA) deficiency with circulating anti-IgA. The disadvantages here are the 24-hour expiration date because of the open system, the special equipment that is necessary, and the overall cost including the disposable washing sets. Caution must also be used with saline washing alone, because although the plasma removal is acceptable, not all automated systems are approved for leukocyte removal using this technique.

FROZEN, DEGLYCEROLIZED RED BLOOD CELLS

In the past 15 years, frozen RBCs have come into widespread general use. They provide an RBC product that is almost free of leukocytes, platelets, and plasma. It has an extended shelf life (10 years or more) in the frozen state, which has made long-term storage of rare units possible and autotransfusions more plausible.

Many procedures are used to freeze and to deglycerolize RBCs. The reader should consult the AABB *Technical Manual*, numerous articles in various journals, the American Red Cross blood service directive on RBC freezing and deglycerolizing, and the manufacturer's directions on the use of their equipment. The three general procedures available are described briefly here.

High Glycerol (40 Percent Weight per Volume)

This method increases the cryoprotective power of the glycerol, thus allowing a slow, uncontrolled freezing process. The freezer used is generally a mechanical freezer that provides storage at −65°C. This particular procedure is probably the most widely used method because the equipment involved is fairly simple and the products require less delicate handling. It does, however, require a larger volume of wash solution for deglycerolizing.

Low Glycerol (14 Percent Weight per Volume)

In this method, the cryoprotection of the glycerol is minimal, and a very rapid, more controlled freezing procedure is required. Liquid nitrogen (N_2) is routinely used for this method. The frozen units must be stored at about −150°C, which is the temperature of liquid N_2 vapor. Because of the minimal amount of protection by the glycerol, temperature fluctuations during storage can cause RBC destruction.

Cytoagglomeration

This method uses the ability of RBCs to agglomerate reversibly in a high sugar concentration. Cytoagglomeration uses a 79.2 percent weight per volume concentration of glycerol with dextrose, fructose, and ethylenediaminetetraacetic acid (EDTA). Like the high glycerol method, cytoagglomeration uses a slow, mechanical freezing and storage process. This method was in very limited use at the writing of the last edition of this book and now may no longer be in use.

The deglycerolizing process varies, depending on the method used to glycerolize the cells. The high-glycerol and low-glycerol methods use similar equipment but slightly different solutions and volumes.

High-Glycerol Method (40 Percent Weight per Volume)

1. Use 150 ml of 12 percent NaCl. Equilibrate for 5 minutes.

2. Wash with 1000 ml of 1.6 percent NaCl.
3. Continue washing with 1000 ml of 0.9 percent NaCl and 0.2 percent dextrose (also functions as the final suspending media).
4. Use batch wash or continuous flow equipment.

Low-Glycerol Method
(14 Percent Weight per Volume)

1. First wash is 300 to 350 ml of 15 percent mannitol in 0.45 percent NaCl or 3 to 3.5 percent NaCl.
2. Continue wash with 1000 to 2000 ml 0.9 percent NaCl or 0.8 percent plus 0.2 g/dl of dextrose.
3. Use automated or manual batch washing only.

Agglomeration

1. In a pH of 5.2 to 6.1, RBCs will agglomerate (reversible reaction).
2. First wash is a 50 percent dextrose plus a 5 percent fructose solution.
3. Cells agglomerate and rapidly settle to the bottom of the bag. The solution is removed.
4. Second wash is 5 percent fructose only. Cells again agglomerate and settle to the bottom. The solution is removed.
5. Final wash solution is 250 ml of normal saline (0.85 percent NaCl).
6. The only equipment that can be used is the cytoagglomerator.

The quality control procedures necessary for RBC freezing include all of the standard procedures for monitoring refrigerators, freezers, water baths, dry thaw baths, and centrifuges. They also include procedures to ensure good RBC recovery (80 percent), good viability (70 percent survival at 24 hours posttransfusion) and adequate glycerol removal (less than 1 percent residual intracellular glycerol).

1. RBC recovery can be determined easily by estimating the recovered RBC mass (final volume × final hematocrit = RBC mass recovered). Compare with the initial (prefreeze) RBC mass.
2. A posttransfusion survival study should be done when the program is first being set up, to ensure the proper use of the equipment and procedure. If the procedure being used is a standard procedure with data already published in the literature, these survival studies are not required.
3. Glycerol must be removed to a level of less than 1 percent residual. The published procedures should accomplish this. It is important, however, to perform this check on each unit before releasing it for transfusion. The procedures are very simple.
   a. Measure the osmolarity of the unit using an osmometer. The osmolarity should be about 420 mOsm (maximum 500 mOsm).
   b. Perform a simulated transfusion. Place one segment (approximately 3 inches) of deglycer-

olized cells into 7 ml of a 0.7 percent NaCl. Mix, centrifuge, and check for hemolysis. Compare with a standard hemoglobin color comparator. If the hue exceeds the 500-mOsm level, hemolysis is too great and the unit is not transferable.

4. Postdeglycerolized tests include confirmation of ABO, Rh, and a direct antihuman globulin test (DAT).
5. Preglycerolizing tests may include the following:
   a. **DAT**. A unit with a positive DAT result should not be used.
   b. **Sickle test**. Cells that carry the sickle trait do not survive routine freezing and deglycerolizing procedures. It is recommended that cells known to carry the sickle trait not be used routinely in a frozen RBC program. If for some reason the cells must be frozen, there is a special deglycerolizing procedure that may be used.[37] If there is a high percentage of black donors in the area, it may be worthwhile to prescreen units before freezing.
   c. **Accurate and complete records**. Good record keeping must be maintained for all phases of the glycerolizing and deglycerolizing procedures.

PLATELET CONCENTRATE

Platelet concentrates are one of the primary products produced during the routine conversion of WB into concentrated RBCs. They have widespread use for a variety of patients: actively bleeding patients who are thrombocytopenic (less than 50,000 μL) due to decreased production or decreased function; cancer patients, during radiation and chemotherapy, because of an induced thrombocytopenia (less than 20,000 μL); and thrombocytopenic preoperative patients (less than 60,000 μL). Prophylactic platelet transfusions are not usually indicated or recommended in disseminated intravascular coagulation (DIC) or idiopathic thrombocytopenic purpura (ITP). In both cases, there is an induced thrombocytopenia owing to increased destruction. ITP is generally thought to be due to an autoantibody, and DIC to mass consumption.

Platelet concentrates prepared from WB are generally referred to as random-donor platelets to distinguish them from single-donor platelets produced by pheresis. Random-donor platelet concentrates contain at least 5.5×10^{10} platelets, are stored at 20°C to 24°C with continuous agitation, contain 50 to 65 ml of plasma, and have a shelf life of 5 days. Single-donor platelet concentrates or "superpack" platelets, as they are sometimes called, are prepared by pheresis (see Chapter 17), contain at least 3.0×10^{11} platelets, are stored at 22°C to 24°C with agitation, contain approximately 300 ml, and generally have a shelf life of 5 days also.

Whole blood used for the preparation of platelet concentrates must be drawn by a single, nontraumatic venipuncture, and the concentrate must be prepared within 6 hours of collection. The following is a general procedure for preparing random donor platelets.

1. Maintain the WB at 20°C to 24°C before and during platelet preparation.
2. Set the centrifuge temperature at 22°C. The rpm and time must be specifically calculated for each centrifuge. It will generally be a short (2- to 3-minute), light (3200-rpm) spin. This spin should separate most of the RBCs but leave most of the platelets suspended in the plasma.
3. Platelet preparation should be done in a closed, multibag system.
4. Express off the platelet-rich plasma into one of the satellite bags. Enough plasma must remain on the RBC to maintain a 70 to 80 percent hematocrit. The hematocrit estimation methods stated in the RBC procedure can be employed here.
5. Seal the tubing between the RBC and the plasma. Disconnect the RBC and store it at 4°C.
6. Recentrifuge the platelet-rich plasma at 22°C using a heavy spin (approximately 3600 rpm for 5 minutes). This will separate the platelets from the plasma.
7. Express the majority of the plasma into the second satellite bag, leaving approximately 50 to 65 ml on the platelets. The volume is important to maintain the pH (above 6.0) during storage.
8. Seal the tubing between the bags and separate. Make segments for both the platelet and the plasma for testing purposes.
9. The plasma can be frozen as fresh frozen plasma (FFP), single-donor plasma frozen within 24 hours (SDP-24), or stored as liquid recovered plasma. Be sure to record the plasma volume on the bag.
10. Allow the platelet concentrate to lie undisturbed for 1 to 2 hours at 20°C to 24°C. Be sure the platelet button is covered with the plasma. Platelets should be resuspended. Gentle manipulation can be used if needed.
11. Store on a rotator, allowing constant, gentle agitation.
12. Shelf life is 5 days from the date of collection. If the system is opened, transfusion must be within 6 hours. The volume, expiration date, and time (if indicated) must be on the label.
13. All of the units for a single dose (typically 6 to 8 units for an adult) can be pooled into a single bag before transfusion. Once pooled, the product must be transfused within 4 hours of pooling. The pooled unit must be given a unique "pool number," which must be on the label.

The quality control procedures must include a platelet count (5.5×10^{10} for random donor, 3.0×10^{11} for single donor); pH (6.0 or greater); and volume (must be sufficient to maintain an acceptable pH until the end of the dating period). These procedures are to be performed regularly—usually 1 to 4 units/month, depending on the production volume—at the end of the product's dating period. Seventy-five percent of all units tested must meet or exceed the minimum standards. Temperature monitoring must be performed during each major stage of production and records maintained of all procedures performed.

Platelets, either random donor or single donor, can be irradiated if the patient's diagnosis indicates it is appropriate. The irradiation requirements are the same as for RBCs (25 to 35 Gy). Irradiation can occur anytime during the platelet shelf life and will not affect or change the expiration date.

SINGLE-DONOR PLASMA: FRESH FROZEN AND FROZEN WITHIN 24 HOURS

Frozen plasma, either FFP or SDP-24, are frequent byproducts of concentrated RBC and platelet concentrate production. It is fresh plasma obtained from a single, uninterrupted, nontraumatic venipuncture. The plasma is then frozen within 6 hours of collection for FFP or within 24 hours of collection for SDP-24, and stored at −18°C or colder. The product is RBC free and contains therapeutic levels of all the plasma clotting factors, including factors V and VIII. FFP contains somewhat higher levels of factors V and VIII, but the levels in SDP-24 are more than adequate and this product is now being used in some areas instead of FFP. FFP production is then used for further manufacture into factor VIII concentrate. The shelf life for FFP or SDP-24 is 12 months in the frozen state (−18°C) and 24 hours after thawing, if stored at 1°C to 6°C.

The use of SDP-24 or FFP is indicated in patients who are actively bleeding and have multiple clotting factor deficiencies. Examples include massive trauma, surgery, liver disease, DIC, or when a specific disorder cannot or has not yet been identified.

Specific deficiencies such as factor VIII or fibrinogen are more appropriately treated with cryoprecipitate. Factor II, VII, IX, and X deficiencies would be better treated using the prothrombin complex concentrates.

A single unit of FFP or SDP-24 should contain 150 to 250 ml of plasma, approximately 400 mg of fibrinogen, and about 1 unit of activity per milliliter of each of the stable clotting factors. FFP also contains the same level (1 unit/ml) of factors V and VIII; SDP-24 contains somewhat less than that level.

If FFP or SDP-24 is to be prepared from WB as part of the production of platelet concentrates, follow the procedure outlined in the platelet concentrate section. At step 9, after the platelet concentrate has been separated from the plasma, proceed in the following manner:

1. Weigh the plasma and determine the volume. Record the volume on the bag.

2. Place the plasma in a protective container and freeze. The plasma must be frozen in such a way that evidence of thawing can be determined. Freezing some sort of indentation into the bag, which is visible as long as the plasma remains frozen, is an easy way to accomplish this. The container is important because the plastic bag becomes quite brittle when frozen at low temperatures and can be cracked or broken easily.

3. The plasma must be frozen solid within the 6-hour time allotment. The lower the temperature of the freezer and the greater the air circulation around the plasma, the faster the freeze. Freezers at −65°C, blast freezers, packing units between dry ice, or the use of an ice-ethanol or ice-antifreeze bath can be used to speed up the freezing process.[39]

4. Before freezing, be sure that any tubing segments and the transfusion ports ("ears") of the bag are tucked in or placed in such a manner as to prevent or minimize possible breakage.

5. The label on the frozen plasma must include all of the standard information required. See Code of Federal Regulations, Title:21 CFR 606.121 for specifics. Frozen plasma also can be produced directly from WB, without preparing platelet concentrates. The procedure changes to eliminate the platelet production section, and the general volume of the plasma will be greater.

There are no specific testing procedures required as part of the quality control program. Specific factor levels are not required. Records must be maintained on the production process to ensure that the product was prepared within the time required and that the product was prepared, frozen, and stored at the appropriate temperatures.

SINGLE-DONOR PLASMA: LIQUID OR FROZEN

Recovered plasma or single-donor plasma (liquid) and single-donor plasma (frozen) can be prepared directly from the WB or as a byproduct of platelet concentrate or cryoprecipitate production. The products can be used as volume expanders or for treatment of stable clotting factor deficiencies. Because of the availability of hepatitis and HIV-free volume expanders, single-donor plasma is not generally used for that purpose. Most recovered plasma is used for the manufacture of plasma fractionation products such as plasma protein fraction (PPF), normal serum albumin (NSA), and immune serum globulin (ISG).

When produced from WB, recovered ("salvaged") plasma can be removed from the cells anytime during the normal dating period and up to 5 days after expiration (26 to 40 days after collection for CPD and CPDA-1, respectively). If SDP (frozen) is being prepared, the plasma is to be stored at −18°C and must be frozen within 6 hours of its transfer to the final container. The shelf life is 5 years in the frozen state.

FFP or SDP-24 that has not been used within the 12-month period can be converted to SDP (frozen). SDP (liquid) is collected in the same manner, stored at 1°C to 6°C, and must be used within 26 to 40 days of whole blood collection.

The production procedure is like that for platelets and FFP, and quality control measures are limited to production and storage temperatures.

CRYOPRECIPITATED ANTIHEMOPHILIC FACTOR

Cryoprecipitate is the cold-precipitated concentration of factor VIII, the antihemophilic factor (AHF). It is prepared from FFP thawed slowly at 4°C. The product contains most of the factor VIII and part of the fibrinogen from the original plasma. It contains at least 80 units of AHF activity and 150 to 250 mg of fibrinogen. Other factors of significance found in cryoprecipitate are factor XIII and von Willebrand factor. Cryoprecipitate has a shelf life of 12 months in the frozen state and must be transfused within 6 hours of thawing or within 4 hours of pooling. Like FFP and SDP-24, cryoprecipitate should be thawed quickly at 37°C. Once thawed, FDA recommends storing at room temperature (22°C to 24°C) until transfused. Cryoprecipitate is indicated in the treatment of classic hemophilia (hemophilia A), von Willebrand's disease, and factor XIII deficiency, and as a source of fibrinogen for hypofibrinogenemia. In recent years, cryoprecipitate has also been used to make "fibrin glue," a substance composed of cryoprecipitate (fibrinogen) and topical thrombin. When combined, they produce an adhesive substance that, applied to a surgical site usually via fine spray, can reduce bleeding. It has been most frequently used in cardiac, otologic, and facial cosmetic surgery. The WB donor requirements and preparation requirements for cryoprecipitate are the same as those for platelets and FFP.

1. The venipuncture must be nontraumatic.
2. The WB can be cooled before and during production inasmuch as platelets are not usually prepared from the units. The volume of plasma required to remain on the RBC and the platelet concentrate will reduce the amount of plasma available for cryoprecipitate production enough to reduce the final AHF activity significantly in the precipitate. At least 200 ml of plasma should be used to ensure that the final product will contain at least 80 AHF units.
3. The plasma must be frozen within 6 hours of collection.
4. The second stage of cryoprecipitate preparation begins by allowing the frozen plasma to thaw slowly in the refrigerator at 1°C to 6°C. This takes 14 to 16 hours when thawed in a standard blood bank refrigerator. If a circulating cryoprecipitate thaw bath (4°C water bath) is used, the thawing time is reduced to about 4 hours. The end point is when the plasma becomes slushy.

5. Centrifuge the plasma at 4°C for a "hard" spin (typically 3400 to 3600 rpm for 3 to 7 minutes, depending on the centrifuge).
6. Express the supernatant plasma into the attached satellite bag. The cryoprecipitate will be a small white mass in the original plasma bag. Leave only 10 to 15 ml of plasma on the precipitate.
7. Separate and refreeze the cryoprecipitate immediately. It should be no longer than 1 hour from the time the plasma reaches the slushy stage until the cryoprecipitate is refrozen. A delay in refreezing, or exposure of the unit to elevated temperatures during processing, will significantly decrease the factor VIII activity level in the final product. The centrifuge temperature must be at 4°C, and it is better if the centrifuge cups are well chilled.
8. The final product should be placed in a protective container because of the brittle nature of the plastic bag at freezer temperatures.
9. Labeling requirements are the same as for other products (see Donor Processing).

The quality assurance requirements mandate that the volume and AHF activity of the final product must be measured on a representative sample of the products prepared and that this be performed regularly. The volume should not exceed 25 ml, and 75 percent of all units tested must show a minimum of 80 IU of AHF activity. Records must be maintained of all quality assurance testing performed.

GRANULOCYTE CONCENTRATES

Granulocyte concentrates are prepared by pheresis (see Chapter 17). Each product should contain 1×10^{10} granulocytes if steroids or HES, or both, are used. Corticosteroids, usually administered to the donor 12 to 24 hours before pheresis, will increase the number of circulating granulocytes by pulling them from the marginating pool. HES is a sedimenting agent that increases the separation between the WBCs and RBCs, thus facilitating a better recovery of the buffy coat. Granulocyte concentrates contain 200 to 600 ml of plasma and should be stored at 20°C to 24°C. The shelf life for this product is 24 hours, but it should be transfused as soon as possible after preparation.

Granulocyte concentrates have very limited application and very narrow success rate. Generally, patients with severe neutropenia (less than 500 polymorphonuclear neutrophils per milliliter), fever that has been unresponsive to antibiotic or other therapy for 24 to 48 hours, and myeloid hypoplasia of the bone marrow and those who have reasonable chance for survival are candidates for granulocyte transfusions. With improvements in antibiotic therapy and chemotherapy, granulocyte transfusions in adults have become almost nonexistent.[40] They are still used in the treatment of neonatal sepsis.

FACTOR VIII CONCENTRATE

Factor VIII concentrates are still generally manufactured from large volumes of pooled plasma but, because of the very high risk for viral disease transmission with this product, a great deal of effort has gone into developing methods that will inactivate or eliminate virus contamination in the final product. The untreated and the dry heat–treated products, both of which were discussed in the last edition of this book, have been completely replaced by newer methods and are no longer available in the United States. A brief description of the product preparation methods now being used follows.

Pasteurization

In this method, stabilizers, usually albumin, sucrose, or glycine, are added to the factor VIII concentrate to prevent denaturation. The concentrate is then heated to 60°C for 10 hours, after which the stabilizers are removed and the product lyophilized. The process is effective in producing a product that is safe from HIV-1 and hepatitis infection, but there is a significant loss of factor VIII activity (30 to 40 percent of the original fraction level) in the final product.[41]

Solvent and Detergent

This method uses a solvent and detergent to disrupt the viral coat chemically, thus inactivating any virus present. The solvents most frequently in use are ethyl ether and tri-(n-butyl) phosphate (TNBP). The detergents are sodium cholate and Tween 80. The concentrate is then purified to remove the solvent and detergent and then lyophilized. Very little of the factor VIII activity is lost (about 10 percent) in this method, and the resulting product is considered safe from viral transmission.[42]

Monoclonal Purification

Immunoaffinity chromatography is used here. A murine monoclonal antibody directed at the factor VIII or von Willebrand factor (vWF) moiety is bound on a solid-phase substrate and used to absorb selectively the factor VIII:vWF complex.[43] The product is then lyophilized. Large concentrations of very pure factor can be obtained with this method, and products produced in this manner have not yet been known to transmit viral disease.

Recombinant Products

With the identification and isolation of the gene for human factor VIII, it has become possible to produce factor VIII using recombinant DNA technology. The products made this way have thus far proved to be safe and effective, although also quite expensive.

Porcine Factor VIII

This product, made from porcine (pig) plasma, has been available for quite some time. It is generally used to treat patients with hemophilia A who have developed inhibitors to human factor VIII. In the past this product has had many adverse side effects, but the newer products, which are better purified, appear to have considerably reduced side effects while still giving good clinical results. Because this is not a product derived from human sources, there is no risk of human virus transmission.[44]

1-Deamino-8-D-Arginine Vasopressin

This is actually not a factor VIII product but a synthetic analog of vasopressin. When injected, it will cause the endothelial cells to release intracellular stores of factor VIII and vWF. If this product is to work, the patient's cells must be able to produce some factor levels. It appears to be suitable for treatment of some types of von Willebrand's disease or mild cases of hemophilia A or both types of disorders. 1-Deamino-8-D-arginine vasopressin can be used in combination with epsilon aminocaproic acid, which will help stabilize clot formation.[45]

For most of the foregoing products, the amount of factor VIII activity is indicated on the bottle or vial. They are usually stored at 1°C to 6°C and require reconstitution before transfusion.

FACTOR IX CONCENTRATE (PROTHROMBIN COMPLEX)

Factor IX concentrates contain significant levels of the vitamin K–dependent clotting factors: II, VII, IX, and X. Like some of the factor VIII products, factor IX concentrate is prepared from large volumes of pooled plasma by adsorbing the factors out using barium sulfate or aluminum hydroxide or by using a cellulose or sephadex column. The concentrate is then lyophilized and viral inactivated. Inactivation is accomplished by various techniques: dry heat at 60°C to 70°C for 20 to 150 hours, depending on the particular manufacturer; heat treated in an organic solvent; or solvent-detergent treatment. All of the products now being made are safe from HIV-1 and HBsAg transmission, but some may not be as good against HCV transmission. The possibility of causing thrombosis, which was always and still is a problem with these products, has led to some manufacturers adding heparin to the product for control of this situation.[46] These products, like factor VIII products, are stored in the refrigerator and, because they are lyophilized, must be reconstituted before infusing.

This product is used primarily to treat patients with factor IX deficiency (hemophilia B or Christmas disease) but is also valuable for treating patients with congenital factor VII and factor X deficiencies.

IMMUNE SERUM GLOBULIN

Immune serum globulin is a concentrate of plasma gamma globulins in an aqueous solution. ISG is prepared from pooled plasma by cold ethanol fractionation. Although the primary serum globulin is IgG, IgA and IgM may also be present.[47]

Plasma found to contain high levels of antibody to special antigens such as hepatitis B or herpes zoster can be used to prepare hyperimmune ISG. ISG is now available in both an intramuscular (IMIg) form and an intravenous (IVIg) form. IMIg is used as a prophylactic for patients who have been exposed to certain diseases and are at risk of infection. It is also used as replacement therapy for patients with primary immunodeficiencies such as congenital agammaglobulinemia, combined variable immunodeficiency, Wiskott-Aldrich syndrome, and severe combined immunodeficiency. IVIg seems to work better for treating at-risk patients with ITP, and exposure prophylaxis in bone marrow transplant patients and AIDS-related thrombocytopenia.[48]

Because of the preparation method for ISG, there appears to be no risk of hepatitis or HIV-1 transmission.

NORMAL SERUM ALBUMIN

Normal serum albumin is prepared from salvaged plasma, pooled and fractionated by a cold alcohol process, then treated with heat inactivation, which removes the risk of hepatitis or HIV infection. It is composed of 96 percent albumin and 4 percent globulin and other proteins.[49] It is available in 25 percent or 5 percent solutions, stored at 1°C or 6°C, and has a shelf life of 5 years. Albumin is used as a colloid volume expander in patients who are hypovolemic and hypoproteinemic.

PLASMA PROTEIN FRACTION

Plasma protein fraction is similar to NSA except that the albumin:globulin ratio is lower—83 percent albumin and 17 percent globulin.[50] It is prepared in a 5 percent solution and can be stored at room temperature for 3 years, or 1°C to 6°C for 5 years. Like albumin, PPF is used as a volume expander in patients who need volume and protein.

SYNTHETIC VOLUME EXPANDERS

These are crystalloids and colloid solutions used as volume expanders alone or in combination with other products. They include normal saline, Ringer's solution, Ringer's lactate, balanced electrolyte solution, dextran (high or low molecular weight), and HES.

RH₀(D) IMMUNOGLOBULIN

Rh immunoglobulin (RhIg) is a solution of concentrated anti-Rh₀(D), which is manufactured from pooled, hyperimmune plasma. It is used to prevent Rh₀(D) immunization of an unsensitized Rh-negative patient after an abortion, miscarriage, or delivery of an Rh-positive baby or after transfusion exposure to Rh-positive cells. It is also routinely given as an antipartum dose at 28 weeks' gestation to reduce the risk of Rh immunization during pregnancy. Like NSA, PPF, and other ISGs, RhIg does not transmit hepatitis, HIV, or the other transfusion-transmitted viruses.

RhIg is available in two concentrations: a 300-μg solution, or "full" dose; and a 150-μg solution, or "micro" or "mini" dose. Both concentrations come in a 1-ml volume suitable for intramuscular injection. The 300-μg dose is used for abortions, miscarriages, or deliveries that occur at 12 weeks' or more gestation; for antipartum injections; and for transfusion accidents or emergencies resulting in the transfusion of an Rh-positive unit to an Rh-negative patient. The 150-μg dose can be used for abortions, miscarriages, or bleeding episodes that occur during the first trimester (less than 12 weeks' gestation).

ANTITHROMBIN III CONCENTRATE

This is a new plasma product since the last edition of this book. It is prepared by fractionation of pools of plasma and then heat treated to reduce the risk of virus transmission. It is used to treat patients who have an inherited deficiency of antithrombin III who are at risk of spontaneous thrombosis.

Review Questions

1. Which of the following information is *not* required for WB donors?
   A. Name
   B. Address
   C. Occupation
   D. Sex
   E. Date of birth

2. Which of the following would be cause for temporary deferral?
   A. Temperature 99.2°F
   B. Pulse 90 beats per minute
   C. Blood pressure 110/70 mm Hg
   D. Hematocrit 37 percent
   E. None of the above; the donor is acceptable

3. Which of the following would be cause for permanent deferral?
   A. History of hepatitis after 10 years of age
   B. Positive hepatitis C test result
   C. Elevated ALT level, above the upper limit of acceptable on two occasions

   D. Positive anti-HBc test result
   E. All of the above

4. Immunization for rubella would result in a temporary deferral for:
   A. 4 weeks
   B. 8 weeks
   C. 6 months
   D. 1 year
   E. No deferral required

5. Which of the following donors is acceptable?
   A. Donor had a first-trimester therapeutic abortion 4 weeks ago.
   B. Donor's husband is a hemophiliac who regularly received cryoprecipitate before 1989.
   C. Donor was treated for gonorrhea 6 months ago.
   D. Donor received HBIg 6 months ago.
   E. Donor had a needlestick injury 10 months ago.

6. Which of the following tests is *not* required as part of the donor-processing procedure?
   A. ABO typing
   B. ALT
   C. STS
   D. Anti-HTLV I/II
   E. Malaria

7. Which of the following is the correct shelf life for the component listed?
   A. Deglycerolized RBCs = 24 hours
   B. RBCs (CPD plus adenine-saline) = 35 days
   C. Platelet concentrate = 7 days
   D. FFP = 5 years
   E. RBCs (CPDA-1) = 21 days

8. Each unit of cryoprecipitate, prepared from WB, should contain approximately how many units of AHF activity?
   A. 40 IU
   B. 80 IU
   C. 120 IU
   D. 160 IU
   E. 180 IU

9. Platelet concentrates prepared by pheresis should contain how many platelets per μL?
   A. 5.5×10^{10}
   B. 6.0×10^{10}
   C. 3.0×10^{11}
   D. 5.5×10^{11}
   E. 6.0×10^{11}

10. The required storage temperature for frozen RBCs is:
    A. 4°C
    B. −20°C
    C. −18°C

D. −30°C

E. −65°C

11. Platelets prepared from a WB donation require which of the following?

A. A light spin, then a hard spin

B. Two light spins

C. A light spin and two heavy spins

D. A hard spin, then a light spin

E. Two heavy spins

12. Once thawed, FFP must be transfused within:

A. 4 hours

B. 6 hours

C. 8 hours

D. 12 hours

E. 24 hours

13. The quality control requirements for RBCs require a maximum hematocrit of:

A. 75 percent

B. 80 percent

C. 85 percent

D. 90 percent

E. 95 percent

14. AHF concentrates are used to treat:

A. Thrombocytopenia

B. Hemophilia B

C. Hemophilia A

D. von Willebrand's disease

E. Hemorrhage secondary to liver disease

15. Prothrombin complex concentrates are used to treat which of the following?

A. Factor IX deficiency

B. Factor VIII deficiency

C. Factor XII deficiency

D. Factor XIII deficiency

E. Factor V deficiency

Answers to Review Questions

1. C (p 200)
2. D (p 202)
3. E (p 202)
4. A (p 205)
5. A (pp 205–206)
6. E (pp 218–221)
7. A (Table 10–2)
8. B (p 231)
9. C (p 230)
10. E (p 228)
11. A (p 230)
12. E (p 230)
13. B (p 221)
14. C (Table 10–2)
15. A (Table 10–2)

References

1. Walker, RH (ed): Technical Manual, ed 10. American Association of Blood Banks, Bethesda, MD, 1990, p 1.
2. Widmann, FK (ed): Standards for Blood Banks and Transfusion Services, ed 14. American Association of Blood Banks, Bethesda, MD, 1991, p 3.
3. Cumor, A: Local Health History Criteria. American Red Cross Blood Services, Chesapeake and Potomac Region, Baltimore, 1985, p 42.
4. Ibid, p 1.
5. Orrell, J (ed): Bulletin #92-4. In News Briefs (Nov/Dec). American Association of Blood Banks, Bethesda, MD, 1992, p 5.
6. Cumor, A, op cit, p 14.
7. Jones, FS (ed): Accreditation Requirements Manual, ed 4. American Association of Blood Banks, Bethesda, MD, 1992, p 29.
8. Walker, RH, op cit, p 3.
9. Cumor, A, op cit, p 18.
10. Ibid, p 21.
11. Orrell, J, op cit, p 5.
12. Jones, FS, op cit, p 29.
13. Walker, RH, op cit, p 7.
14. Jones, FS, op cit, p 29.
15. Orrell, J, op cit, p 7.
16. Walker, RH, op cit, p 434.
17. Ibid, p 443.
18. Ibid, p 444.
19. Gilcher, RO: Autologous blood. In Garner, RJ and Silvergleid, AJ (eds): Autologous and Directed Blood Programs. American Association of Blood Banks, Bethesda, MD, 1987, p 3.
20. Walker, RH, op cit, p 443.
21. Widmann, FK, op cit, p 17.
22. Grant, CJ: Component preparation, donor blood processing and pretransfusion testing. In Chambers, LA and Kaspirisin, CA (eds): Transfusion Therapy From Donor to Patient. American Association of Blood Banks, Bethesda, MD, 1992, p 46.
23. Widmann, FK, op cit, p 17.
24. Stevens, CE, Aach, RD, et al: Hepatitis B virus antibody in blood donors and the occurrence of non-A, non-B hepatitis in transfusion recipients. Ann Intern Med 101:733, 1984.
25. Grant, CJ, op cit, p 44.
26. Ibid, p 45.
27. Busch, MP: Retroviruses and blood transfusions: The lessons learned and the challenge yet ahead. In Nance, SJ (ed): Blood Safety: Current Challenges. American Association of Blood Banks, Bethesda, MD, 1992, p 17.
28. Widmann, FK, op cit, p 45.
29. Walker, RH, op cit, p 637.
30. Anderson, KC: Clinical indications for blood component irradiation. In Baldwin, ML and Jefferies, LC (eds): Irradiation of Blood Components. American Association of Blood Banks, Bethesda, MD, 1992, p 41.
31. Capon, SM: Blood component preparation and therapy. In Chambers, LA and Kasprisin, CA (eds): Transfusion Therapy: From Donor to Patient. American Association of Blood Banks, Bethesda, MD, 1992, p 18.
32. O'Neill, EM: Red blood cell transfusions. In Kasprisin, CA and Rzasa, M (eds): Transfusion Therapy: A Practical Approach. American Association of Blood Banks, Bethesda, MD, 1991, p 18.
33. Ibid, p 19.
34. Ibid, p 20.
35. Ibid, p 20.
36. Capon, SM, op cit, p 20.
37. Meryman, HT, and Hornblower, M: Freezing and deglycerolizing sickle-trait red blood cells. Transfusion 16:627, 1976.
38. Anderson, KC, op cit, p 39.
39. Walker, RH, op cit, p 46.
40. Blaylock, RC: Non-red-cell components. In Kasprisin, CA and Rzasa, M (eds): Transfusion Therapy: A Practical Approach. American Association of Blood Banks, Bethesda, MD, 1991, p 45.

41. Julius, C: Coagulation products for hemophilia A, hemophilia B and von Willebrand's disease. In Hackel, E, Westphal, RG, and Wilson, SM: Transfusion Management of Some Common Heritable Blood Disorders. American Association of Blood Banks, Bethesda, MD, 1992, p 11.
42. Ibid, p 11.
43. Ibid, p 12.
44. Ibid, p 13.
45. Ibid, p 14.
46. Ibid, p 16.
47. Pisciotto, PT, et al (eds): Blood Transfusion Therapy: A Physician's Handbook, ed 3. American Association of Blood Banks, Bethesda, MD, 1989, p 38.
48. Ibid, p 39.
49. Ibid, p 34.
50. Ibid, p 34.

Bibliography

American Red Cross Blood Services: Guidelines for the Management of Reactions and Complications Associated with Blood Donors, ARC Form No. 1783. American Red Cross, Washington, DC, 1984.

Baldwin, ML, and Jefferies, LC (eds): Irradiation of Blood Components. American Association of Blood Banks, Bethesda, MD, 1992.

Baldwin, ML, and Kurtz, SR (eds): Transfusion Practice in Cardiac Surgery. American Association of Blood Banks, Bethesda, MD, 1991.

Chambers, LA, and Kasprisin, CA (eds): Transfusion Therapy: From Donor to Patient. American Association of Blood Banks, Bethesda, MD, 1992.

Garner, RJ and Silvergleid, AJ (eds): Autologous and Directed Blood Programs. American Association of Blood Banks, Bethesda, MD, 1987.

Hackel, E, Westphal, RG, and Wilson, SM (eds): Transfusion Management of Some Common Heritable Blood Disorders. American Association of Blood Banks, Bethesda, MD, 1992.

Jones, FS (ed): Accreditation Requirements Manual, ed 4. American Association of Blood Banks, Bethesda, MD, 1992.

Kasprisin, CA, and Rzasa, M (eds): Transfusion Therapy: A Practical Approach. American Association of Blood Banks, Bethesda, MD, 1991.

Katz, AJ (ed): Fundamentals of a Pheresis Program. American Association of Blood Banks, Bethesda, MD, 1979.

Maffei, LM, and Thurer, RL (eds): Autologous Blood Transfusion: Current Issues. American Association of Blood Banks, Bethesda, MD, 1988.

Milam, JD, et al (eds): Donor Room Procedures. American Association of Blood Banks, Bethesda, MD, 1977.

Nance, ST (ed): Blood Safety: Current Challenges. American Association of Blood Banks, Bethesda, MD, 1992.

Pisciotto, PT, et al (eds): Blood Transfusion Therapy: A Physician's Handbook, ed 3. American Association of Blood Banks, Bethesda, MD, 1989.

Pittiglio, DH, et al: Treating Hemostatic Disorders: A Problem-Oriented Approach. American Association of Blood Banks, Cutter Biologicals, Bethesda, MD, 1984.

Sandler, SG, and Silvergleid, AJ (eds): Autologous Transfusion. American Association of Blood Banks, Bethesda, MD, 1983.

US Department of Health and Human Services, Food and Drug Administration: The Code of Federal Regulations, 21 CFR 600-799. US Government Printing Office, Washington, DC, 1992.

Walker, RH (ed): Technical Manual, ed 10. American Association of Blood Banks, Bethesda, MD, 1990.

Widmann, FK (ed): Standards for Blood Banks and Transfusion Services, ed 14. American Association of Blood Banks, Bethesda, MD, 1991.

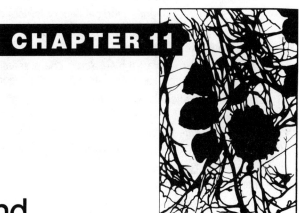

CHAPTER 11

Antibody Detection and Identification

Beth Lingenfelter, MS, MT(ASCP)SBB
Frankie Gillen Gibbs, MS, MT(ASCP)SBB

OBJECTIVES

Upon completion of this chapter, the learner should be able to:

1 Define adsorption, antigram, dosage, eluate, neutralization, and unexpected antibody.

2 Describe the purpose and limitations of the antibody screening tests.

3 List and discuss characteristics of antibody screening cells.

4 List the benefits and risks for using monospecific anti-IgG for routine antibody screening tests.

5 Outline the procedure used for antibody screening tests and describe the purpose of enhancement reagents and Coombs control cells.

6 Properly interpret results of antibody detection and identification tests.

7 Describe how a patient's medical history is useful in antibody identification.

8 Explain the purpose of the autologous control in antibody screening and identification tests.

9 Correlate knowledge of the serologic characteristics of commonly encountered blood group antibodies with antibody identification studies.

10 Describe the rationale for properly ruling out antibody specificities in identification studies.

11 Explain the criteria for conclusive identification of an antibody.

12 Describe the use of selected cells and antigen typing in antibody identification.

13 Given initial panel results, properly select additional cells needed to complete antibody identification.

14 Select appropriate donor units for transfusion to patients with unexpected antibodies.

15 Calculate the approximate number of random donor units needed for screening to find a specific number of compatible units for a patient with unexpected antibodies.

16 List advantages of using enzyme-pretreated panel cells in conjunction with an untreated panel and explain why enzyme-pretreated panels cannot be used alone.

17 Describe the principles of and applications for the following techniques: elution, adsorption, neutralization, and antibody titers.

18 Briefly describe the principles of the three types of elution techniques described in this chapter.

19 Recognize panel results that indicate the presence of multiple alloantibodies and antibodies to high- and low-frequency antigens and list steps to resolve these antibody problems.

20 Compare and contrast the serologic characteristics of warm and cold autoantibodies.

21 List and describe four techniques used to avoid detection of cold autoantibodies in antibody detection tests.

22 Outline the serologic investigation of warm autoantibodies, including the use of elutions, adsorptions, and ZZAP.

Routine pretransfusion testing consists of ABO and Rh typing, antibody screening, and compatibility testing. The purpose of the antibody screen is to detect red blood cell (RBC) antibodies other than anti-A or anti-B. These antibodies are called "unexpected" because only 0.3 to 2 percent[1,2] of the general population have positive antibody screens. Once an unexpected antibody is detected, antibody identification studies are performed to determine the antibody's specificity and clinical significance. An RBC antibody is significant if it causes shortened survival of antigen-positive RBCs. For example, anti-D is a clinically significant antibody because it will bind to D-positive RBCs, resulting in immune destruction or hemolysis.

Proper detection and identification of RBC antibodies is important for the selection of appropriate blood for transfusion and in the investigation of hemolytic disease of the newborn (HDN) (see Chapter 20) and immune hemolytic anemias (see Chapter 21). This chapter will discuss antibody detection and introduce the student to antibody identification studies.

The Antibody Screen

REAGENT RED BLOOD CELLS

Antibody screening tests involve testing patients' serum against two or three reagent RBC samples called screening cells. Screening cells are commercially prepared group O cell suspensions obtained from individual donors that are phenotyped for the most commonly encountered and clinically important RBC antigens. Group O cells are used so that naturally occurring anti-A or anti-B will not interfere with detection of unexpected antibodies. The cells are selected so that the following antigens are present on at least one of the cell samples: D, C, E, c, e, M, N, S, s, P_1, Le^a, Le^b, K, k, Fy^a, Fy^b, Jk^a, and Jk^b. If a set of

CELL	Rh							MNS				Lutheran		P	Lewis		Kell		Duffy		Kidd					
	D	C	E	c	e	f	C^w	M	N	S	s	Lu^a	Lu^b	P$_1$	Le^a	Le^b	K	k	Fy^a	Fy^b	Jk^a	Jk^b				
426509	+	+	+	+	+	0	0	0	+	+	0	0	+	+	+	0	+	+	0	+	0	+				
109632	+	+	+	+	+	0	0	+	0	+	+	0	+	0	0	+	0	+	+	+	+	0				

FIGURE 11–1 Antigram of pooled screening cell.

screening cells did not contain a particular antigen—K for example—then the corresponding antibody would not be detected when serum samples were tested against these cells. An antigram listing the antigen makeup of each cell is provided with each lot of screening cells issued from a manufacturer. It is important that the lot number on the screening cells matches the lot number printed on the antigram, because antigen makeup will vary with each lot. Examples of screening cell antigrams are illustrated in Figures 11–1 to 11–3.

The "ideal" screening cells have RBCs with homozygous expression of as many antigens as possible. An RBC has homozygous expression of an antigen if the donor has two genes that code for the same antigen (e.g., a Jk[a+b−] RBC is usually from a *Jk^{a}Jk^a* donor) and heterozygous expression if the donor has only one copy of the gene (e.g., a Jk[a+b+] RBC is from a *Jk^{a}Jk^b* donor). There is no requirement that screening cells contain RBCs with homozygous expression of antigens; however, most workers prefer that such RBCs are included in screening cell sets because many antibodies, especially Jk and M antibodies, show dosage and give stronger reactions when tested against cells with homozygous expression of their corresponding antigen.[3,4] As a result of dosage, weakly reacting antibody may not be detected if serum samples are not tested against RBCs with homozygous expression of their corresponding antigen. The most notorious example of this is anti-Jk^a and anti-Jk^b. These antibodies are often hard to detect and are capable of causing severe delayed transfusion reactions when the antibodies are not detected and antigen-positive donor units are transfused (see Chapter 8).

Screening cells are available in three forms: (1) a single vial of no more than two donors pooled together in one vial (see Fig. 11–1), (2) two vials each with a different donor (see Fig. 11–2), and (3) three vials representing three different donors (Fig. 11–3). Pooled cells are less sensitive but may be used for detection of antibodies in donor units. Weakly reacting antibodies may be missed, but low levels of anti-

body in the plasma of a donor unit will not harm a recipient.[5] Two- or three-cell screening sets are required for detection of antibodies in pretransfusion testing.[6] Detection of very low levels of antibody in a recipient's serum is important because transfusion of antigen-positive RBCs may result in a secondary immune response with rapid production of antibody and subsequent destruction of transfused RBCs.

ENHANCEMENT REAGENTS

Enhancement reagents are solutions added to serum and cell mixtures to promote antigen-antibody binding or agglutination. There is no requirement for the use of enhancement reagents in antibody detection tests; however, the majority of laboratories use these reagents because they decrease incubation times and increase the sensitivity of the assays. Various enhancement reagents are available but the most widely used are low ionic strength saline (LISS) and bovine albumin. LISS enhances antibody detection tests by increasing the rate at which antibodies bind to RBC antigens.[7,8] Antibody binding to RBC antigen is called sensitization and represents the first phase of a hemagglutination reaction (see Chapter 3). Albumin, on the other hand, is thought to enhance antibody detection tests by reducing the zeta potential, thereby promoting agglutination of sensitized RBCs.[9] Agglutination is the second phase of a hemagglutination reaction.

ANTIHUMAN GLOBULIN REAGENTS

Antihuman globulin (AHG) is used in immunohematology tests to promote agglutination of RBCs sensitized with immunoglobulin G (IgG) or complement molecules (see Chapter 4). The American Association of Blood Banks (AABB) Standards[6] states that tests for unexpected antibodies (antibody screens) must include an AHG test, but there is some flexibility. Many institutions use polyspecific AHG as the concluding step in antibody screening, whereas others have

CELL	Rh							MNS				Lutheran		P	Lewis		Kell		Duffy		Kidd					
	D	C	E	c	e	f	C^w	M	N	S	s	Lu^a	Lu^b	P$_1$	Le^a	Le^b	K	k	Fy^a	Fy^b	Jk^a	Jk^b				
I 420	+	+	+	+	+	0	0	0	+	+	0	0	+	+	+	0	+	+	0	+	0	+				
II 296	+	+	+	+	+	0	0	+	0	+	+	0	+	0	0	+	0	+	+	+	+	0				

FIGURE 11–2 Antigram of a two-cell antibody-screening set.

CELL	Rh D	C	E	c	e	f	V	Cw	MNS M	N	S	s	Lutheran Lua	Lub	P P1	Lewis Lea	Leb	Kell K	k	Duffy Fya	Fyb	Kidd Jka	Jkb				
R1R1-29	+	+	0	0	+	0	0	0	+	0	+	0	0	+	+	+	0	0	+	+	0	+	0				
R2R2-45	+	0	+	+	0	0	0	0	+	+	0	+	0	+	+	0	+	+	+	+	0	0	+				
rr-86	0	0	0	+	+	+	0	0	0	+	0	+	0	+	+	+	0	0	+	0	+	+	+				

FIGURE 11-3 Antigram of a three-cell antibody-screening set.

switched to monospecific anti-IgG. There is a twofold rationale for the use of monospecific anti-IgG:

1. Interference from naturally occurring cold agglutinins in patients' sera is eliminated. Cold agglutinins are clinically insignificant antibodies that are commonly detected in patient sera. Detection of insignificant antibodies in screening tests is not desirable because it does not benefit the patient and may lead to delays in transfusion while the antibody problem is resolved.
2. Some controversy still surrounds the need for the anticomplement component in AHG. There have been reports of clinically significant antibodies detected only by the anticomplement component of polyspecific AHG.[10,11] However, most workers believe that such antibodies are rare and the benefits of using monospecific anti-IgG outweigh the risks.

COOMBS CONTROL CELLS

Coombs control cells are RBCs coated with human IgG antibody. They are used to ensure that AHG tests with negative results are not false negatives owing to inactivation of the AHG reagent. When an AHG test result is negative, there should be free AHG reagent in the test tube. When the Coombs control cells are added, the free AHG in the test should cause agglutination of the sensitized RBCs. If the Coombs control cells do *not* agglutinate, it indicates that the AHG reagent was omitted, inactivated, or neutralized. Such tests are invalid and must be repeated. Neutralization of the AHG reagent is usually the result of inadequate removal of unbound antibodies during the washing procedure. The unbound antibodies bind to the AHG reagent, making it unavailable to cause agglutination of sensitized RBCs.

METHOD

Antibody screening tests are performed in a variety of ways. AABB Standards[6] requires that these tests detect clinically significant antibodies and that they include a 37°C incubation and an AHG test. Generally testing includes the following steps:

1. Appropriately label each tube.
2. Add 2 drops of patient serum to each tube.
3. Add 1 drop of appropriate screening cells to each tube.
4. Centrifuge, then gently resuspend the cell button and read for agglutination or hemolysis. Record results. It should be noted that this step is optional because most significant antibodies are IgG and will not cause agglutination of saline suspended RBCs.
5. Add 2 drops of enhancement reagent to each tube (may vary with enhancement reagent used).
6. Incubate at 37°C for 15 to 30 minutes, according to the manufacturer's recommendation for the enhancement reagent being used. During the incubation, antibody in the patient serum will bind to antigens on the reagent RBC. This is called the sensitization phase.
7. Centrifuge, then gently resuspend the cell button and read for agglutination or hemolysis. Record results.
8. Fill all tubes with saline, centrifuge, and discard supernatant. This is called washing, and it removes unbound IgG that will neutralize the AHG reagent.
9. Repeat step 8 two or three times to remove unbound antibody completely.
10. Add 2 drops of AHG to each tube (polyspecific or anti-IgG).
11. Centrifuge, then gently resuspend the cell button and read for agglutination or hemolysis. Tests that are macroscopically negative are usually checked for microscopic agglutination. Record results.
12. Add one drop of Coombs control cells (or "check cells") to all negative tests.
13. Centrifuge and read for agglutination. Repeat test if agglutination is *not* observed.

GRADING REACTIONS

Agglutination or hemolysis of test RBCs is the visible end point of an antigen-antibody interaction. Test results should be read immediately after centrifugation, as delays in reading may cause elution of antibody and false-negative test results. The first step in reading hemagglutination reactions is inspection of the supernatant for signs of hemolysis (red or pink coloration). Next, the RBCs are resuspended by gently shaking or tilting the tube until the cells no longer adhere to the sides. Agglutination is graded once the RBCs are resuspended. In the blood bank, agglutination reactions are routinely graded as negative (no agglutination), weakly positive, and 1+ through 4+ (see **Color Plate 2**). Scores of 1+ through 4+ may also be described as strong or weak (e.g., $1+^s$, $3+^w$). The degree of the positive reaction generally indicates the amount of antibody present, not its significance. In the other words, an anti-D that reacts weakly will have a lower titer than one that reacts 4+, but they are equally significant. Most workers advocate the use of a light source and optical aid (e.g., agglutination viewer) to enhance observation of weak reactions.

AUTOLOGOUS CONTROL

Many laboratories include an autologous control as part of the antibody screen. The autologous control is performed in parallel with the antibody screen and involves testing the patient's serum against the patient's RBCs. A positive autologous control is an abnormal finding and usually means the patient has a positive direct antiglobulin test (DAT).

The autologous control is not a required test and there is some controversy concerning its use. Positive autologous controls are associated with autoimmune hemolytic anemia, drug-induced hemolytic anemia (see Chapter 21), and hemolytic transfusion reactions (see Chapter 18). However, positive autologous controls and DATs results are also associated with a variety of benign conditions. For example, increased serum protein or blood urea nitrogen is associated with clinically insignificant positive autologous controls and DATs.[12] In addition, several studies have reported that the use of the autologous control or DAT in routine testing rarely provides significant information.[13] As a result, many laboratories have discontinued the routine use of the autologous control, whereas others have streamlined or restricted evaluation of positive autologous controls.

INTERPRETATION

Agglutination or hemolysis at any stage of testing is a positive test result, indicating the need for antibody identification studies. However, evaluation of the antibody screen and autologous control results can provide clues and give direction for the identification and resolution of the antibody or antibodies. The investigator should consider the following questions:

1. In what phase(s) did the reaction(s) occur?

Antibodies of the IgM class will react best at low temperatures and are capable of causing agglutination of saline-suspended RBCs (immediate spin reading). Antibodies of the IgG class will react best at the AHG phase. Of the commonly encountered antibodies, anti-N, -I, and $-P_1$ are frequently IgM, whereas those directed against Rh, Kell, Kidd, and Duffy antigens are usually IgG. Lewis and M antibodies may be IgG, IgM, or a mixture of both.

2. Is the autologous control negative or positive?

A positive antibody screen and a negative autologous control indicate an alloantibody has been de-

tected. A positive autologous control may indicate the presence of autoantibodies, antibodies to medications, or it may be idiopathic. If the patient has been recently transfused, the positive autologous control may be due to alloantibody coating circulating donor RBCs. Evaluation of samples with positive autologous control or DAT results are often complex and may require a lot of time and experience on the part of the investigator.

3. Did more than one screening cell react and, if so, did they react at the same strength and phase?

More than one screening cell will be positive when the patient has multiple antibodies, when the antibodies' corresponding antigen is found on more than one screening cell, or when the patient's serum contains an autoantibody. A single antibody specificity should be suspected when all cells react at the same phase and strength. Multiple antibodies are most likely when cells react at different phases and strengths and autoantibodies are suspected when the autologous control is positive. Figure 11–4 gives several examples of antibody screen results with possible causes.

4. Is hemolysis or mixed-field agglutination present?

Certain antibodies, such as anti-Le^a, $-Le^b$, $-P+P_1+P^k$, and -Vel, are known to cause in vitro he-

RESULTS

cell	IS	37°	AGT (poly)	
SC I	neg	neg	neg	1. Single alloantibody
SC II	neg	neg	2+	2. Two alloantibodies, antigens only present on cell II
auto	neg	neg	neg	3. Probable IgG antibody
cell	IS	37°	AGT	1. Multiple antibodies
SC I	neg	1+	3+	2. Single antibody (dosage)
SC II	neg	neg	1+	3. Probably IgG
auto	neg	neg	neg	
cell	IS	37°	AGT	1. Single or multiple antibodies
SC I	1+	neg	neg	2. Probably IgM antibodies
SC II	2+	neg	neg	
auto	neg	neg	neg	
cell	IS	37°	AGT	1. Multiple antibodies, warm and cold
SC I	2+	neg	1+	
SC II	3+	1+	2+	2. Potent cold antibody binding complement in AGT
auto	neg	neg	neg	
cell	IS	37°	AGT	1. Single warm antibody, antigen present on both cells
SC I	neg	neg	1+	2. Antibody to high-frequency antigen
SC II	neg	neg	1+	
auto	neg	neg	neg	3. Complement binding by a cold antibody not detected at IS
cell	IS	37°	AGT	1. Warm antibody
SC I	neg	neg	3+	2. Transfusion reaction
SC II	neg	neg	3+	3. Probable IgG antibody
auto	neg	neg	3+	

FIGURE 11–4 Examples of reactions that may be observed in antibody detection tests.

molysis. Mixed-field agglutination is associated with anti-Sd^a and Lutheran antibodies.

5. Are the cells truly agglutinated or rouleaux present?

Serum from patients with altered albumin-to-globulin ratios (i.e., patients with multiple myeloma) or who have received high molecular weight plasma expanders (i.e., dextran) may cause nonspecific aggregation of RBCs known as rouleaux. Rouleaux is not a significant finding in antibody screening tests, but it is easily confused with antibody-mediated agglutination. Knowledge of the following characteristics of rouleaux will help in differentiation between rouleaux and agglutination:

1. Cells have a "stacked coin" appearance when viewed microscopically.
2. Rouleaux is observed in all tests containing the patient's serum, including the autologous control and the reverse ABO typing.
3. Rouleaux will not interfere with the AHG phase of testing because the patient's serum is washed away prior to the addition of the AHG reagent.
4. Unlike agglutination, rouleaux is dispersed by the addition of 1 to 3 drops of saline to the test tube.[14]

LIMITATIONS

Antibody screening tests are designed to detect significant RBC antibodies, but they cannot detect all such antibodies. Antigens with frequencies of less than 10 percent (i.e., C^w, Lu^a, Kp^a) are not usually represented on screening cells and, as a result, their corresponding antibodies are not detected in routine screening tests. Antibody screening tests may also yield negative results when the titer or concentration of antibody drops below detectable limits. As described in Chapter 3, antibody levels decrease over time when the individual is no longer exposed to the corresponding antigen. If the level of an RBC antibody drops too low, results of antibody screening tests and crossmatches will appear negative and may lead to transfusion of donor units that carry the corresponding antigen. Reexposure to the RBC antigen will elicit a secondary immune response resulting in a dramatic increase in the antibody titer and possible immunologic destruction of the transfused RBCs. This is called a delayed hemolytic transfusion reaction (DHTR) because it occurs days or weeks after the transfusion. The student should keep in mind that proper performance and interpretation of antibody detection tests will minimize the risk of DHTRs.

Antibody Identification

Antibody identification studies determine the specificity and significance of RBC antibodies. This information is important when selecting donor units for transfusion and for monitoring potential cases of HDN. The majority of patient samples with unexpected RBC antibodies contain single alloantibodies and are relatively simple to identify. Identification studies for samples containing multiple RBC antibodies or autoantibodies may be very complex and require a great deal of time and expertise on the part of the investigator. This section discusses an approach to antibody identification that will resolve the majority of cases and introduces the student to special problems and techniques used to resolve more complex problems.

PATIENT HISTORY

Information concerning the patient's age, sex, race, diagnosis, transfusion and pregnancy history, medication, and intravenous solutions may provide valuable clues in antibody identification studies, especially with complex cases. The patient's race may be valuable because some antibodies are associated with a particular race. For example, anti-U is associated with persons of African descent because most U-negative individuals are found in this race. Transfusion and pregnancy history is helpful because patients that have been exposed to "nonself" RBCs via transfusion or pregnancy are more likely to have immune antibodies (i.e., Rh antibodies). "Naturally occurring" antibodies (e.g., anti-M, Le^b) should be suspected in patients with no transfusion or pregnancy history. The patient's history is especially important when the autologous control or DAT is positive. Certain infections and autoimmune disorders are associated with production of RBC autoantibodies and some medications are known to cause positive DATs (see Chapter 21). Furthermore, in a recently transfused patient (within 3 months), a positive DAT result may indicate a DHTR. Information regarding recent transfusions is also important when antigen typing the patient's RBCs. Antigen-typing results must be interpreted with care when the patient has been recently transfused, because positive reactions may be due to the presence of donor RBCs in the patient's circulation. Positive reactions due to donor RBCs usually show mixed field agglutination, but this will depend on how recently and how much the patient was transfused. A sample of a patient history form is shown in Figure 11–5.

REAGENT RED BLOOD CELLS

Antibody identification is performed in the same manner as the antibody screen except that a panel of reagent RBCs is used in place of screening cells. Panels are expanded versions of antibody screening cells consisting of 8 to 16 group O RBC suspensions. The panel is accompanied by an antigram that lists the antigenic makeup of each panel cell and may also serve as a worksheet to record results (Fig. 11–6). The antigram states whether each donor cell tests positive or negative for the following antigens:

PATIENT'S NAME _____

AGE _____ RACE _____ SEX _____ DR'S NAME _____

DIAGNOSIS _____

PREVIOUS   NUMBER
TRANSFUSIONS _____ OF UNITS _____ DATES _____

    PROBLEMS? _____

                            DUE DATE IF
                            CURRENTLY
PREGNANCIES: NUMBER _____ PREGNANT _____

    PROBLEMS? _____

MEDICATIONS:

1. _____   5. _____

2. _____   6. _____

3. _____   I.V. Solutions _____

4. _____   _____

IMMEDIATE BLOOD NEEDS? _____

_____

FIGURE 11–5 Patient history form.

D, C, Ec, e, and usually V, VS, f, C^w
M, N, S, s
Fy^a, Fy^b
Jk^a, Jk^b
K, k, and usually Kp^a, Kp^b, Js^a, Js^b
Lu^a, Lu^b
Le^a, Le^b
P$_1$
Xg^a

Other blood group antigens may be included, and panel cells with rare phenotypes are usually indicated. Rare phenotypes include cells lacking high-frequency antigens (i.e., U, Vel, Yt^a) or cells possessing low-frequency antigens (i.e., Wr^a, C^w, Co^b). As with screening cells, it is important to match the lot number appearing on the antigram with the lot number on the panel because the pattern of reactions will change with each issue.

The specificity of antibodies in a serum sample is determined by comparing the pattern of positive and negative reactions with the antigram. In other words, a serum sample containing anti-K should react with cells 3, 4, and 7 when tested against the panel shown in Figure 11–6. The remaining cells (1, 2, 5, 6, 8, and 9) should not react with the serum because they do not carry the K antigen. The presence of other antibodies is ruled out when a serum sample does not react with a cell known to carry the corresponding antigen. In our anti-K example, anti-D is ruled out because cell 2 on the panel is D positive but does not react with the serum sample. A well-designed panel will identify most commonly encountered antibodies and eliminate or rule out the presence of antibodies that are not present.

CELL	D	C	E	c	e	f	V	C^w	M	N	S	s	Lu^a	Lu^b	P$_1$	Le^a	Le^b	K	k	Fy^a	Fy^b	Jk^a	Jk^b						
			Rh							MNS			Lutheran		P$_1$	Lewis		Kell		Duffy		Kidd							
1. r'r-2	0	+	0	+	+	+	0	0	+	+	0	+	0	+	0	0	+	0	+	+	0	+	+						
2. R1^{w}R1-1	+	+	0	0	+	0	0	+	+	+	+	0	+	+	+	0	+	0	+	0	+	+	0						
3. R1R1-6	+	+	0	0	+	0	0	0	0	+	0	+	0	+	+	+	0	+	+	0	+	+	0						
4. R2R2-8	+	0	+	+	0	0	0	0	+	+	+	+	0	+	+	0	+	+	0	0	+	0	+						
5. r''r-3	0	0	+	+	+	+	0	0	+	+	+	0	0	+	+	+	0	0	+	0	+	0	+						
6. rr-32	0	0	0	+	+	+	+	0	+	0	+	0	0	+	+	0	0	0	+	+	+	+	0						
7. rr-10	0	0	0	+	+	+	0	0	+	+	+	+	0	+	0	0	+	+	+	0	+	+	+						
8. rr-12	0	0	0	+	+	+	0	0	0	+	0	+	0	+	+	0	+	0	+	+	0	0	+						
9. R$_o$-4	+	0	0	+	+	+	0	0	+	0	0	+	0	+	0	+	0	0	+	0	0	0	+						
Cord cell	/	/	/	/	/	/	/	/	/	/	/	/	/	/	/	0	0	/	/	/	/	/	/						
Patient																													

DIRECT ANTIHUMAN GLOBULIN TEST

Poly	
IgG	
C3	

FIGURE 11–6 Antigram of a panel of reagent red blood cells used in antibody identification.

EVALUATION OF PANEL RESULTS

Evaluation of panel results should be carried out in a logical step by step method to ensure proper identification and avoid missing antibody specificities that may be masked by other antibodies. A logical approach to antibody identification is outlined here, using a series of questions and the example illustrated in Figure 11–7.

1. Is the autologous control positive or negative?

In this case, the autocontrol is negative, indicating the positive reactions are due to alloantibody, not to autoantibody. The presence of autoantibodies complicates the process of antibody identification and will be briefly discussed in Special Problems in Antibody Identification.

2. In what phase(s) and at what strength(s) did the positive reactions occur?

In this case, all positive reactions occurred at the AHG phase and all were 2+, which indicates that a single IgG antibody is present. IgM antibodies are usually detected at the immediate spin reading, whereas reactivity at various strengths and phases indicates the presence of multiple RBC antibodies.

3. What antibodies can be ruled out or eliminated as possibilities?

Antibodies are ruled out when the patient's serum fails to react with a cell known to carry the corresponding antigen. Only cells that gave negative reactions in *all* phases of testing should be used for ruling out antibodies. In addition, it is best to rule out antibodies using panel cells from donors that are homozygous for the corresponding antigen because some weakly reactive antibodies may fail to react with cells from heterozygous donors. For example, a weak anti-Jk^a may not react with a $Jk(a+b+)$ cell because it carries fewer Jk^a antigens than a $Jk(a+b-)$ cell. Using panel cells from homozygous donors to rule out antibody specificities decreases the chance of missing weakly reactive antibodies. In our example, the patient's serum failed to react with cells 4 through 9. The following antibodies can be ruled out using cell number 4 because it is homozygous for the following antigens: D, E, c, Lu^b, Le^b, K, Fy^b, and Jk^b. Continuing with cell 5: f, S, Le^a, and k are ruled out; cell 6: e, V, M, and Jk^a; and cell 8: N, s, and Fy^a. Ruling out specificities makes antibody identification easier because it reduces the possible explanations for the positive results. In this case, ruling out eliminated 20 possible specificities, leaving only anti-C, -C^w, and -Lu^a to be considered.

4. Does the serum reactivity match any of the remaining specificities?

The pattern of reactivity will usually exactly match a pattern when there is a single alloantibody present. In our example, the serum reactivity perfectly matches the C pattern. The serum gave uniform positive results

	Rh								MNS				Lutheran		P₁	Lewis		Kell		Duffy		Kidd			LISS 37C	AHG	check cells
CELL	D	C	E	c	e	f	V	Cw	M	N	S	s	Luᵃ	Luᵇ	P₁	Leᵃ	Leᵇ	K	k	Fyᵃ	Fyᵇ	Jkᵃ	Jkᵇ			
1. r'r-2	0	+	0	+	+	+	0	0	+	+	0	+	0	+	0	0	+	0	+	+	0	+	+		θ	2+	
2. R1ʷR1-1	+	+	0	0	+	0	0	+	+	+	+	0	+	+	+	0	+	0	+	0	+	+	0		θ	2+	
3. R1R1-6	+	+	0	0	+	0	0	0	0	+	0	+	0	+	+	+	0	+	+	0	+	+	0		θ	2+	
4. R2R2-8	+	0	+	+	0	0	0	0	+	+	+	+	0	+	+	0	+	+	0	0	+	0	+		θ	θ	✓
5. r″r-3	0	0	+	+	+	+	0	0	+	+	+	0	0	+	+	+	0	0	+	0	+	0	+		θ	θ	✓
6. rr-32	0	0	0	+	+	+	+	0	+	0	+	0	0	+	+	0	0	0	+	+	+	+	0		θ	θ	✓
7. rr-10	0	0	0	+	+	+	0	0	+	+	+	+	0	+	0	0	+	+	0	+	+	+	+		θ	θ	✓
8. rr-12	0	0	0	+	+	+	0	0	0	+	0	+	0	+	+	0	+	0	+	+	0	0	+		θ	θ	✓
9. Rₒ-4	+	0	0	+	+	+	0	0	+	0	0	+	0	+	0	+	0	0	+	0	0	0	+		θ	θ	✓
Cord cell	/	/	/	/	/	/	/	/	/	/	/	/	/	/	/	/	/	0	0	/	/	/	/				
Patient																									θ	θ	✓

DIRECT ANTIHUMAN GLOBULIN TEST

Poly	negative
IgG	
C3	

FIGURE 11–7 An example of panel results for anti-C antibodies.

with all C-positive cells (1, 2, and 3) and negative results with all of the C-negative cells (4 through 9). Cell 2 is also C^w positive but anti-C^w would not explain the reactions with cells 1 and 3.

The pattern of reactivity will not always match a specific pattern, and there are several reasons for this. The investigator should reexamine the pattern, keeping in mind that weakly reactive antibodies may only give positive results with homozygous cells (i.e., Jk[a+b−]) or cells with strong expression of the antigen (i.e., P$_1$$^{+s}$). Other explanations include the presence of multiple alloantibodies, cold reactive autoantibodies, and antibodies directed at high- and low-frequency antigens. All of these possibilities are more fully discussed in Special Problems in Antibody Identification.

5. Are all commonly encountered RBC antibodies ruled out?

A patient's serum may contain more than one RBC antibody, and the presence of one specificity may mask or interfere with identification of another. In our example, anti-C is identified and all other specificities are ruled out, with the exception of anti-C^w and anti-Lu^a, both of which are antibodies to low-frequency antigens (occurring in less than 5 percent of the population). Antibodies to low-frequency antigens are uncommon because of the small chance of being exposed to the antigen; therefore, it is not necessary to rule them out. On the other hand, if a commonly encountered antibody is not ruled out, it is important to test selected cells that will rule out the presence of the antibody. For example, if anti-K was not ruled out in this case, then an RBC that is C negative and K positive should be tested. A negative result rules out the anti-K, whereas a positive result indicates the presence of anti-C and anti-K.

6. Is there sufficient evidence to prove the suspected antibody?

Conclusive antibody identification requires testing the patient's serum with enough antigen-positive and antigen-negative cells to ensure that the pattern of reactivity is not the result of chance alone. Testing the patient's serum with at least three antigen-positive and three antigen-negative cells will result in a probability (P) value of .05. A P value is a statistic measure of the probability that a certain set of events will happen by random chance. A P value of .05 or less is required for identification results to be considered valid and it means that there is a 5 percent (1 in 20) chance that the observed pattern occurred for reasons other than a specific antibody reacting with its corresponding antigen. Stated another way, it means that the interpretation of the data will be correct 95 percent of the time. Testing of cells selected from other panels is necessary when inadequate numbers of antigen-positive or antigen-negative cells are tested. In our example, the patient's serum reacted with three C-positive cells (1, 2, and 3) but not with six C-negative cells. As a result, selected cells are not required and the identification of anti-C is conclusive.

7. Is the patient lacking the antigen corresponding to the antibody?

Individuals cannot make alloantibodies to antigens that they possess; therefore, the last step in identification studies is to test the patient's cells for the corresponding antigen. A negative result is expected and indicates that identification results are correct. If the patient's RBCs are positive for the corresponding antigen, misidentification of the antibody or a false-positive typing is the most likely explanation.

Antigen typing is also useful in the resolution of complex cases because it eliminates many possibilities. For example, an R$_1$R$_1$, K-negative, Fy(a−b+), Jk(a+b+), M+N+S+s+ patient could only form anti-c, anti-E, anti-K, or anti-Fy^a. It is not practical to do extended typings on all patients with antibodies; however, judicious use of this procedure can be helpful. It is important to know if the patient has been transfused in the last 3 months before using this technique because the presence of donor cells may result in false-positive typings.

Providing Compatible Donor Units

Once an antibody has been identified, the next task is to provide appropriate donor units for transfusion. When clinically insignificant antibodies are detected, use of crossmatch compatible units is appropriate. The AABB *Technical Manual*[14] states that no further testing is needed to confirm compatibility when the antibody is anti-M, anti-N, anti-P$_1$, Le^a, or Le^b. However, when a clinically significant antibody is identified, the blood must be crossmatch-compatible and confirmed as antigen negative with reagent antisera. The most economic way of providing such units is to crossmatch random units and then confirm that the compatible units are antigen negative by typing them with reagent antisera. This approach will not work when the antibody is no longer detectable in the patient's serum and reagent antisera must be used for screening purposes.

Knowledge of the incidence of antigens is useful for determining how many units of blood to screen or crossmatch for patients with antibodies. For example, if a patient with an anti-Jk^a needed four units of blood, how many units would need to be tested to find them? We know that 77 percent of the random population is Jk(a+) or that 23 percent are Jk(a−).[15] As shown here, the number of random units needed for antigen screening is calculated by dividing the number of antigen-negative units desired (four, in this case) by the incidence of antigen-negative individuals in the donor population.

$$Jk\ (a+) = 0.77$$
$$Jk\ (a-) = 0.23$$

$$\frac{4\ units\ Jk(a-)\ blood\ needed}{0.23\ incidence\ of\ Jk(a-)} = 17.4\ units$$

In this case, testing 17 or 18 random units should yield four Jk(a−) units. The same calculations can be used when multiple antibodies are present if the antigen frequencies are first multiplied together. The next example shows that for a patient with an anti-K and anti-Jk^a, 10 random units would need to be tested to find two that are compatible.

$$Jk(a+) = 0.77 \quad K\ positive = 0.09$$
$$Jk(a-) = 0.23 \quad K\ negative = 0.91$$

$$Jk(a-)\ (0.23) \times K\ negative\ (0.91) = 0.20\ Jk(a-)\ and$$
$$K\ negative$$

$$\frac{2\ units\ needed}{0.20\ Jk(a-)\ and\ Kell\ negative} = 10\ units$$

Occasionally it will not be possible to supply a patient with blood by random screening of bank blood. For example, approximately 124 units of blood would need to be screened in order to find two units negative for c, Jk^a, and Fy^a, and 1000 units would need to be tested to find two that are k (cellano) negative. In these cases, blood suppliers or a rare donor registry would be needed. Blood suppliers have more resources and inventory for finding rare units and most have a supply of rare units stored in the frozen state. The main purpose of rare donor registries is to locate blood for the most difficult cases by keeping track of rare units and donors across the country. In the United States, rare donor registries are maintained by the AABB and the American Red Cross. In difficult cases, it is also advisable to test any available siblings because their blood may prove to be compatible.

Special Serologic Techniques

ENZYME TECHNIQUES

Treatment of reagent RBCs with enzymes such as trypsin, bromelin, ficin, and papain enhances the reactivity of some antibody specificities while it eliminates the reactivity of others. Anti-Fy^a, -Fy^b, -M, -N, and -S will not react with enzyme-treated cells because their corresponding antigens are removed or denatured by enzyme treatment. On the other hand, the reactivity of Rh, Kidd, Lewis, P$_1$, and I antibodies is enhanced when the reagent RBCs are treated with enzyme; these antibodies are said to be "enhanced by enzymes." Enzyme techniques are performed by adding a solution of enzyme during testing (one-stage technique), or, more commonly, the cells are treated with enzyme before testing (two-stage technique). The two-stage technique is typically used in antibody identification studies because it is more sensitive than the one-stage technique.

Enzyme-pretreated RBC panels are useful in antibody identification studies because they increase detection of some weakly reactive antibodies, help to separate and identify multiple antibodies, and provide clues to the antibody's identity. Despite these advantages, enzyme techniques cannot be used alone because they will not detect anti-M, -N, -Fy^a, or -Fy^b. In fact, enzyme panels are most informative when the results are compared with the results obtained from the same untreated panel, as illustrated in Figure 11–8. In this example, comparison of the enzyme panel results with the LISS panel results shows that more than one antibody is present because the reactivity of the patient's serum with cells 6 and 8 was eliminated, whereas reactivity with cells 1 through 4 and 9 was enhanced. In addition, clues as to the identity of the antibodies are provided by behavior with the enzyme-treated cells. The reactions with cells 6 and 8 are most likely caused by anti-Fy^a, -Fy^b, -M, -N, or -S because these antibodies do not react with enzyme-treated RBCs, whereas the reactions with cells 1 through 4 and 9 must be caused by an Rh, Kidd, Lewis, P$_1$, or I antibody. The example shown in Figure 11–8 will be more fully discussed in Multiple Antibodies.

ELUTION

A positive DAT result indicates that RBCs were sensitized with antibody in vivo. Positive DAT results may be caused by autoantibodies, alloantibodies (i.e., hemolytic transfusion reactions), antibodies to certain medications, or for nonspecific reasons. Tests with monospecific AHG reagents can determine if IgG complement or both are coating the RBCs, but the antibody specificity cannot be determined while it is bound to the RBC membrane. Elution is a technique used to dissociate IgG antibodies from sensitized RBCs. The recovered antibody is called an eluate and can be tested, like serum, to determine the antibody's specificity. There are numerous elution techniques, but all of them rely on one of the following mechanisms: changing the thermodynamics (temperature), reversing attractive forces between antigen and antibody, or disturbing the structural complementarity of the antigen and antibody.[16] The Landsteiner-Miller heat[17] and Lui freeze-thaw[18] eluates were among the first used to remove antibody from RBCs and to investigate positive DATs. These eluates rely on changes in temperature to disrupt antibody-antigen bonds and alter the complementarity of the antigen and antibody.[16] The Landsteiner-Miller heat[17] eluate involves mixing the patient's washed RBCs with an equal volume of fluid (saline or albumin) and heating the mixture to 56°C. The heat causes antibody to dissociate from RBC antigens, and the antibody is released into the fluid. The antibody containing fluid is the eluate, and it is then separated from the RBCs by centrifuga-

CELL	D	C	E	c	e	f	V	Cw	M	N	S	s	Lua	Lub	P1	Lea	Leb	K	k	Fya	Fyb	Jka	Jkb	LISS 37C	LISS AHG	Ficin 37c	Ficin AHG	check cells Liss/Ficin
1. r'r-2	O	+	O	+	+	+	O	O	+	+	O	+	O	+	O	O	+	O	+	+	O	+	+	0	3+	2+	3+	
2. R1wR1-1	+	+	O	O	+	O	O	+	+	+	+	O	+	+	+	O	+	O	+	O	+	+	O	1+	3+	3+	4+	
3. R1R1-6	+	+	O	O	+	O	O	O	O	+	O	+	O	+	+	+	O	+	+	O	+	+	O	1+	3+	3+	4+	
4. R2R2-8	+	O	+	+	O	O	O	O	+	+	+	+	O	+	+	O	+	+	O	O	+	O	+	1+	3+	3+	4+	
5. r"r-3	O	O	+	+	+	O	O	O	+	+	+	O	O	+	+	+	O	O	+	O	+	O	+	0	0	0	0	✓
6. rr-32	O	O	O	+	+	+	+	O	+	O	+	O	O	+	+	O	+	O	O	+	+	+	O	0	3+	0	0	✓
7. rr-10	O	O	O	+	+	+	O	O	+	+	+	+	O	+	O	O	+	+	+	O	+	+	+	0	0	0	0	✓
8. rr-12	O	O	O	+	+	+	O	O	O	+	O	+	O	+	+	O	+	O	+	+	O	O	+	0	3+	0	0	✓
9. Ro-4	+	O	O	+	+	+	O	O	+	O	O	+	O	+	O	+	O	O	+	O	O	O	+	1+	3+	3+	4+	
Cord cell	/	/	/	/	/	/	/	/	/	/	/	/	/	/	/	O	O	/	/	/	/	/	/					
Patient																								0	0	0	0	✓

DIRECT ANTIHUMAN GLOBULIN TEST

Poly	negative
IgG	
C3	

FIGURE 11-8 An example of panel results for anti-D, anti-C, and anti-Fya antibodies.

tion. Once the eluate is recovered, it is tested against a panel of cells to determine the antibody's specificity. Lui freeze-thaw[18] eluates use the same principle except the RBC-fluid mixture is frozen and then thawed to disrupt the antibody-antigen bond. The next generation of eluates involves mixing the patient's washed RBCs with an organic solvent such as ether, xylene, or dichloromethane. The organic solvent is believed to disrupt antibody-antigen bonds by lowering the surface tension of the liquid media, thereby reversing van der Waal forces needed to hold the antibody and antigen together.[19,20] Organic solvent eluates are more sensitive than the heat or freeze-thaw technique because they remove more antibody from the RBC. However, they are also time consuming and the solvents are hazardous.[21] The third generation of eluates are fast and sensitive and do not use hazardous chemicals.[21] These techniques are called acid eluates because they use acidic solutions to decrease pH and disrupt the complementarity of antibody-antigen bonds.[22] The optimal pH for antibody-antigen binding is 6.8 to 7.2.[21] Acid eluates reduce the pH to 3 or less by mixing sensitized RBCs with an acidic solution. The antibody is released from the RBC membrane and the acidic solution becomes the eluate. The mixture is centrifuged and the acidic eluate separated from the RBCs. Immediately after separation, the pH is returned to neutral by addition of a buffer and the eluate is ready for testing. Citric acid, glycine, and digitonin-acid are three examples of acid elution techniques, and several commercially available kits are based on this principle.

Testing an eluate against a panel of RBCs will help to determine the exact cause of the positive DAT. Eluates containing warm autoantibodies will react with virtually all RBC samples, whereas alloantibodies will be recovered in cases of HDN and hemolytic transfusion reactions. There are many explanations for a nonreactive eluate (all cells negative) such as antibodies to drugs and nonspecific binding of proteins to RBC membranes. The evaluation of samples with positive DAT results can be complex and is beyond the scope of this chapter. The reader is referred to appropriate chapters in this book (e.g., Chapters 18, 20, 21) and sources listed in the references.

ADSORPTION

In blood banking, adsorption is the process of removing antibody from serum by combining a serum sample with appropriate RBCs under optimal conditions. The serum-cell mixture is incubated, and antibody is removed from the serum as it adsorbs (or binds) to the RBC antigens. Following incubation, the mixture is centrifuged and the adsorbed serum is separated from the sensitized RBCs.

Adsorptions are most commonly used to remove autoantibodies from patient serum. Autoantibodies interfere with identification of alloantibodies because they usually react with all reagent and donor cells. Autoadsorptions use the patient's own RBCs to remove the autoantibody from the patient's serum without removing any alloantibodies. The temperature at which an autoadsorption is performed depends on the optimal reactivity of the autoantibody. Warm autoadsorptions are performed at 37°C and are used to remove IgG autoantibodies, whereas cold autoadsorptions are carried out at 4°C and will remove IgM autoantibodies. After the autoantibody has been removed from the serum, the autoadsorbed serum can be used for antibody identification and compatibility testing.

Alloadsorptions use RBCs of known phenotypes to selectively remove alloantibodies or autoantibodies from patient's serum. This technique is especially useful when a serum sample contains multiple antibodies or an antibody to a high-frequency antigen (i.e., anti-Kp^b). For example, it may be difficult to find sufficient numbers of Kp(b−) cells to rule out the presence of other alloantibodies when anti-Kp^b is present. Adsorption with Kp(b+) cells will remove the anti-Kp^b, and the alloadsorbed serum can be tested for other alloantibodies. Cells used in alloadsorptions must be carefully matched to the antibody maker's phenotype in order to avoid removal of other significant alloantibodies.

NEUTRALIZATION

Neutralization uses soluble antigen to inhibit the reactivity of certain antibodies in hemagglutination assays. Soluble antigen is added to serum samples thought to contain the corresponding antibody. The mixture is incubated at room temperature during which time the soluble antigen will neutralize the antibody by occupying its antigen-binding sites. The neutralized serum is then tested against reagent RBCs and inhibition of reactivity indicates successful neutralization. A control of serum and saline must be tested in parallel to ensure the antibody was not simply diluted by the addition of the substance.

Substances containing soluble antigens are only available for a few RBC antibodies. Soluble P_1 antigen can be isolated from many sources such as hydatid cyst fluid, pigeon, and turtledove egg whites and even earthworms![23] Pooled serum or plasma can be used to neutralize anti-Chido and anti-Rodgers as well as Lewis antibodies. In addition, commercial manufacturers sell concentrated P_1 and Lewis substances. Finally, urine, which contains high concentrations of soluble Sd^a antigen, is often used to neutralize anti-Sd^a.

Neutralization can be used to confirm the identity of these antibodies, but it is most useful when the patient's serum contains multiple antibodies. Figure 11–9 demonstrates the use of Lewis substance in the identification of anti-Le^b and anti-K. In this case, the presence of the anti-Le^b is confirmed because Lewis substance successfully inhibits the reactivity and the anti-K pattern is easily recognized once the anti-Le^b is inhibited.

CHLOROQUINE DIPHOSPHATE

Chloroquine diphosphate (CDP) is a reagent used to remove IgG antibodies from the surface of sensitized RBCs without altering the RBC antigens.[24] This reagent is used to accurately antigen type RBCs with positive DATs. RBCs with positive DATs cannot be accurately typed for the Kell, Duffy, Kidd, S, or s antigens because the antisera require an AHG reading. RBCs with positive DATs are already coated with antibody and will always give a positive result when the AHG reagent is added. Antibody can be removed from sensitized RBCs by incubation with CDP for up to 2 hours at room temperature or 30 minutes at 37°C. After incubation, a DAT using monospecific anti-IgG is performed to determine whether or not the antibody was removed. If the DAT result is negative or very weakly positive, the treated RBCs can be phenotyped.

QUANTIFICATION OF ANTIBODY

The relative quantity of an RBC antibody can be determined by testing serial twofold dilutions of serum against an antigen-positive RBC. The reciprocal of the highest serum dilution showing macroscopic agglutination is the antibody titer. Table 11–1 illustrates an example of titration studies. In this example, the titer of the first sample is 16 and the second sample, 64. Titration studies may also be expressed as antibody scores. The score is calculated by assigning specific numeric value to each reaction depending on the reaction strength (4+ = 12, 3+ = 10, 2+ = 8, 1+ = 5, and w+ = 2) and adding the number together.[25] The antibody score reflects variation in reaction strength (2+ versus 3+) as well as the titer of the antibody.

Titers can be used in antibody identification studies but most commonly they are used to monitor the quantity of antibody in a woman's serum during a pregnancy. Increasing titers of maternal antibody indicate that the fetal RBCs possess the corresponding antigen and that the child is at risk for HDN. Significant increases in antibody concentration are indicated when the titer result increases by two tubes (i.e., 4 to 16) or when the score increases by 10 or more.[26]

Titers must be performed in a standardized manner because technical variability greatly influences titer results. The diluent, RBC phenotype, and incubation times must all be the same each time a patient's sample is evaluated. For example, if a K+k+ RBC is used the first time an anti-K is titered, a K+k+ cell must be used for all subsequent evaluations. In addition, parallel testing of previously titered samples will help control for variability in technique from one technologist to the next (e.g., grading reactions, shaking tubes).

CELL	Rh								MNS				Lutheran		P₁	Lewis		Kell		Duffy		Kidd		Albumin		control: serum+saline	serum+Lewis substance
	D	C	E	c	e	f	V	Cʷ	M	N	S	s	Luᵃ	Luᵇ	P₁	Leᵃ	Leᵇ	K	k	Fyᵃ	Fyᵇ	Jkᵃ	Jkᵇ	37C	AHG	AHG	AHG
1. r'r-2	O	+	O	+	+	+	O	O	+	+	O	+	O	+	O	O	+	O	+	+	O	+	+	0	2+	2+	0
2. R1ʷR1-1	+	+	O	O	+	O	O	+	+	+	+	O	+	+	+	O	+	O	+	O	+	+	O	0	2+	2+	0
3. R1R1-6	+	+	O	O	+	O	O	O	O	+	O	+	O	+	+	+	O	+	+	O	+	+	O	0	2+	2+	2+
4. R2R2-8	+	O	+	+	O	O	O	O	+	+	+	+	O	+	+	O	+	+	O	O	+	O	+	0	2+	2+	2+
5. r"r-3	O	O	+	+	+	+	O	O	+	+	+	O	O	+	+	+	O	O	+	O	+	O	+	0	0	0	0
6. rr-32	O	O	O	+	+	+	+	O	+	O	+	O	O	+	+	O	+	O	+	+	+	+	O	0	0	0	0
7. rr-10	O	O	O	+	+	+	O	O	+	+	+	+	O	+	O	O	+	+	+	O	+	+	+	0	2+	2+	2+
8. rr-12	O	O	O	+	+	+	O	O	O	+	O	+	O	+	+	O	+	O	+	+	O	O	+	0	2+	2+	0
9. Rₒ-4	+	O	O	+	+	+	O	O	+	O	O	+	O	+	O	+	O	O	+	O	O	O	+	0	0	0	0
Cord cell	/	/	/	/	/	/	/	/	/	/	/	/	/	/	/	O	O	/	/	/	/	/	/				
Patient																								0	0	0	0

DIRECT ANTIHUMAN GLOBULIN TEST

Poly	*negative*
IgG	
C3	

FIGURE 11–9 Neutralization using Lewis substance for a sample containing anti-Leᵇ and anti-K antibodies.

Following testing, the current sample should be frozen so it can be tested in parallel with the next sample.

Special Problems in Antibody Identification

MULTIPLE ANTIBODIES

The presence of multiple alloantibodies should be considered when one or more of the following is true:

1. The observed pattern of reactivity does not fit that of a single antibody.
2. Variations in reaction strengths occur that cannot be explained based on antigen dosage.
3. Different panel cells react at different phases or the effect of enzyme treatment of the test cell is variable.
4. Unexpected reactions are obtained when attempts are made to confirm the specificity of a single antibody.

As previously discussed, the example shown in Figure 11–8 is an example of a serum with multiple antibody specificities. An enzyme panel has been set up because the reactions in LISS at 37°C fit the pattern for anti-D but reactions at the AHG phase are inconclusive. The first step is to use cells with negative results (cells 5 and 7) to rule out or eliminate possible specificities. Anti-c, -e, -f, -S, -Luᵇ, -P₁, -Leᵃ, -Leᵇ, -K, -k, -Fyᵇ, and -Jkᵇ can be eliminated using homozygous cells. Next, examine the reactions that are positive in

TABLE 11–1 **TITER AND SCORE OF ANTI-D***

	1:2	1:4	1:8	1:16	1:32	1:64	1:128	
Previous sample	2+	2+	1+	±	0	0	0	Titer 1:16
score	8	8	5	2	0	0	0	Score 23
Current sample	3+	3+	2+	2+	1+	±	0	Titer 1:64
score	10	10	8	8	5	2	0	Score 42

*Score values: 4+ = 12; 3+ = 10; 2+ = 8; 1+ = 5; ± = 2.

the AHG phase of LISS but negative in the enzyme panel (cells 6 and 8) to see if they are positive for antigens known to be nonreactive with enzyme-treated RBCs. Cells 6 and 8 are Fy(a+). Finally, the reactions in LISS and ficin with cell 1 are still not explained but may be due to anti-C, which has not been ruled out and is known to be enhanced by enzyme treatment of test RBCs.

After initial evaluation of the panel results, it appears that the patient's serum contains an anti-D, -C, and -Fy^a; however, additional RBCs selected from other panels are needed for conclusive identification. Cells that are used to confirm the presence of antibodies may only be positive for one of the corresponding antigens. For example, panel cell 6 is D−, C−, and Fy(a+) and can be counted as one of the three Fy(a+) cells needed to prove the anti-Fy^a; however, cell 1, which is C+ and Fy(a+), cannot be used to confirm the presence of anti-C or -Fy^a. Figure 11–10 represents a panel of selected cells that validate the suspected findings. Cells 1 and 2 are C+, D− and Fy(a−) and confirm the presence of anti-C. Cells 4 and 5 are D+, C−, and Fy(a−) and prove the presence of anti-D. Cells 6 and 7 are Fy(a+), C−, and D−, confirming the presence of anti-Fy^a. Cell 3 is C−, D−, and Fy(a−) and gives the necessary third negative reaction while also ruling out the presence of anti-s and -Jk^a.

The final step in antibody identification studies is to type the patient's RBCs for the corresponding antigens using commercially available antisera. In our example, it would be expected that the patient's RBCs would be D−, C−, and Fy(a−). Although antigen typing is usually the final step in identification studies, the patient's extended phenotype can be of considerable aid in resolution of samples containing multiple antibodies. For example, if this patient's RBCs are rr (cde/cde), the presence of anti-c and -e could be eliminated from consideration, whereas anti-D, -C, and -E would be suspected.

ANTIBODIES TO HIGH-FREQUENCY ANTIGENS

Antigens such as k, Lu^b, and Vel are called high-frequency antigens because they have an incidence of 98 percent or higher (k 98.8 percent, Lu^b 99.8 percent, Vel greater than 99.9 percent[27]). Antibodies directed against high-frequency antigens are uncommon because only the rare individual lacking one of these antigens (1 percent or less of the general population) can produce antibodies to them. Although these antibodies are uncommon, they should be suspected when the patient's autologous control is negative but the serum reacts in a uniform manner (same phase and strength) with all panel and donor RBCs. Resolution of antibodies to high-frequency antigens requires testing of the patient serum against rare reagent cells that are missing high-frequency antigens. Most laboratories are unable to maintain an adequate inventory of rare cells and a reference laboratory may be needed to resolve such problems. Reference laboratories specialize in resolving difficult antibody problems and therefore maintain extensive inventories of rare RBCs.

As with other antibodies, clues to the identity are provided by its serologic characteristics. Room temperature reactivity suggests a high-frequency IgM antibody such as anti-I, anti-H, and anti-HI, whereas in vitro hemolysis indicates anti-P+P$_1$+P^k, anti-Vel, or anti-Jk^3. The patient's race and extended phenotype may provide important clues to the identity of antibodies to high-frequency antigens. The lack of certain high-frequency antigens is associated with a particular race (e.g., anti-U and anti-Js^b are associated with African decent, whereas anti-Jk^3 is more common among Polynesians). The extended phenotype often provides clues as to which high-frequency antigen the patient is missing (e.g., RBCs from U-negative individuals will type negative for S and s, and those from patients producing anti-Jk^3 will type Jk[a−b−]).

Providing compatible units of blood for patients

SELECTED CELL PANEL

CELL		D	C	E	c	e	f	V	Cw	M	N	S	s	Lu^a	Lu^b	P$_1$	Le^a	Le^b	K	k	Fy^a	Fy^b	Jk^a	Jk^b	Others		37C	AHG	37c	AHG
R268	r'r	0	(+)	0	+	+	+	0	0	+	0	+	+	0	+	0	0	+	0	+	0	+	+	0			0	3+	2+	3+
R043	r'r'	0	(+)	0	0	+	0	0	0	0	+	0	+	0	+	+	+	0	0	+	0	+	0	+			0	3+	2+	3+
R192	rr	0	0	0	+	+	+	0	0	+	+	0	+	0	+	+	+	0	0	+	0	+	+	0			0	0	0	0
R483	R₂r	(+)	0	+	+	+	+	0	0	+	0	+	+	0	+	0	0	+	0	+	0	+	+	+			1+	3+	3+	4+
R276	R₀	(+)	0	0	+	+	+	0	0	+	+	+	+	0	+	+	0	+	0	+	0	0	+	+			1+	3+	3+	4+
R300	rr	0	0	0	+	+	+	0	0	+	0	+	0	0	+	0	+	0	0	+	(+)	0	0	+			0	3+	0	0
R305	rr	0	0	0	+	+	+	0	0	+	+	+	0	0	+	+	0	+	0	+	(+)	0	+	+			0	3+	0	0

FIGURE 11–10 Selected cell panel to confirm anti-D, anti-C, and anti-Fy^a antibodies.

with clinically significant antibodies to high-frequency antigens is often more challenging than identification of the antibody. As previously discussed, blood suppliers, reference laboratories, and rare donor registries are resources used to find rare donor units. In addition, testing the patient's ABO-compatible siblings is useful, as family members are genetically similar and therefore likely to have similar RBC phenotypes.

Some antibodies to high-frequency antigens are not significant because they do not cause shortened survival of antigen-positive units. Antibodies to the Ch[a], Rg[a], Kn[a], McC[a], Cs[a], Yk[a], and JMH antigens will react in vitro with the majority of RBCs tested but will not usually cause RBC destruction in vivo. These antibodies have been referred to as high-titer, low-avidity (HTLA) because they characteristically give very weak reactions (usually microscopic) at the AHG phase but titer to 64 or higher. Although most HTLA antibodies share these serologic characteristics, some investigators find the term misleading because the characteristic weak reactions may be the result of low numbers of antigen sites per RBC not due to antibodies with low avidity. Furthermore, the term may be misleading in identification studies because these antibodies do not always yield weak reactions and they do not always titer to 64. Regardless of what they are called, resolution usually requires testing with reagent RBCs that are missing the corresponding antigens. Enzyme panels can provide clues to the specificity because anti-Ch[a], -Rg[a], and -JMH do not react with enzyme-treated cells and anti-Yk[a] may be weakened. Identification of the specificity is not as important as ruling out the presence of other clinically significant alloantibodies that may be masked or hidden. Approximately 25 percent of samples containing these clinically insignificant antibodies also have underlying alloantibodies that are of clinical significance.[28] Once the antibody problem is resolved, units should be selected that are antigen negative for any clinically significant antibodies and least incompatible by major crossmatch with the clinically insignificant antibody.

ANTIBODIES TO LOW-FREQUENCY ANTIGENS

Reactions between a serum and a single donor or reagent cell sample may be associated with antibodies to low-incidence antigens (i.e., Kp[a], Wr[a]). Other possibilities might be that the donor cells are ABO incompatible or have a positive DAT result. These more common possibilities should be evaluated first. The serum can then be checked against RBCs with known low-frequency antigens, or the reactive cell can be tested with known examples of antibodies to low-frequency antigens. Reference laboratories are available to assist in the resolution. Transfusion therapy should not be delayed because it will be easy to find compatible donor units.

COLD REACTIVE AUTOANTIBODIES

Cold reactive autoantibodies are IgM antibodies that react with antigens found on the patient's own RBCs. Autoanti-I, -H, and -HI are the most common specificities, but many others have also been reported. Most adult sera contain cold autoantibodies, but the overwhelming majority are clinically insignificant or benign because they do not react with their corresponding antigens at body temperatures. Cold autoantibodies that are active at or near body temperature are called pathologic and cause an autoimmune hemolytic anemia known as cold hemagglutinin disease (CHD) (see Chapter 21).

Detection of insignificant autoantibodies is common but undesirable because transfusion must be delayed until the presence of significant antibodies is ruled out. Serologic investigation of cold reactive autoantibodies can be difficult and frustrating owing to their tremendous serologic variability. Cold reactive autoantibodies react with reagent RBCs at low temperatures causing agglutination of saline-suspended RBCs or activation of complement. Cold autoantibodies are easiest to recognize when they cause strong agglutination of all panel cells at the immediate spin reading. Agglutination may also carry over to the 37°C reading, but the reactions usually become weaker with increasing temperature. Cold autoantibodies become difficult to recognize when they bind complement to RBC membranes at low temperatures but do not cause agglutination. In these cases, the immediate spin and 37°C readings will be negative but the anticomplement component of polyspecific AHG reagents will result in weak reactions at the AHG phase with a variable number of panel cells. These cases are difficult to resolve because they appear as weakly reactive IgG antibodies and the reactions are often difficult to reproduce. Cold panels or screens are used to identify or confirm the presence of cold autoantibodies. A cold screen, as shown in Figure 11–11, involves testing the patient's serum at decreasing temperatures with group O adult RBCs, group O cord RBCs, and ABO-compatible reverse grouping RBCs (A$_1$, A$_2$, and B cells). Patient's serum is combined with appropriate reagent RBCs, then the tubes are centrifuged and read for macroscopic agglutination. The tubes are then placed at room temperature for 15 to 30 minutes followed by another reading. Readings are also performed after 15 to 30 minute incubations at 18°C and 4°C. Figure 11–11 gives the typical reactions for an autoanti-HI in a group AB individual.

Although the identification of cold reactive autoantibodies is not of clinical significance, confirmation of their presence will aid in the resolution of the antibody problem. Once the presence of a cold autoantibody has been confirmed, a procedure must be selected to detect significant antibodies while avoiding interference by the autoantibody. The following section describes four of the more commonly used procedures.

CELL	IS	RT	18°C	4°C
A_1	0	0	1+	2+
A_2	1+	2+	4+	4+
B	0	0	2+	3+
O adult	2+	3+	4+	4+
O cord	0	0	1+	2+
Auto	0	0	1+	2+

FIGURE 11-11 A cold antibody screen, illustrating typical reactions for an autoanti-HI in a group AB individual.

Avoiding Detection of Cold Autoantibodies

Use of Monospecific IgG The use of monospecific anti-IgG instead of polyspecific AHG is the simplest way to avoid detection of benign cold autoantibodies because membrane bound complement will not be detected at the AHG phase. As previously discussed in the section on AHG reagents, some laboratories use monospecific anti-IgG for routine testing in order to eliminate detection of insignificant cold reactive antibodies. Other workers believe that significant antibodies may be missed by the routine use of monospecific anti-IgG[10,11] and reserve it only for problem solving.

Prewarm Procedure The prewarm procedure prevents the activation of complement at low temperatures by keeping the test system at 37°C throughout the test procedure. The patient's serum, reagent RBCs, and enhancement media are placed in separate tubes and warmed to 37°C before mixing. Following appropriate incubation at 37°C, the tubes are washed with prewarmed saline (37°C to 45°C) three to four times. The tubes should not be allowed to sit with the warmed saline because significant antibodies may dissociate and give false-negative results. Polyspecific or anti-IgG AHG is added following the washing procedure and the reactions are evaluated as usual. This procedure is simple and easy to use, but significant antibodies may be missed if the procedure is used indiscriminantly.

Cold Adsorption Cold reactive autoantibodies can be selectively removed from patient's serum by adsorption with autologous or rabbit RBCs.[29] Cold autoadsorption involves mixing the patient's serum with an equal volume of packed autologous RBCs and incubating the mixture at 4°C. During the incubation, the autoantibody will bind or adsorb to the RBCs but alloantibodies will remain in the serum. Autologous adsorptions may be performed only when the patient has not been recently transfused (in the last 3 months) because alloantibodies may adsorb to donor RBCs present in the patient's blood sample. Rabbit RBCs are rich in I and H antigen and may be used in place of autologous RBCs to remove autoanti-I, -H, or -HI. Rabbit erythrocyte stroma is commercially available for this purpose, but there are some reports of weak alloantibodies (anti-D, -E, and -Le^b) being adsorbed by these products.[29,30] Following adsorption, the cell-serum mixture is centrifuged and the adsorbed serum separated from the antibody-coated RBCs or stroma. The adsorbed serum can then be used for antibody screening, identification, or crossmatching. Adsorption procedures are time consuming but especially useful for removing strongly reactive cold autoantibodies.

Dithiothreitol and 2-Mercaptoethanol Sulfhydryl compounds such as dithiothreitol (DTT)[31] or 2-mercaptoethanol (2-ME)[32] denature IgM antibodies by breaking the disulfide bonds. A serum that contains cold autoantibodies can be treated with DTT or 2-ME and then evaluated for IgG alloantibodies. IgG agglutinins treated with the sulfhydryl compounds retain their ability to agglutinate RBCs. Equal volumes of DTT or 2-ME and serum are mixed together and incubated for 30 minutes to 3 hours, depending on the strength of the IgM antibody. This mixture is then tested with a panel of RBCs. A control consisting of equal volumes of serum and saline is tested in parallel with the treated serum to ensure that dilution of the antibody is not mistaken for denaturation.

WARM AUTOANTIBODIES

Unlike cold reactive autoantibodies, warm autoantibodies are usually IgG and, active at body temperature. These antibodies are uncommon but usually pathologic because they will sensitize autologous RBCs in vivo. RBCs that are coated with IgG antibodies become targets of immune destruction and may not survive normally. The rate of RBC destruction depends on the quantity and type of antibody present on the RBCs.[33] For example, autoantibodies primarily composed of IgG subclass 3 are more pathologic than those composed of IgG subclass 4. Warm autoimmune hemolytic anemia (WAIHA) results when the rate of RBC destruction exceeds the rate of production by the bone marrow (see Chapter 21).

Warm autoantibodies can interfere with serologic testing because they react with all normal RBCs, including the individual's own RBCs. Patients with warm autoantibodies will have positive autocontrols and DATs because their cells have been sensitized with IgG antibody in vivo. Mixed-field agglutination is not seen, and use of monospecific AHG reagents will give positive results with anti-IgG and variable results (positive or negative) with anti-C3d. Eluates prepared from the patient's sensitized RBCs usually react uniformly with all normal RBCs.

The serum may or may not contain the autoantibody because the antibody binds to the individual's RBCs once it enters the circulation. As a result, the DAT result may be positive and the eluate reacts with all RBCs tested, but results of tests using serum (e.g., the antibody screen) will be negative. Alternately, the autoantibody will be detected in the serum once the amount of antibody produced exceeds the number of

	Rh								MNS				Lutheran		P₁	Lewis		Kell		Duffy		Kidd		*LISS*		*LISS*		check cells
CELL	D	C	E	c	e	f	V	Cʷ	M	N	S	s	Luᵃ	Luᵇ	P₁	Leᵃ	Leᵇ	K	k	Fyᵃ	Fyᵇ	Jkᵃ	Jkᵇ	37C	AHG	37C	AHG	
1. r'r-2	O	+	O	+	+	+	O	O	+	+	O	+	O	+	O	O	+	O	+	+	O	+	+	0	3+	0	1+	
2. R1ʷR1-1	+	+	O	O	+	O	O	+	+	+	+	O	+	+	+	O	+	O	+	O	+	+	O	0	3+	0	2+	
3. R1R1-6	+	+	O	O	+	O	O	O	O	+	O	+	O	+	+	+	O	+	+	O	+	+	O	0	3+	0	2+	
4. R2R2-8	+	O	+	+	O	O	O	O	+	+	+	+	O	+	+	O	+	+	O	O	+	O	+	0	3+	0	0	✓
5. r"r-3	O	O	+	+	+	+	O	O	+	+	+	O	O	+	+	+	O	O	+	O	+	O	+	0	3+	0	0	✓
6. rr-32	O	O	O	+	+	+	+	O	+	O	+	O	O	+	+	O	O	O	+	+	+	+	O	0	3+	0	2+	
7. rr-10	O	O	O	+	+	+	O	O	+	+	+	+	O	+	O	O	+	+	+	O	+	+	+	0	3+	0	1+	
8. rr-12	O	O	O	+	+	+	O	O	O	+	O	+	O	+	+	O	+	O	+	+	O	O	+	0	3+	0	0	✓
9. Rₒ-4	+	O	O	+	+	+	O	O	+	O	O	+	O	+	O	+	O	O	+	O	O	O	+	0	3+	0	0	✓
Cord cell	/	/	/	/	/	/	/	/	/	/	/	/	/	/	/	O	O	/	/	/	/	/	/					
Patient																								0	4+			

Autoadsorbed serum (over the second LISS 37C/AHG columns)

DIRECT ANTIHUMAN GLOBULIN TEST

Poly	4+
IgG	4+
C3	negative

FIGURE 11–12 Warm autoantibody with underlying alloanti-Jkᵃ.

antibody-binding sites on the RBCs. These cases are difficult to resolve because, as illustrated in Figure 11–12, the serum will react with all reagent and donor cells tested. In order to rule out the presence of alloantibodies, the autoantibody must be removed from the serum by adsorption. Warm autoadsorptions are the procedure of choice unless the patient has received a transfusion in the last 3 months. If a patient has been recently transfused, it is necessary to perform multiple alloadsorptions, a procedure that is beyond the scope of this text.

The efficiency of warm autoadsorptions can be enhanced if the RBCs are pretreated with enzymes or ZZAP before use. ZZAP is a mixture of DTT and papain that is used to remove antibody from sensitized RBCs and enzyme treat them at the same time.[34] Removing bound antibody increases the efficiency by increasing the available antibody-binding sites while enzyme pretreatment of adsorbing RBCs increases the quantity of warm autoantibody the cells can adsorb.

Once the autoantibody has been removed from the serum, the adsorbed serum can be used for identification of alloantibodies and for compatibility testing. Figure 11–12 demonstrates a case of a warm autoantibody and anti-Jkᵃ in a patient's serum. The warm autoantibody masked the presence of the anti-Jkᵃ in the initial test but the anti-Jkᵃ pattern is clearly seen in the warm autoadsorbed serum. This patient must receive Jk(a−) units, and crossmatches may be performed with adsorbed serum.

ANTIBODIES TO REAGENTS

Antibodies to a variety of drugs and additives can cause positive results in antibody testing. Several mechanisms may be responsible for this phenomenon. Antibody in the patient's serum can combine with a dye, drug, or chemical in the reagent to form antibody complexes; the chemicals may bind to the cells; or the cell membrane may be modified so that spontaneous agglutination or aggregation occurs. All tests that employ the offending reagent will yield a positive reaction, including the autocontrol. However, the result of the DAT will be negative. Some substances reported to cause this phenomenon are acriflavin, caprylate, thimerosol, LISS, citrate, oxalate, neomycin, and saline.[35] These substances may appear as a portion of the reagent. For example, if a patient has an antibody to caprylate, which is used as a stabilizer in some manufacturers' bovine albumin, all the tubes to which albumin has been added will give a positive reaction. The use of an albumin without caprylate or LISS will produce negative reactions.

Review Questions

1. Based on the following phenotypes, which pairs of cells would make the best screening cells?
   A. Cell 1: Group A, D+C+c−E−e+, K+, Fy(a+b−), Jk(a+b−), M+N−S+s−
      Cell 2: Group O, D+C−c+E+e−, K−, Fy(a−b+), Jk(a−b+), M−N+S−s+
   B. Cell 1: Group O, D−C−c+E−e+, K−, Fy(a−b+), Jk(a+b+), M+N−S+s+
      Cell 2: Group O, D+C+c−E−e+, K−, Fy(a+b−), Jk(a+b−), M−N+S−s+
   C. Cell 1: Group O, D+C+c+E+e+, K+, Fy(a+b+), Jk(a+b+), M+N−S+s+
      Cell 2: Group O, D−C−c+E−e+, K−, Fy(a+b−), Jk(a+b+), M+N+S−s+
   D. Cell 1: Group O, D+C+c−E−e+, K+, Fy(a−b+), Jk(a−b+), M−N+S−s+
      Cell 2: Group O, D+C−c+E+e−, K−, Fy(a+b−), Jk(a+b−), M+N−S+s−

2. Antibodies are ruled out using cells that are homozygous for the corresponding antigen because:
   A. Antibodies show dosage
   B. Multiple antibodies may be present
   C. It results in a *P* value of .05 for proper identification of the antibody
   D. All of the above.

3. A request for 8 units of packed RBCs was received for patient LF. The patient has a negative antibody screen, but one of the 8 units was 3+ incompatible at the AHG phase. Which of the following antibodies may be the cause?
   A. Anti-K
   B. Anti-Le^a
   C. Anti-Kp^a
   D. Anti-Fy^b

4. ES is an Le(a−b−) individual who has produced anti-Le^a and anti-Le^b. If ES's serum were to be mixed with pooled plasma before antibody identification tests, the Lewis antibodies would be:
   A. Enhanced
   B. Destroyed
   C. Neutralized
   D. Unchanged

5. Which of the following antibodies is most likely to be detected at low temperatures?
   A. Anti-Fyb
   B. Anti-Jka
   C. Anti-M
   D. Anti-S

6. A type and screen was ordered for patient DJ. The patient is found to be O Rh positive with a positive antibody screen. A LISS panel was performed, and all the panel cells reacted 3+ at the AHG phase with DJ's serum. The autocontrol was negative. Which of the following would be a possible cause for these results? DJ's serum contains:
   A. Anti-Kp^b
   B. A warm autoantibody
   C. Anti-K and anti-E
   D. Anti-Lu^a

Refer to Figure 11–13 to answer questions 7 through 10.

7. Which of the following antibodies *cannot* be ruled out using the panel results?
   A. Anti-E and anti-K
   B. Anti-V, anti-C^w, anti-Lu^a
   C. Anti-S and anti-Le^a
   D. All of the above

CELL	D	C	E	c	e	f	V	Cw	M	N	S	s	Lua	Lub	P1	Lea	Leb	K	k	Fya	Fyb	Jka	Jkb	IS	37	AHG	AHG
	Rh								MNS				Lutheran		P1	Lewis		Kell		Duffy		Kidd		LISS			Ficin
1.	0	+	0	+	+	+	0	0	+	+	0	+	0	+	0	0	+	0	+	+	0	+	+	0	0	0	0
2.	+	+	0	0	+	0	0	+	+	+	+	0	+	+	+	0	+	0	+	0	+	+	0	0	0	2+	0
3.	+	+	0	0	+	0	0	0	0	+	0	+	0	+	+	+	0	+	+	0	+	+	0	w+	w+	w+	1+
4.	+	0	+	+	0	0	0	0	+	+	+	+	0	+	+	0	+	+	0	0	+	0	+	0	0	2+	0
5.	0	0	+	+	+	+	0	0	+	+	+	0	0	+	+	+	0	0	+	0	+	0	+	w+	w+	3+	1+
6.	0	0	0	+	+	+	+	0	+	0	+	0	0	+	+	0	0	0	+	+	+	+	0	0	0	2+	0
7.	0	0	0	+	+	+	0	0	+	+	+	+	0	+	0	0	+	+	+	0	+	+	+	0	0	2+	0
8.	0	0	0	+	+	+	0	0	0	+	0	+	0	+	+	0	+	0	+	0	+	+	0	0	0	0	0
9.	+	0	0	+	+	+	0	0	+	0	+	0	0	+	0	+	0	0	+	0	0	0	+	w+	w+	w+	1+
10.	+	+	0	0	+	0	0	0	+	0	+	0	0	+	+	0	0	0	+	0	+	+	0	0	0	0	0
AUTO																								0	0	0	0

FIGURE 11–13   Panel for review questions 7 through 10.

8. Which of the following antibodies best explain the panel results?
   A. Anti-E and anti-S
   B. Anti-K, anti-E, and anti-Le^a
   C. Anti-Le^a and anti-S
   D. Anti-Fy^b and anti-Le^a

9. What additional selected cells would need to be tested to complete this antibody identification?
   A. A Le(a−), S−, E+e− RBC to rule out anti-E
   B. A Le(a−), S−, K+ RBC to rule out anti-K
   C. A Le(a+), S− cell to prove anti-Le^a
   D. All of the above

10. What would be the expected results if this patient's RBCs were typed for the Le^a and S antigens?
    A. The patient's RBCs would be S+ and Le(a−).
    B. The patient's RBCs would be S+ and Le(a+).
    C. The patient's RBCs would be S− and Le(a−).
    D. Information is insufficient to indicate the patient's S or Le^a antigen typing.

Answers to Review Questions

1. D (p 239)
2. A (pp 233–234)
3. C (p 251)
4. C (p 248)
5. C (p 241)
6. A (pp 250–251)
7. D (pp 244–245)
8. C (pp 244–245)
9. D (pp 244–245)
10. C (p 245)

References

1. Giblett, ER: Blood group alloantibodies: An assessment of some laboratory practices. Transfusion 17:299, 1977.
2. Boral, LI, and Henry, JB: The type and screen: A safe alternative and supplement in selected surgical procedures. Transfusion 17:163, 1977.
3. Issitt, PD: Applied Blood Group Serology, ed 3. Montgomery Scientific Publications, Miami, 1985, p 309.
4. Ibid, p 324.
5. Widman, FK (ed): Technical Manual, ed 9. American Association of Blood Banks, Arlington, VA, 1985, p 203.
6. Standards for Blood Banks and Transfusion Services, ed 15. American Association of Blood Banks, Bethesda, MD, 1993.
7. Hughes-Jones, NC, Gardner, B, and Telford, R: The effect of pH and Ionic Strength on the Reactions between Anti-D and Erythrocytes. Immunology 7:72, 1964.
8. Atchley, WA, Bhagavan, NV, and Masouredis, SP: Influence of ionic strength on the reactions between anti-D and D positive red cells. Vox Sang 9:396, 1964.
9. Pollack, W, et al: A study of the forces involved in the second stage of hemagglutination. Transfusion 5:158, 1965.
10. Wright, MS, and Issitt, PD: Anticomplement and the indirect antiglobulin test. Transfusion 19:688, 1979.
11. Howard, JE, et al: Clinical significance of the anti-complement component of antiglobulin antisera. Transfusion 22:269, 1982.
12. Toy, PTCY, et al: Factors associated with positive direct antiglobulin tests in pretransfusion patients: A case-control study. Vox Sang 49:215, 1985.
13. Judd, WJ, et al: The evaluation of a positive direct antiglobulin test (autocontrol) in pretransfusion testing revisited. Transfusion 26:220, 1986.
14. Walker, RH (ed): Technical Manual, ed 10. American Association of Blood Banks, 10. Arlington, VA, 1985, p 283.
15. Issitt, PD, op cit, p 279.
16. Judd, JW: Elution of antibody from red cells. In Bell, CA (ed): Antigen-Antibody Reactions Revisited. American Association of Blood Banks, Arlington, VA, 1982, p 175.
17. Landsteiner, K, and Miller, CP: Serologic studies on the blood of primates: II. The blood groups of anthropoid apes. J Exp Med 42:853, 1925.
18. Eicher, CA, et al: A simple freezing method for antibody elution (abstract). Transfusion 18:647, 1978.
19. van Oss, CJ, Absolom, DR, and Neumann, AW: The "hydrophobic effect": Essentially a van de Waals interaction. Colloid Polymer Sci 1:424, 1980.
20. van Oss, CJ, Absolom, DR, and Neumann, AW: Applications of net repulsive van der Waals forces between different particles, macromolecules or biological cells in liquids. Colloid Polymer Sci 1:45, 1980.
21. South, SF: Use of the direct antiglobulin test in routine testing. In Wallace, ME and Levitt, JS (eds): Current Application and Interpretation of the Direct Antiglobulin Test. American Association of Blood Banks, Arlington, VA, 1988, p 25.
22. Howard, PL: Principles of antibody elution. Transfusion 21:477, 1981.
23. Issitt, PD, op cit, 204.
24. Edwards, JM, Moulds, JJ, and Judd, WJ: Chloroquine dissociation of antigen-antibody complexes. Transfusion 22:59, 1982.
25. Marsh, WL: Scoring of hemagglutination reactions. Transfusion 12:352, 1972.
26. Walker, RH, op cit, p 568.
27. Issitt, PD, op cit, p 611.
28. Moulds, MK: Special serologic technics useful in resolving high-titer, low-avidity antibodies. In Recognition and Resolution of High-Titer, Low-Avidity Antibodies: A Technical Workshop. American Association of Blood Banks, Washington, DC, 1979.
29. Waligora, SK, and Edwards, JM: Use of rabbit red cells for adsorption of cold autoagglutinins. Transfusion 23:328, 1983.
30. Orsini, LA, et al: Removal of serum IgG alloantibodies by rabbit erythrocyte stroma (abstract). Transfusion 25:452, 1985.
31. Pirofsky, B, and Rosner, ER: DTT test: A new method to differentiate IgM and IgG erythrocyte antibodies. Vox Sang 27:480, 1974.
32. Deutsch, HF, and Morton, JI: Dissociation of human serum macroglobulins. Science 125:600, 1957.
33. Petz, LD, and Garratty, G: Acquired Immune Hemolytic Anemias. Churchill Livingston, New York, 1980, p 110.
34. Branch, DR, and Petz, LD: A New Reagent Having Multiple Applications in Immunohematology (abstract). Transfusion 20:642, 1980.
35. Issitt, PD, op cit, p 599.

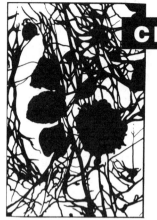

CHAPTER 12

Compatibility Testing

Linda T. Raichle, PhD, MT(ASCP)
Mary E. Paranto, MS, MT(ASCP)SBB

OBJECTIVES

Upon completion of this chapter, the learner should be able to:

1 Recognize the appropriate methods to identify the patient and donor accurately and collect samples for testing.

2 Outline the procedure for testing donor and patient specimens.

3 Select appropriate donor units based on availability, presence or absence of alloantibody in the patient, and unit's age and appearance.

4 Compare and contrast crossmatch procedures.

5 Resolve incompatibilities in the crossmatch.

6 Explain compatibility testing procedures and protocols in special circumstances.

7 State the limitations of compatibility testing procedures.

8 Describe a scheme for effective blood use.

9 List the steps necessary to reidentify the patient before transfusion.

10 Discuss future issues of compatibility testing.

Blood transfusion has been a part of therapy for less than a century. In the past, transfusions were often performed out of desperation with no guarantee that the patients would benefit—or even survive. Donors were chosen based solely on availability and willingness.

Today, transfusion therapy is scientific and successful. The concept of antigens and antibodies was unknown until 1900, when Landsteiner described ABO blood groups and recognized their importance in the success or failure of transfusions. By the early 1940s, there were reports of serious transfusion reactions in cases in which the donor and recipient were ABO compatible.[1] It became obvious that not all incompatible reactions could be prevented by ABO group compatibility alone.

As the knowledge of new blood group systems increased, so did the search for more sensitive pretransfusion compatibility testing methods. Pioneer blood bankers mixed the patient's serum and the donor's red blood cells (RBCs) and observed for direct RBC lysis, agglutination, or both. This became known as the major crossmatch test.

The crossmatch became part of a series of pretransfusion tests known as compatibility testing. The compatibility test as we know it today includes an ABO and $Rh_o(D)$ grouping performed on the donor and recipient samples, screening of the donor's and patient's sera for unexpected antibodies, and a crossmatch. The primary purpose of pretransfusion or compatibility testing is to ensure the best possible results of a blood transfusion. That is, the transfused RBCs will have an acceptable survival rate, and there will be no significant destruction of the recipient's own RBCs. Each of the following is important to ensure safe transfusion therapy and must be considered in any comprehensive review of the process used to select blood for a patient:

1. Identification of the patient and donor and collection of appropriate samples for testing
2. Testing of the donor sample
3. Testing of the patient sample and review of past blood bank records
4. Selection of appropriate donor units
5. Crossmatching
6. Reidentification of the patient before infusion of blood

No testing procedure can prevent sensitization of the recipient to foreign red blood cell antigens or avoid a delayed transfusion reaction caused by antibody present in subdetectable amounts in the pretransfusion serum. Testing cannot guarantee normal survival of transfused cells in the patient's circulation. The potential benefits of transfusion should always be weighed against the potential risks whenever this form of therapy is contemplated. Although adverse responses to transfusion cannot always be avoided, results are much more likely to be favorable if pretransfusion testing is carefully performed and results of laboratory testing show no incompatibility between donor and patient.

Collection and Preparation of Samples

POSITIVE PATIENT IDENTIFICATION

Historically, the major cause of transfusion-associated fatalities have been clerical errors, resulting in incorrect ABO groupings. Today, this fact remains virtually unchanged; 48 percent of transfusion deaths are due to such errors.[2] These disheartening data show that clerical errors remain the greatest threat to safe transfusion therapy. The most common cause of clerical errors, and thus transfusion accidents, is misidentification of the patient involved in the transfusion. Errors have resulted from confusion in identification of the patient when the blood sample was drawn, a mixup of samples during handling in the laboratory, and error in identification of the patient when the transfusion was given.

Exact procedures for proper identification of the patient, patient sample, and donor unit must be established and used by all staff responsible for each aspect of transfusion therapy, in order to prevent errors.

To prevent collection of samples from the wrong patient, the blood request form must be used to confirm the patient's identity before phlebotomy is performed. The request form must state the intended recipient's full name and unique hospital identification number.[3] Other information such as age and date of birth, address, sex, and name of requesting physician can be used to verify patient identity further but is not required on the form. Printing must be legible, and indelible nameplate impressions or computer printouts are preferable to handwritten forms.

The patient's wristband identification must always be compared with the requisition form. Any discrepancies must be completely resolved before the sample is taken. Nameplates on the wall or bed labels must never be used to verify identity, as the patient specified may no longer occupy that bed.

If the patient does not have a wristband or if the patient's identity is unknown, some form of positive identification must be attached to the patient before collection of samples. This may be a temporary tie tag or a wristband or ankleband, but it should not be removed until proper identification has been attached to the patient and verification of identity is made by the phlebotomist.

In some transfusing facilities, if the patient does not have a wristband and is coherent, it is permissible to ask a patient to state his or her full name and spell it out. If the age or home address is printed on the requisition form, the patient might be asked to state this information. Occasional errors can result from two patients with the same name being mistaken for each other. The phlebotomist should never offer a name and ask the patient to confirm that it is correct (e.g., "Are you Mr. Jones?"). Some disoriented patients may answer "yes" to any question. If the patient is very young or is incoherent, some other reliable professional individual who knows the patient must confirm the identity and document this on the requisition form.

Commercially manufactured identification systems using preprinted tags and numbers are especially use-ful in patient and donor verification procedures (Figs. 12–1 to 12–3). In an effort to improve transfusion safety, an identification system that uses a physical barrier to transfusion, in addition to standard identification procedures, has been described.[4] The physical barrier, a plastic combination lock, is applied to a unit of blood intended for a specific recipient. The lock is opened by nursing or medical personnel at the bedside where the combination is obtained from the patient's wristband. This system is reported to eliminate the fatal clerical errors that occur outside of the laboratory.

COLLECTING PATIENT SAMPLES

After positive identification has been accomplished, blood samples should be drawn, using careful technique to avoid mechanical hemolysis. Hemolyzed samples cannot be used for testing because hemolysis caused by activation of complement by antigen-antibody complexes will be masked.

Serum or plasma may be used for pretransfusion testing. Most blood bank technologists prefer serum because plasma may cause small fibrin clots to form, which may be difficult to distinguish from true agglutination. Also plasma may inactivate complement so that some antibodies may not be detected. About 10 ml of blood is usually sufficient for all testing procedures if there are no known serologic problems.

Tubes must be labeled before leaving the patient's bedside. If imprinted labels are used, they must be compared with the patient's wristband and requisition form before use. Labels should be attached to the tubes in a tamper-proof manner that will make re-

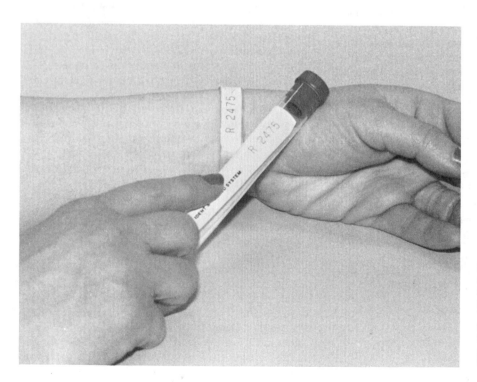

FIGURE 12–1 An example of a commercially manufactured identification system designed to prevent clerical errors in transfusion practice. The patient receives a bracelet at the time the blood sample is drawn. The information printed on the bracelet and on the blood sample tube is identical.

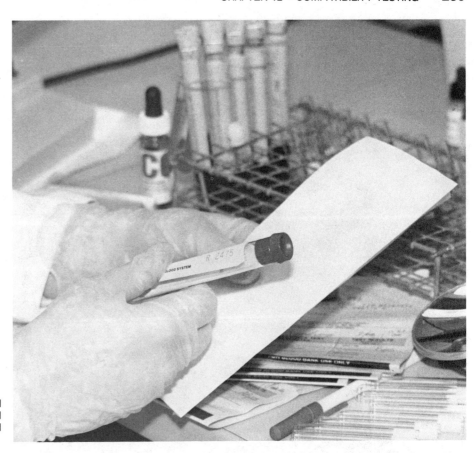

FIGURE 12-2 In the hospital blood bank, the information printed on both the blood sample tube and the requisition is verified.

moval and reattachment impossible. All writing must be legible and indelible, and each tube must be labeled with the patient's full name, hospital identification number, and date of sample collection.[5] The phlebotomist must initial or sign the label and add additional pertinent information as required by the standard procedure of the facility.

Blood samples should not be taken from intravenous tubing lines, in order to avoid contamination with materials that may cause confusing serologic results. Venous samples should not be drawn from above an infusion site but may be drawn from below the site. If a sample must be taken from an intravenous line, the line should be disconnected for 5 to 10 minutes, the first 10 ml of blood drawn should be discarded, and then the sample for testing may be obtained. When a specimen is received in the laboratory, a blood bank technologist must confirm that the information on the sample and requisition form agree. All discrepancies must be resolved before the sample is accepted, and if any doubt exists, a new sample must be drawn. Receipt of an unlabeled specimen requires that a new sample be obtained.

Patient samples should be tested as soon as possible after collection, and the serum should be separated from the patient's RBCs as soon as possible after the sample has clotted. If testing cannot be performed immediately, samples should be stoppered and kept at 1°C to 6°C.

As noted in Chapter 3, recent pregnancy or transfusion indicates an opportunity for a humoral immune response. Antibody production occurs over a predictable range of time, but the exact time will vary from responder to responder (i.e., patient to patient). Specimens used in compatibility testing should ideally be collected during the critical phases of the immune response. In an attempt to capture this important time for each patient, serum obtained from samples less than 72 hours after collection must be used for antibody screening and crossmatch testing if the patient was pregnant or transfused with RBC products within the last 3 months or if these histories are unknown.[6]

Patient RBCs can be obtained from either clotted or anticoagulated samples. They can be washed before use to remove plasma or serum, which may interfere with some testing procedures. A 2 to 5 percent saline suspension of RBCs is used for most serologic testing procedures; however, the manufacturer's directions should be consulted for the proper cell concentration to use for typing tests performed with licensed reagents. A method for preparing a button of washed RBCs suitable for performing one test is given in Procedural Appendix 1 of this chapter.[7]

DONOR SAMPLES

Donor testing samples must be taken when the full donor unit is drawn. Depending on the method used

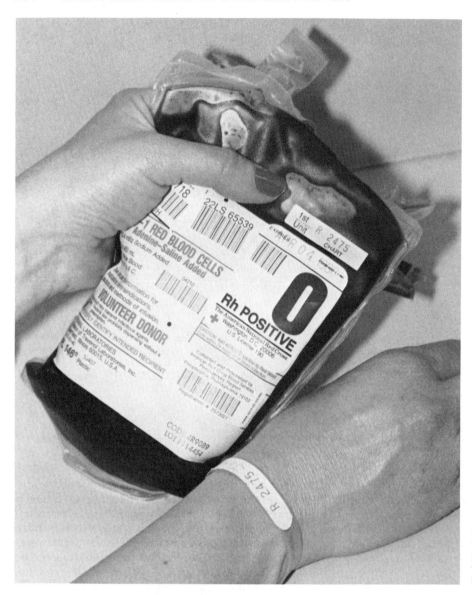

FIGURE 12-3 Before transfusion, the identifying number that was applied to the unit of blood is matched with the number on the patient's bracelet.

for testing, clotted samples, anticoagulated samples, or both, are obtained. The donor information and medical history card, the pilot samples for processing, and the collection bag must all be labeled with the same unique number code before starting the phlebotomy, and the numbers must be verified again immediately after filling. The donor number is used to identify all records of testing and eventual disposition of all component parts of the unit of blood. More detailed information on donor samples can be found in Chapter 10.

Ideal samples for compatibility testing can be prepared from the segmented tubing through which the donor was bled. The tubing segments are attached to the collection bag and each is imprinted with the same numbers. These numbers are different from the donor unit number but, nonetheless, are a positive means of sampling a given unit of blood.

Donor cells can be obtained from the segments in a number of ways that permit several procedures to be performed from the same segment. One technique that works well for sampling is to use a lancet to make a tiny hole in the segment through which a single drop of blood can be expressed easily. The hole is essentially self-sealing, so the rest of the blood in the segment remains uncontaminated. Another technique is to cut the RBC end of the segment and use an applicator stick to remove cells, or express a drop by squeezing the tubing. The segment may be stored with the cut end down in a properly labeled test tube to minimize contamination. The contents of the segment should preferably not be emptied into a test tube for storage because of the increased risk of contamination.

Regardless of the method used to harvest cells from a segment, it is important that engineering or work practice controls, or both, be used to eliminate or minimize aerosol production when the segment is cut or opened. Refer to Chapter 14 for additional information on safety procedures.

Both donor and recipient samples must be stored for a minimum of 7 days following transfusion.[8] The samples should be stoppered and refrigerated at 1°C to 6°C, carefully labeled, and adequate in volume so that they can be reevaluated if the patient experiences an adverse response to the transfusion.

Compatibility Testing Protocols

TESTING OF THE DONOR SAMPLE

According to the Code of Federal Regulations (CFR)[9] and the American Association of Blood Banks (AABB) standards,[10] ABO and Rh grouping (including a test for weak D) and tests intended to prevent disease transmission must be performed on a sample of blood taken at the time of collection of the unit of blood from the donor. A screening test for unexpected antibodies to RBC antigens is required by AABB standards on samples from donors revealing a history of prior transfusion or pregnancy.[11] Testing is performed by the facility collecting the donor unit, and results must be clearly indicated on all product labels appearing on the unit.

The transfusing facility is required by AABB standards[12] to confirm the ABO cell grouping on all units and Rh grouping on units labeled Rh negative. Tests for weak D(D^u) are not required to be repeated. The transfusing facility does not need to repeat any other testing procedure. The sample used for this testing must be obtained from an attached segment on the donor unit.

All testing must be performed using date and licensed reagents, according to manufacturers' directions and protocol established in the written standard operating procedure of the facility. A detailed explanation of the processing of donor blood can be found in Chapter 10.

TESTING OF THE PATIENT SAMPLE

A record of all results obtained in testing patient samples must be maintained. Some large transfusion services keep this information on a computerized retrieval system for ready access. However, during times when computer records are not available, these transfusion services must have a backup system that permits retrieval of patient testing results.[13]

Ideally, the same unique identification number should be assigned each time a patient is admitted for treatment. The number can then be used as a method of positive identification for comparing results of previous and current testing. Verification of previous results helps establish that the current samples were collected from the correct individual. Any discrepancies between previous and current results must be resolved before transfusion is initiated. A new sample should be collected from the patient, if necessary, to resolve the problem.

ABO and Rh grouping results should be included in the file. Notations concerning unusual serologic reactions and the identity of unexpected antibodies in the patient's serum should also be included in the file. This is perhaps the most important information. Sometimes subdetectable amounts of antibody may be present in a patient's serum, and previous records are the only source of information regarding its presence and identity and possible clinical significance.

ABO and Rh grouping and antibody screening of the patient's serum can be performed in advance of or at the same time as the crossmatch. If the patient has had a transfusion or has been pregnant within the last 3 months or if the history is unavailable or uncertain, the sample must be obtained from the patient within 3 days of the scheduled transfusion.[14] An accurate medical history, including information on medications, recent blood transfusions, and previous pregnancies, may help explain unusual results.

ABO Grouping

Determination of the patient's correct ABO group is the most critical pretransfusion serologic test. ABO grouping can be performed on slides or in tubes. Tube tests offer the greater sensitivity. Testing is performed in a manner similar to that described in Chapter 5, using potent licensed reagents according to the manufacturer's directions. If the cell and serum grouping results do not agree, additional testing must be conducted to resolve the discrepancy. Useful information on resolving ABO grouping discrepancies has been presented in Chapter 5. If the patient's ABO group cannot be satisfactorily determined and immediate transfusion is essential, group O packed RBCs should be used.

Rh Grouping

Rh grouping is performed using anti-D blood grouping serum. Tube or slide tests should be performed according to the manufacturer's directions for the reagent, which may or may not include the use of a suitable diluent control. When indicated, these controls must be run in parallel with Rh grouping tests performed on patient samples, to avoid incorrect designation of Rh-negative patients as Rh positive. If the diluent control is positive, the result of the Rh grouping test is invalid.[15] In such a case, a direct antiglobulin test (DAT) should be performed on the patient's RBCs to determine whether uptake of autoantibodies (or alloantibodies, if the patient has been recently transfused) is responsible for the positive control result. If the DAT result is positive, accurate Rh grouping can sometimes be performed using saline-active or chemically modified Rh blood grouping serum with an appropriate diluent or 8 percent albumin control. If the Rh group of the recipient cannot be determined and transfusion is essential, Rh-negative blood should be given.

The test for D[u] is unnecessary when testing transfusion recipients.[16] Individuals typing as Rh negative in direct testing should receive Rh-negative blood, and those typing as Rh positive in direct testing should receive Rh-positive blood. Female patients whose RBCs type as D[u] are considered Rh positive (see Chapters 6 and 20) and may receive Rh-positive blood during transfusion.

Some patients who type as Rh positive, whether it be by direct or indirect testing, may produce anti-D following transfusion of Rh-positive RBC components (see Chapter 6). This occurs rarely and does not justify the routine transfusion of Rh-negative blood to these Rh-positive patients until the antibody is detected.

Antibody Screening

The patient's serum or plasma must be tested for unexpected antibodies. The object of the antibody screening test is to detect as many clinically significant antibodies as possible. In general, the term "clinically significant" antibodies refers to antibodies that are reactive at 37°C or in the DAT or both and are known to have caused a transfusion reaction or unacceptably short survival of the transfused RBCs. Refer to Table 12–1 for a list of these antibodies.[17] The incidence of unexpected antibodies in the patient population is low — 1.64 percent in one large study[18] and 0.78 percent in another.[19]

TABLE 12–1 CLINICAL SIGNIFICANCE* OF ANTIBODIES† DETECTED AT 37°C IN VITRO

Antibodies Regarded as Always Being Potentially Clinically Significant	
ABO	Duffy
Rh	Kidd
Kell	SsU

Antibodies That May Sometimes Be Clinically Significant	
Le[a]	Lutheran (Lu[a], Lub)
MN	Cartwright (Yt[a])
P₁	

Antibodies That Rarely, If Ever, Are Clinically Significant	
Leb	Xg[a]
Chido/Rodgers (Ch[a]/Rg[a])	Bg
York (Yk[a])	HTLA
Sd[a]	

From Garratty,[17] p 209, with permission.

*Clinical significance is defined by proven hemolytic transfusion reactions. This could range from a severe overt reaction to diminished red cell survival as the only sign.

†Very rare antibodies have not been included in this list (e.g., when there is only a single report of a hemolytic transfusion reaction in the literature).

Correct ABO grouping results are much more critical to transfusion safety than antibody screening. Most antibodies, other than anti-A and anti-B, do not cause severe hemolytic transfusion reactions. Therefore, the vast majority of patients would not suffer grave consequences if transfused with blood from ABO group–compatible donors without the benefit of antibody screening tests.

Detection of unexpected antibodies is important, however, for the selection of donor RBCs that are likely to survive maximally in the patient's circulation. Weakly reactive antibodies that are capable of reacting with their antigens at 37°C can cause decreased survival of transfused incompatible red cells. Because large numbers of antibody molecules are present in the patient's circulation compared with the number of RBCs in a unit of blood, incompatible donor cells are highly vulnerable to destruction by patient antibodies.

Antibody screening offers several advantages over direct crossmatch testing for detection of antibodies:

1. Testing is performed using selected group O RBCs that are known to carry optimal representation of important blood group antigens.
2. Testing can be performed well in advance of the anticipated transfusion, allowing ample time for identification of any unexpected antibody and location of suitable donor units lacking the corresponding antigen.

Methods used to detect antibodies in patients' sera must demonstrate all significant coating, hemolyzing, and agglutinating antibodies active at 37°C. Incubation of screening tests at room temperature or below is not advocated because antibodies that react only at lower temperatures in vitro are usually incapable of complexing with their antigens in vivo.

AABB standards stipulate the necessity of performing an antihuman globulin test on patient samples using reagent RBCs obtained from single donors.[20] Single-donor screening cells offer increased sensitivity over pooled cell preparations. They are supplied as sets of individual cell samples from two or more donors whose RBC phenotypes have been carefully matched so that they complement each other.

If an antigen is lacking from one cell sample, it is present on the other. Ideally, one sample in each set should carry the products of homozygous genes for antigens such as Jk[a] and c. Antibodies to these antigens sometimes fail to react with cell samples carrying a single dose of the corresponding antigen.

During the late 1970s and early 1980s, polyspecific antihuman globulin (AHG) reagents, containing adequate levels of anticomplement as well as high levels of anti-IgG activity, were the preferred AHG reagents for patient antibody screening and crossmatch testing.[21] It was shown that detection of complement components bound to RBCs by antigen-antibody complexing was necessary to demonstrate the presence of some weakly reactive antibodies.[22] In addition, Wright and Issitt[23] found that more than 50 percent of antibodies in the Kidd and Duffy blood group systems were detected better when reasonable levels of anti-complement components were present in the AHG serum used. However, polyspecific AHG reagents are known to detect nonspecific proteins, insignificant proteins, or both. When used routinely, spurious reactions were investigated, yielding little relevance to patient care yet increasing costs and consuming valuable technologist time.

The modern blood bank laboratory uses anti-IgG AHG reagents in its compatibility testing procedures. Polyspecific AHG reagents are still used in other tests or procedures. Refer to Chapter 11 for a more complete discussion of the detection and identification of alloantibodies.

In order to detect false-negative AHG tests owing to the inactivation of the anti-IgG in the AHG reagent, AABB standards require the addition of IgG-coated RBCs (i.e., "check cells") to all tubes with negative AHG test results.[24]

The sensitivity of antibody detection tests can be enhanced by increasing the amount of serum added to the test,[25,26] increasing the length of incubation time at $37°C$,[27,28] or adding albumin or another enhancement medium to the test.[29,30] Screening cells can also be treated before use with the proteolytic enzyme solutions such as 0.1 percent papain or ficin to enhance their ability to detect some antibodies.[31,32] However, other antibodies cannot be detected using enzyme-pretreated cell samples, so these cells cannot be used as the only means of screening patients' sera. These serologic factors should be considered when resolving unexpected in vitro results and may be applied to the investigation of incompatible crossmatches, discussed later in this chapter.

Increased sensitivity is especially important when screening the sera of patients who have already formed at least one antibody, since they have proved their ability to produce antibodies in response to foreign RBC antigens.[33,34] Patients who have been recently transfused and those who have experienced previous unexplained adverse reactions to blood transfusion are also candidates for more sensitive antibody screening procedures. These patients may have formed antibodies that are too weak to be demonstrable using routine testing procedures. Reexposure to the corresponding antigens on donor red cells may cause a rapid rise in antibody titer and subsequent destruction of circulating incompatible cells. These additional factors as well as many others may be kept in mind when dealing with unexpected serologic results.

Antibody screening tests should demonstrate the presence of all potentially significant antibodies in the patient's serum and rapidly indicate the need for further studies. All antibodies encountered must be identified in order to determine potential clinical significance and to allow a logical decision to be made as to whether there is a need to select antigen-negative units for transfusion.

SELECTION OF APPROPRIATE DONOR UNITS

In almost all cases, blood and blood components of the patient's own ABO and Rh group should be selected for transfusion. When blood and blood components of the patient's type are unavailable or when some other reason precludes their use, units selected must lack any antigen against which the patient has a significant antibody. It is completely acceptable, however, to use blood and blood components that do not contain all of the antigens carried on the patient's own RBCs (e.g., group A or B packed RBCs can be safely given to a group AB recipient). When transfusions of an ABO group different from the recipient must be given, packed RBCs must be used rather than whole blood, which contains plasma antibodies that are incompatible with the patient's RBCs. Group O packed RBCs can be safely used for all patients; however, conservation of a limited supply of group O blood should dictate its use for patients of other ABO types only in special circumstances. If ABO-specific blood is not available or is in less than adequate supply, alternate blood groups are chosen as summarized in Table 12–2.

Rh-negative blood can be given to Rh-positive patients; however, good inventory management again should conserve this limited resource for use in Rh-negative recipients. However, if the Rh-negative unit is near expiration, the unit should be given rather than wasted. Rh-positive blood should not be given to Rh-negative women of childbearing age. Transfusion of Rh-negative male patients and female patients beyond menopause with Rh-positive blood is acceptable as long as no preformed anti-D is demonstrable in their sera. About 80 percent of Rh-negative patients who receive 200 ml or more of Rh-positive blood may respond to such a transfusion by producing anti-D.[35] However, this outcome must sometimes be weighed against the alternatives of not transfusing at all if the supply of Rh-negative has been exhausted. If the formation of anti-D is unlikely to be of great significance, such as in an Rh-negative elderly surgical patient, use of Rh-positive blood is judicious in the opinion of many technologists. In these situations, approval by or

TABLE 12–2 CHOICE OF ALTERNATIVE BLOOD GROUPS WHEN ABO IDENTICAL DONORS ARE NOT AVAILABLE

Patient's Blood Group	Alternative Blood Group (Given as Packed Cells)
O	None
A	O
B	O
AB	A, B, O*

Adapted from AABB Technical Manual, ed 9. American Association of Blood Banks, Arlington, VA, 1985.

*Packed cell components of any group are acceptable, but only one of the three should be used for a given patient, if possible. Group A is more readily available and thus preferred over group B.

notification of the blood bank's medical director is necessary, according to the laboratory's standard operating procedure.

When an unexpected antibody is found in the patient's serum during antibody screening, randomly selected donor units may be crossmatched with the patient's serum. This may, in fact, help to identify the unexpected antibody. If a clinically significant antibody is identified, the compatible units may be phenotyped with commercial antiserum to verify that they are antigen negative. There is no need to provide antigen-negative RBCs for patients whose sera contain antibodies that are reactive only below 37°C, inasmuch as these antibodies are incapable of causing significant RBC destruction in vivo. Significant or potent examples of anti-P_1, anti -Le^a, anti-Le^b, and other typically cold reactive antibodies in patients' sera can be used to select appropriate donor units that are crossmatch compatible in tests conducted at 37°C.[36]

Potent examples of IgG, warm reactive antibodies in patients' sera, can also be used to select suitable donor units by direct testing. Commercially prepared typing reagents must be used to select blood for patients whose sera contain weak examples of antibodies active at 37°C, antibodies that react well only with cell samples carrying homozygous representation of the corresponding antigens, and for patients whose sera no longer exhibit demonstrable in vitro reactivity but which previously were known to contain clinically significant IgG antibodies such as anti-Jk^a, and anti-K, or anti-E.

Donor units should be selected so that the RBCs are of appropriate age for the patient's needs and will not expire before use. For efficient inventory management, units that will definitely be transfused should be selected from units close to their expiration date.

Packed RBC units should be selected if the patient does not require volume, only increased oxygen-carrying capacity. Whole blood should be reserved for those occasions when the patient genuinely needs volume expansion, such as in major trauma or surgery. Even in these cases, however, support with appropriate crystalloid solutions and blood components usually produces results equal or superior to those achieved by transfusion of whole blood. Donor units should be examined visually before compatibility testing for unusual appearance, correct labeling, and hermetic seal integrity. Donor units showing abnormal color change, turbidity, clots, incomplete or improper labeling information, or leakage of any sort should be returned to the collecting facility.

CROSSMATCHING

The terms compatibility test and crossmatch are sometimes used interchangeably; they should be clearly differentiated. A crossmatch is only part of a compatibility test. Compatibility testing in the United States consists of (1) review of patient's past blood bank history and records; (2) ABO and Rh grouping of the recipient and donor; (3) antibody screening of the recipient's and donor's serum; and finally (4) the crossmatch. The crossmatch has recently undergone much scrutiny, and some workers believe it should be eliminated entirely. However, to many blood bankers the crossmatch still has a definite role.

It is important to note that direct crossmatching preceded antibody screening as part of patient pretransfusion testing by several decades. Selected RBCs were first used in some laboratories during the late 1950s to screen sera from donors.[37,38] Separate antibody screening of patient sera was not popularized as an addition to crossmatching until the early 1960s, when phenotyped RBCs for this purpose were marketed commercially. By that time, direct crossmatching was firmly entrenched as a routine procedure that was necessary to ensure the well-being of the recipient. As early as 1964, however, Grove-Rasmussen[39] questioned the need for an AHG test as part of the crossmatch when antibody screening test results were negative.

Considering that more than 99 percent of significant antibodies in patients' sera will be detected by adequate antibody screening procedures, what then is the value of performing crossmatching between patient and donor samples? Two main functions of the crossmatch test can be cited:

1. It is a final check of ABO compatibility between donor and patient.
2. It may detect the presence of an antibody in the patient's serum that will react with antigens on the donor RBCs but that was not detected in antibody screening because the corresponding antigen was lacking from the screening cells.

The current AABB standards[40] state that tests to detect ABO incompatibility suffice if (1) no clinically significant antibodies were detected in the antibody screening process and (2) no record exists of the detection of clinically significant unexpected antibodies. Elimination of advance crossmatch testing for patients undergoing surgical procedures in which blood is unlikely to be used has been implemented successfully in many facilities, using the "type and screen" approach or the abbreviated crossmatch discussed in more detail later in this chapter.

Major and Minor Crossmatch Tests

Historically, crossmatch testing procedures have been divided into two parts: the major crossmatch test, consisting of mixing the patient's serum with donor RBCs; and the minor crossmatch test, consisting of mixing the donor's plasma with patient RBCs. As the names imply, the major test is much more critical for ensuring safe transfusion than the minor test.

The minor crossmatch test has been completely eliminated in most blood banks, because donor samples are screened beforehand for the more common antibodies. The presence of a low-incidence antibody in the donor's plasma probably would not cause a transfusion reaction because it would be diluted in the recipient's plasma. It is more important to simplify procedures by eliminating the minor crossmatch rather than to perform it in the belief that it might show some unlikely antibody-antigen reaction.[41]

Methods for Major Crossmatch Tests

Many different procedures can be used for crossmatch testing. The objective of testing is to select donor units able to provide maximal benefit to the patient. This fact should be kept in mind when developing the test protocol. Nothing but delay results from detection of in vitro incompatibilities that are not likely to occur in vivo or use of complicated methods that require several tubes for each unit tested. For this reason, incubation of tests at room temperature has been eliminated in many facilities, and a simple crossmatch test of one tube per unit has become the standard. A sample procedure for a one-tube compatibility test is given in Procedural Appendix 2 of this chapter.[42]

Crossmatch methods can be categorized by the test phase in which the procedure ends.

Immediate Spin Crossmatch As mentioned previously, when no clinically significant antibodies are detected nor are there previous records of such antibodies, a serologic test to detect ABO incompatibility is sufficient. This is accomplished by simply mixing patient's serum with donor cells and centrifuging immediately (i.e., immediate spin). Absence of hemolysis or agglutination indicates compatibility.

The type and screen coupled with an immediate spin crossmatch is referred to as an abbreviated crossmatch. Studies of the use of an abbreviated crossmatch show that it is a safe and effective method of pretransfusion testing. It has been calculated to be 99.9 percent effective in preventing the occurrence of an incompatible transfusion.[43] Walker[44] was able to show that the frequency with which an incompatible antiglobulin crossmatch follows a negative screen is very low—0.06 percent. Other studies confirm its safety with similar statistics.[45-48]

Recently, however, the ability of this method to detect all ABO incompatibilities has been challenged.[49] False reactions may be seen in the presence of other immediate spin reactive antibodies (e.g., autoanti-I), in patients with hyperimmune ABO antibodies, when the procedure is not performed correctly (i.e., delay in centrifugation or reading), when rouleaux is observed, or when infants' specimens are tested. Adding ethylenediaminetetra-acetic acid (EDTA) to the test system has been reported to eliminate some of the false-negative reactions, thus improving the sensitivity of the immediate spin crossmatch.[50]

A recent report by Riccardi et al.[51] indicated that an electronic (computer) crossmatch to detect ABO incompatibilities was as safe as the serologic immediate spin test. The computer crossmatch compares recent ABO serologic results and interpretations on file for both the donor and the patient being matched and determines compatibility based on this comparison.

These investigators noted that to decrease the risk of ABO incompatibility further, duplicate patient ABO and Rh groupings were needed.[51] Subsequently, Butch et al.[52] anticipating changes in the AABB standards, produced a model computer crossmatch. Annual savings, reduced sample requirements, reduced handling of biologic materials, and elimination of false reactions associated with the immediate spin crossmatch were additional benefits identified as the result of using the computer crossmatch.[52]

The AABB has indeed changed its standards, which now include statements recognizing the computer crossmatch as an acceptable crossmatch method. The electronic crossmatch may replace the immediate spin crossmatch only when the patient's ABO group has been determined on two occasions. One of the determinations must be done on the current sample. Having a previous ABO result on file many serve as the second occasion. When no results are on file, a second technologist may test the same sample or a second current sample may need to be tested. Additionally, the computer system must be validated to show that it will detect data entry discrepances and ABO incompatibilities between patient and donor.[53]

Antiglobulin Crossmatch The antiglobulin crossmatch procedure begins in the same manner as the immediate spin crossmatch, continues to a 37°C incubation, and finishes with an AHG test. Several methods are used to enhance antigen-antibody reactions. Albumin may be added before incubation at 37°C to enhance reactivity of some antibodies. Low ionic strength solution (LISS) or polyethylene glycol (PEG) may be added in place of albumin to facilitate complexing of antigens and antibodies.[54] For greatest sensitivity, an AHG reagent containing both anti-IgG and anticomplement may be selected for the final phase of this crossmatch method. However, many laboratories routinely use anti-IgG AHG reagents for reasons previously discussed.

The polybrene (P-AHG) test has been shown to be a rapid and sensitive crossmatch technique.[55-57] It has been used as a method for detecting ABO incompatibility when accompanied by a carefully performed negative antibody screen on the patient.

An autocontrol consisting of the patient's own cells and serum may be tested in parallel with the crossmatch test. Although current AABB standards no longer require an autocontrol, some workers still find it useful. Perkins and associates[58] calculated the predictive value of a positive autocontrol (3.6 percent) when the antibody screen was negative and decided to continue using the autocontrol in pretransfusion testing. Results of the autocontrol help clarify possible explanations for positive results in the crossmatches and are discussed later in this chapter.

Interpretation of Results

Tubes should be carefully labeled so that the contents can be identified at any stage of the procedure. After centrifugation of tubes, the supernatant should be examined for hemolysis, which must be interpreted as a positive result. Results should be read against a white or lighted background, and a magnifying mirror or hand lens can be used to facilitate reading if desired. The button of cells should be gently resuspended. A "wiggle-and-tilt" method of resuspension is ideal. Violent shaking or tapping of the tubes may yield false-negative results, as it may disrupt fragile agglutinates. A jagged button edge indicates a positive result, whereas a smooth button edge and swirling free cells indicate the absence of a demonstrable antigen-antibody interaction. After the button has been completely resuspended, the contents of the tube should be interpreted and positive results graded according to a scale used by all technologists in a facility. Uniform grading of reactions allows retrospective analysis of results by supervisory staff as well as comparison of serial results obtained on samples collected from the same patient. Results can be examined microscopically for verification if desired. Review **Color Plate 2** for the grading of typical agglutination reactions.

According to the CFR,[59] all results must be recorded immediately in a permanent ledger using a logical system that allows them to be easily recalled, and actual observations as well as interpretations must be recorded. All work should be signed or initialed by the technologist performing the test. If an incompatibility is found, the record should clearly show the location of results of follow-up studies and additional testing performed.

Resolving Incompatibilities in the Major Crossmatch

The primary objective of the major crossmatch test is to detect the presence of antibodies in the recipient's serum, including anti-A and anti-B, that could destroy transfused RBCs. A positive result in the major crossmatch test requires explanation, and the patient should not receive the transfusion until the cause of the incompatibility has been fully determined. When the crossmatch test result is positive, the results of the autocontrol and antibody screening test should be reviewed to identify patterns that may help determine the cause of the problem.

Causes of Positive Results in the Major Crossmatch

A positive result in the major crossmatch test may be caused by any of the following:

1. **Incorrect ABO grouping of the patient or donor.** ABO grouping should be immediately repeated, especially if strong incompatibility is noted in a reading taken after immediate spin. Samples that bear undisputable identity with the original patient sample and the donor bag should be used for retesting.
2. **An alloantibody in the patient's serum reacting with the corresponding antigen on donor RBCs.** The autocontrol tube will react negatively unless the patient has been recently transfused with incompatible cells. If the antibody screening test result is positive, panel studies should allow identification of antibody specificity, which then permits selection of units lacking the offending antigens for compatibility testing. Chapter 11 provides further discussion of antibody detection and identification as well as examples for study.
   a. If RBCs of all donors tested are incompatible with the patient's serum and the antibody screening test result is positive, suspect either an antibody directed against a high-frequency antigen or multiple antibodies in the patient's serum. Consult a reference laboratory if you are unable to identify the specificity.

      Note: The patient's ABO-compatible brothers and sisters may lack the antigen(s) to which the patient has been sensitized and may be excellent potential donors in an emergency.
   b. If the result of the antibody screening test is negative and only one donor unit is incompatible, an antibody in the patient's serum may be directed against a relatively low-frequency antigen that is present on that donor's RBCs. Panel studies of the patient's serum will usually be noninformative, and identification of the antibody is academic if other compatible units are easily located.
   c. If the antibody screening test is negative, the patient's serum may contain either naturally occurring (e.g., anti-A_1) or passively acquired ABO agglutinins. Passive acquisition of anti-A, -B, or -A,B may occur after transfusion of non-ABO specific blood products (e.g., platelets) or after organ (e.g., liver) or bone marrow transplantation. Checking the serum grouping result to confirm the presence of an unexpected reaction with A_1 cells or checking the patient's transfusion and transplantation histories, or both, will be helpful in the investigation of these cases.
3. **An autoantibody in the patient's serum reacting with the corresponding antigen on donor RBCs.** The autocontrol tube will react positively. The antibody screening test and tests of the patient's serum with donor cells will show positive results. Most autoantibodies have specificity for antigens of relatively high frequency. Panel studies are important to assess whether underlying alloantibodies are also present. Techniques for management of patients with autoantibodies include autoadsorption of the patient's serum to remove autoantibody activity. Compatibility testing should then be performed using the autoadsorbed serum. Chapter 21 provides further discussion of autoantibodies and their serologic activity.
4. **Prior coating of the donor RBCs with protein, resulting in a positive AHG test result.** If one

isolated positive result is obtained, a DAT should be performed on the donor's RBCs. Donor cells that demonstrate a positive DAT result will be incompatible with all recipients tested in the AHG phase because the cells are already coated with immunoglobulin or complement or both.

5. **Abnormalities in the patient's serum.**

   a. Imbalance of the normal ratio of albumin and gamma globulin (A/G ratio), as in diseases such as myeloma and macroglobulinemia, may cause RBCs to stick together on their flat sides, giving the appearance of stacks of coins when viewed microscopically. This is referred to as rouleaux formation (see **Color Plate 2J**). This property of the serum will affect all tests, including the autocontrol. Strong rouleaux may mimic true agglutination; however, clumps are refractile when viewed under the microscope. Rouleaux formation is usually strongest after 37°C incubation, but does not persist through washing before the AHG test. Problems with rouleaux can often be resolved using the saline replacement technique.[60]

   b. The presence of high molecular weight dextrans or other plasma expanders may cause false-positive results in compatibility and other tests. All tests, including the autocontrol, are generally affected equally. Saline replacement may be useful to resolve the problem. However, current studies indicate that the use of dextran does not interfere with pretransfusion testing.[61]

   c. An antibody against additives in the albumin reagents may cause false-positive results in compatibility tests. Rarely, a patient's serum reacts against the albumin in testing reagents. This occurs when the patient has antibodies to the stabilizing substances, such as caprylate, added to the albumin reagents.[62] Thus, caprylate-free albumin solutions should be used in the testing.

6. **Contaminants in the test system.** Dirty glassware, bacterial contamination of samples, chemical or other contaminants in saline, and fibrin clots may produce positive compatibility test results.

Refer to Table 12–3 for suggestions for investigations of incompatible major crossmatches.

Compatibility Testing in Special Circumstances

EMERGENCIES

Urgent need for transfusion may preclude the performance of usual testing protocol. Several approaches can be used in these circumstances. Some laboratorians use an "emergency" compatibility test-

---

TABLE 12–3 INVESTIGATION OF INCOMPATIBLE MAJOR CROSSMATCHES

Observations	Possible Interpretations	Comments
Major crossmatch: + Autocontrol: − Antibody screen: −	Incorrect ABO grouping of patient or donor	Repeat ABO grouping; verify identity of sample.
	Patient's serum may contain an ABO antibody	Check patient's sample for subgroups, check patient's transfusion, and check transplantation histories.
	Alloantibody in patient's serum reacting with antigen donor's red cells but not present on screening cells	Perform antibody identification tests on patient's serum and repeat crossmatch using units negative for the corresponding antigen. If studies are noninformative and patient is incompatible with only 1 unit, locate other compatible units.
	Donor unit may have a positive DAT result	Perform DAT on donor unit; if result is positive, do not use the unit.
Major crossmatch: + Autocontrol: − Antibody screen: +	Alloantibody in patient's serum reacting with antigens on donor's cells and screening cells	Perform antibody identification studies on patient's serum and repeat crossmatch using units negative for the corresponding antigen. If unable to identify antibody specificity, consult a reference laboratory.
Major crossmatch: + Autocontrol: + Antibody screen: +	Both autoantibody and alloantibody may be present in the patient's serum	Perform autoadsorption of patient serum to remove autoantibody (if not recently transfused), perform antibody identification tests, repeat compatibility tests using autoadsorbed serum.
	Abnormalities in patient's serum owing to: 1. Imbalance of A/G ratio	1. If rouleaux formation is seen, use saline replacement technique.
	2. Plasma expanders	2. Obtain new specimen.
	3. Caprylate antibodies	3. Use caprylate-free reagents.
	4. Contaminants	4. Repeat tests using fresh saline, new bottles of reagent, clean test tubes.

ing procedure that employs a shortened incubation time, often with addition of LISS to speed antigen-antibody complexing. Others maintain that regular procedures should be used in all circumstances, and blood should be issued before completion of the standard compatibility testing procedure, if necessary. They feel that there is greater danger is using an unfamiliar procedure under pressure than in releasing blood without completed testing. Although both lines of reasoning have merit, the ideal compromise may be to develop regular testing procedures that are concise, so that they can be used in emergency and routine situations alike. Whatever the approach, the protocol for handling emergencies must be decided in advance of the situation and be familiar to all staff in the transfusion service. Adequate pretransfusion samples should be collected before infusion of any donor blood so that compatibility testing, antibody screening, and identification studies, if necessary, can be performed subsequently.

If blood must be issued in an emergency, the patient's ABO and Rh group should be determined, so that group-compatible blood can be given. In extreme emergencies, when there is no time to obtain and test a sample, group O, Rh-negative packed cells can be used. If the patient is Rh negative and large amounts of blood are likely to be needed, a decision should be made rapidly as to whether inventory allows and the situation demands transfusion of Rh-negative blood. Conversion to Rh positive is best made immediately if the patient is a male or is a woman beyond childbearing age. Injections of Rh immunoglobulin to prevent formation of anti-D may sometimes be appropriate after the crisis has been resolved. This product is discussed in detail in Chapter 20.

Accurate records must be maintained of all units issued in the emergency. A conspicuous tie tag or label must be placed on each unit indicating that compatibility testing was not completed before release of the unit, and the physician must sign a release authorizing and accepting responsibility for the use of incompletely tested products, according to the CFR.[63] Compatibility testing should be completed according to the chosen protocol, and any incompatible result should be reported immediately to the patient's physician and the blood bank medical director.

TRANSFUSION OF NON–GROUP-SPECIFIC BLOOD

When units of an ABO group other than the patient's own type have been transfused, additional units should be selected after analysis of a freshly drawn patient sample for the presence of unexpected anti-A and anti-B in the recipient's serum. Selection of additional units should always be based on this parameter. When serum from the freshly drawn sample is compatible in the AHG phase with RBCs of the patient's own ABO group, then group-specific blood may be given for the transfusion. If the AHG phase reveals incom-

patibility, then additional transfusions should be of the alternate blood group. For example, if a group A patient has been given a large number of units of group O packed cells, anti-A may be demonstrable in the serum in the AHG phase. Group O units should therefore be used for any additional transfusions.

COMPATIBILITY TESTING FOR TRANSFUSION OF PLASMA PRODUCTS

Compatibility testing procedures are not required for transfusion of plasma products. However, for transfusion of large volumes of plasma and plasma products, a crossmatch test between the donor plasma and crossmatch RBCs may be performed, although the current standards do not require a crossmatch test. The primary purpose for testing is to detect ABO incompatibility between donor and patient; therefore, an immediate spin crossmatch is sufficient.

INTRAUTERINE TRANSFUSIONS AND TRANSFUSION OF THE INFANT

Blood for intrauterine transfusion must be selected to be compatible with maternal antibodies capable of crossing the placenta. If the ABO and Rh groups of the fetus have been determined following amniocentesis, chorionic villus sampling, or percutaneous umbilical blood sampling, then group-specific blood could be given provided there is no fetomaternal ABO or Rh incompatibility. If the ABO and Rh groups of the fetus are not known, then group O, Rh-negative RBCs should be selected for the intrauterine transfusion. The group O, Rh-negative cells must lack any other antigens against which the mother's serum contains transfusion (e.g., anti-Kell, anti-Jk^a). Compatibility testing is performed using the mother's serum sample.

Blood for an exchange or regular transfusion of an infant (less than 4 months old) should similarly be compatible with any maternal antibodies that have entered the infant's circulation and are reactive at 37°C. Blood of the infant's ABO and Rh group can be used, provided the ABO and Rh groups are not involved in fetomaternal incompatibility as judged from studies of maternal and cord samples. An initial pretransfusion specimen from the infant must be typed for ABO and Rh groups (only anti-A and anti-B reagents are required to be used for ABO grouping).[64] Antibody detection testing can be performed using the maternal serum or, alternatively, using the infant's serum (e.g., cord serum) or an eluate prepared from the infant's RBCs, or both. In addition, when cells selected for transfusion are not group O, the infant's serum or plasma must be tested to demonstrate the absence of anti-A (using A_1 cells) and anti-B. This testing must include an AHG phase.[65] It is unnecessary to repeat these pretransfusion tests during any one hospital ad-

TABLE 12-4 **COMPATIBILITY TESTING FOR INFANTS**

Once per Admission

Routine
ABO
Rh
Antibody screen
   Using maternal serum *or*
   Using infant's serum, especially when:
      1. No maternal specimen is available
      2. Mother has clinically insignificant antibodies *or*
   Using infant's eluate

Additional
IAT using infant serum and A_1 or B cells or both
   Cells can be reagent or donor (i.e., major crossmatch)
   Must be done if non–group O cells will be transfused
Antigen typing donor unit
   While infant antibody screen is positive
   Donor units must lack antigen corresponding to antibody

Every 3 Days

Same tests as earlier, when:
   ABO- or Rh-incompatible units are transfused *and/or*
   Unexpected antibodies are demonstrated via antibody screen

IAT = indirect antiglobulin test.

mission, provided the infant received only ABO- and Rh-compatible transfusions and had no unexpected antibodies in the serum or plasma.[66] The presence of unexpected clinically significant antibodies, including anti-A and anti-B, indicates that cells lacking the corresponding antigen must be selected for transfusion until the antibody is no longer demonstrable in the infant's serum.[67] A crossmatch is no longer required in these situations. Table 12–4 summarizes the compatibility tests for infants (less than 4 months old) and how frequently they must be performed.

For both intrauterine and infant (less than 4 months old) transfusions, blood should be as fresh as possible and no older than 7 days to reduce the risk and to increase the benefits of the transfusion. Refer to Chapter 20 for additional information on hemolytic disease of the newborn (HDN).

MASSIVE TRANSFUSIONS

When the amount of whole blood or packed cell components infused within 24 hours approaches or exceeds the patient's total blood volume, the compatibility testing procedure may be shortened or eliminated at the discretion of the transfusion service physician following written policy guidelines.[68]

If the patient is known to have an antibody that may be clinically significant, all units infused should be tested and found to lack the offending antigen. The antibody in the patient's serum may not be demonstrable because of dilution with large volumes of plasma and other fluids. However, a rapid rise in antibody titer and subsequent destruction of donor RBCs may occur, if antigen-positive units are infused.

SPECIMENS WITH PROLONGED CLOTTING TIME

Difficulties may be encountered in testing blood samples from patients who have prolonged clotting times caused by coagulation abnormalities associated with disease or medications. A fibrin clot may form spontaneously when partially clotted serum is added to saline suspended screening or donor RBCs. Complete coagulation of these samples can often be prompted by addition of thrombin. One drop of thrombin, 50 units/ml, to 1 ml of plasma (or the amount of dry thrombin that will adhere to the end of an applicator stick) is usually sufficient to induce clotting.[69] A small amount of protamine sulfate can be added to counteract the effects of heparin in samples of blood collected from patients on this anticoagulant.[70]

AUTOLOGOUS TRANSFUSION

Autologous transfusion refers to the removal and storage of blood or components from a donor for the donor's own possible use at a later time, usually during or after a surgical procedure. The ABO and Rh groups of the units must be determined by the facility collecting the blood. Tests for unexpected antibodies and tests designed to prevent disease transmission are not required, when the blood will be used within the collecting facility.[71] These units must be labeled "For Autologous Use Only."[72]

According to AABB standards, the pretransfusion testing and identification of the recipient and the blood sample are required and must conform to the protocols mentioned earlier in this chapter. However, tests for unexpected antibodies in the recipient's serum or plasma and a crossmatch test are optional.

Limitations of Compatibility Testing Procedures

As mentioned in the introduction to this chapter, no current testing procedure can guarantee the fate of a unit of blood that is to be transfused. Even a compatible crossmatch cannot guarantee that the transfused red cells will survive normally in the recipient. Despite carefully performed in vitro testing, some compatible units will be hemolyzed in the patient. In some cases, even limited donor cell survival may help maintain a patient until the patient can begin to produce his or her own cells. Certainly no patient should be denied a transfusion if he or she needs one to survive, and donor cells that appear incompatible by in vitro testing procedures may, in fact, survive quite well in vivo.

In vivo compatibility can be determined using donor RBCs labeled with radioactive chromium (^{51}Cr) or technetium (^{99m}Tc) to measure the likelihood of successful transfusion when standard in vitro testing procedures are inconclusive.[73,74] If a transfusion is needed to save a patient's life and all units are incompatible, and if the ^{51}Cr studies indicate adequate survival of donor RBCs, then transfusion of an in vitro incompatible unit may need to be considered. This decision should be made in consultation with the blood bank medical director and the patient's physician. The blood should be transfused slowly and the patient monitored carefully.[75]

Effective Blood Use

Many blood bankers are keenly aware of the need to use blood efficiently, owing to limited blood resources and increasing demands for blood. Technologists observed that there were many surgical procedures, such as dilatation and curettage, and cholecystectomy, for which blood was routinely ordered but rarely used. Blood bankers also pointed out that for many other surgical procedures more units were ordered than used.

The maximum surgical blood order schedule (MSBOS) was developed to promote more efficient use of blood. The goal of MSBOS is to establish realistic blood ordering levels for certain procedures. Inasmuch as variation exists in the surgical requirements of institutions, the standard blood orders should be based on the transfusion pattern of each institution and should be agreed on by the staff surgeons, anesthesiologists, and the blood bank medical director. Table 12–5 provides a sample MSBOS.

Use of a type and screen policy is another method to manage blood inventory levels efficiently and to reduce blood banking operating costs.[76–78] With the type and screen methods, the patient's blood sample is completely tested for ABO and Rh groups and unexpected antibodies. The specimen is refrigerated for immediate crossmatching if the need arises. The blood bank must make sure appropriate donor blood is available in case it is needed. If the patient has blood group alloantibodies, donor blood lacking the corresponding antigens must be available and should be fully crossmatched before surgery or transfusion.

If this type and screen policy is part of the standard operating procedure and if blood is needed quickly, the blood bank must be prepared to release blood of the same ABO and Rh group of the patient and perform the immediate spin (or computer) phase of the crossmatch test before release of the unit, provided the patient has no unexpected antibodies. Once the blood is issued, both a 37°C incubation and an AHG crossmatch is performed using the same tube employed for the immediate spin crossmatch, provided the AHG crossmatch is the standard protocol used by the laboratory. If either the 37°C incubation or the AHG phase of testing reacts positively, the patient's physician is notified immediately and the transfusion of the unit of blood is stopped.

TABLE 12–5 **TRANSFUSION SERVICE GUIDELINES FOR ELECTIVE SURGICAL PROCEDURES**

Type of Surgery	Transfusion Guidelines
General	
Aneurysm resection	6 units
Breast biopsy	T&S
Colon resection	2 units
Exploratory laparotomy	4 units
Femoropopliteal bypass	T&S
Hernia	T&S
Mastectomy—radical	1 unit
Pancreatectomy	4 units
Splenectomy	2 units
Thyroidectomy	T&S
Gynecologic	
AP repair	1 unit
D & C	T&S
Hysterectomy—abdominal	T&S
Hysterectomy—radical	2 units
Obstetric	
C-Section, hysterectomy	2 units
C-Section	T&S
L & D admission	HOLD
Thoracic-Cardiac	
Bypass procedures—adult	6 units
Bypass procedures—children	4 units
Vascular	
Aortic bypass	6 units
Endarterectomy	1 unit
Renal artery repair	6 units
Orthopedic	
Arthroscopy	T&S
Laminectomy	T&S
Spinal fusion	8 units
Total hip	5 units
Total knee	T&S
Urology	
Prostatectomy—perineal	2 units
Prostatectomy—transurethral	T&S
Renal transplant	2 units
TURP	T&S

From AABB Technical Manual, ed 10. Arlington, VA, 1990, p 516, with permission.

*T&S = Type and antibody screen

Reidentification of the Patient Before Transfusion

The final link in the chain of events leading to safe transfusion is reestablishment of the identity of the intended recipient and selected donor product. The same careful approach used to identify the patient before sample collection must be used to verify that the patient is indeed the same person who provided the blood for testing. In addition, the actual product and accompanying record of testing must be verified as relating to the same donor number.

After compatibility testing is completed, two special documents must be prepared in addition to the laboratory log entry. A statement of compatibility must be retained as part of the patient's permanent record if the blood is transfused, and a label or tie tag must be attached to the unit stating the identity of the intended recipient, the results of compatibility testing, and the donor number.[79] This identification must remain on the unit throughout the transfusion.

The original blood request form can be used conveniently to accomplish one or both of these record-keeping requirements. A multipart form is used in some facilities to record the entire history of pretransfusion testing and infusion of the unit. Useful information might include the initials or signature of the phlebotomist taking the sample, the donor numbers, results of compatibility testing, the initials or signature of the technologist performing the test, and the signatures of the persons who verify identity of the patient before infusion and who start the infusion. One copy of the form can be placed on the patient's chart after the transfusion is completed and the other returned to the blood bank, if desired, for filing. The last copy of the form might be printed on heavier stock and perforated so that it can be torn off and attached to the unit in the laboratory. The most important feature of this system is that the patient's nameplate impression, rather than a handwritten transcription, identifies all forms used to identify the patient-donor combination.

Other useful systems, mentioned earlier in this chapter, employ numbered strips or other unique coding systems that can be attached to the patient's wristband and to the compatibility form and donor unit. Bar-coded identification symbols verified by portable laser scanner devices may be the system of choice in the near future for linking sample, patient, and donor products.

Whatever system is used, the information should be verified at least twice before infusion of the product actually takes place. A copy of the original blood requisition form, placed on the patient's chart after samples are collected, can be used as the request for release of the units from the blood bank. This allows another check of the nameplate impressions on all forms.

Before blood is taken from the blood bank to the patient treatment area, the following records must be checked: ABO and Rh groupings, clinically significant unexpected antibodies, and adverse reactions to transfusion.[80] In addition, the person releasing and the person accepting the units should verify agreement between the donor numbers and ABO and Rh groups on the compatibility form and on the products themselves. The unit should also be inspected visually for any abnormalities in appearance indicating contamination. If any abnormality is seen, the unit should not be issued unless specifically authorized by the medical director.[81]

Before transfusion is initiated, a reliable professional (and preferably two professionals) must once again verify identity of the patient and donor products. A system of positive patient identification by comparison of wristband identification and compati-

bility forms must be followed strictly. This is the most critical and yet the most fallible check because the transfusion may occur in the operating suite or emergency room, where the person responsible for identification may be involved with many other duties as well.

If a unit is returned to the blood bank for any reason, within the specified time frame for that laboratory, it should not be reissued if the container closure was opened or if the unit was allowed to warm above 10°C or to cool below 1°C.[82]

The Future of Compatibility Testing

Modern transfusion medicine is a rapidly progressing science. Recent technologic advances will certainly affect the future practice of blood banking.

Recent developments include the use of RBC substitutes such as modified hemoglobin solutions, currently under investigation.[83,84] These substitutes can provide oxygen-carrying capacity and, because they are biologically inert and nonimmunogenic, can be administered with no requirements for crossmatching. They have been used in coronary angioplasty procedures[85] and could be used instantly at the scene of an accident or in the emergency room.[86] However, further research is needed to develop viable substitutes for blood products, and a range of products targeted at specific clinical indications, rather than one generic product, will most likely emerge from this research.

The continued use and development of monoclonal antibodies is having a decisive impact on transfusion medicine and patient care. Progress in the knowledge of blood group substances may result in the biochemical modification of all non-O blood groups to a "phenotypically universal donor blood."[87] This could possibly solve the problem of disproportions in certain blood group supplies.

Automation with pretransfusion testing instruments, such as continuous flow and batch analyzers, has streamlined compatibility testing, especially in large blood centers. Two of the most successful approaches have employed microplates to perform either liquid agglutination tests or solid-phase RBC adherence tests. These methods provide efficient and economic compatibility testing to process large numbers of donor specimens.[88] Similar innovations are emerging to streamline blood banking services in hospital transfusion services.

The technologies of galvanic testing and gel testing are in the development stages. With a galvanic biosensor, the energy exploited in an antigen-antibody reaction may be measured.[89] This electrochemical procedure could be applied to all immunohematologic tests dependent on antigen-antibody binding, and subsequently to automation.

Europeans and Canadians currently use a gel test for blood typing and for direct and indirect antiglobulin tests, including the crossmatch. The gel test is sensitive for both antigen testing and antibody detection, is reproducible, and has the potential to be converted to automation.[90,91] Commercially prepared gel test kits are not yet available in the United States.

Dipstick tests for determining ABO blood groups represent an important step toward streamlining services for the hospital transfusion service. These tests, which are based on the principles of dot immunobinding assays, have sensitivity and specificity equal to those of conventional agglutination tests and are fast, stable, inexpensive, and easy to interpret.[92,93]

Researchers from England have identified a dry plate method of ABO and Rh grouping for use in the field or at the patient's bedside. This method, in which monoclonal blood grouping antibodies are dried in a microplate and rehydrated before use, is 99.8 percent accurate and may best be used in developing countries lacking effective refrigeration and in situations requiring point-of-care testing (e.g., trauma sites).[94]

Preparing for clinical care in space, National Aeronautics and Space Administration (NASA) scientists showed that ABO and Coombs-sensitized standard blood grouping tests can be performed under microgravity. This was done using a closed self-operating system that automatically performed the tests and fixed the results onto filter paper for analysis on earth. Agglutinates were smaller than usual; however, reaction end points were clear.[95] While these researchers noted that additional experiments in space were needed to confirm and quantify their results, these preliminary findings indicate yet another method to perform compatibility testing that is "out of this world."

Perhaps, in what may further seem to be like a scene from a science fiction movie, all aspects of patient care, including compatibility testing, may be computerized. In addition to performing an electronic crossmatch, future computer systems will include electronic identification of the patient, automated testing, and electronic transfer of data. The success of this system lies on interfacing automated testing instruments with bar-code readers and a laboratory computer. The advantages of the system include the issue of blood products that are as safe as, if not safer than, current methods of compatibility testing, and reduction of costs and workload.

Our knowledge of compatibility testing is in a dynamic state, and we look forward to continuing developments in technical procedures to streamline and safeguard transfusion practice. The challenge of modern blood banking will be to merge new technology with the assurance of beneficial results and positive outcomes for the patient.

Review Questions

1. Compatibility testing will:
   A. Prove that the donor's plasma is free of all irregular antibodies
   B. Detect most irregular antibodies on the donor's RBCs that are reactive with patient's serum
   C. Detect most errors in the ABO groupings
   D. Ensure complete safety of the transfusion

2. Which of the following is not true of rouleaux formation?
   A. It is a stacking of RBCs to form aggregates.
   B. It can usually be dispersed by adding saline.
   C. It occurs in conditions in which the albumin-globulin serum protein balance is disturbed.
   D. It can occur in normal blood owing to the presence of multiple antibodies.

3. What type of blood should be given in an emergency transfusion when there is no time to type the recipient's sample?
   A. O Rh(D) negative whole blood
   B. O Rh(D) positive whole blood
   C. O Rh(D) positive packed cells
   D. O Rh(D) negative packed cells

4. A patient developed an anti-Jk^a 5 years ago. The antibody screen is negative now. To obtain suitable blood for transfusion, the best procedure is to:
   A. Type the patient for the Jk^a antigen as an added part to the crossmatch procedure.
   B. Crossmatch donors with the patient's serum and release the compatible units for transfusion to the patient.
   C. Type the donor units for the Jk^a antigen and crossmatch the Jk^a-negative units for the patient.
   D. Crossmatch the patient with type O Rh-negative, low-titer donor units, because the patient has developed an anti-Jk^a antibody and is a prime candidate to develop many other blood group antibodies.

5. A 26-year-old woman with group B Rh(D)-negative blood requires a transfusion. There are no type B Rh(D)-negative donor units available. Which of the following should be chosen for transfusion?
   A. A Rh(D)-negative whole blood
   B. O Rh(D)-negative red cells
   C. AB Rh(D)-negative whole blood
   D. A Rh(D)-negative red cells

6. If all the crossmatches and screening cells react positively but the autocontrol reacts negatively, the cause could be:
   a. A mixture of antibodies
   b. An antibody to a high-frequency antigen
   c. An antibody to a low-frequency antigen
   A. a and c
   B. a, b, and c

C. c only

D. a and b only

7. In crossmatching 5 units of packed cells on a patient, 4 units were compatible and results of both the autocontrol and the antibody screen were negative, but 1 unit was weakly incompatible on the major side of the crossmatch at the AHG phase. What is the most probable explanation for this problem?
   A. A high-frequency antigen-antibody reaction occurred.
   B. The patient had a positive DAT result.
   C. The donor unit had a positive DAT result.
   D. A caprylate antibody is suspected.

8. What percentage of Rh-negative individuals would be expected to develop anti-D after transfusion with one unit of Rh-positive blood?
   A. 0 to 25 percent
   B. 26 to 50 percent
   C. 51 to 75 percent
   D. 76 to 85 percent

9. Predict compatibility or incompatibility for the following situation. (Assume the patient has negative antibody screen and autocontrol results.)

	Group	Rho(D)
Patient	B	Positive
Donor	O	Positive

   A. Compatible major side crossmatch
   B. Compatible minor side crossmatch
   C. Incompatible major side crossmatch
   D. Not enough information to predict

10. Blood donor and recipient samples used in crossmatching must be stored for a minimum of _____ days following transfusion.
    A. 2
    B. 5
    C. 7
    D. 10

11. Which of the following is *true* regarding compatibility testing for infants under age 4 months?
    A. A DAT is required.
    B. A crossmatch is not needed when unexpected antibodies are present.
    C. Maternal serum cannot be used for antibody detection.
    D. To determine the infant's ABO group, RBCs must be tested with reagents anti-A, anti-B, and anti-A,B.

Answers to Review Questions

1. C (p 264)
2. D (p 267)
3. D (p 268)
4. C (p 264 and Table 12–3)
5. B (p 268 and Table 12–2)
6. D (p 266 and Table 12–3)
7. C (pp 266–277)
8. D (p 263)
9. A (p 263)
10. C (p 261)
11. B (pp 268–269 and Table 12–4)

References

1. Wiener, AS, and Peters, HR: Hemolytic reactions following transfusions of blood of the homologous group, with three cases in which the same agglutinogen was responsible. Ann Int Med 13:2304, 1940.
2. Sazama, K: Analysis of causes of blood transfusion fatalities. ASCP Teleconference, December 3, 1992.
3. Widmann, F (ed): Standards for Blood Banks and Transfusion Services, ed 15. American Association of Blood Banks, Bethesda, MD, 1993, p 23, F1.000.
4. Wenz, B, and Burns, ER: Improvement in transfusion safety using a new blood unit and patient identification system as part of safe transfusion practice. Transfusion 31:401, 1991.
5. Standards for Blood Banks and Transfusion Services, op cit, p 23, F2.000.
6. Ibid, p 24, G2.000.
7. Pittiglio, DH (ed): Modern Blood Banking and Transfusion Practices. FA Davis, Philadelphia, 1983, p 266.
8. Standards for Blood Banks and Transfusion Services, op cit, p 28, H2.000.
9. Code of Federal Regulations (CFR), Title 21, Food and Drug Administration. Office of the Federal Register, National Archives and Records Service, General Services Administration, revised April 1, 1992, Part 610, section 40; and Part 640, section 5.
10. Standards for Blood Banks and Transfusion Services, op cit, p 11, B5.000.
11. Ibid, p 12.
12. Ibid, p 24, G1.000.
13. Ibid, p 39, M1.300.
14. Ibid, p 24, G2.000.
15. White, WB, Issitt, CH, and McGuire, D: Evaluation of the use of albumin controls in Rh typing. Transfusion 14:67, 1974.
16. Standards for Blood Banks and Transfusion Services, op cit, p 24, G2.000.
17. Garratty, G: Mechanisms of immune red cell destruction, and red cell compatibility testing. Hum Pathol 14:204, 1983.
18. Giblett, ER: Blood group alloantibodies: An assessment to some laboratory practices. Transfusion 17:299, 1977.
19. Spielmann, W, and Seidl, S: Prevalence of irregular red cell antibodies and their significance in blood transfusion and antenatal care. Vox Sang 26:551, 1974.
20. Standards for Blood Banks and Transfusion Services, op cit, p 24, G2.000.
21. Engelfriet, CP, and Giles, CM: Working party on the standardization of antiglobulin reagents of the expert panel of serology. Vox Sang 38:178, 1980.
22. Petz, LD, and Garratty, G: Antiglobulin sera—past, present and future. Transfusion 18:257, 1978.
23. Wright, MS, and Issitt, PD: Anticomplement and the antiglobulin test. Transfusion 19:688, 1979.
24. Standards for Blood Banks and Transfusion Services, op cit, p 24, G2.000.
25. Beattie, KM: Control of the antigen-antibody ratio in antibody detection and compatibility test. Transfusion 20:277, 1980.
26. Hughes-Jones, NC, et al: Optimal conditions for detecting blood group antibodies by the antiglobulin test. In Pittiglio, DH

(ed): Modern Blood Banking and Transfusion Practices. FA Davis, Philadelphia, 1983, p 252.

27. Issitt, PD, and Issitt, CH: Applied Blood Group Serology, ed 2. Spectra Biologicals, Oxnard, CA, 1975, p 41.

28. Steane, EA: The interaction of antibodies with red cell surface antigens: Kinetics, noncovalent bonding and hemagglutination. In Dawson, RD (ed): Blood Bank Immunology. American Association of Blood Banks, Washington, DC, 1977, pp 61–63.

29. Stroup, M, and MacIlroy, M: Evaluation of the albumin antiglobulin technic in antibody detection. Transfusion 5:184, 1965.

30. Reckel, RP, and Harris, J: The unique characteristics of covalently polymerized bovine serum albumin solutions when used as antibody detection media. Transfusion 18:397, 1978.

31. Moulds, JJ: Multiple antibodies and antibodies to high incidence blood group factors. In Dawson, RB (ed): Troubleshooting the Crossmatch. American Association of Blood Banks, Washington, DC, 1977, pp 67–84.

32. McKeever, BG: Antibody screening and identification. In Treacy, M (ed): Pre-Transfusion Testing for the '80s. American Association of Blood Banks, Washington, DC, 1980, pp 409–450.

33. Issitt, PD: On the incidence of second antibody populations in the sera of women who have developed anti-Rh antibodies. Transfusion 5:355, 1965.

34. Issitt, PD, et al: Three examples of Rh-positive good responders to blood group antigens. Transfusion 13:316, 1972.

35. Mollison, PL: Blood Transfusion in Clinical Medicine, ed 7. Blackwell Scientific Publications, Oxford, 1983, p 353.

36. Walker, RH (ed): Technical Manual, ed 10. American Association of Blood Banks, Arlington, VA, 1990, p 194.

37. Mollison, PF: Factors determining the relative clinical importance of different blood group antibodies. Br Med Bull 15:92, 1959.

38. Giblett, ER: Blood group alloantibodies: An assessment of some laboratory practices. Transfusion 17:299, 1977.

39. Grove-Rasmussen, M: Routine compatibility testing: Standards of the AABB as applied to compatibility tests. Transfusion 4:200, 1964.

40. Standards for Blood Banks and Transfusion Services, op cit, pp 24–25, G3.000.

41. Weisz-Carrington, P: Principles of Clinical Immunohematology. Year Book Medical Publishers, Chicago, 1986, p 212.

42. Pittiglio, DH, op cit, p 266.

43. Henry, JB: Type and Screen. In Polesky, HF and Walker, RH (eds): Safety in Transfusion Practices, CAP Conference, Aspen, 1980. Skokie, IL, College of American Pathologists, 1982, p 191.

44. Walker, RH: On the safety of the abbreviated crossmatch. In Polesky, HF and Walker, RH (eds): Safety in Transfusion Practices, Aspen, 1980. Skokie, IL, College of American Pathologists, 1982, p 75.

45. Shulman, IA, et al: Experience with the routine use of an abbreviated crossmatch. Am J Clin Pathol 82:178, 1984.

46. Dodsworth, H, and Dudley, HAF: Increased efficiency of transfusion practice in routine surgery using pre-operative antibody screening and selective ordering with an abbreviated crossmatch. Br J Surg 72:102, 1985.

47. Garratty, G: Abbreviated pretransfusion testing (editorial). Transfusion 26:217, 1986.

48. Shulman, IA, et al: Experience with a cost-effective crossmatch protocol. JAMA 254:93, 1985.

49. Judd, WJ: Are there better ways than the crossmatch to demonstrate ABO incompatibility? (editorial) Transfusion 31:192, 1991.

50. Shulman, IA, and Calderon, C: Effect of delayed centrifugation or reading on the detection of ABO incompatibility by the immediate-spin crossmatch. Transfusion 31:197, 1991.

51. Riccardi, D, et al: Risk of ABO and non-ABO incompatibility by using type and screen and electronic crossmatch. (Abstract) Transfusion 31:60S, 1991.

52. Butch, SH, et al: The computer crossmatch. (abstract) Transfusion 32:5S, 1992.

53. Standards for Blood Banks and Transfusion Services, op cit, p 25, G3.000.

54. Slater, JL, et al: Evaluation of the polyethylene glycol-indirect antiglobulin test for routine compatibility testing. Transfusion 29:686, 1989.

55. Mentz, PD, and Anderson, G: Comparison of a manual hexadimethrine bromide-antiglobulin test with saline and albumin-antiglobulin tests for pretransfusion testing. Transfusion 27:134, 1987.

56. Steane, EA, et al: A proposal for compatibility testing incorporating the manual hexadimethrine bromide (Polybrene) test. Transfusion 25:540, 1985.

57. Mentz, PD, and Anderson, G, op cit.

58. Perkins, JT, et al: The relative utility of the autologous control and the antiglobulin test phase of the crossmatch. Transfusion 30:503, 1990.

59. CFR, op cit, Part 606, section 160.

60. Green, TS: Rouleaux and autoantibodies (or things that go bump in the night). In Treacy, M (ed): Pre-Transfusion Testing for the 80s. American Association of Blood Banks, Washington, DC, 1980, p 93.

61. Bartholomew, JR, et al: A prospective study of the effects of dextran administration on compatibility testing. Transfusion 26:431–433, 1986.

62. Golde, DW, et al: Serum agglutinins to commercially prepared albumin. In Weisz-Carrington, P: Principles of Clinical Immunohematology. Year Book Medical Publishers, Chicago, 1986, p 214.

63. CFR, op cit, Part 606, section 160.

64. Standards for Blood Banks and Transfusion Services, op cit, p 26, G6.100.

65. Ibid, p 26, G6.200; p 27, G6.300.

66. Ibid, p 26, G6.110; p 26, G6.210; p 27, G6.310.

67. Ibid, p 27, G6.320.

68. Ibid, p 26, G5.000.

69. General laboratory procedures: Treatment of incompletely clotted specimens. In Walker, RH (ed): Technical Manual. American Association of Blood Banks, Arlington, VA, 1990, p 523.

70. Ibid.

71. Standards for Blood Banks and Transfusion Services, op cit, p 36, L1.320.

72. Ibid, p 36, L1.400.

73. Mollison, PL: Blood Transfusion in Clinical Medicine, op cit, pp 606–608.

74. Holt, JT, et al: A technetium-99m red cell survival technique for in vivo compatibility testing. Transfusion 23:148, 1983.

75. Garratty, G: Mechanisms of immune red cell destruction and red cell compatibility testing. Hum Pathol 3:211, 1983.

76. Shulman, IA, et al: Experience with a cost-effective crossmatch protocol. JAMA 254:93, 1985.

77. Davis, SP, et al: Maximizing the benefits of type and screen by continued surveillance of transfusion practice. Am J Med Technol 49:579, 1983.

78. Issitt, PD: Applied Blood Group Serology, ed 3. Montgomery Scientific Publications, Miami, 1985, pp 489–492.

79. Standards for Blood Banks and Transfusion Services, op cit, p 28, H1.000.

80. Ibid.

81. Ibid, p 28, H3.000.

82. Ibid, p 28, H4.000.

83. Rudowski, W: Blood transfusion: Yesterday, today, and tomorrow. World J Surg 11:86, 1987.

84. Allen, RW, Kahn, RA, and Baldassare, JJ: Advances in the production of blood cell substitutes with alternate technologies. In Walls, CH, and McCarthy LJ (eds): New Frontiers in Blood Banking. American Association of Blood Banks, Arlington, VA, 1986, p 21.

85. Ibid.

86. Rudowski, op cit, p 88.

87. Greenwalt, TJ: Research in transfusion medicine. In Wallis, C and Simon, TL (eds): Educational Progress in Transfusion Medicine. American Association of Blood Banks, Arlington, VA, 1985, pp 55–69.

88. Plapp, V: New techniques for compatibility testing. Arch Pathol Lab Med 113(3):262, 1989.
89. Moulds, JJ: Galvanic testing. In Levitt, JS and Brecher, ME (eds): Emerging Trends in Technology. American Association of Blood Banks, Bethesda, MD, 1992, p 1–3.
90. LaPierre, Y, et al: The gel test: A new way to detect red cell antigen-antibody reactions. Transfusion 30:109, 1990.
91. Weiland, D: The gel technology—a new approach to blood group serology. In Levitt, JS and Brecher, ME (eds): Emerging Trends in Technology. American Association of Blood Banks, Bethesda, MD, 1992, p 3–1.
92. Plapp, FV, Rachel, JM, and Sinor, LT: Dipsticks for determining ABO blood groups. Lancet 1:1465, 1986.
93. Plapp, 1989, op cit.
94. Blakely, D, et al: Dry instant blood typing plate for bedside use. Lancet 336:854, 1990.
95. Morehead, RT, et al: Erythrocyte agglutination in microgravity. Aviat Space Environ Med 60:235, 1989.

PROCEDURAL APPENDIX 1

Preparation of Washed "Dry" Button of Red Cells for Serologic Tests

1. Transfer a small amount of red cells using an applicator stick into a 10×75 mm test tube filled with saline. Tube should be prelabeled to identify contents.
2. Centrifuge at high speed, until red cells are collected into a tight button at the bottom of the tube.
3. Decant saline by quick inversion of the tube over a receptacle. Flick last drop saline from cells by giving tube a quick shake while still inverted. (Reduce aerosol production by using engineering controls or work practice controls or both.)
4. Add serum directly to "dry" button of cells. Method can be used for antibody screening of identification procedures, compatibility testing, and cell typing using a tube technique.

PROCEDURAL APPENDIX 2

Model One-Tube Per Donor Unit Compatibility Testing Procedure

NOTE: No minor side compatibility test is performed.

1. Into an appropriately labeled, 10×75 mm test tube, dispense 1 drop of a washed, 2 to 5 percent suspension of donor red cells. (Alternatively, prepare a washed "dry" button of donor red cells, using the technique in Procedural Appendix 1.)
2. Add 2 or 3 drops of serum to the tube to achieve an approximate $2:1$ ratio of serum to red cell. (Droppers used to dispense red cells and serum should be of equivalent size.)
3. Centrifuge at a speed and for a time that has been previously shown to give clear-cut differentiation between positive and negative results (15 seconds in a Serofuge is usually adequate).
4. Observe supernatant for hemolysis that must be considered indicative of an antigen-antibody interaction. Resuspend cell button by *gentle* manipulation of the tube. Grade all positive results. Record observations. STOP HERE FOR IMMEDIATE SPIN CROSSMATCH.
5. Add 2 drops of 22 percent bovine albumin (or other enhancement medium, such as LISS) to the tube (may be omitted, if desired). Mix and incubate for 30 minutes at 37°C.

NOTE: If LISS is added to tests at this stage in place of albumin, decrease incubation time to 10 minutes and refer to manufacturer's directions for additional directions.

6. Centrifuge as previously, observe supernatant, resuspend cells, and record results.
7. Wash three to four times using an automated instrument or manual washing technique. Decant saline completely from last wash.
8. Add 1 to 2 drops of antiglobulin serum to tube. (Follow manufacturer's directions for use of reagent selected.) Centrifuge, resuspend cells, and record results.
9. Add 1 drop IgG-sensitized red cells to each test having a negative result. Centrifuge and examine. Test result must be *positive*, or results of procedure are invalid and test must be repeated.

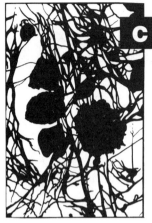

CHAPTER 13

Orientation to the Routine Blood Bank Laboratory

Judith Ann Sullivan, BS, MT(ASCP)SBB

OBJECTIVES

Upon completion of this chapter, the learner should be able to:

1 Describe the various functional areas of a blood bank.
2 Specify the tests that are performed on a unit of blood during donor processing.
3 Describe the criteria that must be met before a blood product can be labeled.
4 List the components that can be prepared from a unit of whole blood.
5 Compare the methods used for ABO and Rh testing and antibody screening on donor sample versus patient samples.
6 Discuss the tests performed by the reference section of the blood bank laboratory.

The chapters in this book have, up to this point, been organized into individual units dealing with specific topics in immunohematology. However, it is important to realize that none of these topics exists in a vacuum. In order to translate theory into reality, it is necessary to see how these various pieces interrelate in the actual setting of a blood bank.

To the first-time visitor, a blood bank can be a very confusing and intimidating place. The pressured pace, unfamiliar equipment, and strange and abbreviated terminology can make even those with the theoretic knowledge of immunohematology feel like "strangers in a strange land." However, all blood banks do share common characteristics that, if identified, can serve as points of orientation. Procedure manuals may differ from blood bank to blood bank, reflecting a response to workload, services, and patient population, but all blood banks follow guidelines established by the Food and Drug Administration (FDA) in its *Code of Federal Regulations*[1] and by the American Association of Blood Banks in its *Standards for Blood Banks and Transfusion Services.*[2]

The purpose of this chapter is to serve as a tour through the typical blood bank and to describe the various sections in each department and the procedures that are performed there. I hope this will help you better understand how the theory you have learned in this book is applied practically in order to achieve the goals of high-quality patient care and safe transfusion practice.

Organization

For ease of discussion, it will be assumed that the blood bank is divided into distinct departments, each with its own purpose and function. In reality, with the exception of very large hospitals, these departments tend to overlap within the overall structure of the laboratory. These departments include the following:

1. **Component preparation and storage.** In this area, units of whole blood are separated into their various components and stored under optimal conditions for survival.
2. **Donor processing.** Here, the testing that is required to determine the suitability of a blood product for transfusion is performed.
3. **Main laboratory.** This is the heart of the blood bank, where patient samples are received, testing is performed, and blood and blood components are issued for transfusion.
4. **Reference laboratory.** Any discrepancies in testing are resolved here.

Component Preparation and Storage

Hospitals vary widely in their capabilities to prepare blood components. The hospital that has its own blood

collection facility has a greater need to prepare a wider range of components than does the hospital that receives its blood products from an outside facility. We will examine these two situations separately.

BLOOD BANKS WITHOUT COLLECTION FACILITIES

Blood banks that depend on an outside source for their blood supplies usually receive their products in component form. However, situations do arise in which products must be modified (Fig. 13–1). For example, a unit received as whole blood may be needed as packed red blood cells. Often, this procedure is as simple as allowing the unit to rest undisturbed until the red cells have settled and then removing the supernatant plasma. However, when time is of the essence, the procedure may be accelerated through centrifugation. Large floor model refrigerated centrifuges are used for this purpose (Fig. 13–2).

In some clinical situations, washed red blood cells may be the product of choice for transfusion therapy. A variety of automated cell washers, which operate in similar fashions, are available to prepare this product. A unit of blood is introduced into a sterile disposable bowl that has tubing connected to a normal saline solution. A portion of this saline is added to the bowl, the cells and saline are mixed, the mixture is centrifuged, and the supernatant is removed through waste tubing. Multiple washes can be performed in this manner.

Blood components such as platelet concentrates and cryoprecipitate may be received as individual units but are more easily administered if pooled before infusion. Such product manipulation is a common occurrence in most blood banks.

If freezers capable of maintaining temperatures below −65°C are available, blood banks may choose to freeze rare or autologous units in 40 percent glycerol for long-term storage. The same automated cell washers just mentioned for washing cells can be used to remove the glycerol from these units before transfusion by adding increasingly diluted concentrations of saline to the cells during the procedure (Fig. 13–3).

BLOOD BANKS WITH COLLECTION FACILITIES

In addition to the foregoing situations blood banks that collect their own units of blood can use their

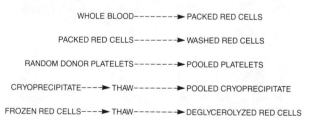

FIGURE 13-1 Modifications that blood banks without collection facilities can make to various blood components.

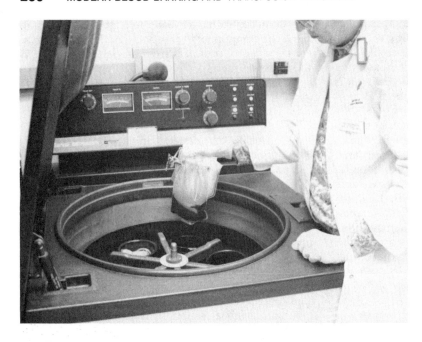

FIGURE 13-2 Units of whole blood may be centrifuged in order to separate plasma from packed cells. (Courtesy of National Institutes of Health, Bethesda, MD.)

blood resources more efficiently by separating them into various components including platelets, plasma, cryoprecipitate, and packed red blood cells (see Chapter 10).

To maximize the number of components derived from one unit of blood, processing must occur within 6 hours of collection. Within this period, the blood

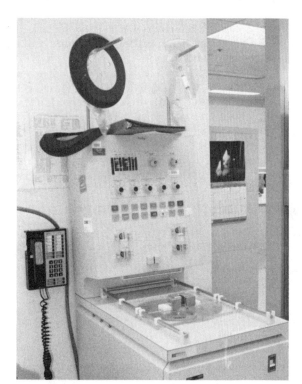

FIGURE 13-3 An automated cell washer such as this may be used to prepare washed red cells or to deglycerolize frozen red cells. (Courtesy of National Institutes of Health, Bethesda, MD.)

can be centrifuged to pack the red blood cells as previously described, and the plasma can be expressed and frozen. This is the process by which fresh frozen plasma is made. If the unit of blood is maintained at room temperature throughout this process and the appropriate centrifugation times and speeds are observed, a platelet concentrate can also be derived from the expressed plasma before it is frozen. In addition, through a controlled thawing process, the frozen plasma can be further manipulated to yield cryoprecipitate.

Various blood components may also be prepared through a procedure known as apheresis. In apheresis, a donor's blood is removed sterilely through tubing connected to an automated machine that then processes the blood; removes the desired component (platelets, plasma, or white blood cells); and returns the remainder of the components back to the donor via another set of connected tubing. High concentrations of specific components can be removed in this way with minimal removal of red cells (see Chapter 17).

Regardless of the method used to obtain blood and blood components, all blood banks must follow certain guidelines in the storage of their blood products. Thus, in any blood bank you will see:

1. Refrigerators maintained at 1°C to 6°C for the storage of packed red blood cells and whole blood
2. Freezers maintained at −18°C or lower for the storage of fresh frozen plasma and cryoprecipitate
3. Freezers maintained at −65°C or lower for the storage of red blood cells frozen in 40 percent glycerol
4. Platelet rotators that provide constant gentle agi-

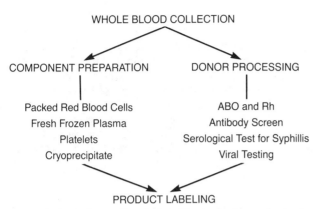

FIGURE 13-4 Processing of whole blood units from collection to labeling. Note that component preparation and donor processing may occur concurrently.

tation at room temperature for the storage of platelet concentrates

Donor Processing

Before a unit of blood can be placed into the general inventory (rendering it available to be used for crossmatching purposes), testing must be performed to determine its suitability for transfusion. This is the responsibility of the donor processing area (Fig. 13-4). Blood banks that collect their own units of blood are required to perform extensive testing to determine the suitability of each of these units. These tests must be performed at each donation regardless of the number of times a donor has previously donated. A separate tube of blood is collected from the donor at the time of donation for this purpose. Required tests include ABO and Rh testing, antibody screen, serologic test for syphilis (STS), and viral testing.

ABO AND Rh TESTING

This involves forward grouping with anti-A and anti-B, reverse grouping with A_1 and B cells, and Rh typing with anti-D (including D^u testing when indicated). Some blood banks using human sources of anti-A and anti-B choose to include anti-A,B in their forward groups because of its increased sensitivity over anti-A for detecting weaker subgroups of A. Others choose monoclonal anti-A reagents that have demonstrated ability to detect weak subgroups for this purpose.[3] A_2 cells may be included in the reverse group in order to differentiate a weak subgroup of A with anti-A_1 from a group O (see Chapter 5). Because this situation occurs so rarely, many blood bankers feel comfortable with eliminating A_2 cells from their reverse group tests.

Because of the potential for false-positive reactions due to the high viscosity of slide and modified tube test anti-D, an Rh-hr control is usually run in parallel with the anti-D reagent and must have a negative re-

sult for the test to be considered valid. Because an Rh-negative unit of blood mistaken for Rh-positive would be transfused only to an Rh-positive patient, which would cause no adverse clinical consequences, a blood bank may choose to eliminate the use of an Rh-hr control for donor processing. Some blood banks avoid the problem of false-positive Rh types by using anti-D reagents that are blends of monoclonal and polyclonal antibodies. These reagents have a lower protein concentration than the slide and modified tube test reagents, and thus are not prone to the same false-positive reactions (see Chapter 6).

The ABO and Rh results of the current donation are compared with the results from any previous donations. All discrepancies must be resolved before any products are labeled.

ANTIBODY SCREEN

Donor units must be screened in such a way as to detect clinically significant antibodies, because red cell destruction may occur if a large amount of plasma containing a high-titered clinically significant antibody is transfused to a patient whose cells contain the corresponding antigen (see Chapter 10). Some blood banks choose a pooled screening cell for donor antibody detection. This reagent is a pool of two donors chosen so that, between the two, all commonly encountered antigens are expressed. Although not adequately sensitive for routine patient antibody screens, this pooled screening cell is acceptable for detecting donor antibodies that may cause clinical problems. All units that are identified as containing clinically significant antibodies must be transfused as packed cells, and all plasma-containing components discarded or used only for reagent or research purposes.

SEROLOGIC TEST FOR SYPHILIS

Blood bankers may choose to perform this test themselves or send it to another hospital laboratory for completion.

VIRAL TESTING

Viral testing includes detection of hepatitis B surface antigen (HBsAg), antibodies to hepatitis B core antigen (anti-HBc) and to human immunodeficiency virus (anti-HIV) and human T-cell lymphotropic virus types I and II (anti-HTLV-I/II), and measurement of alanine aminotransferase (ALT). These tests may be performed in a laboratory other than that of the blood bank (see Chapter 19). As tests are developed to detect additional viral agents that can be transmitted through blood products, the number of required viral tests that must be performed on donor blood will increase.

Labeling of blood products may occur only after a careful review of all test results shows the unit to be suitable for transfusion. Suitability requirements include:

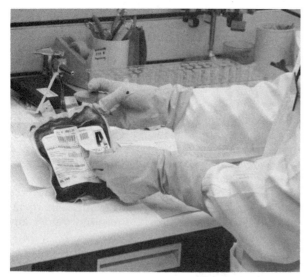

FIGURE 13–5 When all testing requirements are met, units of blood are labeled with ABO group and Rh type and expiration date. (Courtesy of National Institutes of Health, Bethesda, MD.)

1. No discrepancies in the ABO and Rh testing
2. Absence of detectable antibodies in plasma-containing components
3. Nonreactive STS and viral testing
4. ALT values within established limits

When the established criteria are met, the red cells and any other components are labeled with the appropriate ABO, Rh, and expiration date, and the products are stored at their proper temperatures (Fig. 13–5).

It is important to note that the requirements for processing autologous units are different from those just described (see Chapter 10 for additional information).

Units received from an outside source have already undergone the aforementioned required testing and have been deemed suitable for transfusion by the shipping facility. However, because of the serious consequences of transfusing ABO-incompatible blood, the blood bank to which this blood is shipped is required to reconfirm the ABO of each red cell–containing product received. As a cost containment measure, many blood banks confirm group O units using only anti-A,B and other blood groups using anti-A and anti-B. Because of the potential sensitization that may occur if Rh-positive blood is transfused to an Rh-negative patient, the Rh type of all Rh-*negative* units must be reconfirmed. Because no harm will be done if an Rh-negative unit incorrectly labeled as Rh-positive is transfused to an Rh-positive patient, the Rh type of Rh-positive units need not be reconfirmed.

The manner in which donor processing laboratories perform ABO and Rh testing and antibody screening reflects the particular needs of each institution. Thus, hospitals with minimal donor processing may perform all testing using tube methodologies. Microplate methods may suit the needs of blood banks that main-tain large blood supplies or collect a large portion of their own blood inventory because these methods are time efficient and conserve reagents when performing batch testing. Expensive automated machinery can usually be justified only by very large donor centers.

Computers have become an integral part of many donor processing laboratories. Computers may be used for such functions as donor deferral, comparison of ABO and Rh testing with previous donations, input, storage and retrieval of test results, labeling, and product inventory.

Main Laboratory

Patient care is the primary mission of the main laboratory. Here the testing is performed that determines the compatibility between a patient requiring transfusion and the unit of blood to be transfused. Because of the severe adverse reaction that may occur if the wrong unit of blood is transfused to a patient, great care must be taken not only in the testing performed, but also in specimen and unit identification and paperwork. Common approaches are evident in the pretransfusion testing protocols that are established by different blood banks to ensure the orderly, timely, and accurate processing of patient samples (Fig. 13–6).

SAMPLE ACCEPTANCE

Proper patient identification is crucial for any specimen used in blood bank testing. Consequences may be fatal if a blood specimen is labeled with the wrong patient's name. Thus, each specimen and request form the blood bank receives is carefully examined for proper spelling of the patient's name, correct hospital number, correct date, and identification of the phlebotomist. Some hospitals employ commercially available systems that provide additional safeguards for proper patient identification.

ROUTINE TESTING

Once a patient sample has been judged acceptable, the testing requested by the patient's physician can be performed. Tests are usually requested as a group, and, for ease in ordering, a shorthand notation designates a group. Orders you may see include those that follow.

Type and Screen

Many surgical procedures have a very low probability of requiring blood transfusion. To make better use of their blood supplies, blood bankers may choose not to crossmatch units of blood for these procedures but, instead, to use type-and-screen protocol. ABO and Rh testing and antibody screening are performed using a current patient specimen.

SAMPLE ACCEPTABILITY

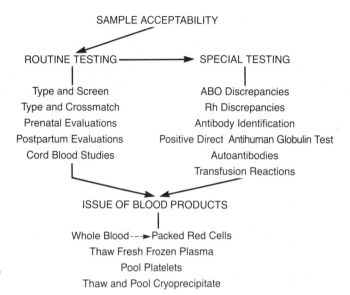

ROUTINE TESTING ──────────────▶ SPECIAL TESTING

Type and Screen	ABO Discrepancies
Type and Crossmatch	Rh Discrepancies
Prenatal Evaluations	Antibody Identification
Postpartum Evaluations	Positive Direct Antihuman Globulin Test
Cord Blood Studies	Autoantibodies
	Transfusion Reactions

ISSUE OF BLOOD PRODUCTS

Whole Blood -- ➤ Packed Red Cells
Thaw Fresh Frozen Plasma
Pool Platelets
Thaw and Pool Cryoprecipitate

FIGURE 13-6 Processing of patient samples from acceptance into the laboratory until issuance of blood products.

Because only a small percentage of individuals who type as Rh-negative using an immediate spin technique are shown to be D^u positive, many hospitals choose to contain cost and utilize time more efficiently by eliminating D^u testing of patient samples and to determine patient Rh types based on immediate spin results only (see Chapter 6).

In order to increase the sensitivity of the antibody screen, some blood banks use a three-cell antibody screening set that provides homozygous antigen expression in all major blood group systems. If the blood is needed on an emergency basis during surgery, blood can be released using an abbreviated crossmatch (see farther on). If an antibody is detected, identification of that antibody is performed and compatible units are reserved for the patient. A blood bank may decide to include or eliminate an autocontrol or direct antiglobulin test (DAT) in a type-and-screen protocol (see Chapter 12). This decision is based on the patient population of the facility, the time and cost involved in the testing, and the amount of useful information the test is expected to provide.[4]

Type and Crossmatch

When a physician orders units to be crossmatched for a patient, more testing is necessary than the order to crossmatch implies. ABO and Rh testing and antibody screening must be performed on a current patient specimen. The same specimen is also used to crossmatch with a segment of the unit intended for transfusion. In the absence of extreme emergency, the unit of blood can be issued for transfusion only if all testing discrepancies are resolved and the crossmatch is compatible (Fig. 13 – 7). If the result of the antibody screen is positive, the antibody must be identified, and if the antibody is clinically significant, antigen-negative units must be chosen for transfusion.

Abbreviated crossmatch protocols have been adopted by some blood banks for routine crossmatching and by others for only emergency situations. In these protocols, ABO and Rh testing and antibody screening are performed. In the absence of clinically significant antibodies, blood is issued following an immediate spin crossmatch that serves as a confirmation of ABO compatibility. (Compare this with a conventional crossmatch in which an indirect antiglobulin test is performed following incubation at 37°C.)

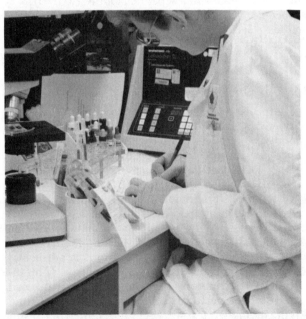

FIGURE 13-7 Extensive compatibility testing is performed before a unit of blood is issued for transfusion to the designated recipient. (Courtesy of National Institutes of Health, Bethesda, MD.)

Prenatal Evaluation

Accurate serologic testing of obstetric patients is an essential component in the prevention and treatment of hemolytic disease of the newborn (HDN). Maternal blood samples are evaluated during the pregnancy to determine the Rh status of the mother and the presence of serum antibodies that have the potential to cause HDN.[5] If the woman is Rh negative and D^u negative, she may be a candidate for antenatal Rh Immune Globulin. If the result of the antibody screen is positive, the antibody must be identified. Serial titrations may be performed during the course of the pregnancy if the antibody is considered potentially harmful to the fetus. The obstetrician uses laboratory results in conjunction with other methods for evaluating the fetal condition in order to determine the need for clinical intervention, such as intrauterine transfusion or early delivery (see Chapter 20).

Postpartum Evaluation

All women admitted for delivery must be tested to determine their Rh status.[1] A D^u test is performed on any specimen that shows a negative reaction on immediate spin. If the mother is Rh negative and her baby Rh positive, the maternal sample is further evaluated in order to detect a fetomaternal hemorrhage (FMH) in excess of 30 ml of whole blood. (One vial of Rh Immune Globulin prevents maternal Rh immunization from exposure to up to 30 ml of fetal whole blood.[6]) Commercial kits using rosetting techniques are commonly used for this purpose. Once an FMH has been detected, quantitation is performed using a Kleihauer-Betke test (see Chapter 20). This may be performed in the blood bank or in a separate laboratory. If HDN is suspected, an antibody screen is performed on the mother's serum, and if the result is positive, attempts are made to identify the antibody.

Cord Blood Studies

Protocols to evaluate cord blood specimens can vary widely from blood bank to blood bank. Cord blood from infants born to Rh-negative mothers is tested for Rh (including a D^u test) to determine the mother's candidacy for Rh Immune Globulin prophylaxis. ABO and Rh typing and DAT are performed on cord samples from infants born to women with clinically significant antibodies. Additional tests may also be performed. Many blood banks follow published guidelines[5] recommending that, beyond these circumstances, routine testing of cord samples is not necessary unless the clinical situation warrants it. If an infant develops symptoms that suggest HDN, a full cord blood study is performed that may include ABO and Rh (including D^u) testing, DAT, and, if the DAT result is positive, an eluate and subsequent antibody identification (see Chapter 20).

REQUESTS FOR OTHER BLOOD COMPONENTS

When components such as granulocyte concentrates, which contain large amounts of red blood cells, are requested, pretransfusion testing is identical to that performed for red cell requests (see the previous section). Orders for platelets and fresh frozen plasma may be filled once the ABO group of the recipient has been determined.

ISSUE OF BLOOD PRODUCTS

When all pretransfusion testing has been completed, blood components may be released for transfusion to the designated recipient. *It is essential that all serologic discrepancies be resolved before issue of blood products, except in extreme emergency.* The individual in the blood bank who will issue the blood product inspects the unit for any abnormal appearance and verifies that all required transfusion forms and labels are complete and adequately identify the transfusion recipient. If another individual is responsible for delivering the blood product to the appropriate location, he or she may also verify that all information is complete. If there are no discrepancies, the component may be released. Some form of documentation is used to record the transaction.

Some component preparation may be necessary before the issue of blood products. Fresh frozen plasma may be thawed in a constant-temperature (37°C) water bath, individual platelet concentrates may be pooled into a single bag for ease of transfusion, and individual units of cryoprecipitate may be thawed and then pooled. Because these manipulations shorten the expiration date of the products, it is best that they be performed as close to the time of issue as possible (see Chapter 10).

Blood products may be irradiated before issue in order to prevent passenger lymphocytes from causing graft-versus-host disease. Blood banks in large medical centers may have an irradiator on the premises; smaller facilities may make arrangements to have the needed products irradiated elsewhere.

Computers have become an essential part of many transfusion services. Computers may be used for such functions as input, storage, and verification of test results; inventory management; issue of blood products; and training of blood bank personnel.

Reference Laboratory

Whether it is an entity separate from the main laboratory or, as in most cases, an integrated part, the reference laboratory is the problem-solving section of the blood bank (Fig. 13–8). The responsibility here is to ensure that any discrepancies that are detected in routine testing are resolved in an accurate and time-efficient manner. Other chapters in this book discuss in depth the various problems encountered in sero-

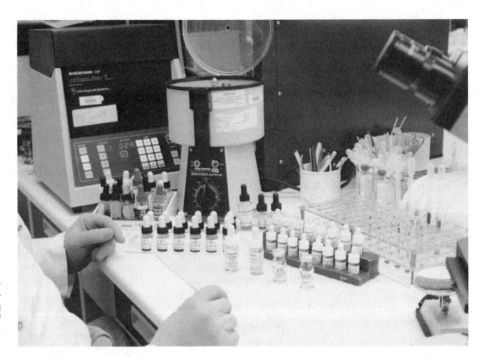

FIGURE 13-8 Reference laboratories employ a variety of techniques and reagents in resolving serologic problems. (Courtesy of National Institutes of Health, Bethesda, MD.)

logic testing and strategies for resolving them. Here, then, is a brief summary of some problem situations and their investigation. It should be noted that before any serologic testing is performed, special testing always includes an investigation of patient diagnosis, age, and pregnancy, drug, and transfusion history.

ABO DISCREPANCIES

All inconsistencies between forward and reverse group test results must be resolved before an ABO interpretation can be made (see Chapter 5). ABO investigations may include:

1. Variations in incubation times and temperatures
2. Testing with A_2 cells or anti-A_1 lectin
3. Room temperature antibody identification
4. Adsorption and elution using anti-A or anti-B
5. Autoadsorption
6. Removal of red cell–bound cold autoantibodies (see farther on)
7. Secretor studies

Rh DISCREPANCIES

Problems in Rh typing may occur because of certain clinical conditions or as inherited characteristics (see Chapter 6). Rh investigations may include:

1. Rh phenotyping using antisera with low-protein concentrations
2. Adsorption and elution using Rh antisera
3. Isolation of cell populations
4. Use of rare antisera and cells

ANTIBODY IDENTIFICATION

A positive antibody screen in the absence of a positive autocontrol or DAT result indicates possible alloantibody immunization through blood transfusion or pregnancy (see Chapter 11). In order to establish the identity and clinical significance of an antibody and provide appropriate blood for transfusion, antibody investigations may include:

1. Antibody identification panels employing various enhancement media (such as albumin, low ionic strength solution [LISS], polybrene, polyethylene glycol [PEG], or enzymes) and test systems (such as tubes, microplates, or capillaries)
2. Neutralization using such substances as plasma, saliva, urine, or human milk
3. Antigen typing
4. Titration
5. Adsorption and elution
6. Treatment of serum with dithiothreitol (DTT) or 2-mercaptoethanol (2-ME)
7. IgG subclassing
8. Monocyte monolayer assay (MMA)
9. Use of rare antisera and cells

POSITIVE DIRECT ANTIGLOBULIN TEST

A positive DAT may be a result of an immune reaction to a drug, a disease state, or a delayed hemolytic transfusion reaction (see Chapters 4 and 18). The investigation of a positive DAT may include:

1. Use of monospecific reagents (anti-IgG, anti-C3)

2. Elution techniques
3. Antibody identification
4. Removal of red cell–bound antibody using chloroquine diphosphate or other reagents
5. Red cell phenotyping
6. Drug studies

WARM AUTOANTIBODIES

In addition to causing a positive DAT result (see previous section), the presence of a warm autoantibody in a patient's serum may mask the presence of clinically significant alloantibodies (see Chapter 21). Tests performed in the investigation of warm autoantibodies may include:

1. Removal of red cell–bound autoantibody followed by autoadsorption
2. Heterologous or differential adsorptions
3. Elution techniques
4. Autoantibody identification
5. Reticulocyte enrichment

COLD AUTOANTIBODIES

Potent cold autoantibodies may cause discrepancies in ABO testing as well as a positive DAT result (see previous section) and may mask the presence of clinically significant alloantibodies (see Chapter 21). The management of cold autoantibodies may include:

1. Removal of red cell–bound autoantibody using 37°C saline
2. Prewarmed technique
3. Antibody identification
4. Autoadsorption
5. Adsorption using rabbit erythrocyte stroma
6. Treatment of serum or cells with DTT or 2-ME

TRANSFUSION REACTIONS

Any adverse reactions to transfusion must be investigated to determine if the reaction was antibody mediated (see Chapter 18). The extent of transfusion reaction investigations varies widely, depending on policies established by a particular blood bank and the result of initial testing. If there is strong evidence of an antibody-mediated transfusion reaction, further investigations may include:

1. Elution, followed by antibody identification
2. Use of more sensitive techniques for antibody detection including enzymes, polybrene, PEG, or enzyme-linked antiglobulin test (ELAT)
3. Cell separation techniques

Summary

On cursory examination, one blood bank may appear to have very little in common with any other blood bank. As we have seen, though, many common themes become apparent with a more thorough investigation. With varying patient needs, changing technologies, and fluctuating economies, future blood banks may look nothing like the blood banks of today. However different they may appear at first glance, the same commitment to patient care and excellence in testing will ensure that common themes will still be evident on closer scrutiny.

Review Questions

1. All of the following criteria must be met before a unit of blood can be labeled, *except*:
   A. ABO and Rh test results must agree with results from previous donations.
   B. STS results must be nonreactive.
   C. ALT results must be nonreactive.
   D. Viral testing results must be nonreactive.

2. Freezers that maintain a temperature of −65°C or below must be used for the storage of:
   A. Fresh frozen plasma
   B. Red cells frozen in 40 percent glycerol
   C. Cryoprecipitate
   D. Red cells frozen in 20 percent glycerol

3. Which of the following is *not* required for a type and crossmatch?
   A. ABO testing
   B. Rh testing
   C. D^u testing
   D. Antibody screening
   E. Compatibility testing

4. Which of the following products is least likely to cause graft-versus-host disease?
   A. Whole blood
   B. Irradiated packed red cells
   C. Granulocyte concentrates
   D. Platelets prepared by apheresis

5. Cryoprecipitate is made by:
   A. Fractionation of plasma
   B. Apheresis
   C. Filtration of fresh frozen plasma
   D. Controlled thawing of fresh frozen plasma

6. Pooled screening cells may be used for antibody screening of:
   A. Donors
   B. Surgical patients
   C. Obstetric patients
   D. Neonates

Answers to Review Questions

1. C   (p 282)
2. B   (p 279)

3. C (p 283)
4. B (p 284)
5. D (p 280)
6. A (p 281)

References

1. Code of Federal Regulations. Food and Drug Administration, Title 21. US Government Printing Office, Washington, DC, 1993.
2. Widmann, FK (ed): Standards for Blood Banks and Transfusion Services, ed 15. American Association of Blood Banks, Arlington, VA, 1993.
3. Stroup, M: A review: the use of monoclonal antibodies in blood banking. Immunohematology 6:30–36, 1990.
4. Laird-Fryer, B: Application and interpretation of direct antiglobulin test results as applied to healthy persons and selected patients. In Wallace, E and Levitt, JS (eds): Current Applications and Interpretations of the Direct Antiglobulin Test. American Association of Blood Banks, Arlington, VA, 1988, pp 105–144.
5. Judd, WJ, et al: Prenatal and perinatal immunohematology: recommendations for serologic management of the fetus, newborn infant, and obstetric patient. Immunohematology 30:175–183, 1990.
6. Bowman, JM: Historical overview: Hemolytic disease of the fetus and newborn. In Kennedy, MS and Kelton, JG (eds): Perinatal Transfusion Medicine. American Association of Blood Banks, Arlington, VA, 1990, pp 1–52.

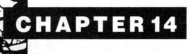

CHAPTER 14

Modern Principles of Blood Banking Compliance with Food and Drug Administration Regulations

Mary Ann Tourault, MA, MT(ASCP)SBB

OBJECTIVES

Upon completion of this chapter, the learner should be able to:

1　Describe briefly the regulation of the biologics industry.
2　Discuss the significant milestones in the Food and Drug Administration's regulation of biologics.
3　List the inspectional authorities.
4　List the biologic products regulated by the Food and Drug Administration.
5　Discuss short supply agreements.
6　Describe the licensing activities pertaining to recovered plasma.
7　Discuss various aspects of the inspection process.
8　Characterize regulatory sanctions such as product recalls.

9 Describe administrative actions such as warning letters, injunctions, and prosecution.

10 State the Food and Drug Administration requirements regarding quality assurance.

The Food and Drug Administration (FDA) enforces regulations to ensure the safety and efficacy of biologics, drugs, and devices that include blood and blood components and diagnostic reagents used or manufactured by blood establishments. This chapter describes the history of the regulatory and inspection process, requirements of the FDA, and selected quality assurance issues. The applicable regulations for blood and blood products promulgated under the Public Health Service Act and the Federal Food, Drug, and Cosmetic (FD&C) Act are found in Parts 211 to 680 of Title 21, *Code of Federal Regulations* (CFR).[1] These regulations mandate adherence to current good manufacturing practices (CGMPs) by following the guidance detailed in written standard operating procedures (SOPs). Applicable additional standards for the manufacture of blood and blood products must also be followed. In addition, the regulations address the statutory requirements regarding establishment and product licensing and registration as well as product-specific standards for bacterial products, viral vaccines, and human blood and blood products.

Separate federal licenses are issued (concurrently) for the biologic product and for the establishment manufacturing the biologic product. Such licenses are issued by the Center for Biologics Evaluation and Research (CBER)* following a comprehensive review of the license applications and an establishment inspection that are intended to determine and ensure that both entities meet applicable standards to ensure the continued safety, purity, and potency of such product. Within the United States and at foreign establishments holding a US license, on-going compliance with the FD&C Act is secured through inspections of the facilities and products, analysis of product samples, educational activities, and legal proceedings.

The FDA has a number of administrative and legal sanctions available to address deviations from the regulations or violations of the law. These include license suspension or revocation, or both, warning letters, seizure, injunction, and prosecution.

History and Overview of Biologics Regulation

Laws regulating the handling of food and some drug substances have been described in the histories of the early Hebrews and Egyptians.[2] Early Greek and Roman laws prohibited merchants from adding water to wine and selling short measures for grain and cooking oil. More complex protection became necessary as civilization advanced. During the Middle Ages, trade guilds were created to combat the adulteration of spices and drugs. These organizations conducted inspections to monitor the incidence of the problem and to encourage corrective action.

Early in the 1900s, biologic drugs were coming into widespread use in the United States after having met with great success in Europe and Russia. Countries such as France, Germany, Italy, and Russia had instituted regulatory controls for such biologics as early as 1895. The regulation of biological products in the United States began when Congress passed the Biologics Control Act of 1902 (also known as the Virus Toxin Law).[3]

This act was passed following the deaths of 10 children who had received injections of diphtheria antitoxin contaminated with tetanus.[4] In 1901, there was a serious epidemic of diphtheria resulting in a great demand for the diphtheria antitoxin. At the time, the manufacturing process was not controlled properly. There was no requirement for safety testing, and, therefore, none was performed. The tetanus contamination was traced to an infected horse whose serum was used in producing the antitoxin.

The 1902 act required that biologics be manufactured in a manner that ensured safety, purity, and potency.[5] Provisions of the act included:

Establishment license requirements
Product license requirements
Labeling requirements
Inspection requirements
Suspension or revocation of licenses, or both
Penalties for violations

The responsibility for implementing this new law was placed under the hygienic laboratory for the Public Health Service (PHS). In 1903, the PHS expanded the regulations to include, among other provisions, that inspections would be unannounced and that licenses were to be issued on the basis of an annual inspection.[6] Today, this act is known as the PHS Act, 42 USC 262, and serves as the legal basis for the CBER's premarket approval activities for biological products. Section 351 of the PHS Act requires that any establishment that manufactures or prepares biological products shipped in interstate commerce (including internationally) for sale, barter, or exchange must be licensed.

---

*The history of CBER is taken from a draft manual for CBER inspectors, with the permission of the author, Margaret A. Tart.

The 1902 act was amended in 1944. One change included a requirement that a biologic product license could be issued only on demonstrating that both the *product* and the *establishment* met standards to ensure the continued safety, purity, and potency of such products. This evaluation was to be made during inspections by federal officials. Another change that occurred at this time involved the focal point for administering the act. This responsibility was delegated to the National Microbiological Institute at the National Institutes of Health (NIH).

Changes in the focal point for administering the PHS Act occurred in the mid-1950s with the advent of polio vaccines.[7] From 1955 to 1972, biological products were regulated within the NIH in the Division of Biologics Standards (DBS). In 1972, biologics regulation was transferred to the FDA, Bureau of Biologics (BOB), which in turn added a regulatory impetus to an organization that had previously emphasized a research function.

The transfer for the oversight of biologics to the FDA began a merger of the regulatory requirements of the PHS Act and the FD&C Act (21 USC 301 et seq). Biologics were viewed as biological products under the PHS Act and as drugs under the FD&C Act, subject to inspection according to the good manufacturing practices (GMPs) regulations for drugs. During this era, the reagent manufacturers were also inspected under the drug GMPs because the device amendments to the FD&C Act were not enacted until 1976. As a result, administration of the regulatory powers inherent in each of the acts had to be approached with the knowledge that they do not in any way modify each other. Therefore, it was possible for a biological product to be adulterated or misbranded as a drug or device within the meaning of the FD&C Act. Included among the significant changes that occurred as a result of the FDA assuming regulatory responsibility for biological products was the requirement that biologic establishments, including blood banks, were required to register with the FDA. GMPs for blood and blood products were promulgated under the FD&C Act as well as the PHS Act. Today, one of the major programs is to ensure the safety of the nation's blood supply.

In 1982, the FDA merged the BOB and the Bureau of Drugs into the Center for Drugs and Biologics (CDB). In 1988, this organization was divided into two distinct entities, the CBER and the Center for Drug Evaluation and Research (CDER). Significant events that led to the division of the CDB into the current entities included the pandemic outbreak of the acquired immunodeficiency syndrome (AIDS) and a perceived drugs approval lag in the United States for traditional pharmaceuticals, and the advent of bioengineering- and biotechnology-derived products. CBER has grown in its responsibilities since its beginning in 1902 as the Hygienic Laboratory for the PHS, when the technologies for producing biological products were in their infancy and when its primary function was regulation of vaccines.

Today the regulation of a wide variety of novel biologic products and their use as therapeutics requires knowledge of new developments in manufacturing technology, as well as updated approaches to basic research in the relevant biologic disciplines. Even with the infusion of technologic advances into biologics, CBER recognizes that the establishment inspection that was first used in 1902 will continue to be an integral part of the surveillance effort in regulating new biotherapeutics and monitoring future scientific efforts.

Milestones in the Food and Drug Administration's Regulation of Biologics

Biologic products are defined in Section 351 of the PHS Act as ". . . any virus, therapeutic serum, toxin, antitoxin, vaccine, blood, blood component or derivative, allergenic product, or analogous product applicable to the prevention, treatment, or cure of diseases or injuries of man."[8] The original statute did not list blood, blood components, or blood derivatives in the definition.

In July 1940, the first federal license for manufacturing normal human plasma was issued. At that time, blood was considered analogous to a therapeutic serum, which was one of the products explicitly covered by Section 351 of the PHS Act. The first license for Whole Blood was issued in May 1946.

Blood and blood products were considered to be within the ambit of the statutory authority of the FD&C Act as the administrator of the Federal Security Agency (predecessor of Health, Education, and Welfare) ruled on May 31, 1945, that in order to avoid a duplication of effort, one agency should be responsible for requiring biologic manufacturers to comply with all applicable provisions of the FD&C Act as well as the provisions of the PHS Act.

Carrying out this responsibility, the provisions of the FD&C Act were often applied to manufacturers of blood and blood products. For example, pursuant to Section 503(b) of the act, blood labels were required to carry the legend "Caution: Federal Law prohibits dispensing without prescription." In addition, pursuant to Section 502 of the FD&C Act, blood banks were required to supply a package enclosure along with the blood that provided instructions for use, indications, contraindications, side effects, and precautions. Since the effective date of their implementation, the regulations issued pursuant to such provisions have been applied to all biologic drugs, including blood products.

Another milestone in the history of blood bank regulation occurred in 1968 in a legal action brought by the federal government against a commercial blood bank (*United States versus Charles and Maxine Blank*).[9] Maxine Blank and her codefendants were found guilty of false labeling of blood products under Section 351 of the PHS Act and of misbranding a drug (blood) under the FD&C Act. On appeal in 1968, her conviction for violations of the PHS Act was reversed on grounds that the products involved were not within the scope of the statute. That is, Congress in 1902 could not have considered blood products to come under the ambit of the PHS Act statute. The appellate court upheld the conviction for violations of the FD&C Act, which charged misbranding a drug.

As a result of this ruling, an amendment was made in 1970 to Section 351 of the PHS Act specifically to include blood, blood components, or blood derivatives, making it clear that Congress intended blood and blood products to be subject to provisions of the PHS Act.

On August 26, 1972, a notice of proposed rule making was published in the *Federal Register* requiring registration pursuant to Section 510 of the FD&C Act. In Section 510(b), Congress clearly indicated that "every person who owns or operates any establishment in any State engaged in the manufacture, preparation, propagation, compounding, or processing of a drug or drugs shall register with the Secretary his name, places of business, and all such establishments." It was questioned whether Congress intended to classify blood as a drug. An analysis of Section 201(g)(s) of the FD&C Act (21 321) reveals that blood and blood products fall within the definitions recognized in the *United States Pharmacopoeia* (USP), XV Edition (December 15, 1955) and have been included in each USP since that edition. Federal courts that have had occasion to consider the issue have held without exception that blood is a drug within the meaning of the FD&C Act. The registration requirement applies not only to establishments that collect or process blood for transfusion but also to those that collect blood and use it or its components in the manufacture of diagnostic laboratory reagents and controls. The notice provided the opportunity for interested parties to comment on the proposal within 60 days of the date of publication. Only 100 persons and organizations availed themselves of the opportunity to comment on the proposed rule.

In 1976, the FD&C Act was amended to strengthen the FDA's authority to regulate medical devices. The FDA now requires manufacturers of class III medical devices to demonstrate that their products are safe and effective prior to marketing them. Before this time, FDA's authority was limited only to removing hazardous or falsely represented products from the market. Among the several changes were that blood banks were now required to register their establishments with the FDA and to list the products they prepared, and GMPs for blood and blood products were promulgated.

There were also changes in inspectional responsibilities. The FDA has a large network of field offices at the regional, district, and resident post levels across the United States. These field offices are staffed with investigators who perform the inspection and investigation work required of FDA. Because the FDA was charged with inspection of all the blood banks (licensed and unlicensed) in the United States, the field inspectional force was used to share the increased workload. At one time, the inventory of blood-related firms encompassed approximately 7000 locations. However, since 1980, the number FDA is obligated to inspect has been significantly reduced owing to an agreement with the Health Care Financing Administration (HCFA). The 1980 Memorandum of Understanding (MOU) between HCFA and FDA reduced the number of federal agencies inspecting the same facility. If units of blood are drawn on a routine basis, including the collection of autologous units, blood banks are required to register with, and be inspected by, the FDA. Those facilities that do not routinely collect blood or do not prepare blood components are generally inspected under the auspices of HCFA. The preparation of blood components for which a facility would register includes washing, rejuvenating, freezing, and deglycerolyzing red blood cells (RBCs) but not separating plasma from RBCs. Inspectors from FDA's headquarters staff (CBER) were responsible for inspecting the licensed military establishments.

At present, the inventory of registered blood establishments that are inspected by FDA is approximately 2800. The field offices are responsible for the routine inspections of these blood bank and plasmapheresis establishments.

The CBER inspectors conduct all prelicense and preapproval inspections of blood establishments and annual inspections of manufacturers of related categories of biologic products such as blood bank reagents and plasma derivatives.

Inspection Authorities and Guidance

Licensed manufacturers of biologic products are inspected under the authorities found in both the PHS Act [42 USC 262(c)] and the FD&C Act [21 USC 374]. As discussed earlier, most biological products also meet the definition of a drug under the FD&C Act. For this reason, the applicable portions of both acts, as well as their implementing regulations, are enforced for biological products. The preamble to the 1978 regulation covering CGMP for drug products discusses and defines how the drug regulations apply to biological products.

There are also several licensed biological products such as blood grouping reagents and viral marker test kits that meet the definition of a device under the FD&C Act. The premarket approval over these licensed diagnostic products continues within the licensure mechanism of the PHS Act.

However, the emphasis focused on in vitro products has differed somewhat in approach. The reasons for this include (1) the strict premarket clearance associated with licensure and (2) a policy decision in 1982 to continue to regulate the products as devices by CBER.

The regulations in 21 CFR 600.20 to 600.22 describe the establishment inspection for licensed, biological product manufacturers, including time of inspections and duties of inspectors. In addition, the regulations for finished pharmaceuticals found in 21 CFR 210 and 211 et seq are applicable to biologic drugs including blood and blood products. The device CGMPs contained in 21 CFR 820 et seq apply to in vitro diagnostic test kits and any biologic devices regulated by CBER.

Guidance in the form of memoranda issued to all registered blood establishments, and the FDA's checklist and instructions for inspections are available on request from the Congressional and Consumer Affairs Staff, HFM-12, FDA, 1401 Rockville Pike, Rockville, MD 20852-1448 (301-594-2000). The Compliance Program and Compliance Policy Guides are available through the Freedom of Information Act (FOIA) and may be obtained by writing to FOI Officer, 5600 Fishers Lane, Rockville, MD 20856.

Biological Products Regulated by CBER

The FDA inspections of firms manufacturing the following categories of licensed biologic products are conducted by FDA staff. The list has been divided into the product lines that correspond to the organizational structure of CBER.

1. Blood and Blood Products
   a. Whole Blood and Blood Components
   b. Source Plasma
   c. Plasma Derivatives (e.g., Antihemophilic Factor [AHF], Plasma Protein Fraction [PPF], Normal Serum Albumin [NSA], Immune Serum Globulin [ISG])
   d. Streptokinase
   e. Antilymphocyte Globulin
   f. Licensed in vitro reagents (e.g., Blood Grouping Sera, Monoclonal Antibodies/Recombinant DNA Products)
   g. Blood Group Substances
   h. Fibrinolysin
2. Bacterial and Viral Products
   a. Toxoids (e.g., Tetanus Toxoids)
   b. Antitoxins (e.g., Tetanus Antitoxin)
   c. Bacterial Vaccines (e.g., Diphtheria and Tetanus Toxoids and Pertussis Vaccine [DPT])
   d. Viral Vaccines (e.g., Poliovirus Vaccine, Live, Oral, Trivalent)
   e. Allergenic Products
   f. Tuberculin
   g. Antiviral Serum (e.g., Antirabies Serum)
3. In Vitro Test Kits
   a. Anti-HIV, Anti–HTLV-I
   b. Hepatitis B, Antihepatitis C Virus

4. New Technology Biotherapeutic Products (Biotechnology Derived)
   a. Interferons
   b. Granulocyte Colony-Stimulating Factor (GCSF)
   c. Granulocyte Macrophage Colony-Stimulating Factor (GMCSF)
   d. Erythropoietin (EPO)
   e. OKT3-Monoclonal Antibody
5. New Drug Application Products
   a. Anticoagulants in Blood Collection Bags
   b. Plasma Volume Extenders
   c. Urokinase
   d. Perfluorochemicals (e.g., Fluosol)
6. Miscellaneous Products (products often reviewed within CBER by individuals with particular scientific expertise and not necessarily assigned within a strict division context)
   a. Antivenin
   b. Collagenase
   c. Limulus Amebocyte Lysate/Tachypleus Tridentata

Licensing Activities

Applications for blood and blood product licenses may be obtained from CBER, Division of Blood Establishment and Product Applications (HFM-370). Initially the establishment license and at least one product license must be requested and issued simultaneously; thereafter, additional product licenses may be requested as long as the establishment license remains unsuspended and unrevoked.

Before granting a license, CBER personnel review applications and, if all necessary data and information are found satisfactory, conduct a prelicense inspection. The application will be reviewed for safety and efficacy, product labeling, and compliance with all applicable regulations. Sample lots must be submitted to CBER for some products and samples may be required from each lot for lot release testing for new products.

The CBER will conduct the prelicense inspections accompanied by a field investigator. The prelicense inspection is an in-depth review of the physical facilities; manufacturing methods; SOP manual, records, and equipment; as well as an evaluation of the training of staff involved in manufacturing. This inspection is announced, and the establishment must be operational for at least 30 days before the inspection and capable of fully manufacturing the product for which they have requested a license. The inspection is intended to determine the firm's ability to meet commitments made in the license applications and to operate in compliance with applicable regulations. If the results of the prelicense inspection show the firm to be operating in a satisfactory manner, and the product meets applicable standards and regulations for safety and efficacy, then establishment and product licenses will be issued. Licenses must be amended before changing any significant step in manufacturing or making any substantive modification to the facility. Having a US license allows the establishment to ship products interstate and internationally for sale, barter, or exchange. Unlicensed firms may not ship products across state lines, nor may licensed firms ship products for which they do not hold a federal license, except in documented medical emergency situations. Compliance Policy Guide No. 7134.11 provides guidance to FDA investigators to explain the regulatory aspects of these shipments.

An establishment must designate a Responsible Head, who will represent the manufacturer in all pertinent matters (21 CFR 600.10[a]). The Responsible Head must also exercise control of the establishment in all matters relating to compliance. The person designated as Responsible Head has the authority to represent the manufacturer with FDA. He or she must have the authority to enforce, or to direct enforcement of, discipline and the performance of assigned functions; the understanding of scientific principles and techniques involved in the manufacturing process; and the responsibility for training and informing employees of policy. The concept of a Responsible Head is unique to US licensed establishments, and it has not been the policy of CBER to approve more than one individual as responsible head. If the Responsible Head is not located at the site of the establishment, there must be a qualified on-site manager. The supporting documentation for the candidates will be reviewed and approved by CBER, Division of Blood Establishment and Product Applications (HFM-370).

The Responsible Head should not be responsible in name only but should have and use the authority to effect change. He or she may delegate tasks or functions but not the responsibility.

A manufacturer must file amendments to the product license application if the licensed product is to be prepared at locations separate from the original licensed establishment. After review of the amendments by CBER and a satisfactory prelicense inspection, the establishment license is reissued to include the additional location(s); separate license numbers for locations are not issued. Such locations are generally fully operating facilities, although they may not manufacture all of the products prepared by the main establishment.

SHORT SUPPLY

One of the most frequently misunderstood areas is the concept of short supply. Short supply was introduced in 1948, and the provisions governing short supply are found in 21 CFR 601.22. The short supply provisions of the regulations constitute an exemption from licensure in limited areas and under controlled conditions.

The concept is that certain products, such as Factor VIII, are designated by CBER to be in short supply. The short supply provision allows unlicensed source material to be shipped interstate and to be used to manufacture a licensed product. For example, for Factor VIII, the source material may be Recovered Plasma, which is not a licensed product. The Recovered Plasma is not the product in short supply. The short supply provisions allow manufacturers to use an unlicensed or another licensed establishment to perform the initial and partial manufacturing step of collecting blood or plasma. In order for Recovered Plasma to be shipped to a fractionator for further manufacture into injectable products, a short supply agreement must exist. The written agreement should be current and state the use of the product, as well as which tests are performed on the units. The use of the product is a key element in being able to label the product correctly. If the product will be used for further manufacture into an injectable product, the label should bear the statement: "Caution: For Manufacturing Use Only." If the product will be used for further manufacture into a noninjectable product, the label statement should be: "For Use in Manufacturing Non-injectable Products Only." If there is no short supply agreement, the label should read: "Caution: For Use in Manufacturing Non-injectable Products Only," and the following statement should also be used: "Not for use in products subject to license under Section 351 of the Public Health Service Act."

To use the short supply provisions, the manufacturer holding a US license to prepare the finished biological product must establish with the suppliers the procedures, inspections, tests, or other arrangements necessary to ensure full compliance with the applicable regulations for blood establishments. (The short supply agreement must be between the licensed fractionator and the collecting facility. This agreement *cannot* be between the licensed fractionator and the broker.) The written agreement should be updated annually and signed by all parties, including the broker. The responsibility for compliance with standards for the source material rests with the licensed manufacturer (i.e., the fractionator) of the final product, as well as with the supplier. Noncompliance may result in revocation of the short supply exemption as well as other enforcement activities by the FDA.

RECOVERED PLASMA REGULATIONS AND REQUIREMENTS

Recovered Plasma is derived from single units of expired or unexpired Whole Blood, or Plasma, or is a byproduct of the preparation of blood components from single units of blood as defined in 21 CFR 606.3(c). It is an unlicensed source material intended for use in the manufacture of both licensed and unlicensed products, such as licensed fractionated products for injection, licensed diagnostic products, and unlicensed diagnostic products, including clinical

DEPARTMENT OF HEALTH AND HUMAN SERVICES
PUBLIC HEALTH SERVICE
FOOD AND DRUG ADMINISTRATION
BLOOD BANK INSPECTION CHECKLIST AND REPORT

1.   GENERAL INFORMATION

a. NAME OF INVESTIGATOR(S)	b. DATE(S) OF INSPECTION

c. TOTAL INSPECTION TIME IN THE BLOOD BANK	d. LEGAL NAME OF THE BLOOD BANK	e. DBA

f. ADDRESS OF ESTABLISHMENT BEING INSPECTED	g. TELEPHONE NUMBER	h. REGISTRATION NUMBER/MEDICARE NUMBER/CLIA NUMBER

i. U.S. LICENSE NUMBER AND LOCATION NUMBER	j. TYPE OF OPERATION (Check all applicable)	k. TYPE OF INSPECTION (Check all applicable)
	☐ BLOOD BANK ☐ TRANSFUSION SERVICE	☐ SCHEDULED ☐ FOLLOW-UP
	☐ DONOR CENTER ☐ TESTING LABORATORY	☐ PRELICENSE ☐ INVESTIGATION
	☐ MOBILE SITE	

l. ARE THERE CORRECTIONS TO BE MADE ON FORM FDA 2830, "BLOOD ESTABLISHMENT REGISTRATION AND PRODUCT LISTING"?
　　　　　☐ YES (If "YES" specify in comments)　　　☐ NO

m. ARE ALL FIXED LOCATIONS REGISTERED? ☐ YES ☐ NO	n. HAS FORM FDA 483, "INSPECTION OBSERVATIONS" BEEN ISSUED? ☐ YES ☐ NO

o. HAVE DEVIATIONS CITED IN THE PREVIOUS INSPECTION BEEN CORRECTED?
　　　　　☐ YES　　　☐ NO (If "NO" list continuing deviations in comments)

2.   RESPONSIBLE INDIVIDUALS AND PERSON(S) INTERVIEWED

a. NAME OF DIRECTOR, IF NOT LICENSED [606.20(a)]	b. NAME OF RESPONSIBLE HEAD, IF LICENSED [600.10(a)]	c. NAME OF SUPERVISOR(S)

d. NAME AND TITLE OF INDIVIDUAL(S) INTERVIEWED	e. NAME OF PERSON(S) WITH WHOM OVERALL INSPECTION WAS DISCUSSED

3.   RESOURCE DATA

a. APPROXIMATELY HOW MANY UNITS OF WHOLE BLOOD ARE COLLECTED EACH YEAR? _____ (1) HOW MANY OF THESE ARE AUTOLOGOUS?_____ (2) HOW MANY OF THESE ARE DIRECTED? _____	b. APPROXIMATELY HOW MANY UNITS OF WHOLE BLOOD AND RED BLOOD CELLS ARE RECEIVED FROM OUTSIDE SOURCES EACH YEAR? _____ (1) HOW MANY OF THESE ARE AUTOLOGOUS?_____ (2) HOW MANY OF THESE ARE DIRECTED? _____

c. APPROXIMATELY HOW MANY UNITS OF WHOLE BLOOD AND RED BLOOD CELLS ARE TRANSFUSED EACH YEAR?
_____

4.   OPERATIONS (Circle products prepared and activities conducted)

a. DONOR SUITABILITY AND COLLECTION (Whole Blood)

　(1) HOMOLOGOUS

　(2) AUTOLOGOUS

　(3) DIRECTED DONORS

　(4) THERAPEUTIC

b. LABORATORY (For establishments which collect blood and/or prepare components, includes ABO & Rh and viral testing of blood components)

c. RED BLOOD CELLS

　(1) ADDITIVE SOLUTIONS

　(2) RED BLOOD CELLS, FROZEN

　(3) RED BLOOD CELLS, DEGLYCEROLIZED

　(4) REJUVENATING SOLUTIONS

　(5) RED BLOOD CELLS, LEUKOCYTES REMOVED

　(6) IRRADIATED BLOOD

d. PLASMA, LIQUID PLASMA, FRESH FROZEN PLASMA, AND RECOVERED PLASMA (If plasmapheresis or therapeutic plasma exchange is performed, also complete form FDA 2722, "Plasmapheresis Checklist and Report")

e. PLATELETS

f. CRYOPRECIPITATED AHF/POOLED (If plasmapheresis or therapeutic plasma exchange is performed, also complete form FDA 2722, "Plasmapheresis Checklist and Report")

g. LABELING

h. COMPATIBILITY TESTING AND TRANSFUSION REACTIONS

i. STORAGE, DISTRIBUTION

j. PLATELETS, PHERESIS

k. COMPUTERIZATION

FORM FDA 2609 (5/91)   PAGE 1 OF 27 PAGES

FIGURE 14-1　The FDA blood bank inspection checklist.

ITEM	CFR NO	YES	NO	COMMENTS - IDENTIFY BY NUMBER
5. STANDARD OPERATING PROCEDURES (SOP's):				
a. For all operations performed by the Blood Bank, are SOP's maintained as required?	606.100			
b. Is there a written procedure to minimize the spread of infectious agents?				
c. Is there evidence of periodic review and updating of procedures?	606.100(b)			
d. Do personnel appear familiar with current SOP's?	606.100(b) 606.20(b)			
e. Are SOP's readily available to personnel?	606.100(b)			
f. Is there documentation of personnel review of SOP's	606.160			
6. RECORDS:				
a. Is a record of unsuitable donors used to prevent the distribution of products collected from such individuals?	606.160(e)			
b. Are all distribution and disposition records complete as required?	606.160(b)(3) (i)			
c. Do distribution records readily enable a unit of whole blood and all of its components to be traced?	606.165 (a)&(b)			
d. Destruction Records:	606.160(b)(3) (i)			
(1) Are destruction records maintained?				
(2) Do records indicate reason for destruction?	606.160(a)(1)			
(3) Do records include all components prepared from an HBsAg/anti-HIV reactive or otherwise unsuitable unit?	606.160(a)(1)			
(4) Do records indicate method of destruction?	606.160(a)(1)			
e. Are records retained after processing for at least five years or six months after the latest expiration date for the individual product (whichever represents a later date)?	606.12(b) 606.160(d)			
f. Are they traceable to the donor?	606.160(c)			
7. ERRORS AND ACCIDENTS/REPORTABLE INCIDENTS:				
a. Have there been any fatal donor and/or recipient reactions since the last inspection?				
b. If yes, was the Director, Office of Compliance, CBER, notified as soon as possible?	606.170(b)			
c. Have there been any shipments or distribution of unsuitable blood products, or laboratory, or labeling errors affecting product quality since the last inspection?				
d. If yes, and the firm is licensed, has the Director, Office of Compliance, CBER, been notified?	600.14(a)			
e. If yes, has the firm notified the users and attempted to retrieve unsuitable products? Has the local FDA district office been notified?				
f. Were appropriate records maintained of such incidents?	606.160(b)(7) (iii) 606.170(a)			
g. Was the firm's review and investigation of the error/accident and corrective action adequate to prevent a recurrence?				
8. FACILITIES, EQUIPMENT, AND PERSONNEL:				
a. Are all facilities clean, orderly and suitable?	606.40			
b. Is equipment used in collection, processing, compatibility testing, storage, and distribution of blood and blood components:	606.60(a)			
(1) Maintained in a clean and orderly manner?				

FIGURE 14-1 *Continued*

chemistry controls. A license is not required to manufacture, distribute, relabel, pool, or repack recovered plasma.

Brokers frequently act as an intermediary between the collector and the licensed manufacturer of the final product. Selling plasma to a broker does not relieve the collector of the responsibility of obtaining a short supply agreement if needed or from correctly labeling the product. It is in the best interest of the establishment to obtain a letter from the broker stating the intended use of the product. The short supply agreement is between the collector and the licensed fractionator, not the broker. Plasma brokers may act as authorized agents and should be identified in the agreement. Brokers that take physical possession of plasma must register with the FDA.

TESTING LABORATORIES

The FDA regulations require that US licensed blood establishments have testing performed on products at US licensed facilities. Written contracts between the two facilities should designate the number of times a test will be performed and that all viral marker tests will follow the manufacturer's package insert. Strict adherence to an algorithm (manufacturer's instructions and FDA guidance requiring that units be discarded if two of three tests are reactive) is often not fully understood and continues to cause product recalls.

Overview of the Inspection Process

A compliance program is written by the CBER to give guidance to the FDA headquarters and field personnel concerning surveillance and enforcement activities involving blood establishments.[10] The objective of the compliance program is to ensure that blood and blood products are safe, effective, and adequately labeled. This guidance manual includes regulatory and administrative guidance for inspecting licensed and unlicensed blood banks. Each inspection covers the manufacturing operation of the blood bank to ensure that GMPs are being followed. Use of the blood bank inspection checklist (Fig. 14–1) is encouraged so that inspections will follow a uniform approach. The checklist is designed to follow a unit of blood through the system or from donor to patient. The checklist uses a systems approach to perform inspections. Questions elicit information about each of the areas in the blood bank, blood center, or transfusion service. The sections of the checklist are:

1. Donor suitability and collection
2. Laboratory
3. RBCs
4. Plasma
5. Platelets

```
                INSTRUCTION BOOKLET

                       FOR

     BLOOD BANK INSPECTION CHECKLIST AND REPORT

                 FORM FDA-2609


               TABLE OF CONTENTS
```

(5/91)

FIGURE 14–2 Table of contents of the instruction booklet for the FDA blood bank inspection checklist and report.

6. Cryoprecipitated AHF
7. Labeling
8. Compatibility testing and transfusion reactions
9. Storage and distribution
10. Platelets, Pheresis
11. Computerization

A set of instructions outlined in the table of contents that accompany the checklist gives additional information about the meaning of the questions (Fig. 14–2). The checklist is designed so that adequate performance will be documented if most of the answers to the questions are "yes"; usually "no" answers require an explanation and would mean that regulations or recommendations have not been followed.

The first page of the checklist asks questions about SOPs; records of distribution or destruction or both; errors; accidents and fatalities; facilities; equipment; personnel; and disposal of infectious waste. These questions are placed in the beginning of the checklist to focus attention on evaluating important areas at the start of the inspection.

In 1991, a CBER review of inspectional findings, error and accident reports, blood product recalls, and enforcement actions indicated a substantial increase in these areas compared with those of the past five years, which prompted the issuance of a memorandum on March 21, 1991 to all registered blood establishments, entitled "Deficiencies Relating to the Manufacture of

Blood and Blood Components." This memorandum listed the most significant deficiencies observed and was provided so that blood establishments could use this information to perform audits to ensure they did not have deficiencies in these areas and, if they did, to correct them promptly. The significant deficiencies in the donor deferral systems were:

Deferral records were incomplete, not current, or did not provide for accurate identification of the donor as required by 21 CFR 606.160.

Donors were not recognized as having multiple reasons for deferral (e.g., hepatitis B surface antigen and serologic test for syphilis)

Computer systems contributed to the loss of donor records or did not recognize all reasons for deferrals.

Blood bank directors as well as supervisors were urged to review SOPs and manufacturing operations with regard to the potential for errors in testing and donor deferral lists. The information was provided so it could be used for self-audits. The number of recalls and errors reported to the FDA increased dramatically in 1987, and the upward spiral continues at the time of writing this chapter. Figure 14–3 illustrates how the number of recalls stayed at the same low level from 1981 to 1985. With the advent of anti–human immunodeficiency virus (anti-HIV) testing and additional donor suitability criteria associated with signs and symptoms of AIDS and behaviors that would place donors at increased risk, the number of recalls increased in 1986. A sharp increase was again noted in 1988. FDA Commissioner Frank Young requested workshops for FDA investigators, which focused on inspection of viral marker testing. In 1988, the schedule for inspection of blood establishments was changed to annually rather than every 2 years. The workshops as well as the additional testing requirements for blood products for transfusion resulted in further increases in the number of recalls in 1989, 1991, and 1992.

In addition to an increase in the number of recalls,

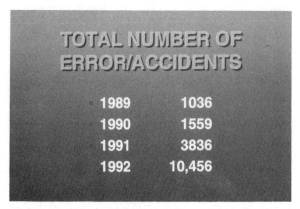

FIGURE 14–4 Total number of error/accident reports submitted to the CBER from 1989 to 1992.

an increase in the number of errors reported to the FDA has also been observed (Fig. 14–4). The increase in error reports is due in part to the memorandum that reminded the blood bank community of 21 CFR 600.14, which requires licensed establishments to report errors to FDA by licensed establishments. Registered establishments that do not hold a US license are required to keep a record of errors as well as any necessary corrective action, per 21 CFR 606.100(c), but they are not required by regulation to report these errors to the FDA. The FDA requested voluntary reporting by registered establishments in the March 20, 1991 memorandum; however, only a few institutions have chosen to send the reports to the CBER. The sharp increase to more than 10,000 reports (Fig. 14–5) in 1992 is due to information received from donors at a subsequent donation and to donors calling back after their donation to give information that would have been cause for deferral if the donor had given the information at the time of donation (Fig. 14–6). Both categories are due, in part, to the direct questioning of donors concerning risk behaviors. Guidance concerning which reports should be sent to the CBER has lowered the number of reports.

Another area addressed during an inspection is fa-

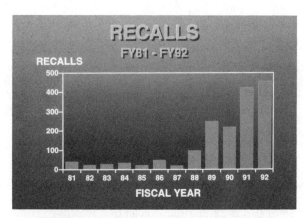

FIGURE 14–3 Biologics recalls from 1981 to 1992.

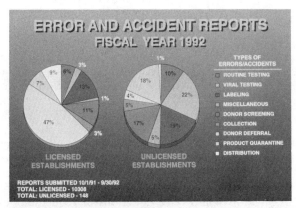

FIGURE 14–5 Error and accident reports submitted to the CBER from October 1, 1991 to September 30, 1992.

ERROR REPORTS

	1989 %	1990 %	1991 %	1992 %
ROUTINE TESTING	24.5	17.8	13.3	7.0
VIRAL TESTING	4.1	4.0	7.0	2.9
COLLECTION	6.0	4.3	3.8	2.0
LABELING	18.7	17.4	18.0	14.2
DONOR SCREENING	12.5	10.4	8.4	12.2
DONOR DEFERRAL	0.5	21.0	24.5	41.9
PRODUCT QUARANTINE	3.2	9.6	9.4	7.5
DISTRIBUTION	26.4	14.6	13.8	11.3
MISCELLANEOUS	4.1	0.7	1.8	1.0

FIGURE 14–6 Error and accident reports by category from 1989 to 1992.

talities. When a death occurs after transfusion, or in the rare case of blood collection, blood bank staff are often uncertain about which fatalities must be reported to the CBER.[11] Many patients die while receiving blood and blood components or immediately afterward, but it is not the intent of 21 CFR 606.170 to require that each of these deaths be reported to the CBER. The death of the patient or donor may have only a temporal relationship to the transfusion or collection of blood. This regulation requires reporting only actions related to a transfusion that may have contributed to the death of a patient or a blood collection error that may have caused a donor fatality. Purposes of this reporting are (1) to ensure that the incidents are thoroughly investigated; (2) to determine if appropriate corrective action has been taken to prevent a recurrence; and (3) to evaluate reports for trends that may warrant action by the FDA or HCFA, such as new recommendations or policies or the review of existing approvals or policies.

Inspection Outcomes

Administrative and legal actions such as license suspension, injunction, and prosecution are rare occurrences, and voluntary compliance is the usual course of action and the goal of the FDA.

One frequent question is what to do when an inspection does not come to a happy conclusion. There are a number of examples that come to mind. What should be done if you disagree with an item that has been written on the list of observations of objectionable conditions (form FDA-483)? First, you must be certain that you are not in violation of FDA regulations, and then you should respond to the Form FDA-483 in writing to the local district office. Each Form FDA-483 has the address and telephone number of the local FDA office in the upper righthand corner. The FDA Form-483 is a list of observations that the investigator believes are deviations of regulations or CGMPs. This is the opinion of the investigator and, prior to any regulatory action, the FDA Form-483 and

the narrative report will be reviewed by a supervisory investigator in the district office. If the supervisor is convinced that the observations made by the investigator are serious enough to warrant regulatory action, the report will be referred to the district compliance branch, which will obtain CBER concurrence if the violations concern viral marker testing, donor reentry, computers and labeling, or promotional advertising. A copy of the written report may be obtained by requesting it through the FOIA. Although not required, a letter of corrective action should be sent to the local district office. Sending a letter to the FDA describing the corrective action indicates that prompt action has been taken, and will be taken into consideration if regulatory action is being considered. It is no guarantee that regulatory action will not be pursued, but it could tip the scales and prevent further action by the FDA.

Another question is what can be done when you believe that an investigator is being unfair and is not listening to your responses? In this case the responsible staff should make an appointment to discuss the situation with the local director of investigations or by calling the investigator's supervisor.

Differences of opinion will always exist in inspection programs, but such differences can usually be discussed and resolved—however, perhaps not to everyone's satisfaction. You will always get an answer to your prayers; it just may not be the answer you expected.

Regulatory Sanctions and Administrative Actions

If an establishment is found violating any of the laws that the FDA enforces, it is usually given a chance to correct the problem voluntarily before the FDA pursues legal action. When an establishment cannot or will not correct a public health problem voluntarily, the FDA can invoke legal sanctions. The regulatory remedies available to the FDA to obtain compliance with the regulations are Warning Letters and Suspension or Revocation of operations under US license. Legal actions include Seizure, Injunction, and Prosecution.

Product recalls are voluntary actions taken by establishments, or in rare instances, requested by the FDA, to remove violative products from the market or correct the labeling of such products. The regulations governing recalls are found in 21 CFR, Part 7.

PRODUCT RECALLS

This is the most frequent administrative action used by the FDA. The FDA classified 2858 recalls in fiscal year 1991 and 2922 in 1992 (Fig. 14–7). Recalls of biologics accounted for 423 of the 2858 in 1991 and 456 of the 2922 in 1992. Recall of a violative product from the market by the manufacturer on its own initia-

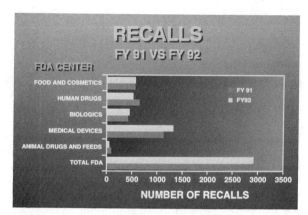

FIGURE 14–7 Recalls classified by the FDA for fiscal years 1991 and 1992 for biologics, food and cosmetics, human drugs, medical devices, animal drugs, and total FDA figures.

tive, or as requested by the FDA, is usually the quickest and most effective way to remove a violative product from the market. Why is recall necessary when the product has already been transfused? The purpose is to notify the consignee that the product was not what it was purported to be. Recall does not always mean that you literally get the product back. It can be a simple label correction such as an extended expiration date, or it could be a serious label correction such as notification that the viral marker tests were reactive. The most frequent causes of blood establishment recalls are due to mistakes in viral marker testing, donor deferral problems, and donor suitability errors. For example, a donor may admit to having been an intravenous drug user or to having traveled in an area endemic for malaria and the information was not used to defer the donor.

WARNING LETTERS

When violative conditions are documented during an establishment inspection, the report is reviewed in the local FDA district office by supervisory investigators and the district's compliance branch. Any significant deviation from the regulations that indicates a failure to assure donor protection and product safety or that represents a continuing pattern of noncompliance may result in the issuance of a Warning Letter by the local district office. In cases when the violations concern viral marker testing, donor reentry, product advertising, computer issues, and labeling, CBER concurrence is required before issuing a Warning Letter. A Warning Letter is the agency's threat to take further legal action indicating that the FDA has enough evidence to invoke additional and more severe regulatory sanctions such as injunction, license suspension, license revocation, seizure, or prosecution without further notice. After a Warning Letter has been issued, a follow-up inspection will occur to determine if corrective action has been effected. If appropriate corrective action has not been taken, the agency will consider how best to achieve compliance with the regulations.

LICENSE SUSPENSION OR REVOCATION

The suspension of a license prevents interstate shipment of all biological products under an establishment's control by requiring the immediate cessation of the authority to ship interstate. Suspension of a license is considered when conditions jeopardize donor health or product safety, and immediate correction is necessary. Suspension may also be an intermediate step to license revocation. Unlike license revocation, which can be a lengthy procedure, suspension is a summary action that is very quick and effective in stopping the danger to public safety or health. This administrative sanction is a very powerful tool and is used with great caution. The number of establishment license suspensions has been approximately three to 10 each year since 1977, most involving plasmapheresis centers rather than blood establishments. Only three blood establishment licenses have been suspended from 1972 to 1993. Such action by the agency against blood establishments is generally accompanied by adverse publicity leading to significant curtailment of overall activities by the firm and immediate correction of the violative conduct leading to the suspension.

The primary basis for revocation of a license is noncompliance with standards in the regulations as well as those in the license application. If it is determined that the violations of the law were willful or that corrective actions have not been taken during the period of license suspension, FDA will notify the firm of the intent to revoke the license. The violations must be determined to be a danger to the health of the donor or the recipient of the product. Revocation is the complete and final decision of a firm's authority to operate in interstate commerce.

SEIZURE

Seizure is a civil action to condemn the products, take custody of products, and remove them from distribution channels. After seizure, the products may not be tampered with, except by permission of the federal court. The owner or claimant of the seized products is usually given 30 days by the court to decide on a course of action. If nothing is done, the products will be disposed of by the court. The charges may be contested, and the case will be scheduled for hearings or trial. The owner of the products is required to provide a monetary deposit (i.e., bond to ensure that the orders of the court will be carried out) and must pay for FDA supervision of any compliance procedure.

INJUNCTION

The traditional injunction used by the FDA is the prohibitory injunction. Once ordered by the court, this action prohibits the firm from operating *unless and until* adequate corrections are made and verified by the FDA. The effect of such action is significant and ordinarily results in the complete shutdown of the firm, except in a hospital environment where the firm's transfusion services would continue to process blood from outside sources.

The other type of injunction used by the FDA is mandatory injunction, in which the court orders the affected firm to address certain specified conditions while the firm continues to operate.

Injunction is considered when there is a current health hazard or the establishment has a history of uncorrected deviations despite past warnings and the evidence suggests that serious violations will continue. Injunction may be considered as a legal remedy if there is no US license to suspend. Injunction may also be the legal remedy with a US licensed facility. Violation of an injunction is punishable as contempt of court. Any or all of these types of procedures may be used, depending on the circumstances. Since 1972, there have been three injunctions of volunteer blood establishments. The first injunction of a blood bank was in 1975, the second in 1979. The 1975 injunction followed a cease and desist letter sent from the FDA commissioner. The FDA filed a Complaint for Injunction on July 23, 1975, and the firm signed a Consent Decree of Permanent Injunction on August 18, 1975. The inspections revealed deviations from GMPs in the testing, storage, and adequate control over expired reagents.

The 1979 mandatory injunction *US versus John Elliott Blood Bank* charged that the methods, facilities, and controls used for collecting, manufacturing, processing, testing, labeling, and distribution of whole blood and blood components failed to comply with the CGMP regulations for drugs found in 21 CFR 211.1 to 211.115 and the biologic products regulations found in 21 CFR 600.3 to 680.16.[12] Injunction was chosen as the legal remedy to enable the blood supply for the area to continue and to ensure that the regional blood supply would be safe.

PROSECUTIONS

When fraud, health hazards, or continuing significant violations are encountered, it is the FDA's policy to consider prosecution. Before initiating a prosecution, the FD&C Act provides in Section 305 that individuals be given an opportunity to present their views with regard to the contemplated action. Only under limited and defined conditions will the FDA consider proceeding with prosecution without issuing such notice (e.g., if the violations are fraudulent or if those responsible are likely to flee). Prosecution is a criminal action directed against the firm or responsible individuals or both. It is punitive with the view of punishing past behavior and obtaining future compliance. The courts take a dim view of willful violations of the law and have imposed significant sentences, including incarceration of responsible individuals.

Quality Assurance: The Future

If anything can define the 1990s for the blood banking community it has to be quality assurance, total quality management, or process engineering. These are the current buzzwords that are in vogue, but what does this mean to the FDA?

The FDA sponsored an open public meeting in January 1991 that addressed quality assurance concerns. The workshop was held in response to a significant increase in the number of deficiencies observed during blood bank inspections relating to the release of unsuitable blood and blood products. The purpose of the workshop was to inform the public of FDA's expectations and to have dialogue with the blood bank community to learn of their quality assurance programs and views of quality assurance. FDA published proposed quality assurance guidelines in the *Federal Register*. Appropriate comments and suggestions offered at the workshop will be included in the document. These guidelines will be finalized after the comments received following publication of the proposed guideline in the *Federal Register* have been considered and the appropriate comments incorporated into the guidelines.

The promulgation of regulations and guidelines by the federal government should be monitored by each blood bank, transfusion service, or blood center. When proposals appear in the *Federal Register* these should be dissected and discussed to determine how they will affect your firm. The final regulation or guideline will be changed by the comments received following publication of a proposal.

Good Manufacturing Practices

There are many definitions of GMPs. The following definition is proposed by CBER's Office of Compliance: A GMP is the part of quality assurance that ensures that products are consistently manufactured according to, and controlled by, the quality standards appropriate for their intended use. It encompasses both manufacturing and quality control procedures.

There have been numerous discussions about the FDA's drug GMPs, which are found in 21 CFR 211. These regulations were written with the manufacture of drugs in mind and were not specifically written for the manufacture of blood or blood products. There is a noticeable difference in the language found in Part 600 as these regulations specifically address procedures that are commonly performed in a blood bank or transfusion service or blood center.

The drug GMPs require that each firm must have a quality control unit, which, in the current terminology would be called a "quality assurance (QA) unit." This is not found in the blood GMPs. The blood GMPs have requirements for quality control and set specific quality control requirements. The drug regulations also specify that this quality control unit must be separate from production or manufacturing and not reportable to the production group.

The responsibilities of the quality control unit are

1. To review and approve procedures, specifications, production records, and final release of the product
2. To analyze and test raw materials, bulk, in-process product, finished product, and postmarket stability
3. To audit by reviewing procedures, records, complaints, and recalls, thereby determining compliance with GMPs and SOPs, and to provide findings to production supervisors
4. To review and approve SOPs, record-keeping systems, incoming materials, and equipment validation and maintenance programs
5. To monitor SOPs and reagents; verify production at critical control points; and monitor complaints, errors or accidents, and adverse reactions
6. To audit the systems at critical control points, determine compliance with SOPs and GMPs, and reinspect for results of corrective action
7. To maintain previous SOPs and labels, records of quality control and release testing, investigations of errors or accidents, adverse reactions, complaints, and internal reviews
8. To review and approve training programs and employee position descriptions, and to monitor employee training and performance

Quality assurance is thought by some to be an elusive concept. How can a blood bank or transfusion service assure quality? The cornerstone of QA is a review of systems and the parts of each system to see how each part works and how the parts work together. One of the concepts discussed is how to foolproof the system. The idea is that if mistakes keep occurring, the procedure must be examined to see why it does not work. The previous way of addressing mistakes was to place blame on the employee and counsel, threaten, or fire that individual.[13] QA shifts the focus to looking at systems to see why they do not work and to fix the system, procedure, or SOP. This is not to say that there will never be human errors by employees who do not follow SOPs, but QA should cause an evaluation by asking: "Is this a good procedure and have staff been adequately trained to be able to understand and follow the procedure?"

When CBER staff reviews error reports, they are looking at the corrective action to see if steps have been taken to prevent the error from recurring. These reports are forwarded to the district offices, which will follow up at the time of the next inspection to ensure that the corrective action reported has, in fact, been implemented.

Compliance Policy Guide 7151.02, "FDA Access to Results of Quality Assurance Program Audits and Inspections," was revised to express the following policy: FDA will not review or copy reports and records that result from audits and inspections of a written QA program.[14] This policy applies to any regulated entity that has a written QA program that provides for periodic audits or internal inspections.

The FDA may seek written certification that such audits and inspections have been implemented, performed, and documented and that any required corrective action has been taken.

In addition, the FDA will continue to review and copy records and reports related to investigations of product failures and manufacturing errors as required by GMP regulations.

Chapter 15 describes how to implement a QA program in your institution.

Review Questions

1. Which of the following is responsible for establishing and maintaining the safety, purity, and potency of biological products for human use?
   A. Occupational Safety and Health Administration
   B. College of American Pathologists
   C. FDA
   D. Health Care Financing Administration
   E. Joint Commission on Accreditation of Healthcare Organizations

2. The regulations for blood and blood products are found in:
   A. The AABB *Technical Manual*
   B. The *Code of Federal Regulations*
   C. The AABB *Standards*
   D. The NIH Biosafety Manual
   E. The Interstate Commerce Regulations

3. The regulation of biological products in the United States began with:
   A. The Public Health Service Act of 1903
   B. The establishment of NIH in 1910
   C. The CLIA 67 guidelines
   D. The establishment of OSHA in 1980
   E. The Biologics Control Act of 1902

4. This law was passed in response to the deaths of:
   A. Ten children who died after receiving contaminated diphtheria antitoxin
   B. Two patients who died following transfusions with the wrong ABO group blood
   C. Five men in San Francisco who died of HIV complications
   D. Three neonates who died of Rh hemolytic disease of the newborn
   E. Two women who received contaminated flu shots

5. Responsibility for implementing this law was placed under:
   A. The National Institutes of Health
   B. The Office of Safety and Health Administration
   C. The Public Health Service
   D. The Office of the Surgeon General
   E. The Federal Bureau of Investigation

6. Which of the following is *not* part of the FDA blood bank inspection checklist?
   A. Donor suitability and collection
   B. Credentials of FDA inspectors
   C. Platelets
   D. Storage and distribution
   E. Labeling

7. GMPs refers to:
   A. General manufacturing products
   B. Good marketing practices
   C. Generic monoclonal products
   D. Good manufacturing practices
   E. Genetically manufactured products

8. Which of the following is *not* true about recovered plasma?
   A. A license is not required to distribute it.
   B. It is intended for use in unlicensed diagnostic products.
   C. It is intended for use in licensed fractionated products.
   D. It is intended for use in chemistry controls.
   E. A license is required to distribute it.

Answers to Review Questions

1. C   (p 289)
2. B   (p 289)
3. E   (p 289)
4. A   (p 289)
5. C   (p 289)
6. B   (p 296)
7. D   (p 300)
8. E   (p 296)

References

1. Code of Federal Regulations, Title 21 Parts 1–800, FDA, US Government Printing Office, Washington, DC, 1992.
2. Janssen, WF: The US Food and Drug Law: How It Came, How It Works. HHS Publication No (FDA) 79-1054, US Department of Health and Human Services, Public Health Service, FDA, Rockville, MD.
3. The Coroner's Verdict in the St Louis Tetanus Cases. 1901 New York Medical Journal 74; Special Article: Fatal results from diphtheria antitoxin. Minor comments: Tetanus from anti-diphtheria serum. JAMA 37:1255; 1260, 1901.
4. Milestones in US Food and Drug History, An FDA Consumer Memo. HHS Publication No (FDA) 85-1063, US Department of Health and Human Services, FDA, Office of Public Affairs, Rockville, MD.
5. Brady, R, and Kracov, DA: From diphtheria to cytokine products: A remarkable scientific journey/An ageing regulatory framework. Regulatory Affairs 3:105, 1991.
6. Timm, EA: 75 Years Compliance with Biological Product Regulations. Food Drug Cosmetic Law Journal, May 1978, Washington, DC, p 225.
7. Pittman, M: The regulations of biologics standards. 1902–1972. In Greenwald, HR, Harden, VA (eds): National Institute of Allergy and Infectious Diseases: Intramural Contributions, 1887–1987. US Department of Health and Human Services, Washington, DC, 1987, pp 61–70.
8. Legislative History of the Regulation of Biological Products, US Department of Health, Education, and Welfare; Public Health Service, FDA Bureau of Biologics, Washington, DC, 1978.
9. Blank vs US 400 Federal Supplement and 302 (CA 5, 1968).
10. FDA Compliance Program 7342.001—Inspection of Licensed and Unlicensed Blood Banks. Form FDA 2438f (8/90), insert TN 92-67, Washington, DC, (08/03/92).
11. Tourault, MA: Fatality reports. AABB News Briefs 15:12, 1992.
12. US vs John Elliott Blood Bank, Inc, et al, Civil No. 79-1807 (SD FLA 1979).
13. Gambino, R: Most laboratory errors are system dependent—not people dependent. Lab Med 20:123, 1989.
14. FDA Compliance Policy Guides. Chapter 61: Inspectional, FDA Access to Results of Quality Assurance Program Audits and Inspections. Form FDA 2678 a, Washington, DC, (6/3/89).

Bibliography

Bachner, P: Quality assurance: An accreditation perspective. Lab Med 20:159, 1989.
House of Representatives (Report No. 2713) in HR 15289, June 27, 1902: April 16, 1902 letter from acting chairman. The Medical Society of Washington, Washington, DC.

Organization-Wide Quality Assurance

Bonnie Lupo, MS, SBB(ASCP)

OBJECTIVES

Upon completion of this chapter, the learner should be able to:

1 Describe the difference between quality assurance and compliance.
2 Define organization-wide quality assurance.
3 List the components of organization-wide quality assurance.
4 Describe the need for and function of a process improvement team.

5 Solve problems or improve processes by using the Focus-Analyze-Develop-Execute (FADE) cycle.

6 Discuss the purpose of total process control.

7 List the components of total process control.

8 Explain the cause of variations in processes.

9 Explain a process or procedure utilizing a flow chart.

10 Understand current good manufacturing procedures.

11 Describe the essential features of an incident, error, and accident report.

12 State the purpose of an internal audit.

Webster defines quality as "the level of excellence of something; as, a product of high quality"; and defines assurance as "a promise, guarantee."[1] In a blood bank, the definitions of quality and assurance are combined to become the activity of providing the evidence needed to establish confidence that quality functions are performed at an elevated level. Quality functions include quality management, quality planning, and quality improvement. (Table 15–1 is a list of some of the many acronyms associated with the subject of quality assurance.) Quality management is a continuous managerial process that will ensure the quality of a product by using critical observations and studies of the processes, materials, and finished products. Quality management becomes synonymous with organization-wide quality assurance (OWQA), in that quality cannot be ensured in a product unless the process is properly managed.

Quality Assurance versus Compliance

Organization-wide quality assurance is not synonymous with compliance. Organization-wide quality assurance is active and continuous; compliance, like a snapshot, is the state of a program at a single point in time.

Compliance programs are designed to evaluate efficiency and effectiveness, by searching for and correcting errors, deficiencies, and any deviations from the norm. Compliance inspections are conducted every 1 to 2 years. Although this seems like the logical process, recent findings prove that compliance programs alone are inadequate due to the accelerated pace at which modern blood banks (which are complex and highly technologic) change. No longer can laboratories, blood banks, or medical services afford themselves the luxury of the standard 1- to 2-year interval between evaluations of the efficiency and effectiveness of their operations.

Programs that simply require the correction of obvious or identifiable deviations or deficiencies, or both, in manufacturing may leave the facility with a false conclusion that it has been brought into a temporary state of compliance. Compliance inspections characteristically do no more than provide an occasional opportunity to expose new and different problems. More time and effort must be invested in preventing deficiencies and errors, particularly with respect to blood collections and processing. Structural problems that underlie the deficiencies should be identified and corrected in order to minimize errors or accidents in a blood bank.

TABLE 15–1 ACRONYMS ASSOCIATED WITH QUALITY ASSURANCE

Acronym	Source Words
CAT	Corrective Action Team
CFR	Code of Federal Regulations
CGMP	Current Good Manufacturing Procedures
FADE	Focus-Analyze-Develop-Execute
FDA	Food and Drug Administration
HR	Human Resources
JCAH	Joint Commission on Accreditation of Hospitals
OWQA	Organization-Wide Quality Assurance
PIT	Process Improvement Teams
PM	Preventive Maintenance
QA	Quality Assurance
QAT	Quality Action Team
QC	Quality Control
QMB	Quality Management Board
SOP	Standard Operating Procedure

Quality Management Process

All blood bank activities require constant attention to achieve theoretical OWQA. In a blood bank, OWQA denotes programs or a quality management process that continuously monitors the performance of operations in three areas: (1) manufacturing, (2) administration, and (3) transfusion practice.

Manufacturing includes the collection, processing, testing, storage, and distribution of blood and blood components for transfusion or further manufacturing.

Administration includes all nontechnical functions and support services in the facility.

Transfusion practice includes clinical use of blood and blood components, patient-informed consent, autologous and directed donor programs, patient apheresis policies and procedures, intraoperative salvage, post-transfusion follow-up, investigation of transfusion reactions or infections, and reports to and meetings of the hospital transfusion committee.[2]

Organization-Wide Quality Assurance

The definition of OWQA is a customer-focused, strategic, and systematic approach to continuous improvement involving all persons in the organization. Organization-wide quality assurance provides the opportunity for all staff to be part of the team approach to continuous improvement. Organization-wide quality assurance provides a common structure for improvement of problems, processes, and issues that are shared by many persons from different departments and divisions. Organization-wide quality assurance is important not only for a blood bank but also for an entire organization. Everyone must be involved, from the top down and from the bottom up, to ensure success. Organization-wide quality assurance directs attention to serving customers. A customer can be the next person in a process (internal or external). Internal customers may include personnel on other shifts, nursing staff, housekeeping staff, transport personnel, purchasing department staff, etc. External customers may include donors, hospitals (other than your employer), physicians, patients, etc. Customers' needs must be satisfied with quality products and services, on time, with the correct order the first time, and supplied at the best possible cost. By working together, both internal and external customers can be satisfied.

Implementing OWQA requires an infrastructure in the organization: a foundation for *Quality*. Figure 15–1 is a suggested infrastructure.

QUALITY COUNCIL

A quality council should be composed of top-level management from the various departments ensuring total organizational representation. This council is responsible for developing the OWQA philosophy and policy, developing strategies for OWQA implementation, providing resource support, identifying projects and determining their priorities, and providing support for cross-functional process improvements.

QUALITY MANAGEMENT BOARD OR STEERING COMMITTEE

Each department within the organization has or is part of a Quality Management Board (QMB). These

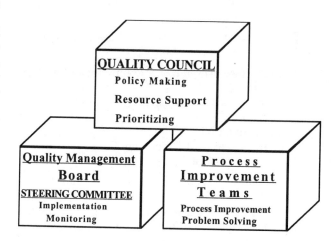

FIGURE 15–1 Organization-Wide Quality Assurance Infrastructure.

boards include senior managers and line representatives. The QMBs provide a structure to operationalize OWQA implementation strategies and to ensure continuous process improvement.

PROCESS IMPROVEMENT TEAMS, QUALITY ACTION TEAMS, OR CORRECTIVE ACTION TEAMS

Process Improvement Teams (PIT), Quality Action Teams (QAT), and Corrective Action Teams (CAT) are interchangeable terms; however, PIT and QAT are related to continuous improvement, whereas CAT suggests action taken as a result of a problem. In either case, teams are composed of individuals working on a specific process or problem. The teams are specifically formed to address a particular concern and disband when their work is completed. PITs should focus on opportunities to improve processes affecting:

1. Quality of product
2. Quality and reliability of service (to both internal and external customers)
3. Efficiency and accuracy of job performance
4. Waste reduction, scrap, rework, and operating costs
5. Equipment performance, up-time, and reliability
6. Intradepartment and interdepartment communications
7. Process control and improvement
8. Safety, hygiene, and work environment
9. Learning new skills, upgrading knowledge of the business, and developing personal capabilities
10. System improvement, procedures, and information transfer
11. Becoming "team players"

12. Scheduling, improved planning, and response time

Process Improvement Teams should *not* work on solving any issue concerning:

1. Problems covered by or directly related to union contracts
2. Grievances and grievance procedures
3. Seniority
4. Job assignments
5. Rates of pay and fringe benefits
6. Job classification

The Quality Council should set the general policy for PIT activity. Quality Management Boards should oversee formation of teams and ongoing PIT activities. The teams should identify processes for improvement, validate through measurement, propose solutions, implement solutions, and monitor processes for continuous improvement. To ensure success, a team leader is assigned to each PIT. This person is trained as a team leader. With newly established OWQA units it is advisable to have team leaders trained by outside agencies that are experts in the field. A formalized process (discussed in the next section) must be used to ensure success of these teams.

FADE (FOCUS-ANALYZE-DEVELOP-EXECUTE) CYCLE

When an opportunity for improvement has been identified, the FADE cycle (Fig. 15–2) can be used to manage the problem-solving process:

Focus on and define the right problems.
Analyze those problems.
Develop realistic and worthwhile solutions.
Execute new procedures and systems.

Total Process Control

A process is a systematic series of actions directed to the achievement of a goal. Process control is the activity that ensures a process will keep operating in a state that continuously is able to meet process goals without compromising the process itself. Total process control is the evaluation of the performance of a process, comparing actual performance with goal, and then taking action on the difference. Process measures or quality indicators are activities that are repeatable and measurable over a period of time.

Current Good Manufacturing Practices (CGMPs) are Food and Drug Administration (FDA) requirements that are sited in the *Code of Federal Regulations* (CFR), Title 21, Sections 200 and 600. They require that policies be developed to ensure that products are consistently manufactured to meet the quality standards appropriate to their intended use. Process controls are intended to reduce the amount of time spent on final inspection. The intent is to build quality into

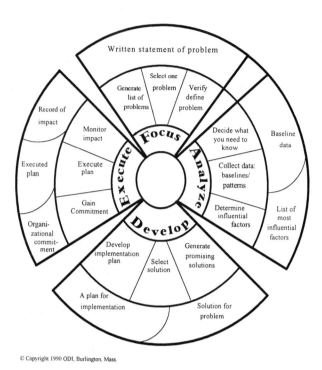

© Copyright 1990 ODI, Burlington, Mass.

FIGURE 15–2 The FADE cycle. (From Quality Action Teams. Organizational Dynamics Inc., Burlington, MA, 1990, with permission. Copyright 1990, ODI, Burlington, MA.)

the process from the very beginning, not only to inspect for quality into the final product.

Quality Control (QC) has been a part of blood banking since the early 1960s. It has evolved into a manageable process that is used to determine if reagents and equipment are functioning prior to testing. Controls run with the test validate that the assay has been performed correctly. Unacceptable results require an investigation to determine the cause and corrective action. What caused the unacceptable results? Did the process from beginning to end have process controls in place? Was the reagent deteriorating, were there weakly reactive results that were not detectable, did the instrument fail to operate correctly or had the technician not worked in that area for several months? If the process was completely detailed, including Standard Operating Procedure (SOP), process flow charts, critical control points, and process measures, the investigation would be inclusive. A process flow chart is used to visualize steps in a process. Critical control points must be identified. A critical control point is a step in the process that must be executed properly to ensure the final outcome is not compromised. Process measures are used to determine: the frequency of failure, potential cause(s) of failure, and the effect of any changes to the process.

Process measures or QC indicators are not limited to tests with measurable results. Indicators selected should be able to demonstrate that all systems are

TABLE 15-2 TRANSFUSION SERVICE INDICATORS

Number of blood products released and returned unused
Reason for return of blood products
Number of blood bags returned with needles still attached
Adequacy of blood supply
Availability of blood before surgery
Number of autologous and directed donors drawn
Accurately completed transfusion request forms
Labeling errors on specimens sent to the blood bank
Patient wristband identification errors
Turnaround time on antibody identification
Complaints concerning laboratory service

functioning within acceptable limits. Quality indicators can also be used to determine if a problem exists or to monitor effectiveness of corrective action. Once data are collected, they must be reviewed to be useful and thresholds must be set that will identify a drift in the system or process. After a change in procedure, measurements will visualize the impact of the change. Once it is determined that a process is in control, the frequency of recording measurements can be evaluated.

The transfusion service is required by the Joint Commission on Accreditation of Healthcare Organizations (JCAHO) to monitor patient care and efficacy of transfused products. The laboratory traditionally monitors technical or clerical errors, transfusion reactions, crossmatch-to-transfusion ratio, outdating of blood and blood products, and transfusion-transmitted disease. In a blood bank any process or event that is repeatable and has a measurable outcome can be monitored. Table 15-2 lists suggestions for indicators that may be monitored in a transfusion service.

VARIATIONS IN A PROCESS

It is essential to monitor a process to ensure that it is performing as required, to correct process problems before they affect output, and to improve process(es) to meet changing needs and technology.

The performance of a process can vary from day to day, but not all variation is cause for concern. Some minor variation is normal and results from causes you cannot easily control or change; however, other variations that exceed normal limits are the result of specific problems or influences that you can do something about.

If your process is affected by random, uncontrollable variations, you may be observing common causes, and as long as only common causes are at work your process is in control (e.g., employee illness). Common causes result from many factors, each of which may affect your process to a small degree. Common causes are often due to design and operating limitations and may be impractical or difficult to remove from the process. In fact, the slight daily variation you experience from common causes usually has a minimal effect

on your overall process. Removing these causes may not be necessary. Over time the process performs normally, and the status quo is maintained.

Certain factors, such as changes in the marketplace, sharper competition, and technologic advances, may direct you to fine-tune your process even though it is functioning normally. You may have reached a point where common causes are limiting competitive advancement. Under such circumstances, it may make sense to identify and remove these common causes. The only way to get rid of common causes is to redesign the process from the ground up.

If the process exceeds certain statistically determined operating limits, it is out of control, and you must act quickly to determine the specific cause of the variation and correct it. Special causes make a process go out of control. Unlike common causes, special causes:

1. Have a significant effect on a process
2. Affect a process in unpredictable ways
3. Provide immediate opportunities for improving the performance of the process.[3]

CONTROL CHARTS

Control charts and trend analysis are tools that offer ways to measure and monitor a process. When you develop process measures and use a control chart, you will be able to determine whether your process is in control or out of control and will identify opportunities for improvement.

Laboratories have used control charts to monitor assay performance. Standards or controls with known values are run periodically and entered on a chart. Statistical processing is used to determine the upper and lower limits for the control. Each time controls are run it is determined whether or not the process is in control. If the values are within range (i.e., they do not exceed the upper or lower limits), then the process is said to be in control. If the values exceed the range, then the process is considered out of control. An investigation is performed to determine the cause, and corrective action is decided on. Any tests performed associated with the out-of-range controls are repeated after the process is brought back into control.

Control charts can be used for any repeatable process that can be measured over time. Figure 15-3 is an example of a control chart that was used to track the number of sample labeling errors and the effectiveness of staff retraining.

FLOW CHARTS

Flow charts illustrate the actual sequence of events that occur during a process. Flow charts help develop a common understanding of the process. Mapping a situation helps uncover bottlenecks, missing steps, decision points, processing choices, and critical control points and acts as a reference for following a process.

SAMPLE LABELING ERRORS

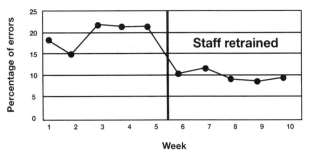

FIGURE 15-3 An example of a control chart used to monitor a process.

It is advantageous to use several charts to illustrate a process clearly. A flow chart can be constructed only after the process has been divided into a logical sequence of events. The last box of one chart would become the first box of another chart. It is easier for staff to follow if the flow chart can be limited to one page for each process or step.

Figure 15–4 is a basic flow chart for processing a unit of whole blood collected in a double bag. It illustrates decision points and processing choices and is an overview of the process.

Components of Total Process Control

Several factors must be considered when analyzing a process. A list of requirements and resources should be available for each process in the laboratory. In addition to the SOP for each process, several key elements to Total Process Control must be considered before performing the process (Table 15–3).

STAFF

Education. Human Resources (HR) department must evaluate and certify employee credentials and determine the literacy of the employee. The job description includes educational and license requirements for the posted position. Federal, state, and/or local regulations must be followed.

Skills. If the position requires a skilled employee, a competency test must be given before training in a given area (e.g., the ability to use a computer spreadsheet program).

Training. The program must be comprehensive, structured, mandatory, and appropriate for employee job responsibilities and duties.

Competency. Direct observation, record review, and tests (written, verbal, and/or practical) are used to determine employee competency. A minimum passing grade is required to take the proficiency test.

Proficiency. A panel of samples with known reactivity will be given to an employee to test. The only acceptable score is 100 percent.

Recertification. Once an employee is certified to work in an area, a competency and proficiency evaluation will be given yearly. Employees who have not worked in an area for 30 consecutive days must be recertified before working in that area again.

Each laboratory is required to document its policies. The criteria listed are recommendations and do not represent regulatory requirements.

EQUIPMENT

Equipment and instruments can be purchased or supplied by the manufacturer. Equipment does not require hardware, firmware, or software to function. Calibration, preventive maintenance (PM), and QC programs are designed to test the equipment for its intended use. Frequency of testing is determined by regulatory requirements, manufacturer's recommendations, frequency of use, testing volume, and reliability of apparatus. QC is required for critical steps. A critical step is any part of a process that will significantly change the expected outcome of the process if performed incorrectly.

INSTRUMENTS

Instruments include any apparatus that requires hardware, firmware, or software to function. Automated analyzers, readers, pipettors, and washers are included in this category. In addition to the items listed under equipment, instruments must also be validated. The complexity and decision-making functions of each instrument must be challenged during the validation. Instruments must be validated when installed and after upgrades to hardware, firmware, or software. A PM and QC system should be one that is manageable and meaningful for the intended use of the instrument.

ASSAY

An assay is a test system that is chosen based on an evaluation process that requires both technical and operational input. Sensitivity, specificity, and operational ease of use are the factors considered. Operations staff should also evaluate all factors in conjunction with the assay (i.e., the supplies, equipment, instrumentation, work flow, and staff requirements). A new assay requires a field validation. Operational data on an assay's performance can vary significantly due to size of laboratory, quality of samples tested, and environmental conditions. Lot-to-lot testing of both the new and the old lot number of a reagent or kit must be performed in order to determine equivalency. Daily or run QC is essential in order to monitor assay performance continuously.

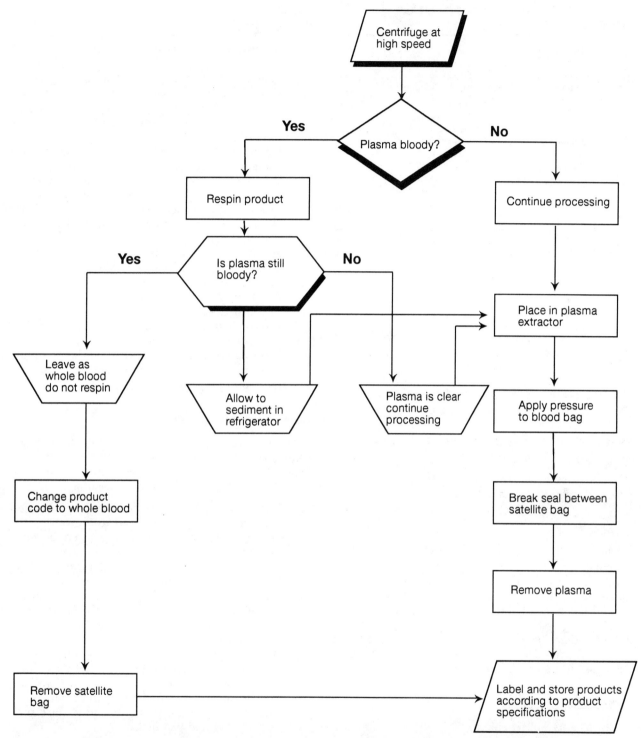

FIGURE 15-4 An example of a flow chart for processing a unit of whole blood collected in a double bag.

DOCUMENTATION

Documentation includes SOPs, manufacturer's directions on use of equipment, instruments or reagents, computer entry (inclusive of audit trail), software versions used, hard copy documents from instruments, manual test records, training records, competency testing, lot-to-lot testing, etc. Systems designed for manual entry of data must incorporate a manageable review process to ensure compliance to SOPs. An archive system for SOPs and other data should be in place to allow for easy retrieval. SOPs and records must be kept for a minimum of 5 years or 6 months past the product expiration date (21 CFR

TABLE 15–3 **COMPONENTS OF TOTAL PROCESS CONTROL**

Staff	*Assay*
Education	Sensitivity
Skills	Specificity
Training	Field validation
Competency	Lot to lot
Proficiency	QC
Recertification	
	Documentation
Equipment	SOP
Calibration	Test data
PM and QC	QC records
	Proficiency records
Instruments	Monitoring reports
Validation	
Calibration	
PM and QC	

PM = preventive maintenance; QC = quality control; SOP = standard operating procedure.

606.160). State and local requirements for record storage must be adhered to.

NYBC (New York Blood Center) Production and Process Controls[4]

PRODUCTION AND PROCESS CONTROL PLAN

The following is an outline from the New York Blood Center's (NYBC) CGMP training program on production and process controls.

Purpose

This module will provide a general application and rationale for production and process controls for a production system to ensure that process and procedures are conducted within established criteria for acceptance. Specific process control requirements for an operating system, pertaining to written SOP, batch records, time restrictions, in-process tests, criteria used, and adequate supervision will be reviewed and examined using applicable case studies.

Instructional Objectives

Participants will be able to:

1. Identify and name process controls now in place at their respective work areas
2. Identify work areas that may need process controls and make recommendations.

Preevaluation

Participants given pretest to determine current level of understanding

Definitions

1. *Production and process controls:* Activity (or series of activities) to manage the production of a product through all steps of manufacturing to eliminate the necessity of reliance on final inspection
2. *Control:* Activities related to evaluating the performance of a process, comparing actual performance with goal, and taking action on the difference
3. *SOP:* Directives issued by quality assurance for communicating established methods for performing and administering the work relative to ensuring and controlling the quality of NYBC products and services
4. *Batch:* Products identified and traceable to a specific production period
5. *In-process test:* Examinations to ensure standards, specifications, and characteristics are met for products being produced
6. *Deviation:* Activity that represents changes from established methods
7. *Process:* Systematic series of actions directed to the achievement of a goal
8. *Process control:* Activity of keeping the operating process in a state that continues to be able to meet process goals

Laboratory requirements

The *Code of Federal Regulations* (CFR), Section 21, code 211.100 (a) and (b) and 606.100 of Subpart F, Production and Process Controls, state the following:
211.100 Written procedures; deviations.

1. There shall be written procedures for production and process control designed to assure that the drug products have the identity, strength, quality, and purity they purport or are represented to possess. Such procedures shall include all requirements in this subpart. These written procedures, including any changes, shall be drafted, reviewed, and approved by the appropriate organizational units and reviewed and approved by the QC unit.
2. Written production and process control procedures shall follow in the execution of the various production and process control functions and shall be documented at the time of performance. Any deviation from the written procedure shall be recorded and justified.

606.100 Standard operating procedures. Written standard operating procedures shall be maintained and shall include all steps to be followed in the collection, processing, compatibility testing, storage, and distribution of blood and blood components for homologous transfusion, autologous transfusion, and further manufacturing purposes. Such procedures shall be available to the personnel for use in the areas where the procedures are performed. . . . [5]

PRODUCTION PROCESS CONTROLS FOR A UNIT OF BLOOD

Production process controls (PPCs) make certain that a unit of blood is not adversely affected by the process and that the process will identify and reject unsuitable blood from further manufacturing. To achieve this, written procedures for process controls must be available to personnel responsible for production. The staff must be qualified and adequately trained to perform the procedures as they were intended to be performed. Identify critical control points that must be strictly adhered to in order to avoid compromising the final product.

To ensure proper collection, processing, testing, labeling, and distribution of blood and blood products at NYBC, the following SOPs contain the required PPCs: NYBC Nursing Manual, NYBC Central Laboratory Manual, SafeBlood Operators Manual (SafeBlood is the NYBC laboratory computer system), and the NYBC Distribution Manual. The following are process (critical) control points at NYBC:

Donor Suitability

1. The health historian conducts the interview, performs donor qualifying tests and measurements, and ensures all predonation requirements are met before phlebotomy is performed.
   a. Donor must be a volunteer donor.
   b. The consent is signed, the signature verified, and a confidential donor decision label is affixed on the form.
   c. Donor must indicate that he or she is in good health, has an acceptable medical history, and passes qualifying tests and measurements.
2. Health historian reviews form for completeness, verifies that the donor has met the criteria for an acceptable donation, and signs registration form to that effect.

Blood Collection

In the donor collection area, the phlebotomist must verify that:

1. The donor is identified and a unique donor identification number is affixed to the registration form, each blood bag, and test tubes.
2. Collection scale devices are adjusted and set to measure accurately the quantity of blood removed from the donor.
3. Schedules and procedures for equipment maintenance and calibration are maintained.
4. The site of phlebotomy is scrubbed effectively for 30 seconds with an appropriate solution to give maximum assurance of a sterile container of blood.
5. The blood bag is agitated thoroughly to mix the blood with the anticoagulant.
6. The bleeding time does not exceed 20 minutes.

7. The phlebotomist who collected the blood signs the health history form.
8. The storage temperature requirements for the unit of blood are maintained.

Component Processing

On arrival in the laboratory:

1. Blood transportation temperature and storage requirements are checked.
2. SafeBlood donor form input is performed.
3. SafeBlood bag check-in is performed.
4. Not-for-transfusion (NFT) units are quarantined immediately.
5. Temperature requirements for component preparation are met.
6. Volume requirements and time restrictions for component preparation are met.
7. Temperature requirements for component are maintained during processing.
8. Schedules and procedures for equipment maintenance and calibration are maintained: centrifuges, scales, refrigerators, freezers, etc.
9. Quality control for product meets standards: platelets, fresh frozen plasma (FFP), cryoprecipitate (Cryo), red blood cells (RBCs), etc.
10. Rejected in-house materials such as incomplete, contaminated, overweight, and NFT units are identified and quarantined.

Testing

The testing laboratory ensures:

1. Sample tube identification and volume requirements are met.
2. Quality control procedures for reagents and equipment are within acceptable limits.
3. Required test and repeat tests are performed for each uniquely identified sample. The following tests are currently required: ABO Rh; alanine aminotransferase (ALT); antibody screening; hepatitis B surface antigen (HBs Ag); hepatitis B core antibody (HBc); hepatitis C antibody (HCV); human immunodeficiency virus types 1 and 2 (HIV-1, HIV-2); human T-cell lymphotropic virus type 1 (HTLV-1); and syphilis.
4. Schedules and procedures for equipment maintenance and calibration are maintained.
5. Divisions and laboratories are notified by the central laboratory after completion of the quality assurance review of test results.

Review and Labeling

1. Labeling takes place after all required tests are completed and the SafeBlood laboratory unit exception report is reconciled.
2. Blood and blood products are labeled through

SafeBlood after all process requirements are completed:

  a. Donor decision has been scanned.
  b. Nursing audit is completed.
  c. Unit withdrawal registry (donor deferral database) has been checked.
  d. ABO Rh prior history is checked.
  e. Test results, retrospective, and general hold interdictions are identified.
  f. All tests have been completed as required by testing profile.
  g. The temporary test table in SafeBlood has been checked for unscheduled tests that were performed (cytomegalovirus, hemoglobin S).
  h. ABO Rh discrepancy report has been reviewed and any discrepancies have been investigated.
  i. Processing date and time for platelets are within 8 hours of blood collection date and time.
  j. Processing date and time for FFP and Cryo (placed in freezer) are within 8 hours from blood collection date and time.
  k. The plasma volume in the final platelet product is between 40 and 60 ml.
  l. Expiration date on final product is displayed on computer screen and verified with product label.
  m. Alert codes entered during processing are displayed at labeling and product handled accordingly.

3. Length of expiration dates are checked and assigned for each product produced.
4. Labeling reconciliation reports are checked before product is released to inventory.
5. Products are released from work in progress and physically transferred to distribution area holding refrigerators, freezers, and room temperature incubators.

Inventory Storage and Distribution

Component storage: Storage temperatures and methods of controlling storage temperatures for all blood products are maintained.

Distribution: Whole blood and RBC products are visually inspected before issue for bacterial contamination, clots, icteric plasma, lipemic plasma, and correct product labeling. Frozen products are inspected for evidence of thawing and correct product labeling.

The Process

Staff training is an integral part of OWQA. The CGMP course is required and is intended to be informational and create an awareness of the complexity of our laboratories. In order to succeed, the process must be adopted by the entire organization and all employees must be trained. Depth of training will vary according to job responsibilities.

Figure 15–5 illustrates the cyclic process that encourages continuous improvement.

Incident Reporting

Regulatory agencies require the reporting of any error or accident in the manufacture of products that may affect the safety, purity, or potency of any product, or that compromises the safety of the donor or the recipient. Each facility must have a system for detecting, reporting, evaluating, and correcting errors and accidents. Procedures should be in place to ensure that donor and recipient adverse reactions are investigated. Donor or recipient adverse reactions may be life threatening, permanently disabling, or fatal. A

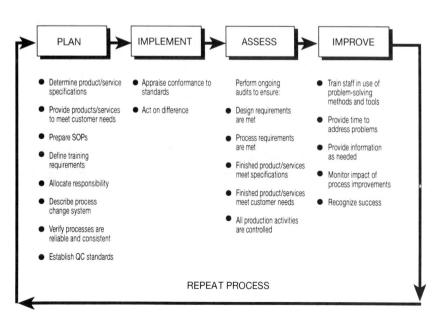

PLAN	IMPLEMENT	ASSESS	IMPROVE
• Determine product/service specifications	• Appraise conformance to standards	Perform ongoing audits to ensure:	• Train staff in use of problem-solving methods and tools
• Provide products/services to meet customer needs	• Act on difference	• Design requirements are met	• Provide time to address problems
• Prepare SOPs		• Process requirements are met	• Provide information as needed
• Define training requirements		• Finished product/services meet specifications	• Monitor impact of process improvements
• Allocate responsibility		• Finished product/services meet customer needs	• Recognize success
• Describe process change system		• All production activities are controlled	
• Verify processes are reliable and consistent			
• Establish QC standards			

REPEAT PROCESS

FIGURE 15–5 The process of Organization-Wide Quality Assurance.

program should be in place to train donor and patient care staff to recognize symptoms of adverse reactions so that appropriate intervention can be taken.

Investigation of complaints and error or accident feedback into the system are essential elements of quality assurance. If there is no investigation of complaints or errors, then factors that contributed to the problem cannot be identified and corrected. Errors and accidents in manufacturing may be identified either by employees in the course of routine activities or by supervisors during review of activities. Quality Assurance must assess all errors that occur during manufacturing, including those identified before products are released. There should be thresholds for initiating retraining related to errors and accidents. Quality Assurance procedures should be in place to ensure that all complaints regarding product quality are investigated to determine whether the complaint is related to an error or accident in manufacturing or to a patient or donor adverse reaction.[6]

In addition to the regulatory requirements, OWQA requires a reporting system that will allow the organization to track all incidents that occur. An incident is an occurrence or event that affects the quality of the laboratory's products and services and includes (but is not limited to) the following:

Accident: An unfortunate happening
Adverse reaction: Complication that occurred during the donation process to the donor or recipient of transfused blood or blood product
Complaint: Expression of dissatisfaction from an internal or external customer
Deviation: Variation from an approved SOP
Discrepancy: Difference or inconsistency in a process, procedure, or test results
Error: Variation from accuracy or correctness
Retrospective call: Call or letter from a donor with additional information regarding their donation

All employees are encouraged to participate in incident reporting. It is essential that incident reporting is not depicted as a tool for disciplining or finger pointing. Instead, it is a process improvement tool that is used to identify problems, analyze the cause, develop solutions, execute the solution, and track the effectiveness. Corrective action is required for error and accident reports and is usually connected to a process improvement activity.

The incident reporting process must be clearly defined so that the information is tracked and acted on, and feedback is provided (Fig. 15–6). A standard report can be used to capture all incidents. The Quality Assurance (QA) Officer (person responsible for performing quality assurance function in a facility) reviews all incidents, assigns an accession number, and forwards the incident to the department(s) that will be involved in the investigation. The completed report is returned to the QA Officer. The report is reviewed for completeness and appropriateness of corrective action. If the incident is reportable, it is sent to the Responsible Head or the Regulatory Affairs Officer,

QUALITY ASSURANCE INCIDENT REPORT

ORIGINATOR ACCESSION # ____________ TODAY'S DATE ______________

UNIT #(s) ______________________

DEPARTMENTS(s) ______________________________________

NAME OF ORIGINATOR ______________________________________

BRIEF DESCRIPTION OF INCIDENT (Attach additional paper, if needed) ________________

DATE SENT TO QA ______________________________________

INVESTIGATING DEPARTMENT ______________________________________

DATE RECIEVED __________ NAME OF INVESTIGATOR(s) ________________

ADDITIONAL DESCRIPTION OF INCIDENT ______________________________

INDICATE CORRECTIVE ACTION TO BE TAKEN (Attach additional paper if needed) ______

QUALITY ASSURANCE

SIGNATURE OF QA OFFICER ____________________________ DATE __________

__________ REPORTABLE __________ NON-REPORTABLE

DATE SENT TO REGULATORY (If Reportable) ______________________________

REGULATORY AFFAIRS

DATE RECIEVED ____________ DATE INCIDENT REPORTED ____________

RETURN FORM TO RESPONSIBLE QA OFFICER

FIGURE 15–6 Incident Report Form.

or both, and the appropriate forms are completed and submitted to the regulatory agencies. Completed reports and forms are returned to the QA Officer. Figure 15–7 is a suggested process flow for incident reporting.

Internal Audits

Previously, it was stated that quality assurance is active and continuous. . . . Internal audits are a useful approach for continuously monitoring the effectiveness of the total quality systems in place. Audits should be conducted by QA Officers sufficiently knowledgeable and trained to identify problems (critical control point deviations) in the areas under review. The QA Officers should not be responsible for performing the procedures that they are required to audit. Compliance and accrediting agency inspection checklists can be compiled and used as a guide for the area under audit. Unlike compliance inspections, internal audits should be scheduled; however, the internal audit should follow the same format as a compliance inspection. The audit is considered complete when an exit interview is held and the auditor outlines their findings. Observations noted require a response and corrective action. A process should be in place for the evaluation and review of the audit. In order to ensure that the corrective actions will be implemented, the Responsible Head and top management must be

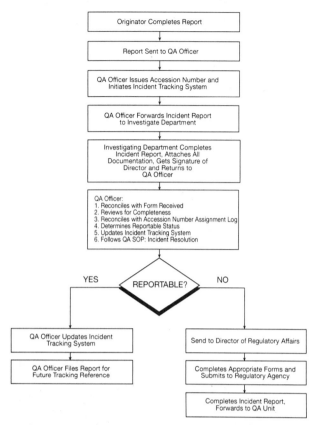

FIGURE 15-7 Flow chart for the incident reporting process.

QUALITY ASSURANCE INTERNAL AUDIT

Area/Function Assessed	
Subject Area	Date:
Key Positive Findings:	
Key Opportunity Areas:	
Recommendations for Improvement:	
Auditors:	Date:
Response: Planned Actions and Completion Dates	
Area Mgmt.:	Date:
Approved By:	Date:

FIGURE 15-8 Internal Audit Form.

involved. Figure 15-8 is an example of an internal audit form.

According to the FDA's Compliance Policy Guide 7151.02, internal reports that meet the guidelines in this policy will not be reviewed routinely by the FDA. The policy states, "This policy applies to any regulated entity which has a written quality assurance program that provides for periodic audits and inspections. FDA may seek written certification that such audits and inspections have been implemented, performed, and documented, and that any required corrective action has been taken. In addition, FDA may seek access to reports and records of such audits and inspection during a 'directed' or 'for cause' inspection of a sponsor or monitor of a clinical investigation, during litigation (under applicable procedural rules), or by an inspection warrant where access to records is authorized by statute. FDA will continue to review and copy records related to quality control investigations of product failures and manufacturing errors."[7]

Summary

If blood banking establishments are to achieve the standards of excellence needed to survive changes facing the blood banking industry today, quality assurance will be a requirement, not a luxury. Future vendors will be required to show documented proof that their facility is involved in an OWQA program. Only those facilities demonstrating OWQA will be approved for the purchasing of products and services. This cultural change will take time, so facilities that have not started must begin immediately. Noncompliant facilities will not pass compliance or accrediting agency's inspections, and consumers of hospital and laboratory services will accept no less than the total quality offered by those facilities already in compliance.

Review Questions

1. Organization-Wide Quality Assurance is:
   A. Synonymous with compliance
   B. Active and continuous
   C. A snapshot
   D. Evaluation of efficiency

2. Process Improvement Teams should focus on:
   A. Rates of pay and fringe benefits
   B. Efficiency and accuracy of job performance
   C. Grievances and grievances procedures
   D. Job assignments

3. The FADE cycle process is:
   A. Failure, analyze, disasters, effectiveness
   B. Future, academic, decisions, evaluate
   C. Focus, analyze, develop, execute
   D. Focus, achievement, decisions, efficiency

4. Common causes of variation are:
   A. Constant, controllable
   B. Random, uncontrollable
   C. Constant, uncontrollable
   D. Random, controllable

5. Flow charts are used to illustrate:
   A. Organization chart
   B. Educational objectives
   C. A sequence of events
   D. A sequence of objectives

6. Current Good Manufacturing Practices refer to:
   A. Regulations pertaining to laboratory safety
   B. Validation of testing
   C. Incident reports
   D. CFR regulations pertaining to manufacturing of products to meet quality standards

7. All of the following are components of Total Process Control *except*:
   A. Documentation
   B. Instruments
   C. Discipline
   D. Staff

8. The purpose of an internal audit is:
   A. Punitive: to punish employees
   B. Argumentative: to show employees they are always wrong
   C. Combative: to keep employees on their toes
   D. Improvement: for continuous improvement of the process

9. Organization-Wide Quality Assurance:
   A. Is a new European approach to quality
   B. Involves all persons in an organization
   C. Does not apply to hospitals or blood banks
   D. Refers to external customers only

10. Total Process Control is:
   A. Validation of instruments
   B. A systematic series of actions directed to the achievement of a goal
   C. Calibration of equipment
   D. A system in which management mandates controls and all activities

Answers to Review Questions

1. B (p 304)
2. B (p 305)
3. C (p 306)
4. B (p 307)
5. C (p 307)
6. D (p 306)
7. C (Table 15–2)
8. D (p 313)
9. B (p 312)
10. B (p 306)

References

1. *Webster's Dictionary*. Merriam-Webster, Springfield, MA, 1985.
2. Solomon, J: Expansion and redirection of the AABB Inspection and Accreditation Program. Rockville, MD, 1990.
3. Organizational Dynamics Inc.: The Quality Advantage. Training Handouts, Burlington, MA, 1989.
4. Fiorello, J: Section Y—Production/Process Controls. New York Blood Center GMP Training Program. Unpublished material, 1992.
5. *Code of Federal Regulations*. 21 CFR 211.100, 21 CFR 606.100, April 1, 1991.
6. FDA: *Compliance Policy Guide*. 7151.02, Chapter 51, Inspectional. Office of Enforcement, Division of Compliance Policy, US Government Printing Office, Washington, DC, 1989.
7. Robins, JL: Redefining and expanding quality assurance. Clin Lab Med 12:805, 1992.

Bibliography

Accreditation Manual for Pathology and Clinical Laboratory Services. Joint Commission on Accreditation of Healthcare Organizations, Oakbrook, IL, 1993.
American Association of Blood Banks: FDA enforcement legislation will strengthen FDA inspection sanctions. Blood Bank Week 8:1, 1991.
Committed to quality: An introduction to the Joint Commission on Accreditation of Healthcare Organizations. Joint Commission on Accreditation of Healthcare Organizations, Oakbrook, IL, 1990.
Department of Health and Human Services: Clinical laboratory improvement amendments of 1988: Final rule. Federal Register 57:7002–7288, US Government Printing Office, Washington, DC, 1992.
Feigenbaum, A: Total Quality Control. McGraw-Hill, New York, 1983, p 91.
Guideline on General Principles of Process Validation. Center for Drugs and Biologics and Center for Devices and Radiological Health. FDA, May 1987.
Ratliff, TA, Jr: The Laboratory Quality Assurance System: A Manual of Quality Procedures with Related Forms. Van Nostrand Reinhold, New York, 1990.

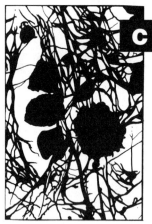

CHAPTER 16

Transfusion Therapy

Melanie S. Kennedy, MD
Carmen Julius, MD

OBJECTIVES

Upon completion of this chapter, the learner should be able to:

1 Describe the blood components currently available for therapeutic use.

2 Discuss the composition of each blood component and product, including the approximate volume of each product.

3 Select the appropriate blood product for patients with specific disorders.

4 State the expected incremental increase of a patient's:
    a Hematocrit following transfusion of each unit of packed red cells
    b Platelet count following transfusion of each unit of platelets

5 List the protocol necessary for preparation of each blood component and plasma derivative.

6 Compare and contrast the two types of filters used for blood transfusion.

7 Relate the groups of recipients at highest risk of infection from transfusion of cytomegalovirus-positive red blood cells or platelets.

8 Discuss the role of irradiation in the prevention of post-transfusion graft versus host disease.

9 Recognize the significance of the maximum surgical blood-ordering schedule as it relates to the reduction in unnecessary crossmatching.

10 State the main advantage of autologous transfusion.

11 Review the most important factors to consider when emergency transfusion is indicated.

12 Define "massive transfusion."

13 Differentiate the various transfusion requirements of oncology and transplantation patients.

14 Compare and contrast hemophilia A and von Willebrand's disease.

15 State the respective blood components of choice for treatment of von Willebrand's disease and hemophilia A.

16 Specify the steps involved in the proper administration of blood.

Blood Components

Blood and blood components are considered drugs because of their use in treating diseases. As with drugs, adverse effects may occur, necessitating careful consideration of therapy. The transfusion of blood cells is also transplantation, in that the cells must survive and function after transfusion in order to have a therapeutic effect. The transfusion of red blood cells (RBCs) is the best-tolerated form of transplantation, but it may cause rejection, as in a hemolytic transfusion reaction. The rejection of platelets, as shown by refractoriness to platelet transfusion, is relatively common in multiply transfused patients. Table 16–1 is a summary of the blood components and products discussed in this chapter.[1]

WHOLE BLOOD

The blood collected from a donor is considered whole blood; however, the blood circulating in the donor's blood vessels is not the same as that which is labeled "whole blood." In this sense, whole blood is the donor blood mixed with the anticoagulant and preservative solution, and thus diluted in the proportion of eight parts blood to one part anticoagulant. The citrate in the anticoagulant chelates ionized calcium, preventing activation of the coagulation system. The glucose, adenine, and phosphate (if present) serve as substrates for RBC metabolism during storage (see Chapter 1).

Although at one time whole blood was the principal product transfused, the development of component therapy has limited the use of whole blood to a few clinical conditions. Whole blood should be used to replace the loss of both RBC mass and plasma volume.[1] Thus, rapidly bleeding patients can receive whole blood, although most commonly RBCs are used and are equally effective clinically.

Whole blood is used for donor-specific transfusions. In this case, organ transplant recipients (mostly kidney) are sensitized to donor tissue antigens after exposure to donor whole blood[2-4] and eventually develop a tolerance to donor antigens. White blood cells (WBCs) are the bearers of these tissue antigens in the form of HLA and other cell membrane histocompatibility antigens.

A definite contraindication to the use of whole blood is severe chronic anemia. Patients with chronic anemia have a reduced amount of RBCs but have compensated by increasing their plasma volume to restore their total blood volume. Thus, these patients do not need the plasma in the whole blood and, in fact, may adversely respond to the unneeded plasma by developing pulmonary edema and heart failure. This volume overload is more likely to occur in patients with kidney failure or preexisting heart failure.

For the typical 70-kg (155-lb) human, each unit of whole blood should increase the hematocrit 3 to 5 percent or hemoglobin 1 to 1.5 g/dl. After transfusion, the increase may not be apparent for 48 to 72 hours while the patient's blood volume adjusts to normal. For example, a patient with a 5000-ml blood volume and 25 percent hematocrit has 1250 ml of RBCs. With transfusion of 500 ml whole blood, the blood volume will be 5500 ml, or 26.4 percent hematocrit. But when the patient's blood volume readjusts to 5000 ml, the hematocrit will be 29 percent (1450 ml divided by 5000 ml). The increase is greater in a smaller person and less in a larger one.

TABLE 16–1 **BLOOD COMPONENTS AND PLASMA DERIVATIVES**

Component or Product	Composition	Approximate Volume	Indications
Whole blood	RBC; plasma; WBC; platelets	500 ml	Increase both RBC mass and plasma volume (WBC and platelets not functional; plasma deficient in labile clotting factors V, VIII)
RBCs	RBC; reduced plasma, WBC	250 ml	Increase RBC mass in symptomatic anemia (WBC and platelets not functional)
RBCs, adenine-saline added	RBC; reduced plasma, WBC and platelets; 100 ml of additive solution	330 ml	Increase RBC mass in symptomatic anemia (WBC and platelets not functional)
Leukocyte-poor RBC (prepared by filtration, centrifugation, or saline washing)	RBC; $<5 \times 10^8$ WBC and few platelets; minimal plasma	200 ml	Increase RBC mass; minimize febrile reactions owing to leukocyte antibodies or decrease likelihood of alloimmunization to leukocyte or HLA antigens. If washed, prevent allergic reactions to plasma proteins
RBC deglycerolized	RBC; low numbers of WBC; no plasma	180 ml	Increase RBC mass; minimize febrile or allergic transfusion reactions; used for rare blood storage
Granulocyte pheresis	Granulocytes ($>1.0 \times 10^{10}$ PMN/unit); lymphocytes; platelets ($>2.0 \times 10^{11}$ platelets/unit); some RBC	220 ml	Provide granulocytes for selected patients
Platelets	Platelets ($>5.5 \times 10^{10}$ platelets/unit); some WBC; plasma; some RBC	50 ml	Bleeding owing to thrombocytopenia or thrombocytopathy (5-day shelf life)
Plateletpheresis	Platelets ($>3 \times 10^{11}$ platelets/unit); some WBC; plasma; some RBC	300 ml	Bleeding owing to thrombocytopenia or thrombocytopathy. However, most often used in patients with HLA or antiplatelet antibodies; product often HLA matched (5-day shelf life)
Fresh frozen plasma	Plasma; all coagulation factors; complement; no platelets	220 ml	Treatment of some coagulation disorders
Plasma	Plasma; stable clotting factors; no platelets	220 ml	Treatment of stable clotting factor deficiencies (II, VII, IX, X, XI)
Cryoprecipitated AHF	Fibrinogen; factors VIII and XIII, vWF	15 ml	Deficiency of factor XIII, fibrinogen; treatment of von Willebrand's disease
Factor VIII concentrate	Factor VIII	25 ml	Hemophilia A (VIII deficiency)
Factor IX complex concentrate	Factors II, VII, IX, X	25 ml	Hereditary factor IX deficiency
Albumin	Albumin, (5% or 25% solution)	Varies	Volume expansion; fluid mobilization
Plasma protein fraction	Albumin, some α, β globulins	Varies	Volume expansion
Immunoglobulin	IgG antibodies	Varies	Treatment of hypogammaglobulinemia or agammaglobulinemia; disease prophylaxis
Antithrombin III	Antithrombin III; trace amounts of other plasma proteins	10 ml	Treatment of antithrombin III deficiency

From Pisciotto,[1] pp 2–3, with permission.

RED BLOOD CELLS

Red blood cells are indicated for increasing the RBC mass in patients who require increased oxygen-carrying capacity.[1] These patients typically have pulse rates greater than 100 beats per minute; respiration rates greater than 30 breaths per minute; and may have dizziness, weakness, angina (chest pain), and difficulty thinking. The decreased RBC mass may be caused by decreased bone marrow production (leukemia or aplastic anemia), decreased RBC survival (hemolytic anemia), or surgical or traumatic bleeding.

Transfusion of RBCs is contraindicated in patients who are well compensated for the anemia, such as in chronic renal failure. RBCs should not be used to treat nutritional anemia, such as iron-deficiency or pernicious anemia, unless the patient shows signs of decom-

pensation (need for increased oxygen-carrying capacity).

There are no set hemoglobin levels that indicate a need for transfusion. Although the level of 10 g/dl has been used for many years for surgical and leukemic patients, the critical level is 7.0 g/dl or lower, except for patients with heart, lung, or cerebral vascular disease.[5] Most renal dialysis patients can tolerate 7 g/dl. In fact, healthy individuals could tolerate hemoglobin levels as low as 5.0 g/dl with minimal effects,[6,7] especially if they are placed at bed rest or at decreased levels of activity. Consensus committees suggest trigger values of hemoglobin of less than 7.0 g/dl in the absence of disease and between 8 and 10 g/dl with disease.[8]

Each unit of transfused RBCs is expected to increase the hemoglobin 1 to 1.5 g/dl and the hematocrit 3 to 5 percent in the typical 70-kg (155-lb) human. The increase in hemoglobin and hematocrit will be evident more quickly than with 1 unit of whole blood, because the adjustment in blood volume is less. In the previous example, the RBC volume would be increased the same, to 1450 ml, but the blood volume is increased only 300 ml to 5300 ml. The hematocrit is increased immediately to 27.2 percent.

Red blood cells prepared with additive solutions such as additive solution 1 (AS-1) have greater volume than with citrate-phosphate-dextrose (CPD) or citrate-phosphate-dextrose-adenine (CPDA-1) (330 ml versus 250 to 275 ml) (see Chapter 1), but the AS-1 unit has less plasma. The RBC mass is the same. Therefore, the hematocrit differs from 70 to 80 percent for CPDA-1 red cells to 55 to 60 percent for AS-1 red cells. The shelf life for CPD RBCs is 21 days; for CPDA-1, 35 days; and for AS-1, 42 days. AS-1, containing no protein and a minimal amount of oncotic material (mannitol), is quickly eliminated from the body. All types of RBC products are stored at 1°C to 6°C for the duration of their shelf lives. Neonatal exchange transfusion is still performed using CPDA-1 anticoagulated blood, for there is very little knowledge as to how a neonate's system (cardiovascular, renal, etc.) deals with the AS-1.

LEUKOCYTE-REDUCED AND LEUKOCYTE-POOR RED BLOOD CELLS

Most febrile transfusion reactions are due to leukocytes in the transfused blood unit. Removing 70 to 90 percent of the leukocytes by any of several methods (centrifuging, washing, and deglycerolizing) prevents nearly all febrile reactions. More efficient removal (greater than 99 percent) can be effected by the use of third-generation leukodepletion filters.[9] Patients who have repeated (two or more) febrile reactions are candidates for leukocyte-poor RBCs.[1,10] The expected increase in the patient's hematocrit may be smaller using those methods in which 20 to 30 percent of RBCs are lost (centrifuging and washing). The cost of leukocyte-poor RBCs varies with the method, with deglycerolized RBCs being the most expensive.

Standards currently exist regarding leukocyte counts on RBC units. A level of less than 5×10^8 will prevent febrile nonhemolytic transfusion reactions.[11] Many blood filters currently guarantee a level of less than 1×10^6 or even 1×10^4.[12,13] Low levels of leukocytes may prevent or delay sensitization to HLA antigens or possibly may prevent the transmission of cytomegalovirus (CMV) infection. These last two issues are still being evaluated.[14,15]

WASHED RED BLOOD CELLS

Patients who have febrile or allergic transfusion reactions to ordinary units of RBCs may benefit from receiving washed RBCs.[1] The washing process removes about 90 percent of contaminating leukocytes, the cause of most febrile reactions, and plasma, the cause of most allergic reactions. The use of filters, however, is the most efficient method for removing WBCs and preventing febrile reactions. Washed RBCs are used for the rare patient with IgA deficiency and anti-IgA antibodies. Frozen deglycerolized RBCs can be substituted for washed RBCs. The expected response in hematocrit is the same as that of unwashed RBCs.

The blood container must be entered to wash the RBCs. This step shortens the shelf life to 24 hours. Therefore, washing is reserved for IgA-deficient or highly allergic patients, rather than for patients needing leukocyte-depleted RBCs.

FROZEN AND DEGLYCEROLIZED RED BLOOD CELLS

Freezing RBCs allows the long-term storage of rare blood donor units, autologous units, and units for special purposes, such as intrauterine transfusion. Because the process needed to deglycerolize the RBCs removes nearly all leukocytes and plasma, these units, although more expensive, can be used interchangeably with washed RBCs. The 24-hour outdate of deglycerolized RBCs severely limits the use of these products. The expected hematocrit increase in the patient is the same as that with regular RBC units.

PLATELETS AND PLATELETPHERESIS

Platelets prepared from whole blood units (random-donor platelets) are indicated for patients who are bleeding owing to thrombocytopenia (low platelet count) or, in a few cases, owing to abnormally functioning platelets.[16] Thrombocytopenia may be caused by decreased platelet production by the bone marrow (e.g., aplastic anemia or chemotherapy for malignancy). Massive transfusion, which is discussed later in this chapter, may also cause thrombocytopenia owing to the rapid use of platelets for hemostasis and the dilution of the platelets by resuscitation fluids and stored blood.

Each unit of platelets should increase the platelet count 5,000 to 10,000/μl in the typical 70-kg human. Each unit of platelets must contain at least 5.5×10^{10} platelets.[11] Pools of 6 units, then, will contain roughly 3×10^{11} platelets. Massive splenomegaly, high fever, sepsis, disseminated intravascular coagulation (DIC), and platelet or HLA antibodies can cause less than expected platelet count increment and survival. The 1-hour posttransfusion platelet count increment is less affected by splenomegaly, high fever, and DIC than by the presence of platelet or HLA antibodies.[17] If the 1-hour increment is less than 50 percent of expected, the patient is considered refractory and should be screened for HLA antibodies and be typed for HLA antigens. An HLA-compatible donor can then be selected for platelet donation by apheresis.

A plateletpheresis product (also called platelets pheresis) is prepared from one donor and must contain a minimum of 3×10^{11} platelets.[11] As such, one plateletpheresis product is equivalent to one dose of random platelet concentrates (i.e., a pool of 6 units). Products procured by apheresis can be given as random products or, because of their HLA type, as HLA-matched products. Random apheresis products have the potential of preventing HLA sensitization and limiting donor exposure (i.e., exposure to multiple donors). Although this has been theorized,[18,19] it remains to be thoroughly tested.[14] A corrected count increment—using a 1-hour postinfusion platelet count—can provide invaluable information about patient response to a platelet product.[17] The platelet count increment can be corrected for differences in body size so that more reliable estimates of expected platelet increment can be determined.[20] The minimum expected corrected platelet increment is $10,000/\mu l$ per m^2. One formula for corrected count increment is

$$\frac{\text{Absolute platelet increment}/\mu l \times \text{Body surface area (m}^2\text{)}}{\text{Number of platelets transfused } (10^{11})}$$

in which the absolute platelet increment is the posttransfusion platelet count minus the pretransfusion platelet count, the body surface area is expressed as square meters, and the number of platelets transfused is determined by multiplying the number of units (bags) of platelets by 0.55 (the number of platelets in each unit expressed in 10^{11}).

For example, a patient with $10,000/\mu l$ platelet count has a body surface area of $2.3 \ m^2$. Six units of platelets are given. The 1-hour posttransfusion platelet count is $50,000/\mu l$. Put these into the formula:

$$\frac{(50,000/\mu l - 10,000/\mu l) \times 2.3}{6 \text{ units} \times 0.55/\text{unit}} = 15,758 \ \mu l$$

The answer shows that the patient has a good increment and is not refractory to platelets. An answer of less than $5000/\mu l$ indicates refractoriness. The formula can be used for plateletpheresis by using 3 (times 10^{11}) as the number of platelets in each unit.

GRANULOCYTE PHERESIS AND BUFFY COAT

Patients who have received intensive chemotherapy for leukemia or bone marrow transplant or both may develop severe neutropenia and serious bacterial or fungal infection. Without neutrophils (granulocytes), the patient may have difficulty controlling an infection even with appropriate antibiotic treatment. Criteria have been developed to identify those patients who are most likely to benefit from granulocyte transfusions: fever, neutrophil counts less than $500/\mu l$, septicemia or bacterial infection unresponsive to antibiotics, reversible bone marrow hypoplasia, and a reasonable chance for patient survival.[1] Prophylactic use of granulocyte transfusions is of doubtful value for those patients who have neutropenia but no demonstrable infection.

Newborn infants may develop overwhelming infection with neutropenia because of their limited bone marrow reserve and neutrophil production. In addition, neonatal neutrophils have impaired function. Recent studies have shown granulocyte transfusions to be beneficial for these patients.[21] Buffy coats prepared from a unit of fresh whole blood also are effective.

For an adult, the usual dose is one granulocyte pheresis product daily for 4 or more days. For neonates, a buffy coat or a granulocyte pheresis unit is usually given once or twice.

These products are stored at $20°C$ to $24°C$.[11] They should be administered as soon as possible and, at most, within 24 hours of collection.[11] In most instances, the granulocyte products need to be crossmatched because of a significant content of RBCs.[11] The patient must be followed for resolution of symptoms and clinical evidence of efficacy, for the granulocyte count will not noticeably increase in response to infusion of this product.[22]

FRESH FROZEN PLASMA

Fresh frozen plasma can be used to replace all coagulation factors, so it is especially useful to treat multiple coagulation deficiencies occurring in patients with liver failure, DIC, vitamin K deficiency, warfarin toxicity, or massive transfusion.[23]

Vitamin K deficiency or warfarin toxicity should be treated with vitamin K infusion (intravenously or intramuscularly) if liver function is adequate and if enough time exists before a major or minor hemostatic challenge such as surgery. Fresh frozen plasma is given in these situations if there is active bleeding or if no time is afforded for warfarin reversal before surgery.

Congenital coagulation factor deficiencies also may be treated with fresh frozen plasma, although the requirement for surgical procedures and serious bleeding may be so great as to cause pulmonary edema owing to volume overload, even in a young individual with a healthy cardiovascular system. Factor concentrates (see following discussion) currently offer more effective modes of therapy. Factor XI deficiency, however, is still treated by plasma infusion. This disease is milder than hemophilia A or hemophilia B. Factor XI also has a long half-life, so treatment is not needed on a daily basis.

A coagulation factor unit is defined as the activity in 1 ml of pooled normal plasma, so 100 percent activity is 1 unit/ml or 100 units/dl. Less than 50 percent activity of any of the coagulation factors is required for adequate hemostasis. Thus no more than half of the plasma volume, or about 5 to 6 units, is required to correct a hemostatic deficiency. Repeated transfusions, however, would be required for surgical patients until healing has occurred. For example, factor IX has a half-life of 18 to 24 hours, warranting the need for daily transfusions.

Fresh frozen plasma is sometimes used as a replacement fluid in the setting of plasma exchange (plasmapheresis). In cases of thrombotic thrombocytopenic purpura, hemolytic uremic syndrome, and the syndrome of hemolysis, elevated liver enzymes, and low platelets (HELLP)[25] (i.e., preeclampsia and hemolysis), fresh frozen plasma provides an unknown substance that the patient's plasma lacks, thus reversing the symptoms.[24-26] HELLP syndrome occurs in a subgroup of pregnant women who have preeclampsia (pregnancy-induced hypertension and proteinuria). It is manifested by thrombocytopenia and liver enzyme derangement and usually occurs in the postpartum period. Plasmapheresis is used when the disease does not remit on its own.[25]

Fresh frozen plasma should not be used for blood volume expansion or protein replacement because safer products are available for these purposes—serum albumin, synthetic colloids, and balanced salt solutions—none of which transmits disease or causes severe allergic reactions.

LIQUID PLASMA AND PLASMA

Liquid plasma was formerly known as single-donor plasma. Liquid plasma contains variable (usually small) amounts of the labile coagulation factors V and VIII and thus is not recommended for treatment of patients who have deficiency of either or both of these clotting factors. The plasma can be used for treatment of stable coagulation deficiency, especially factor XI deficiency, or as the only source of plasma for patients undergoing extensive plasma exchange with plasma replacement. However, for surgical procedures and serious bleeding, the required coagulation factor level may be difficult to achieve owing to volume overload in the patient. Plasma should not be used for blood volume expansion or protein replacement for the same reasons as for fresh frozen plasma.

CRYOPRECIPITATED ANTIHEMOPHILIC FACTOR

Antihemophilic factor (AHF) is also called factor VIII. The cryoprecipitated AHF also contains fibrinogen, von Willebrand factor (vWF), and factor XIII (Table 16–2); thus this product can be used to correct deficiency of some of these coagulation factors.[27] However, mild or moderate factor VIII deficiency (hemophilia A) is usually treated with desmopressin acetate (1-deamino-[8-D-arginine]-vasopressin [DDAVP]) or factor VIII concentrates, or both, whereas severe factor VIII deficiency is treated with factor VIII concentrates. For the most part, cryoprecipitate is routinely given for treatment of von Willebrand's disease

or fibrinogen deficiency (e.g., DIC). Each bag of cryoprecipitated AHF contains only about 15 ml, so large numbers of units may be given without blood volume overload.

Cryoprecipitated AHF can also be used as a source of fibrin glue,[28] which consists of a unit of cryoprecipitate as the source of fibrinogen. Bovine thrombin is mixed with the contents of the bag of cryoprecipitate at the tip of a spray gun (atomizer). The fibrinogen is thus activated by the thrombin as it is expelled from the bag. The glue is applied topically on prosthetic vascular grafts as well as vascular tissue planes in surgery. The activated fibrinogen thus acts as a fibrin sealant in the area to which it is applied.

Each unit of cryoprecipitate must contain at least 80 units of factor VIII.[11] This is a carryover from the days when cryoprecipitate was used exclusively for the treatment of hemophilia A. Recent literature has challenged this with the idea that cryoprecipitate is used mostly for fibrinogen now.[29] Each unit contains approximately 250 mg of fibrinogen (see following discussion).

If there is a need for factor VIII, and no concentrate preparation is readily available, cryoprecipitate can provide the necessary factor. The dose of cryoprecipitated AHF can be calculated by using the minimum level of factor VIII per bag (80 units), the patient's plasma volume, and the initial and desired factor VIII levels in the patient. For example, if a 50-percent level (50 units/dl or 0.5 unit/ml) is desired in a patient with less than a 1-percent level and a plasma volume of 3000 ml, the AHF units required is 0.5 unit/ml × 3000 ml = 1500 units. (The amount can also be calculated by changing the 3000 ml to 30 dl, dividing by 100, and then multiplying the result by 50 units/dl.)

The number of bags required is 1500 units divided by 80 units/bag or 18.74 bags, rounded to 19. The dose is repeated every 12 hours for serious hemorrhage and surgical procedures. In trauma cases, the level is assumed to be 0 percent, and calculations are made from this point.

Cryoprecipitated AHF is a blood product of choice for von Willebrand's disease, because the level of vWF varies considerably with the manufacturer's lot of factor VIII concentrate. Cryoprecipitate is used after treatment with DDAVP (a synthetic vasopressin analog) has failed to release adequate amounts of endogenous vWF and after treatment with some virus-safe, sterilized factor VIII concentrates has been tried. In this case, cryoprecipitate provides exogenous vWF to a patient who needs it for a hemostatic challenge (e.g., trauma, surgery).

Currently, cryoprecipitated AHF is the only concentrate available for fibrinogen replacement. Fibrinogen replacement may be required in patients with liver failure or DIC and in rare patients with congenital fibrinogen deficiency. Each bag of cryoprecipitated AHF contains approximately 250 mg of fibrinogen. A plasma level of at least 50 mg/dl of fibrinogen is required for adequate hemostasis with surgery or

TABLE 16–2 **CRYOPRECIPITATED AHF**

Constituents	Amount
Factor VIII	80–120 units/concentrate
Fibrinogen	150–250 mg/concentrate
vWF	40–70% of original FFP
Factor XIII	20–30% of original FFP

From Kennedy,[27] with permission.

trauma. For example, a patient's fibrinogen must be increased from 30 mg/dl to 100 mg/dl, or 70 mg/dl (100 − 30). To calculate the amount to be infused, first convert milligrams per deciliter to milligrams per milliliter by dividing by 100 (100 ml/dl). Multiplying this figure, 0.7 mg/ml, by the plasma volume, 3000 ml, we thus require 2100 mg (0.7 mg/ml × 3000 ml). To calculate bags, divide 2100 mg by 250 mg/bag to get 8.4 bags. The number here may be rounded up. (One can convert the plasma volume to deciliters, instead, by dividing by 100 ml/dl).

FACTOR VIII CONCENTRATE

Factor VIII concentrate is prepared by pharmaceutical firms by fractionation and lyophilization of pooled plasma. The plasma is usually obtained from paid donors by plasmapheresis or from volunteer whole blood donors. The concentrate is stored at refrigerator temperatures and is reconstituted with saline at the time of infusion. This ease of handling allows home therapy for individuals with hemophilia.

Factor VIII concentrate is now treated to reduce the risk of transmission of infectious diseases. Factor VIII concentrate is prepared in a variety of ways, including anion exchange chromatography, monoclonal antibody purification, and recombinant DNA techniques. More and more pure concentrates are prepared today, with DNA technology providing the purest product.[30] Factor VIII concentrates can also be sterilized in different ways including pasteurization and solvent-detergent treatment. All of the sterilization methods used ensure sterility for human immunodeficiency virus (HIV) and hepatitis C virus (HCV).[30] Cases of hepatitis B still occur but are rare. The recombinant DNA product is the safest because it is not human-derived.

Using the factor VIII content on the vial label, the dose of factor VIII is calculated by the method described earlier for cryoprecipitated AHF. Although some preparations contain effective, intact von Willebrand's multimers and have been used in von Willebrand's disease,[30] the majority of products should not be used for most patients with von Willebrand's disease because the content of vWF varies considerably.

FACTOR IX CONCENTRATE

Factor IX concentrate is prepared by barium sulfate or aluminum hydroxide adsorption and lyophilization of pooled plasma. The concentrate contains the "prothrombin complex," factors II, VII, IX, and X; however, the product is recommended only for factor IX–deficient patients (hemophilia B), patients with factor VII or X deficiency (rare), or selected patients with factor VIII inhibitors.[31] Activated coagulation factors in the product may cause thrombosis, especially in patients with liver disease. Some, therefore, contain heparin.[30] Factor IX concentrate is also sterilized by a variety of methods, reducing the risk of transmissible

disease. New *isolated* factor IX concentrates (e.g., affinity chromatography- and monoclonal antibody-purified) are being developed.[30] These concentrates, containing mostly, or only, factor IX, would not be useful in cases of factor VIII deficiency with inhibitors. They would only be of use in factor IX deficiency.[30]

The dose is calculated in the same manner as that for cryoprecipitated AHF, using the assayed value of factor IX on the label with the caveat that one half of any dose of factor IX will rapidly diffuse into tissues, whereas the remaining one half will remain within the intravascular space.

ANTITHROMBIN III AND PROTEIN C CONCENTRATES

Antithrombin III is a protease inhibitor with activity toward thrombin.[32] Binding and inactivation of thrombin is enhanced by giving the patient heparin. Antithrombin III deficiency can be hereditary or acquired. The hereditary deficiency is manifested by venous thromboses, whereas the acquired deficiency is seen most frequently in those with DIC. Antithrombin III concentrates are licensed for use in the United States for patients with hereditary deficiency of antithrombin III. The product is pasteurized to eliminate the risk of HIV or HCV infections.[33,34] Use in acquired deficiency is currently being evaluated.

Protein C is a vitamin K–dependent factor and a serine protease inhibitor. Protein C inactivates factors V and VIII, thus preventing thrombus formation. Deficiency (hereditary or acquired) leads to a hypercoagulable state (i.e., prethrombotic state). Protein C concentrates are currently approved for use only in hereditary deficiency states.

ALBUMIN AND PLASMA PROTEIN FRACTION

Albumin and plasma protein fraction are prepared by chemical fractionation of pooled plasma. Albumin is available as a 5-percent or a 25-percent solution, of which 96 percent of the protein content is albumin. Plasma protein fraction is available only as a 5-percent solution, containing 83 percent albumin and 17 percent globulins. All products are heat treated, eliminating the risk of infectious disease transmission. They have proved virus-safe over many years.

These products may be used to treat patients requiring blood volume replacement. Controversy surrounds whether these products or crystalloid (i.e., saline or electrolyte) solutions are better for treating hypovolemia. Albumin is used routinely as the replacement fluid in many plasmapheresis procedures. It adequately replaces the colloid that is removed during the procedures. It is used in the treatment of burn patients for replacement of colloid pressure as well.

Albumin and plasma protein fraction can be used with diuretics to induce diuresis in patients with low total protein owing to severe liver or protein-losing disease. The 25-percent solution brings enough extravascular water into the vascular space to dilute the solution to 5 to 6 percent. Thus, patients receiving 25 percent albumin need to have adequate extravascular water and compensatory mechanisms to deal with the expansion of the blood volume.

IMMUNOGLOBULIN

Immunoglobulin (Ig) prepared from pooled plasma is primarily IgG. Although small amounts of IgM and IgA may be present in some preparations, others are free of these contaminating proteins.[35] Products are available for intramuscular or intravenous administration. The intramuscular product must not be given intravenously because a severe anaphylactic reaction may occur. The intravenous product must be given slowly to lessen the risk of reaction.

Immunoglobulin is used for patients with congenital hypogammaglobulinemia and for patients exposed to diseases such as hepatitis A or measles. For hypogammaglobulinemia, monthly injections are usually given because of the 22-day half-life of IgG. The recommended dose is 0.7 ml/kg intramuscularly or 100 mg/kg intravenously. For hepatitis A prophylaxis, 0.02 to 0.04 ml/kg intramuscularly is recommended.

Various hyperimmune globulins are available for prevention of diseases such as hepatitis B, varicella zoster, rabies, mumps, and others. These are prepared from the plasma of donors who have high antibody titers to the specific virus causing the disease. The dose is recommended in the package insert. It should be remembered that preparations such as hepatitis B hyperimmune globulin provide only passive immunity after an exposure. They do not confer permanent immunity and so must be accompanied by active immunization.

Rh immunoglobulin (RhIg) was developed to protect the Rh-negative mother who is pregnant with or gives birth to an Rh-positive infant (see Chapter 20). Much of the IgG in this preparation is directed against the D antigen within the Rh system. Administration of this preparation allows for attachment of anti-D to any Rh-positive cells of the infant that have entered the maternal circulation. The sensitized cells are subsequently removed by the reticuloendothelial system of the mother, preventing active immunization or sensitization.

Special Restrictions of Transfusion

FILTERS FOR BLOOD COMPONENTS

Two types of filters are typically used for blood transfusion: a 170-μm filter and a leukocyte-depletion filter. The 170-μm filter is a "clot-screen" filter that removes gross clots from any blood product and is used in routine blood administration sets. A standard blood administration filter must be used for transfusion of all blood components.

The leukocyte-depletion, or leukopoor, filter is designed to remove viable WBCs from cellular blood products (RBCs and platelets).[9] This filter can be used to prevent febrile nonhemolytic transfusion reactions. Prevention or delay of the development of HLA antibodies by this filter is currently being studied by several investigators. Because HLA antibodies can cause poor recovery of transfused platelets, the filters could be valuable in patients requiring repeated platelet transfusions. These filters can reduce the risk of transfusion of CMV, because CMV is carried in polymorphonuclear leukocytes (PMNs) and monocytes, which are removed or reduced in number when the product is filtered.[36,37] Therefore, a filter can be used in place of a CMV-seronegative unit if none is available. Clinical trials are presently ongoing to address the issue of the equivalence of filtered and CMV-seronegative cellular blood products. Filtration and filtered products will most likely require laboratory-based quality control on a lot-to-lot basis for adequate evaluation of efficacy.[38]

CYTOMEGALOVIRUS AND BLOOD COMPONENTS

Cytomegalovirus is carried, in a latent or infectious form, in PMNs and monocytes. Infusion of these virus-infected cells in a cellular product such as RBCs or platelets can transmit infection. Infection of the patients can be prevented by the removal of leukocytes by filtration or by administering a unit from a donor who is CMV antibody negative. CMV-negative products should be administered to recipients who are CMV negative and at risk for severe sequelae of CMV infection.[39] These recipients are not those healthy adults, children, or newborn infants receiving only 1 or 2 units of blood components. Instead, those at established risk include CMV-negative pregnant women (mainly for the sake of the fetus), CMV-negative bone marrow transplant recipients, and CMV-negative premature infants.[40] Other risk groups are being assessed with regard to the need for CMV-negative products.[41-43]

IRRADIATED BLOOD COMPONENTS

Graft-versus-host (GVH) disease requires three prerequisites to occur: (1) transfusion or transplantation of immunocompetent T lymphocytes, (2) histocompatibility differences between graft and recipient (major or minor HLA or other histocompatibility antigens), and (3) usually an immunocompromised recipient.[44] GVH disease, common after allogeneic bone marrow transplantation, is a syndrome affecting skin, liver, and gut.[45]

Posttransfusion graft-versus-host (PTGVH) disease, occurring less frequently,[45] is caused by viable T lymphocytes in cellular blood products (e.g., RBCs and platelets). Mortality is high;[46,47] therefore, prevention is key. Prevention centers on irradiation of cellular components before administration to significantly immunocompromised individuals. Irradiation doses range from 1500 to 5000 rads, with the higher doses being more effective.[48] Irradiation decreases or eliminates the mitogenic (blastogenic) response of the transfused T cells, rendering these donor T cells immunoincompetent.

Recipients at risk for PTGVH disease are individuals with congenital immunodeficiencies (severe combined immunodeficiency [SCID], DiGeorge syndrome, Wiskott-Aldrich syndrome); individuals with Hodgkin's lymphoma; bone marrow transplant recipients (allogeneic or autologous); fetuses undergoing intrauterine transfusion; neonates undergoing exchange transfusion; and individuals, regardless of immune status, receiving products from all blood relatives.[11,47,48] In the last case, healthy recipients have experienced PTGVH disease after receiving nonirradiated blood components as directed donations primarily from first-degree relatives. Rejection of donor lymphocytes is absent because HLA-type similarities in these related individuals prevents the healthy host (patient) from rejecting the T lymphocytes from the graft (donor). The donor lymphocytes thus reject the host.[49] Other than the foregoing recommended individuals, indications for other patients remain empiric, as no one knows whether current practices have significantly reduced disease incidence or whether cases simply remain rare or underreported. At this time, neither the level of immunosuppression necessary for a recipient to develop PTGVH disease (although the severe immunosuppression cases listed previously are at most risk) nor the dose of lymphocytes needed for PTGVH disease to occur is known. For the latter reason, prevention is dependent on irradiation and *not* reduction of lymphocytes by filtration. Other patient groups at risk continue to be evaluated.[47,48]

Transfusion Therapy in Special Conditions

MAXIMUM SURGICAL BLOOD ORDER SCHEDULE; TYPE AND SCREEN

Reviews of blood transfusion practices have found that most surgical procedures do not require blood transfusion. Crossmatching for procedures with a low likelihood of transfusion increases the number of crossmatches performed, increases the amount of blood inventory in reserve and unavailable for transfusion, and contributes to the aging and possible outdating of the blood products. These patients can be better served by performing only a type and antibody screen (Table 16–3). If, in a rare instance, blood is required for transfusion, ABO– and Rh–type specific blood may be released, in the absence of a positive antibody screen, after an immediate spin crossmatch.

TABLE 16-3 MAXIMUM SURGICAL BLOOD ORDER SCHEDULE

Purpose	Two units crossmatched
Reduce unnecessary crossmatching	Pulmonary lobectomy
Examples	Hemicolectomy
Type and screen	
Vagotomy and pyloroplasty	
Exploratory laparotomy	
Cholecystectomy	

From Kennedy,[27] with permission.

For a patient who is likely to require blood transfusion, the number of units crossmatched should be no more than twice those usually required for that surgical procedure. Thus, the crossmatch-to-transfusion (C/T) ratio will be between 2:1 and 3:1, which has been shown to be optimal practice. Although individual institutions may vary, general outlines are available concerning the maximum surgical blood-ordering schedule.[50]

AUTOLOGOUS TRANSFUSION

Autologous (self) transfusion is the donation of blood by the intended recipient.[51] In contrast, the infusion of blood from another donor is homologous transfusion. The patient's own blood is the safest blood possible, reducing or eliminating the possibility of transfusion reaction or the transmission of infectious disease.

One type of autologous transfusion is the predeposit of blood by the patient (Fig. 16–1). The blood, collected by regular blood donation procedure, can be stored liquid or, for longer storage, frozen. Patients may donate several units of blood over a period of weeks. They should take iron supplements to replace lost iron and to stimulate erythropoiesis during the time of donation. Predeposit autologous donation is usually reserved for those patients anticipating a need for transfusion, such as scheduled surgery; however, patients with multiple RBC antibodies or antibodies to high-incidence antigens may store frozen units for unanticipated future need.

Another type of autologous transfusion, intraoperative hemodilution, is the collection of 1 or 2 units of blood from the patient just before the surgical procedure, replacing the blood volume with crystalloid or colloid solution. Then, at the end of surgery, the blood units are infused into the patient. Care must be taken to label and to store the blood units properly and to identify the blood units with the patient before infusion. This has proved useful in the setting of liver transplantation.[52]

Salvage of shed blood may be performed intraoperatively and/or postoperatively for autologous transfusion (see Fig. 16–1). Several types of equipment are available for collecting, washing, and filtering the shed blood before reinfusion. Washing of intraoperative salvage blood is generally recommended to remove

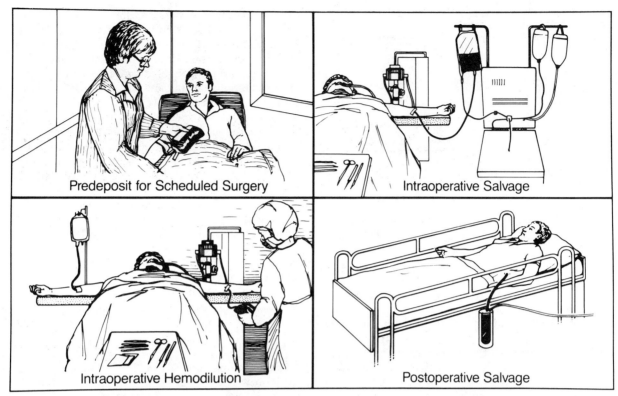

FIGURE 16-1   Types of autologous transfusions. (From Kennedy,[27] with permission.)

cellular debris, fat, and other contaminants. Heparin or citrate solutions may be used for anticoagulation of the shed blood, although postoperative salvage of thoracotomy blood may not require anticoagulation. For unknown reasons, blood exposed to serosal surfaces, such as the pleural lining, is defibrinated. Meticulous salvage of shed blood has allowed surgical procedures that once required many units of blood to be performed without the need for any homologous blood.

Recombinant erythropoietin (EPO) is available for the treatment of the anemia of chronic renal failure as well as the anemia caused by azidothymidine (AZT) therapy in acquired immunodeficiency syndrome (AIDS) patients.[53] This preparation is derived from recombinant DNA technology and not from humans.

In the indications listed here, the use of EPO may avoid the transfusion of homologous RBC products. Current research is being conducted to evaluate the efficacy of EPO for autologous transfusion.[54] Here, EPO is being used to collect more blood than the usual 2 to 3 units before surgery.[54] The use of EPO may allow a patient to donate more often under the established guidelines for autologous donation.

EMERGENCY TRANSFUSION

Patients who are rapidly or uncontrollably bleeding may require immediate transfusion. Group O RBCs are selected for those patients in whom transfusion cannot wait until the ABO and Rh type of the patient

can be determined. Group O–negative RBC units should be used, especially if the patient is a woman of childbearing age. A male patient or an older female patient can be switched from Rh-negative to Rh-positive RBCs if few O-negative units are available and massive transfusion is required. These instances should be rare, even in a large hospital with a busy emergency room.

Patients should be resuscitated with crystalloid or colloid solutions, and transfusions should be reserved for those patients losing more than 20 percent of their blood volume. The condition of most patients allows for the determination of ABO and Rh type and selection of ABO– and Rh–type specific blood for transfusion. Delaying blood transfusion in emergency situations may be more dangerous than the small risk of transfusing incompatible blood before the antibody screen and crossmatch are completed. After issuing O blood or type-specific blood, the antibody screen can be completed, and decisions can then be made for the selection of additional units of blood. If the patient has been typed and screened for a surgical procedure and his or her antibody screen is negative, ABO– and Rh–type specific blood can be selected and given with an immediate spin crossmatch.

MASSIVE TRANSFUSION

Massive transfusion is defined as the replacement of one or more blood volume(s) within 24 hours or about

TABLE 16–4 TREATMENT STRATEGY FOR MASSIVE HEMORRHAGE

Condition	Treatment
Low blood volume*	Crystalloid or colloid
Low oxygen-carrying capacity*	RBCs
Hemorrhage owing to:	
Thrombocytopenia	Platelet concentrates
Coagulopathy	Fresh frozen plasma, cryoprecipitate (if fibrinogen is low)

From Kennedy,[27] with permission.
*If these occur simultaneously, whole blood may be indicated.

10 units of blood in an adult. The strategy for treatment of massive hemorrhage is outlined in Table 16–4. Analysis of the patient's clinical status and laboratory tests is essential for deciding appropriate transfusion therapy. Patients receiving less than one blood volume replacement rarely require platelet or plasma transfusion. Patients receiving two blood volumes may require platelet transfusion and, in some instances, plasma.[55] If the patient is actively bleeding, platelets are required if the platelet count is less than $50,000/\mu l$, and plasma is needed if the prothrombin time (PT) is greater than 16 seconds or the activated partial thromboplastin time (PTT) exceeds 60 seconds. Fibrinogen levels should also be monitored as replacement by cryoprecipitate may be indicated. Replacement by cryoprecipitate is efficient and is usually indicated when the fibrinogen level is less than 100 mg/dl.[8] Maintenance of the blood volume is of utmost importance in preventing tissue damage and worsening of thrombocytopenia and coagulopathy because of shock.[56] Extensive monitoring of PT, PTT, platelet count, fibrinogen, and hemoglobin and hematocrit can help direct the choice of the best and most indicated products during the duration of the massive transfusion.[57]

A critical patient and a finite supply of type-specific blood may, sometimes, eventuate a change in ABO or Rh types. An Rh-negative male patient or postmenopausal female patient may be switched from Rh-negative to Rh-positive blood if there is concern about exhausting the inventory of Rh-negative blood. However, an Rh-negative potentially childbearing woman should receive Rh-negative RBC products as long as possible.

NEONATAL TRANSFUSION

Premature infants frequently require transfusion of small amounts of blood to replace blood drawn for laboratory tests. Various methods are available to prepare small aliquots for transfusion. Small aliquots of donor blood can be transferred from the collection bag to a satellite bag or transfer bag, or blood can be withdrawn from the collection bag or transfer bag using an injection site coupler, needle, and syringe.

The aliquot must be labeled clearly with the name and identifying numbers of the patient and donor. The blood must be as fully tested as blood for adult transfusion. Blood units less than 5 days old are preferred to lessen the risk of hyperkalemia and to maximize the 2,3-diphosphoglycerate (2,3-DPG) levels, although, in some instances, CPDA-1 RBCs 14 to 21 days old are used routinely.

For very low birthweight infants, the blood should be selected to be CMV seronegative to prevent CMV infection, which can be serious in premature infants. Indeed, pregnant women and new mothers should be given CMV-negative cellular components if they test negative for CMV.

Irradiation of the blood is recommended to prevent possible GVH disease when blood is used for intrauterine transfusion, for an exchange transfusion, or for transfusion of a premature (less than 1200 g) neonate. Routine transfusions in a full-term newborn infant do not require routine irradiation.[45,46]

Infants who are hypoxic or acidotic should receive blood tested and negative for hemoglobin S.

ONCOLOGY AND TRANSPLANTATION

The bone marrow of oncology patients may function poorly because of chemotherapy, radiation therapy, or infiltration and replacement of the bone marrow with malignant cells. Repeated RBC and platelet transfusions may require rare RBC units and/or HLA-matched plateletpheresis products because of incompatibility problems. Platelet use, as well, may necessitate a change from Rh-negative to Rh-positive products. This may be in an emergency or in the everyday setting of prophylactic platelet transfusion. RhIg may be given to a woman with childbearing potential to protect against immunization by the 5 ml or less of Rh-positive RBCs present in each transfused Rh-positive plateletpheresis product or pool of platelet concentrates. One 300-μg dose of RhIg can neutralize the effects of up to 30 ml of Rh-positive cells. Thus, one dose could be used for up to six doses of platelets.

In addition, some malignancies such as chronic lymphocytic leukemia and lymphoma are frequently complicated by autoimmune hemolytic anemia, increased destruction of RBCs, and pretransfusion testing problems.

Because of immunosuppression therapy, bone marrow transplant patients are at risk for PTGVH disease. Chronic PTGVH disease can cause severe deformity and both acute and chronic PTGVH are usually fatal. Thus irradiation of every blood product containing lymphocytes is essential. Patients receiving transplants other than bone marrow do not require irradiated blood.

Patients having transplants—including bone marrow, kidney, heart, and other organs—may develop severe CMV disease. CMV-negative blood units should be selected for transplant patients who are CMV seronegative.

Liver transplant patients require plasma as well as

RBCs during the transplant procedure because of their liver failure (see the next section of this chapter). The plasma must be transfused judiciously, however, because liver function is necessary to metabolize the citrate anticoagulant in the plasma. High citrate levels can result in hypocalcemia, causing disturbed heart contraction and deteriorating heart function.

Renal transplant patients have been shown to benefit from deliberate transfusion before transplant, whether donor-specific or random. Blood transfusion causes immune suppression and has been reported to increase the survival of the grafted kidney. Donor-specific transfusions require whole blood infusions over the course of 2 to 4 weeks before transplant. Immune tolerance to the graft is thus induced.[2,4] Many theories exist to explain the efficacy of the donor-specific transfusion.[2,4]

Transfusion may be contraindicated in patients with certain cancers, apparently because the immune suppression allows the cancer to grow and metastasize more easily.[3] Studies are continuing to explore the mechanisms of this effect of blood transfusion.

COAGULATION FACTOR DEFICIENCIES

Bleeding disorders can be caused by dysfunction of the blood vessels or deficiency or dysfunction of platelets or coagulation factors.

Factor VIII is a complex of two proteins: the procoagulant protein (factor VIII) and vWF (Fig. 16–2). Both proteins are necessary for normal hemostasis. Hemophilia A, or classic hemophilia, is a deficiency of the procoagulant portion of the factor VIII complex. The procoagulant portion is measured in functional (clotting) assays of factor VIII. Hemophilia A is generally not apparent unless the factor VIII level is less than 10 percent (normal 80 to 120) (Table 16–5). Those individuals with a level less than 1 percent have severe and spontaneous bleeding, typically into muscles and joints. The vWF level is usually normal.

Von Willebrand's disease is characterized by a deficiency of vWF. Type I von Willebrand's disease is manifested by a reduced amount of all sizes of vWF multimers and is milder than type III, in which little or

TABLE 16–5 DIFFERENTIAL DIAGNOSIS OF HEMOPHILIA A AND VON WILLEBRAND'S DISEASE

	Hemophilia A	von Willebrand's Disease
Typical coagulation values	VIII <30%, vWF 50–150%	VIII 2–50%, vWF <40%
Bleeding time	Usually normal	Prolonged
Clinical course	Bleeding into joints and muscles	Mucosal bleeding
	Bleeding with trauma or surgery	Bleeding with trauma or surgery

From Kennedy,[27] with permission.

no vWF is produced. Type IIA is characterized by a deficient release of high-molecular weight multimers whereas type IIB is manifested by abnormal high-molecular weight multimers that have an increased avidity for binding to platelets. Type I and IIA patients have the ability to make the full spectrum of vWF multimers but do not release them into the circulation in normal amounts (as mentioned previously). DDAVP, a synthetic vasopressin analog, can stimulate release of the vWF in type I patients as well as in Type IIA patients. Cryoprecipitated AHF is the only blood product that reliably provides high concentrations of vWF. Cryoprecipitated AHF can be used in type III von Willebrand's disease, or in type I disease when DDAVP treatment has failed (see earlier).

Hemophilia B is the congenital deficiency of factor IX. Factor IX is activated by factors XIa and VIIa (Fig. 16–3). The activated factor IX (IXa), along with factor VIII, ionized calcium, and phospholipid, promotes the activation of factor X. Factor IX deficiency can be treated with factor IX concentrates.[30] Treatment is more difficult with plasma because hypervolemia limits the level of factor IX that can be achieved. Factor IX concentrates are more potent and are made virus-safe by a multitude of sterilization techniques.[30]

All coagulation factors except vWF are made in the liver. With severe liver failure, multiple coagulation factor deficiencies occur. In addition, some of the

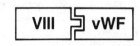

VIII—Procoagulant protein, active in clotting

vWF—von Willebrand Factor

FACTOR VIII COMPLEX

FIGURE 16–2 Factor VIII complex. (From Kennedy,[27] with permission.)

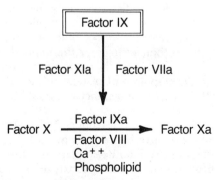

FIGURE 16–3 Factor IX deficiency. (From Kennedy,[27] with permission.)

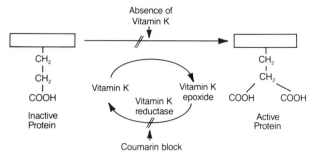

FIGURE 16-4 Mechanism of action of coumarin. (From Kennedy,[27] with permission.)

intravascular release of procoagulant activity

intravascular coagulation

ischemic tissue damage | consumption of fibrinogen, platelets and labile clotting Factors V and VIII | microangiopathic hemolytic anemia

hemorrhagic coagulopathy

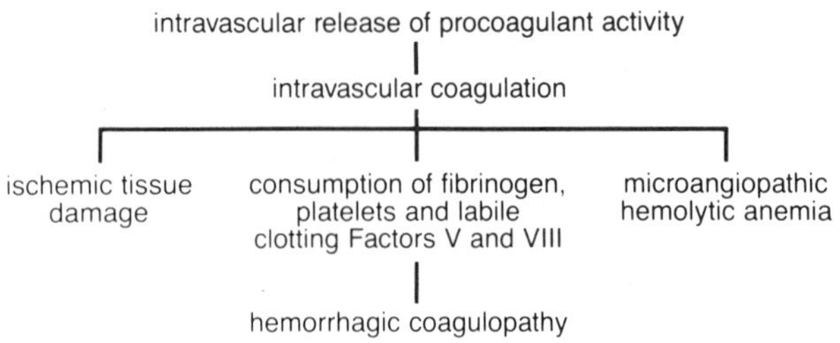

FIGURE 16-5 Pathogenesis of disseminated intravascular coagulation. (From Kennedy,[27] with permission.)

coagulation factors produced may be abnormal. The liver also produces many of the thrombolytic proteins, leading to imbalance between the coagulation process and the control mechanism. Fresh frozen plasma, having normal amounts of all these proteins, can be used to treat these patients.

Vitamin K aids in the carboxylation of factors II, VII, IX, and X (Fig. 16-4). With the absence of vitamin K or the use of drugs, such as coumarin, that interfere with vitamin K metabolism, the inactive coagulation factors cannot be carboxylated to active forms. Administration of vitamin K is preferred to fresh frozen plasma administration in order to correct vitamin K deficiency or coumarin overdose. Because several hours are required for vitamin K effectiveness, signs of hemorrhage may require transfusion of fresh frozen or single-donor plasma. However, in the absence of hemorrhage, vitamin K should have adequate time to work.

Disseminated intravascular coagulation is the uncontrolled activation and consumption of coagulation proteins, causing small thrombi within the vascular system throughout the body (Fig. 16-5). Treatment is aimed at correcting the cause of the DIC: sepsis, disseminated malignancy, obstetric complications, or shock. In some cases, transfusion of fresh frozen plasma, platelets, or cryoprecipitate may be required. Monitoring of the PT, PTT, platelet count, fibrinogen, and hemoglobin and hematocrit helps to direct therapy and helps with the choice of the next product to be used during the treatment.

Platelet functional disorders may be caused by drugs, uremia, or congenital abnormalities. Platelet transfusions in these patients should be reserved for the treatment of hemorrhage or the impending need for normal hemostasis (such as a surgical procedure) to decrease development of platelet refractoriness. In uremia, DDAVP may be beneficial as would be dialysis or even platelet transfusions.[58] DDAVP helps to release fresh, functional vWF from endothelial cells. Dialysis helps to remove byproducts of protein metabolism that degrade vWF and coat platelets, thus making both nonfunctional. Platelet transfusions provide a source of fresh and (at least for a while, in the absence of dialysis) functional platelets.

General Transfusion Practices

BLOOD ADMINISTRATION

Blood must be administered properly for patient safety (Fig. 16-6). The proper identification of the patient, the patient's blood specimen, and the blood unit for transfusion are essential. Careful identification procedures prevent a major cause of transfusion-related deaths: ABO incompatibility. Still today, clerical errors represent the main cause of transfusion-related deaths and acute hemolytic transfusion reactions.[59] The identification process begins with proper identification of the patient; that is, asking patients to state or spell their name while one reads their wristband. A patient identification label is prepared at the bedside after the specimen is drawn. This prevents an empty specimen tube from being labeled with a patient name and potentially being used for the collection of a specimen from another patient. The labels are applied to the specimen tubes before leaving the bedside to avoid labeling the wrong tube.

Proper identification is carried out in the laboratory as worklists (computer or handwritten) are drafted. Another clerical check is performed as blood is issued from the blood bank. At the issue of blood products, two individuals verify the affixing of the proper labels to the properly selected and tested blood products. The final clerical check is performed at the patient bedside when the nurse uses the patient armband to compare the patient identification to the patient crossmatch and issuance tags attached to the components to be transfused.

The patient with difficult veins should have the intravenous infusion device in place before the blood is issued from the transfusion service. All blood components must be filtered (170 μm filter) because clots and cellular debris develop during storage. Blood components are infused slowly for the first 10 to 15 minutes while the patient is closely observed for signs of a transfusion reaction. The blood components should then be infused as quickly as tolerated or, at most, within 4 hours. The patient's vital signs (pulse, respiration, blood pressure, and temperature) should be monitored periodically during the transfusion to detect signs of transfusion reaction promptly. These

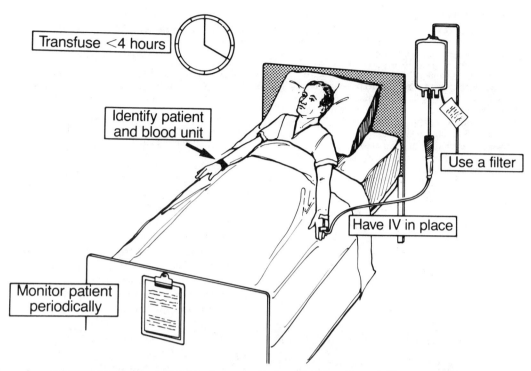

FIGURE 16-6 Blood administration and patient safety. (From Kennedy,[27] with permission.)

signs are fever with back pain (acute hemolytic transfusion reaction), anaphylaxis, hives/pruritus (urticarial reaction), congestive heart failure (volume overload), and fever alone (febrile nonhemolytic transfusion reaction). A delayed hemolytic transfusion reaction (jaundice, decreasing hematocrit) may only be diagnosed 1 to 10 days after transfusion and thus is not considered an immediate reaction.

Rapid transfusion, including exchange transfusion, requires blood warming because the cold blood can cause hypothermia in the patient. Patients with paroxysmal cold hemoglobinuria or with cold agglutinins reactive at 37°C during pretransfusion testing may also require blood warming. The blood warmer should have automatic temperature control set for 37°C with an alarm that will sound if that temperature is exceeded (Fig. 16-7). Blood units must not be warmed by immersion in a water bath or by a microwave oven because uneven heating, damage to blood cells, and denaturation of blood proteins may occur.

Only isotonic (0.9 percent) saline or 5 percent albumin should be used to dilute blood components because other intravenous solutions may damage the RBCs and cause hemolysis (dextrose solutions such as 5 percent dextrose in water [D5W]) or initiate coagulation in the infusion set (calcium-containing solutions such as lactated Ringer's solution).[60] In addition, many drugs will cause hemolysis if injected through the blood infusion set.

Leukodepletion filters may be used to prepare leukocyte-poor products for patients having repeated febrile transfusion reactions or as a preventive mechanism against HLA sensitization.

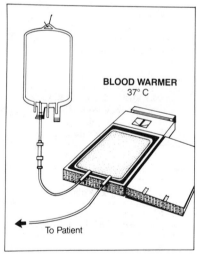

FIGURE 16-7 Blood warming. (From Kennedy,[27] with permission.)

HOSPITAL TRANSFUSION COMMITTEE

The Joint Commission for Accreditation of Hospital Organizations (JCAHO) requires that all blood transfusions be reviewed for appropriate use. A hospital transfusion committee, although not required by JCAHO, may serve as the peer review group for transfusions. Another alternative is blood usage review in which the blood bank director directly interacts and corresponds with the chair of individual hospital departments in regard to medical staff blood component usage patterns. Appropriate criteria for blood transfusion have been published (Table 16-6), serving as a

TABLE 16-6 **CRITERIA FOR TRANSFUSION AUDIT**

All Blood Components
Review of patients with transfusion reactions of hemolysis, severe allergic signs or anaphylaxis, circulatory overload, or infection
Review of patients with abnormal liver function or diagnosis of hepatitis or abnormal liver function within 6 months of transfusion
Charts of patients with adverse reaction or transfusion-transmitted disease must contain physician evaluation

Whole Blood	
Indications:	Actively bleeding *and* blood loss >25% total blood volume *or* actively bleeding and received 4 units RBCs
Outcome:	H/H <24 hours after transfusion
	Surgical procedures: postoperative H/H < preoperative H/H
	Review of patients dying within 72 hours of transfusion

Red Blood Cells	
Indications:	Hypovolemia and decreased oxygen-carrying capacity secondary to bleeding
	or acute loss of 15% blood volume
	or hemoglobin <8 g/dl or hematocrit <24%
	or symptoms related to anemia *and* a specific chronic anemia, leukemia, lymphoma, Hodgkin's disease, aplastic anemia, thalassemia, or dialysis for renal disease
	Review of patients with hemoglobin <8 g/dl, without hypovolemia or hypoxia, *and* iron deficiency anemia, pernicious anemia, nutritional deficiency anemia, intestinal malabsorption, or hereditary hemolytic anemia
Exceptions:	Patients with chronic disease or specified anemia listed above and hemoglobin >8 g/dl *and* coronary artery disease, chronic pulmonary disease, or cerebral vascular disease
Outcome:	H/H <24 hours after transfusion
	Surgical patients: postoperative hemoglobin < preoperative hemoglobin
	Review of transfusion reactions and complications

Platelets	
Indications:	Platelet count <20,000/μl
	or operative procedure in <12 hours and platelet count <50,000/μl
	Review of patients receiving platelets and with idiopathic (autoimmune) thrombocytopenia purpura, DIC, thrombotic thrombocytopenia purpura, or hemolytic uremic syndrome
	Review of adults receiving >12 units or <4 units
Outcome:	Platelet count immediately before and <18 hours after transfusion
	Review of transfusion reactions and complications

Fresh Frozen Plasma	
Indications:	Activated PTT >60 seconds
	or PT >16 seconds
	or documented coagulation factor deficiency *and* significant bleeding
Outcome:	PT, activated PTT, or coagulation factor assay immediately before and fewer than 4 hours after transfusion
	Review of transfusion reactions and complications

TABLE 16-6 **CRITERIA FOR TRANSFUSION AUDIT** *Continued*

Cryoprecipitated AHF	
Indications:	Hemophilia A *or* von Willebrand's disease *or* fibrinogen deficiency *or* factor XIII deficiency
Outcome:	Factor VIII, fibrinogen, or factor XIII determination after transfusion

Modified from the Consensus Development Panel,[16,23] and Sazama[59]. H/H = hemoglobin and hematocrit.

guide for review.[61] The results of the review can be used by the transfusion committee to recommend changes in practice by the hospital staff, to improve patient care. The transfusion committee also reviews each transfusion reaction to ensure that adverse reactions are unavoidable. In addition, the transfusion committee ensures that appropriate procedures (such as blood administration) are in place and are followed by hospital personnel.

The transfusion committee is most effective if the various groups who order and administer blood, such as surgeons, anesthesiologists, and oncologists, are represented on the committee. The transfusion committee must have a mechanism for reporting activities and recommendations to the medical staff and hospital administration. Optimally, the transfusion committee ensures that the most appropriate, efficient, and safe use of the blood supply is achieved.

Review Questions

1. Select the appropriate product for the indicated patient or need:

I. Hemophilia A	A. Factor VIII concentrate
II. Hemophilia B	B. Cryoprecipitate
III. Fibrinogen deficiency	C. Fresh frozen plasma
IV. Bone marrow transplant patient with anemia unresponsive to iron and vitamin B_{12} therapy	D. Irradiated red blood cells
	E. Red blood cells
V. Increasing oxygen-carrying capacity	F. Granulocyte pheresis
	G. Leukocyte-poor red cells
VI. Vitamin K deficiency and hemorrhage	H. Washed or deglycerolized red blood cells
VII. Also called AHF	I. Immunoglobulin
VIII. Directed donation from a first-degree relative	J. Hepatitis B immunoglobulin
	K. 0.9 percent saline
IX. Repeated febrile	L. Lactated Ringer's solution

transfusion reactions
X. IgA deficiency H
XI. Life-threatening neutropenia F
XII. Needlestick accident with infectious blood (hepatitis B) J
XIII. Immunodeficiency I
XIV. Used for dilution of red blood cells K

M. 5 percent dextrose and water solution
N. Factor IX concentrate

2. Leukopoor filters can do all of the following *except*:
   A. Reduce the risk of CMV infection
   B. Prevent or reduce the risk of HLA allo-immunization
   C. Prevent febrile, nonhemolytic transfusion reactions
   D. Prevent PTGVH disease

3. Albumin should *not* be given for:
   A. Burns
   B. Shock
   C. Nutrition
   D. Plasmapheresis

4. Of the following, which blood type is selected when a patient cannot wait for ABO matched blood?
   A. A
   B. B
   C. O
   D. AB

5. Which patient does not need an irradiated product?
   A. Bone marrow transplant recipient (autologous)
   B. Bone marrow transplant recipient (allogeneic)
   C. Healthy adult receiving a 1–red cell unit transfusion
   D. Healthy adult receiving a 1–red cell unit transfusion from a first-degree relative

6. Red blood cell transfusions should be:
   A. Accomplished within 4 hours
   B. Routinely mixed with lactated Ringer's
   C. Carried out always using a washed product
   D. Carried out always using an irradiated product

7. Which type of transplantation requires all cellular blood products to be irradiated?
   A. Bone marrow
   B. Heart
   C. Liver
   D. Pancreas
   E. Kidney

8. Deglycerolized red blood cells are all of the following *except*:
   A. Expensive
   B. A product with a 24-hour expiration date
   C. A product used for rare antigen type donor blood
   D. A product used for IgA-deficient recipients
   E. The best type of leukodepleted (leukopoor) product

Answers to Review Questions

1. I A (p 322)
   II N (p 322)
   III B (p 321)
   IV D (pp 323–324)
   V E (pp 318–319)
   VI C (pp 320–321)
   VII B (p 321)
   VIII D (pp 323–324)
   IX G (p 323)
   X H (p 319)
   XI F (p 320)
   XII J (p 323)
   XIII I (p 323)
   XIV K (p 329)

2. D (p 323)
3. C (pp 322–323)
4. C (p 325)
5. C (pp 323–324)
6. A (p 328)
7. A (pp 323–324)
8. E (p 319)

References

1. Pisciotto, PT (ed): Blood Transfusion Therapy: A Physician's Handbook, ed 3. American Association of Blood Banks, Arlington, VA, 1989, pp 2–3.
2. Brunson, ME and Alexander, JW: Mechanisms of transfusion-induced immunosuppression. Transfusion 30:651, 1990.
3. Blumberg, N, Triulzi, DJ, and Heal, JM: Transfusion-induced immunomodulation and its clinical consequences. Transfus Med Rev 4:24, 1990.
4. Meryman, HT: Transfusion-induced alloimmunization and immuno-suppression and the effects of leukocyte depletion. Transfus Med Rev 3:180, 1989.
5. Gould, SA, Rice, CL, and Moss, GS: The physiologic basis of the use of blood and blood products. Surg Annu 16:13, 1984.
6. Graettinger, JS, Parsons, RL, and Campbell, JA: A correlation of clinical and hemodynamic studies in patients with mild and severe anemia with and without congestive failure. Ann Intern Med 58:617, 1963.
7. Kruskall, MS: Clinical management of transfusions to patients with red cell antibodies. In Nance, SJ (ed): Immune Destruction of Red Blood Cells. American Association of Blood Banks, Arlington, VA, 1989, p 263.
8. Silberstein, LE: Strategies for the review of transfusion practices. JAMA 262:1993, 1989.

9. Miyamoto, M, et al: Leukocyte-poor platelet concentrates at the bedside by filtration through Sepacell-PL. Vox Sang 57:164, 1989.

10. Brand, A: White cell depletion. In Nance, SJ (ed): Transfusion Medicine in the 1990's. American Association of Blood Banks, Arlington, VA, 1990, p 35.

11. Widmann, FK (ed): Standards for Blood Banks and Transfusion Services, ed 15. American Association of Blood Banks, Arlington, VA, 1993, p 10.

12. Pall Rc 50 and Rc 100 Leukocyte-Removal Filters for Blood Transfusion at Bedside (product information). Pall Biomedical Products, Glen Cove, NY, 1990.

13. Pall Rc 400 High-Efficiency Rapid Flow Leukocyte Removal Filter for Blood (product information). Pall Biomedical Products, East Hills, NY, 1991.

14. Kao, KJ and Berthof, MF: Leukocyte-depleted blood components for patients with leukemia or aplastic anemia-CON. In Kurtz, SR, Baldwin, ML, and Sirchia, G (eds): Controversies in Transfusion Medicine: Immune Complications and Cytomegalovirus Transmission. American Association of Blood Banks, Arlington, VA, 1990, p 13.

15. Kickler, TS, et al: Depletion of white cells from platelet concentrates with a new adsorption filter. Transfusion 29:411, 1989.

16. Consensus Development Panel: Platelet transfusion therapy. Consensus conference. JAMA 257:1777, 1987.

17. Daly, PA, et al: Platelet transfusion therapy: One-hour posttransfusion increments are valuable in predicting the need for HLA-matched preparations. JAMA 243:435, 1980.

18. Kickler, TS: The challenge of platelet alloimmunization: Management and prevention. Transfus Med Rev 4:8, 1990.

19. Nemo, GJ and McCurdy, PR: Prevention of platelet alloimmunization (editorial). Transfusion 31:584, 1991.

20. Theil, KS and Kennedy, MS: Corrected count increment: A measure to prevent platelet alloimmunization. Diagn Med 7:8, 1984.

21. Cairo, MS, et al: Role of circulating complement and polymorphonuclear leukocyte transfusion in treatment and outcome in critically ill neonates with sepsis. J Pediatr 110:935, 1987.

22. Boral, LI and Henry, JB: Transfusion medicine. In Henry, JB (ed): Clinical Diagnosis and Management by Laboratory Methods, ed 18. WB Saunders, Philadelphia, 1991, p 930.

23. Consensus Development Panel: Fresh-frozen plasma: Indications and risks. Consensus conference. JAMA 253:551, 1985.

24. Brain, MC and Neame, PB: Thrombotic thrombocytopenic purpura and the hemolytic uremic syndrome. Semin Thromb Haemost 8:186, 1982.

25. Martin, JN, et al: Plasma exchange for preeclampsia: I. Postpartum use for persistently severe preeclampsia-eclampsia with HELLP syndrome. Am J Obstet Gynecol 162:126, 1990.

26. Shepard, KV and Bukowski, RM: The treatment of thrombotic thrombocytopenic purpura with exchange transfusions, plasma infusion, and plasma exchange. Semin Hematol 24:178, 1987.

27. Kennedy, MS (ed): Blood Transfusion Therapy: An Audiovisual Program. American Association of Blood Banks, Arlington, VA, 1987.

28. Casali, B, et al: Fibrin glue from single-donation autologous plasmapheresis. Transfusion 32:641, 1992.

29. Howard, PL, Bovill, EG, and Golden, E: Postthaw stability of fibrinogen in cryoprecipitate stored between 1 and 6 C. Transfusion 31:30, 1991.

30. Julius, CJ: Coagulation products for hemophilia A, hemophilia B, and von Willebrand's disease. In Hackel, E, Westphal, RG, and Wilson, SM (eds): Transfusion Management of Some Common Heritable Blood Disorders. American Association of Blood Banks, Bethesda, MD, 1992, p 1.

31. Brettler, DB: Inhibitors of factor VIII: Detection and treatment. In Hackel, E, Westphal, RG, and Wilson, SM (eds): Transfusion Management of Some Common Heritable Blood Disorders. American Association of Blood Banks, Bethesda, MD, 1992, p 37.

32. Jandl, JH: Thrombotic and fibrinolytic disorders (Chapter 33). In Jandl, JH: Blood. Little, Brown, Boston, 1987, p 1147.

33. Menache, D, Grossman, BJ, and Jackson, CM: Antithrombin III: Physiology, deficiency, and replacement therapy. Transfusion 32:580, 1992.

34. Hoffman, DL: Purification and large-scale preparation of antithrombin III. Am J Med 87 (Suppl 3B):23S, 1989.

35. Immune Globulin, Intravenous (Human): Polygam (product information). Baxter Healthcare/Hyland Div, Glendale, CA, 1990.

36. de Graan-Hentzen, YCE, et al: Prevention of primary cytomegalovirus infection in patients with hematologic malignancies by intensive white cell depletion of blood products. Transfusion 29:757, 1989.

37. Gilbert, GL, et al: Prevention of transfusion-acquired cytomegalovirus infection in infants by blood filtration to remove leukocytes. Lancet 2:1228, 1989.

38. Chambers, LA and Garcia, LW: White blood cell content of transfusion components. Lab Med 22:857, 1991.

39. Reusser, P, et al: Cytomegalovirus infection after autologous bone marrow transplantation: Occurrence of cytomegalovirus disease and effect on engraftment. Blood 75:1888, 1990.

40. Sayers, MH, et al: Reducing the risk for transfusion-transmitted cytomegalovirus infection. Ann Intern Med 116:55, 1992.

41. Braine, HG: Cytomegalovirus infection in clinical transplantation: The role of transfusion support using donors seronegative for cytomegalovirus. In Kurtz, SR, Baldwin, ML, and Sirchia, G (eds): Controversies in Transfusion Medicine: Immune Complications and Cytomegalovirus Transmission. American Association of Blood Banks, Arlington, VA, 1990, p 81.

42. Preiksaitis, JK: Cytomegalovirus-seronegative blood support for perinatal patients-CON. In Kurtz, SR, Baldwin, ML, and Sirchia, G (eds): Controversies in Transfusion Medicine: Immune Complications and Cytomegalovirus Transmission. American Association of Blood Banks, Arlington, VA, 1990, p 103.

43. Dock, NL: Cytomegalovirus-seronegative blood support for perinatal patients-PRO. In Kurtz, SR, Baldwin, ML, and Sirchia, G (eds): Controversies in Transfusion Medicine: Immune Complications and Cytomegalovirus Transmission. American Association of Blood Banks, Arlington, VA, 1990, p 131.

44. Sacher, RA and Luban, NLC: Transfusion-associated graft-versus-host disease. In Rossi, EC, Simon, TL, and Moss, GS (eds): Principles of Transfusion Medicine. Williams & Wilkins, Baltimore, 1991, p 649.

45. Leitman, SF and Holland, PV: Irradiation of blood products: Indications and guidelines. Transfusion 25:293, 1985.

46. Anderson, KC and Weinstein, HJ: Transfusion-associated graft-versus-host disease. N Engl J Med 323:315, 1990.

47. Linden, JV and Pisciotto, PT: Transfusion-associated graft-versus-host disease and blood irradiation. Transfus Med Rev 6:116, 1992.

48. Anderson, KC, et al: Variation in blood component irradiation practice: Implications for prevention of transfusion-associated graft-versus-host disease. Blood 77:2096, 1991.

49. Otsuka, S, et al: The critical role of blood from HLA-homozygous donors in fatal transfusion-associated graft-versus-host disease in immunocompetent patients. Transfusion 31:260, 1991.

50. Henry, JB, Mintz, P, and Webb, W: Optimal blood ordering for elective surgery. JAMA 237:451, 1977.

51. Autologous transfusion. In Walker, RH (ed): Technical Manual, ed 10. American Association of Blood Banks, Arlington, VA, 1990, p 433.

52. Stehling, L and Zauder, HL: Acute normovolemic hemodilution. Transfusion 31:857, 1991.

53. Zanjani, ED and Ascensao, JL: Erythropoietin. Transfusion 29:46, 1989.

54. Goodnough LT, et al: Preoperative red cell production in patients undergoing aggressive autologous blood phlebotomy with and without erythropoietin therapy. Transfusion 32:441, 1992.

55. Leslie, SD and Toy, PTCY: Laboratory hemostatic abnormalities in massively transfused patients given red blood cells and crystalloid. Am J Clin Pathol 96:770, 1991.

56. Kruskall, MS, et al: Transfusion therapy in emergency medicine. Ann Emerg Med 17:327, 1988.

57. Nelson, CC, Otteson, SP, and Johnson, R: Massive transfusion. Lab Med 22:94, 1991.

58. Mannucci, PM, et al: Deamino-8-d-arginine vasopressin shortens the bleeding time in uremia. N Engl J Med 303:8, 1983.

59. Sazama, K: Reports of 355 transfusion-associated deaths: 1976 through 1985. Transfusion 30:583, 1990.

60. Weisz-Carrington, P: Incompatible intravenous fluids: Their potential effect on blood and blood transfusion. Immunohematology ASCP Check Sample 31:1, 1988.

61. Grindon, AJ, et al: The hospital transfusion committee: Guidelines for improving practice. JAMA 253:540, 1985.

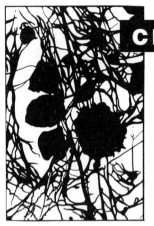

CHAPTER 17

Apheresis

Estrellita Culotta, MHS, MT(ASCP)SBB
Francis R. Rodwig, Jr., MD, MPH

OBJECTIVES

Upon completion of this chapter, the learner should be able to:

1 Define apheresis, leukapheresis, plateletpheresis, plasmapheresis, cytapheresis, and plasma exchange.

2 Describe the procedures of continuous-flow centrifugation and intermittent-flow centrifugation.

3 Discuss the use of membrane filtration technology in the separation of blood components.

4 State the American Association of Blood Banks requirements for apheresis donation.

5 Estimate the approximate platelet count in a patient that will necessitate platelet transfusion.

6 State the shelf life of platelet concentrate and granulocyte concentrate.

7 List the therapeutic indications for hemapheresis, differentiating between those conditions requiring plasma exchange and those necessitating cytapheresis.

8 Describe the different types of adsorbents and their clinical application.

9 Identify the factors that can be removed by plasmapheresis.

10 Discuss the possible adverse effects of apheresis.

History and Development

Apheresis (or hemapheresis) is derived from a Greek word that means to separate or to take away. Thus, the process of separating or taking away the white blood cells (WBCs) from the blood becomes leukapheresis. Similar terms are given to the removal of the other blood components, including platelets (plateletpheresis or thrombocytapheresis), red blood cells (RBCs) (erythrocytapheresis), and plasma (plasmapheresis).

In the early 1900s, apheresis first emerged as a possible treatment modality. The procedures were performed laboriously by a manual technique and had limited acceptance and success. Broader acceptance has occurred in the last 25 years owing to advances in technology. These advances were contingent on the development of the necessary equipment and software that could selectively remove one or more blood components from the blood and return the remainder to the individual. When anticoagulated blood is centrifuged in a test tube, it will separate into RBCs, WBCs, platelets, and plasma because of the different weights (specific gravities) of these components (Fig. 17–1).

By placing a pipette at the appropriate level in the test tube, any of these components can be aspirated. The most widely used apheresis equipment applies the same concept, using a machine with a centrifuge bowl or belt. Blood is removed from an individual — usually with a large-bore needle — anticoagulated, and transported directly to the separation mechanism where it is separated into specific components. Once the components have been separated, any component can be withdrawn. The remaining portions of the blood are then remixed and returned to the donor or patient (Fig. 17–2).

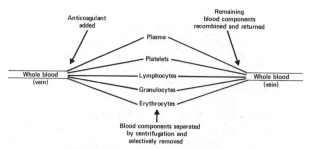

FIGURE 17–2 Principles of apheresis.

Depending on the goal of the individual procedures (e.g., collecting platelets, removing RBCs), the instruments must be adjusted appropriately. The variables are (1) centrifuge speed and diameter, (2) length of dwell time of the blood in the centrifuge, and (3) type of solutions added, such as anticoagulants or sedimenting agents. By manipulating these variables, the operator can harvest plasma, platelets, WBCs, or RBCs for commercial or therapeutic purposes.

Methodology

Procedures for performing apheresis vary according to the particular component of the blood to be harvested and equipment used. Manufacturers' instructions should always be consulted for specific techniques. The amount of time for a particular procedure can range from 90 to 150 minutes. Machines that are currently available require the use of disposable software, which includes sterile bags, tubing, and collection chambers unique to the machine. Platelets col-

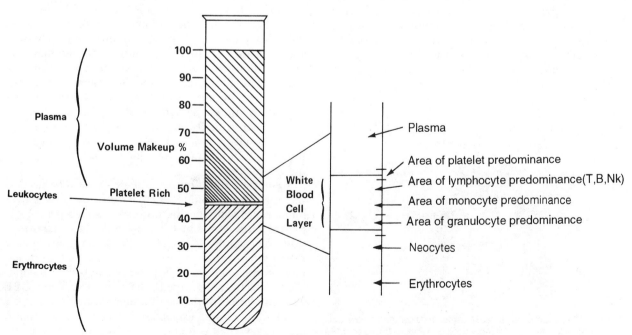

FIGURE 17–1 Sedimented blood sample. (Courtesy of IBM.)

lected using these systems are considered "closed," with a 5-day dating period. Other sets are composed of sterile tubing and bowls that have to be assembled on the machine before use. Such sets are considered an "open" system; therefore, the product has a 24-hour dating period.

The most commonly used instruments employ the centrifugation method of separation. These can be divided into the two basic categories of intermittent-flow centrifugation (IFC) and continuous-flow centrifugation (CFC). A newer technology now being employed involves the use of membrane filtration.

EQUIPMENT

Intermittent-flow centrifugation procedures are performed in cycles (or passes). Blood is drawn from an individual with the assistance of a pump. To keep blood from clotting, an anticoagulant (acid-citrate-dextrose [ACD]) is added to the tubing. The blood is pumped into the centrifuge bowl through the inlet port. The bowl rotates at a fixed speed, separating the components according to their specific gravities. The RBCs, which have greater mass, are packed against the outer rim of the bowl, followed by the WBCs, platelets, and plasma. The separated components flow from the bowl through the outlet port and are harvested as desired into separate collection bags (Fig. 17–3). The centrifuge is stopped, and the pump reversed. The undesired components are diverted into a reinfusion bag and returned to the individual. Reinfusion completes one cycle. The cycles are repeated until the desired quantity of product is obtained. A platelet-pheresis procedure usually takes six to eight cycles to collect a therapeutic dose.

One of the advantages of the IFC procedure is that it can be done with only one venipuncture (a one-arm procedure; that is, the blood is drawn and reinfused through the same needle). The amount of time for the process can be reduced if both arms are used: one for phlebotomy and one for reinfusion (two-arm procedure). The most widely used machines of this type are

manufactured by the Haemonetics Corporation. The semiautomated model 30 was extremely popular in the 1980s. The updated, fully automated model V50 is versatile, easy to operate, and capable of efficient component collections (Fig. 17–4). A computerized control panel allows the operator to select the desired procedure and collection parameters. The machine is equipped with optical sensors, which detect plasma-cell interfaces and divert components according to the preselected mode.

Continuous-flow centrifugation procedures withdraw, process, and return the blood to the individual simultaneously. This is in contrast to IFC procedures, which complete one cycle before beginning the next one. Because blood is drawn and returned continuously during a procedure, two venipuncture sites are necessary. Blood is drawn from the phlebotomy site with the assistance of a pump, mixed with anticoagulant, and collected in a chamber or belt, depending on the machine. Separation of the components is achieved through centrifugation, and the component is diverted and retained in a collection bag. The remainder of the blood is reinfused to the individual via the second venipuncture site. The process of phlebotomy, separation, and reinfusion is uninterrupted, or continuous. Examples of machines employing this concept are the Fenwal CS-3000 (Fig. 17–5) and the COBE Spectra (Fig. 17–6).

The IFC and CFC machines have individual advantages and disadvantages.[1] The IFC equipment has the advantage of being more mobile, owing to the smaller size of the machine. A single venipuncture may be used with IFC procedures, whereas two venipunctures are required with the CFC procedures. New protocols are being developed to allow the CFC equipment to operate with single access. The extracorporeal volume (the amount of blood out of the individual in the centrifuge bowl and tubing) is greater with IFC than with CFC. This may be an important consideration in individuals with small blood volumes (e.g., children and the elderly). The extra volume removed may lead to difficulties in maintaining proper fluid volume in the individual and cause adverse effects during the procedure. Because CFC procedures are uninterrupted, the time a person spends on the machine may be less than with IFC machines. The choice of equipment should be based on the functions and needs of the institution and the donor (or patient) requirements.

Membrane filtration technology can also be used to separate blood components. Blood that passes over membranes with specific pore sizes allows passage of plasma through the membrane, while the cellular portion passes over it. Filtration has several advantages over centrifugation, including the collection of a cell-free product and the ability to remove plasma components selectively by varying the pore size. The COBE TPE employs continuous-flow membrane filtration for therapeutic plasma exchanges.[2] A new cell separation technology that combines centrifugation and mem-

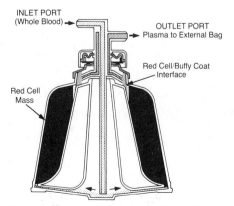

INLET PORT (Whole Blood)

OUTLET PORT Plasma to External Bag

Red Cell/Buffy Coat Interface

Red Cell Mass

FIGURE 17–3 Cross-section of Haemonetics centrifuge bowl (IFC procedure). (Courtesy of Haemonetics Corporation, Braintree, MA.)

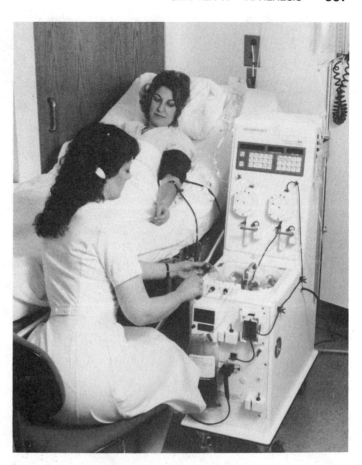

FIGURE 17–4 A therapeutic apheresis procedure using the Haemonetics V-50 (IFC procedure). (Courtesy of Haemonetics Corporation, Braintree, MA.)

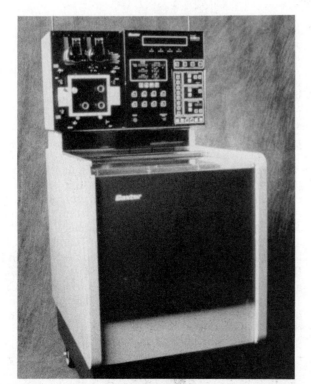

FIGURE 17–5 The Fenwal CS-3000 continuous-flow blood cell separator. (Courtesy of Baxter Healthcare Corporation, Deerfield, IL.)

brane filtration for plasma collection is found in the Fenwal Autopheresis-C. This intermittent-flow machine collects blood in a small cylinder that is rotating, forcing plasma through a polycarbonate membrane (Fig. 17–7).[3] This system has recently been modified to collect apheresis platelets with a 5-day storage. Platelet-rich plasma (600 to 700 ml) is collected in the first step, and then the platelets are concentrated to a smaller volume of plasma by using a second rotating membrane plasma separation device integrally attached to the processing unit.[4]

Apheresis products may be collected manually, using a refrigerated centrifuge and a specialized multiple plastic bag system, available from commercial sources. In this procedure, whole blood is collected into a plastic bag, which is then separated from the collection set and centrifuged. The desired component is retained, and the remainder reinfused. The process is then repeated.[5] Figure 17–8 shows a manual plasmapheresis. The procedure is simple and inexpensive because sophisticated equipment is not required. However, the method has its disadvantages. The amount of component harvested per procedure is far less than the yield with the automated devices. Because the whole blood must be separated from the collection set to be centrifuged, there is the added risk of returning the RBCs to the wrong individual. Consequently, stringent methods to identify the RBC unit

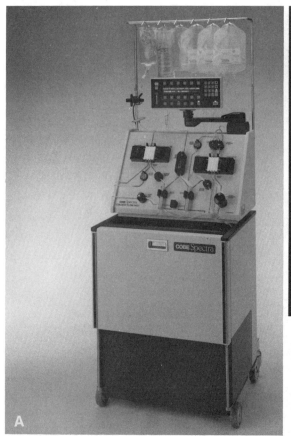

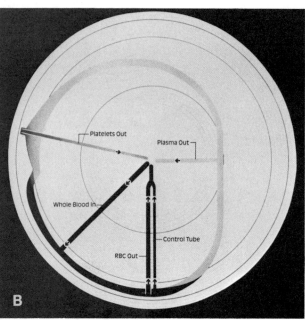

FIGURE 17-6 (*A*) The COBE Spectra apheresis system. (*B*) The separation chamber uses a unique asymmetric design to minimize contamination from red and white blood cells.

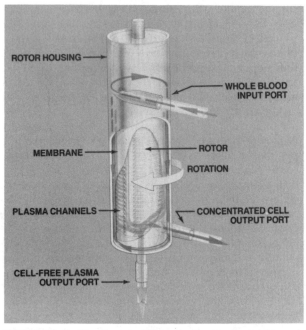

FIGURE 17-7 The Plasmacell-C separation device of the Fenwal Autopheresis-C. (Courtesy of Baxter Healthcare Corporation, Deerfield, IL.)

with the donor must be implemented. This technique is a viable alternative when a person's veins cannot withstand the demands of automated equipment or when such equipment is not available.

FLUIDS

All apheresis procedures use anticoagulants to keep the blood from clotting as it enters the separation mechanism. The most common anticoagulant is ACD. Normal saline is used to prime the system, keep the line open, and help maintain fluid volume. For granulocyte collection, a sedimenting agent is added to the blood so that better separation between the WBCs and RBCs is achieved (because RBC and WBC specific gravities are very similar—1.093 to 1.096 for RBCs; 1.087 to 1.092 for granulocytes).[6] The most commonly used sedimenting agent is hydroxyethyl starch (HES). This solution causes RBCs to form rouleaux, thus allowing WBCs to be harvested more efficiently.

In therapeutic plasmapheresis procedures, large volumes of a patient's plasma are retained. The fluid must be replaced to maintain appropriate intravascular volume and oncotic pressure. Several solutions are available, and the choice is determined by each institu-

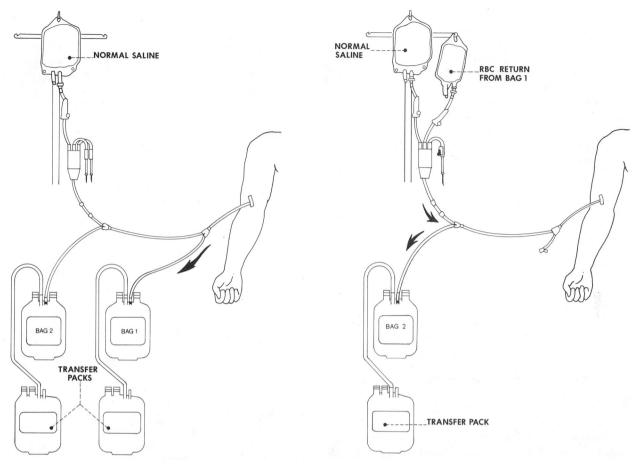

FIGURE 17-8 Venous blood is collected into bag 1 and mixed with anticoagulant (*left*). Bag 1 and its transfer bag are sealed off and taken to a centrifuge for separation into plasma and red blood cells. In the meantime, the needle and tubing are kept open with normal saline. The red blood cells are attached to the administration set and infused (*right*). The process is then repeated using bag 2. (From Kennedy, MS and Domen, RE: Therapeutic Apheresis. Vox Sang 45:261, 1983, with permission.)

tion. Crystalloids such as normal saline may be used. Because saline provides less oncotic pressure than plasma, it has the disadvantage that two to three times the volume removed must be used in replacement. Normal serum albumin (NSA) in a 5 percent solution and plasma protein fraction (PPF) are alternatives that may be replaced in a 1:1 ratio. These products provide the proper oncotic properties but increase the cost of the procedure. Plasma protein fraction has been associated with hypotensive reactions[7] and is generally not used in most centers. Neither NSA nor PPF have been implicated in transmission of transfusion-transmitted viruses. Mixtures of normal saline and NSA have also been used. Fresh frozen plasma (FFP) contains all the constituents of the removed plasma and thus would appear to be the optimal replacement fluid. FFP has the disadvantages of possible disease transmission, ABO incompatibility, citrate toxicity, and sensitization to plasma proteins and cellular antigens.[8] It has been implicated in fatal reactions and is now recommended primarily for the treatment of patients with thrombotic thrombocytopenic purpura (TTP) or hemolytic uremic syndrome (HUS). FFP may provide some factor that patients with TTP or HUS

are missing, such as a precursor for prostacyclin or other antithrombotic factors.[9] Recently, reports of an unusually large von Willebrand factor (vWF) as a proposed etiology of TTP or HUS has prompted the use of cryosupernatant fraction of plasma as the replacement fluid, a component deficient in vWF.[10]

GENERAL REQUIREMENTS

Good equipment and a well-trained, motivated staff are essential to an effective apheresis program. Operators of automated machines must be knowledgeable in all aspects of operation and troubleshooting. Individuals hired to perform these procedures may be medical technologists or nurses. In some institutions technicians are trained on the job. Medical technologists relate well to the technical aspects of the program but may feel uncomfortable in dealing with infusion of fluids and therapeutic procedures in which patient care may be required. The education background of nurses includes administering resuscitative procedures and dealing with adverse reactions, but nurses may not be as comfortable with automated equipment. In many units, technicians function satisfactorily under the supervision of a medical technologist or nurse. Regardless of the professional background of the apheresis staff, operators must participate in an intensive orientation program dealing with all aspects of apheresis. This training should include machine operation and quality control, donor selection, familiarity with the American Association of Blood Banks (AABB) standards and the *Code of Federal Regulations* (CFR), documentation, management of complications, and venous access. An apheresis operator should be a people-oriented person. Inasmuch as the procedures are often lengthy, complications may be avoided by the operator's ability to relieve the donor's or patient's boredom and anxiety. It is preferable to have two operators per procedure. However, if this is not possible, it is essential to have another qualified individual immediately available to assist in case of emergencies. A physician does not have to be in the room but should be within reach if complications should occur.

Written, informed consent must be obtained from donors and patients. The procedure, possible risks and benefits, tests performed to reduce the risk of transfusion-transmitted infectious diseases, and alternative modes of therapy must be explained in understandable language. Prospective donors must be given educational materials regarding the risks of infectious diseases transmitted by blood transfusion. The individual must then be given the opportunity to ask questions and to accept or reject the procedure.

The apheresis unit must contain an operator's manual with detailed instructions concerning the following:

1. Informed consent process
2. Standardized protocols and policies for component collection (donors) and therapeutic procedures (patients)
3. Quality control of the equipment and apheresis products (component collections)
4. Management of adverse reactions
5. Postapheresis care
6. Proper record keeping; documentation should comply with all accrediting agencies

Applications

Blood banks were established primarily to provide compatible and viable RBCs to restore oxygen-carrying capacity to the tissues. Anticoagulant and preservative solutions and plastic bags were developed that allowed maximum RBC storage with acceptable post-transfusion survival and function. Later, as advances were made in medicine, particularly in chemotherapy, blood banks were faced with the demands for products to overcome the effects of bone marrow depression caused by these drugs. Patients needed platelets and WBCs to survive the period of intensive drug therapy. The doses of blood components required to treat such patients effectively could not be met by products prepared from single whole blood donations. New tech-

nology had to be developed to collect larger quantities of a component from a single donor. In addition, increasing concern about transfusion-transmitted diseases and alloimmunization led to the development of programs to reduce the number of donor exposures to the patient. Automated or semiautomated apheresis equipment was the answer to the new demands placed on the blood banks. Component collection thus was the primary application of apheresis equipment.

It was soon realized that the machines also could be used therapeutically to treat patients with certain diseases. The rationale for the procedure was to remove the pathologic component from the blood or patient. Therefore, the use of apheresis technology can be divided into two categories: component collections and therapeutic procedures.

COMPONENT COLLECTIONS

In component collections, a normal healthy donor undergoes a procedure to obtain a specific blood component that will be transfused to a patient. Apheresis donors must meet the requirements established by the standards of the AABB.[11] Donors undergoing an occasional procedure (performed no more frequently than once every 8 weeks) must meet the same criteria as a whole blood donor. Exceptions to the requirements are allowed if the product would be of particular value to the patient. In such cases, a physician must verify in writing that the donor's health would not be compromised. More stringent regulations govern the donor who participates in a serial apheresis program (procedure performed more frequently than once every 8 weeks). Careful monitoring of weight, blood cell counts, serum protein levels, and quantitation of immunoglobulins are required. The interval between apheresis procedures should be at least 48 hours, and the amount of RBC loss should not exceed 25 ml per week. The maximum amount of plasma that can be retained during a procedure should not exceed the amount approved by the Food and Drug Administration (FDA). Apheresis procedures shall not be performed more than two times in a week or 24 times in a year unless approved by the blood bank physician. If the donor's RBCs during a procedure were not reinfused, or if the participant donates a unit of whole blood, 8 weeks should elapse before a subsequent cytapheresis procedure, unless the hemoglobin requirement is met and the donor is found acceptable by a blood bank physician. In component collections, replacement fluids are usually not required. However, careful monitoring of fluid volume in and out is required to prevent complications from shifts in blood volume. Extracorporeal blood volume should not exceed 15 percent of the donor's estimated total blood volume at any time during the procedure. The donor's total blood volume may be obtained from a chart by using the height, weight, and gender of the individual. The extracorporeal volume (volume out of the donor) is calculated from the volume of the apheresis chamber, the donor's hematocrit, and the total blood volume. Several of the modern apheresis machines perform these calculations automatically. If not, the manufacturer must be consulted for the formulas used for each specific machine. Testing of the apheresis donor's blood must be identical to the testing for whole blood donation. If the cytapheresis donor is dedicated to the support of a specific patient, routine testing for ABO, Rh, unexpected antibodies, and tests to prevent disease transmission must be performed before the first apheresis component is transfused, and at least every 10 days thereafter.

Plateletpheresis

Random platelets are harvested from routine whole blood donations, resulting in 1 unit of platelets (5.5×10^{10}) per unit of whole blood. The usual dose prescribed is 6 to 10 units of platelets for an adult and 1 unit/10 kg body weight for a child. The clinical indications for platelet transfusions include bleeding caused by thrombocytopenia (platelet counts between 20,000 and 50,000/μl). However, the platelet count that triggers an order varies significantly. A platelet count less than 20,000/μl in the absence of bleeding ordinarily requires platelet transfusions, although many patients tolerate lower counts. A platelet count greater than 50,000/μl is desired when surgery or an invasive procedure is performed.

Random pooled platelet concentrates are the component of choice in patients who achieve the expected increment 1 hour after transfusion. One unit of platelets should increase the count by 5,000 to 10,000/μl in a 70-kg adult, and 1 unit of apheresis platelets should increase the platelet count 30,000 to 60,000/μl.[12] However, patients with leukemia or aplastic anemia who receive multiple, long-term platelet transfusions may become alloimmunized to HLA antigens on platelets, thus leading to a refractory or unresponsive state. HLA-matched platelets can be collected from selected donors for patients with alloimmunization during bleeding episodes. Reducing the number of leukocytes in the product may prevent febrile, nonhemolytic transfusion reactions and prevent or delay the development of HLA alloimmunization and platelet refractoriness.[13] A number of methods have been developed to reduce the leukocyte contamination during the collection and processing of an apheresis platelet product. Most software currently in use has this capability.

Plateletpheresis is the removal of the platelets from a donor with the return of the donor's RBCs, WBCs, and plasma. Sedimenting agents are not necessary for this procedure. The platelets are selectively separated from the whole blood and retained in a collection bag while the remainder of the components are reinfused to the donor. The platelet yield is related to the donor's initial platelet count and the amount of blood processed. An apheresis donor for platelets must not have taken aspirin-containing medication within the last 3 days. Aspirin, by inhibiting the enzyme cyclooxy-genase in the prostaglandin pathway, prevents adequate platelet aggregation and the release of platelet adenosine disphosphate (ADP). Because an apheresis product would be the sole source of platelets for the patient, careful screening of potential donors is essential for obtaining a therapeutically effective product. A platelet count shall be obtained before the platelet-pheresis procedure on all individuals donating more frequently than once every 8 weeks and must be greater than 150×10^9/liter. The concentrate obtained from a single procedure must contain a minimum of 3×10^{11} platelets in 75 percent of the units tested. A routine procedure to produce such a product takes 1 to 3 hours. The product is usually prepared in a closed system, which is approved for 5 days' storage. If the product is prepared in an open system, it must be transfused within 24 hours. Platelets stored at room temperature (20°C to 24°C) should be maintained with continuous, gentle agitation. The pH at the end of the storage period must be 6.0 or greater. If RBC contamination in the product is negligible (less than 5 ml), compatibility testing is not required, but it is recommended that the donor plasma be ABO compatible with the recipient, especially in the case of an infant.[11]

Side effects to the donor during plateletpheresis procedures are commonly attributed to citrate toxicity. Citrate, used to anticoagulate the blood as it enters the separation chamber, is metabolized quickly in the liver. However, if the amount of citrate infused exceeds the body's ability to metabolize it, the donor may feel numbness or tingling around the mouth. The problem can be solved by decreasing the reinfusion rate of the returned components or giving the donor exogenous calcium. Complications also may occur owing to improper monitoring of fluid volumes, particularly if IFC equipment is used to perform the procedure.

Leukapheresis

Plateletpheresis therapy rapidly became so successful in treating patients with bone marrow suppression that bleeding was no longer the cause of death in these patients. Instead, they died from sepsis. The next logical step was to develop techniques for collecting leukocytes by apheresis. Leukapheresis is defined generically as the removal of WBCs with the return of RBCs, plasma, and platelets to the donor. The specific cell product that is required for treating sepsis is the neutrophil, or granulocyte. It was soon realized that the unique characteristics of this cell presented technical problems that differed from those of RBCs and platelets. The collection of RBCs and platelets was easier because the volume of these cells in the intravascular space is larger and the daily consumption less. Neutrophils comprise a small portion of the cellular components of the blood, yet 50 percent of the bone marrow is dedicated to their production. The proportion is understandable in view of the daily consumption of neutrophils. Production in a normal adult is about 10^{11} cells per day. These cells have a half-life of approximately 6 hours in the blood. A patient with sepsis can increase production to 10^{12} cells per day.[14] It is estimated that approximately 230 percent of the neutrophils are replaced daily in a healthy adult, compared with only 1 percent of the RBCs and 10 percent of platelets.[15] The situation thus presented a dual problem: More cells had to be harvested from a pool of fewer cells.

Automated collection procedures provided the means to process large quantities of blood to obtain minimum doses for patients. The equipment can process several liters of blood over a period of hours and concentrate the product for transfusion. The actual procedure involves the same basic steps as platelet-pheresis. Owing to the similar specific gravities of the RBCs and WBCs (Fig. 17–1), however, sedimenting agents such as HES are recommended for better separation.[6] HES is added to the donor's blood along with the anticoagulant as it enters the separation chamber. Donors can also be premedicated with steroids to produce a greater yield of granulocytes.[16,17] Steroids are believed to increase the vascular pool of granulocytes either by stimulation of the bone marrow to increase cellular output or by causing a shift of the cells from the tissues to the blood. Distribution of polymorphonuclear leukocytes in the body is approximately 96 percent in the bone marrow, 1.7 percent in the circulation, and 1.9 percent in the marginal pool. However, steroids may exacerbate certain medical conditions, and their use must be evaluated by the blood bank physician.

The granulocyte concentrate must contain a minimum of 1.0×10^{10} granulocytes in at least 75 percent of the units tested. The product has a shelf life of 24 hours, but should be transfused as soon as possible after collection for optimal therapeutic effectiveness. The product should be stored at room temperature (20°C to 24°C), without agitation. Because of the large numbers of viable lymphocytes, granulocyte preparations must be irradiated to prevent GVH disease in immunocompromised recipients. The function of the granulocytes is not affected by irradiation. Microaggregate filters are not recommended for administration. Owing to the inherent RBC contamination in the procedure, the RBCs of the donor should be ABO compatible with those of the recipient. Compatibility testing is required in products containing greater than 5 ml of RBCs.[11] Because of the necessity of going into the RBC layer to obtain a good granulocyte product, compatibility testing is often required. Contamination of the product with lymphocytes, and to a lesser degree platelets, cannot be avoided, owing to the collection technique.

Donors undergoing leukapheresis may experience citrate toxicity. Of more concern is the potential long-term effect of HES on the donor. Donors undergoing consecutive procedures may experience a buildup of HES because of incomplete excretion in the urine.

HES has been reported in a donor 1 year after a procedure. The possibility exists that accumulation of this product could block the reticuloendothelial system and interfere with the antigen processing by the macrophages. A low molecular weight preparation of HES with rapid excretion rates has been shown to be an efficacious and safe RBC sedimenting agent for leukapheresis by centrifugation.[18]

Once methods for granulocyte collection were developed, questions arose concerning the therapeutic effectiveness achieved versus the possible risks to the donors from HES and steroids. Clinical applications of granulocyte transfusions yielded disappointing results except in the treatment of neonatal sepsis. Success in this select group of patients may be related to the comparatively larger doses that can be transfused per body surface area with the same apheresis product.[19] Some authors have indicated that a component with 1×10^9 granulocytes is sufficient for the treatment of the neonate. The development of new technology is needed to increase the dose of granulocytes that can be given to adults. Methods aimed at collecting neutrophils specifically may be beneficial. The trend has been to move away from the use of granulocyte transfusions for the septic patient, particularly with newer and better antibiotics constantly appearing on the market. Granulocytes may still be prepared for the neonate using techniques that do not involve the expense of apheresis or the risk to the donor. The buffy coat from a unit of whole blood less than 12 hours old may be harvested with a yield of approximately 0.5×10^9 granulocytes. It has been reported that 1×10^9 granulocytes may be obtained from the buffy coat of a unit of whole blood if HES is added.[20]

Neocytapheresis

Patients with thalassemia major require continuous RBC transfusion therapy in order to survive. Homozygous inheritance of a genetic defect results in the inability of the patient to manufacture β-globin chains essential for the production of normal adult hemoglobin. Consequently, insufficient hemoglobin is produced, and severe anemia occurs early in life. Unless treated, the survival time of these patients is very short, only a few years.

Chronic transfusion therapy has increased the life-span of these patients considerably. This treatment, however, produces its own characteristic pathology: siderosis. The increased iron from transfused RBCs cannot be excreted quickly and efficiently, leading to iron deposition in tissues.

Traditional therapy for this complication is iron-chelating agents that enhance the urinary excretion of iron. Another approach uses a form of apheresis termed *neocytapheresis*. The method involves the selective removal of the donor's neocytes, or reticulocytes found in the upper portion of the RBC layer (Fig. 17–1).

A unit of neocytes has a half-life approximately

twice that of a regular unit of RBCs, thus reducing the frequency of transfusions in these patients.[21] Various techniques have been developed to collect neocytes, some of which do not use apheresis equipment. However, the preparation of these units is time consuming and costly and has not gained wide acceptance.

Plasmapheresis

In a plasmapheresis procedure, the plasma is separated from the cellular components in a collection bag and retained, and then the cells are reinfused to the donor. The procedure may be performed by the manual method described in this chapter or by using automated equipment. For the clinical setting, plasmapheresis may be used to increase the inventory of FFP of a particular ABO group (such as group AB) or to decrease donor exposures by collecting "jumbo" plasma from a single donor. The procedure may be used to collect immune plasma for immunosuppressed patients who have been exposed to varicella zoster or herpes zoster. Reference laboratories perform apheresis to collect rare RBC and WBC antibodies. Commercially, plasma centers use serial plasmapheresis to draw plasma for manufacturing into such products as plasma derivatives, hepatitis immunoglobulin, and Rh immune globulin.

If the procedure is performed no more than once every 8 weeks, the same criteria that apply to whole blood donation should be used. However, if the donor is participating in a serial plasmapheresis program (plasma is donated more frequently than once every 8 weeks), AABB standards require additional and continuous assessment of the donor's health. The procedure should not be performed if the total serum protein is less than 6.0 g/dl. Unexplained weight loss (greater than 10 lb) is a reason for deferral. Every 4 months all records and laboratory tests must be reviewed and evaluated by a physician, and a serum protein electrophoresis or immunoglobulin level determined. If the donor's RBCs during a procedure were not reinfused, or if the participant donates a unit of whole blood, 8 weeks should elapse before the donor may be reinstated in the program, unless the hemoglobin requirement is met and the donor found acceptable by a blood bank physician.

Proper identification of the RBC reinfusion bag is essential, particularly during manual procedures when the bag is separated from the donor. The RBCs must be returned within 2 hours of the phlebotomy. RBC loss must not be greater than 25 ml per week. The amount of whole blood that can be processed during a plasmapheresis procedure must not be greater than 500 ml at one time or 1000 ml in any 48-hour period (600 ml or 1200 ml, respectively, if the donor weighs at least 176 lb); or 2000 ml (2400 ml if the donor weighs at least 176 lb) in a 7-day period. When plasmapheresis is performed by an automated procedure, the amount of plasma collected should not exceed the amount approved by the FDA for that instrument.[11]

THERAPEUTIC PROCEDURES

When therapeutic apheresis was originally introduced as a treatment modality, it generated enormous enthusiasm and excitement. It was hoped that this new technology would be the answer to many problems, particularly in diseases involving immune-mediated mechanisms. Expectations far exceeded the therapeutic abilities of the procedure. Assessment of effectiveness was difficult because reports in the literature presented data from uncontrolled studies. Most clinical trials were retrospective rather than prospective. However, the last decade has provided the medical field with sufficient data to evaluate apheresis as a form of therapy more realistically and to define its role in the treatment of disease (Table 17–1).[22,23]

Apheresis cannot cure a disease but can be very effective in alleviating the symptoms produced by the underlying disease state. Efficacy of the procedure is enhanced by concomitant drug therapy, particularly immunosuppressive therapy in immune-mediated problems. Duration of the effects of the procedure varies with the individual. The course of therapy may last from several days to months and is based on the response and tolerance of the patient.

Therapeutic apheresis has placed blood banks in the position of direct medical care for the patient. This situation has necessitated a change in the perspective of the medical director and the technical staff. Clearly defined policies must delineate the responsibility of the blood bank and the attending physician. Issues such as who makes the decision about vascular access; who orders laboratory tests to evaluate and to monitor the patient; and who chooses replacement fluids must be resolved. The medical director should be involved with the attending physician in deciding whether there are clinical indications for the procedure. The technical staff must be properly trained to care for very ill patients. Confidence in handling emergency situations is essential. Attention must be given to the patient's medication schedule. Apheresis may dangerously lower plasma levels of medications given before the procedure. Proper documentation of all facets of the procedure is required. Written informed consent must be properly obtained from the patient.

The rationale of therapeutic apheresis is based on the following:

1. A pathogenic substance exists in the blood that contributes to a disease process or its symptoms.
2. The substance can be more effectively removed by apheresis than by the body's own homeostatic mechanisms.

The apheresis procedures that reduce the level of the substance involved, and thus improve the symptoms, are classified by the component removed: cytapheresis if the component is cellular and plasma exchange (or immunoadsorption) if the substance circulates in the plasma.

TABLE 17–1 **GUIDELINES FOR THERAPEUTIC HEMAPHERESIS***

Category I	Category II	Category III	Category IV
Coagulation factor inhibitors	Chronic inflammatory	ABO-incompatible organ or	AIDS (for symptoms of
Cryoglobulinemia	demyelinating	marrow transplantation	immunodeficiency)
Goodpasture's syndrome	polyneuropathy	Maternal treatment of maternal	Amyotrophic lateral sclerosis
Guillain-Barré syndrome	Cold agglutinin disease	fetal incompatibility	Aplastic anemia
Homozyguous familial	Drug overdose and poisoning	(hemolytic disease of the	Fulminant hepatic failure
hypercholesterolemia	(protein bound toxins)	newborn)	ITP (chronic)
Hyperviscosity syndrome	HUS	Thyroid storm	Lupus nephritis
Myasthenia gravis	Pemphigus vulgaris	Multiple sclerosis	Polymyositis/dermatomyositis
Posttransfusion purpura	Rapidly progressive	Progressive systemic sclerosis	Psoriasis
Refsum's disease	glomerulonephritis	Pure RBC aplasia	Renal transplant rejection
TTP	Systemic vasculitis (primary or	Transfusion refractoriness due	Rheumatoid arthritis
	secondary to rheumatoid	to alloantibodies (RBC,	Schizophrenia
	arthritis or systemic lupus	platelet, HLA)	
	erythematosus)	Warm autoimmune hemolytic	
		anemia	

Cytapheresis			
Leukemia with	Cutaneous T-cell lymphoma	Life-threatening hemolytic	Leukemia without
hyperleukocytosis syndrome	(cytoreduction or	transfusion reactions	hyperleukocytosis syndromes
Sickle cell syndrome (also see	photopheresis)	Multiple sclerosis	Hypereosinophilia
category III)	Hairy cell leukemia	Organ transplant rejection (also	Polymyositis/dermatomyositis
Thrombocytosis, symptomatic	Hyperparasitemia (e.g., malaria)	photopheresis)	
	Peripheral blood stem cell	Sickle cell disease (prophylactic	
	collections for hemopoietic	use in pregnancy)	
	reconstitution		
	Rheumatoid arthritis		

From Guidelines for Therapeutic Hemapheresis, American Association of Blood Banks Extracorporeal Therapy Committee, with permission.
*The indications have been divided into four categories as follows: Category I, standard and acceptable under certain circumstances, including primary therapy; category II, sufficient evidence to suggest efficacy, acceptable therapy on an adjunctive basis; category III, inconclusive evidence for efficacy, uncertain benefit/risk ratio; and category IV, lack of efficacy in controlled trials.
HUS = hemolytic uremic syndrome; ITP = idiopathic thrombocytopenic purpura; TTP = thrombotic thrombocytopenic purpura.

Cytapheresis

Plateletpheresis (thrombocytapheresis) can be used to treat patients who have abnormally elevated platelet counts with related symptoms.[24] This condition has been reported in patients with myeloproliferative disorders such as polycythemia vera. Patients having counts greater than 1,000,000/μl may develop thrombotic or hemorrhagic complications. During a routine apheresis procedure, the platelet count can be decreased by as much as one-third to one-half the initial value.[25] The procedure can be repeated as frequently as necessary until drug therapy becomes effective and the symptoms disappear.

Leukapheresis has been used to treat patients with leukemia. This therapy is particularly indicated in patients with impending leukostasis, in which leukocyte aggregates and thrombi may interfere with pulmonary and cerebral blood flow. Leukocyte counts in excess of 100,000/μl are considered appropriate indications for instituting apheresis therapy. The greatest therapeutic benefits are seen in acute cases under each of the following conditions: (1) Drug therapy was just started and has not yet taken effect; (2) drug therapy is contraindicated; or (3) patients have become refractory to drug treatment. Lymphocytapheresis (the removal of lymphocytes) has been investigated as a means of producing immunosuppression in diseases with a cellular

immune mechanism such as rheumatoid arthritis, systemic lupus erythematosus, kidney transplant rejection, and autoimmune and alloimmune diseases. These procedures are not used routinely, and further studies are required to determine efficacy and to assess possible long-term complications from the procedure.

The therapeutic uses of cytapheresis mentioned earlier involve depletion of cellular constituents without replacement. Erythrocytapheresis, however, is considered an exchange procedure. A predetermined quantity of RBCs is removed from the patient and replaced with homologous blood. The procedure has been used successfully to treat various complications of sickle cell disease, such as priapism and impending stroke.[26] Other indications are rare. Successful therapy has been reported in patients with severe parasitic infections from malaria and babesiosis.[27,28]

Plasma Exchange

Plasmapheresis is the removal and retention of the plasma with return of all cellular components to the patient. This therapeutic procedure has become synonymous with the term *plasma exchange*, which describes the protocol more accurately. The purpose is to remove the offending agent in the plasma causing the clinical symptoms. The plasma that is removed

TABLE 17-2 **FACTORS REMOVED BY PLASMAPHERESIS**

1. Immune complexes (e.g., systemic lupus erythematosus)
2. Autoantibodies or alloantibodies (e.g., factor VIII inhibitors)
3. Antibodies causing hyperviscosity (e.g., Waldenström's macroglobulinemia)
4. Inflammatory mediators (e.g., fibrinogen and complement)
5. Antibody blocking the normal function of the immune system
6. Protein-bound toxins (e.g., barbiturate poisoning)
7. Lipoproteins
8. Platelet-aggregating factors (e.g., possible role in TTP)

TTP = thrombotic thrombocytopenic purpura.

must be replaced or exchanged; hence the term *plasma exchange*. It has been postulated that beneficial effects of the procedure, particularly in diseases that involve malfunction of the immune system, may be attributed to the removal of the factors listed in Table 17-2.[29]

The efficiency of a plasma exchange is related to the amount of plasma removed. This effect is diluted by the necessity to replace the plasma to maintain the patient's fluid volume. A procedure that removes an amount of plasma equal to the patient's plasma volume is called a one-volume exchange. The actual amount of plasma removed may vary from 2 to 4 liters, depending on the patient's size. A one-volume exchange should reduce the unwanted plasma component to approximately 30 percent of its initial value. If a second plasma volume is removed as part of the same procedure, the procedure becomes less efficient, reducing the component to only approximately 10 percent.[8] Because of the diminishing effect of increased plasma removal, it is recommended that approximately 1 to 1.5 plasma volumes be exchanged per procedure.[30]

Synthesis and catabolism of the pathologic component as well as its distribution between the extravascular and the intravascular spaces are factors affecting the outcome of a plasma exchange. If the antibody causing the patient's symptoms is IgM, apheresis can be an effective therapeutic tool. IgM is primarily intravascular and is synthesized slowly, whereas IgG is equally distributed in the intravascular and extravascular spaces. Reappearance of IgG in the plasma occurs more quickly owing to reequilibration. Removal of IgG with apheresis can lead to increased antibody synthesis (rebound phenomena). Because of this effect, therapeutic procedures performed to remove IgG antibodies are most effective when combined with immunosuppressive drugs.

Immunoadsorption

Immunoadsorption refers to a method in which a specific ligand is bound to an insoluble matrix in a column or filter. Plasma is then perfused over the column, with selective removal of the pathogenic substance and return of the patient's own plasma. The removal is usually mediated by an antigen-antibody or chemical reaction. Both off-line and on-line procedures have been developed using the current apheresis equipment. A diagram of the process is shown in Figure 17-9.

A number of adsorptive matrices have been used with varying specificity. Table 17-3 lists some of the adsorbents, the substance removed, and the clinical applications for each.

Staphylococcal protein A as an immunoadsorbent has gained greater acceptance in clinical use. This ligand has an affinity for IgG classes 1, 2, and 4 as well as IgG immune complexes. The immunoaffinity column currently has federal licensure to treat patients with idiopathic thrombocytopenic purpura (ITP).[31] The column has also shown promise in the treatment of a variety of other disease processes, including human immunodeficiency virus [HIV]–associated thrombocytopenia,[32] chemotherapy-induced TTP/HUS,[33] and alloimmunization resulting in platelet refractoriness.[34] A number of adverse reactions, including fever, chills, and rash, have been reported, as have several fatalities.[35]

The mechanism of action of these columns is not well established. Removal of IgG and immune complexes alone cannot explain the clinical benefit of the treatment. There appears to be a significant immunomodulatory effect of this treatment, with enhanced anti-idiotypic antibody regulation and activated cellular immune function.[35]

Adverse Effects

Apheresis is accepted as a relatively safe procedure, but complications do occur. These effects may be observed in component collections as well as therapeutic procedures. In the latter case, it is sometimes difficult to evaluate whether the deleterious effects were caused by the procedure or the underlying disease entity. Some of the problems encountered are listed in Table 17-4.

Citrate toxicity is usually observed during cytapheresis component collections when anticoagulated plasma is returned at a rapid rate. If FFP is used as replacement fluid during a therapeutic plasma exchange, this phenomenon will more likely occur. Decreasing the reinfusion rate usually alleviates the symptoms. Some centers have switched to using a lower percent citrate solution. The most common initial complaint of citrate toxicity is tingling around the mouth. Citrate binds to calcium, and the lowering of the body's ionized calcium leads to the symptoms. Intravenous calcium is not recommended on a routine basis, although exogenous calcium may be useful. If unattended, the symptoms can lead to tetany and cardiac arrhythmia.

Vasovagal reactions often can be avoided by attentive, receptive apheresis operators. Individuals undergoing these procedures require assurance from the operators. Hypovolemia is observed more frequently

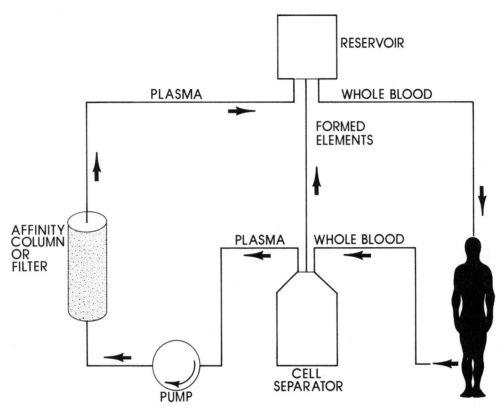

FIGURE 17–9 Perfusion of plasma over columns or filters. (From Berkman, EM and Umlas, J (eds): Therapeutic Hemapheresis: A Technical Workshop. American Association of Blood Banks, p 142, with permission.)

TABLE 17–3 TYPES OF ADSORBENTS AND THEIR CLINICAL APPLICATION

Adsorbent	Substance Removed	Application
Charcoal	Bile acids	Cholestatic pruritus
A and B antigens	Anti-A, anti-B	Transplantation
Anti-LDL, heparin	LDL	Hypercholesterolemia
DNA	ANA, immune complexes	Systemic lupus erythematosus
Protein A	IgG, immune complexes	ITP, cancer, HUS

ANA = antinuclear antibodies; HUS = hemolytic uremic syndrome; ITP = idiopathic thrombocytopenic purpura; LDL = low-density lipoproteins.

with IFC equipment. These machines require a greater extracorporeal volume than the CFC machines (fluid volume out of the individual and into the separation chamber and tubing must not exceed 15 percent of the patient's total blood volume). Careful monitoring of the volume in and out is necessary to prevent not only hypovolemia but also hypervolemia. Allergic reactions are related to the replacement fluids. This is generally observed in cases in which FFP is administered, but it has also been reported with albumin. Hemolysis is usually caused by a mechanical problem with the equipment, such as a kink in the plastic tubing. Observing the return line is critical to avoid the problem. Air embolism and clotting factor deficiencies are not commonly observed. Normal proteins and immunoglobulins may be reduced following plasma exchanges.

Deaths due to therapeutic apheresis procedures have been reported.[36] The majority of these have been caused by circulatory (cardiac arrest) or respiratory distress. Of the 50 deaths reported, 25 had received plasma as part or all of the replacement fluid. Because plasma has been associated with fatalities, its use is recommended only in cases of TTP/HUS in which there is a specific indication for its use. Plasma is also

TABLE 17–4 ADVERSE EFFECTS OF APHERESIS

1. Citrate toxicity
2. Hematoma
3. Vasovagal reactions
4. Hypovolemia
5. Allergic reactions
6. Hemolysis
7. Air embolus
8. Depletion of clotting factors
9. Circulatory and respiratory distress
10. Transfusion-transmitted diseases
11. Lymphocyte loss
12. Depletion of proteins and immunoglobulins

capable of transmitting diseases such as hepatitis and HIV.

Donors undergoing multiple plateletpheresis procedures in a short period of time may experience significant decreases in lymphocyte counts.[9] The long-term effects of lymphocyte reduction following plateletpheresis are minimal.[37]

Adoptive Immunotherapy

Adoptive immunotherapy refers to an antitumor therapy in which autologous immunocompetent mononuclear cells, when stimulated by cytokines, can lead to tumor regression when reinfused to the patient. The lymphokine-activated killer (LAK) cell phenomenon, first described in 1982,[38] indicated that a population of human lymphocytes, when incubated with interleukin-2 (IL-2), a T-cell lymphokine, produced a cell population that could lyse malignant cells. A novel application of apheresis technology has thus placed the cancer patient in the role of a cytapheresis donor. The protocols involve infusing the patient-donor with recombinant IL-2 (either intermittently or continuously), followed by daily leukapheresis for several days. The harvested cells are then cultured in IL-2 for several more days before reinfusion to the patient. The side effects of the therapy are considerable, including pancytopenia, hepatic dysfunction, and massive fluid shifts, leading to severe hypotension and fluid retention with weight gain. This therapy has shown some tumor regression in patients with renal cell carcinoma, melanoma, and colorectal cancer, although clinical trials have been unable to reproduce the results of the original studies.[39] Attempts to reduce the toxicity of the treatment and improve its effect are continuing.

A new adaptation of this therapy involves extracting the lymphocytes within a portion of the surgically removed tumor (tumor-infiltrating lymphocytes [TIL]). These lymphocytes, which appear to have increased tumor-specific activity, are then placed in cell culture with IL-2 before reinfusion to the patient. Initial trials are encouraging.[39] This therapy does not involve apheresis.

Apheresis technology is used in a third form of immunotherapy, which involves autologous peripheral blood monocytes. These cells, when stimulated by the cytokine interferon gamma (activated killer monocytes [AKM]), develop specific antitumor activity.[40] The collection, culture, and reinfusion process is adapted from the LAK cell protocols. Limited data are available on the clinical benefit of this therapy.

The concept of adoptive immunotherapy has the potential for growth as the molecular biology of the immune response to malignancy becomes more evident. It has been theorized that the blood bank, especially apheresis, will be important in the development of specialized blood components composed of the different subsets of T lymphocytes.[41]

New Technology and Techniques

The equipment discussed thus far has used primarily the principle of differential centrifugation. In therapeutic plasma exchange, large volumes of plasma are removed and replaced with certain fluids. This nonspecific method can reduce levels of nonpathogenic proteins, can result in transfusion-transmitted diseases, and is expensive. Ideally, only the pathogenic substance should be removed, and the remaining plasma returned to the patient.

A number of techniques have been developed to achieve this selective removal. Cascade filtration uses filters in a sequential fashion to select out plasma components based on molecular weight. Although promising, the technique needs refinement before it becomes widely accepted. It is likely that immunoadsorption technology (described earlier in Plasma Exchange) will continue to evolve as the mechanism of immunoadsorption becomes better understood. As larger numbers of patients are treated, clinical indications will be firmly established. New ligands are certain to be developed to treat diseases currently treated by other modalities.

Apheresis techniques have been applied to the field of bone marrow transplantation (BMT). BMT has been used more frequently in the past several years for various hematologic diseases including thalassemia major, leukemia, and aplastic anemia. In the procedure, autologous or allogeneic bone marrow is collected from the donor, and following a period of chemotherapy or radiation therapy, or both, the marrow is reinfused. This marrow provides pluripotential hematopoietic progenitor cells that can develop into mature blood cells. Once harvested, the marrow must undergo extensive processing before storage and reinfusion. The processing can require cell separation, with RBC removal, buffy coat concentration, and mononuclear cell purification. In addition, malignant cells in the bone marrow may be purged by monoclonal antibodies. Techniques have been developed using the currently available apheresis equipment to perform these tasks.[42]

The hemopoietic progenitor cells that eventually repopulate the bone marrow also circulate in the blood and are called peripheral blood stem cells (PBSCs). A number of studies have shown that these cells, when collected from the peripheral blood and reinfused following marrow ablative therapy, can successfully engraft. These cells can be isolated from patients using procedures that collect the mononuclear cells with standard apheresis equipment. Multiple procedures are required to collect an equal number of cells that can be collected by bone marrow aspiration. The technique is useful when standard bone marrow collection cannot be done, such as when the marrow is involved with malignancy, the marrow is damaged owing to infection or radiation therapy, or the patient cannot tolerate general anesthesia.[43]

Photopheresis is a recently developed leukocytapheresis technique, requiring a special intermittent-flow machine using the bowl technology. This treatment has been shown to be efficacious against cutaneous T-cell lymphoma, a malignant skin disorder characterized by an abnormal proliferation of CD4 lymphocytes. Before the procedure, the patient ingests the drug psoralen, which binds to the DNA of all nucleated cells. Following the leukocytapheresis, the collected WBCs are exposed to ultraviolet light, which activates the psoralen and prevents replication. These treated cells are then returned to the patient, inducing an immune response against the abnormal lymphocyte clone.[44] Photopheresis has been used in a number of other immunologically mediated diseases, including scleroderma,[45] rheumatoid arthritis,[46] and chronic heart transplant rejection.[47]

The field of apheresis continues to evolve, as do all areas of transfusion medicine. Emerging technology, especially monoclonal antibodies, have resulted in dramatic advances in the understanding of the immune response, and the diseases associated with immune abnormalities. Transfusion and transplantation practices have benefited from this knowledge and will continue to rely on the collection of cellular or plasma components by apheresis, for transfusion or therapeutic purposes.

Review Questions

1. American Association of Blood Bank standards require that plateletpheresis products:
   A. Prepared in a closed system be transfused within 24 hours
   B. Contain 3×10^{11} platelets in 75 percent of the units tested
   C. Have a compatibility test performed before transfusion
   D. Have a pH of 6.0 or greater on the day of collection

2. Therapeutic cytapheresis is used in patients with:
   A. Sickle cell disease to alleviate painful crises
   B. Systemic lupus erythematosus to remove immune complexes
   C. Leukemia to help increase granulocyte production
   D. Polycythemia vera to decrease the RBC count

3. The minimum interval allowed between apheresis component collection procedures is:
   A. 24 hours
   B. 48 hours
   C. 7 days
   D. 8 weeks

4. A donor weighing 75 kg is undergoing a plasmapheresis procedure. What is the maximum amount of plasma that can be retained over a 7-day period?
   A. 500 ml
   B. 600 ml
   C. 1000 ml
   D. 1200 ml

5. In a plasma exchange, the therapeutic effectiveness is:
   A. Greatest with the first plasma volume removed
   B. Affected by the type of replacement fluid used
   C. Enhanced if the unwanted antibody is IgG rather than IgM
   D. Independent of the use of concomitant immunosuppressive therapy

6. The replacement fluid indicated during plasma exchange for TTP or HUS is:
   A. Normal (0.9%) saline
   B. HES
   C. FFP
   D. PPF
   E. NSA (5%)

7. The most common adverse effect of collection plateletpheresis is:
   A. Allergic reactions
   B. Hepatitis
   C. Hemolysis
   D. Citrate toxicity
   E. Air embolism

8. Apheresis can be used to collect all of the following *except*:
   A. Leukocytes
   B. Macrophages
   C. Neocytes
   D. Platelets
   E. Lymphocytes

9. Platelets collected in a closed apheresis system have a shelf life of:
   A. 35 days
   B. 24 hours
   C. 5 days
   D. 21 days
   E. 7 days

10. Peripheral blood stem cells are:
    A. Incubated with IL-2 to become LAK cells
    B. Removed during erythrocytapheresis
    C. Pluripotential hemopoietic precursors that circulate in the blood
    D. Immature RBCs used for transfusion in patients with thalassemia
    E. Lymphocytes involved with the immune response

11. Adoptive immunotherapy refers to:
    A. Antibody-mediated response to infection

B. Cytokine-stimulated mononuclear cells used to treat malignancies
C. Processing of bone marrow–derived mononuclear cells by apheresis technology
D. Immunosuppressive drug therapy
E. Vaccines

12. Advantages of CFC over IFC include:
A. Portability
B. Greater extracorporeal volume
C. Two venipunctures needed
D. Single venipuncture needed
E. Lower extracorporeal volume

Answers to Review Questions

1. B (p 341)
2. A (p 344)
3. B (p 340)
4. C (pp 341, 343)
5. A (p 344–345)
6. C (p 339)
7. D (p 341)
8. B (p 335)
9. C (p 341)
10. C (p 347)
11. B (p 347)
12. E (p 336)

References

1. Price, TH: Centrifugal equipment for the performance of therapeutic hemapheresis procedures. In MacPherson, JL and Kaspirisin, DO (eds): Therapeutic Hemapheresis. Vol 1. CRC Press, Boca Raton, FL, 1985, p 123.
2. Grossman, L, et al: Clinical evaluation of a flat-plate membrane plasma exchange system. J Clin Apheresis 1:225, 1983.
3. Rock, G, Tittley, P, and McCombie, N: Plasma collection using an automated membrane device. Transfusion 26:269, 1986.
4. Simon, T, et al: Storage and transfusion of platelets collected by an automated two-stage apheresis procedure. Transfusion 32:624, 1992.
5. Blood collection, storage and component preparation. In Walker, RH (ed): Technical Manual, ed 10. American Association of Blood Banks, Arlington, VA, 1990, pp 642–644, 1990.
6. Heustis, DW, et al: Use of hydroxyethyl starch to improve granulocyte collection in the Latham blood processor. Transfusion 15:1559, 1975.
7. Alving, BM, et al: Hypotension associated with prekallikrein activator (Hageman-factor fragments) in plasma protein fraction. N Engl J Med 299:66, 1978.
8. McCullough, J and Chopek, M: Therapeutic plasma exchange. Lab Med 12:745, 1981.
9. Westphal, RG: Complications of hemapheresis. In Westphal, RG and Kaspirisin, DO (eds): Current Status of Hemapheresis: Indications, Technology and Complications. American Association of Blood Banks, Arlington, VA, 1989, p 87.
10. Byrnes, JJ, et al: Effectiveness of the cryosupernatant fraction of plasma in the treatment of refractory thrombocytopenic purpura. Am J Hematol 34:169, 1990.
11. Standards for Blood Banks and Transfusion Services, ed 15. American Association of Blood Banks, Bethesda, MD, 1993.
12. Blood Transfusion Therapy: A Physician's Handbook, ed 3. American Association of Blood Banks, Arlington, VA, 1989.
13. Murphy, MF, et al: Use of leukocyte poor blood components and HLA matched platelet donors to prevent HLA alloimmunization. Br J Haematol 62:529, 1986.
14. Klock, JC: Granulocyte transfusion physiology. In Mielke, CH (ed): Apheresis: Development, Applications, and Collection Procedures. Alan R Liss, New York, 1981, p 14.
15. Wright, DG: Leucocyte transfusions: Thinking twice. Am J Med 76:637, 1984.
16. Ford, JM and Cullen, MH: Prophylactic granulocyte transfusions. Exp Hematol (Suppl)5:65, 1977.
17. Winton, EF and Vogler, WR: Development of a practical oral dexamethasone premedication schedule leading to improved granulocyte yields with the continuous-flow centrifugal blood cell separator. Blood 52:249, 1978.
18. Strauss, RG, et al: Selecting the optimal dose of low-molecular weight hydroxyethl starch (Pentastarch) for granulocyte collection. Transfusion 27:350, 1987.
19. Herzig, RH: Granulocyte transfusion therapy: Past, present and future. In Garratty, G (ed): Current Concepts in Transfusion Therapy. American Association of Blood Banks, Arlington, VA, 1985, p 267.
20. Rock, G, et al: Simple and rapid preparation of granulocytes for the treatment of neonatal septicemia. Transfusion 24:510, 1984.
21. Propper, RD: Neocytes and neocyte-gerocyte exchange. In Volger, WR (ed): Cytapheresis and Plasma Exchange Clinical Indications. Alan R Liss, New York, 1982, p 227.
22. Report of the AMA Panel on Therapeutic Plasmapheresis: Current status of therapeutic plasmapheresis and related techniques. JAMA 253:819, 1985.
23. Guidelines for Therapeutic Hemapheresis, American Association of Blood Banks, Bethesda, MD, 1992.
24. Taft, EG: Therapeutic apheresis. Hum Pathol 14:235, 1983.
25. Goldfinger, D: Clinical applications of therapeutic cytapheresis. In Berkman, EM and Umlas, J (eds): Therapeutic Hemapheresis. American Association of Blood Banks, Washington, DC, 1980, p 67.
26. Kleinman, SH and Goldfinger, D: Erythrocytapheresis (ERCP) in sickle cell disease. In MacPherson, JL and Kaspirisin, DO (eds): Therapeutic Hemapheresis. Vol 2. CRC Press, Boca Raton, FL, 1985, p 129.
27. Yarrish, RL, et al: Transfusion malaria. Treatment with exchange transfusion after delayed diagnosis. Arch Intern Med 142:187, 1982.
28. Cahill, KM, et al: Red cell exchange: Treatment of babesiosis in a splenectomized patient. Transfusion 21:193, 1981.
29. Patten, E: Pathophysiology of the immune system. In Kolins, J and Jones, JM (eds): Therapeutic Apheresis. American Association of Blood Banks, Arlington, VA, 1983, p 13.
30. Klein, HG: Effect of plasma exchange on plasma constituents: Choice of replacement solutions and kinetics of exchange. In MacPherson, JL and Kaspirisin, DO (eds): Therapeutic Hemapheresis. Vol 2. CRC Press, Boca Raton, FL, 1985, p 5.
31. Snyder, HW Jr, et al: Experience with protein A-immunoadsorption in treatment-resistant adult immune thrombocytopenia purpura. Blood 79:2237, 1992.
32. Mittelman, A, et al: Treatment of patients with HIV thrombocytopenia and hemolytic uremic syndrome with protein A (Prosorba Column) immunoadsorption. Semin Hematol 26 (Suppl 1):15, 1989.
33. Snyder, HW Jr, et al: Successful treatment of cancer-chemotherapy associated thrombotic thrombocytopenic purpura/hemolytic uremic syndrome (TTP/HUS) with protein A immunoadsorption. Blood 76(Suppl 1):4679, 1990.
34. Christie, DJ, Howe, RB, and Lennon, SS: Protein A column therapy in the treatment of immunologic refractoriness to platelet transfusion. Blood 76(Suppl 1):396a, 1990.
35. Pineda, AA: Immunoaffinity apheresis columns: Clinical applications and therapeutic mechanisms of action. In Sacher, RA, et al: Cellular and Humoral Immunotherapy and Apheresis, American Association of Blood Banks, Arlington, VA, 1991, p 31.

36. Heustis, DW: Risks and safety practices in haemapheresis procedures. Arch Pathol Lab Med 113:273, 1989.

37. Boogaerts, MA: Side effects of hemapheresis. Trans Med Rev 1:186, 1987.

38. Grimm, EA, et al: Lymphokine-activated killer cell phenomenon. Lysis of natural killer-resistant fresh solid tumor cells by interleukin-2 activated autologous human peripheral blood lymphocytes. J Exp Med 155:1823, 1982.

39. Fefer, A, et al: The future of cellular immunotherapy of cancer. In Sacher, RA, et al: Cellular and Humoral Immunotherapy and Apheresis. American Association of Blood Banks, Arlington, VA, 1991, p 99.

40. Klein, HG: Therapeutic mononuclear cell transfusion: Adoptive immunotherapy. In Rossi, RC, Simon, TL, and Moss, GS: Principles of Transfusion Medicine. Williams & Wilkins, Baltimore, 1991, p 295.

41. McCullough, J: A new generation of blood components. Transfusion 32:299, 1992.

42. Areman, EM and Sacher, RA: Bone marrow processing for transplantation. Trans Med Rev 5:214, 1991.

43. Lasky, LC: Peripheral blood stem cell collection and use. In Sacher, RA, et al: Cellular and Humoral Immunotherapy and Apheresis. American Association of Blood Banks, Arlington, VA, 1991, p 73.

44. Edelson, R, et al: Treatment of cutaneous T-cell lymphoma by extracorporeal photochemotherapy—preliminary results. N Engl J Med 316:297, 1987.

45. Rook, AH, et al: Treatment of systemic sclerosis with extracorporeal photochemotherapy. Arch Dermatol 128:337, 1992.

46. Malawista, SE, Trock, DH, and Edelson, RL: Treatment of rheumatoid arthritis by extracorporeal photochemotherapy—a pilot study. Arthritis Rheum 34:646, 1991.

47. Constanza-Nordin, MR, et al: Successful treatment of heart transplant rejection with photopheresis. Transplantation 53:808, 1992.

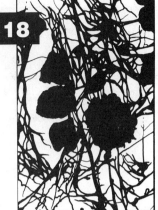

CHAPTER 18

Adverse Effects of Blood Transfusion

Patricia Joyce Larison, MT(ASCP)SBB, MA
Lloyd O. Cook, MD

OBJECTIVES

Upon completion of this chapter, the learner should be able to:

1 Define what transfusion reaction means.

2 Explain risks of transfusions.

3 Compare and contrast immediate hemolytic transfusion reactions from delayed hemolytic transfusion reactions.

4 List the types of immediate and delayed transfusion reactions.

5 Differentiate clinical signs and symptoms of each described transfusion reaction.

6 List antibodies most associated with immediate and delayed hemolytic transfusion reactions.

7 Identify procedures to follow at a patient's bedside in the event of a suspected transfusion reaction.

8 Discuss the importance of the patient's history in relationship to medications, transfusions, and pregnancies.

9 List logical steps and procedures to follow in a laboratory investigation of transfusion reactions.

10 Discuss reporting of transfusion reaction work-ups.

11 List accreditation agencies involved in determining policies regarding transfusion reactions.

12 State record retention, comparison requirements, and procedure to follow in reporting of a fatal transfusion reaction.

Transfusion is an irreversible event that carries potential benefits and risks to the recipient. A transfusion reaction is any unfavorable transfusion-related event occurring in a patient during or after transfusion of blood components.[1] In addition to proper recognition, appropriate therapy and prevention of transfusion reactions require that the clinical and laboratory staff understand the various types of reactions. Transfusion reactions are divided into immune- and non–immune-mediated and are categorized according to their relationship to the time of transfusion: immediate or delayed. By knowing rapidity of onset and mechanism of action, transfusionists can better assess current and future risks along with providing proper treatment and preventive measures.

Risks of Transfusion

As with any medical or technical procedure, the act of blood component transfusion has the potential for both benefit and risk to the patient. Table 18–1 lists specific adverse consequences of transfusions. The risk of fatality from noninfectious causes was analyzed using transfusion-associated death reports from registered blood establishments submitted to the Food and Drug Administration (FDA) from 1976 through 1985.[2] Table 18–2 lists typical causes of transfusion-associated deaths. Of the 256 immediate hemolysis deaths reported to be due to noninfectious complications, clerical error was the prime factor determined as the fundamental flaw. This is consistent with pre-

TABLE 18-1 IMMEDIATE AND DELAYED NONINFECTIOUS TRANSFUSION REACTION EFFECTS

Immediate	Delayed
Immune Effects	
IHTR	DHTR
FNHTR	Alloimmunization
Allergic reaction	PTP
Anaphylaxis and anaphylactoid reactions	GVH disease
NCPE	
Nonimmune Effects	
Bacterial contamination	Iron overload
Circulatory overload	
Physical RBC damage	
Depletion and dilution of coagulation factors and platelets	

TABLE 18-3 DISEASES SIMULATING TRANSFUSION REACTIONS

1. Paroxysmal nocturnal hemoglobinuria
2. Autoimmune hemolytic anemia
3. Glucose-6-phosphate dehydrogenase (G-6-PD) deficiency
4. Malignant hyperthermia
5. Hemoglobinopathies
6. RBC membrane defects

ERROR ANALYSIS

An internal study of the 355 reports received by FDA of transfusion-associated fatality cases for the period 1976 through 1982 sought to identify where errors occurred in preventable transfusion-associated deaths.[7] Table 18-5 identifies transfusion locations where errors associated with transfusion reactions have occurred. Four leading causes of preventable laboratory errors were (1) improper specimen identification, (2) improper patient identification, (3) antibody identification error, and (4) crossmatch procedure error. For nursing, anesthesia, and medical staff errors, improper patient identification was by far the major cause of transfusion death. Thus, adherence to proper transfusion standards, policies, and procedures is essential to reducing transfusion-associated fatalities. Table 18-6 summarizes frequent error causes associated with transfusion reactions.

Some studies have demonstrated a wide variance in the rate of occurrence of DHTR,[8,9] which can be attributed to reduced clinical recognition of DHTR and the nonspecific clinical evidence of DHTR in complicated patient cases with fever, jaundice, anemia, etc., that may be linked to other disease processes. Al-

vious reviews of transfusion-associated deaths.[3] Diseases that can cause red blood cell (RBC) hemolysis and might be misinterpreted for a hemolytic transfusion reaction are listed in Table 18-3.

RATES OF RISKS

Occurrence rates of the various transfusion reaction types, along with their signs and symptoms, are useful in determining the most probable reaction type a patient may be experiencing. Table 18-4 categorizes relative occurrence rates of transfusion reaction effects.

A National Institutes of Health (NIH) Consensus Conference panel[4] reviewed occurrence data for common immune transfusion reactions and assigned the following rates of occurrence per unit transfused: (1) nonhemolytic febrile transfusion reaction (NHFTR), 1 to 2 percent; (2) allergic, 1 to 2 percent; (3) immediate hemolytic transfusion reaction (IHTR) and delayed hemolytic transfusion reaction (DHTR), 1:6000; (4) fatal immediate, 1:100,000. The risk of alloimmunization sensitization to foreign RBC antigens appears to be 1.0 to 1.6 percent, except for $Rh_o(D)$ antigen, which is more antigenic.[5] Immunization to $Rh_o(D)$ antigen has been documented with blood volumes of as little as 0.1 ml.[6]

TABLE 18-2 SOME TYPICAL CAUSES OF TRANSFUSION-ASSOCIATED DEATHS

Acute hemolysis (ABO-incompatible blood components)
Acute pulmonary edema
Bacterial contamination of product
Delayed hemolytic reactions
Anaphylaxis
External hemolysis (e.g., temperature exceeded 40°C)
Acute hemolysis; damaged blood component (e.g., nondeglycerolized, improper solution)
GVH disease

TABLE 18-4 RELATIVE OCCURRENCE OF TRANSFUSION REACTION EFFECTS

Type of Reaction	Common	Less Common	Unusual
Febrile reaction	X		
Allergic reaction	X		
Alloimmunization	X		
Circulatory overload		X	
Delayed hemolytic transfusion reactions		X	
Depletion and dilution of coagulation factors and platelets		X	
Immediate hemolytic transfusion reactions			X
Noncardiogenic pulmonary edema			X
Iron overload			X
Anaphylaxis and anaphylactoid reactions			X
Bacterial contamination			X
Physical RBC damage			X
Posttransfusion purpura			X
GVH disease			X

TABLE 18–5 LOCATIONS OF PREVENTABLE TRANSFUSION-ASSOCIATED DEATHS, IN ORDER OF OCCURRENCE

Laboratory
Nursing service
Anesthesia service
Clinical staff

though rare, DHTR single case reports of death have been reported, with the incidence of DHTR fatalities about one sixth (1 : 600,000) that of IHTR fatalities.[10]

Anaphylactic and anaphylactoid reactions are immediate immune reactions.[11] About 1 in 700 of healthy individuals in the general population is IgA deficient.[12] Despite this relatively large risk group, anaphylactic and anaphylactoid reactions occur at very low rates, about 1 in 20,000 transfusions.[13] Errors in clinical diagnosis and case reporting do not allow calculation of an accurate risk rate.[14]

Acute pulmonary injury accounted for 15 percent of the fatal transfusion-associated reports and was the third most reported cause of transfusion-associated deaths.[15] Bacterial contamination of blood components and nonimmune hemolysis accounted for the next largest number of cases reported to the FDA during the 1976 to 1985 period.[6]

Hemolytic Transfusion Reactions

Hemolytic transfusion reactions (HTR) can occur either at the time of transfusion (immediate) or a few days after the transfusion (delayed).

IMMEDIATE HEMOLYTIC TRANSFUSION REACTION

Definition

Most commonly, an IHTR occurs very soon after the transfusion of incompatible RBCs. The cells are rapidly destroyed, releasing hemoglobin and RBC stroma into the circulation. In an anesthetized patient, hemoglobinuria, abnormal bleeding at the surgical wound site, and hypotension may be the only warning signs of IHTR. The reaction period varies from 1 or 2 hours[16] to 24 hours following transfusion.[17] However, signs and symptoms can occur within minutes after

TABLE 18–6 SUMMARY OF FREQUENT ERROR CAUSES ASSOCIATED WITH TRANSFUSION REACTIONS

1. Patient misidentification
2. Sample error
3. Wrong blood issued
4. Transcription error
5. Administration error
6. Technical error
7. Storage error

starting the transfusion. ABO-incompatible transfusions may be life threatening causing shock, acute renal failure, and disseminated intravascular coagulation (DIC). Prompt diagnosis and treatment are essential.

Pathophysiology

The underlying causative factor of immune IHTR is transfusion of an immunologically incompatible whole blood or RBC product to a recipient. The four most commonly identified RBC antibody specifities causing IHTR are anti-A, anti-Kell, anti-Jk[a], and anti-Fy[a].[18] These four antibodies are traditionally considered strong binders of complement to RBC surfaces and have efficient in vitro lytic properties. Immune-mediated IHTR can destroy RBCs by one of two mechanisms: (1) intravascular hemolysis or (2) extravascular hemolysis.[19] In both, the initial event is binding of patient antibody to the transfused, incompatible RBCs, which forms an antigen-antibody (Ag-Ab) complex on the RBC surface. Intravascular RBC lysis releases hemoglobin, RBC stroma, and intracellular enzymes manifesting in hemoglobinemia and hemoglobinuria. Figure 18–1 is an overall view of the gross pathology of kidneys demonstrating sclerotic glomeruli, fibrosis of the cortex, and tubular necrosis. Figure 18–2 is an overall view of gross pathology of the liver demonstrating portal fibrosis and necrotic hepatocytes. Both organs are from a patient who experienced acute intravascular hemolysis.

Extravascular immune-mediated IHTR is characterized by Ag-Ab complex formation on RBCs with incomplete activation of complement. Because RBC lysis does not occur intravascularly, there is no release into the circulation of free hemoglobin, RBC enzymes, or RBC stroma.

Signs, Symptoms, and Clinical Work-up

For immune-mediated IHTR with intravascular hemolysis, signs and symptoms can be profound. Table 18–7 lists clinical signs and symptoms that can occur in IHTR and can usually be observed in a conscious patient. Several important clinical findings:[20,21]

1. 35 percent of patients with IHTR experience fever or fever with chills.
2. 34 percent experience oliguria with complete recovery.
3. 13 percent develop anuria.
4. 10 percent die with sustained hypotension being the primary clinical finding.
5. 8 percent experience coagulopathy.

Signs and symptoms associated with extravascular IHTR are usually mild and not life threatening. Fever, chills, jaundice, unexpected anemia, and decreased haptoglobin are usual findings. Once an immune-mediated IHTR is suspected, immediate action is mandatory. Table 18–8 abbreviates guideline bedside procedures for handling suspected IHTRs.

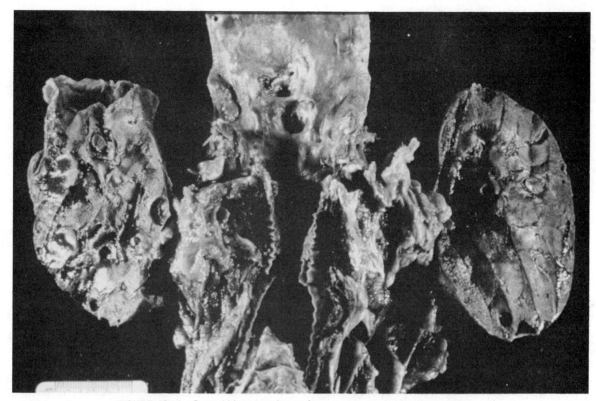

FIGURE 18-1   Gross kidney specimens from a patient experiencing hemolysis.

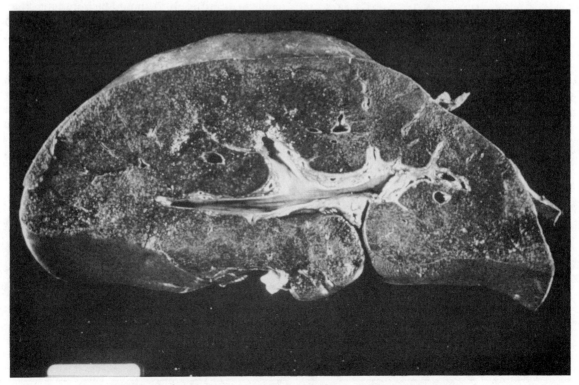

FIGURE 18-2   Gross liver specimen from a patient experiencing hemolysis.

TABLE 18–7 CLINICAL SIGNS AND SYMPTOMS THAT MAY BE CAUSED BY IMMEDIATE HEMOLYTIC TRANSFUSION REACTIONS

Fever	Hemoglobinemia
Chills	Hemoglobinuria
Facial flushing	Shock
Chest pain	Anemia
Back or flank pain	Oliguria or anuria (renal failure)
Hypotension	Pain at transfusion site
Abdominal pain	Generalized bleeding
Nausea	Urticaria
Dypsnea	Diarrhea
Vomiting	Disseminated intravascular coagulation

Therapy and Prevention

Patient care in IHTRs is focused on prevention and supportive measures. The physician should closely monitor the patient for risk factors to DIC, hypotension, and acute renal failure.[22] Traditionally, mannitol has been the agent of choice to induce renal diuresis and prevent renal failure.[23] More recent investigations using ethacrynic acid and furosemide indicate that these agents both improve renal blood flow and induce diuresis.[24,25] Hypotension is treated with intravenous fluids and vasoactive drugs (e.g., dopamine) as necessary. Blood component therapy, such as fresh frozen plasma, cryoprecipitate, and platelet concentrates, should be used in patients having a bleeding diathesis or significant coagulation abnormalities. Extravascular IHTR usually does not require therapeutic intervention. To ensure the patient's welfare, the vital signs, coagulation status, and renal output should be monitored.

Inasmuch as most IHTRs are due to clerical (i.e., human) error, they are potentially preventable. All policies and procedures should be followed to ensure proper patient identification, sample collection and labeling, unit identification, patient testing, handling, and correct transfusion at the bedside. Table 18–9 lists preventive measures to minimize transfusion reactions.

DELAYED HEMOLYTIC TRANSFUSION REACTION

Definition

Delayed hemolytic transfusion reaction most often is due to an anamnestic response in a patient who has

TABLE 18–8 IMMEDIATE TRANSFUSION REACTION BEDSIDE PROCEDURES

1. *Stop the transfusion.*
2. Keep intravenous line open with physiologic saline.
3. Notify patient's physician and transfusion service.
4. Take care of patient per physician's orders.
5. Perform bedside clerical checks.
6. Return unit, set, and attached solution to blood bank.
7. Collect appropriate blood specimens for evaluation.
8. Document reaction.

TABLE 18–9 PREVENTIVE TRANSFUSION REACTION MEASURES

Store RBCs only in blood bank–monitored refrigerators.
Never warm RBCs above 37°C for transfusion.
Do not transfuse blood if patient or donor identification is not accurate.
Never sign out blood by name only.
Do not add medications to blood.
Follow procedures for issuing blood components.
Follow protocol for specimen collection, labeling, and testing.
Follow transfusion policies and procedures.

previously been sensitized by transfusion or pregnancy and in whom antibody is not detectable by standard pretransfusion methods.[26] Clinical signs and symptoms are usually mild, and severe DHTR cases and fatalities are uncommon. Unexpected or unexplained decreases in hemoglobin or hematocrit values following transfusion should be investigated as possible DHTR.

Pathophysiology

Two different types of DHTR have been identified: (1) secondary (anamnestic) response to transfused RBCs and (2) primary alloimmunization. In DHTR due to a secondary response, a period of about 3 to 7 days from the time of transfusion is necessary for enough antibody to be produced by the patient to cause clinical signs and symptoms of extravascular RBC hemolysis.[27] In DHTR due to primary alloimmunization, the patient has no past history of pregnancy or transfusion. It should be noted that the time from transfusion to the onset of clinical signs and symptoms of hemolysis and detection of the causative antibody is longer for DHTR than for IHTR.[28]

Extravascular hemolysis is the mechanism of RBC destruction for both types of DHTR. Patient antibody attaches to the specific foreign donor RBC antigen, causing sensitization of RBCs, which are removed by the reticuloendothelial system (RES). Table 18–10 groups common and uncommon antibodies implicated in DHTR.[29] DHTR is also reportedly associated with bone marrow transplantation and may be caused by HLA antibodies in some cases.[30]

TABLE 18–10 ANTIBODIES IMPLICATED IN DHTR

Common Antibodies	Uncommon Antibodies
Anti-Jk^a	Anti-A$_1$
Anti-E	Anti-P$_1$
Anti-D	
Anti-C	
Anti-K	
Anti-Fy^a	
Anti-M	

TABLE 18-11 **CLINICAL SIGNS AND SYMPTOMS OF DHTR**

Common Signs and Symptoms	*Unusual Signs and Symptoms*
Fever	Hemoglobinemia
Anemia	Hemoglobinuria
Mild jaundice	Shock
	Renal failure

Signs, Symptoms, and Clinical Work-up

Clinical signs and symptoms of DHTR are mild compared with those of IHTR because of the extravascular hemolysis. In DHTR complement is not activated; therefore, no intravascular hemolysis occurs, as is observed in IHTR.[31] Most commonly, DHTR is manifested by mild fever or fever with chills, and moderate jaundice may be observed. Oliguria and DIC are rare.[32] Table 18-11 lists signs and symptoms that have been observed in DHTRs.

When DHTR is suspected, blood specimens (both clotted and anticoagulated) should be sent to the blood bank for posttransfusion reaction investigation. Other laboratory testing for DHTR may include hemoglobin, hematocrit, coagulation studies, and renal function tests. The patient should be closely observed for signs and symptoms indicating severe complications.

Therapy and Prevention

The goal of therapy is to prevent and, if necessary, treat severe complications of DHTR. Renal function can be supported with intravenous fluid therapy to maintain a normovolemic status.[33] Only symptomatic anemia should be treated with RBC transfusions. Clinical signs and symptoms of hemolysis or DIC should be monitored to reduce risk of renal failure.

Because DHTRs are usually due to an anamnestic response, a thorough medical history including previous transfusions, pregnancies, and transfusion reactions should be taken. The blood bank should be alerted to any previously reported complicating factors. Ideally a type and screen should be performed at the time of admission on patients who may need transfusion, who have previously received blood, or who have known risk factors.

Immediate Nonhemolytic Transfusion Reactions

The common types of immediate nonhemolytic transfusion reactions are febrile, allergic, anaphylaxis and anaphylactoid, and noncardiogenic pulmonary edema. Although the immune system is a common pathway for each of these reactions, intravascular or extravascular RBC hemolysis does *not* occur.

FEBRILE NONHEMOLYTIC TRANSFUSION REACTION

Definition

Febrile nonhemolytic transfusion reaction (FNHTR) occurs in about 1 percent of transfusions. Along with allergic reactions, FNHTR is the most commonly encountered type of transfusion reaction. Several common definitions are used regarding FNHTR, based on increases in temperature after transfusion. The American Association of Blood Banks (AABB) *Technical Manual*[34] defines FNHTR as a 1°C temperature rise associated with transfusion and having no medical explanation other than blood component transfusion. Others[35] define FNHTR as (1) any 1°C or greater temperature increase above the patient's baseline temperature, during or within 24 hours after transfusion with a minimum recorded temperature of 38°C; or (2) a 1°C temperature increase above the patient's baseline pretransfusion temperature during or within 8 hours after the end of the transfusion.

Pathophysiology

Febrile nonhemolytic transfusion reactions are caused by antileukocyte antibodies present in the patient's plasma. The antileukocyte antibodies are commonly directed against antigens present on monocytes, granulocytes, and lymphocytes.[36] Alloimmunization by prior blood transfusion, tissue transplantation, or pregnancy is the causative stimulus for antibody formation. These antibodies are predominantly HLA or lymphocytotoxic antibodies.[37]

The febrile mechanism still remains to be fully elucidated. The febrile reaction may follow activation of the complement system, producing C5a, which causes production and release of the pyrogen interleukin-1 (IL-1) from the patient's macrophages and monocytes.[38] IL-1 may initiate synthesis of prostaglandins (PGE_2) in the hypothalamic cells, resulting in an additional pyrogenic effect.[39] Release of pyrogens from the transfused white blood cells (WBCs) also plays a role in fever development and other clinical signs and symptoms.[40]

Signs, Symptoms, and Clinical Work-up

The most frequent expressions of FNHTRs are fever with or without chills and, rarely, hypotension. Most symptoms are mild and benign. Occasionally, a patient may exhibit pronounced pallor briefly. Severe reactions may include hypotension, cyanosis, tachycardia, tachypnea, dyspnea, cough, limited fibrinolysis, and transient leukopenia.[41]

FNHTR is a diagnosis of exclusion, as the nonspecific signs and symptoms can be due to many other causes. For example, fever can be caused by IHTR, bacteremia, drugs taken by the patient, or another underlying illness. Past medical history for transfusion, transplantation, pregnancy, and drug therapy is important for accurate diagnosis. Tests to evaluate FNHTRs may vary from one laboratory to another. When an FNHTR is suspected the transfusion should be stopped, but the intravenous line should be kept open with normal saline to support treatment in the event of a severe complication.

Therapy and Prevention

Because leukocyte antibodies are the primary cause of FNHTR, leukocyte-poor blood components are indicated. A variety of methods have been developed that effectively remove enough leukocytes from blood components to prevent FNHTR, including laboratory or bedside filtration using leukopoor blood filters, washed RBCs, deglycerolized RBCs, or centrifugation.[42] Inasmuch as approximately one in eight patients will react to the next unit transfused following an FNHTR, many recommend documenting two or more FNHTRs before ordering leukocyte-poor blood components.[43] Antipyretics such as aspirin or acetaminophen can be used to premedicate a patient before transfusion. It should be noted that aspirin is contraindicated in patients with thrombocytopenia and thrombocytopathy.

Even with WBC reduction in blood components, not all FNHTRs can be prevented. Premedication may be beneficial to patients with documented histories of FNHTR. As leukopoor filter cost declines, more aggressive use of these bedside filters will eventually reduce the incidence of FNHTR.

ALLERGIC (URTICARIAL) TRANSFUSION REACTIONS

Definition

Allergic, or urticarial, transfusion reactions are as commonly reported as are FNHTRs. If clinical signs and symptoms appear within minutes of exposure, the allergic reaction is of the immediate hypersensitivity type. Anaphylactic and anaphylactoid reactions are also of the immediate hypersensitivity type but are more clinically severe and are discussed later.

Pathophysiology

Despite the fact that allergic reactions are one of the two most commonly reported transfusion reactions, the definitive causes are still not known. Two possible etiologies have been proposed[44] based on the passive transfer of donor plasma to a patient after transfusion of a blood component:

1. The donor plasma has a foreign protein (allergen) with which immunoglobulin E (IgE) or IgG or both antibodies (reagin) in patient plasma react.
2. The donor plasma has reagins (IgE or IgG or both) that combine with allergens in the patient plasma.

Histamine appears to be the primary mediator of the allergic response.[45] Histamine is released when the allergen-reagin complex attaches to the surface of tissue mast cells. Upon release from mast cells, histamine increases vascular dilation and permeability, allowing vascular fluids to escape into tissues. This causes swelling and raised red weals that may itch (pruritus). Another group of mediators that may participate in allergic reactions are leukotrienes, which have been estimated to be about 1000 times more potent than histamine.[46]

Signs, Symptoms, and Clinical Work-up

The majority of allergic reactions are mild and not life threatening. Most common signs and symptoms include local erythema (redness), pruritus (itching), and hives (raised, firm, red weals). Fever may or may not be present. Rarely, allergic reactions can be severe with angioneurotic edema, laryngeal edema, and bronchial asthma.

No reliable laboratory tests are available to identify the offending allergens or reagins causing an allergic reaction. Bedside observation focuses on identifying the manifestations of an allergic reaction, monitoring for severe effects, and instituting supportive care.

Therapy and Prevention

Treatment with an antihistamine such as diphenhydramine (Benadryl) is often sufficient for mild forms of allergic reactions. In patients with histories of repeated allergic reactions, removal of plasma from blood components is often used (washed RBCs; washed platelets). Premedication with antihistamines before transfusion is also common. For severe allergic reactions, the use of aminophylline, epinephrine, or corticosteroids may be necessary. Some clinicians permit temporary cessation of blood component transfusion when a mild allergic reaction is observed, while antihistamine treatment is given. Following antihistamine administration, the same component transfusion is resumed. Because some allergic reactions can be severe, some blood banks recommend following the same transfusion reaction protocol as in other transfusion reactions and observing the patient for any severe reaction effects.

Allergic reactions cannot be completely prevented. For patients with suspected or documented histories of allergic reactions, premedication or plasma-deficient blood components or both are the usual prevention strategies.

ANAPHYLACTIC AND ANAPHYLACTOID REACTIONS

Definition

Anaphylactic and anaphylactoid reactions are of the immediate hypersensitivity type of immune system response. Anaphylaxis can range from mild urticaria (hives) and pruritus to severe shock and death. Any organ of the body can be involved such as lungs, blood vessels, nerves, skin, and gastrointestinal tract.[47] Two significant features distinguish anaphylactic and anaphylactoid reactions from other types of transfusion reactions: (1) fever is absent; and (2) clinical signs and symptoms occur after transfusion of just a few milliliters of plasma or plasma-containing blood components.

Pathophysiology

Anaphylactic and anaphylactoid reactions are attributed to IgA-deficiency in patients who have developed anti-IgA antibodies by sensitization from transfusion or pregnancy.[48] Despite the fact that about 1 of 700 people have some level of IgA deficiency, anaphylactic and anaphylactoid reactions are quite rare.[49]

As discussed previously in allergic transfusion reactions, immune hypersensitivity reactions are mediated by histamines and leukotrienes.

Signs, Symptoms, and Clinical Work-up

These hypersensitivity reactions have been divided into two categories[50]: (1) anaphylactic, patients deficient in IgA who have class-specific IgA antibodies; and (2) anaphylactoid, patients having normal levels of IgA but a limited type-specific anti-IgA that reacts with light chain (kappa or lambda) of the donor's IgA. Anaphylactic reactions are sudden in onset with pronounced symptoms that may include coughing, dyspnea, nausea, emesis, bronchospasm, flushing of skin, chest pain, hypotension, abdominal cramps, diarrhea, possibly shock, loss of consciousness, and death. Anaphylactoid reactions are usually less severe and are characterized by urticaria, periorbital swelling, dyspnea, or perilaryngeal edema.

There is no predictive test to determine who is at risk for either anaphylactic or anaphylactoid reactions. If either type of reaction is suspected, a patient serum sample can be immunoelectrophoresed to determine IgA levels, or immunodiffusion techniques may identify subclass antibodies.

Therapy and Prevention

Treatment measures must be prompt:

1. Stop the transfusion, and do not restart transfusion of the blood component.
2. Keep the intravenous line open with normal saline.
3. Immediately give epinephrine (usually about 0.5 ml of 1:1000 solution).
4. For severe reactions, corticosteroids or aminophylline or both may be indicated. Airway patency must be maintained, along with stabilizing vital signs by appropriate means.

Because the diagnosis of anaphylactic and anaphylactoid reactions is retrospective, patients with documented or suspected histories of these reactions must be provided special measures. If a plasma-containing blood component has been implicated in the anaphylactic or anaphylactoid reactions and the patient requires transfusions, two transfusion approaches may be considered: (1) remove all plasma from the blood component before transfusion, or (2) transfuse blood components from donors lacking IgA.[51] Even a small amount of plasma found in fibrin glue preparation may cause anaphylactic reactions.[52] In a prospective study colloid transfusion products also carried a risk of anaphylactoid reactions (plasma-protein solutions, 0.003 percent; hydroxyethyl starch (HES), 0.006 percent; dextran, 0.008 percent; and gelatin solution, 0.038 percent.[53] Therefore, any transfusable source of IgA antigenic material can precipitate anaphylactic or anaphylactoid reactions.

NONCARDIOGENIC PULMONARY EDEMA REACTIONS

Definition

Several terms have been used to identify pulmonary complications associated with blood component transfusion: noncardiogenic pulmonary edema (NCPE),[54] transfusion-related acute lung injury (TRALI),[22] pulmonary hypersensitivity reaction,[55] and allergic pulmonary edema.[56] The clinical picture of NCPE is similar to that of adult respiratory distress syndrome (ARDS).

Pathophysiology

Although the cause of NCPE is not well understood, the most consistent finding is antileukocyte antibodies in donor or patient plasma.[24] Several mechanisms for lung injury have been postulated and include (1) antileukocyte antibodies in donor or patient plasma could initiate complement-mediated pulmonary capillary endothelial injury[25]; and (2) antileukocyte antibodies could react with leukocytes to trigger the complement system to produce C3a and C5a. This in turn causes tissue basophils and platelets to release histamine and serotonin, resulting in leukocyte emboli aggregating in the lung capillary bed.[57] Whatever the mechanism, capillary damage induces interstitial edema and fluid in alveolar air spaces causing decreased gas exchange and hypoxia.

Signs, Symptoms, and Clinical Work-up

Noncardiogenic pulmonary edema is usually characterized by chills, cough, fever, cyanosis, hypotension, and increasing respiratory distress shortly after transfusion of blood component volumes that usually do not produce hypervolemia. Clinical signs and symptoms may be mild, resolving after a few days, or severe, resulting in rapidly progressive pulmonary failure. Sera from both the donor and patient should be tested for antileukocyte antibodies. The diagnosis of NCPE is a diagnosis of exclusion. Conditions that should be excluded are heart failure, volume overload, bacterial sepsis, and myocardial infarction.

Therapy and Prevention

If clinical signs and symptoms occur during the transfusion, the transfusion should be discontinued and not restarted. Explicit instructional procedures should be followed for handling the transfusion reaction. With adequate respiratory and hemodynamic supportive treatment, NCPE pulmonary infiltrates usually clear after several days.[58]

If NCPE is due to patient antileukocyte antibodies, then leukopoor blood component preparations should be used. If NCPE is due to donor antileukocyte antibodies, then no special blood component preparations appear to be indicated for the patient in the future. Deferral of donors associated with an NCPE case is a complicated and controversial issue. At present, no standard has been set for acceptance or deferral of donors associated with NCPE.

CIRCULATORY OVERLOAD

Definition

Circulatory overload is a good example of an iatrogenic (physician-caused) transfusion reaction. Patients at significant risk include pediatric groups, geriatric populace, chronic normovolemic anemia, cardiac disease, thalessemia major, and sickle cell disease.[59]

Pathophysiology

The most frequent cause of circulatory overload is transfusion of a unit at too fast a rate. Hypervolemia associated with transfusion leads to congestive heart failure, and pulmonary edema (which may or may not be reversible).[60]

Signs, Symptoms, and Clinical Work-up

Clinical circulatory overload effects include dyspnea, coughing, cyanosis, orthopnea, chest discomfort, headache, restlessness, tachycardia, systolic hypertension (greater than a 50 mm Hg increase), and abnormal electrocardiograms.

The transfusion should be stopped *immediately*. If transfusion is critical to patient therapy, then the slowest possible infusion rate must be used. The intravenous line should be maintained, and the patient may be placed in a sitting position. Electrocardiogram and chest x-ray examinations to assess cardiac and pulmonary status should be considered. If possible, central venous pressure, along with peripheral vital signs, should be closely monitored.

Therapy and Prevention

Rapid reduction of hypervolemia and patient respiratory and cardiac support are primary goals. Oxygen therapy and intravenous diuretics should be used appropriately. If more rapid fluid volume reduction is necessary, therapeutic phlebotomy can be used. Cardiac arrhythmias or decreased myocardial function should be corrected.

The usual rate of transfusion is about 200 ml per hour. In patients at risk or patients with histories of circulatory overload, 100 ml per hour or less is appropriate.[61] Donor units should be split into aliquots to permit transfusion for longer time periods. RBCs should be used instead of whole blood. Washed or frozen-washed RBCs have been advocated to reduce plasma oncotic load to the patient.[62] In some patients with chronic normovolemic anemia having hematocrits in the range of 10 to 20 percent, a therapeutic phlebotomy to reduce plasma volume equal to the intended transfusion volume should be considered.

BACTERIAL CONTAMINATION REACTIONS

Definition

Although the frequency of bacterial contamination of blood components is rare, this type of septic reaction can have a rapid onset and lead to death. Cases have been reported with transfused RBCs,[63] platelets,[64] and other blood components as well as manufactured products such as intravenous solutions and HES.[65]

Pathophysiology

Transfusion reactions due to bacterial contamination reactions are commonly caused by endotoxin produced by bacteria capable of growing in cold temperatures (psychrophilic) such as *Pseudomonas* species, *Escherichia coli*, and *Yersinia enterocolitica*.[66,67]

Signs, Symptoms, and Clinical Work-up

Clinical signs and symptoms of septic reactions usually appear rapidly during transfusion or within about 30 minutes after transfusion. Clinically this type of reaction is termed *warm* and is characterized by dryness and flushing of the patient's skin. Additional manifestations include fever, hypotension, shaking chills, muscle pain, vomiting, abdominal cramps, bloody diarrhea, hemoglobinuria, shock, renal failure, and DIC.

Rapid recognition of sepsis due to bacterial contamination is essential. At the first sign of the reaction, the transfusion must immediately be stopped, the intravenous line kept open, and instructions for handling transfusion reactions followed. The blood component unit and any associated fluids and transfusion equipment should be sent immediately to the blood bank for visual inspection, Gram's stain, and cultures.[68] In addition, blood cultures should be drawn from the patient as soon as possible for detection of aerobic or anaerobic organisms.

Therapy and Prevention

Broad-spectrum antibiotics should be immediately administered intravenously. Therapy for shock, steroids and vasopressors such as dopamine, fluid support, respiratory ventilation, and maintenance of renal function may be indicated.

Bacterial contamination of blood components usually occurs at the time of phlebotomy, during the component preparation or processing, or during thawing of blood components in water baths.[69] Strict adherence to policies and procedures regarding blood component collection, storage, handling, and preparation is essential to reducing risk. Visual observation of RBC units for color change at the time of issue for transfusion is required, but this step alone cannot guarantee that there is no bacterial contamination.[70] Visual inspection of components prior to release from the blood bank includes looking for the presence of brown or purple, visible clots, or hemolysis. However, gross observation is often inadequate in detecting the presence of bacterial contamination. One preventive measure is to make sure the blood components are infused within standard allowable maximum time limits (usually 4 hours). Adherence to good component production methods and prudent transfusion practices is currently the best strategy to reduce the risk of bacterial contamination and sepsis.[71]

PHYSICALLY OR CHEMICALLY INDUCED TRANSFUSION REACTIONS

Definition

Patients are at risk of experiencing a transfusion reaction owing to a broad range of physical or chemical factors that either affect a blood component or is a consequence of the transfusion event. Physically or chemically induced transfusion reactions (PCITRs) are a heterogeneous group and can include physical RBC damage, depletion and dilution of coagulation factors and platelets, hypothermia, citrate toxicity, and hypokalemia or hyperkalemia (decreased or increased ionized serum potassium level in the patient). Because the clinical signs and symptoms of PCITRs can be subtle, the transfusionist must be alert to identify and correct these reaction effects.

Pathophysiology

Red cells are susceptible to membrane damage and intravascular lysis by hypertonic or hypotonic solutions, heat damage from blood warmers, freeze damage in absence of a cryoprotective agent, or mechanical damage such as roller pumps in a blood pump.[68,72] During massive transfusion (replacement of patient's total blood volume within a 24-hour period), rapid depletion and dilution of platelets and plasma coagulation factors can occur.[73] Hypothermia, a core body temperature of less than 35°C, usually is associated with large volumes of cold fluid transfusions.[74] Excess citrate from transfusions can act on the patient's plasma free ionized calcium and may result in hypocalcemia.[75] Transfusion-associated hyperkalemia can be caused by the intracellular loss of potassium from RBCs during storage into the blood unit plasma.[76] Transfusion-induced hypokalemia is most likely due to infusion of intracellular potassium-depleted RBC blood components, such as washed RBCs or frozen-washed RBCs.[77]

Mechanical or chemical damage of transfused RBCs can result in intravascular hemolysis. The resulting free hemoglobin is rapidly cleared by the kidneys. Usually the resulting RBC stroma does not induce DIC, but DIC is a possibility.[78] Coagulation factors, especially factor VIII, decline in activity level during blood component storage, and factor levels can be reduced by use of fluid replacement solutions such as colloids and crystalloids during massive transfusions.[79] Hypothermia inhibits the immune system function, intensifies lactic acidosis and cardiac arrhythmias, and can cause coagulopathies.[80] Citrate toxicity is caused by the rapid lowering of plasma free calcium ions due to chelation with citrate. Massive transfusion is seldom a cause of citrate toxicity, but automated apheresis procedures using large amounts of citrate anticoagulant are a more likely cause.[81] Hyperkalemia and hypokalemia can cause cardiac arrhythmias and seizures.

Signs, Symptoms, and Clinical Work-up

Many of the clinical signs and symptoms of PCITR are nonspecific. The more common signs and symptoms include facial numbness, chills, numbness, muscle twitching, cardiac arrhythmias, nausea, vomiting, perioral tingling, altered respirations, and anxiety. Laboratory tests for PCITRs investigation may include electrolyte levels, serum ionized calcium, blood pH, blood glucose, urinalysis, hemoglobin, hematocrit, platelet count, prothrombin time, and activated partial thromboplastin time.

Therapy and Prevention

Treatment is directed at correcting the underlying cause of the signs and symptoms. For example, hypothermia could be treated by placing the patient on a warming blanket and giving supportive care to any cardiac arrhythmias or electrolyte imbalance. Heparin might be indicated for DIC due to physical RBC lysis. Citrate toxicity is often rapidly self-correcting, but administration of a calcium-rich product such as milk or an antacid containing calcium gluconate (e.g., Tums) is usually adequate.

Precautionary measures are the best strategies to avoid PCITR. Blood warmers can be used to avoid hypothermia. Prudent use of platelet concentrates and fresh frozen plasma may avoid rapid depletion and dilution of coagulation factors during massive transfusion. Monitoring the patient's mental status and vital signs may prove valuable in detecting rapid changes in levels of calcium and potassium. The close monitoring of RBCs transfused through blood pumps can avoid mechanical destruction. In general, attention to proper transfusion practices can greatly reduce the risk of PCITRs.

Delayed Nonhemolytic Transfusion Reactions

ALLOIMMUNIZATION

Definition

Alloimmunization may result from prior exposure to donor blood components. As an adverse effect of blood component transfusion, alloimmunization is a significant complication. Even very small amounts of donor antigenic RBCs can elicit an alloimmune response.[82] Adverse effects may include difficulty in finding compatible RBC units owing to the presence of clinically significant RBC antibodies; transfusion reactions; or platelet refractoriness.[83]

Pathophysiology

Because no two humans (except identical twins) have the same genetic inheritance, exposure to foreign antigens by blood component transfusions, tissue transplantation, or pregnancy may cause a patient's immune system to produce alloantibodies.

With the first exposure to foreign antigen, lymphocyte memory is invoked. This results in a moderate production of IgM and IgG antibodies. Secondary exposure elicits rapid production of large amounts of IgG class antibody rising rapidly in the first 2 days after reexposure to the antigen. Antibody produced attaches to the antigenic surface and may interact with the complement system or RES.[84]

Signs, Symptoms, and Clinical Work-up

Clinical signs and symptoms may be mild, including slight fever and falling hemoglobin and hematocrit, or severe, including platelet refractoriness with bleeding. To detect an alloimmunization state in a patient, several tests can be of benefit. The antibody screen test in the blood bank is used to detect clinically significant RBC antibodies. If HLA antibodies are suspected, lymphocyte panels and lymphocytotoxic antibody procedures can be performed on the patient's serum. However, a thorough patient history of past transfusions, transplantations, and pregnancy is important.

Therapy and Prevention

Treatment depends on the type and severity of the transfusion reaction. Most reactions are mild and often missed clinically. Severe reactions should be treated promptly, as appropriate. Alloimmunization cannot be completely prevented. With the advent of third-generation bedside leukocyte filters, delay if not prevention of antileukocyte antibody production is now possible.[85] The matching of donor and patient RBC phenotypes to avoid sensitization in chronically transfusion-dependent patient populations has also been recommended to prevent the formation of RBC antibodies by the patient.[86]

POSTTRANSFUSION PURPURA

Definition

A rare complication of blood transfusion, usually involving platelet concentrates (PC), posttransfusion purpura (PTP) is characterized by a rapid onset of thrombocytopenia due to anamnestic production of platelet alloantibody.[87] PTP usually occurs in multiparous females. The lagtime between transfusion and onset of thrombocytopenia is approximately 7 to 14 days.

Pathophysiology

The platelet antibody specificity most frequently identified is anti-PL^A1. Other implicated antibody specificities are HLA-A2 and lymphocytotoxic antibodies.[88] About 2 percent of people are negative for the PL^A1 platelet-specific antigen.

Platelet alloantibody attaches to the platelet surface, which permits extravascular destruction by the RES in the liver and spleen. The patient's autologous platelets are destroyed, enhancing the thrombocytopenia. The exact mechanism of platelet destruction is still not fully explained.[89]

Signs, Symptoms, and Clinical Work-up

Purpura and thrombocytopenia occur at about 1 to 2 weeks after transfusion. Thrombocytopenia can be severe, as platelet counts of less than 10,000/mm^3 have been reported.[90] Hematuria, melena, and vaginal bleeding have also been reported. Diagnosis is retrospective because the purpura and thrombocytopenia start a week or two after transfusion. Platelet counts and coagulation support should be considered. The thrombocytopenia is usually self-limited. Platelet transfusions should be reserved for severe cases, as they usually are *not* beneficial. Patient sera should be tested for platelet-specific antibodies, HLA antibodies, and lymphocytotoxic antibodies.

Therapy and Prevention

Three types of therapy have been advocated: corticosteroids, exchange transfusions, and plasmapheresis.[91,92] Intravenous immunoglobulin therapy has also been advocated.[93] Review of the PTP literature does not yield a strong consensus of opinion on treatment of PTP. In an acute, bleeding patient with concomitant lesions, the most likely therapeutic regimen would be moderate-dose corticosteroids (prednisone), intravenous immunoglobulin (IVIgG), and plasmapheresis (personal communication, L. Lutcher, MD). Exchange transfusions would be reserved for cases in which initial therapy was considered a failure. Platelet transfusion should be avoided as much as possible during the PTP treatment period. Further, there are no good means to prevent posttransfusion purpura. A thorough patient history of prior transfusion and any adverse reactions should be taken before all blood component therapy. In suspicious cases with possible risk, appropriate antibody studies should be considered.

GRAFT-VERSUS-HOST DISEASE

Definition

Transfusion-associated graft-versus-host (GVH) disease is a complication of blood component therapy or bone marrow transplantation. Although GVH disease is a rare complication of transfusion, there are significant populations of patients at risk, and mortality is significant. Some of the at-risk groups include patients experiencing lymphopenia or bone marrow suppression, fetuses receiving intrauterine transfusions, newborn infants receiving exchange transfusions, individuals with congenital immunodeficiency syndromes, patients with certain hematologic and oncologic disorders, and those receiving blood components from first-degree relatives.[94,95] The fatality rate for transfusion-associated GVH disease has been documented at 84 percent with a median survival period of 21 days after transfusion.[96] Death is usually due to infection or hemorrhage secondary to bone marrow aplasia.

Pathophysiology

Graft-versus-host disease is caused by a proliferation of T-cell lymphocytes derived from the donor blood immunologically responding to major and minor histocompatibility antigens in the patient.[97] Patients with cell-mediated immunodeficiency are at risk of not being able to reject transfused lymphocytes. Another risk group includes patients who have an HLA type that is haploidentical with that of the donor; these are usually first-degree relatives.[98] The mechanism of GVH disease has not been fully explained.

Signs, Symptoms, and Clinical Work-up

Most clinical signs and symptoms of transfusion-associated GVH disease appear in about 3 to 30 days after transfusion.[99] Pancytopenia is a clinically significant indication of GVH disease. Other effects include fever, elevated liver enzymes, copious watery diarrhea, erythematous skin rash progressing to erythroderma, and desquamation.

Tissue biopsies and laboratory tests assessing liver function status should be considered if histologic changes indicative of GVH disease are found in the liver, gastrointestinal tract, skin, and bone marrow. Close observation for infection or coagulation abnormalities should be monitored because these complications are responsible for most GVH disease fatalities. HLA cell typing to confirm the presence of donor cells in the patient's circulation is used to confirm diagnosis.[100]

Therapy and Prevention

Various therapeutic treatments have been used in patients with GVH disease including corticosteroids, cyclosporine, methotrexate, azathioprine, and antithymocyte globulin. To date, clinical efficacy of these and other experimental agents has not proved adequate in transfusion-associated GVH disease. As there is no adequate therapy for transfusion-associated GVH disease, prevention is the only method of avoiding potential fatalities. Blood component gamma irradiation has been demonstrated as the best current technology to reduce risk of GVH disease.[101] The usual dosage range is 25 to 35 Gy (1 gray [Gy] = 100 rads).[102] Irradiation of the blood component before transfusion will result in inactivation of the lymphocytes in the blood components, inhibiting lymphocyte blast transformation and mitotic activity.

IRON OVERLOAD

Definition

A long-term complication of RBC transfusion is iron overload, also known as transfusion hemosiderosis. Each unit of RBCs has about 225 mg of iron as part of the hemoglobin molecules. Patients with certain diseases are chronically dependent on RBC transfusion support as part of therapy. Some of these diseases include congenital hemolytic anemias, aplastic anemia, and chronic renal failure.

Pathophysiology

Accumulated iron begins to affect the function of heart, liver, and endocrine glands. The full mechanism of iron overload leading to hemosiderosis is not yet fully elucidated. A likely pathologic effect is interference of mitochondrial function by excess iron accumulation.

Signs, Symptoms, and Clinical Work-up

Clinical signs and symptoms of hemosiderosis may include muscle weakness, fatigue, weight loss, mild jaundice, anemia, mild diabetes, and cardiac arrhythmias. A long history of chronic RBC transfusion should be a strong clinical indicator for diagnosis of iron overload. Assessment of storage iron levels such as ferritin levels and other iron studies should be performed. Tissue stains specific for iron in tissue biopsies should be considered.

Therapy and Prevention

Removal of accumulated tissue iron stores without lowering patient hemoglobin levels is the treatment of choice. Subcutaneous infusion of desferrioxamine, an iron-chelating agent, has been tried with some success.[103] Chronically transfusion-dependent patients should be exposed to as few units of RBCs as possible. One promising strategy is hypertransfusion using units rich in neocytes (young RBCs) to reduce the frequency of transfusion.[104]

Transfusion Reaction Investigation

Adverse clinical manifestations after transfusion of blood components must be evaluated promptly and to the extent considered appropriate by the medical director. The exception to this rule is circulatory overload and allergic reactions, which do not have to be evaluated to the same extent as hemolytic transfusion reactions.[105] The transfusionist must first recognize that a transfusion reaction is occurring, and then must take action immediately initiating appropriate established procedures for transfusion reaction responses. Investigations of transfusion reactions are necessary for (1) diagnosis, (2) selection of appropriate therapy, (3) transfusion management, and (4) prevention of future transfusion reactions. Investigation should include correlations of clinical data with laboratory results.[106] Transfusion reaction protocols may vary, depending on clinical signs and symptoms of the patient, federal regulations, and assessment of the medical director and patient's physician. In the investigation, one should remember that absence of evidence is *not* evidence of the absence of a transfusion reaction!

Any investigation of a suspected transfusion reaction must include investigation of clinical data to include (1) diagnosis, (2) medical history of pregnancies and previous transfusions, (3) current medications, and (4) clinical signs and symptoms of the reaction. The transfusion history may give clues as to the possible cause of the transfusion reaction.[107] During the investigation, the following questions related to the transfusion and medical information may be included:

1. How many milliliters of RBCs or blood component were transfused?
2. How fast and for how long was the unit transfused?
3. Were RBCs given cold or warmed?
4. Was the transfusion given under pressure, and what size needle was used?
5. How was it given? Was a filter used, and if so, what type? What other solutions were given?
6. Were any drugs given at the time of transfusion?

A transfusion reaction form should be completed for each reaction and include the patient's pretransfusion and posttransfusion vital signs, type of reaction,

time of occurrence, amount transfused, and other pertinent information.[108]

The transfusion service must have a procedure manual detailing instructions to follow when a transfusion reaction occurs.[109,110] Table 18–12 details procedures to include in manuals. To investigate a suspected HTR the blood bank should receive promptly after the transfusion a clotted blood sample properly collected (avoiding hemolysis) and labeled, along with a nonclotted ethylenediaminetetraacetic acid (EDTA) specimen. Tests considered appropriate for an investigation are determined by the blood bank medical director, indicated by the patient's clinical signs and symptoms, or ordered by the patient's physician.[111]

Depending on the preliminary investigation results, more specimens may be required:

1. A clotted blood specimen drawn 5 to 7 hours after transfusion for unconjugated indirect bilirubin determination[112]
2. The first voided posttransfusion urine collection[113]
3. Other specimens collected at various times that are considered appropriate to the transfusion reaction investigation[114]

IMMEDIATE LABORATORY INVESTIGATIVE PROCEDURES

Laboratory transfusion reaction investigative procedures will vary but begin with immediate preliminary procedures. Based on the preliminary investigative results and the patient's clinical condition, further testing may be necessary. Table 18–13 outlines immediate procedures, additional procedures that may be required, and other extended testing that may be performed in investigating an HTR.[115,116] Immediate transfusion reaction procedures include clerical checks, visual inspection, and direct antiglobulin test (DAT).

Clerical Checks

Because many of the transfusion reactions reported have resulted from clerical errors (mislabeling and misidentification causes), immediate investigation should always begin with clerical checks.[117] Clerical checks should identify any possible errors or discrep-

TABLE 18–12 TRANSFUSION REACTION PROCEDURE MANUAL REQUIREMENTS

1. Specimen requirements
2. Reporting policies
3. Clerical and technical check procedures
4. Return of bag, solutions, filter-set, intact tubing
5. Immediate investigation procedure
6. Extended investigation procedure
7. Specimen test procedures
8. Physician notification policies
9. Results reporting policies

TABLE 18-13 LABORATORY INVESTIGATION OUTLINE FOR HTR

Immediate Procedures
Clerical checks
Visual inspection of serum and plasma for free hemoglobin
  (pretransfusion and posttransfusion)
Direct antiglobulin test—posttransfusion EDTA sample

"As Required" Procedures
ABO grouping and Rh typing, pretransfusion and posttransfusion
Antibody screen test, pretransfusion and posttransfusion
Major compatibility test, pretransfusion and posttransfusion, with
  donor RBCs from segment or container
Alloantibody identification
Free hemoglobin in first voided urine after transfusion
Unconjugated (indirect) bilirubin 5 to 7 hours after transfusion

Extended Procedures (As Indicated)
Gram's stain and culture of unit
Free hemoglobin
Serum haptoglobin, pretransfusion and posttransfusion
Hemoglobin and hematocrit
Platelet counts; peripheral blood smear
Coagulation and renal output studies
Electrophoresis

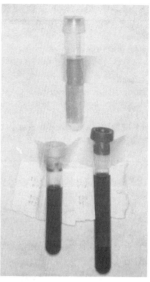

FIGURE 18-3 Comparison of a pre- and posttransfusion blood specimen from a sickle cell patient experiencing a delayed hemolytic transfusion reaction. The pretransfusion specimen (top tube) is clear, with no hemolysis; the posttransfusion specimens (bottom tubes) demonstrate hemolysis.

ancies in patient or donor identification.[118] Clerical checks may include patient and specimen identification data, blood unit inspection, tubing, filter, and solution examination, along with label and record checks. Table 18–14 itemizes posttransfusion verification procedures.

Visual Inspection

Visually observe the serum of the patient's pretransfusion and posttransfusion reaction blood specimens. Color of pretransfusion reaction serum and immediate posttransfusion recipient serum or plasma should be compared for evidence of RBC hemolysis. This is critical to investigation of an HTR. Normal serum or plasma appears pale yellow. If plasma or serum contains 0.2 g/liter (20 mg/dl) of free hemoglobin, it will appear pink. If free hemoglobin exceeds 1 g/liter (100 mg/dl), the plasma or serum will appear red.[119] During visual color observation, if only the posttransfusion specimen shows pink or red discoloration, a hemolytic process can be presumed. The posttransfusion plasma sample should be spectrophotometrically measured to quantitate the amount of free plasma hemoglobin. If the sample was not collected immediately after the transfusion, hemoglobin can be converted to

TABLE 18-14 POSTTRANSFUSION REACTION VERIFICATIONS

Rule out that the patient received the wrong blood component.
Verify that the appropriate blood component was selected,
  accurately tested, and properly issued within expiration period.
Verify accuracy of patient and donor ABO and Rh type.
Verify accuracy of labels and records.
Rule out that any other patient or blood component was involved.

bilirubin and change the plasma color to a bright yellow. The maximum bilirubin concentration occurs usually 3 to 6 hours after a hemolytic transfusion episode.[120] Myoglobin can cause serum to appear pink. If crush injuries exist, differentiation of myoglobin from hemoglobin should be determined. In the absence of extensive muscle trauma myoglobin is unlikely.[121] Figure 18–3 depicts pretransfusion and posttransfusion reaction specimens from a patient with sickle cell disease experiencing a DHTR that demonstrates visually discernible free hemoglobin in the posttransfusion specimen.

A visual inspection of the return blood bag(s), solution(s), and attached tubing and filter set(s) may rule out hemolysis from nonimmunologic causes.[122] RBC hemolysis has been reported from open-heart bypass surgery machines, blood pumps, infusion through small-bore needles,[123] infusion of blood under high pressure, drugs or solutions added to blood lines,[68] heating or freezing blood improperly, and bacterial contamination.[124]

Direct Antiglobulin Test

In suspected immediate or delayed hemolytic reactions, a DAT should be performed on the posttransfusion specimen. The DAT result may be negative if the incompatible transfused cells have been immediately destroyed. In both immediate and delayed reactions, the DAT result may be positive, show mixed-field reactions, or be negative. When the DAT result appears as mixed-field agglutination, there are mixtures of agglutinated transfused donor cells along with unagglutinated patient cells.[125] Table 18–15 summarizes some approaches to DAT.[126]

TABLE 18-15 **APPROACHES TO DAT**

DAT Result Positive
Perform an elution and determine specificity.
Repeat DAT on several specimens to detect rising antibody titers.

DAT Result Negative
Perform an elution, if clinical hemolysis is present.
If there exist too few antibody molecules to detect, perform an elution and concentrate antibody
If all incompatible RBCs are destroyed, screen serum, perform clerical and technical checks, and repeat DAT later with new specimen.

TABLE 18-16 **CAUSES OF FALSE-NEGATIVE ANTIBODY SCREEN RESULTS**

Failure to detect antibody in original test procedure
Test not sensitive enough to detect antibody
Clerical or technical error
Antibody screening cells represented a single dose of antigen (donor cells from a heterozygote)
Antibody identified in posttransfusion specimen only (may represent anamnestic response or patient sample identification problem)

ADDITIONAL TESTING, AS INDICATED

If the immediate procedures suggest hemolysis, or if the results are misleading or negative but the patient's signs and symptoms suggest immune hemolysis, then additional testing is necessary and may include the following tests.

ABO Grouping and Rh Typing

The recipient pretransfusion and posttransfusion reaction blood specimens and donor segments should be tested and misidentification of any other patient sample or donor unit ruled out.[127]

Compatibility Test

When indicated, testing should include the pretransfusion and posttransfusion reaction samples tested with RBCs from donor units involved.[128] An incompatible crossmatch with the pretransfusion sample indicates an original error (clerical or technical) with recipient or donor specimens. Incompatibility with only the posttransfusion specimen indicates a possible anamnestic response (as seen in DHTR) or a patient sample identification problem.[129]

Antibody Screen and Alloantibody Identification

To determine if the transfusion reaction was the result of an antibody, the antibody screening tests should be repeated on the pretransfusion and posttransfusion reaction specimen and donor unit.[130] Table 18-16 identifies causes of false-negative antibody screen results that should be considered in transfusion reaction investigations. Unexpected alloantibodies found in the patient's serum should be identified and any posttransfusion reaction positive DAT result investigated.[131,132] If the pretransfusion or posttransfusion antibody screening tests are reactive, identification is essential to determine antibody specificity to avoid another reaction when the patient requires further transfusion. Once antibody specificity is determined, all donor units must be tested for the corresponding antigen before additional transfusions are performed.

Urine Tests

The first voided posttransfusion reaction specimen should be examined for the presence of free hemoglobin. Intact RBCs (hematuria) represents bleeding, not hemolysis. When unexplained hemoglobinemia occurs, the urine can be examined for hemoglobinuria. Table 18-17 indicates responses when using reagent strips to test urine for free hemoglobin and urobilinogen in suspected HTRs.

A week or more following suspected HTR investigation, urine can be examined for hemosiderinuria. Hemosiderin can appear in urine when the level exceeds 0.5 g/liter (50 mg/dl) as free hemosiderin.[133]

Bilirubin Test

A change from a pretransfusion normal pale-yellow serum to a post-transfusion reaction bright- or deep-yellow serum should prompt an investigation for RBC hemolysis. The maximum concentration of bilirubin following hemolysis is not evident until approximately

TABLE 18-17 **URINE REAGENT STRIP (MULTISTIX) CHART FOR SUSPECTED HTR**

	Reaction	Identify Reason	Microscopic (Rule Out Intact RBCs)	Monitor Patient's Renal Function	Test Sensitivity
Free hemoglobin	Positive	✓	✓	✓ Evaluate further	0.0015-0.0062 mg/dl Equivalent to 5-10 intact RBCs
Urobilinogen (<1 Ehrlich unit† is normal)	Positive (pink-red color)*	✓		✓ Evaluate further	0.02-1.0 Ehrlich unit† Test immediately or store in dark container*

*Reagent strips using *p*-dimethylaminobenzaldehyde are subject to interference by Ehrlich unit.
†1 mg/dl = 1 Ehrlich unit.

TABLE 18-18 LABORATORY EVIDENCE SUGGESTING DHTRs

Positive DAT result after transfusion; pretransfusion DAT result negative
Posttransfusion indirect bilirubin elevation
Posttransfusion hemoglobin decrease 2 g/dl or more
Hemoglobinuria or hemosiderinuria
Antibody present 3 to 5 days (or more) after transfusion; antibody absent before transfusion

3 to 6 hours after transfusion.[134] The posttransfusion reaction result for indirect bilirubin should be compared with the pretransfusion result. Bilirubin excretion may return to normal within 24 hours.[135]

Hemoglobin and Hematocrit

Hemoglobinemia results when large excesses of free hemoglobin are released into the blood. The hemoglobin and hematocrit can be monitored to detect a drop in hemoglobin or failure of the transfusion to raise the hematocrit. Table 18-18 summarizes laboratory evidence supporting a diagnosis of DHTR. Hemoglobinemia immediately after a transfusion reaction confirms hemolysis, provided an acceptable blood specimen was collected. Serial hematocrit and hemoglobin testing may be necessary to demonstrate therapeutic or nontherapeutic responses.[136] Table 18-19 lists suggested times that some tests may be performed when investigating a possible HTR.

Extended testing will depend on analysis and interpretations of tests performed and the patient's clinical condition.

REPORTING OF TRANSFUSION REACTION WORK-UPS

If the laboratory evaluation or test interpretations suggest an HTR or a bacterial contamination, the patient's physician and blood bank medical director must be immediately notified. After the medical director of the transfusion service has evaluated the laboratory results, interpretations must be recorded in the patient's chart. The transfusion service must maintain the testing results, interpretations, and reaction classification for referral if the patient requires further transfusion therapy.[137] The AABB standards require that transfusion reaction records be retained for a minimum of 5 years, and that prior to issue of blood components for transfusion, ABO and Rh typing during the past 12 months, difficulty in blood typing, and clinically significant unexpected antibodies must be compared with current test interpretations.[138]

Both federal regulatory and voluntary accreditation agencies require investigation and reporting of recipient adverse transfusion reactions. The FDA states in the *Code of Federal Regulations* (CFR) requirements for transfusion reaction reporting. If a reaction results in a fatality, the Director of the Office of Compliance for the Center of Biologic Evaluation and Research must be notified by telephone or telegraph as soon as possible. A required written report to the Director must follow within 7 days of the investigation.[139] Voluntary agencies requiring investigation and internal reporting of transfusion reactions include the College of American Pathologists (CAP),[140] the AABB,[141] and the Joint Commission on Accreditation of Healthcare Organizations (JCAHO).[142] All of these agencies require that written policies and procedures include steps for detection, evaluation, and reporting of adverse transfusion reactions.

Summary

This chapter has outlined posttransfusion difficulties associated with blood components. The transfusion service should establish policies and procedures that optimize transfusion practices and provide safety to transfusion recipients with reduced risk of morbidity and mortality. Continuous quality improvement of transfusion practices for the patient's safety requires

TABLE 18-19 TIMES TO PERFORM LABORATORY TEST TO INVESTIGATE IHTRs AND DHTRs

	Immediate	1-3 Hours	3-6 Hours	24 Hours	Days
Blood					
Antibody IHTR	✓	✓	✓	✓	✓
Antibody DHTR					✓
Direct Coombs IHTR	✓				May need to repeat
Direct Coombs DHTR					✓
Hemoglobinemia	✓	✓	✓		
Haptoglobin			✓	✓	✓
Bilirubin			✓		✓
			3-12 hours		
Methemalbumin		✓	✓	✓	✓
					1-2 days
Urine					
Hemoglobin	✓	✓	✓		
Urobilinogen				✓	✓
Hemosiderin					✓

constant review and surveillance of procedures, practices, and standards.

Transfusion Reaction Case Studies

Case 1

CLINICAL HISTORY

A 45-year-old white man was admitted to the hospital with gastrointestinal bleeding from recurrent peptic ulcers. The patient had been transfused 4 months earlier for the same symptoms.

Hospital Course

His hemoglobin upon admission was 70 g/l (7 g/dl). Four units of blood were ordered and crossmatched, were found to be compatible, and were transfused. Five days after the transfusion the patient appeared pale and mildly jaundiced, and had a fever of 39°C (102.2°F). A complete blood count (CBC) and a blood culture was ordered by the physician.

LABORATORY FINDINGS

Hematology Test Results

The patient's 5-day posttransfusion hemoglobin was 50.0 g/l (5 g/dl); hematocrit 0.15 (15 percent). Spherocytes were present on the peripheral blood smear. Because of the low hemoglobin, 2 units of blood were ordered by the patient's physician.

Blood Bank Test Results

Five days after the transfusion 2 units of blood were crossmatched and found to be incompatible. The antibody screen was positive at this time. Five days previously the antibody screen test result had been negative. A transfusion reaction work-up was initiated.

Clerical Checks

No clerical errors were revealed.

Technical Results

Repeat ABO and Rh typings on pretransfusion and posttransfusion reaction specimens confirmed original results. Repeat crossmatch test on pretransfusion and posttransfusion patient specimens with donor units revealed no incompatibility. The pretransfusion DAT result was negative, but the posttransfusion DAT result was positive owing to IgG sensitization. Panels completed on the patient's serum and eluate revealed the following antibody identification:

Serum: Anti-Jkᵃ by enzyme technique
Eluate: Anti-Jkᵃ by enzyme technique
Phenotyping of patient's RBCs for Jkᵃ antigen (pretransfusion specimen)
Patient's test results: Jkᵃ negative

Microbiology Results

Results of the patient's blood culture, Gram's stain, and culture of the donor unit were negative.

Interpretation

This case illustrates the laboratory results of a DHTR. Anti-Jkᵃ is known for its transient properties of appearing and disappearing and for its enhancement by enzymes. The reaction occurred at a time when transfusion was least suspected as the causative reason. The transfusion caused a secondary immune stimulus, resulting in rise in antibody titer. In DHTR transfused donor RBC, destruction is usually gradual. The patient experienced anemia, fever, and mild jaundice 3 to 7 days after the transfusion. If the patient should require future transfusion, blood lacking Jkᵃ antigen would be required.

CONCLUSION

The patient had DHTR caused by Jkᵃ antibody.

Case 2

CLINICAL HISTORY

A 55-year-old man was hospitalized to have abdominal surgery for carcinoma. The patient had no previous history of transfusion.

Hospital Course

The patient's admission hemoglobin was 100 g/l (10 g/dl). Two units of RBCs were ordered for the surgery. The patient was blood group O positive. The antibody screen result was negative. Two units of RBCs were crossmatched and found compatible. During surgery, following receipt of the first unit of RBCs, the patient experienced oozing at the surgical site. The patient's blood pressure fell from a pretransfusion level of 120/70 mm Hg to 80/40 mm Hg after the transfusion. The transfusion was immediately stopped, and the hypotension treated. A new blood sample was sent to the blood bank requesting four more units of RBCs immediately.

Laboratory Findings

The blood bank technologist, upon typing the new posttransfusion sample, obtained the following results:

Reactions of Cells with		Reaction of Serum with RBCs		
Anti-A	Anti-B	A1	B	O
+mf	neg	++	+++	neg
mf = mixed field; + = positive; neg = negative.				

Repeat typing of the patient's pretransfusion blood specimen confirmed the blood group as originally designated O positive.

The posttransfusion reaction specimen revealed mixed-field agglutination when tested with anti-A and anti-B antisera. The surgeon was notified by the medical director that a potential immune hemolytic reaction may be in progress.

Clerical Checks

Clerical checks were performed both in the blood bank and in the operating room. Upon completion of the clerical checks, it was determined that the wrong unit of blood had been selected for this patient. Two patients were undergoing surgery who had similar names. The unit had been selected from the operating room refrigerator by name only, and had not been checked to include hospital identification number prior to transfusion. It was additionally determined that two persons had not checked the unit before transfusion, as the hospital transfusion policy required. Investigation eliminated that any other patient was at risk for a similar incident at that time. The unit inadvertently transfused was determined to be group A positive.

Laboratory Investigation

The postreaction DAT result was negative indicating rapid destruction of the incompatible transfused RBCs. The pretransfusion and posttransfusion antibody screen test results were negative. The crossmatch on the pretransfusion specimens with the original group O donor units revealed no incompatibility. Hemoglobinemia and hemoglobinuria was present with free hemoglobin demonstrated in the first posttransfusion urine specimen.

The patient developed a hemorrhagic coagulopathy with afibrinogenemia. The patient's platelets became decreased with a concomitant increase in fibrinogen and fibrin degradation products. Shortly the patient became anuric, producing only 50 ml of urine in 12 hours. The patient's condition deteriorated despite attempts to control the hemorrhagic process. Autopsy findings 4 days posttransfusion revealed hemoglobin casts in the renal tubules of the patient's kidneys.

Interpretation

In an anesthetized patient the only symptoms of an HTR may be oozing, bleeding, or hypotension, as experienced by this patient. The erroneously transfused group A donor unit RBCs reacted with the patient's anti-A antibody, resulting in destruction of the transfused donor cells. The coagulation system was activated, resulting in a hemorrhagic diathesis with resultant acute renal failure and death. To prevent HTRs identity of the patient and donor blood component by two persons is essential to ensure that the appropriate blood component will be transfused. Blood must never be released relying only on a patient's name. Not only must there be verification policies, but monitoring must occur to ensure that established policies are adhered to. At the first sign of a transfusion reaction, the transfusion must be stopped, a line left open for normal saline administration, the patient immediately attended to, and an immediate investigation initiated. Most errors in ABO mismatch of blood transfusion are misidentification of either the patient or blood sample. Human errors resulting in serious or fatal transfusion reactions are often litigated, not excused.

CONCLUSION

This patient had an immune acute hemolytic transfusion reaction due to ABO incompatibility.

Case 3

CLINICAL HISTORY

A 45-year-old woman was admitted to the hospital for a hysterectomy. The patient had been pregnant four times previously with no history of transfusions. She was taking no medications.

The patient's admission CBC revealed a low hemoglobin of 80 g/l (8.0 g/dl). The physician ordered a unit of RBCs to be given before surgery to correct her anemia in time for an elective hysterectomy.

Laboratory Test

A unit of group O Rh-positive RBCs was crossmatched and found compatible. The patient's antibody screen test result was negative.

Hospital Course

A transfusion of group O Rh-positive compatible RBCs was begun at 1:45 PM and given through a standard 170 μm blood infusion set. After receiving approximately half of the RBCs, the patient experienced chills and had a temperature elevation to 39.4°C (103°F) from a pretransfusion temperature of 37.2°C (99°F). She had a severe headache, and felt anxious and uncomfortable. The blood transfusion was stopped and the patient's physician notified. A transfusion reaction investigation was initiated.

LABORATORY FINDINGS

Clerical Checks

No clerical errors were detected. Donor and patient identification was verified.

Serologic Findings

Examination of the patient's pretransfusion and posttransfusion blood and urine specimens revealed no visible hemolysis. The DAT result on the posttransfusion blood specimen was negative. No RBC alloantibodies were detected in the serum of patient or donor. Repeat blood typings and crossmatch tests on the pretransfusion and posttransfusion specimens and donor unit confirmed the original test results. No incompatibility was demonstrated. Results of the serum bilirubin test 5 hours after the transfusion were normal. Bacterial contamination was ruled out by a negative culture and Gram's stain.

Interpretation

Because serologic test results did not indicate a hemolytic reaction, or blood group incompatibility, or bacterial contamination, other causes were considered. The patient's four pregnancies and transfusion reaction signs and symptoms suggested that a reaction to donor leukocytes had occurred. Leukocytes in RBC and platelet transfusions have been associated frequently with adverse effects (1 to 3 percent) when transfused to recipients who are alloimmunized from previous pregnancies, transfusions, or organ transplantation. The reactions are frequently associated with alloimmunization to HLA class I or leukocyte-specific antigens. RBC transfusions contain approximately 2 to 5×10^9 leukocytes. Using adsorption RBC filters to transfuse the RBCs through, leukocyte removal can achieve up to a 3-log (99.9 percent) leukocyte reduction. This reduction can prevent recurrent NHFTRs and delay alloimmunization to leukocyte antigens in select patients requiring long-term transfusion therapy.

CONCLUSION

This patient had an NHFTR. If she should experience two or more similar reactions, leukocyte-poor prepared blood or an in-line leukocyte-reduction filter should be used. Although there are a number of ways to prepare leukocyte-poor blood, the third-generation adsorption filters removing leukocytes by adherence can achieve profound leukocyte reduction.

Case 4

CLINICAL HISTORY

A 38-year-old man arrived at the hospital emergency room complaining of abdominal pain. A CBC was ordered. His hemoglobin level was found to be 70 g/l (7 g/dl). The physician determined evidence of bleeding and ordered 2 units of RBCs immediately. The patient had no history of prior transfusion and was taking no medications.

Laboratory Findings

Two units of RBCs were crossmatched and found compatible. The patient's antibody screen test result was negative. One compatible donor unit was released to the emergency room.

Hospital Course

After proper identification of the unit of RBCs with the patient by two persons, vital signs were checked and recorded, and the transfusion was initiated. Thirty minutes after the transfusion had begun, the patient experienced a slight rash and itching. No other associated adverse effects were noted. The patient was given diphenhydramine (Benadryl). While the medication took effect, the transfusion was discontinued and normal saline transfused. Once the symptoms subsided (15 to 20 minutes), the transfusion was continued with no ill effects noted.

Interpretation

Urticarial reaction is the only immediate immunologic adverse effect of transfusion in which the transfusion can continue, provided no other adverse effects are manifested. These reactions are likely caused by the passive transfer of IgE or IgG antiatopen, or both, from the donor plasma to the recipient. Histamine is presumed the mediator, as it is released from antigen attached to the mast cell along with the IgE antibody. If the signs and symptoms are more severe (pulmonary edema,

asthma, facial edema, hives over entire body), or become more severe after medicative treatment, the transfusion must be stopped immediately and investigated.

CONCLUSION

This patient had an urticarial reaction, treated effectively with Benadryl.

Review Questions

1. Plasma that contains free hemoglobin in quantities of 100 mg/dl has a color that appears as:
   A. Straw yellow
   B. Faint pink
   C. Deep, bright yellow
   D. Red
   E. Blue

2. Transfused plasma constituents resulting in immediate erythema, itching, and hives best describes which of the following transfusion reactions?
   A. HTR
   B. DHTR
   C. Allergic
   D. Iron overload
   E. Alloimmunization

3. Which listed transfusion reaction may result from an anamnestic response following a secondary exposure to donor RBCs?
   A. IHTR
   B. Alloimmunization
   C. Anaphylactoid reaction
   D. Circulatory overload reaction
   E. GVH disease reaction

4. Transfused patients at greater risk of developing circulatory overload may include:
   A. Pediatric groups
   B. Geriatric groups
   C. Chronic normovolemic anemia patients
   D. Sickle cell disease patients
   D. All of the above

5. Which listed transfusion reaction is most associated with transfused patients lacking IgA immunoglobulin?
   A. Anaphylactic
   B. Hemolytic
   C. Febrile
   D. Circulatory overload
   E. Allergic

6. The result of the direct antiglobulin test after a delayed transfusion reaction may be:
   A. Positive
   B. Mixed field

C. Positive, owing to complement coating only

D. Negative

E. All of the above

7. A transfusion reaction that usually appears rapidly during transfusion termed "warm" and may result in fever, shock, or death, is which one of the following listed reactions?

A. Hemolytic

B. Bacterial contamination

C. Circulatory overload

D. Allergic

E. FNHTR

8. Following a hemolytic transfusion reaction the recipient's serum bilirubin may return to normal in:

A. 5 hours

B. 12 hours

C. 48 hours

D. 3 hours

E. 24 hours

9. Which of the following antibodies is most responsible for immediate hemolytic transfusion reactions?

A. Anti-Le^a

B. Anti-N

C. Anti-A

D. Anti-M

E. Anti-D

10. Fatal transfusion reactions are most frequently caused by:

A. Clerical errors

B. Improper refrigeration

C. Overheating blood

D. Mechanical trauma

E. Filters

11. When a suspected hemolytic reaction occurs, the first thing to do is:

A. Slow the transfusion rate, and call the physician.

B. Administer medication to stop the reaction.

C. Stop the transfusion, but keep the intravenous line open with saline.

D. First inform the laboratory to begin an investigation.

E. Begin technical checks.

12. Which of the following statements best describes febrile nonhemolytic transfusion reaction symptoms?

A. Shock, hemoglobinuria, hypotension

B. Respiratory distress, vascular instability, shock

C. DIC, renal failure, hemoglobinuria

D. Temperature rise of 1°C with transfusion

E. Temperature rise of 2°C or more with transfusion

13. If a patient experiences two or more FNHTRs, with each reaction becoming more severe, the easiest preventative approach for transfusion of RBCs is to:

A. Administer the RBCs slowly.

B. Use specialized filters that remove most of the WBCs.

C. Use washed RBCs.

D. Administer smaller amounts of RBCs.

E. Use phenotypically matched RBCs.

14. FNHTRs are characterized by which of the following descriptions?

A. Hemolysis, DIC, thrombocytopenia

B. Local erythema, hives, itching

C. 1°C temperature rise associated with the transfusion

D. Respiratory distress, vascular instability, nausea, shock

E. Generalized bleeding, shock, hemoglobinuria

15. Delayed hemolytic transfusion reactions from anamnestic responses usually occur within which time period?

A. 5 hours

B. 24 hours

C. Several weeks after transfusion

D. 7 to 10 days after transfusion

E. 48 hours after transfusion

16. Pretransfusion irradiation of all blood products in certain patients is done to prevent which of the following?

A. CMV

B. GVH disease

C. FNHR

D. PNHA

E. HTR

17. If a fatality results directly from a transfusion complication, who must be notified within 24 hours of the fatality?

A. FDA

B. CAP

C. AABB

D. CDC

E. JCAHO

18. The most common reason for transfusion of leukocyte-poor blood is because the recipient:

A. Has RBC alloantibodies

B. Has a positive DAT result

C. Has been pregnant

D. Has experienced an urticaria reaction

E. Has had two or more FNHTRs

19. When a patient receiving platelet transfusion experiences purpura, the most likely cause is:

A. RBC alloantibodies

B. Platelet antigens

C. Contaminating leukocytes in the platelet component
D. Platelet antibodies
E. Plasma proteins in product

20. Symptoms of an HTR in an anesthetized patient may present only as:
A. Unexplained hypotension and abnormal bleeding
B. Unexplained hypertension and thrombocytopenia
C. Pale skin color
D. Abdominal distention
E. Respiratory distress

Answers to Review Questions

1. D (p 365)
2. C (p 358)
3. B (p 362)
4. E (p 360)
5. A (p 359)
6. E (p 365)
7. B (p 360)
8. E (p 367)
9. C (p 354)
10. A (p 352)
11. C (Table 18–8)
12. D (p 357)
13. B (p 358)
14. C (p 357)
15. D (p 356)
16. B (p 363)
17. A (p 367)
18. E (p 353)
19. D (p 362)
20. A (p 354)

References

1. Standards for Blood Banks and Transfusion Services, ed 14. American Association of Blood Banks, Arlington, VA, 1991, p 41, K2.000.
2. Sazama, K: Reports of 355 transfusion associated deaths: 1976 through 1985. Transfusion 30:583, 1990.
3. Edinger, SE: A closer look at fatal transfusion reactions. Medical Laboratory Observer 14:41, 1985.
4. NIH Consensus Conference: Perioperative red cell transfusion. JAMA 260:2700, 1988.
5. Lostumbo, MM, et al: Isoimmunization after multiple transfusions. N Engl J Med 175:141, 1966.
6. Ascari, WO, et al: Incidence of maternal immunization by ABO compatible and incompatible pregnancies. Br Med J 1:399, 1969.
7. Pritchard, E: Transfusion-associated fatalities: Review of Bureau of Biologic Reports 1976–1982. Health Care Finance Administration Regional Office, Philadelphia 1982.
8. Pineda, AA, et al: Delayed hemolytic transfusion reaction. An immunologic hazard of blood transfusion. Transfusion 18:1, 1978.
9. Moore, SB, et al: Delayed hemolytic transfusion reactions. Evidence of the need for an improved pretransfusion compatibility test. Am J Clin Pathol 74:94, 1980.
10. Sazama, K, op cit, p 585.
11. Walker, RH (ed): Technical Manual, ed 10. American Association of Blood Banks, Arlington, VA, p 412.
12. Backman, R: Studies on the seven YA-globulin level. III. The frequency of A-YA globulinemia. Scand J Clin Lab Invest 17:316, 1965.
13. Pineda, AA and Taswell, HF: Transfusion reactions associated with anti-IgA antibodies: Report of four cases and review of the literature. Transfusion 15:10, 1975.
14. Taswell, HF: Hemolytic transfusion reactions: Frequency and clinical and laboratory aspects. In Bell, CA (ed): A Seminar on Immune Mediated Cell Destruction. American Association of Blood Banks, Washington, DC, 1981, p 71.
15. Sazama, K, op cit, p 583.
16. Holland, PV: The diagnosis and management of transfusion reactions and other adverse effects of transfusion. In Petz, LD and Swisher, SN (eds): Clinical Practice of Transfusion Medicine, ed 2. Churchill Livingstone, New York, 1989, p 714.
17. Popovsky, MA: Immune-mediated transfusion reactions. In Nance, SJ (ed): Immune Destruction of Red Blood Cells. American Association of Blood Banks, Arlington, VA, 1989, p 201.
18. Taswell, HF, op cit, p 76.
19. Pisciotto, PT (ed): Blood Transfusion Therapy—A Physician's Handbook, ed 3. American Association of Blood Banks, Arlington, VA, 1989, p 77.
20. Pineda, AA, Brzica, SM, and Taswell, HF: Hemolytic transfusion reaction. Recent experience in a large blood bank. Mayo Clin Proc 53:378, 1978.
21. Gralnick, HR, Marchesi, S, and Grivelber, H: Intravascular coagulation in acute leukemia: Clinical and subclinical abnormalities. Blood 40:709, 1972.
22. Popovsky, MA, Abel, MD, and Moore, SB: Transfusion-related acute lung injury associated with passive transfer of antileukocyte antibodies. Am Rev Respir Dis 128:185, 1983.
23. Barry, KG and Malloy, JP: Oliguric renal failure. Evaluation and therapy by the intravenous infusion of mannitol. JAMA 179:510, 1962.
24. Wolf, CFW and Canale, VC: Total pulmonary hypersensitivity reaction to HLA incompatible blood transfusion: Report of a case and review of the literature. Transfusion 16:135, 1976.
25. Hammerschmidt, DE and Jacob, HS: Adverse pulmonary reactions to transfusion. Adv Intern Med 27:511, 1983.
26. Mollison, PL: Blood Transfusion in Clinical Medicine, ed 7. Blackwell Scientific Publications, Oxford, 1983, p 658.
27. Walker, RH, op cit, p 424.
28. Patten, E, et al: Delayed hemolytic transfusion reaction caused by a primary immune response. Transfusion 22:248, 1982.
29. Furling, MB and Monaghan, WP: Delayed hemolytic episodes due to anti-M. Transfusion 21:45, 1981.
30. Panzer, S, et al: Haemolytic transfusion reactions due to HLA antibodies. Lancet 1:474, 1987.
31. Chaplin, H, Jr: The implication of red-cell bound complement in delayed hemolytic transfusion reactions. Transfusion 24:185, 1984.
32. Holland, PV and Wallerstein, RO: Delayed hemolytic transfusion reaction with acute renal failure. JAMA 204:1007, 1968.
33. Levin, MW: Furosemide and ethacrynic acid in renal insufficiency. Med Clin North Am 55:107, 1971.
34. Walker, RH, op cit, p 420.
35. Wenz, B: Microaggregate blood filtration and febrile transfusion reaction: A comparative study. Transfusion 23:95, 1983.
36. Gleichmann, H and Greininger, J: Over 95% sensitization against allogenic leukocytes following single massive blood transfusion. Vox Sang 28:66, 1975.
37. Moore, SB, et al: Transfusion-induced alloimmunization in patients awaiting renal allografts. Vox Sang 47:354, 1984.
38. Okusawa, S, et al: C5a induction of human interleukin-1: Synergistic effect with endotoxin or interferon-α. J Immunol 139:2635, 1987.

39. Dinnarello, CA and Wolff, SM: Molecular basis of fever in humans. Am J Med 72:799, 1982.
40. Brittingham, TE and Chaplin, H: Febrile transfusion reactions caused by sensitivity to donor leukocytes and platelets. JAMA 165:819, 1957.
41. Brubaker, DB: Immunologically mediated immediate adverse effects of blood transfusions (allergic, febrile nonhemolytic, and noncardiogenic pulmonary edema). Plasma Ther Transfus Technol 6:19, 1985.
42. Wenz, B: Clinical and laboratory precautions that reduce the adverse reactions, alloimmunization, infectivity, and possibly immunomodulation associated with homologous transfusions. Transfusion Medicine Reviews 4:3, 1990.
43. Kevy, SV, et al: Febrile, non-hemolytic transfusion reactions and the limited role of leukoagglutinin in their etiology. Transfusion 2:7, 1962.
44. Seldon, TH: Untoward reactions and complications during transfusions and infusions. Anesthesiology 22:810, 1961.
45. Thompson, JS: Urticaria and angioedema. Ann Intern Med 69:361, 1968.
46. Dahler, SE, et al: Leukotrienes promote plasma leakage and leukocyte adhesion in postcapillary venules: In vivo effects with relevance to the acute inflammatory response. Proc Natl Acad Sci USA 78:3887, 1981.
47. Bochner, BS and Lichtenstein, LM: Anaphylaxis. N Engl J Med 324:1785, 1991.
48. Vyas, GN, et al: Serologic specificity of human anti-IgA and its significance in transfusion. Blood 34:573, 1969.
49. Mollison, PL: Blood Transfusion in Clinical Medicine, ed 8. Blackwell Scientific Publications, Oxford, 1987, p 605.
50. Vyas, GN, Perkins, HA, and Fudenberg, HH: Anaphylactoid transfusion reactions associated with anti-IgA. Lancet 2:312, 1968.
51. Yap, PL, Pryde, EAD, and McClelland, DBL: IgA content of frozen-thawed-washed red blood cells and blood products measured by radioimmunoassay. Transfusion 22:36, 1982.
52. Milde, LN: An anaphylactic reaction to fibrin glue. Anesth Analg 69:684, 1989.
53. Ring, J and Messmer, K: Incidence and severity of anaphylactoid reactions to colloid volume substitutes. Lancet 1:466, 1977.
54. Culliford, AT, Thomas, S, and Spencer, FC: Fulminating noncardiogenic pulmonary edema. J Thorac Cardiovasc Surg 80:868, 1980.
55. Ward, HN, Lipscomb, TS, and Cawley, LP: Pulmonary hypersensitivity reaction after blood transfusion. Arch Intern Med 122:362, 1968.
56. Kernoff, PBA, et al: Severe allergic pulmonary oedema after plasma transfusion. Br J Haematol 23:777, 1972.
57. Hammerschmidt, DE, et al: Association of complement activation and elevated plasma-C5a with adult respiratory distress syndrome. Lancet 1:947, 1980.
58. Holland, PV: Other adverse effects of transfusion. In Petz, LD and Swisher, SN (eds): Clinical Practice of Blood Transfusion. Churchill Livingstone, New York, 1981, p 783.
59. Barton, JC: Noninfectious transfusion reactions. In Dutcher, JP (ed): Modern Transfusion Therapy. CRC Press, Boca Raton, FL, 1990, p 71.
60. Goldfinger, D: Adverse reactions to blood transfusion. In Mayer, K (ed): Guidelines to Transfusion Practices. American Association of Blood Banks, Washington, DC, 1980, p 144.
61. Marriott, HL and Kekwick, A: Volume and rate in blood transfusion for relief of anemia. Br Med J 1:1043, 1940.
62. Goldfinger, D and Lowe, C: Prevention of adverse reactions to blood transfusion by the administration of saline washed red blood cells. Transfusion 21:277, 1981.
63. Tipple, MA, et al: Sepsis associated with transfusion of red cells contaminated with *Yersinia enterocolitica*. Transfusion 30:207, 1990.
64. Braine, HG, et al: Bacterial sepsis secondary to platelet transfusion: An adverse effect of extended storage at room temperature. Transfusion 26:391, 1986.
65. Braudle, A: Transfusion reactions from contaminated blood —their recognition and treatment. N Engl J Med 258:1289, 1958.
66. Tabor, E and Geraty, RJ: Five cases of Pseudomonas species transmitted by blood transfusions. Lancet 1:1403, 1984.
67. Buckholz, DH, et al: Detection and quantitations of bacteria in platelet products stored at ambient temperature. Transfusion 13:268, 1985.
68. Davey, RJ, Lee, BJ, and Coles, SM: Acute intraoperative hemolysis following rapid infusion of hypotonic solution. Lab Med 17:282, 1986.
69. Elin, RJ, Lundberg, WB, and Schmidt, PJ: Evaluation of bacterial contamination in blood processing. Transfusion 15:260, 1975.
70. Kim, DM, et al: Visual identification of bacterially contaminated red cells. Transfusion 32:221, 1992.
71. Hoppe, PA: Interim measures for detection of bacterially contaminated red cell components. Transfusion 32:199, 1992.
72. Linden, JV, et al: In vitro and in vivo evaluation of an electromechanical blood infusion pump. Lab Med 19:574, 1988.
73. Miller, RD, et al: Coagulation defects associated with massive blood transfusion. Ann Surg 174:794, 1971.
74. Reuler, JB: Hypothermia: Pathophysiology, clinical settings, and management. Ann Intern Med 89:519, 1978.
75. Gibson, JG, Gregory, CB, and Button, LN: Citrate-phosphate-dextrose solutions for preservation of human blood: A further report. Transfusion 1:280, 1961.
76. Valeri, C: Viability and function of preserved red cells. N Engl J Med 284:81, 1971.
77. Mammen, E and Walt, A: Eight years of experience with massive blood transfusion. J Trauma 11:275, 1971.
78. Quick, AJ: Influence of erythrocytes on the coagulation of blood. Am J Med Sci 239:101, 1960.
79. Barton, JC: Massive transfusion: Complications and their management. J Tenn Med Assoc 68:895, 1975.
80. Best, R, Syverud, S, and Novak, RM: Trauma and hypothermia. Am J Emerg Med 3:48, 1985.
81. Silberstein, LE, et al: Calcium homeostasis during therapeutic plasma exchange. Transfusion 26:151, 1986.
82. Wolfowitz, E and Shechter, Y: More about alloimmunization by transfusion of fresh-frozen plasma. Transfusion 24:544, 1984.
83. Cox, JV, et al: Risk of alloimmunization and delayed hemolytic transfusion reactions in patients with sickle cell disease. Arch Intern Med 148:2488, 1988.
84. Salama, A and Mueller-Eckhardt, C: Delayed hemolytic transfusion reactions. Evidence for complement activation involving allogeneic and autologous red cells. Transfusion 24:188, 1984.
85. Kooy, MVM, et al: Use of leukocyte-depleted platelet concentrates for the prevention of refractoriness and primary HLA alloimmunization: A prospective, randomized trial. Blood 77:201, 1991.
86. Vichinsky, EP, et al: Alloimmunization in sickle cell anemia and transfusion of racially unmatched blood. N Engl J Med 322:1617, 1990.
87. Mueller-Eckhardt, C, et al: Posttransfusion purpura: Immunological and clinical studies in two cases and review of the literature. Blut 40:249, 1980.
88. Soulier, JP, et al: Posttransfusion immunologic thrombocytopenia. Vox Sang 37:21, 1979.
89. Kickler, TS, et al: Studies on the pathophysiology of posttransfusion purpura. Blood 68:347, 1986.
90. Farboody, GH, Clough, JD, and Hoffman, GC: Posttransfusion purpura. Cleve Clin Q 45:241, 1978.
91. Cimo, PL and Aster, RH: Posttransfusion purpura: Successful treatment by exchange transfusion. N Engl J Med 287:290, 1980.
92. Abramson, N, Eisenberg, PD, and Astor, RH: Posttransfusion purpura: Immunologic aspects and therapy. N Engl J Med 291:1163, 1974.
93. Mueller-Eckhardt, C, et al: High-dose intravenous immunoglobulin for posttransfusion purpura. 18th Congress of the

International Society of Blood Transfusion, Abstract, P12-21, 1984, p 194.

94. Brubaker, DB: Human posttransfusion graft-versus-host disease. Vox Sang 45:401, 1983.
95. Parkman, R, et al: Graft-versus-host disease after intrauterine and exchange transfusion for hemolytic disease of the newborn. N Engl J Med 290:359, 1974.
96. Anderson, KC and Weinstein, HJ: Transfusion-associated graft-versus-host disease. N Engl J Med 323:315, 1990.
97. Thomas, ED, et al: Bone-marrow transplantation. N Engl J Med 292:832, 1975.
98. Linden, JV and Pisciotto, PT: Transfusion-associated graft-versus-host disease and blood irradiation. Transfusion Medicine Reviews 6:116, 1992.
99. Rosen, RC, Huestis, DW, and Corrigan, JJ: Acute leukemia and granulocyte transfusion: Fatal graft-versus-host disease following transfusion of cells obtained from normal donors. J Pediatr 93:268, 1981.
100. Siimes, MA and Hoskimies, S: Chronic graft-versus-host disease after blood transfusions confirmed by incompatible HLA antigens in bone marrow. Lancet 1:42, 1982.
101. Button, LN, et al: The effects of irradiation on blood components. Transfusion 21:419, 1981.
102. Anderson, KC, et al: Variation in blood component irradiation practice: Implications for prevention of transfusion-associated graft-versus-host disease. Blood 77:2096, 1991.
103. Hoffbrand, AV, et al: Improvement in iron status and liver function in patients with transfusional iron overload with long-term subcutaneous disferrioxamine. Lancet 1:947, 1979.
104. Propper, RD, Button, LN, and Nathan, DG: New approach to transfusion management of thalessemia. Blood 55:55, 1980.
105. Standards for Blood Banks and Transfusion Services, op cit, p 42, K2.000.
106. Judd, WJ: Investigation and management of immune hemolysis—autoantibodies and drugs. In Wallace, ME and Levitt, JS (eds): Current Applications and Interpretations of the Direct Antiglobulin Test. American Association of Blood Banks, Arlington, VA, 1988, p 47.
107. Laird-Fryer, B: Application and interpretation of direct antiglobulin test results as applied to healthy persons and selected patients. In Wallace, ME and Levitt, JS (eds): Current Applications and Interpretations of the Direct Antiglobulin Test. American Association of Blood Banks, Arlington, VA, 1988, p 123.
108. Baker, RJ, Moinichen, SL, and Myhus, LM: Transfusion reaction: A reappraisal of surgical incidence and significance. Ann Surg 169:684, 1969.
109. Accreditation Requirement Manual of the American Association of Blood Banks, ed 4. Bethesda, MD, 1992, p 154.
110. Larison, J, et al: How to write a procedure manual. In Kutt, S and Mobley, R (eds): The Learning Laboratorian Series. Academic Publishing Services, Augusta, GA, 1992.
111. Walker, RH, op cit, p 411.
112. Mollison, PL, op cit, p 651.
113. Walker, RH, op cit, p 415.
114. Ibid, pp 413–416.
115. Accreditation Requirement Manual of the American Association of Blood Banks, op cit, p 157.
116. Sherwood, GK: Hemolytic transfusion reactions: In Dawson, RB (ed): New Approaches to Transfusion Reactions: A Technical Workshop. American Association of Blood Banks, Washington, DC, 1974, p 1.
117. Sacher, RA, McPherson, RA, and Campos, JM: Transfusion Medicine. In Sacher, RA (ed): Widmann's Clinical Interpretation of Laboratory Tests. FA Davis, Philadelphia, 1991, p 299.
118. Bacon, JM and Young, IF: ABO incompatible blood transfusion. Pathology 21:181, 1989.
119. Mollison, PL, op cit, p 670.
120. Ibid, p 671.
121. Miller, WV: Transfusion Reactions. In: Blood Group Immunology Theoretical and Practical Concepts. Dade Division American Hospital Supply Corporation, Miami, p 132.
122. Seldon, TH, op cit, p 813.
123. Masooril, ST and Piercy, S: A step-by-step guide to trouble-free transfusions. Registered Nurse 47:34, 1984.
124. Spurling, CL: Transmissible disease and blood transfusion. In Dawson, RB (ed): New Approaches to Transfusion Reactions: A Technical Workshop. American Association of Blood Banks, Washington, DC, 1974, p 57.
125. Issitt, PD: Applied Blood Group Serology, ed 3. Montgomery Scientific Publications, Miami, 1985, p 507.
126. Reid, ME and Ellisor, SS: Resolution of a positive antibody screen and a positive direct antiglobulin test. Clin Lab Sci 2:174, 1989.
127. Walker, RH, op cit, p 413.
128. Ibid.
129. Oberman, HA: The crossmatch. Transfusion 21:645, 1981.
130. Walker, RH, op cit, p 415.
131. Ibid, p 414.
132. Kutt, SM, Larison, PJ, and Kessler, L: Antibody Detection and Identification. Ortho Diagnostic Systems, Academic Publishing Services, Augusta, GA, 1991.
133. Mollison, PL, op cit, p 631.
134. Ibid, p 671.
135. Walker, RH, op cit, p 415.
136. Ibid, p 416.
137. McCord, RG and Myhre, B: A method for rapid and thorough work-up of febrile and allergic transfusion reactions. Lab Med 9:39, 1978.
138. Standards for Blood Banks and Transfusion Services, op cit, pp 50, 51.
139. Code of Federal Regulations, Title 21, Part 606.170. FDA, US Government Printing Office, Washington, DC, 1991.
140. Inspection Checklist Transfusion Medicine. CAP Commission on Laboratory Accreditation, Northfield, IL, 1991, p 25.
141. AABB Inspection and Accreditation Program Inspection Report Form. American Association of Blood Banks, Bethesda, MD, 1991, p 36.
142. Accreditation Manual for Hospitals (AMH). Joint Commission on Accreditation of Healthcare Organizations, Oakbrook Terrace, IL, 1992, p 97.

Bibliography

Ciavarella, D (ed): Symposium On Leukocyte-Depleted Blood Products. Transfusion Medicine Reviewers 4(Suppl) 1–41, 1990.
Dutcher, JP (ed): Modern Transfusion Therapy. Vols I and II. CRC Press, Boca Raton, FL, 1990.
Harmening, D (ed): Modern Blood Banking and Transfusion Practices, ed 2. FA Davis, Philadelphia, 1989.
Miale, JB (ed): Laboratory Medicine: Hematology, ed 6. CV Mosby, St Louis, 1982.
Petz, LD and Swisher, SN (eds): Clinical Practice of Transfusion Medicine, ed 6. Churchill Livingstone, New York, 1989.
Rutnam, RC and Miller, WV (eds): Transfusion Therapy: Principles and Procedures. Aspen Systems Corp, Rockville, MD, 1981.
Turgeon, ML: Fundamentals of Immunohematology: Theory and Technique. Lea & Febiger, Philadelphia, 1989.

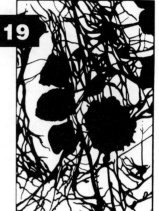

CHAPTER 19

Transfusion-Transmitted Viruses

Herbert F. Polesky, MD

OBJECTIVES

Upon completion of this chapter, the learner should be able to:

1 List the criteria for donor selection.
2 List the tests performed on donor blood.
3 Describe procedures for look-back and recipient follow-up.
4 Describe the nature of various hepatitis viruses and the diseases they cause.
5 Discuss the current theories regarding transfusion-associated hepatitis.
6 Characterize the human immunodeficiency virus.
7 Discuss the nature of the acquired immunodeficiency syndrome and its relation to blood products.
8 Name and describe the laboratory tests performed on donor blood to detect human immunodeficiency virus infection.

9 Describe the dangers of cytomegalovirus and Epstein-Barr virus contamination of blood components.

10 Discuss the various laboratory tests for the detection of viruses with reference to their sensitivity and accuracy.

The decision to transfuse must be based on weighing the therapeutic benefits against any potential risks to the recipient. Although small, the possibility of transmitting one or more viruses to the recipient continues to be one of the major complications of transfusion. In spite of this possible risk, if the use of blood and blood components is limited to individuals who meet carefully chosen clinical criteria, the safety of giving blood greatly exceeds the harm of not transfusing.

Donor Selection

The most important step in ensuring that transfused blood will not transmit a pathogenic virus is careful selection of the donor. Part of this selection process is the inducement used to motivate the donation. Before the availability of tests to detect hepatitis B surface antigen (HBsAg) it was clearly shown that eliminating donors motivated by cash payment significantly decreased the risk of hepatitis B virus infection in recipients.[1] With the recognition that acquired immunodeficiency syndrome (AIDS) might be transmitted by transfusion, and in the absence of any serologic screening test, requesting potential donors to self-defer based on predonation information about activities that could increase their chance of being infected with human immunodeficiency virus (HIV) had a major impact on the safety of blood.[2]

Selection of blood and organ donors to prevent disease transmission includes evaluation of the individual's medical history. Potential donors who have (1) had an exposure in the past 12 months to individuals with a viral illness that could be transfusion-transmitted (TTV), (2) been implicated as a donor in a case of TTV, (3) a past history of hepatitis after age 10, (4) engaged in risk behaviors that are associated with infection by HIV, (5) signs and symptoms suggestive of hepatitis or AIDS, or (6) received pituitary growth hormone of human origin (possible source of Creutzfeldt-Jakob disease) may need to be deferred. Direct questions about possible risk behaviors and review of past deferrals are essential parts of the donor evaluation process. The current edition of the American Association of Blood Banks (AABB) Standards and memoranda from the Food and Drug Administration (FDA) should be consulted to determine specific criteria for disqualifying donors.[3,4]

The brief donor physical examination should include inspection of both arms for possible signs of intravenous drug use and evaluation of the donor's health status. During the donor interview it is important to be sure the donor understands the importance of self-rejection if he or she might be putting a recipient at risk. A mechanism for privately indicating that the donated blood is not suitable for transfusion, confidential unit exclusion (CUE), may be used to allow self-deferral for those who feel compelled by peer pressure to donate.

Donor Testing

Testing donor blood for specific and surrogate markers of TTV is the final step in ensuring the safety of a unit of blood and its component parts. Specific tests that will be discussed later in this chapter include HBsAg, antibody to hepatitis C virus (anti-HCV), anti-HIV, antibody to cytomegalovirus (anti-CMV), and antibody to human T-cell lymphotropic virus types I and II (anti–HTLV-I/II). Surrogate tests that are also used to prevent TTV include antibody to hepatitis B core antigen (anti-HBc) and alanine aminotransferase (ALT) levels. In doing these tests, appropriate quality-control methods and documentation must be used. These tests are screening procedures that determine whether a unit can be released. Most blood banks require additional confirmation tests to establish the specificity of the result. A system must be in place to ensure that only units tested and found negative for all mandated markers are released for transfusion.[4] Although most of the tests are very sensitive (true-positive/true-positive and false-negative [TP/TP + FN]) and have good specificity (true-negative/true-negative and false-positive [TN/TN + FP]), none will detect all carriers of a virus. The efficacy of each test can be determined by calculating the predictive value of a positive or negative test result. For example, in the case of anti-HCV screening, if 95 of 100 reactive tests are confirmed as true positives by supplementary testing, the predictive value of a positive test (chance that the donor is an HCV carrier) is 95/100, or 0.95 (95 percent). In the case of anti-HIV testing by enzyme-linked immunosorbent assay (ELISA), which has a sensitivity of 99 percent and a specificity of 98 percent, most positive test results will be false-positives because the prevalence of the disease in the population is very low. If the prevalence of disease in the tested population is 1 percent, the ratio of true-positives to false-positives will be 1 : 2 and the predictive value of a positive test result equal to 33 percent.[5]

Recipient Follow-up

Another way to increase the safety of the blood supply is to eliminate from the donor pool individuals who have negative test results but who are implicated in TTV. The AABB Standards[3] require that the donor of blood or component given to a recipient who develops clinical or laboratory evidence of transfusion-associated hepatitis (TAH), HIV infection, or HTLV-I/II infection must be permanently deferred if his or her unit was the only unit administered. Identifying recipients who have developed viral complications after transfusion is not easy. Many of the patients transfused at tertiary care facilities may not be followed up at the same hospital or by the physician who ordered the transfusions. Patients may die of complications of their primary illness during the incubation period of the TTV illness. In addition the long incubation time between infection and disease recognition may result in failure to consider transfusion as the source of infection. Good communication between the hospital infection control service and the blood bank is one of the best ways to find these cases. Treating physicians should be reminded periodically of the need to suspect and report cases of TTV.

Look-Back (Inventory, Donor, Recipient)

When a donor is found to have a reactive test for a TTV or reports development of a transfusion-transmissible disease, it is important to determine the status of any prior units donated by the individual. If components are still in inventory, these may need to be quarantined, discarded, or both.

As discussed earlier, when a recipient develops a transfusion-associated viral infection it is important to identify implicated donors. Inasmuch as most patients get units from multiple donors and donors who give frequently are at a greater risk of being implicated, the decision to defer all or some of the donors is often difficult. A mathematical approach taking into account the total number of donors and other factors in the case allows assignment of a risk factor to each donor.[6,7] This is particularly useful when the same donor is implicated in more than one case.

If an individual who develops HIV infection (detected because of seroconversion on a subsequent donation or by clinical history) has been a blood donor, it is necessary to determine prior recipients of components from this donor and notify them of the risk of infection. Look-back and recipient notification are also necessary when there is a possibility of HTLV-I/II infection in the donor. It is also important to initiate tracing of other potential recipients when a patient with a transplant develops a viral disease that may have been transmitted by the tissue. In many cases organs and tissues from the donor have been used for multiple patients.

Transfusion-Associated Hepatitis

At least five viruses have been associated with hepatitis occurring after transfusion:

1. Hepatitis A virus (HAV)
2. Hepatitis B virus (HBV)
3. Hepatitis C virus (HCV)
4. Hepatitis delta virus (HDV)
5. Non-A, non-B, non-C (NANBNC) hepatitis virus

A sixth hepatitis virus, hepatitis E virus, has been identified as the cause of epidemic hepatitis associated with contaminated water. This agent, found in many underdeveloped areas of the world, has not been associated with TAH.[8] The frequency with which hepatitis occurs after transfusion is difficult to establish. Many patients who develop TAH will be asymptomatic and are likely to be recognized only if they are prospectively followed or if they are incidentally found to have an abnormal test result such as an elevated ALT. It is estimated that less than one third of patients with TAH develop clinical signs and symptoms of the disease, which can include jaundice, abdominal tenderness, nausea, vomiting, weakness and fatigue, dark urine, and acholic (light) stools. The frequency of this transfusion complication has been variously reported to be as high as 18 percent of recipients to as low as 0.1 percent.[9] Several factors influence the rates reported. These include geographic differences in the frequency of hepatitis carriers in the population, the tests used to screen the donor blood, and the adequacy of reporting of cases. Recent data suggest that less than 1 in 3000 (0.03 percent) of recipients of blood screened for HBsAg, anti-HBc, anti-HCV, and ALT will develop TAH.[10]

The severity of TAH is also quite variable. A majority of patients will be asymptomatic. Of those who develop acute illness, most will recover; however, about 1 to 2 percent of this group may die from the disease. Table 19–1 indicates that both mortality and morbidity are increased when hepatitis occurs in individuals over the age of 40. A very rare occurrence is the development of acute fulminant hepatitis. About 70 percent of these patients die during their acute illness. Another severe form of TAH is superinfection by HDV. This fulminant form of hepatitis is a special problem in chronically transfused individuals who are also carriers of HBV.

Sequelae of TAH include the development of chronic active hepatitis (CAH) or chronic persistent hepatitis (CPH). This occurs more commonly when there is infection with HCV and can, over many years, progress to cirrhosis or hepatocellular carcinoma or both.[1] The chronic liver problems can occur in asymptomatic patients as well as those with acute disease that appears to resolve. In a large group of patients followed for 18 years after a diagnosis of non-A, non-B TAH, there was no difference in mortality compared with that of control subjects who were selected from transfused patients who did not develop TAH.[11] There

TABLE 19–1 EPIDEMIOLOGIC AND CLINICAL CHARACTERISTICS OF PATIENTS WITH HEPATITIS*

Patient Characteristics	HEPATITIS B (%)		NANB HEPATITIS (%)	
	All Ages (9309 Patients)	Age >40 y (1987 Patients)	All Ages (2083 Patients)	Age >40 y (702 Patients)
Blood transfusion	1.2	4.0	7.7	20.8
Jaundice	79.6	71.2	78.2	72.4
Hospitalized	29.6	40.6	33.5	44.3
Died	1.1	2.8	2.6	5.6

Data from Hepatitis Surveillance Report No. 53, Centers for Disease Control, Atlanta, GA, 1990, pp 18–31.
*Centers for Disease Control Viral Hepatitis Surveillance Program, 1988.
NANB = non-A, non-B hepatitis.

was a slight excess of deaths due to liver disease in the TAH group compared with controls, but in both groups 70 percent of the liver-related deaths occurred in patients with chronic alcoholism.

Characteristics of Hepatitis Viruses

HEPATITIS A VIRUS

The virus causing hepatitis A or infectious hepatitis is a 27-nm RNA virus in the family *Picornaviridae*. The virus replicates in infected liver cells and may be shed in the stools of acutely ill patients.[12] These is no chronic carrier state in humans. Infection is usually spread by the oral-fecal route. Outbreaks usually can be traced to contamination of food or water or person-to-person spread where hygiene is compromised (e.g., daycare centers).

Transfusion-transmitted HAV infection has occurred but is very rare.[13] Infection by transfusion requires that the donor have viremia and the recipient be susceptible to the virus. Viremia, if it occurs, is usually brief, occurring at the onset of acute illness. Antibodies to hepatitis A regularly appear after infection (Fig. 19–1); thus, a large percent of the popula-

tion has immunity. The frequency with which anti-HAV is found increases with age and is inversely related to the level of sanitation.

Hepatitis A infection can be prevented by vaccination, with intramuscular immune serum globulin (IG) given either after exposure (ideally within 2 weeks) or prophylactically to individuals traveling to endemic areas. The rarity of infection after transfusion does not warrant routine testing of donors or the use of IG in recipients.

HEPATITIS B VIRUS

HBV is in the family *Hepadnaviridae*. These DNA viruses have been found in the Peking duck, woodchuck, and some ground squirrels.[14] In humans the virus is a 42-nm particle consisting of a 28-nm core with double-stranded circular DNA and DNA polymerase. The core is surrounded by a coat protein—HBsAg—which also occurs free in the serum as 22-nm spheres and 22- to 200-nm filaments (Fig. 19–2). There are several polypeptides associated with this virus, including the hepatitis B e antigen (HBeAg). The polypeptide making up the coat protein was described by Blumberg[15] in 1965, when he discovered a precipitin line between serum from a multitransfused

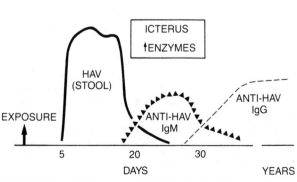

FIGURE 19–1 Markers in acute HAV infection. The typical pattern of HAV infection includes early shedding of virus in the stool, appearance of IgM anti-HAV with the onset of symptoms, and development of IgG anti-HAV and immunity on recovery.

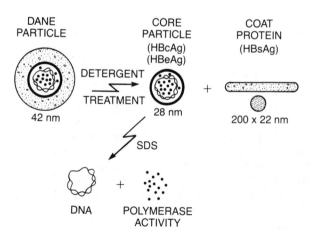

FIGURE 19–2 Diagram of the intact Dane particle (HB virion) as seen by electron microscopy. Detergent treatment disrupts the particle, releasing DNA (double- and single-stranded) and DNA polymerase activity.

TABLE 19-2 **SEROLOGIC TESTS IN THE DIAGNOSIS OF VIRAL HEPATITIS**

Hepatitis Agent	Diagnostic Test						Interpretation
HAV	Total (IgM + IgG) and/or IgM anti-HAV						Acute hepatitis A
	Total (IgM + IgG) only						Previous hepatitis A

	HBsAg	Anti-HBs	Anti-HBc Total	Anti-HBc IgM	HBeAg	Anti-HBe	
HBV	+	−	(+/−)	(+/−)	−	−	Early acute hepatitis B, before symptoms
	+	−	+	+	+	−	Acute hepatitis B
	−	−	++	(+)	(+/−)	+	Early convalescence from hepatitis B or "low-level" carrier state
	+	(−/+)	+	(−)	+	−	Chronic HBsAg carrier
					−	+	or
	−	+	+	(−)	−	(−/+)	Previous hepatitis B (recovered)
	−	+	−	(−)	−	−	Distant previous hepatitis B or vaccination with HBsAg
	−	−	+	(−)	−	−	Distant previous hepatitis B

Hepatitis Agent	Diagnostic Test	Interpretation
HDV	Anti-HDV Total (IgG) +/− low titer + high titer (persistent) +	IgM (not available commercially) + low titer (rising) acute delta + high titer (persistent) −
		Chronic delta hepatitis Previous delta hepatitis
	ELISA RIBA	
HCV	+ +	Acute or chronic
	+ − or	Possible false-positive
	Ind*	Acute or chronic
NANBNC	None available Exclude HAV, HBV, HCV, HDV, HEV, CMV, EBV	Acute and chronic

*Indeterminate.

hemophiliac patient and a sample from an Australian aborigine. Initially this antigen was called Australia Antigen (Au) and was thought to be associated with leukemia. Its subsequent association with hepatitis led to the terms hepatitis-associated antigen (HAA) and HBsAg.

When an individual is infected by HBV, several of the antigens and antibodies can be detected by serologic tests (Table 19–2). Usually the first marker of HBV to appear is HBsAg (Fig. 19–3). This marker is also found in the 5 to 10 percent of infected patients who become chronic carriers of HBV. This polypeptide is very complex, and several antigenic variants known as subtypes have been defined. The subtypes occur with different frequencies in various parts of the world and can be helpful in epidemiologic studies. The subtypes are related to the viral strain, not the host. In addition, all strains have a common determinant.

Shortly after infection and before clinical signs and symptoms or biochemical changes in liver function can occur, two other markers—HBeAg and anti-HBc—are usually detectable in serum from infected individuals. Initially the anti-HBc is an immunoglobulin M (IgM) antibody; however, as the infection progresses, IgG antibody appears. This latter antibody persists in persons who recover from HBV infection (Table 19–2). HBeAg usually disappears when the patient enters the convalescent phase. In individuals who do not develop immunity to HBV (usually those infected ver-

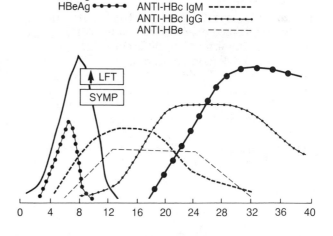

FIGURE 19-3 Markers in HBV infection.

tically [transplacentally] or with immunosuppression), HBeAg, HBsAg, and anti-HBc can be present. In others with chronic infection (persistence of HBsAg for longer than 6 months), HBeAg is cleared and anti-HBe found. This group of patients, unlike those with HBsAg, are more likely to have normal liver function test results and minimal histologic evidence of disease.

Immunity to HBV develops in most individuals who

have acute or asymptomatic infection. As with HAV infection, immunity to HBV is specific; individuals do not have a second infection with the HBV, although they will not be immune to infection from another hepatitis virus, such as HAV or HCV. Individuals who have recovered from HBV infection will have anti-HBs or anti-HBc or both in their sera. The frequency of these markers depends on the population studied.

Two approaches have been used to prevent HBV infection. An immune globulin prepared from persons with a high titer of anti-HBs called hepatitis B immunoglobulin (HBIG) has been used to provide passive immunity to healthcare workers and others who are exposed to patients with HBV infection. Extensive studies of HBIG after accidental needlestick exposure showed that its effect was to prolong the incubation and reduce the severity of the disease. In 1982 a vaccine made from HBsAg isolated from human plasma was licensed.[16] This material has been shown to be very effective in preventing HBV infection in cases of accidental needlestick, in infants whose mothers are positive for both HBsAg and HBeAg and in homosexual men. About 90 to 95 percent of those given vaccine in the deltoid muscle (it is less effective if given in the gluteal muscle) develop anti-HBs, which can subsequently be detected for several years. In 1987 a recombinant vaccine prepared from common baker's yeast (*Saccharomyces cereversiae*) infected with a plasmid containing the gene for HBsAg was licensed.[17] This vaccine has minimal side effects and is recommended for all healthcare workers who are likely to be exposed to blood or body fluid containing HBV. Usually the vaccine is given in three doses. In individuals lacking immunity who are exposed to HBV (needlestick or newborn), it is recommended that both HBIG and the vaccine be administered in different sites. Follow-up vaccine is given 1 month and 6 months later.

Prevention of HBV infection through universal vaccination is a goal of several current public health initiatives.[18] Because this virus is often sexually transmitted, early vaccination can eliminate the morbidity associated with acute disease, prevent long-term sequelae (in endemic areas, long-term HBV infection is associated with a high incidence of hepatoma [primary liver cell cancer]), and eliminate the risk of vertical transmission.

HEPATITIS DELTA VIRUS

The delta agent, first described by Rizzetto in 1977, is a particle about 35 nm in diameter.[19] This RNA virus can infect and replicate but appears to require HBV virus to cause hepatocellular damage.[20] Infection with HDV can occur simultaneously with HBV infection (coinfection) or in a carrier of HBV (superinfection). This latter infection is of particular concern in chronically transfused patients who may have been previously exposed to HBV.

Most delta infections occur in drug addicts. At least one report documents the occurrence of HDV infec-

tion in a small percent of patients with TAH.[21] The illness associated with delta infection is usually severe, and antibody to HDV occurs more frequently than expected in patients with fulminant hepatitis.

The diagnosis of delta hepatitis depends on finding anti-delta in the serum or demonstrating the antigen (HDAg) by use of immunofluorescence on liver biopsy material. Individuals who recover after HDV infection usually become seronegative. Methods that prevent HBV infection should effectively reduce the risk of HDV infection as well.

HEPATITIS C VIRUS

In 1989 after an extensive testing of a gene library with serum taken from a chimpanzee infected with non-A, non-B hepatitis (NANB), a fusion peptide that represents a portion of the HCV genome was identified.[22] Further characterization of this material revealed it to be an RNA virus of about 3000 base pairs. A diagram of the proposed genome is shown in Figure 19-4. This virus, which has not been cultured or isolated, is probably part of the family *Flaviviridae*. Using recombinant technology and peptide synthesis, several test systems were developed that made it possible to identify an antibody, anti-HCV, that is present in more than 80 percent of patients having transfusion-associated or community-acquired NANB hepatitis.[23-25] Initial studies with anti-HCV 1.0 showed that some patients with TAH did not have detectable antibody for up to 30 weeks after onset of acute illness or a significant rise in ALT.[26] Recent modifications of the test systems (anti-HCV 2.0) make it possible to detect seroconversion earlier. Routine screening of blood donors in the United States with anti-HCV 1.0 started in May 1990. Second-generation reagents (anti-HCV 2.0) became routinely available in March 1992. A major problem with donor screening for anti-HCV has

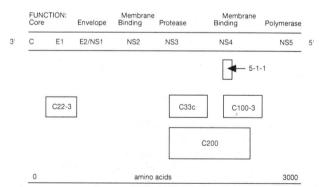

FIGURE 19-4 The proposed HCV genome and the recombinant proteins used to test for HCV. The HCV 1.0 test detects antibody to C100-3. The HCV 2.0 test detects antibody to C200 (including C33c and C100-c) and C22-3. Supplementary tests, such as the recombinant immunoblot assay (RIBA), detect antibody to specific gene products including C22-3, C33c, C100-3, and 5-1-1. (Adapted from the package insert for the HCV 2.0 test. Ortho Diagnostic Systems, Raritan, NJ.)

been the lack of confirmatory assays for further evaluation of reactive donors. Two supplemental tests, one of which is licensed in the United States, have been available. One is based on a neutralization of antibody. The other, known as recombinant immunoblot assay (RIBA), is based on reaction of specific antibodies with antigen fixed to a membrane.

There is probably at least one other viral agent that causes some of the clinical disease formerly called NANB hepatitis. Thus, the 10 to 20 percent of NANB hepatitis that tests negative for anti-HCV will now be considered to be NANBNC hepatitis.

In the United States, before the routine screening of donated blood for anti-HCV, between 5 and 10 percent of NANB hepatitis was found in individuals with a history of blood transfusion, about 40 percent in drug addicts, and less than 5 percent in individuals having household or occupational exposure.[27] Thus, a large percentage of NANB hepatitis cases seem to have no identified risk factor. Studies have shown that unlike HBV and HIV, heterosexual and homosexual transmission of HCV is rare. One epidemiologic study has shown a correlation between HCV-positive NANB hepatitis and low socioeconomic status.[24]

The time from infection by HCV to onset of symptoms is quite variable. In transfusion recipients, the HCV incubation period is 40 to 60 days, which is considerably shorter than the 90 to 180 days associated with HBV infection. Many patients are asymptomatic and may be identified as having HCV infection only by the presence of mild liver function abnormalities such as an elevated ALT or by a positive anti-HCV test result. A major problem with HCV is that 40 to 60 percent of infected individuals may develop chronic liver disease. In some people this results in cirrhosis and or hepatocellular carcinoma or both. The time lag between the acute infection and recognition of the chronic liver disease may be as long as 20 years. In selected patients with chronic liver disease due to HCV infection, treatment with recombinant alpha interferon may induce both biochemical and histologic improvement.[28]

Before the development of a specific test for anti-HCV, surrogate test systems were introduced in an attempt to reduce this transfusion complication. ALT and anti-HBc have been used to screen donors. If a donor has an ALT above an established cutoff level (e.g., mean ALT plus 2 standard deviations [SD]), his or her unit is not used. If the level is twice this cutoff, the donor usually is deferred for 1 year. The evidence that ALT testing will reduce NANB-TAH was reported in a prospective study in which recipients of blood with ALT levels above the cutoff value were several times more likely to develop elevated ALT levels after transfusion.[29] It is thought that this mild liver function abnormality reflects ongoing inflammation caused by the virus. Continued use of ALT screening has been recommended as a method to detect HCV-infected donors who have not seroconverted.

Prospective studies showed that NANB-TAH was also more likely to occur if the recipient was given anti-HBc–positive donor blood.[30] Epidemiologic studies suggest that in some groups individuals with prior HBV infection also are likely to be carriers of NANB hepatitis. Several studies of donors with anti-HCV have failed to show a correlation with this marker and the presence of anti-HBc. If a donor has both anti-HBc and an elevated ALT, or an ALT twice the cutoff value, then anti-HCV is often present. It has also been suggested that anti-HBc may be present in some donors capable of transmitting HBV whose test result is negative for HBsAg.[31] The impact of these surrogate tests (ALT and anti-HBc) on the safety of transfusion is unclear. What is clear is that many donors with a long history of safe donation are no longer eligible because of these tests. It is also clear that ALT can be transiently elevated because of alcohol ingestion and other physiologic factors. Testing for anti-HBc yields a positive result in a large number of healthy donors who have recovered from an asymptomatic infection with HBV. These donors also will be anti-HBs positive. Another group of donors will be anti-HBc positive with the screening test used, but when tested with another manufacturer's reagent they are usually nonreactive.[32] Both of these tests led to blood centers discarding from 1 to 5 percent of units collected and a need to notify many donors that they are no longer eligible to donate.

The Human Immunodeficiency Virus Types 1 and 2

The HIV, of the family *Retroviridae*, is a lentivirus that causes chronic infection and grows slowly. The HIV organism is a 100-nm sphere with an envelope consisting of a lipid membrane through which glycoproteins protrude. The core of the virus contains the genomic RNA and reverse transcriptase (Fig. 19–5).[33] Various types of HIV, such as HIV-1 and HIV-2, have different envelope and core proteins (Table 19–3) and can produce different clinical and serologic responses in the host.

SEROLOGIC RESPONSE TO HIV INFECTION

Figure 19–6 is a schematic representation of the usual serologic findings in an individual who develops HIV-1 infection.[34] Shortly after exposure, the core protein, p24, has been found in some individuals. Within a few weeks to up to 6 months antibody to both envelope (gp41) and core (p24) proteins appear. During the early phase of infection, a nonspecific acute "viral illness" may occur. There is some controversy as to which antibody, anti-p24 or anti-gp41, appears first. Once antibody appears it seems to increase in titer even though the host is asymptomatic. During this phase of infection, viral cultures of isolated lymphocytes will demonstrate the presence of virus. As

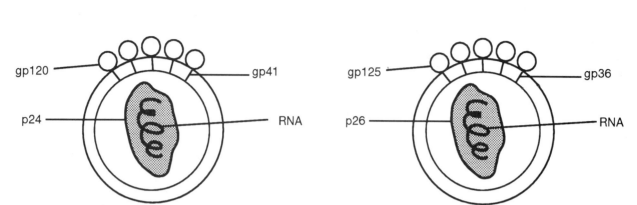

FIGURE 19–5   Schematic representation of the human immunodeficiency viral genomes, HIV-1 and HIV-2.

TABLE 19–3   **COMPONENTS OF THE HIV VIRUS**

| Gene | BANDS OBSERVED | | Protein |
	HIV-1	HIV-2	
Gag	p18, p24, p15	p16, p26, p55	Core
Pol	p31		Endonuclease
	p51, p65	p68	Reverse transcriptase
Env	gp41	gp36	Transmembrane protein
	gp120, gp160	gp140, gp125	Envelope unit

p = protein;   gp = glycoprotein (number indicates molecular weight).

infection progresses, changes in the ratio of T lymphocytes with specific surface markers, CD4 (helper) to CD8 (suppressor) cells, will be observed. The number or percent of CD4-positive (CD4+) T cells in an HIV-seropositive individual is useful as a guide to clinical

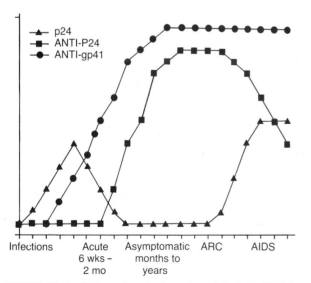

FIGURE 19–6   Pattern of serologic markers detected in HIV infection. ARC = AIDS-related condition.

and therapeutic management. Under classification guidelines recently issued by the Centers for Disease Control (CDC), HIV-positive persons with fewer than 200 CD4+ T cells per μL are considered as having AIDS, even in the absence of symptoms and/or opportunistic infection.[35] Depending on the host and other as yet unidentified factors, the type of symptoms and length of time before severe illness occurs varies. In patients with a terminal illness, antibody to the core proteins may fall in titer and even disappear.

TRANSFUSION-ASSOCIATED AIDS (TAA)

There is no question as to the infectivity of blood and components from individuals infected with HIV.[36] Recipients have developed AIDS after receiving a single contaminated unit of whole blood or any of its components. Derivatives from human blood such as albumin and immunoglobulins have not been reported to transmit HIV infection. Coagulation concentrates if heat treated or purified by chemical or antibody methods have little risk of transmitting HIV infection when these products are made from donor plasma that has been screened for anti-HIV.

As of January 1, 1993, transfusion or tissue transplantation had been reported as the only identifiable risk in 5286 AIDS cases reported to the CDC.[37] In addition, 2214 cases have occurred in patients with hemophilia. Although TAA represents about 2 percent of all AIDS cases, it accounts for 7 percent of cases among women and in individuals less than 13 years of age. Except for a very few cases (21 reported as of December 31, 1992), the transfusions were given before routine testing for anti-HIV was available. All cases reported from blood collected in the United States have been due to HIV-1.

The mean incubation period between the time of transfusion and diagnosis of AIDS was estimated to be 4.5 years with a range of 2 to 14 years.[38] This long incubation period and a high mortality among transfusion recipients (approximately 50 percent within 6 months) makes it difficult to determine the actual risk of TAA from blood and components collected before the availability of serologic tests for anti-HIV. Estimates of the risk from blood collected since testing has been available place the risk in the range of 1 case per 250,000 units transfused.[10]

HUMAN T-CELL LYMPHOTROPIC VIRUS TYPE I

Human T-cell lymphotropic virus type I is an oncogenic retrovirus that causes adult T-cell leukemia (ATL) and several neuromuscular wasting syndromes. This RNA virus is endemic in southern Japan and the Caribbean basin. It has rarely been associated with transfusion-transmitted disease; however, seroconversion (development of anti–HTLV-I) has been observed in recipients of fresh blood components prepared from seropositive donors.[39] Seropositivity has also been found in drug addicts.

A study of about 40,000 US blood donors, using an ELISA and confirmation by Western blotting and radio immunoprecipitation assay (RIPA), found six confirmably positive donors.[40] All of these were residents of the southeastern United States, and most were black women. Routine testing of all donors was instituted because of concerns related to the long incubation period of ATL and the possibility of transmission of HTLV-I infection by blood transfusion.

Cytomegalovirus and Epstein-Barr Virus

Two viruses in the family *Herpesviridae*—cytomegalovirus (CMV) and Epstein-Barr virus (EBV)—can cause disease following transfusion.[41] These are DNA viruses that can persist in the host and cause latent infection. Antibodies to these agents are found with high frequency, indicating that they are prevalent in many populations (CMV, 40 to 90 percent; EBV, 90 percent). Inasmuch as a large percentage of recipients are carriers of these viruses, transmission by donor blood should not be a significant route of infection. This is true for EBV, which rarely causes infectious mononucleosis–like illness following cardiopulmonary bypass.

Transfusion-associated CMV infection is a problem, particularly in neonates and immunosuppressed patients. Convincing evidence exists that low birth weight infants (less than 1250 g) born to anti-CMV–negative women have less morbidity and mortality when they are transfused with blood and components lacking anti-CMV or from which white cells have been removed (e.g., filtering, freeze-thawing, washing).[42] The effects of CMV on transplant recipients is less clear. In some patients immunosuppression can reactivate latent infection, in others the organ is the source of infection, and in still others transfusion plays a role.

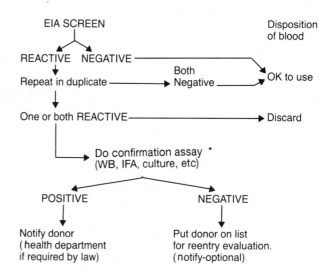

* If the screening test is a combination anti-HIV-1, HIV-2 additional testing with anti-HIV-1 and anti-HIV-2 reagents is indicated.

FIGURE 19–7 Flow diagram for testing donor samples for anti-HIV.

CMV infection is a serious complication in patients given an allogeneic bone marrow transplant.

Prevention of CMV complications requires testing of donors and patients. If the blood of the mother of a low birth weight infant is found to have anti-CMV, giving blood tested for anti-CMV is not worthwhile. The use of tested blood in transplant patients depends on the protocol and the CMV status of the recipient.

Testing for Viral Markers

Several test systems are available to detect the presence of markers of viral infection. Each test varies in sensitivity and specificity and requires careful quality control. Confirmation of a reactive screening test is also important, particularly when it is found in a healthy blood donor. The general scheme shown in Figure 19–7 for anti-HIV testing can also be applied to other markers. The general principles of the tests are shown in Table 19–4. In almost all systems detection is based on a labeled antibody or antigen. In the case of HBV and HIV, although the tests are very sensitive, not all infectious units will be detectable. It is also possible that an infectious individual early in the incubation phase of the disease may not have been seroconverted when tested (see Figs. 19–4 and 19–6).

Testing for HIV

The ELISA systems developed to screen blood donors (Table 19–5) for anti-HIV have been based on

TABLE 19–4 TESTS FOR VIRAL HEPATITIS MARKERS: PRINCIPLES AND CALCULATIONS

Principle	Method	Calculation Radioimmunoassay/ELISA*		Test for
Direct	Antibody-coated solid phase + Unknown + Labeled antibody	— ↑cpm ↑OD	A/A	HBsAg HBeAg
Sandwich	Antigen-coated solid phase + Unknown + Labeled antigen	— ↑cpm ↑OD	A/A	Anti-HBs
Antigen capture	Anti-IgM–coated solid phase + Unknown (specific antibody-IgM class) + Antigen + labeled antibody	— ↑cpm ↑OD	B/B	IgM Anti-HAV
Indirect	Antigen-coated solid phase + Unknown + labeled antibody	— ↓cpm ↓OD	C/C	Anti-HBc Anti-HBc Anti-HAV
Competitive	Antibody-coated solid phase + Unknown + antigen	— ↓cpm ↓OD	C/C	Anti-HBe

*Method of calculating negative cutoff value: Radioimmunoassay Tests

A Factor (e.g., 2.1) × mean negative control counts per minute (cpm).
B Mean negative control cpm + 0.1 (mean positive control cpm)
C $\dfrac{\text{Mean negative control cpm} + \text{mean positive control cpm}}{2}$

EIA Tests:

A Factor (e.g., 0.05) + mean negative control optical density (OD)
B Factor (mean positive control OD) + mean negative control OD
C Factor (mean negative control OD) + factor (mean positive control OD)

TABLE 19–5 **PRINCIPLES OF TEST METHODS—DETECTION OF HIV ANTIBODIES AND ANTIGENS**

Enzyme-Labeled Antiglobulin	Western Blot	Antigen Capture
Antigen on solid phase*	Separate viral lysate in SDS—PAGE Transblot to a membrane	Anti-HIV on solid phase
Diluted unknown serum	Incubate with unknown serum	Unknown sample Antibody to specific HIV protein (probe)
Labeled antihumn Ig or antigen	Labeled antihuman Ig	Labeled antiprobe Ig
Substrate-chromogen	Substrate-chromogen	Substrate-chromogen
Measure color (proportional to amount of anti-HIV)	Evaluate bands present	Measure color (proportional to amount of captured antigen)

*Viral lysate, recombinant, or synthetic peptide.

indirect detection of antibody similar to the antihuman globulin method for detecting red cell antibodies. Material containing the appropriate viral epitopes is coated onto a solid phase such as a bead or microtiter well. Antigen is derived from viral cultures by disruption of the infected host cell. This material is then purified and treated to eliminate the risk of infectivity. Other approaches to obtaining antigen are the use of recombinant material or synthesizing polypeptides containing the desired epitope. Reagents that detect donor antibody bound to the antigen on the solid phase are polyspecific or monospecific antihuman immunoglobulin (goat, murine monoclonal) labeled with enzyme (horseradish peroxidase, alkaline phosphatase). A chromogenic substrate is used to obtain a colorimetric reaction that can be read in a spectrophotometer. Most tests also require a blocking agent to be used as part of the sample diluent. These include combinations of various animal proteins, powdered milk, and proprietary substances, which are intended to prevent nonspecific attachment of immunoglobulin in the unknown to the coated solid phase. A stop solution (1N sulfuric acid, sodium hydroxide) is usually used to terminate the color development after a specified time interval. Also available are direct testing systems, which also depend on antibody in the unknown attaching to the antigen on the solid phase. Detection of bound antibody depends on binding of labeled purified antigen. These methods are often referred to as sandwich systems.

Because the number of false-positive test results compared with true-positives is high when screening normal donors with a low prevalence of disease and because there can be lot-to-lot variation in the specificity of the test reagents, FDA protocols have been developed to allow reentry of donors whose subsequent anti-HIV, anti-HCV, or HBsAg tests are nonreactive.[43,44] These reentry schemes require a defined interval between the reactive test and the subsequent test. This is based on the observation that seroconverters whose initial test was weakly positive will show increased reactivity over time. Other requirements for reentry include use of multiple reagents and negative results with specified confirmation assays.

CONFIRMATION ASSAYS: WESTERN BLOTTING, IMMUNOFLUORESCENCE, AND POLYMERASE CHAIN REACTION

Transblotting, first described by E.M. Southern (Southern blots) as a method to study DNA, when applied to proteins is referred to as Western blotting (WB). This technique is useful in detecting the presence of anti-HIV and determining with which viral components the antibodies react. This test is both sensitive and specific, but its technical complexity precludes using it as a screening test.

The various components of a purified, heat-treated, viral lysate dissolved in sodium dodecyl sulfate (SDS) are separated electrophoretically on polyacrylamide gel (PAGE). The viral components are distributed according to their molecular weights. The proteins are then transferred (transblotted) by use of electrophoresis from the gel to a nitrocellulose membrane. Commercially prepared transblotted membranes are available. The membrane is divided into multiple strips, which are incubated with blocking agents before the sample is added. Incubation and rotation of the unknown with the strip is followed by washing. If antibodies in the unknown have reacted with the viral proteins, the bands will be detected by the indicator system (i.e., biotinylated antihuman IgG). After incubation and washing, avidin-labeled alkaline phosphatase is added. This is followed by a nitro blue tetrazolium, 5-bromo-4-chloro-3-iodophosphate substrate and stain. Known anti-HIV–positive and –negative samples must be run with each membrane. It is also useful to run molecular weight standards when doing electrophoresis and transblotting. Interpretation of WB results depends on the bands detected (see Table 19–3).[44] Most patients with AIDS and donors with anti-HIV show multiple bands, including p17/18, p24, p31, gp41, p65, gp120, and gp160; however, in some cases very few bands are seen. Usually these blots are called indeterminate, and repeat samples are requested. In healthy donors without other risk factors, indeterminate blots that do not change over 6 months are considered false-positive, although the individual is not eligible as a donor.

Immunofluorescence assays (IFA) based on the reaction of unknown sera with cells infected with HIV have been shown to have good sensitivity and specificity. Reactive samples are detected by using a fluorescent labeled antibody that gives a distinct pattern when anti-HIV reacts with the cells on a coated slide.

The most sensitive assay for the detection of HIV infection is the polymerase chain reaction (PCR).[45] This test depends on the amplification of HIV integrated in the DNA of infected cells. PCR systems require several cycles with a thermostable polymerase at carefully controlled temperatures and need specific primers present as templates for the amplified DNA. The detection of the amplification product is by a labeled probe in an immunoblot assay. This method, although extremely sensitive, requires careful control to ensure that positive reactions are specific.

Review Questions

1. What is the most important step in ensuring that transfused blood is safe?
   A. Using the most sensitive testing techniques available
   B. Using the most specific testing techniques available
   C. Carefully selecting the donor
   D. Carefully selecting the recipient

2. Infection of which virus is usually by the oral-fecal route?
   A. HAV
   B. HBV
   C. HDV
   D. HCV

3. Which of the following should be given to a low birth weight infant if the mother is anti-CMV negative?
   A. Whole blood from a donor with anti-CMV
   B. Red cells from a donor who is anti-CMV negative
   C. It does not matter whether anti-CMV is present or not
   D. None of the above

4. Testing donors for anti-HBc was thought to prevent transmission of which of the following infections?
   A. Hepatitis A
   B. AIDS
   C. Hepatitis B
   D. Non-A, non-B hepatitis

5. Which of the following test or tests is useful to confirm that a patient or donor is infected with HCV?
   A. ALT + anti-HBc
   B. Anti–HIV-1/2

C. Lymph node biopsy
D. RIBA

Answers to Review Questions

1. C (p 376)
2. A (p 378)
3. B (p 383)
4. D (p 381)
5. D (p 381)

References

1. Alter, HJ: You'll wonder where the yellow went: A 15-year retrospective of post transfusion hepatitis. In Moore, SB (ed): Transfusion Transmitted Viral Disease. American Association of Blood Banks, Arlington, VA, 1987, pp 53–86.
2. Pindyk, J, et al: Measures to decrease the risk of acquired immunodeficiency syndrome transmission by blood transfusion. Evidence of volunteer blood donor cooperation. Transfusion 25:3, 1985.
3. Widmann, F (ed): Standards for Blood Bank and Transfusion Services, ed 15. American Association of Blood Banks, Bethesda, MD, 1993.
4. Code of Federal Regulations: Current edition. 21 Food and Drugs, parts 600–700. US Government Printing Office, Washington, DC, 1993.
5. Galen, RS and Gambino, SR: Beyond Normality: The Predictive Value and Efficiency of Medical Diagnosis. John Wiley & Sons, New York, 1975.
6. Hanson, M and Polesky, HF: A method for calculating the risk of donors implicated in transfusion-associated hepatitis. Proceedings of the International Hepatitis Workshop, Stirling, Scotland, 1982, pp 99–100.
7. Ladd, DJ and Hillis, A: A new method for evaluating the hepatitis risk of the multiply-implicated donor. Transfusion 24:80, 1984.
8. Chauhan, A, et al: Hepatitis E virus transmission to a volunteer. Lancet 341:149, 1993.
9. Polesky, HF and Hanson, M: Transfusion-associated hepatitis: A dilemma. Lab Med 14:717, 1983.
10. Dodd, RY: The risk of transfusion-transmitted infection. N Engl J Med 327:419, 1992.
11. Seef, LB, et al: Long-term mortality after transfusion-associated non-A, non-B hepatitis. N Engl J Med 327:1906, 1992.
12. Aach, RD: Primary hepatic viruses: Hepatitis A, hepatitis B, delta hepatitis and non-A, non-B hepatitis. In Insalaco, SJ and Menitove, JE (eds): Transfusion-Transmitted Viruses: Epidemiology and Pathology. American Association of Blood Banks, Arlington, VA, 1987, pp 17–40.
13. Hollinger, FB, et al: Posttransfusion hepatitis type A. JAMA 250:2313, 1983.
14. Mason, WS, Seal, G, and Summers, J: Virus of Peking ducks with structural and biological relatedness to human hepatitis B virus. J Virol 36:829, 1980.
15. Blumberg, BS, Alter, HJ, and Visnich, S: A "new" antigen in leukemia sera. JAMA 191:541, 1965.
16. Szmuness, W, et al: Hepatitis B vaccine: Demonstration of efficacy in a controlled clinical trial in a high risk population in the United States. N Engl J Med 303:833, 1980.
17. Stevens, CE, et al: Yeast-recombinant hepatitis B vaccine: Efficacy with hepatitis B immune globulin in prevention of perinatal hepatitis B virus transmission. JAMA 257:2612, 1987.
18. Centers for Disease Control: Immunization Practices Advisory Committee recommendations for hepatitis B virus: A comprehensive strategy for eliminating transmission in the United States through universal childhood vaccination. MMWR 40:11, 1991.

19. Rizzetto, M: Biology and characterization of the delta agent. In Szmuness, W, Alter, H, and Maynard, J (eds): Viral Hepatitis 1981 International Symposium. Franklin Institute Press, Philadelphia, 1982, pp 355–362.

20. Craig, JR: Hepatitis delta virus: No longer a defective virus. Am J Clin Pathol 98:552, 1992.

21. Rosina, F, Saracco, G, and Rizzetto, M: Risk of post transfusion infection with the hepatitis delta virus: A multi-center study. N Engl J Med 312:1488, 1985.

22. Choo, Q-L, et al: Isolation of a clone derived from blood-borne non-A, non-B viral hepatitis genome. Science 244:359, 1989.

23. Kuo, G, et al: An assay for circulating antibodies to a major etiologic virus of human non-A, non-B hepatitis. Science 244:363, 1989.

24. Alter, MJ, et al: The natural history of community-acquired hepatitis C in the United States. N Engl J Med 327:1899, 1992.

25. Aach, RD, et al: Hepatitis C virus infection in post-transfusion hepatitis: An analysis with first- and second-generation assays. N Engl J Med 325:1325, 1991.

26. Esteban, JI, et al: Evaluation of antibodies to hepatitis C virus in a study of transfusion-associated hepatitis. N Engl J Med 323:1107, 1990.

27. Alter, MJ, et al: Risk factors for acute non-A, non-B hepatitis in the United States and association with hepatitis C virus infection. JAMA 264:2231, 1990.

28. Davis, GL, et al: Treatment of hepatitis C with recombinant interferon alfa: A multicenter randomized, controlled trial. N Engl J Med 321:1501, 1989.

29. Aach, RD, et al: Serum alanine aminotransferase of donors in relation to the risk of non-A, non-B hepatitis in recipients: The transfusion-transmitted viruses study. N Engl J Med 304:989, 1981.

30. Stevens, CE, et al: Hepatitis B antibody in blood donors and occurrence of non-A, non-B hepatitis in transfusion reagents: An analysis of the transfusion-transmitted viruses study. Ann Intern Med 104:488. 1984.

31. Hoofnagle, JH: Posttransfusion hepatitis B. Transfusion 30:384, 1990.

32. Hanson, MR and Polesky, HF: Evaluation of routine anti-HBc screening of volunteer blood donors: A questionable surrogate test for non-A, non-B hepatitis. Transfusion 27:107, 1987.

33. Smith, TF: Structure, classification and replication of viruses. In Insalaco, SJ and Menitove, JE (eds): Transfusion-Transmitted Viruses: Epidemiology and Pathology. American Association of Blood Banks, Arlington, VA, 1987, pp 1–16.

34. Allain, JP, et al: Serologic markers in early stages of human immunodeficiency virus infection in haemophiliacs. Lancet ii:1233, 1986.

35. Centers for Disease Control and Prevention: 1993 revised classification system for HIV infection and expanded surveillance case definition for AIDS among adolescents and adults. MMWR 41/RR-17:1, 1992.

36. Busch, MP: Retroviruses and blood transfusions: The lessons learned and the challenge yet ahead. In Nance, SJ (ed): Blood safety: Current challenges. American Association of Blood Banks, Bethesda, MD, 1992, pp 1–44.

37. Centers for Disease Control and Prevention: HIV/AIDS surveillance report. 1, 1993.

38. Lui, KJ, et al: A model-based approach for estimating the mean incubation period of transfusion-associated acquired immunodeficiency syndrome. Proc Natl Acad Sci 83:3051, 1987.

39. Okachi, K, Sato, H, and Himuma, Y: A retrospective study in transmission of adult T cell leukemia virus by blood transfusion: Sero-conversion in recipients. Vox Sang 46:245, 1984.

40. Williams, AE, et al: Seroprevalence and epidemiological correlates of HTLV-I infection in US blood donors. Science 240:643, 1988.

41. Tegtmeier, GE: The role of blood transfusion in the transmission of herpes viruses. In Insalaco, SJ and Menitove, JE (eds): Transfusion-Transmitted Viruses: Epidemiology and Pathology. American Association of Blood Banks, Arlington, VA, 1987, pp 41–68.

42. Eisenfeld, L, Silver, H, and McLaughlin, J: Prevention of transfusion-associated cytomegalovirus infection in neonatal patients by removal of white cells from blood. Transfusion 32:205, 1992.

43. Zoon, KC: Revised recommendations for prevention of human immunodeficiency virus (HIV) transmission by blood and blood products. FDA, Center for Biologics Evaluation and Research, Bethesda, MD, 1992, pp 1–21.

44. Centers for Disease Control: Interpretative criteria used to report Western blot results for HIV-1–antibody testing—United States. MMWR 40:692, 1991.

45. Jackson, JB: The polymerase chain reaction in transfusion medicine. Transfusion 30:51, 1990.

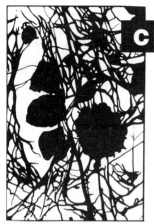

CHAPTER 20

Hemolytic Disease of the Newborn and Fetus

Melanie S. Kennedy, MD
Abdul Waheed, MS, MT(ASCP)SBB

OBJECTIVES

Upon completion of this chapter, the learner should be able to:

1 State the definition and characteristics of hemolytic disease of the newborn.
2 Describe the role of the technologist in the diagnosis and clinical management of hemolytic disease of the newborn.

3 Compare and contrast ABO versus Rh hemolytic disease of the newborn in terms of:

   a Pathogenesis

   b Incidence

   c Blood types of mother and baby

   d Severity of disease

   e Laboratory data: anemia, direct antiglobulin test, bilirubin

   f Prevention and treatment

4 Define Rh immune globulin and describe its function.

5 Identify the requirements that must be met before a woman can receive Rh immune globulin.

6 List the tests used for detection of fetomaternal hemorrhage.

7 Outline the protocol for testing of maternal and cord blood in cases of suspected hemolytic disease of the newborn.

8 Given maternal and infant ABO blood group phenotypes, state the possible ABO donor blood group(s) you would select for an exchange transfusion. Be specific as to donor blood groups for both the plasma and red blood cells.

9 State the blood components, and the maximum age of the donor unit preferred, for intrauterine or exchange transfusions.

10 State with whom (mother and child) the crossmatch for a neonate must always be compatible.

Hemolytic disease of the newborn and fetus (HDN) is the destruction of the red blood cells (RBCs) of the fetus and neonate by antibodies produced by the mother. The mother can be stimulated to form the antibodies by previous pregnancy or transfusion; a small number occur during the pregnancy itself. Previously, about 95 percent of the cases were due to antibodies in the mother directed against the Rh antigen D or Rh_o. The incidence of the disease due to anti-D has steadily decreased since 1968 with the introduction of Rh immune globulin (RhIg). Currently, $Rh_o(D)$ incompatibility is still the most common, although other RBC incompatibilities are increasing in incidence at referral centers.[1] Because $Rh_o(D)$ incompatibility was the major concern for many years, the diagnosis and treatment of HDN due to anti-D has been the emphasis of much investigation. These findings can be applied to other clinically significant RBC antibodies causing HDN, except for ABO antibodies, which will be discussed separately.

In addition to the use of RhIg, many other advances have been made in the diagnosis and treatment of HDN. Ultrasound and percutaneous umbilical blood sampling have greatly increased the success of accurately diagnosing and adequately treating this disease.

Etiology

HISTORIC OVERVIEW

Although the changes in the fetus and newborn were noted as early as the 17th century, it was not until 1939 that Levine and Stetson reported a transfusion reaction from transfusing the husband's blood to a postpartum woman. They postulated the mother had been immunized to the father's antigen through the fetus.

Then in 1940, Landsteiner and Wiener conducted the experiments immunizing rabbits and guinea pigs to rhesus monkey RBCs. Levine, using the serum from these experiments, demonstrated the mother who had the transfusion reaction was rhesus negative and the father rhesus positive. In addition, the mother's serum agglutinated the father's RBCs.

DISEASE MECHANISM

Hemolytic disease of the newborn and fetus is caused by the destruction of the RBCs of the fetus by antibodies produced by the mother. Only antibodies of the immunoglobulin G (IgG) class are actively transported across the placenta; other classes, such as IgA and IgM, are not. Most IgG antibodies are directed against bacterial, fungal, and viral antigens, so the transfer of IgG from the mother to the fetus is beneficial. However, in HDN, the antibodies are directed against paternal antigens on the fetal RBCs.

Rh HEMOLYTIC DISEASE OF THE NEWBORN AND FETUS

Usually in the case of Rh disease, the Rh-positive first-born infant of an Rh-negative mother is unaffected because the mother has not yet been immu-

Pathogenesis

Fetomaternal Hemorrhage
↓
Maternal Antibodies Formed Against
Paternally Derived Antigens
↓
During Subsequent Pregnancy, Placental
Passage of Maternal IgG Antibodies
↓
Maternal Antibody Attaches
to Fetal Red Blood Cells
↓
Fetal Red Blood Cell Hemolysis

FIGURE 20–1 Pathogenesis of hemolytic disease of the newborn and fetus.

nized. During gestation, and particularly at delivery when the placenta separates from the uterus, variable numbers of fetal RBCs enter the maternal circulation (**see Color Plate 15**). These fetal cells, carrying Rh antigen inherited from the father, immunize the mother and stimulate the production of anti-D. Once the mother is immunized to Rh antigen, all subsequent offspring inheriting the D antigen will be affected. The maternal anti-D will cross the placenta and bind to the fetal Rh-positive cells (Fig. 20–1). The sensitized RBCs are destroyed by the fetal reticuloendothelial system, resulting in anemia.

FACTORS AFFECTING IMMUNIZATION AND SEVERITY

Antigenic Exposure

Transplacental hemorrhage of fetal RBCs into the maternal circulation occurs in some women during gestation.[2] This may occur in from 0.4 percent to 7.0 percent of pregnant women. In addition, interventions such as amniocentesis and chorionic villus sampling, as well as trauma to the abdomen, increase the number of women with fetomaternal hemorrhage. At delivery, the incidence is more than 50 percent. However, as little as 1 ml of fetal RBCs can immunize the mother.

Fetomaternal hemorrhage during pregnancy can cause significant increases in maternal antibody titers, leading to increasing severity of HDN. In addition, the number of antigenic sites on the fetal RBCs corresponds to heterozygous RBCs, as all fetal antigens incompatible with the mother must have been inherited from the father, who can give only one gene to the fetus. Generally heterozygous RBCs have fewer antigenic sites than homozygous RBCs.

Host Factors

The ability of individuals to produce antibody in response to antigenic exposure varies depending on complex genetic factors. In Rh-negative individuals who are transfused with 1 unit of Rh-positive red blood, about 80 percent will form anti-D.[3] Nearly all of the nonresponders will fail to produce anti-D even with repeated exposures to Rh-positive blood. On the other hand, the risk of immunization is only about 10 percent for an Rh-negative mother after an Rh-positive pregnancy if RhIg is not administered.

Immunoglobulin Class

Immunoglobulin class and subclass of the maternal antibody affect the severity of the HDN. Of the immunoglobulin classes (IgG, IgM, IgA, IgE, and IgD), only IgG is transported across the placenta. The active transport of IgG begins in the second trimester and continues until birth. The IgG molecules are transported via the Fc portion of the antibodies.

Of the four subclasses of IgG antibody, IgG_1 and IgG_3 are more efficient in RBC hemolysis than are IgG_2 and IgG_4. Therefore, the subclass(es) in the mother can affect the severity of the hemolytic disease.

Antibody Specificity

Of all the RBC antigens, Rh(D) is the most antigenic. For this reason, only Rh-negative blood is transfused to Rh-negative women of childbearing age. Other antigens in the Rh system, such as C(rh′), E(rh″), and c(hr′), are also potent immunogens (although less potent than D); these antibodies are encountered in transfused patients frequently and in pregnant patients less often. These other Rh antibodies have been associated with moderate to severe cases of HDN. Anti-E in particular has caused HDN severe enough to require intervention and treatment.

Of the non–Rh-system antibodies, anti-Kell is considered the most clinically significant in its ability to cause HDN. Almost any IgG RBC antibody is capable of causing HDN, although the disease caused by these antibodies is usually moderate in severity. Nevertheless, all pregnant women with IgG RBC antibodies should be followed closely for HDN. Vengelen-Tyler[4] lists and discusses 64 different RBC antibody specificities reported to cause HDN.

Influence of ABO Group

When the mother is ABO incompatible with the fetus (major incompatibility), the incidence of detectable fetomaternal hemorrhage decreases. Investigators noted many years ago that the incidence of Rh immunization is less in those mothers with major ABO incompatibility with the fetus. The ABO incompatibility protects somewhat against Rh immunization apparently by the hemolysis in the mother's circulation of

ABO-incompatible Rh-positive fetal RBCs before the Rh antigen can be recognized by the mother's immune system.

Pathogenesis

HEMOLYSIS AND ERYTHROPOIESIS

Hemolysis (RBC destruction) occurs when maternal IgG attaches to specific antigens of the fetal RBCs (see Fig. 20–1 and **Color Plate 16**). The antibody-coated cells are then removed from the circulation by the macrophages of the spleen. Depending on the amount of antibody, specificity, avidity, and other antibody characteristics, the amount of fetal RBCs destroyed can cause anemia. The fetal bone marrow and other hemopoietic tissues in the spleen and liver increase the amount of RBCs produced, even to the point of releasing immature (nucleated) RBCs into the circulation. The term "erythroblastosis fetalis" was used to describe this finding.

ANEMIA

The fetal anemia may range from mild to severe, depending on the amount of fetal RBCs that are destroyed and the capacity of the fetal erythropoiesis to compensate. If the anemia becomes severe, the fetus may develop hydrops fetalis: severe edema, effusions, and ascites from the extremely enlarged liver and spleen, causing portal hypertension and hepatocellular damage. In the past, hydrops fetalis was almost uniformly fatal; currently, most of these fetuses can be successfully treated.[1,5]

The process of RBC destruction goes on even after such an infant is delivered alive—in fact, as long as maternal antibody persists in the newborn infant's circulation. The rate of RBC destruction after birth decreases because no more maternal antibody is entering the infant's circulation through the placenta. However, IgG is distributed both extravascularly and intravascularly and has a half-life of 25 days, so sensitization and hemolysis of RBCs continues for several days to weeks after delivery.

BILIRUBIN

The RBC destruction releases hemoglobin, which is metabolized to bilirubin (Fig. 20–2). This bilirubin is called "indirect," in that indirect methods are required to measure the bilirubin in the laboratory. The indirect bilirubin is transported across the placenta and conjugated in the maternal liver to "direct" bilirubin. The conjugated bilirubin is then excreted by the mother. Although levels of total bilirubin in the fetal circulation and in the amniotic fluid may be elevated, these do not cause clinical disease in the fetus. However, after birth, accumulation of metabolic by-products of RBC destruction can become a severe problem for the newborn infant. The newborn liver is unable to

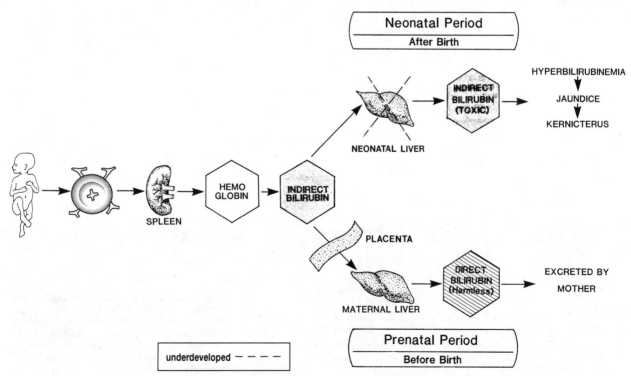

FIGURE 20–2 Metabolism of bilirubin in the fetus and newborn. (Courtesy Ortho Diagnostic Systems, Raritan, NJ.)

conjugate bilirubin efficiently, especially in premature infants. With moderate to severe hemolysis, the unconjugated or indirect bilirubin can reach levels toxic to the infant's brain (generally >18 mg/dl), which, if left untreated, can cause kernicterus or permanent damage to parts of the brain.

Diagnosis and Management

The diagnosis and management of HDN require close cooperation among the pregnant patient, her obstetrician, her spouse or partner, and the personnel of the clinical laboratory performing the serologic testing. Serologic and clinical tests performed at appropriate times during the pregnancy can accurately determine the level of antibody in the maternal circulation, the potential of the antibody causing hemolytic disease, and the severity of RBC destruction during gestation (Fig. 20–3). If clinical and serologic data indicate the fetus is becoming severely anemic, interventions such as intrauterine transfusion can be used to treat the anemia and prevent the development of severe disease.

SEROLOGIC TESTING

The recommended obstetric practice is to perform a type and antibody screen at the first prenatal visit, preferably during the first trimester. At that time, the pregnant woman can be asked about previous pregnancies and their outcomes. Previous severe disease and poor outcome predict similar findings in the current pregnancy.

ABO and Rh Testing

The testing of the specimen should include ABO and Rh testing for D and, if immediate spin is nonreactive for D, for D^u antigen, or weakened expression of D. The patient's RBCs should also be tested simultaneously with Rh control reagent while testing for D^u. If D^u positive, the patient can be considered Rh positive. In rare cases, D^u phenotype is caused by missing a part of the Rh antigen. Such patients may produce anti-D, as an alloantibody, which has been reported to cause HDN.

Antibody Detection Test (Antibody Screen)

The test conditions must be able to detect all clinically significant IgG alloantibodies that are reactive at 37°C and in the antiglobulin phase. At least two separate reagent screening cells, covering all common blood group antigens, should be used. An antibody-enhancing medium such as albumin or low ionic strength saline solution (LISS) can increase sensitivity of the assay. Many prenatal patients produce clinically insignificant antibodies, such as Lewis specificities. Therefore, many workers in this field encourage omitting immediate spin and room temperature incubation phases and using anti-IgG, rather than broad-spectrum, antiglobulin reagent. These steps reduce detection of IgM antibodies, which cannot cross the placenta.

If the antibody screen is nonreactive, repeat testing is recommended at 20 to 24 weeks' gestation and again at delivery.

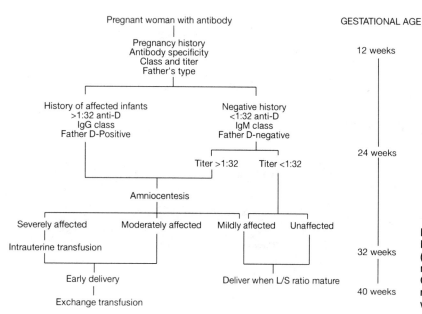

FIGURE 20–3 Diagnosis and management of hemolytic disease of the newborn and fetus. (From Kennedy, MS: Essentials of immunohematology and blood therapy. In Zuspan, FP and Quilligan, EJ (eds): Practical Manual of Obstetrical Care. CV Mosby, St Louis, 1982, p 119, with permission.)

Antibody Specificity

If the antibody screen is reactive, the antibody specificity must be determined. Follow-up testing will depend on the antibody specificity.

Cold reactive IgM antibodies such as anti-I, anti-IH, anti-Le^a, anti-Le^b, and anti-P$_1$ can be ignored. As mentioned earlier, Lewis system antibodies are rather common in pregnant women but have not been reported to cause HDN.

Antibodies such as anti-M and anti-N can be IgM, IgG, or a combination of both. Both anti-M and anti-N can cause mild to moderate HDN. To establish the immunoglobulin class, the serum can be treated with sulfhydryl reagents such as dithiothreitol (DTT) or 2-mercaptoethanol, and then retested with appropriate controls. IgM antibodies will be destroyed by this treatment; IgG antibodies will remain.

Many Rh-negative pregnant women will have weakly reactive anti-D, particularly during the third trimester. Most of these women will have received RhIg (see farther on), either after an event with increased risk of fetomaternal hemorrhage or at 28 weeks' gestation. The passively administered anti-D will be weakly reactive in testing and will remain demonstrable for 2 to 3 months or longer. This must be distinguished from active immunization. A titer of 1:4 or higher almost always indicates active immunization. With a titer under 1:4, active immunization cannot be ruled out but is less likely.

If the antibody specificity is determined to be clinically significant and the antibody is IgG, further testing is required. Other than anti-D, the most common and most significant antibodies are anti-K, anti-E, anti-c, anti-C, and anti-Fy^a.

Paternal Phenotype

A specimen of the father's blood should be obtained and tested for the presence and zygosity of the corresponding antigen. If the mother has anti-D and the father is D positive, a complete Rh phenotype can help determine his chance of being homozygous or heterozygous for the D antigen. The information is helpful in planning further testing of the mother and in counseling her.

In cases of antibody specificity other than D, testing the father can save a great deal of time, expense, and worry if he is shown to lack the corresponding antigen. The mother must be counseled in private as to the paternity of the fetus.

Antibody Titers

The relative concentration of all antibodies capable of crossing the placenta and causing HDN must be determined by antibody titration. The patient serum is serially diluted and tested against appropriate RBCs to determine the highest dilution at which a reaction occurs. The method must include the indirect antiglobulin phase using anti-IgG reagent. The result is expressed as either the reciprocal of the titration end point or as a titer score.

The titration must be performed exactly the same way each time the patient's serum is tested. The RBCs used for each titration should be of the same genotype (preferably from the same donor), approximately the same storage time, and the same concentration. The first serum specimen should be frozen and run in parallel with later specimens. Only a difference of greater than two dilutions or a score change of more than 10 should be considered as a significant change in titer.

Each laboratory should develop its own critical titer levels by reviewing the outcome of a number of pregnancies complicated by HDN. In general, a titer of 32 is considered significant. If the initial titer is 32 or higher, a second titer should be done at about 18 to 20 weeks' gestation. A titer reproducibly and repeatedly at 32 or above represents an indication for amniocentesis or percutaneous umbilical blood sampling between 20 and 24 weeks' gestation.

When the titer is 16 or less, the titer should be repeated monthly during the second trimester, beginning at 18 to 20 weeks' gestation, and biweekly during the third trimester. The last determination should be made within a week of the expected date of delivery.

Antibody titer in itself cannot predict the severity of HDN. In some sensitized women, the antibody titer may remain moderately high throughout pregnancy while the fetus is becoming more and more severely affected. Similarly, a previously sensitized woman may have consistently high antibody titer whether pregnant or not and, if pregnant, whether the fetus is Rh positive or Rh negative. In others, the titer may rise rapidly, which portends increasing HDN. However, antibody titers consistently below the laboratory's critical level throughout the pregnancy reliably predict an unaffected or only moderately affected fetus.

AMNIOCENTESIS AND CORDOCENTESIS

At about 24 weeks' gestation, further diagnosis and treatment is begun. Patients with a history of a severely affected fetus or early fetal death may require earlier intervention. Under ultrasound guidance, amniocentesis or cordocentesis or both is done to assess the status of the fetus. The amniotic fluid is subjected to a spectrophotometric scan at steadily increasing wavelengths, so that the change in the optical density (ΔOD) at 450 nm (the absorbance of bilirubin) can be calculated. The measurement is plotted on the Liley graph (Fig. 20–4) according to gestational age. The optical density of the amniotic fluid is high in the second trimester and steadily decreases until delivery. An increasing or unchanging ΔOD 450 as pregnancy proceeds predicts worsening of the fetal hemolytic disease and the need for frequent monitoring and

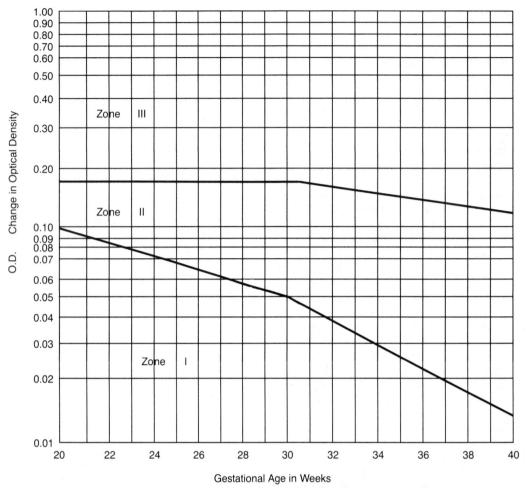

FIGURE 20-4 Liley graph (modified by The Ohio State University Prenatal Laboratory).

intervention if indicated. Values in zone III indicate severe and often life-threatening hemolysis and require urgent intervention. In zone II, most fetuses will have moderate disease that may require intervention. Values in zone I predict mild or no disease, which do not require intervention.

Cordocentesis is performed by cannulating the umbilical vein under ultrasound guidance (Fig. 20–5). The fetal blood sample can be then tested for hemoglobin and hematocrit, blood type, and direct antiglobulin test, and inspected for nucleated RBCs on stained smear. The cordocentesis technique also allows for direct fetal transfusion.

INTRAUTERINE TRANSFUSION

Intrauterine transfusion can also be performed by injecting the RBCs into the fetal peritoneal cavity. The RBCs are then absorbed into the circulation. The peritoneal method is less effective and efficient than cordocentesis in severely ill infants.[1] Cordocentesis is becoming the preferred method in all cases because it is a direct method of assessment and treatment.[5] Ultrasound is also useful in assessing the presence of

edema, effusions, and ascites, which portend severe disease and require urgent intervention.

Amniocentesis and cordocentesis have several risks, among them trauma to the placenta, which may cause increased antibody titers because of antigenic challenge to the mother through fetomaternal hemorrhage.

PLASMA EXCHANGE AND INTRAVENOUS IMMUNE GLOBULIN

Other therapies include repeated high-volume plasma exchange or intravenous immune globulin, or both, for the pregnant woman. The procedures, which are carried out during the second and third trimesters, have had varying success.[1] These therapies may be beneficial in delaying severe hemolytic disease until the fetus is large enough for treatment with intrauterine transfusion.

EARLY DELIVERY

Early delivery was used for many years for moderate to severe disease to interrupt the transport of mater-

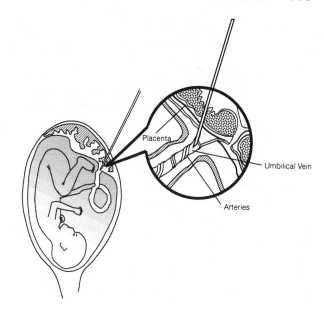

FIGURE 20–5 Technique of percutaneous umbilical blood sampling. (From Ludomirski,[5] p 91, with permission.)

nal antibody to the fetus and allow exchange transfusion. With the use of repeated and frequent intravenous transfusions in the fetus, delivery before the lungs are mature usually can be avoided.

PHOTOTHERAPY

After delivery, phototherapy with ultraviolet light can be used. In infants with mild to moderate hemolysis, the use of phototherapy may avoid the need for exchange transfusion to treat hyperbilirubinemia.

SEROLOGIC TESTING OF THE NEWBORN INFANT

ABO Grouping

ABO antigens are not fully developed in newborn infants and thus may give weak reactions. In addition, the infant does not have his or her own isoagglutinins but may have those of the mother, so reverse grouping cannot be used to confirm the ABO group.

Rh Typing

If the direct antiglobulin test result is strongly positive, Rh reagents with high-protein media can give false-positive results. Therefore, saline reagents are recommended for all RBCs with a positive direct antiglobulin test. In addition, red cells heavily sensitized with anti-D can give a false-negative Rh type, or what has been called, "blocked Rh." An eluate from these red cells will reveal anti-D, and typing of the eluted red cells will show reaction with anti-D.

Direct Antiglobulin Testing

The most important serologic test for diagnosis of HDN is the direct antiglobulin test with anti-IgG re-

agent. The positive test result indicates antibody is coating the infant's RBCs; however, the strength of the reaction does not correlate well with the severity of the HDN. A positive test result may be found in infants without clinical or other laboratory evidence of hemolysis.

Elution

The preparation of an eluate may be helpful when the cause of HDN is in question. The routine preparation of an eluate of all infants with a positive direct antiglobulin test result is unnecessary. As noted earlier, the resolution of a case of "blocked Rh" will require an eluate.

NEWBORN TRANSFUSIONS

The newborn infant may receive small aliquot transfusions or exchange transfusions, or both. Small aliquots can be used to correct anemia when the bilirubin level is not high enough to warrant an exchange transfusion. Exchange transfusions are primarily used to remove high levels of unconjugated bilirubin and thus prevent kernicterus. Premature newborn infants are more likely than full-term infants to require exchange transfusions for elevated bilirubin because their livers are less able to conjugate bilirubin. Other advantages of exchange transfusion include the removal of part of the circulating maternal antibody, removal of sensitized RBCs, replacement of incompatible RBCs with compatible RBCs, and suppression of erythropoiesis (Table 20–1). All of these help interrupt the bilirubin production owing to hemolysis; however, the suppression of erythropoiesis by small aliquot or exchange transfusions may cause anemia to occur after the immediate neonatal period.

Although full-term newborn infants normally have

TABLE 20-1 **BENEFICIAL EFFECTS OF EXCHANGE TRANSFUSION**

Removal of bilirubin
Removal of sensitized RBCs
Removal of incompatible antibody
Replacement of incompatible RBCs with compatible RBCs
Suppression of erythropoiesis (reduced production of incompatible RBCs)

rather high hemoglobin levels (14 to 20 g/dl), below 12 g/dl is considered anemia that may require transfusion. Below 8 g/dl is considered severe anemia and corresponds to zone III of the Liley graph, whereas 8 to 12 g/dl corresponds to zone II. A cord blood sample closely correlates with the levels during gestation. If the obstetrician infuses placenta blood after delivery, the infant's hemoglobin level will be higher than the cord sample.

SELECTION OF BLOOD

Most centers handling HDN use group O RBCs for intrauterine as well as neonatal transfusions. Donors are usually cytomegalovirus (CMV) seronegative, as well. Physicians in these centers are usually transfusing neonates for other indications, such as RBC replacement for blood samples taken for laboratory tests. This allows a small inventory of group O, CMV-seronegative donor units to be set aside for intrauterine and neonatal transfusions. Rh-negative units are selected for those fetuses and neonates whose blood type is unknown or is Rh negative.

For exchange transfusions, a good practice is to prepare RBCs from the whole blood units and then replace the plasma with group AB plasma to reduce the amount of blood group antibodies transfused. This procedure may be avoided if both the fetus or neonate and the mother are the same ABO group.

Blood transfused to the fetus and premature infant should also be gamma irradiated to prevent graft-versus-host disease. It is also recommended that blood be selected that does not contain hemoglobin S, as the decreased oxygen tension that may occur during gestation or early in the neonatal period may cause hemoglobin S–containing blood to sickle. Blood units should be less than 7 days from collection from the donor, except in special circumstances, such as the need for units of mother's blood when high-incidence antibodies are involved.

Rh Immune Globulin

Active immunization induced by RBC antigen can be prevented by the concurrent administration of the corresponding RBC antibody. This principle has been used to prevent immunization to Rh(D) antigen by the use of high-titered RhIg.

During pregnancy and delivery, mixing of fetal and maternal blood occurs. If the mother is Rh negative and the fetus Rh positive, the mother has up to a 9 percent chance of being stimulated to form anti-D.[2] As little as 1 ml of fetal RBCs can elicit a response. Before delivery, the risk of sensitization is 1.5 to 1.9 percent of susceptible women, indicating that a significant amount of fetal RBCs can enter the maternal circulation during pregnancy.[1] However, the greatest risk of immunization to Rh is at delivery.

MECHANISM OF ACTION

The administered RhIg attaches to the fetal Rh-positive RBCs in the maternal circulation. The antibody-coated RBCs are trapped in the maternal spleen where they take up more antibody from the circulating plasma. This activates suppressor cells, the production of blocking antibody, or both. The amount of antibody necessary for the suppressor effect has been determined experimentally and is known to be less than that required to saturate all D antigen sites.[1]

INDICATIONS

Postpartum

The Rh-negative unsensitized mother should receive RhIg soon after delivery of an Rh-positive infant. The recommended time interval is within 72 hours after delivery, based on experiments conducted many years ago. Even if more than 72 hours have elapsed, RhIg should still be given, as it may be effective and is not contraindicated.

The mother should be D negative as well as D^u negative (Fig. 20-6). The infant should be D or D^u positive. If the type of the infant is unknown (e.g., if the infant is stillborn), RhIg should also be administered. Antibody titers are not recommended because the amount of circulating RhIg does not correlate with effectiveness of the immune suppression nor with the amount of fetomaternal hemorrhage.[6]

Antenatal

Because of the known risk of Rh immunization during pregnancy, RhIg should be given early in the third trimester, or at about 28 weeks' gestation. The dose does not pose a risk to the fetus, as this amount will cause a titer of only 1 : 1 or 1 : 2 in the mother.[1] However, a positive direct antiglobulin test result may be observed in the newborn.

If the infant is Rh positive, a second dose is indicated after delivery. The half-life of IgG is about 25 days, so only about 10 percent of the original dose will be present at 40 weeks' gestation. It is essential that the anti-D from antenatal RhIg present at delivery is not interpreted erroneously as active rather than passive immunization. Omission of the indicated dose after delivery may lead to active immunization.

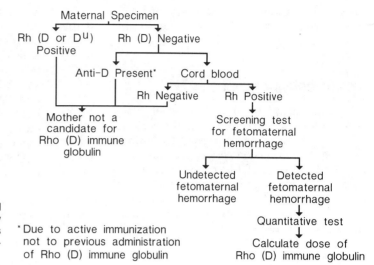

Maternal Specimen

Rh (D or D^U)   Rh (D) Negative
Positive

Anti-D Present*   Cord blood

Rh Negative   Rh Positive

Mother not a
candidate for
Rho (D) immune
globulin

Screening test
for fetomaternal
hemorrhage

Undetected
fetomaternal
hemorrhage

Detected
fetomaternal
hemorrhage

Quantitative test

Calculate dose of
Rho (D) immune globulin

FIGURE 20-6 Decision tree for the indications and dose of Rh immune globulin as determined by laboratory test results. If the cord or neonatal blood specimen is unavailable, assume the fetus is D positive. (From Kennedy,[7] p 235, with permission.)

*Due to active immunization not to previous administration of Rho (D) immune globulin

Other conditions may pose a risk of Rh immunization and therefore require RhIg administration (Table 20–2). The microdose can be used for abortions and ectopic pregnancies before the 12th week of gestation.[7]

DOSE AND ADMINISTRATION

The regular dose vial in the United States contains sufficient anti-D to protect against 15 ml of packed RBCs or 30 ml of whole blood. This is equal to 300 μg of the World Health Organization (WHO) reference material. The regular dose vial in the United Kingdom contains about 100 μg, which appears to be adequate for postpartum prophylaxis.

The microdose (equivalent to 50 μg) is sufficient for abortion, amniocentesis, and ectopic rupture up to 12 weeks' gestation. The total fetal blood volume is estimated to be less than 5 ml at 12 weeks.

Massive fetomaternal hemorrhages of more than 30 ml of whole blood occur in less than 1 percent of deliveries. These massive hemorrhages can lead to immunization if adequate RhIg is not administered. Massive fetomaternal hemorrhages can be detected by the routine use of a screening test such as the rosette technique. Quantitation of the actual amount of hemorrhage must be done by a test such as the Kleihauer-Betke. In this test, a maternal blood smear is treated with acid (or alkali) and then stained with a counterstain. Fetal cells contain hemoglobin resistant to acid or alkali, and will remain red. The maternal cells will appear as ghosts. After several hundred cells are counted, the percentage of fetal cells is determined and the volume of fetal hemorrhage is calculated using the formula:

The calculated volume of fetomaternal hemorrhage is then divided by 30 to determine the number of required vials of RhIg.

In the third trimester, many women will have variable amounts of fetal hemoglobin in their RBCs. It is important to distinguish these cells having smaller amounts of fetal hemoglobin from true fetal RBCs.

The number of vials for transfusion accidents is calculated by dividing the volume of Rh-positive packed RBCs transfused by 15 ml, the amount of RBCs covered by one vial. The number of vials can be large, so the entire dose is often divided and administered in several injections at separate sites. Another approach is to perform an exchange transfusion with Rh-negative blood and then calculate the dose based on the number of Rh-positive RBCs remaining in the circulation.

For platelet concentrates, one vial is sufficient for 30 or more units (bags), because each unit contains less than 0.5 ml RBCs. The dose for leukocyte concentrates can be calculated by obtaining the hematocrit and volume of the product from the supplier.

RhIg as available in the United States must be injected intramuscularly only. Intravenous injections of

TABLE 20-2 ADDITIONAL INDICATIONS FOR RhIg

Amniocentesis
Chorionic villus sampling
Abortion (spontaneous and induced)
Ectopic pregnancy
Abdominal trauma
Accidental or inadvertent transfusion

$$\frac{\text{No. of fetal cells} \times \text{Maternal blood volume}}{\text{No. of maternal cells}} = \text{Volume of fetomaternal hemorrhage}$$

these preparations can cause severe anaphylactic reactions owing to the anticomplementary activity of the products.

OTHER CONSIDERATIONS

Rh immune globulin is of no benefit once a person has been actively immunized and has formed anti-D. Care must be taken, however, to distinguish those women who have been passively immunized by antenatal administration of RhIg from those who have been actively immunized by exposure to Rh-positive RBCs.

Care must also be taken so that fetal Rh-positive RBCs in the maternal circulation not be interpreted as maternal, because then the mother would be assumed erroneously to be D^u positive. The difference is distinguished by a quantitative test, such as the Kleihauer-Betke.

RhIg is not indicated for the mother if the infant is found to be D and D^u negative. The blood type of abortions, stillbirths, and ectopic pregnancies usually cannot be determined; therefore, RhIg should be administered in these circumstances. RhIg must not be given to the newborn infant.

There is no risk of transmission of the viral diseases hepatitis A and B and human immunodeficiency virus (HIV).[8] Several investigators have reported transmission of non-A, non-B hepatitis, however. RhIg has been reported to contain antibody to hepatitis A, B, and C, and thus may cause false-positive hepatitis serology.[9]

ABO Hemolytic Disease of the Newborn

ABO incompatibility between the mother and newborn infant can cause HDN. Maternal ABO antibodies that are IgG can cross the placenta and attach to the ABO-incompatible antigens of the fetal RBCs. However, destruction of fetal RBCs leading to severe anemia is extremely rare. More commonly, the disease is manifested by the onset of hyperbilirubinemia and jaundice within 12 to 48 hours of birth. The increasing levels of bilirubin can be treated with phototherapy. Severe cases requiring exchange transfusion are extremely rare.

As the incidence of HDN caused by Rh$_o$(D) has declined, ABO incompatibility has become the most common cause of hemolytic disease. Statistically, mother and infant are ABO incompatible in one of every five pregnancies.

FACTORS AFFECTING INCIDENCE AND SEVERITY

ABO antibodies are present in the sera of all individuals whose RBCs lack the corresponding antigen. These antibodies, the result of environmental stimulus, occur more frequently as high-titered IgG antibodies in group O individuals than in group A or B individuals. Hence, ABO HDN is nearly always limited to A or B infants of group O mothers with potent anti-A,B. Most cases occur in group A infants in white populations. In the black population, however, group B infants are more often affected, and the overall incidence of ABO HDN is several times greater than in other groups.

The mother's history of prior transfusions or pregnancies seems unrelated to the occurrence and severity of the disease. Thus, ABO HDN may occur in the first pregnancy and in any, but not necessarily all, subsequent pregnancies. However, tetanus toxoid administration and helminth parasite infection during pregnancy have been linked to the production of high-titered IgG ABO antibodies and severe HDN.

Even high-titered IgG antibodies that are transported across the placenta seem incapable of causing significant RBC destruction in an ABO-incompatible fetus. These infants are delivered with mild anemia or normal hemoglobin levels. The mild course of ABO HDN is related more to the slow development of ABO antigens on fetal RBCs than the characteristics of the maternal antibody. That ABO antigens are not fully developed until after the first year of life is well demonstrated by the A antigen. Group A infant RBCs are serologically more similar to A$_2$ adult cells, with group A$_2$ infant RBCs much weaker. The weakened A antigen on fetal and neonatal RBCs is more readily demonstrable with human than with monoclonal anti-A reagents. As expected, group A$_2$ infants are less likely to have ABO HDN.

The laboratory findings in ABO HDN differ from those in Figure 20–3 for Rh disease. Microspherocytes and increased RBC fragility in the infant are characteristic of ABO HDN but not of Rh HDN. The severity of the disease is independent of the presence of a positive direct antiglobulin test result or demonstrable anti-A, anti-B or anti-A,B in the eluate of the infant's RBCs.

The bilirubin peak is later, at 1 to 3 days, as well. Phototherapy is usually sufficient for slowly rising bilirubin levels. With rapidly increasing bilirubin levels, exchange transfusion with group O RBCs may be required. The serious consequences of Rh and other blood groups causing HDN, such as stillbirth, hydrops fetalis, and kernicterus, are extremely rare in ABO HDN.

PRENATAL SCREENING

Many workers have tried to use the immunoglobulin class and titer of maternal ABO antibodies to predict ABO HDN. These tests are laborious and at best demonstrate the presence of IgG maternal antibody but do not correlate well with the degree of fetal RBC destruction. Consequently, detection of ABO HDN is best done after birth.

POSTNATAL DIAGNOSIS

No single serologic test is diagnostic for ABO HDN. When a newborn infant develops jaundice within 12 to 48 hours after birth, various causes of jaundice need to be investigated, of which ABO HDN is only one. The direct antiglobulin test (DAT) on the cord or neonatal RBCs is the most important diagnostic test. In all cases of ABO HDN requiring transfusion therapy, the DAT result has been positive.[10] On the other hand, the DAT result can be positive even in the absence of signs and symptoms of clinical anemia in the newborn infant. However, these infants may have compensated anemia or the RBCs may not be destroyed by the reticuloendothelial system.

Collecting cord blood samples on all delivered infants is highly recommended. The sample should be collected by venipuncture to avoid contamination with Wharton's jelly and maternal blood and should be anticoagulated for storage. If the neonatal infant develops jaundice, then ABO, Rh, and DAT results can be assessed. The DAT result is neither strongly nor consistently positive, although 90 percent of the cases complicated by jaundice will be positive.[11] When the DAT result is negative but the infant is jaundiced, other causes of jaundice should be investigated. In the rare cases in which ABO incompatibility can be the only cause of neonatal jaundice but the DAT result is negative, the eluate of the cord RBCs always reveals ABO antibodies. The eluate can also be helpful when the mother's blood specimen is not available.

Case Study

At a rural hospital near a migrant farm camp, a 32-year-old Hispanic woman has just delivered a sick infant. At 6 weeks' gestation, she was typed as A negative, with positive antibody screen. The antibody was identified as anti-D, titer 1:256. A report stated she had had an intrauterine transfusion 3 weeks earlier at a university hospital in another state. The cord blood collected at delivery was typed as A negative. On a heelstick specimen, the infant's hemoglobin was reported as 4.3 g/dl, and bilirubin 3.9 mg/dl. Typing results of this specimen are as follows:

Anti-A	Anti-B	Anti-A,B	Anti-D	Dᵘ	DAT
0	0	0	0	+	+/−

What is the infant's blood type? Why is the infant so anemic? What further testing is indicated?

First of all, the blood types of the cord blood and heelstick specimens are different—A negative versus O Dᵘ positive. The severely anemic infant could have HDN, although the cord blood results do not indicate severe disease (DAT +/−). On the other hand, a large fetomaternal hemorrhage could have occurred. Further testing showed the following:

	Cord Blood	Heelstick
Anti-I	4+	3+
Kleihauer-Betke	0/1000	23/1000

The results indicate that the cord blood specimen is all adult blood and the heelstick specimen is nearly all adult blood. How could that happen?

Cord blood should be collected by needle and syringe from the umbilical cord vein. Collecting the specimen by allowing blood from the placenta or cord to drip into the tube can contaminate the specimen with maternal blood. In this case, the tube marked "cord blood" could have been a mislabeled maternal blood sample.

The heelstick is nearly all adult blood because of the recent intrauterine transfusion. Group O blood is usually used. As discussed in this chapter, transfusion causes suppression of erythropoiesis and therefore the production of few fetal RBCs. Those cells produced are being hemolyzed by the high-titered maternal antibody. This leads to anemia, in this case quite severe, with elevated bilirubin levels indicating hemolysis is occurring.

Further testing was done on the heelstick specimen.

	Anti-A	Anti-B		RBC Eluate
4° C	0	+		Anti-D

These results indicate the infant is probably B positive and has HDN caused by anti-D.

Review Questions

1. Hemolytic disease of the newborn is characterized by:
   A. IgM antibody
   B. Nearly always anti-D
   C. Different RBC antigens between mother and father
   D. Antibody titer less than 1:32

2. The main difference between the fetus and the newborn is:
   A. Bilirubin metabolism
   B. Maternal antibody level
   C. Presence of anemia
   D. Size of RBCs

3. Kernicterus is due to the effects of:
   A. Anemia
   B. Unconjugated bilirubin
   C. Antibody specificity
   D. Antibody titer

4. The advantages of cordocentesis include all of the following *except*:
   A. Allows measurement of fetal hemoglobin and hematocrit levels

B. Allows antigen typing of fetal blood
C. Allows direct transfusion of fetal circulation
D. Decreases risk of trauma to the placenta

5. Amniocentesis is used to:
   A. Measure bilirubin in milligrams per deciliter
   B. Determine fetal blood type
   C. Determine change in optical density
   D. Measure hemoglobin in grams per deciliter

6. Blood for intrauterine transfusion should be all of the following *except*:
   A. More than 7 days old
   B. Screened for CMV
   C. Gamma irradiated
   D. Compatible with maternal serum

7. Rh immune globulin is indicated for:
   A. Mothers who have anti-D
   B. Infants who are Rh negative
   C. Infants who have anti-D
   D. Mothers who are Rh negative

8. Rh immune globulin is given without regard for fetal Rh type in all of the following conditions *except*:
   A. Ectopic pregnancy rupture
   B. Amniocentesis
   C. Induced abortion
   D. Full-term delivery

9. A Kleihauer-Betke test indicates 10 fetal cells per 1000 adult cells. For a woman with a 5000-ml blood volume, the proper dose of RhIg is:
   A. One regular-dose vial
   B. Two regular-dose vials
   C. One microdose vial
   D. Two microdose vials

10. Rh immune globulin is indicated in the following circumstance:
    A. Mother D^u positive
    B. Infant D and D^u positive
    C. Mother D and D^u positive
    D. Infant D and D^u negative

11. ABO HDN is usually mild because
    A. ABO antigens are poorly developed in fetus
    B. ABO antibodies prevent the disease
    C. ABO antibodies readily cross the placenta
    D. ABO incompatibility is rare

Answers to Review Questions

1. C (p 389)
2. A (pp 391–392)
3. B (p 392)
4. D (p 394)
5. C (p 393)
6. A (p 396)
7. D (p 396)
8. D (p 398)
9. B (p 397)
10. B (p 396)
11. A (p 398)

References

1. Bowman, JM: Historical overview: Hemolytic disease of the fetus and newborn. In Kennedy, MS, Wilson, S, and Kelton, JG (eds): Perinatal Transfusion Medicine. American Association of Blood Banks, Arlington, VA, 1990, p 1.
2. Mollison, PL, Engelfriet, CP, and Contreras, M: Blood Transfusion in Clinical Medicine, ed 9. Blackwell Scientific, London, 1993, p 543.
3. Mollison, PL, Engelfriet, CP, and Contreras, M: Blood Transfusion in Clinical Medicine, ed 9. Blackwell Scientific, London, 1993, p 218.
4. Vengelen-Tyler, V: The serological investigation of hemolytic disease of the newborn caused by antibodies other than anti-D. In Garratty, G (ed): Hemolytic Disease of the Newborn. American Association of Blood Banks, Arlington, VA, 1984, p 145.
5. Ludomirski, A: The anemic fetus: Direct access to the fetal circulation for diagnosis and treatment. In Kennedy, MS, Wilson, S, and Kelton, JG (eds): Perinatal Transfusion Medicine. American Association of Blood Banks, Arlington, VA, 1990, p 89.
6. Ness, PM and Salamon JL: The failure of postinjection Rh immune globulin titers to detect large fetal-maternal hemorrhages. Am J Clin Pathol 85:604, 1986.
7. Kennedy, MS: Rho(D) immune globulin. In Rayburn, W and Zuspan, FP (eds): Drug Therapy in Gynecology and Obstetrics, ed 3. CV Mosby, St Louis, 1991, p 297.
8. Lack of transmission of human immunodeficiency virus through Rho(D) immune globulin (human). MMWR 36:728, 1987.
9. Tabor, E, Smallwood, LA, and Gerety, RJ: Antibodies to hepatitis A and B virus antigen in Rho(D) immune globulin. Lancet 1:322, 1986.
10. Issitt, PD: Applied Blood Group Serology, ed 3. Montgomery Scientific, Miami, 1985, p 588.
11. Walker, RH: Relevancy in the selection of serologic tests for the obstetric patient. In Garratty, G (ed): Hemolytic Disease of the Newborn. American Association of Blood Banks, Arlington, VA, 1984, p 173.

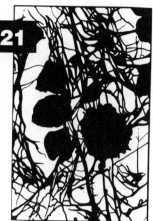

CHAPTER 21

Autoimmune Hemolytic Anemias

Denise M. Harmening, PhD, MT(ASCP), CLS(NCA)
Lee Ann Prihoda, BS, MT(ASCP)SBB

OBJECTIVES

Upon completion of this chapter, the learner should be able to:

1 Define autoantibody and compare the types of immune hemolytic anemias with respect to thermal amplitude, red cell destruction, and the type of protein (antibody or complement) coating the red cells.

2 Characterize autoantibodies that react at temperatures less than 37°C and discuss problems encountered in laboratory testing of specimens containing cold autoagglutinins.

3 Identify the common specificities of benign cold autoagglutinins and outline laboratory testing that can differentiate among these specificities.

4 Discuss pathologic cold autoagglutinins, including laboratory testing and treatment.

5 Differentiate between idiopathic warm autoimmune hemolytic anemia and drug-induced immune hemolytic anemia.

6 Illustrate the clinical and laboratory findings in warm autoimmune hemolytic anemia, including red cell hemolysis, difficulties in serologic testing, and selection of blood for transfusion.

7 Compare the four proposed mechanisms for drug-induced hemolysis and give examples of medications causing each type.

Immune hemolytic anemia is defined as shortened red blood cell (RBC) survival mediated through the immune response, specifically by humoral antibody. Immune hemolysis represents the result of an acquired extracorpuscular abnormality associated with demonstrable antibodies, as opposed to intracorpuscular defects, which represent intrinsic abnormalities of the patient's RBCs.

Numerous classifications of immune hemolytic anemias have been proposed; however, three broad categories are generally used:

1. Alloimmune
2. Autoimmune
3. Drug-induced

In an alloimmune response, patients produce alloantibodies to foreign RBC antigens introduced into their circulation through either transfusion or pregnancy. For more information on alloantibody production, refer to Chapters 18 and 20.

This chapter focuses on the latter two categories, autoimmune hemolytic anemia and drug-induced hemolytic anemia. An autoimmune response occurs when a patient produces antibodies against his or her own RBC antigens. Drug-induced hemolytic anemia is the result of a patient's production of antibody to a particular drug or drug complex, with ensuing damage to the patient's RBCs.

Autoantibodies

DEFINITION

Antibodies that are directed against the individual's own RBCs are autoantibodies or autoagglutinins. Most autoantibodies react with high-incidence antigens; they will agglutinate, sensitize, or lyse RBCs of most random donors in addition to autologous cells. RBC survival is shortened by the humoral antibody.

It is currently believed that production of antibodies against "self" occurs because there is a failure of the mechanisms regulating the immune response. Briefly,

under normal circumstances, immunoglobulins (Ig) are made by B lymphocytes. Another type of lymphocyte, the T lymphocyte, modulates the activity of the antibody-producing cells. Helper T cells assist immunocompetent B cells in making antibody against foreign antigens. Another population of T lymphocytes, suppressor T cells, has the opposite effect on B-cell activity; they prevent excessive proliferation of B cells and overproduction of antibodies. Suppressor T cells are thought to act through a feedback mechanism. An increasing concentration of antibody activates these T cells and suppresses further antibody production.[1]

Autoantibody production may be prevented through a similar mechanism. Suppressor T cells induce tolerance to self antigens by inhibiting B-cell activity. Conversely, loss of suppressor T-cell function could result in autoantibody production. Support for this concept comes from animal models[2] and in patients taking the drug methyldopa.[3] The cause of dysfunction of the regulatory system in not understood, but microbial agents and drugs have been suggested.[4] For more discussion of the immune response, see Chapter 3.

Autoantibodies are important for two reasons. First, they can cause destruction of RBCs in vivo. In addition, when an individual's cells are coated with autoantibody and the serum contains autoantibody reactive with the cells of most random donors, it may be difficult to interpret correctly routine cell typing, antibody detection and identification, and compatibility tests. The effect of autoantibodies on routine testing and techniques to resolve the difficulties are discussed subsequently. It is important to note that the serologic and clinical problems can be found separately or together.

CHARACTERIZATION

The presence of autoantibodies in a patient's serum or coating a patient's cells may indicate autoimmune hemolytic anemia (AIHA), but additional information is needed before this conclusion should be drawn.

One must establish that RBCs are being destroyed by an immune-mediated process. Individuals who are experiencing immune RBC destruction may or may not be anemic (decreased hemoglobin and hematocrit levels), depending on whether RBC production has increased to compensate for the loss. The reticulocyte count and the unconjugated bilirubin levels will be increased, and the haptoglobin levels will be decreased. If RBC destruction is predominantly intravascular, hemoglobinemia and hemoglobinuria may occur. There are other causes of hemolysis (e.g., hereditary spherocytosis and hemoglobinopathies); therefore, AIHA must be confirmed by additional serologic testing. Diagnostic tests include (1) the direct antiglobulin test (DAT) using polyspecific and monospecific antiglobulin reagents and (2) characterization of the autoantibody in the serum and eluate. Based on these results and the clinical evaluation of the patient, AIHA can be diagnosed and classified as cold reactive, warm reactive, or drug-induced. The expected laboratory findings for each type are discussed later. Petz and Garratty[5] devote one chapter in their book, *Acquired Immune Hemolytic Anemias*, to the diagnosis of the hemolytic anemias and another to drug-induced immune hemolytic anemia. The reader is referred to this text for a complete discussion.

Individuals with autoantibodies in their sera and on their RBCs may display no evidence of decreased RBC survival. For example, the incidence of positive DAT results in normal healthy blood donor populations has been reported to be as high as 1 in 1000 in the US population,[6] whereas the incidence in hospitalized patients ranges from 0.3 to 1 percent (using anti-IgG antiglobulin reagent)[7,8] to 15 percent (using polyspecific antiglobulin reagent).[9] Many of these individuals have only anticomplement bound to the RBCs. The differences between individuals who are affected (i.e., have AIHA) and those who are unaffected by autoantibodies are not clearly understood. Possibly significant factors include the following:

1. Thermal amplitude of antibody reactivity[10]
2. IgG subclass of the antibody[11]
3. Amount of antibody bound to the RBCs[12]
4. Ability of the antibody to fix complement in vivo[12]
5. Activity of the individual's macrophages[5]

The opposite situation also occurs; there are patients with hemolytic anemia in whom autoantibodies cannot be demonstrated by routine techniques. Some patients have more IgG on their RBCs than normal but less than the amount detectable by the routine antiglobulin test.[13] In other cases the patient's RBCs are sensitized with anti-IgA.[14,15] Because polyspecific antihuman globulin reagents must contain only anti-IgG and anti-C3d,[16] anti-IgA is not consistently present and IgA-sensitized cells may not yield a positive test result. Finally, before the current requirements for polyspecific antiglobulin reagents, many commercial reagents did not agglutinate cells coated with complement components.[17] Therefore, finding a negative DAT result was not unusual in patients with cold agglutinin hemolytic anemia. The reader is cautioned, however, to note the date of a publication in which AIHA associated with a negative DAT result is reported.

As stated earlier, autoantibodies can be divided into two main groups, depending on the optimal temperature of reactivity. About 70 percent of the reported cases of AIHA are those that react best at warm temperatures (37°C), with cold reactive (4°C to 30°C) autoagglutinins accounting for about 18 percent. Drug-induced autoagglutinins are present in about 12 percent of the reported AIHA cases. Characterization of autoantibodies is important because treatment of the patient and resolution of the serologic problems differ according to the optimal temperature of reactivity. The clinical and laboratory aspects of cold reactive, warm reactive, and drug-induced autoantibodies are discussed subsequently.

Cold Reactive Autoantibodies

BENIGN COLD AUTOAGGLUTININS

The most commonly encountered autoantibody is a benign cold agglutinin that is demonstrable in the serum of most normal, healthy individuals when testing is done at 4°C. It usually does not present a serologic problem because routine tests are not done at this temperature. The typical cold agglutinin has a relatively low titer; at 4°C it is less than 64. Occasionally, the antibody has increased thermal amplitude and will agglutinate cells at room temperature (20°C to 24°C). However, even in this situation one obtains the strongest reactions at 4°C. Table 21–1 compares the characteristics of benign (normal) cold autoantibodies with those of pathologic cold autoagglutinins. Most cold agglutinins react best with enzyme-treated cells; therefore, cold agglutinins are quite likely to be detected when using ficin-treated cells. Cold autoantibodies are of the IgM class and can activate complement in vitro. Reactions may be seen in the antiglobulin phase when using polyspecific antiglobulin reagents. Table 21–2 shows reactions typical of cold autoagglutinins.

Laboratory Tests Affected by Cold Agglutinins

Cold agglutinins sometimes interfere with routine serum and cell testing. The degree to which they cause problems depends on how strongly the antibody reacts at room temperature (i.e., the concentration and thermal amplitude of the antibody). Although the normal cold autoantibody found in the serum of most people usually does not interfere with testing, it is one of the more common causes of serologic problems. Therefore, one should be familiar with the recognition and methods of resolution of problems associated with these antibodies.

ABO Grouping If an individual's RBCs are heav-

TABLE 21–1 **COMPARISON OF CHARACTERISTICS OF NORMAL COLD AUTOANTIBODIES AND PATHOLOGIC COLD AUTOANTIBODIES**

Characteristic	Normal	Pathologic
Thermal amplitude	<22°C	Broad; up to 32°C
Spontaneous autoagglutination (in anticoagulated tube of blood)	None	Significant degree, which disperses upon warming to 37°C
Titer	<64 (seldom >16 at 4°C)	>1000 at 4°C
Enhancement by albumin	None	Enhances reactivity
Clonality of antibody	Polyclonal	Idiopathic = monoclonal Secondary to infection = polyclonal
Clinical significance	None	Causes cold AIHA
Common antibody specificity	Anti-I	Anti-I
DAT	Negative or weakly positive with polyspecific antiglobulin reagent	2+ to 3+ with polyspecific antiglobulin reagent

Adapted from Harmening,[54] p 204.

TABLE 21–2 **SEROLOGIC REACTIONS OF A TYPICAL COLD AUTOAGGLUTININ**

Serologic Reactions	O Cells (Screening Cells)	Autologous Cells
4°C	4+	4+
RT	+	+
37°C	0	0
AHG (poly)	w+	w+
AHG (anti-IgG)	0	0

RT = room temperature reactions, 20°C to 24°C; AHG = antihuman globulin phase.

ily coated with cold agglutinins, they may agglutinate spontaneously. Consequently, one can obtain false-positive reactions with the routine ABO reagents. In most cases, valid results can be obtained using cells washed once or twice with normal saline warmed to 37°C. The cold autoantibody elutes from the cells during washing. For example, group O cells coated with cold autoantibody might give the following reactions before and after washing:

	Anti-A	Anti-B
Serum-suspended RBCs	+	+
Saline-washed, suspended RBCs	0	0

If more potent agglutinins are present, the specimen can be kept at 37°C after collection and the cells washed with 37°C to 45°C saline to remove the autoantibody.[18] In the very rare situation in which washing with warm saline is not effective, thiol reagents (e.g., dithiothreitol) can be used to disperse the autoagglutination.[19] (See Procedure A of the Procedural Appendix at the end of this chapter.)

Because ABO serum grouping is done at room temperature, cold autoagglutinins can cause discrepancies in the reverse typing also. In the following example, the forward typing results indicate the cells to be group AB. Therefore, one does not expect the serum

to agglutinate the A_1 or B cells. Although a number of explanations exist for this discrepancy, a cold agglutinin is a likely cause. Autologous cells should also be tested and will be positive if a cold autoagglutinin is present.

	Anti-A	Anti-B	
RBCs	4+	4+	

	A_1 Cells	B Cells	Autologous Cells
Serum	+	+	+

Such a discrepancy is easily resolved if the serum is prewarmed before testing, or if the cold reactive autoantibody is removed by an autoabsorption technique, and the tests with the A_1 and B cells are repeated with autoabsorbed serum. (See Procedure B of the Procedural Appendix.)

	A_1 Cells	B Cells	Autologous Cells
Autoabsorbed serum	0	0	0

Rh Typing As in ABO cell grouping, one can find false-positive reactions with Rh reagents when testing RBCs coated with cold autoagglutinins. In typing with anti-D (high-protein reagent), the Rh control will be positive, rendering the test invalid. Today, the commonly used chemically modified or monoclonal blend Rh (low-protein) reagents will usually yield valid results. When using these types of reagents, a negative reaction with any of the ABO reagents serves as the control for the Rh typing. As stated earlier, if a discrepancy exists in the ABO typing, washing the cells in warm saline will usually result in acceptable results. This also holds true when testing with low-protein anti-D. Thiol reagents may be used when washing with warm saline is ineffective.

Cold autoagglutinins can activate the complement cascade in vitro, causing complement components to be bound to the RBC, leading to false-positive reactions in the D^u test when polyspecific antiglobulin reagents are used. The control reaction will also be positive. As shown in the following example, monospecific anti-IgG can be used for D^u testing. The problem can also be avoided if the RBCs are collected into ethylenediaminetetraacetic acid (EDTA), so that complement cannot bind in vitro.

	Anti-D	Rh Control	Comments
Immediate spin	0	0	
Antihuman globulin (polyspecific)	+	+	Detects complement components
Antihuman globulin (anti-IgG)	0	0	Does not detect complement
RBCs collected in EDTA	0	0	Complement not bound

Similar problems can be encountered in other phenotyping tests (e.g., K, Fy^a) that require the use of an antiglobulin test.

Direct Antiglobulin Test When a properly collected specimen is used (EDTA), the result of the DAT on a patient with benign cold autoagglutinins is negative. However, a positive result is frequently obtained when using a clotted specimen because complement can be activated in vitro. If monospecific reagents are used, these cells are agglutinated by anti-C3 but not by anti-IgG. As discussed in the previous section, false-positive antigen typings can be obtained when clotted specimens and polyspecific antiglobulin reagents are used.

Antibody Detection and Identification The frequency with which cold autoagglutinins interfere with detection and identification of RBC alloantibodies depends to a large extent on the routine procedures used in patient testing. As shown in Table 21–2, cold agglutinins react best at 4°C but are not detected because routine testing is not done at this temperature. Room temperature reactive autoantibodies usually will not be detected if the laboratory no longer performs routine testing at this phase. Antibodies reactive only at room temperature are usually not clinically significant. Benign cold autoagglutinins do not react at 37°C but may interfere with testing at the antiglobulin phase if polyspecific antiglobulin reagent is used. They bind to cells at lower temperatures when the serum and cells are mixed together initially or during centrifugation after the 37°C incubation, and complement is activated. The antibody elutes during the incubation or washing phases, but complement remains attached. Polyspecific antiglobulin reagent will agglutinate the cells coated with C3. When enzyme-treated cells are used, reactions in all phases may be stronger.

Many antibodies capable of causing accelerated RBC destruction are detected by the antiglobulin test; therefore, reactions in this phase may be significant and must be investigated. The reactions caused by a cold autoagglutinin can mask those of an alloantibody. The use of anti-IgG antiglobulin reagent will eliminate most problems with cold autoagglutinin reactivity in the antiglobulin phase.

Other techniques useful in differentiating between cold autoantibodies and alloantibodies are prewarming tests or preforming tests with autoabsorbed serum.[18] By prewarming the cells and serum before mixing, avoiding room temperature centrifugation after 37°C incubation, and washing with 37°C to 45°C saline, one can prevent the reaction between the cold autoagglutinin and the antigen, thus preventing complement activation. Alloantibodies reactive at 37°C, however, can bind to the cells and cause agglutination at the antiglobulin phase. (See Procedure C of the Procedural Appendix.) An example of the results of testing a serum that contains a cold autoagglutinin and an anti-Fy^a by routine antiglobulin technique and by the prewarmed technique is shown in Table 21–3. Reactions are present at the antiglobulin phase (using a polyspecific antiglobulin reagent) with both Fy^a(+) and Fy^a(−) cells. In a prewarmed test, only the reactions expected of the anti-Fy^a are evident. The weak reactions of the cold autoagglutinin are eliminated by prewarming the test. The simple prewarming technique is successful in most cases. If the autoantibody is very potent, it may be difficult to keep the cells and serum at a high enough temperature through each phase of testing to avoid the antigen-antibody interaction and complement activation.

When strong cold autoantibodies are present or if one wishes to identify a room temperature–reactive alloantibody, an absorption must be done to remove the autoantibody. An autologous absorption may be done if the patient has not been recently transfused. An aliquot of the patient's cells is incubated with an equal aliquot of the patient's serum at 4°C. Autoantibody is removed, and alloantibody remains in the serum. It may be necessary to repeat the absorption several times if the autoantibody is particularly strong. The patient's RBCs may be treated with enzymes before absorption to increase the amount of autoantibody removed by the absorption. (See Procedure B of the Procedural Appendix.) Special precautions must

TABLE 21–3 REACTIONS OBSERVED WITH A SERUM CONTAINING ANTI-Fy^a AND A COLD AUTOAGGLUTININ

Reagent RBCs	Standard Antiglobulin Technique*	Prewarmed Antiglobulin Technique
Fy(a+)	+	+
Fy(a−)	w+	0
Fy(a+)	+	+
Fy(a−)	+	0
Fy(a−)	w+	0
Fy(a+)	+	+

*Using polyspecific antiglobulin reagent.

be taken if a patient has been recently transfused because donor RBCs will be present in the patient's circulation. Alloantibodies as well as autoantibodies will be absorbed if an autoabsorption is performed. In this situation, it is best to use the prewarmed technique.

If anti-IgG reagent is used, one can avoid the problem caused by most cold agglutinins. However, one can miss very rare clinically significant alloantibodies that are detected only because they bind complement. Use of anti-IgG reagents is an attractive alternative when prewarming is not effective and there is not enough time to absorb the serum.

Compatibility Testing The difficulties encountered in antibody detection and identification tests are also found in compatibility tests because the most commonly encountered autoantibody (autoanti-I) is directed against an antigen that is found on the RBCs of most random donors as well as on most reagent RBCs. Compatibility tests, like antibody identification tests, can be done with prewarmed or autoabsorbed serum or with anti-IgG.

Two of the other common cold autoagglutinins, anti-IH and anti-H, distinguish between reagent RBCs and random donor cells. As discussed in the following section on specificity, anti-IH and anti-H react best with group O cells; they react less well with group A_1 and A_1B cells. Anti-IH and anti-H are found most often in the serum of group A_1 and A_1B persons; therefore, the units selected for compatibility testing are those which will give the weakest, if any, reactivity. On the other hand, group O cells give the strongest reactions.

Specificity of Cold Autoagglutinins

Anti-I, Anti-i Most cold reactive autoantibodies have anti-I specificity. The I antigen is fully expressed on virtually all adult RBCs but only weakly expressed on cord RBCs. At birth, the infant has the i antigen on the cells. As an infant matures, the i antigen is converted to I antigen; the amount of I antigen increases until the adult levels are reached at about 2 years of age.[18] Very rarely adults may lack the I antigen; these individuals are termed "i adults."

The reactivities of several examples of anti-I are given in Table 21–4. As shown, anti-I specificity may

TABLE 21–4 REACTIONS OF SERA CONTAINING ANTI-I WITH ADULT AND CORD CELLS

| Sera | Serum Dilution | RBCs | |
		Adult	Cord
Serum 1	Neat	3+	0
Serum 2	Neat	4+	2+
	1:2	4+	+
	1:4	3+	0
	1:8	2+	0

TABLE 21–5 RELATIVE STRENGTHS OF SEROLOGIC REACTIONS OF COLD AUTOAGGLUTININS AT 4°C*

RBC Phenotype	Anti-I	Anti-i	Anti-H	Anti-IH
O I (adult)	4+	+	4+	4+
A_1 I (adult)	4+	+	+	+
A_2 I (adult)	4+	+	2+	2+
O_h I (adult)	4+	+	0	2+
O i (cord)	+	3+	4+	+
O i (adult)	+	4+	4+	+
A_1 i (adult)	+	4+	+	0
A_2 i (adult)	+	4+	2+	+
O_h i (adult)	+	4+	0	0

*Sera are ABO compatible with RBCs.

be apparent when a serum is tested with adult and cord cells. Serum 1, for example, reacts with adult cells but not with cord cells. Serum 2 reacts with both adult and cord cells, but the preference for the adult cells is still obvious. Alloanti-I is frequently present in the serum of i adults.[20]

Anti-i is a relatively uncommon autoantibody. As shown in Table 21–5, this antibody reacts antithetically to anti-I. Cord cells and i adult cells have the most i antigen, adult I cells the least.

Anti-H, Anti-IH Cold agglutinins found in the sera of group A_1 and A_1B individuals (and rarely group B) may have the specificity of an anti-H. This antibody distinguishes among cells of various ABO groups. Group O and A_2 cells react best because they have the most H substance. Group A_1 and A_1B cells have the least H antigen, so they react weakly. The pattern of reactivity seen with anti-H is shown in Table 21–5. (See Chapter 5 for a discussion of the ABO system and H substance.)

It is very important not to confuse cold reactive anti-H with the anti-H found in the serum of O_h (Bombay) individuals who are H negative. Cold reactive anti-H is an autoantibody, even though the cells of the antibody maker (A_1 or A_1B) may give considerably weaker reactions. The anti-H in the O_h person is a potent alloantibody, reacts at 4°C to 37°C, and is capable of causing rapid RBC destruction.

Anti-IH, another of the usually harmless cold autoagglutinins, is also found more commonly in the serum of group A_1 and A_1B individuals. This antibody agglutinates only RBCs that have both the I and H antigens. As with anti-H, group O and A_2 cells react best. The difference between these two antibodies is that group O i_{cord} cells and group O i_{adult} cells react as strongly as group O I_{adult} cells with anti-H but not with anti-IH (Table 21–5).

OTHER COLD REACTIVE AUTOANTIBODIES

A number of other, less commonly encountered, cold agglutinins have been described, such as anti-Pr, anti-Gd, and anti-Sd* (anti-R_x). (See the review by

Marsh[21] for additional information.) Most workers agree that specificity of cold reactive autoantibodies is primarily of academic interest and not clinically important.

PATHOLOGIC COLD AUTOAGGLUTININS

Cold Hemagglutinin Disease (Idiopathic Cold AIHA)

In most cases cold autoagglutinins do not cause RBC destruction, but in some patients they can cause hemolytic anemia that varies in severity from mild to life-threatening intravascular lysis. Cold reactive immune hemolytic anemia may be a chronic, idiopathic (no identifiable cause) condition or an acute, transient disorder that is usually associated with an infectious disease, such as *Mycoplasma pneumoniae* infection or infectious mononucleosis. Cold agglutinin syndrome, also called cold hemagglutinin disease (CHD) or idiopathic cold AIHA, represents approximately 16 percent of AIHA cases. A moderate chronic hemolytic anemia is produced by a cold autoantibody that optimally reacts at 4°C but also reacts between 25°C and 31°C. The antibody is usually IgM, which quite efficiently activates complement.

Clinical Picture Cold hemagglutinin disease occurs predominantly in older individuals, with a peak incidence beyond 50 years of age. Antibody specificity in this disorder is almost always anti-I, less commonly anti-i, and rarely anti-Pr. It is rarely severe and is usually seasonal, inasmuch as the winter months often precipitate the signs and symptoms of a chronic hemolytic anemia. Acrocyanosis of the hands, feet, ears, and nose is frequently the patient's main complaint, along with a sense of numbness in the extremities. Changes take place when the person is exposed to the cold, because the cold autoantibody will cause agglutination of the patient's RBCs in the skin capillaries, resulting in localized blood stasis. During cold winter weather, the temperature of an individual's blood falls to as low as 28°C in the extremities, activating the cold autoantibody in these patients. The antibody then agglutinates the RBCs and fixes complement as the cells flow through the capillaries of the skin, causing autoagglutination and signs of acrocyanosis. These patients may also experience hemoglobinuria, because the complement fixation may result in intravascular hemolysis. However, this intravascular hemolytic episode is not associated with fever, chills, or acute renal insufficiency, which is characteristic of patients with paroxysmal cold hemoglobinuria (PCH) or severe warm AIHA.

Patients usually display weakness, pallor, and weight loss, which are characteristic signs and symptoms of chronic anemia. Cold hemagglutinin syndrome usually remains quite stable, and if it does progress in severity, it is insidious in intensity. Physical findings such as hepatosplenomegaly are infrequent owing to the mechanism of hemolysis. Other clinical features of CHD include jaundice and Raynaud's phenomenon (symptoms of cold intolerance, such as pain and bluish tinge in the fingertips and toes owing to vasospasm). Patients with severe CHD usually do well in warmer climates.

Laboratory Findings Laboratory findings in CHD include reticulocytosis and a positive DAT result caused by complement coating only. A simple serum-screening procedure should be performed initially to test the ability of the patient's serum to agglutinate autologous saline-suspended RBCs at 18°C to 20°C. If this test result is positive, further steps must be taken to determine the titer and thermal amplitude of the patient's cold autoantibody. If the result is negative, the diagnosis of CHD is unlikely. The peripheral smear of a patient with CHD may show agglutination, polychromasia, a mild to moderate anisocytosis, and poikilocytosis (**see Color Plate 17**). Autoagglutination of anticoagulated whole blood samples is characteristic of CHD and occurs quickly as the blood cools to room temperature, causing the binding of cold autoantibodies to the patient's RBCs. As a result of this autoagglutination, performance of blood counts and preparation of blood smears are extremely difficult with these patient samples. Leukocyte and platelet counts are usually normal.

Table 21-6 summarizes the clinical criteria for diagnosis of CHD.

Selection of Blood for Transfusion Most patients with CHD do not require transfusion, but when they do it is sometimes difficult to select blood. As previously described, potent cold autoantibodies interfere with most routine tests. Perhaps the most difficult problem is to detect and identify alloantibodies. Procedures to manage these problems have been described earlier in this chapter. It is important that RBCs compatible with clinically significant alloantibodies are given. Most patients are transfused with blood positive for the autoantibody. Units of i_{adult} RBCs are extremely rare and should be reserved for patients with alloanti-I.

TABLE 21-6 CLINICAL CRITERIA FOR THE DIAGNOSIS OF COLD AGGLUTININ SYNDROME

1. Clinical signs of an acquired hemolytic anemia, with a history (which may or may not be present) of acrocyanosis and hemoglobinuria upon exposure to cold
2. Positive DAT result using polyspecific antisera
3. Positive DAT result using monospecific anti-C3 antisera
4. Negative DAT result using monospecific anti-IgG antisera
5. Presence of reactivity in the patient's serum owing to a cold autoantibody
6. Cold agglutinin titer of 1000 or greater in saline at 4°C with visible agglutination of anticoagulated blood at room temperature

From Harmening,[54] p 205, with permission.
DAT = direct antiglobulin test.

Cold Autoantibodies Related to Infection (Secondary Cold AIHA)

Cold hemagglutinin disease also can occur as a transient disorder that is secondary to infections. Episodes of cold AIHA often occur after upper respiratory infections. Approximately 50 percent of patients suffering from pneumonia due to *M. pneumoniae* have cold agglutinin titers greater than 64. In the second or third week of the patient's illness, CHD may occur in association with the infection, with a rapid onset of hemolysis. Pallor and jaundice are characteristically present. Acrocyanosis and hemoglobinuria are uncommon and not consistently present. Usually, resolution of the episode occurs within 2 to 3 weeks because the hemolysis is self-limiting. The offending cold autoantibody is IgM with a characteristic anti-I specificity. Very high titers of cold autoagglutinins are seen almost exclusively in patients with *M. pneumoniae* infection. The cold agglutinin produced in this infection may be an immunologic response to the mycoplasma antigens, and this antibody may cross-react with the RBC I antigen.

The antibodies produced in CHD and in this disorder secondary to *M. pneumoniae* infection both have anti-I specificity, and the RBCs are sensitized with complement components. If the complement cascade does not proceed to C9 (cell death by lysis), the macrophages of the reticuloendothelial system can still clear the sensitized RBCs through their receptors for C3b fragments, thereby causing hemolysis.

Infectious mononucleosis also may be associated with a hemolytic anemia due to a cold autoantibody. Although occurring infrequently, it has been well documented that a high-titered IgM anti-i with a wide thermal range plays a major role in hemolytic anemia associated with this viral infection. Acute illness with a sore throat and a high fever, followed by weakness, anemia, and jaundice, are characteristic features of infectious mononucleosis.

Lymphadenopathy and hepatosplenomegaly are common findings. A larger percentage of patients with infectious mononucleosis have been reported to develop anti-i, but only a small number of these patients develop the antibody of sufficient titer and thermal amplitude to induce in vivo hemolysis. Table 21–7 lists the cold autoantibody specificity most commonly found in the various infections that cause secondary CHD.

Treatment Therapy for CHD is generally unsatisfactory. Most patients require no treatment and are instructed to avoid the cold, to keep warm, or to move to a milder climate. Patients with moderate anemia are given the same instructions, urging them to tolerate the symptoms rather than to use drugs on a therapeutic trial basis. There is some advantage to the use of plasma exchange in more severe cases, inasmuch as IgM antibodies have a predominantly intravascular distribution. However, response to plasma exchange is still variable in this patient population. Corticosteroids also have been used but generally have a poor effect. In some patients whose RBCs are strongly coated with C3, use of corticosteroids has been successful. Some favorable responses also have been reported with the alkylating drug chlorambucil. Splenectomy is generally considered ineffective.

Paroxysmal Cold Hemoglobinuria

Paroxysmal cold hemoglobinuria is the least common type of AIHA, with an incidence of about 1 to 2 percent. It is, however, more common in children in association with viral illnesses such as measles, mumps, chickenpox, infectious mononucleosis, and the ill-defined "flu syndrome."

Originally, PCH was described in association with syphilis, with an autoantibody formed in response to the *Treponema pallidum* infection. However, with the discovery and use of antibiotics to treat syphilis, PCH is no longer a common disorder related to this disease.

Red cell destruction is due to a cold autoantibody referred to as an autohemolysin, which binds to the patient's RBCs at low temperatures and fixes complement. Hemolysis occurs when the body temperature rises to 37°C and the sensitized cells undergo complement-mediated intravascular lysis. In contrast to the other cold reactive autoagglutinins, the antibody in PCH is IgG with biphasic activity; therefore, it is termed a biphasic hemolysin. The classic antibody produced in PCH is called the Donath-Landsteiner antibody and has the specificity of an autoanti-P. Other specificities have been reported, including anti-i[22] and anti-Pr-like.[23]

To confirm the diagnosis of PCH, the Donath-Landsteiner test is performed in the laboratory. This test involves the collection of two blood specimens from the patient. One specimen is used as a control and kept at 37°C for 60 minutes. The second sample is cooled at 4°C for 30 minutes and then incubated at 37°C for an additional 30 minutes. Both samples are then centrifuged and observed for hemolysis. In a positive Donath-Landsteiner test result, hemolysis will be demonstrable in the sample placed at 4°C and then at 37°C, whereas no hemolysis is observed in the control sample. Table 21–8 summarizes the reactions of the Donath-Landsteiner test.

As the name PCH implies, paroxysmal or intermittent episodes of hemoglobinuria occur upon exposure to cold. These acute attacks are characterized by a sudden onset of fever, shaking chills, malaise, abdominal cramps, and back pain. All of the signs of intravas-

TABLE 21–7 SECONDARY COLD AIHA

Type of Infection	Cold Autoantibody Specificity
Mycoplasma pneumoniae	Anti-I
Infectious mononucleosis	Anti-i
Lymphoproliferative disorder	Anti-i

From Harmening,[54] p 206, with permission.

TABLE 21-8 **DONATH-LANDSTEINER TEST**

	Whole Blood Sample 1 (Control)	Whole Blood Sample 2
Procedure		
1. 30 minutes	37°C	4°C
2. 30 minutes	37°C	37°C
3. Centrifuge and observe.		
Results		
Positive	No hemolysis	Hemolysis
Negative	No hemolysis	No hemolysis
Inconclusive	Hemolysis	Hemolysis

From Harmening,[54] p 206, with permission.

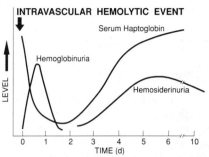

FIGURE 21-1 Indicator of acute intravascular hemolysis. Within a few hours of an acute hemolytic event, free hemoglobin is cleared from plasma and the serum haptoglobin falls to undetectable levels. Hemoglobinuria ceases soon after this. If no further hemolysis occurs, the serum haptoglobin level recovers and methemalbumin disappears within several days. The urinary hemosiderin can provide more lasting evidence of the hemolytic event. (From Hillman, RS and Finch, CA: Red Cell Manual, ed 6. FA Davis, Philadelphia, 1992, p 103, with permission.)

cular hemolysis are evident, along with hemoglobinemia, hemoglobinuria, and bilirubinemia, depending on the severity and frequency of the attack (Fig. 21-1). This results in a severe and rapidly progressive anemia with hemoglobin values frequently 4 to 5 g/dl. Polychromasia, nucleated RBCs, and poikilocytosis are demonstrated in the peripheral smear, findings that are consistent with hemolytic anemia. These signs and symptoms, as well as hemoglobinuria, may resolve in a few hours or persist for days. Splenomegaly, hyperbilirubinemia, and renal insufficiency may also develop.

Paroxysmal cold hemoglobinuria is an acute hemolytic anemia occurring almost exclusively in children and young adults, and almost always represents a transient disorder. Table 21-9 compares and contrasts PCH with CHD.

Treatment For chronic forms of PCH, protection from cold exposure is the only useful therapy. Acute postinfection forms of PCH usually terminate spontaneously following resolution of the infectious process. Steroids and transfusion may be required, depending on the severity of the attacks.

Paroxysmal nocturnal hemoglobinuria (PNH) is often confused with PCH because of the similarity of the names and acronyms. RBC destruction in PNH is complement mediated, but the mechanism is not clearly understood. An autoantibody has not been implicated in PNH; a membrane defect is thought to be involved. The only reason for this comment is to alert the reader to a common error in relating PCH and PNH.

Warm Reactive Autoantibodies

Autoantibodies that react best at 37°C are not found as often as the almost ubiquitous cold autoanti-I. However, many more of the AIHAs are of the warm type (70 percent) than of the cold reactive type (16 percent).[5] As with the cold reactive antibodies, there are individuals who have apparently harmless warm reactive autoantibodies. The harmless autoantibodies are serologically indistinguishable from the harmful ones. No diagnostic tests can be performed to determine which autoantibodies will cause RBC destruction. When a warm reactive autoantibody is encoun-

TABLE 21-9 **COMPARISON OF PCH AND COLD AGGLUTININ SYNDROME**

	PCH	Cold Agglutinin Syndrome
Patient population	Children and young adults	Elderly or middle-aged
Pathogenesis	Following viral infection	Idiopathic; lymphoproliferative disorder; following *Mycoplasma pneumoniae* infection
Clinical features	Hemoglobinuria; acute attacks upon exposure to cold (symptoms resolve in hours or days)	Acrocyanosis; autoagglutination of blood at room temperature
Severity of hemolysis	Acute and rapid	Chronic and rarely severe
Hemolysis	Intravascular	Extravascular; intravascular
Autoantibody	IgG (anti-P specificity) (biphasic hemolysin)	IgM (anti-I/i), monophasic
DAT	3+ (polyspecific antiglobulin); neg IgG; 3-4+ C3 monospecific antiglobulin	3+ (polyspecific antiglobulin); neg IgG; 3-4+ C3 monospecific antiglobulin
Thermal range	Moderate (<20°C)	High (up to 30°C to 31°C)
Titer	Moderate (<64)	High (>1000)
Donath-Landsteiner test	Positive	Negative
Treatment	Supportive (disorder terminates when underlying illness resolves)	Avoid cold

From Harmening,[54] p 207, with permission.

tered, it should be characterized as such and reported to the patient's physician. The antibody may alert the physician to an underlying autoimmune disease.

CLINICAL FINDINGS

Patients with warm AIHA present a different problem to the blood bank than those with cold AIHA. A significant percentage of patients suffer from an anemia of sufficient severity to suggest the possible need for transfusion. The degree of anemia is variable; however, hemoglobin levels less than 7 g/dl are not uncommon. The onset of warm AIHA is usually insidious and may be precipitated by a variety of factors such as infection, trauma, surgery, pregnancy, or psychologic stress. In other patients the onset is sudden and unexplained.

Warm AIHA may be idiopathic, with no underlying disease process, or may be secondary to a pathologic disorder. Table 21–10 lists the disorders associated with AIHA.

Signs and symptoms appear when a significant anemia has developed. Pallor, weakness, dizziness, dyspnea, jaundice, and unexplained fever occasionally are presenting complaints. Hemolysis is usually acute at onset and may stabilize or continue to accelerate at a variable rate.

The blood smear usually displays polychromasia, reflecting reticulocytosis, which is characteristic of a hemolytic anemia (see Color Plate 18). Spherocytosis and occasionally RBC fragmentation, indicating extravascular hemolysis, can be demonstrated along with nucleated RBCs. An uncommon manifestation of warm AIHA is reticulocytopenia. It is usually seen in the presence of a hyperplastic marrow, although it may also be associated with a hypoplastic marrow that is secondary to underlying disease state. Because antigenic determinants on erythrocyte precursors also can react with the patient's RBC autoantibodies, reticulocytes can be destroyed as they are released from the bone marrow. Reticulocytopenia at the time of intense hemolysis, therefore, is associated with a high mortality. Products of hemolysis such as bilirubin (particularly the unconjugated or indirect fraction) and urinary urobilinogen are increased. In severe cases, depleted serum haptoglobin, hemoglobinemia, hemoglobinuria, and increases in lactic dehydrogenase (LDH) may be demonstrated.

RED CELL HEMOLYSIS

In 80 percent of cases of warm AIHA, the antibody causing the hemolysis is IgG, with IgG subclasses 1 and 3 found in patients demonstrating clinical signs of hemolytic anemia.

The subclasses or isotypes of IgG are distinguished by the number of disulfide bonds present in the hinge region of the molecule. This accounts for their different electrophoretic mobility and biologic properties. (See Chapter 3 for a complete discussion of the properties of the IgG subclasses.) All IgG subclasses possess the ability to bind complement via the classic pathway of activation, with IgG_3 being more efficient than IgG_1, which in turn is more efficient than IgG_2. Macrophages possess receptors for the Fc fragment of IgG_1 and IgG_3.

Immune RBC destruction resulting from sensitization with IgG antibody is primarily extravascular, taking place in the fixed reticuloendothelial system (RES) cells, primarily those of the liver and spleen. However, the spleen has been demonstrated to be 100 times more efficient in removal of Rh IgG-sensitized RBCs. The macrophages are equipped with two important biologic receptors on their membranes: (1) a receptor for the Fc fragments of IgG_1 and IgG_3 and (2) a receptor for the C3b fragment of complement. Sensitized RBCs are phagocytized by interaction with RES mononuclear phagocytes, depending on which protein coats the erythrocytes. If only IgG is coating the RBCs, phagocytosis of the erythrocytes occurs. If both IgG and C3b are coating the RBCs, there is a rapid phagocytosis, because the C3b fragment augments the action of IgG, enhancing sequestration and phagocytosis of the coated erythrocytes. If only C3b is coating the RBCs, then transient immune adherence occurs. It has been estimated that greater than 100,000 molecules of the complement fragment would be required to induce phagocytosis. Therefore, the activity of the macrophages and the severity of hemolysis via phagocytosis of sensitized RBCs are dependent on various factors, summarized in Table 21–11.

TABLE 21–10 DISORDERS REPORTED TO BE FREQUENTLY ASSOCIATED WITH WARM AIHA

1. Reticuloendothelial neoplasms, such as chronic lymphocytic leukemia, Hodgkin's disease, non-Hodgkin's lymphomas, thymomas
2. Collagen disease such as SLE, scleroderma, and rheumatoid arthritis
3. Infectious diseases such as viral syndromes in childhood
4. Immunologic diseases such as hypogammaglobulinemia, dysglobulinemia, and other immunodeficiency syndromes
5. Gastrointestinal diseases such as ulcerative colitis
6. Benign tumors such as ovarian dermoid cysts

Adapted from Petz and Garratty,[5] p 32.
AIHA = autoimmune hemolytic anemias; SLE = systemic lupus erythematosus.

TABLE 21–11 FACTORS AFFECTING ACTIVITY OF MACROPHAGES

1. Subclass of IgG
2. Presence of complement (C3b) fragments
3. Quantity of Ig or complement
4. Number and activity of helper T cells (T_4)
5. Number and activity of suppressor T cells (T_8)

From Harmening,[55] p 153, with permission.

SEROLOGIC CHARACTERISTICS

Because warm reactive autoantibodies are typically IgG, they react best by the antiglobulin technique. As a rule, these autoantibodies do not agglutinate saline-suspended RBCs after 37°C incubation. However, if albumin or another agglutination potentiator is added to the reaction mixture, agglutination may be observed in this phase. Warm reactive autoantibodies may activate complement and are usually enhanced by enzyme techniques. Most of these autoantibodies react with a high-incidence antigen and have a general specificity within the Rh blood group system, but autoantibodies have been associated with most of the other blood group systems. Identification of autoantibodies is discussed in the following section. The typical reactions of warm autoantibodies are shown in Table 21–12.

Laboratory Tests Affected by Warm Reactive Autoantibodies

Warm reactive autoantibodies can interfere with most routine blood bank tests, possibly presenting more of a problem than cold autoagglutinins. Most cold autoantibodies can be avoided if testing is performed at 37°C or if anti-IgG is used. In the case of warm AIHA, however, both significant alloantibodies and the autoantibodies react best at 37°C. Therefore, more complicated procedures may have to be used to resolve the problems encountered.

ABO Typing Because warm reactive autoantibodies are not direct agglutinins, ABO grouping is usually not affected. Even though the patient's cells may be heavily coated with antibody, they do not agglutinate spontaneously when reagent anti-A and anti-B are added. Similarly, warm autoantibodies in the serum usually do not agglutinate saline-suspended A_1 and B cells.

Rh Typing False-positive Rh typing test results can be a problem when the patient's cells are coated with warm reactive autoantibodies. Agglutination potentiators are added to many Rh-typing reagents (the slide–modified tube reagents) so that D-positive cells, once coated with anti-D, will agglutinate. Potentiators are beneficial because they allow one to perform an immediate-spin Rh (anti-D) test. The disadvantage of adding potentiators is that cells coated with any anti-

body may be agglutinated, including D-negative cells coated with autoantibody. For this reason a control test, consisting of patient cells and the Rh diluent, must be performed in parallel with the Rh test when using the high-protein (slide–modified tube) reagents. The results of the Rh typing are valid only when the control result is negative.

Similar problems that occur with cold autoagglutinins can be easily resolved by washing the cells with warm saline. Warm reactive autoantibodies cannot be easily removed from the cells, so other approaches must be used. Most of the time a low-protein anti-D reagent (chemically modified IgG, the monoclonal-polyclonal blend IgG, or saline IgM) can be used to obtain valid results. As stated earlier, a negative reaction among the ABO forward typing results serves as a control for the low-protein anti-D reagents. If the patient types as AB, Rh positive (all tubes in the ABO forward and Rh typings are positive), a separate Rh control of 6 percent albumin must be tested along with the anti-D to ensure the validity of the Rh typing (see Chapter 6). In an extreme situation, the cells can be treated with chloroquine disulfate according to the procedure by Edwards et al.[24] to remove the IgG antibody from the cells before typing. (See Procedure D of the Procedural Appendix.)

If one wishes to test for the weak expression of the D antigen, D^u, one must use special techniques for removal of the autoantibody before performance of the D^u test. Monospecific anti-IgG is of no help in this situation because the autoantibody is IgG in nature. Chloroquine-treated cells, as described earlier, may be used. Another technique, the rosette test commonly used in detection of fetomaternal hemorrhage, may also be used to detect Rh-positive cells. (See Chapter 20, for discussion of the rosette test.) This screening test, used to detect fetal Rh-positive cells in the circulation of the Rh-negative mother, will also detect Rh-positive cells in any cell population. If the patient's cells are D positive, the rosette test result will be strongly positive. Because the rosette test does not incorporate an antiglobulin phase, a patient with a positive DAT result can be accurately typed for the D antigen by this method. It is important to note that it is not absolutely necessary to determine the correct D typing of a patient with warm AIHA because D-negative RBCs can be transfused if necessary.

Direct Antiglobulin Test A positive DAT result is expected in association with warm reactive autoantibodies. The RBCs may be coated with IgG alone (20 percent), IgG and complement (67 percent), or complement alone (13 percent).[5] In rare cases, the DAT result may be negative or only IgA[14] may be present.

Antibody Detection and Identification The serum of a patient with warm autoagglutinins may contain only autoantibody or a mixture of autoantibody and alloantibody, if the patient has been previously transfused or pregnant. When smaller amounts of autoantibody have been produced, all of the autoantibody may be absorbed onto the patient's cells in

TABLE 21–12 **SEROLOGIC REACTIONS OF TYPICAL WARM AUTOANTIBODIES**

Reaction Phase	Screening Cells	Autologous Cells
RT	0	0
37°C*	0	0
AHG	2–3+	4+

*Agglutination may be observed if the RBCs are suspended in albumin or low ionic strength solution or if they are enzyme treated.
AHG = antihuman globulin; RT = room temperature.

vivo and no free autoantibody will be detectable in the serum.

When warm reactive autoantibodies are present in the serum or on the patient's cells, the extent of the testing should be based on the patient's history. It must be determined that the antibody coating the patient's cells is an autoantibody, and limited testing should be performed to determine the specificity. If the patient has been previously transfused or pregnant, efforts must be made to detect clinically significant alloantibodies that might be masked by the autoantibody.

Evaluation of Autoantibody A positive DAT result can be caused by RBC alloantibodies or drug-induced antibodies, as well as by RBC autoantibodies. IgG may be present on the cells in each case and antibody may not be present in the serum. It is important to differentiate the reasons for a positive DAT result, as selection of RBCs for transfusion and treatment protocols may differ. To make the distinction between these causes, the patient's medical history, including previous transfusions and pregnancies, diagnosis, and medications, must be known. When a patient has been recently transfused, alloantibodies may be coating the transfused donor's cells. In most cases, by examining the DAT microscopically for mixed-field agglutination and by determining the specificity of the antibody in the eluate, alloantibodies can be established as the cause (see Chapter 18). Because warm autoantibodies are frequently associated with certain diseases such as systemic lupus erythematosus (SLE) and with medications such as methyldopa, the patient's diagnosis and drug history are informative. As discussed subsequently, the specificity of the antibody may help differentiate between autoantibody and alloantibody.

To identify the specificity of a warm reactive autoantibody, one must test an eluate prepared from the patient's RBCs and the serum against a panel of reagent RBCs. (See Procedure E of the Procedural Appendix for instruction in preparing a digitonin-acid eluate.) If the patient has not been transfused recently (within the past 2 to 3 months), any antibody activity in the eluate can be assumed to be autoantibody. The serum may contain alloantibody in addition to autoantibody.

The reactions of an autoantibody may be different in the serum and in the eluate. Warm autoantibodies may have an apparent autoanti-e specificity in the serum but may show panagglutination of RBCs tested with the eluate because the concentration of antibody removed from the cells in the elution process may be greater than that in the serum. Table 21–13 illustrates an example of such reactivity. Differing elution techniques may also yield varying results in testing eluate (i.e., a heat eluate usually reacts more weakly than an acid eluate or one of the chemical eluates such as dichloromethane or ether).

Many warm reactive autoantibodies have a complex Rh-like specificity similar to those shown in Table 21–14. They may react with all RBCs of normal Rh pheno-

TABLE 21–13 SEROLOGIC REACTIONS OF SERUM AND ELUATES CONTAINING WARM AUTOANTIBODIES

RBC Phenotype	ANTIGLOBULIN REACTIONS		
	Serum	Acid Eluate	Heat Eluate
DCe/DCe	+	4+	2+
DcE/DcE	0	3+	+
dce/dce	+	4+	2+
DCe/dce	+	4+	2+
dcE/dcE	0	3+	+

type (e.g., cde/cde, CDe/cDE, etc.). To categorize them as anti-nl (normal), anti-pdl (partially deleted), or anti-dl (deleted), one must use very rare RBCs—for example, partially deleted (−D−/−D−) and fully deleted (Rh$_{null}$).[25]

There are numerous reports of autoantibodies with specificities other than Rh. Among the other specificities are autoanti-U, −Wr^a, −En^a, −Kp^b, −Vel[26], and −Ge[27]. Chapter 7 of Petz and Garratty[5] gives a detailed discussion of autoantibody specificity.

It is not necessary to do extensive studies to identify autoantibodies, but limited testing is recommended. By testing a commercial RBC panel, an antibody of simple specificity can be identified. This information may be useful in evaluating whether the antibody is autoantibody or alloantibody. On the other hand, an antibody reactive with all cells is probably an autoantibody. There are, however, many exceptions to these interpretations. The need to consider the medical history cannot be overemphasized. Specificity may also be helpful in selecting blood for transfusion. Some workers prefer to transfuse RBCs that are compatible with the autoantibody when, for example, the specificity is e-like.

Detection and Identification of Alloantibodies Detection and identification of all alloantibodies are of primary concern when a patient with warm AIHA must be transfused, especially when that patient has been previously transfused or pregnant. When autoantibody is found in the serum, it will typically mask any alloantibodies present. In this situation one can use several techniques:

TABLE 21–14 SEROLOGIC REACTIONS OF WARM AUTOANTIBODIES WITH RBCs OF SELECTED Rh PHENOTYPES

	RBC PHENOTYPE		
	Normal (cde/cde, etc.)	Partially Deleted (−D−/−D−, etc.)	Fully Deleted (Rh$_{null}$)
Anti-nl	+	0	0
Anti-pdl	+	+	0
Anti-dl	+	+	+

1. If the autoantibody shows a specificity, test a panel of cells negative for the corresponding antigen and positive for other selected antigens.
2. If the patient has not been transfused recently (within the past 2 to 3 months), absorb the autoantibody with autologous RBCs.
3. If the patient has been recently transfused or is severely anemic, absorb the autoantibody with RBCs of selected donors (i.e., homologous absorption).

If the autoantibody has a demonstrable specificity, such as anti-e, a panel of antigen-negative (e-negative, in this case) cells can be selected that are positive for the other important antigens such as Kell, Duffy, Kidd, S, and s.

When autoantibodies have a broader specificity, an absorption technique must be used. (A discussion follows of difficulties involved in using an autoabsorption procedure.) In an autoabsorption, the patient's serum and autologous cells are incubated at 37°C, allowing the autoantibody to be bound to the autologous cells and leaving the alloantibody in the serum. To improve the uptake of autoantibody, some of the antibody that has coated the cells in vivo can be removed by a gentle elution at 45°C, or the cells can be treated with the ZZAP reagent (a mixture of proteolytic enzyme and thiol reagent). If there is a large amount of autoantibody in the serum, more than one absorption may be necessary (see Procedure F of the Procedural Appendix). Table 21–15 gives an example of antibody-detection tests using unabsorbed, once-absorbed, and twice-absorbed serum. In this example, one absorption did not remove all the autoantibody, but two absorptions were effective. No underlying alloantibodies are present in this example.

There are several problems to consider with autoabsorptions. First, if the patient has been recently transfused, donor RBCs in the patient specimen may remove alloantibody during the procedure. Autoabsorption would not be recommended in this instance. Second, if the patient is severely anemic, one may not be able to obtain enough autologous cells for multiple absorptions. Third, whenever an absorption is done, whether with autologous or homologous cells, the serum is diluted to some degree. Some saline is present in packed RBCs. A weakly reactive alloantibody could be missed if multiple absorptions are performed.

When the patient has been recently transfused or is

TABLE 21–16 DIFFERENTIAL ABSORPTION TECHNIQUE FOR DETECTING ALLOANTIBODIES IN THE SERUM OF A PATIENT WITH WARM REACTIVE AUTOANTIBODIES

Donor	RBC Phenotype of Absorbing Cells	Antibody Remaining in Absorbed Serum
A	R1R1, Ss, Fy(a−b+), Jk(a+b−), kk	c, E, Fyᵃ, Jkᵇ, K
B	R2R2, ss, Fy(a+b+), JK(a−b+), kk	C, e, S, Jkᵃ, K
C	rr, SS, Fy(a+b−), Jk(a+b+), kk	C, D, E, s, Fyᵇ, K

severely anemic, cells of selected phenotypes can be used for absorption. They should lack the antigens for the more commonly encountered clinically significant alloantibodies (e.g., Rh, Kell, Duffy, Kidd, Ss). As shown in Table 21–16, if one absorbs the patient's serum with cells from donors A, B, and C and then tests the absorbed sera, one can detect many important alloantibodies. It is important to detect *all* clinically significant alloantibodies, like those directed against high-incidence antigens. For example, an anti-k (Cellano) would be absorbed onto virtually all random donor cells because the k antigen is present on the cells of more than 99 percent of the population (such as cells A, B, and C).

When alloantibodies are found or suspected in the serum of a patient with warm AIHA, it is necessary to test the patient's RBCs for the absence of the corresponding antigen. Because the patient has a positive DAT result, usually with IgG coating the cells, antigen typing using an antiglobulin test (such as typing for Kell, Duffy, or Kidd antigens) will be invalid. Chloroquine-treated cells may be used in these situations to obtain valid antigen typings. Chloroquine diphosphate will remove much of the coating IgG while leaving the antigens intact. Careful attention should be paid to the procedure, following instructions on the package insert of commercially available chloroquine reagents, in order to ensure that certain antigens will not be destroyed or weakened.

SELECTION OF BLOOD FOR TRANSFUSION

Many patients with warm AIHA never require transfusion; they can be managed with medical treatment. Occasionally, however, the anemia is so severe

TABLE 21–15 ANTIBODY DETECTION USING UNABSORBED AND AUTOABSORBED SERUM

Reagent Red Cells	UNABSORBED		ABSORBED × 1		ABSORBED × 2	
	37°C	AHG	37°C	AHG	37°C	AHG
I	+	3+	0	+	0	0
II	+	3+	0	+	0	0

AHG = antihuman globulin.

that transfusion cannot be avoided.[5] Patients who have a nonhemolytic warm AIHA pose problems when blood is needed for a surgical procedure. In these cases compatibility with any alloantibodies in the patient's serum is the main concern. Compatibility with the autoantibody is controversial. If the autoantibody shows a simple specificity, such as anti-e, local practice may be to select donor units negative for the corresponding antigen. However, one must ensure that the cells selected do not possess an antigen likely to result in stimulation of the patient to form alloantibodies. For example, an Rh-negative patient with autoanti-e specificity should not be transfused with D-positive RBCs in order to have cells lacking the e antigen.[28] Finding compatible units for patients with a broad specificity warm autoagglutinin is virtually impossible. "Least-incompatible" RBCs may be selected for transfusion. In all cases, the transfused donor cells will likely be destroyed as rapidly as are the patient's own RBCs. Units compatible with any present alloantibodies should be selected using the techniques described in the previous section.

TREATMENT

The aim is to treat the underlying disease first, if one is present. General measures to support cardiovascular function are important in severely anemic patients. Transfusion is usually avoided, if possible, inasmuch as this may only accelerate the hemolysis instead of ameliorating the anemia. However, transfusion is used in life-threatening situations.

The three forms of treatment described here are used, according to the severity of the disorder.

Corticosteroid Administration

This form of therapy involves the use of corticosteroids, such as prednisone. Initially, high doses of 100 to 200 mg of prednisone are maintained until the patient's hematocrit stabilizes. Patients who are not transfused respond to steroid therapy more rapidly than those who are transfused. Several mechanisms have been proposed for the action of prednisone, including (1) reduction of antibody synthesis, (2) alteration of antibody activity, and (3) alteration of macrophage receptors for IgG and C3, which reduces the clearance of antibody-coated RBCs.

The dosage of prednisone should be reduced when the hematocrit begins to rise and the reticulocyte count drops. Finally, the steroids are withdrawn slowly over 2 to 4 months. A beneficial response to the administration of prednisone is demonstrated in 50 to 65 percent of all patients with warm AIHA. An androgenic steroid, danazol, has also been beneficial in prednisone-resistant cases.[29]

Splenectomy

If steroid therapy fails or if a patient requires large doses of steroids to control hemolysis, splenectomy is usually recommended. The decision to perform splenectomy requires clinical evaluation and judgment. The three reasons for performing splenectomy are (1) failure of steroid therapy, (2) need for continuous high-dose steroid maintenance, and (3) complications of steroid therapy. Splenectomy accomplishes two functions: (1) It decreases the production of antibody, and (2) it removes a potent site of RBC damage and destruction. Patients who had a good initial response to steroid therapy respond better with splenectomy than do those who failed to respond initially to steroid therapy.

As many as 60 percent of patients with warm AIHA benefit from splenectomy if steroid dosages greater than 15 mg/day are also used to maintain remission.

Immunosuppressive Drugs

This is usually the last approach used in management of warm AIHA. Azathioprine (Imuran) and cyclophosphamide are examples of immunosuppressive drugs that interfere with antibody synthesis by destroying dividing cells.

Experience in using this therapy is limited. The most detrimental side effect that threatens the common use of these drugs is the potential for neoplastic growth resulting from the defective immune surveillance of immunosuppressed patients.

Table 21–17 reviews and compares the characteristics of cold and warm autoimmune hemolytic anemias.

Drug-Induced Immune Hemolytic Anemia

Drugs can cause a variety of side effects, including immune destruction of RBCs and other blood cells, although the incidence of drug-induced immune hemolytic anemia is rare. Hemolytic anemia, thrombocytopenia, and agranulocytosis can occur separately, but in some patients more than one cell line can be af-

TABLE 21–17 COMPARISON OF WARM AND COLD AUTOIMMUNE HEMOLYTIC ANEMIAS

	Warm AIHA	Cold AIHA
Optimal reactivity	>32°C	<30°C
Ig class	IgG	IgM
Complement activation	May bind complement	Binds complement
Hemolysis	Usually extravascular (no cell lysis)	Usually intravascular (cell lysis)
Frequency	70–75% of cases	16% of cases (PCH: 1–2%)
Specificity	Frequently Rh	Ii system (PCH: anti-P)

From Harmening,[54] p 207, with permission.
AIHA = autoimmune hemolytic anemias; PCH = paroxysmal cold hemoglobinuria.

fected. The cells may be coated with antibody, antibody and complement, or complement alone. The discussion in this section is limited to RBC problems, but many of the same principles apply to platelets and leukocytes also.

Drug-mediated problems may come to the attention of the blood bank technologist in one of two ways:

1. A request for diagnostic testing on a patient with a possible hemolytic anemia
2. Unexpected results in routine testing (e.g., a positive autologous control reaction in the antiglobulin phase of antibody screening or compatibility testing or a positive DAT result)

Drugs should be suspected as a possible explanation for immune hemolysis or a positive DAT result when there is no other reason for the serologic and hematologic findings and if the patient has a history of taking the drug. Other causes should be considered first because, with the exception of methyldopa-induced problems, drug-induced positive DAT results or hemolytic anemia is relatively rare. Petz and Garratty[5] review four different mechanism by which drugs can induce problems: immune complexes, drug adsorption, membrane modification, and autoantibody formation. Each mechanism has characteristic serologic and clinical features. Specific drugs are commonly associated with one particular mechanism but may work by another.[30–32]

IMMUNE COMPLEX (INNOCENT BYSTANDER) MECHANISM

Although the occurrence is rare, the largest variety of drugs causing immune-mediated problems work by the immune complex mechanism. First described in the early 1960s, it was thought that drugs operating through this mechanism combine with plasma proteins to form immunogens.[33] The antibody (IgG or IgM) subsequently produced recognizes determinants on the drug. If the patient ingests the same drug (or a drug bearing the same haptenic group) following immunization, the formation of a drug-antidrug complex may occur. Following antigen-antibody interaction, the complement cascade may be activated. RBCs are thought to be involved in this process only as "innocent bystanders."[34] The soluble drug-antidrug complex nonspecifically adsorbs loosely to the RBC surface. Complement, when activated, sensitizes the cell and may cause lysis (Fig. 21–2).

More recently, however, Garratty[35] has suggested that attachment of immune complex to the RBC may be specific. The resulting antibody may react with the drug-RBC complex, the RBC antigens alone, or both in the same patient, but not with the normal cell without the drug complex. Drugs associated with the immune complex mechanism are listed in Table 21–18.

Because complement activation is involved in the immune complex, clinically affected patients frequently present with acute intravascular hemolysis.[36] When other causes for hemoglobinemia and hemoglo-

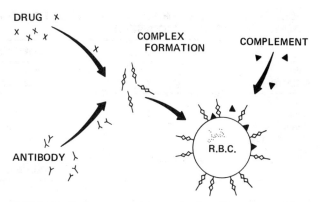

FIGURE 21–2 Immune complex mechanism. (From Petz and Garratty,[5] p 272, with permission.)

binuria have been excluded (e.g., ABO hemolytic transfusion reactions or cold AIHA), a drug-antidrug reaction should be considered. When obtaining the drug history it is important to realize that this group of patients need take only small doses of the drug to be affected. The patient recovers rapidly once the drug is withdrawn.

The DAT result on the patient's RBCs will usually be positive. If monospecific reagents are used, agglutination usually occurs with anticomplement but not with anti-IgG. Test results using anti-IgG are negative, even when the antibody is of the IgG class, because the drug-antidrug complex is thought to elute from the cell during the washing procedure before the antiglobulin test. Results from other routine blood bank tests are negative in all phases; the antibody is directed against a drug, not against an RBC antigen. Therefore, the antibody screen and compatibility test results are negative, unless an alloantibody is also present. An eluate tested against reagent RBCs will also react negatively. Typical serologic results are summarized in Table 21–19.

To confirm that a drug-antidrug reaction through this mechanism is responsible for a positive DAT result, one must demonstrate the antibody in the patient's serum. The patient's serum can be incubated with a solution of the drug in question and ABO-compatible RBCs. Complement activation is the usual indicator of an antigen-antibody reaction; therefore, one should observe for hemolysis after incubation and use reagents containing anti-C3 activity for the antiglobulin test. A general procedure for demonstrating antibodies reacting by the immune complex mechanism, suggested by Garratty,[37] is given in Procedure G of the Procedural Appendix.

For the test results to be interpreted correctly, adequate control tests must be performed. The patient's serum must not react with the cells when saline or the diluent used to dissolve the drug is substituted for the drug solution, and the drug solution must not hemolyze the suspension of cells nonspecifically. Examples of typical reactions with the patient's serum and control are given in Table 21–20.

An eluate from the patient's cells is usually nonreactive even if the drug and a source of complement are

TABLE 21–18 **DRUGS THAT HAVE CAUSED POSITIVE DAT RESULTS AND SOMETIMES HEMOLYTIC ANEMIA**

MECHANISMS		
Auto Antibody	Drug Absorption	Membrane Modification
Methyldopa	Penicillins	Cephalosporins
Levodopa	Cephalosporins	
Mefenamic acid	Carbromal*	
Procainamide	Erythromycin*	
Ibuprofen*		
IMMUNE COMPLEXES		
I†	II‡	Not Yet Defined
Stibophen	Sulphonamides	Methadone
Quinidine	Pyramidon	Methysergide
Quinine	Dipyrone	Hydralazine
p-aminosalicyclic acid	Melphalan	Inosine dialdehyde
Phenacetin	Insulin	Cisplatin
Chlorinated hydrocarbons (insecticides)	Acetaminophen	Methotrexate
Antihistamines	Probenecid	Podophyllotoxin derivatives
Isoniazid	Triamterene*	Zomepirac
Chlorpromazine	9-Hydroxy-methyl elliptinium*	Tolmetin
Sulphonylurea derivatives	Sodium pentothal	Furosemide
Rifampin		Butizide metabolite
Hydrochlorothiazide		
Streptomycin		
Tetracycline		
Nomifensine		

From American Red Cross: Immunohematology. Journal of Blood Group Serology and Education 2:1, 1985, with permission.
*Suggested but more evidence is needed.
†Described more than once in the medical literature.
‡One case only in the medical literature.

added. Very little antibody, if any, remains on the cells after washing.

In most blood banks, confirmatory testing is done only when the patient has hematologic complications and not when the patient simply has a history of taking the drug and a positive DAT result. Some of the drugs known to cause immune complex–mediated problems are in frequent use, and there are a large number of patients with a positive DAT result and no evidence of hemolysis. Therefore, a full work-up is done only for academic interest and is not required before release of RBCs for transfusion.

Treatment is aimed at stopping the use of the drug. Although hemolysis by this mechanism is rare, the onset is usually sudden and characterized by intravascular hemolysis and renal failure. Therefore, immediate cessation of the drug is essential. Steroid treatment also may be given.

DRUG-ADSORPTION (HAPTEN) MECHANISM

Unlike drugs acting through the immune-complex mechanism, drugs operating through the drug-adsorption mechanism bind firmly to proteins, including

TABLE 21–19 **SEROLOGIC REACTIONS OBSERVED WITH DRUG-INDUCED POSITIVE DAT RESULTS**

Mechanism	DAT			Serum	Eluate
	Polyspecific	Anti-IgG	Anti-C3		
Immune complex	+	0*	+	Routine antibody screens negative	
				Antibody demonstrable if serum, complement, drug incubated with RBCs	Antibody not demonstrable even in presence of drug
Drug adsorption	+	+	0*	Routine antibody screens negative	
				High-titered antibody demonstrable if serum tested with drug-coated RBCs	Antibody demonstrable using drug-coated RBCs
Membrane modification	+	+	+	Routine antibody screens negative; nonimmunologic mechanism	
Autoantibody formation	+	+	0*	Autoantibody reactive with normal RBCs may or may not be present	Eluate reactive with normal RBCs

*May occasionally be positive.

TABLE 21-20 INTERPRETATION OF TESTS TO CONFIRM PRESENCE OF ANTIDRUG ANTIBODY ACTING BY IMMUNE COMPLEX MECHANISM

	Patient's Serum	Fresh Serum (Complement)	Drug	RBCs	Results*	Interpretation
Tests	X	X	X	X	Positive	Antidrug antibody present if controls working
	X	X	X	X	Negative	Antidrug antibody not present; drug not present in proper concentration
Controls						
Patient's serum	X	0	0	X	Negative	No alloantibody against these RBC antigens present
Fresh serum	0	X	X	X	Negative	No alloantibody against RBC or drug present in serum of random donor (complement)
Drug solution	0	0	X	X	Negative	Drug solution does not cause RBCs to agglutinate or lyse

*Based on presence of hemolysis, agglutination.

the proteins of the RBC membrane (Fig. 21-3). Presumably because of their ability to bind to proteins, these drugs are better immunogens. For example, antibodies to penicillin, the drug most commonly associated with this mechanism, are found in about 3 percent of hospitalized patients receiving large doses of penicillin; of these, less than 5 percent will develop a hemolytic anemia.[18] Even with the relatively high incidence of antipenicillin antibodies and the ability of the drug to bind to the RBC membrane, penicillin-induced positive DAT results are rare.[9] The low incidence may reflect the fact that the patient must receive massive doses (10 million units/day) of penicillin for the cells to be coated adequately. Also most penicillin antibodies are IgM and therefore are not detected by the antiglobulin test. The penicillin antibody responsible for a positive DAT result is IgG. Complement activation does not occur.

The laboratory results are consistent with this description of the mechanism (Table 21-19). Cells from patients with a positive DAT result are usually coated with IgG alone. However, sometimes both IgG and complement are present on the cells. The patient's serum and eluate are nonreactive with reagent RBCs and random donor cells. Therefore, the antibody screen is negative and crossmatches are compatible in all phases. However, if the serum and eluate are tested against penicillin-coated cells, agglutination does occur in the antiglobulin phase. The procedure for preparing the penicillin-coated cells is given in Procedure H of the Procedural Appendix.[37] Because many patients have penicillin antibodies, Garratty emphasizes that the serum antibody must be high titered and the eluate positive before the findings are definitive.[37] Interpretation of the confirmatory tests to demonstrate antipenicillin antibodies is outlined in Table 21-21.

Only a small percentage of those patients with penicillin-induced positive DAT results exhibit hematologic complications. The clinical features of such a hemolytic episode differ from those of immune complex–mediated problems in several ways. Because the complement cascade is usually not activated, cell destruction is predominantly extravascular rather than intravascular. Therefore, the anemia develops more slowly and is not life threatening unless the cause for the hemolysis is not recognized and the penicillin therapy is continued. Penicillin-induced hemolysis occurs only when the patient receives massive doses of the antibiotic, in contrast to the small amounts of drug that are necessary for hemolysis due to immune complexes. The patient improves once the drug is withdrawn, but hemolysis continues at a decreasing rate until cells heavily coated with penicillin are removed. The DAT result may remain positive for several weeks. Mixed-field agglutination will be seen in the DAT result because some cells will be penicillin coated and others will not. The antibody may cross-react with ampicillin and methicillin.

Other drugs cause a positive DAT result and hemolytic anemia by this mechanism (see Table 21-18). Among these are cephalothin (Keflin) and quinidine.[5] Distinguishing between Keflin-induced problems and penicillin-induced problems is technically difficult because the drugs have antigenic determinants in common, and antipenicillin is frequently in the serum. Antipenicillin will react with Keflin-treated cells; anti-Keflin with penicillin-coated cells. Garratty[37] suggests that comparing the strength of the reactivity of the serum or eluate (titer or score) with penicillin- and Keflin-coated cells may be of value.

Additional difficulties are involved with using Keflin-treated cells. As discussed in the next section, Keflin-treated cells may adsorb protein nonspecifically

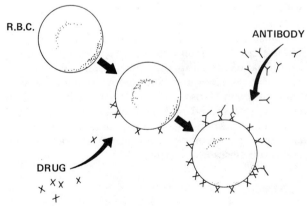

R.B.C.

ANTIBODY

DRUG

FIGURE 21-3 Drug adsorption mechanism. (From Petz and Garratty,[5] p 280, with permission.)

TABLE 21-21 INTERPRETATION OF SCREENING TESTS FOR PRESENCE OF ANTIDRUG ANTIBODIES ACTING BY DRUG ABSORPTION MECHANISM

	Patient's Serum or Eluate	Drug-Coated RBCs	Uncoated RBCs*	Results†	Interpretation
Test	X	X	0	Positive	Antidrug antibody present if controls working; antibody in serum usually high titered
	X	X	0	Negative	Antidrug antibody not present
Controls					
Patient's serum	X	0	X	Negative	No alloantibody against these RBC antigens present in serum or eluate
Drug-coated RBCs	0	X	0	Negative	Drug-coated RBCs do not spontaneously agglutinate or lyse

*Same RBCs as those coated with drug.
†Based on presence of agglutination (or hemolysis with serum).

and give a positive indirect antiglobulin test result with a serum that contains no anti-Keflin antibodies.

MEMBRANE MODIFICATION (NONIMMUNOLOGIC PROTEIN ADSORPTION)

It is hypothesized that the cephalosporins, in addition to operating through the drug-adsorption mechanism, are able to modify RBCs so that plasma proteins (e.g., IgG, IgM, IgA, and complement) can bind to the membrane (Fig. 21-4).[38] Consequently, RBCs from approximately 3 percent of patients receiving cephalosporins (e.g., Keflin) may exhibit a positive DAT result with polyspecific and monospecific reagents. The uptake of immunoglobulins or complement components is not the result of an antigen-antibody reaction, so this mechanism is nonimmunologic. Inasmuch as antibody is not involved, results of tests with the patient's serum and eluate are negative (see Table 21-19). Several cases of cephalosporin-associated hemolytic anemia have been reported, but destruction seems to have been mediated through the drug adsorption mechanism rather than the membrane modification mechanism.[39-42] There is no treatment approach because hemolytic anemia associated with the ingestion of these drugs has not been described in relation to membrane modification.

AUTOANTIBODY FORMATION

Unlike the drugs acting through the previously described mechanisms, which induce production of an *allo*antibody against a determinant on a drug, methyldopa (Aldomet) induces the production of an *auto*antibody that recognizes RBC antigens.[42,43] The antibodies produced are serologically indistinguishable from those seen in patients with warm AIHA (see previous section). Methyldopa-induced positive DAT results are frequently encountered. Approximately 10 to 20 percent of patients receiving this antihypertensive drug develop a positive DAT result. However, very few (0.5 to 1 percent) of this group of patients subsequently develop immune hemolytic anemia.[5] Other drugs that also cause autoantibody production are L-dopa, mefanamic acid, procainamide, and ibuprofen (see Table 21-18).[35]

Several mechanisms by which methyldopa causes the production of autoantibodies have been proposed (Table 21-22).[44-46] The most attractive suggestion is that of Kirtland, Horwitz, and Mohler,[3] who propose that methyldopa alters the function of T-suppressor cells and suggest that this upset in the immune system would allow production of antibody against "self."

The serologic features of this type of drug-induced problem are very different from those of the other drug-related immune hemolytic anemias. As shown in Table 21-19, the antibody in the eluate *will* react with normal RBCs in the absence of the drug. Antibody of similar specificity and reactivity may be found in the serum. Patients' RBCs are usually coated with IgG, rarely with complement components.

Because the serology of methyldopa-induced positive DAT result and immune hemolytic anemia is identical to that of the idiopathic warm AIHA, one cannot establish in the laboratory that methyldopa is the cause of the problem. However, if the patient is receiving the drug, one should be highly suspicious. If methyldopa is withdrawn, autoantibody production will eventually stop, but it may be several months before the DAT result becomes negative.

TREATMENT

Discontinuation of the drug is the treatment of choice for patients with a drug-induced hemolytic ane-

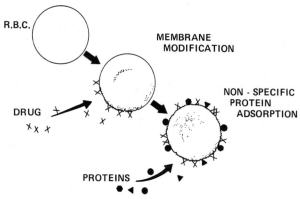

FIGURE 21-4 Membrane modification mechanism. (From Petz and Garratty,[5] p 284, with permission.)

TABLE 21–22 **PROPOSED THEORIES FOR METHYLDOPA-INDUCED MECHANISM OF IMMUNE HEMOLYTIC ANEMIA**

1. Normal RBC antigens are altered by the drug and are no longer recognized as "self," resulting in production of autoantibodies to these RBC antigens.
2. The drug acts as a hapten, resulting in the production of antibodies, which cross-react with normal RBC antigens.
3. The drug produces aberrations in the proliferation of normal lymphocytes, producing clones of abnormal immunologically competent cells, which produce antibodies against normal RBC antigens.
4. The drug affects the synthesis of IgG, exerting a direct effect on T lymphocytes, which results in a loss of suppressor function and subsequent proliferation of autoantibodies by B lymphocytes.

From Harmening,[54] p 209, with permission.

mia. The presence of a positive DAT result does not necessarily imply that the drug must be discontinued, if the effects of the drug are therapeutically beneficial. In general, however, other drugs should be substituted and the patient observed for resolution of the anemia to confirm a drug-induced hemolytic process. If the patient has a positive DAT result without hemolysis, continued administration of the drug is optional.

Generally, the prognosis for patients with drug-induced hemolytic anemia is excellent. In Table 21–23, the four recognized mechanisms leading to the development of drug-related antibodies are compared. Table 21–24 contrasts the antibody characteristics of the various types of AIHAs.

Summary

By understanding the mechanisms by which drugs can cause a positive DAT result or immune hemolytic anemia, one can quickly decide which laboratory tests are most likely to be informative. (Table 21–18 lists problem drugs.) Other drugs cited are fluclozacillin,[47] probenecid,[48] diclofenac,[49] sulfasalazine,[50] glafenine,[51] latamoxef,[51] teniposide,[52] ticarcillin,[53] and nalidixic acid.[53] Before any special testing is done, one should proceed in the following manner:

1. Obtain the patient's medical history, including

TABLE 21–23 **MECHANISMS LEADING TO DEVELOPMENT OF DRUG-RELATED ANTIBODIES**

Mechanism	Prototype Drugs	Ig Class	DAT Result	Eluate	Frequency of Hemolysis
Immune complex formation ("innocent bystander")	Quinidine Phenacetin	IgM or IgG	Positive (often to complement only; however, IgG may be present)	Often negative	Small doses of drugs may cause acute intravascular hemolysis with hemoglobinemia and hemoglobinuria; renal failure common
Drug adsorption (hapten)	Penicillins Cephalosporins Streptomycin	IgG	Positive (strongly, owing to IgG)	Often negative	3–4% of patients taking large daily doses (10 million units) of penicillin, which is one of the most common causes of immune hemolysis, usually extravascular in nature
Membrane modification (nonimmunologic protein adsorption)	Cephalosporins	Numerous plasma proteins (nonimmunologic sensitization)	Positive, owing to various serum proteins	Negative	No hemolysis; however, 3% of patients receiving the drug develop a positive DAT result
Methyldopa-induced (unknown)	Methyldopa (Aldomet)	IgG	Strongly positive (owing to IgG sensitization)	Positive (warm autoantibody identical to that found in warm AIHA)	0.8% of patients receiving the drug develop hemolytic anemia that mimics a warm AIHA (depends on drug dose); 15% of patients receiving methyldopa develop positive DAT result

Adapted from Harmening,[54] p 210.
AIHA = autoimmune hemolytic anemias.

TABLE 21–24 SUMMARY OF ANTIBODY CHARACTERISTICS IN AUTOIMMUNE HEMOLYTIC ANEMIAS

	Warm Reactive Autoantibody	Cold Reactive Autoantibody	Paroxysmal Cold Hemoglobinuria	Drug-Related Autoantibody
Ig characteristics	Polyclonal IgG, IgM, and IgA may be present; rarely IgA alone	Polyclonal IgM infection; monoclonal kappa chain IgM in cold agglutination disease	Polyclonal IgG	Polyclonal IgG
Complement activity	Variable	Always	Always	Depends on mechanism of drug, antibody, and RBC interaction
Thermal reactivity	20°C to 37°C (optimum 37°C)	4°C to 32°C; rarely to 37°C (optimum 4°C)	4°C to 20°C; biphasic hemolysin	20°C to 37°C (optimum 37°C)
Titer of free antibody	Low (<32); may be detectable only with enzyme-treated cells	High (>512 at 4°C)	Moderate to low (<64)	Depends on mechanism of drug, antibody, and RBC interaction
Reactivity of eluate with antibody screening cells	Usually panreactive	Nonreactive	Nonreactive	Panreactive with methyldopa type; nonreactive in all other cases
Most common specificity	Anti-Rh precursor; anti-common Rh; anti-LW; anti-Enᵃ/Wrᵇ; anti-U	Anti-I	Anti-P	Anti-'e'-like; methyldopa antidrug
Site of RBC destruction	Predominantly spleen with some liver involvement	Predominantly liver, rarely intravascular	Intravascular	Intravascular and spleen

From Harmening,[54] p 211, with permission.

transfusions, pregnancies, medications, and diagnosis.

2. Perform a DAT using RBCs collected in EDTA. Test the cells with a polyspecific antiglobulin reagent and monospecific reagents.

3. Screen the patient's serum for RBC alloantibodies.

4. Prepare and test an eluate for RBC alloantibodies if the patient has been recently transfused.

After evaluating this information, one can decide whether drugs are a possible cause of the problem and which of the mechanisms is involved. Then, when other causes (e.g., transfusion reaction) have been excluded and if the clinical situation warrants additional testing, drug-coated cells or solutions of the drug can be prepared for confirmatory tests.

Case Studies

Case 1

PART A

A 45-year-old black man was admitted to the hospital with complaints of extreme fatigue and back pain. Admission testing results are as follows:

Hemoglobin	4.5 g/dl
Reticulocyte count	30 percent
Total bilirubin	6.8 mg/dl

The attending physician ordered 4 units of packed RBCs for transfusion as soon as possible. Records indicate that the patient was transfused 3 years ago with 4 units of RBCs following an automobile accident. No serologic problems were noted at that time. Initial testing results follow:

Antisera			Cells	
−A	−B	−D	A₁	B
0	0	3+	4+	4+

		IS	AHG
Antibody screen	I	0	3+
	II	0	3+
	III	0	3+
Crossmatches	1	0	3+
	2	0	3+
	3	0	3+
	4	0	3+

IS = immediate spin; AHG = antihuman globulin.

1. In light of the patient history and results, what kinds of problems might be present in this patient?

2. What further information or testing would be helpful?

PART B

Direct antiglobulin testing was performed on the patient's cells:

Anti-IgG   4+
Anti-C3d   Negative

A panel was performed on the patient's serum and all cells reacted (3+). An autocontrol was also 4+, as expected.

The patient's history was investigated and the following points were noted:

Only known transfusion was that contained in previous record (3 years ago).

Patient has had problems with hypertension and is currently taking methyldopa.

1. What explanation for the serologic problems can you now give?

2. What additional testing must be done in order to provide blood for this patient, if the physician decides to transfuse?

3. What advice might you give the patient's physician regarding transfusion?

PART C

The patient's cells were treated with ZZAP reagent and an autoabsorption was performed. The antibody screen and crossmatches were repeated with the following results:

Absorbed Serum		IS	AHG
Antibody screen	I	0	0
	II	0	2+
	III	0	0
Crossmatches	1	0	0
	2	0	0
	3	0	3+
	4	0	0

IS = immediate spin; AHG = antihuman globulin.

A panel was performed, and the results are given in the Case Answers Section that follows.

1. What antibody specificities are evident?

2. What further testing must be done before release of blood for transfusion?

3. What additional tests might be helpful in providing blood for transfusion to this patient in the future?

Case 1 Answers

PART A

1. With the significantly decreased hemoglobin and increased reticulocyte count, this patient may be experiencing a hemo-lytic episode. The serologic results indicate a panagglutinin, reactive with all cells tested thus far. This may indicate that the patient has a warm autoantibody and is suffering from warm AIHA.

2. A DAT should be performed to determine if the antibody is an alloantibody or autoantibody (warm AIHA). Anti-IgG and anti-C3 should be tested for to determine which protein is coating the cells. We know that the patient has not been recently transfused. We need to know the patient's diagnosis and medications that he has been taking. A panel should be tested to determine if the antibody shows any specificity.

PART B

1. From the serologic results and the history of methyldopa therapy, it is evident that the patient must have a methyl-dopa-associated warm AIHA.

2. Because the patient has a history of transfusion, it is essential to ensure that he has no underlying alloantibodies before providing blood for transfusion. We can perform a warm autoabsorption because the patient has not been recently transfused to remove the autoantibody, leaving any alloanti-bodies to be identified.

3. Transfuse this patient only as a last resort. Transfusion of a patient with warm AIHA will only complicate the serologic picture, and the transfused cells will be destroyed as quickly as the patient's own cells. If the patient stops taking methyl-dopa, the clinical status will improve, although not rapidly. The autoantibody may be present in the patient's serum for up to 2 years.

PART C

1. An alloanti-E is present in this patient's serum.

2. Any units released for transfusion to this patient must be E negative. The units will, of course, be incompatible owing to the autoantibody if crossmatched using the unabsorbed serum. The patient should also be tested for the lack of the E antigen to prove that this antibody is truly an alloantibody. Because the patient has a positive DAT result, a low-protein antisera (chemically modified) must be used in order to obtain a valid E antigen typing. An autologous control using patient cells and 6 percent bovine albumin should be tested along with the antigen typing to ensure that the patient's cells are not spontaneously agglutinating. An alternate method would be chloroquine treatment of the patient's cells, as discussed subsequently.

3. It may be helpful to determine the patient's complete RBC phenotype using chloroquine-treated cells to know what anti-bodies the patient is capable of making. When using the chloroquine method of removing IgG from RBCs, one must keep in mind the evidence that some antigens may be weak-ened by chloroquine treatment. Cells should be treated in a 2-hour, room temperature incubation, not in a 30-minute, 37°C incubation, to minimize the weakening of significant antigens.

Panel Performed Using Absorbed Serum

	D	C	E	c	e	M	N	S	s	K	k	Fy^a	Fy^b	Jk^a	Jk^b	Xg^a	37°	AHG
1	0	+	0	+	+	0	+	+	+	0	+	+	+	+	+	+	0	0
2	+	+	0	0	+	0	+	0	+	0	+	+	+	+	0	+	0	0
3	+	+	0	0	+	+	0	+	0	0	+	+	+	0	+	+	0	0
4	+	0	+	+	0	+	+	0	+	+	+	0	+	0	+	+	0	2+
5	0	0	+	+	+	+	0	+	0	0	+	0	0	+	0	0	0	2+
6	0	0	0	+	+	0	+	0	+	0	+	+	0	+	0	+	0	0
7	0	0	0	+	+	0	+	0	+	+	0	+	0	+	+	+	0	0
8	0	0	0	+	+	+	+	0	+	0	+	0	0	+	+	+	0	0
9	+	0	0	+	+	0	+	0	+	0	+	0	+	0	+	+	0	0
10	+	+	0	+	+	+	+	+	+	0	+	+	+	+	0	+	0	0

AHG = antihuman globulin.

Case 2

PART A

A 77-year-old woman is admitted for treatment of a severe upper respiratory infection. Her past medical history is unremarkable, and she had been in excellent health for many years, until 12 days before admission, when she developed "a bad cold." Her symptoms have progressively worsened until today when she felt "too weak to get out of bed," and she is noted to be slightly jaundiced. She had three uneventful pregnancies and normal deliveries and has never been transfused.

Her admission laboratory results follow:

Hemoglobin:	7.5 g/dl	WBC differential:	
Hematocrit:	23.2 percent	Segmented	
		neutrophils:	56
White blood cells	15.3 × 10³/mm³	Immature	
(WBCs):		neutrophils:	8
Platelets:	125,000/mm³	Lymphocytes:	33
RBC morphology:		Eosinophils:	2
Normocytic, normochromic, few		Basophils:	1
spherocytes, rare schistocytes			

The physician orders a crossmatch for 2 units of packed RBCs. The initial transfusion service results are:

Antisera			Cells	
−A	−B	−D	A₁	B
4+	0	3+	1+	4+

		IS	AHG (Anti-IgG)
Antibody screen	I	1+	0
	II	1+	0
	III	1+	0
Crossmatches	1	w+	0
	2	w+	0

IS = immediate spin; AHG = antihuman globulin.

1. What problem do you note in the initial testing results?
2. What are possible explanations for these results?
3. What further testing must be performed before blood is released for transfusion?
4. Does the patient history give any clues as to the cause of the testing results?

PART B

An autocontrol is tested at immediate spin, along with repeating the reverse grouping, with the following results:

A₁ cells:	1+
B cells:	4+
Autologous cells:	1+

A DAT is also tested to obtain more information about this apparent autoantibody:

Polyspecific antiglobulin:	3+
Anti-IgG:	0
Anti-C3d:	3+

The reverse grouping, antibody screen, and compatibility testing are repeated using a prewarmed technique. The immediate spin results are:

Cells	IS
A₁	0
B	4+
Auto	0
SC I	0
II	0
III	0
XM 1	0
XM 2	0

IS = immediate spin.

1. What is the patient's true ABO type and the result of the antibody screen?
2. What conclusions can you draw regarding the clinical significance of this antibody?
3. Is this antibody likely to cause hemolysis of the transfused RBCs?

Case 2 Answers

PART A

1. The forward and reverse typing do not match. The forward result is that typical of a group A, whereas the reverse is that of a group O (with a weak reaction between the patient's serum and the A₁ cells). There is also an unexpected reaction in the immediate spin phase of the antibody screening test and the compatibility testing.

2. a. The patient may be a subgroup of A with anti-A₁ in the serum. This antibody would not, however, explain the reactions with the antibody screening cells.

   b. The patient may have an alloantibody reactive at room temperature, such as anti-Leᵃ or −Leᵇ, −M, −N, or −P1. The reverse grouping cells are quite likely to be positive for any of these antigens because those cells are produced from pools of donors. An RBC panel must be tested to determine if one of the antibodies might be responsible for the reactions.

   c. The patient may have a cold autoantibody that reacts with the reverse grouping cells as well as with the antibody screening cells and the donor units. An autocontrol would be helpful in determining if this might be the case. If the autocontrol result is positive, a DAT is indicated to determine the nature of the protein coating the patient's RBCs.

3. As mentioned earlier, an autocontrol, tested at immediate spin, and possibly an antibody identification panel must be performed in order to resolve the discrepancy. If the autocontrol result is positive, a prewarmed technique may be used to obtain valid reactions without interference from the cold autoantibody.

4. The patient has an upper respiratory infection. It is known that infections with *Mycoplasma pneumoniae* are associated with CHD due to anti-I. The patient's clinical symptoms and laboratory evidence of anemia would also be consistent with CHD.

PART B

1. The patient is A positive, and the antibody screen is negative for clinically significant antibodies.

2. This antibody is most likely an autoanti-I produced in response to infection by *M. pneumoniae*. The antibody will cause hemolysis of the autologous cells, on some occasions resulting in a clinical anemia. Because the antibody is IgM, causing sensitization of the cells with complement, there is no reaction in the antibody screen or compatibility testing with anti-IgG antiglobulin. In this case, the use of a prewarmed technique eliminates all aberrant reactions and allows the provision of crossmatch-compatible RBCs for transfusion if needed.

3. If it is determined that this patient truly needs transfusion, the RBCs may be administered through a blood warmer. If the RBCs are kept at 37°C, there should be little hemolysis. It should be remembered, however, that the hemolytic process is transient and will resolve within 2 to 3 weeks with treatment of the primary disease. Supportive care and avoiding cold are the best therapy.

Review Questions

1. Immune hemolytic anemias may be classified in which of the following categories?
   A. Alloimmune
   B. Autoimmune
   C. Drug-induced
   D. All of the above

2. Which of the following blood groups reacts best with an anti-H or anti-IH?
   A. A₁B
   B. B
   C. A₂
   D. A₁

3. Cold AIHA is often associated with infection by:
   A. *Staphylococcus aureus*
   B. *Mycoplasma pneumoniae*
   C. *Escherichia coli*
   D. Group A *Streptococcus*

4. The blood group involved in the autoantibody specificity in paroxysmal cold hemoglobinuria is:
   A. P
   B. ABO
   C. Rh
   D. Lewis

5. Problems in routine testing caused by cold reactive autoantibodies can usually be resolved by all of the following *except*:
   A. Prewarming
   B. Washing with warm saline
   C. Using anti-IgG serum
   D. Collecting only clotted specimens

6. Many warm reactive autoantibodies have a broad specificity within which of the following blood groups?
   A. Kell
   B. Fy
   C. Rh
   D. Jk

7. Valid Rh typing can be usually obtained on a patient with warm AIHA using all of the following reagents *except*:
   A. Slide and modified tube anti-D
   B. Chemically modified anti-D
   C. Saline (IgM) anti-D
   D. Monoclonal blend anti-D

8. In pretransfusion testing for a patient with warm AIHA, the primary concern is:
   A. Treating the patient's cells with chloroquine for reliable antigen typing
   B. Adsorbing out all antibodies in the patient's serum to be able to provide compatible RBCs
   C. Determining the exact specificity of the autoantibody so that compatible RBCs can be found
   D. Discovering any existing significant alloantibodies in the patient's circulation

9. By which mechanism does penicillin given in massive doses cause hemolysis?
   A. Immune complex

B. Drug adsorption

C. Membrane modification

D. Autoantibody formation

10. A patient has a positive DAT result with anti-IgG. The indirect antiglobulin test result is also positive with all cells tested. Which of the following drugs is most likely responsible for these reactions?

A. Penicillin

B. Quinidine

C. Methyldopa

D. Cephalothin

Answers to Review Questions

1. D (p 402)
2. C (p 406)
3. B (p 408)
4. A (p 408)
5. D (pp 403–406)
6. C (p 411)
7. A (p 411)
8. D (pp 412–413)
9. B (p 417)
10. C (pp 418–419)

References

1. Banacerraf, B and Unanue, ER: Textbook of Immunology. Williams & Wilkins, Baltimore, 1979.
2. Barthold, DR, Kysela, S, and Steinberg, AD: Decline in suppressor T cell function with age in female NZB mice. J Immunol 112:9, 1974.
3. Kirtland, HH, Horwitz, DA, and Mohler, DN: Inhibition of suppressor T cell function by methyldopa: A proposed cause of autoimmune hemolytic anemia. N Engl J Med 302:825, 1980.
4. van Loghem, JJ: Concepts on the origin of autoimmune diseases: The possible role of viral infection in the etiology of idiopathic autoimmune diseases. Semin Hematol 9:17, 1965.
5. Petz, LD and Garratty, G: Acquired Immune Hemolytic Anemias. Churchill Livingstone, New York, 1980.
6. Allan, J and Garratty, G: Positive direct antiglobulin tests in normal blood donors (abstr). Proceedings of the 16th Congress of the International Society of Blood Transfusion, Montreal, 1980.
7. Okuno, T, Germino, F, and Newman, B: Clinical significance of autologous control (abstr). Am Soc Clin Pathol 16, 1984.
8. Lau, P, Haesler, WE, and Wurzel, HA: Positive direct antiglobulin reaction in a patient population. Am J Clin Pathol 65:368, 1976.
9. Judd, WJ, et al: The evaluation of a positive direct antiglobulin test in pretransfusion testing. Transfusion 20:17, 1980.
10. Garratty, G, Petz, LD, and Hoops, JK: The correlation of cold agglutinin titrations in saline and albumin with haemolytic anaemia. Br J Haematol 35:587, 1977.
11. Engelfriet, CP, et al: Autoimmune hemolytic anemias. I. Serological studies with pure anti-immunoglobulin reagents. Clin Exp Immunol 3:605, 1968.
12. Rosse, WF: Quantitative immunology of immune hemolytic anemia. II. The relationship of cell-bound antibody to hemolysis and the effect of treatment. J Clin Invest 50:734, 1971.
13. Gilliland, BC, Baxter, E, and Evans, RS: Red cell antibodies in acquired hemolytic anemia with negative antiglobulin serum tests. N Engl J Med 285:252, 1971.
14. Stratton, F, et al: Acquired hemolytic anemia associated with IgA anti-e. Transfusion 12:197, 1972.
15. Sturgeon, P, et al: Autoimmune hemolytic anemia associated exclusively with IgA of Rh specificity. Transfusion 19:324, 1979.
16. Hoppe, PAH: The role of the Bureau of Biologics in assuring reagent reliability. In Considerations in the Selection of Reagents. American Association of Blood Banks, Washington, DC, 1979, pp 1–33.
17. Garratty, G and Petz, LD: An evaluation of commercial antiglobulin sera with particular reference to their anticomplement properties. Transfusion 11:79, 1971.
18. Walker, RH (ed): Technical Manual, ed 10. American Association of Blood Banks, Arlington, VA, 1990, pp 315–339.
19. Reid, ME: Autoagglutination dispersal utilizing sulfhydryl compounds. Transfusion 18:353, 1978.
20. Chaplin, H, et al: Clinically significant allo-anti-I in an I negative patient with massive hemorrhage. Transfusion 26:57, 1986.
21. Marsh, WL: Aspects of cold-reactive autoantibodies. In Bell, CA (ed): A Seminar on Laboratory Management of Hemolysis. American Association of Blood Banks, Washington, DC, 1979, pp 79–103.
22. Shirey, RS, et al: An anti-i biphasic hemolysin in chronic paroxysmal cold hemoglobinuria. Transfusion 26:62, 1986.
23. Judd, WJ, et al: Donath-Landsteiner hemolytic anemia due to an anti-Pr-like biphasic hemolysin. Transfusion 26:423, 1986.
24. Edwards, JM, Moulds, JJ, and Judd, WJ: Chloroquine dissociation of antigen-antibody complexes: A new technique for typing red blood cells with a positive direct antiglobulin test. Transfusion 22:59, 1982.
25. Weiner, W and Vos, GH: Serology of acquired hemolytic anemias. Blood 22:606, 1963.
26. Becton, DL and Kinney, TR: An infant girl with severe autoimmune hemolytic anemia: Apparent anti-Vel specificity. Vox Sang 51:108, 1986.
27. Reynolds, MV, Vengelen-Tyler, V, and Morel, PA: Autoimmune hemolytic anemia associated with auto anti-Ge. Vox Sang 41:61, 1981.
28. Wilkinson, SL: Serological approaches to transfusion of patients with allo- or autoantibodies. In Nance, ST (ed): Immune Destruction of Red Blood Cells. American Association of Blood Banks, Arlington, 1989, pp 227–261.
29. Anderson, DR and Kelton, JG: Mechanisms in intravascular and extravascular cell destruction. In Nance, ST (ed): Immune Destruction Red Blood Cells. American Association of Blood Banks, Arlington, VA, 1989, p. 39.
30. Kerr, RO, et al: Two mechanisms of erythrocyte destruction in penicillin-induced hemolytic anemia. N Engl J Med 298:1322, 1972.
31. Ries, CA, et al: Penicillin-induced immune hemolytic anemia. JAMA 233:432, 1975.
32. Freedman, J and Lim, FC: An immunohematologic complication of isoniazid. Vox Sang 35:126, 1978.
33. Shulman, NR: Mechanism of blood cell destruction in individuals sensitized to foreign antigens. Trans Assoc Am Phys 76:72, 1963.
34. Dameshek, W: Autoimmunity: Theoretical aspects. I. Ann NY Acad Sci 124:6, 1965.
35. Garratty, G: Drug-induced immune hemolytic anemia and/or positive direct antiglobulin tests. Immunohematology. Journal of Blood Group Serology and Education 2:6, 1985.
36. Worlledge, SM: Immune drug-induced haemolytic anemias. Semin Haematol 6:181, 1969.
37. Garratty, G: Laboratory Investigation of Drug-Induced Immune Hemolytic Anemia and/or Positive Direct Antiglobulin Tests. American Association of Blood Banks, Washington, DC, 1979.
38. Spath, P, Garratty, G, and Petz, LD: Studies on the immune response to penicillin and cephalothin in humans. II. Immunohematologic reactions to cephalothin administration. J Immunol 107:860, 1971.
39. Kaplan, K, Reisburg, B, and Weinsteins, L: Cephaloridine stud-

ies of therapeutic activity and untoward effects. Arch Intern Med 121:17, 1968.

40. Gralnick, HR, McGinniss, MH, and Elton, W: Hemolytic anemia associated with cephalothin. JAMA 217:1193, 1971.
41. Forbes, CD, Craig, JA, and Mitchell, R: Acute intravascular hemolysis associated with cephalexin therapy. Post Grad Med J 48:186, 1972.
42. Jeannet, M, et al: Cephalothin-induced immune hemolytic anemia. Acta Haematol 55:109, 1976.
43. Carstairs, KC, et al: Incidence of a positive direct Coombs' test in patients on alpha-methyldopa. Lancet ii:33, 1966.
44. Worlledge, SM, Carstairs, KC, and Dacie, JV: Autoimmune hemolytic anemia associated with methyldopa therapy. Lancet ii:135, 1966.
45. Gottlieb, AJ and Wurzel, HA: Protein-quinone interaction: In vivo induction of indirect antiglobulin reactions with methyldopa. Blood 43:85, 1974.
46. Dameshek, W: Alpha-methyldopa red cell antibody: Cross reaction or forbidden clone. N Engl J Med 276:1382, 1967.
47. Tuffs, L and Mancharan, A: Flucloxacillin-induced haemolytic anaemia. (Letter) Med J Aust 144:559, 1986.
48. Kickler, TS, et al: Probenecid induced immune hemolytic anemia. J Rheumatol 13:208, 1986.
49. Kramer, MR, Levine, C, and Hershko, C: Severe reversible autoimmune haemolytic anaemia and thrombocytopenia associated with diclofenac therapy. Scand J Haematol 36:118, 1986.
50. Mechanick, JI: Coombs' positive hemolytic anemia following sulfasalazine-therapy in ulcerative colitis: Case reports, review, and discussion of pathogenesis. Mt Sinai J Med (NY) 52:667, 1985.
51. Habibi, B: Drug induced red blood cell autoantibodies codeveloped with drug specific antibodies causing haemolytic anaemias. Br J Haematol 61:139, 1985.
52. Seldon, MR, et al: Ticarcillin-induced immune haemolytic anaemia. Scand J Haematol 28:459, 1982.
53. Tafani, O, et al: Fatal acute immune haemolytic anaemia caused by nalidixic acid. Br Med J 285:936, 1982.
54. Harmening, DM: Clinical Hematology and Fundamentals of Hemostasis, ed 2. FA Davis, Philadelphia, 1991.
55. Pittiglio, D and Sacher, RA: Clinical Hematology and Fundamentals of Hemostasis. FA Davis, Philadelphia, 1987.

Bibliography

Calvo, R, et al: Acute hemolytic anemia due to anti-i; frequent cold agglutinins in infectious mononucleosis. J Clin Invest 44:1033, 1965.

Carter, P, Koval, JJ, and Hobbs, JR: The relation of clinical and laboratory findings to the survival of patients with macroglobinaemia. Clin Exp Immunol 28:241, 1977.

Chaplin, H and Avioli, LV: Autoimmune hemolytic anemia. Arch Intern Med 137:346, 1977.

Dacie, JV: Autoimmune hemolytic anemia. Arch Intern Med 135:1293, 1975.

Evans, RS, Baxter, E, and Gilliland, BC: Chronic hemolytic anemia due to cold agglutinins: A 20-year history of benign gammopathy with response to chlorambucil. Blood 42:463, 1973.

Frank, MM, Atkinson, JP, and Gadek, J: Cold agglutinins and cold agglutinin disease. Annu Rev Med 28:291, 1977.

Garratty, G: Target antigens for red-cell-bound autoantibodies. In Nance, ST (ed): Clinical and Basic Science Aspects of Immunohematology. American Association of Blood Banks, Arlington, VA, 1991, pp 33–72.

Harmening-Pittiglio, DM: Warm auto immune hemolytic anemia: A review of clinical and laboratory considerations. Immunohematology. Journal of Blood Group Serology and Education 1, 1984.

Leddy, JP and Swisher, SN: Acquired immune hemolytic disorders (including drug-induced immune hemolytic anemia). In Samter, M (ed): Immunological Diseases, ed 3, Vol 2. 1978, p 1187.

Petz, LD and Branch, DR: Immune Hemolytic Anemias. Churchill Livingstone, Edinburgh, 1985.

Tanowitz, HB, Robbins, N, and Leidich, N: Hemolytic anemia: Associated with severe mycoplasma pneumoniae pneumonia. NY State J Med 78:2231, 1978.

Wallace, ME and Green, TS (eds): Selection of Procedures for Problem Solving. American Association of Blood Banks, Arlington, VA, 1983.

Wallace, ME and Levitt, JS: Current Applications and Interpretations of the Direct Antiglobulin Test. American Association of Blood Banks, Arlington, VA, 1988.

PROCEDURAL APPENDIX

A. Use of Thiol Reagents to Disperse Autoagglutination[18,19]

APPLICATION

Thiol reagents, which cleave the intersubunit disulfide bonds of pentameric IgM molecules, can be used to disperse agglutination caused by cold-reactive autoantibodies. Treating spontaneously agglutinated RBCs with 2-mercaptoethanol (2-ME) or dithiothreitol (DTT) provides a nonagglutinated specimen for use in blood grouping tests.

MATERIALS

1. 0.01 M DTT or 0.1 M 2-ME
2. Phosphate-buffered saline (PBS) at Ph 7.3
3. Packed washed RBCs to be treated

METHOD

1. Dilute washed RBCs to a 50 percent concentration in PBS.
2. Add an equal quantity of 0.01 M DTT in PBS, or 0.1 M 2-ME in PBS, to the RBCs.
3. Incubate at 37°C for 15 minutes for DTT or 10 minutes for 2-ME.
4. Wash RBCs three times.
5. Dilute the treated RBCs to a 3 to 5 percent concentration in saline and use in blood grouping tests.

B. Cold Autoabsorption[18]

APPLICATION

Autoabsorption can be used to remove cold reactive autoantibodies, allowing detection of clinically significant alloantibodies.

MATERIALS

1. 1 percent ficin or 1 percent papain
2. 2 ml of serum to be absorbed
3. 3 ml of packed autologous RBCs

METHOD

1. Wash the RBCs four times in saline and divide into three equal aliquots in 13 × 100 mm test tubes.
2. Add 0.5 ml of 1 percent ficin or 1 percent papain to each tube.
3. Mix, and incubate at 37°C for 15 minutes.
4. Wash the RBCs three times in saline. Centrifuge the last wash for 5 minutes at 1000 g, and remove as much of the supernatant saline as possible.

NOTE: To avoid dilution of the serum and possible loss of weak alloantibody activity during the absorption process, it is important to remove as much of the residual saline as possible in step 4. Placing a narrow strip of filter paper into the packed RBCs helps remove saline that surrounds the packed cells.

5. To one tube of enzyme-treated RBCs add 2 ml of the autologous serum.

6. Mix, and incubate at 4°C for 30 to 40 minutes.
7. Centrifuge at 1000g for 5 minutes, and transfer the serum into a second tube of enzyme-treated autologous RBCs.
8. Mix, and incubate at 4°C for 30 to 40 minutes.
9. Repeat steps 7 and 8 for the third tube of enzyme-treated RBCs.
10. Following the final absorption, test the serum for alloantibody activity.

C. Prewarmed Technique for Testing Serum Containing Cold Agglutinins[18]

1. Prewarm a bottle of saline to 37°C.
2. Label one tube for each reagent or donor sample to be tested.
3. Add 1 drop of the appropriate 2 to 4 percent cell suspension to each tube.
4. Place the tubes containing the RBCs and a tube containing a small amount of patient's serum at 37°C for 5 to 10 minutes.
5. Transfer 2 drops of prewarmed serum into each tube containing prewarmed RBCs. Mix without removing the tubes from the incubator.
6. Incubate at 37°C for 30 minutes.
7. Without removing the tubes from the incubator, fill all tubes with prewarmed saline (37°C). Centrifuge and wash two to three more times with warm saline.
8. Add anti-IgG reagent, centrifuge, and record reactions.

COMMENTS: Most problems encountered in compatibility testing, antibody detection, and identification tests that are caused by cold agglutinins can be resolved with the use of this technique. By preventing the reaction between the cold agglutinin and the RBC at room temperature (during centrifugation, and so on), one prevents complement activation. Use of the anti-IgG antiglobulin reagent ensures that positive reactions due to cold autoagglutinins with complement binding only will not be detected. Most significant antibodies will react in the antiglobulin phase with anti-IgG reagent.

D. Dissociation of IgG by Chloroquine[18,24]

APPLICATION

Red cells with a positive DAT result cannot be used directly for blood grouping with antisera, such as anti-Fy^a, that require the use of an indirect antiglobulin technique. Under controlled conditions, chloroquine diphosphate dissociates IgG from RBCs with little or no damage to the RBC membrane. Use of this procedure permits complete phenotyping of RBCs coated with warm reactive autoantibody, including tests with antisera solely reactive by the indirect antiglobulin test.

MATERIALS

1. Chloroquine diphosphate solution prepared by dissolving 20 g of chloroquine diphosphate in 100 ml of saline
2. Test RBCs with a positive DAT result due to IgG coating
3. Control RBCs heterozygous for the antigen for which the test sample is to be phenotyped
4. Anti-IgG reagent (need not be specific for heavy chains)

METHOD

1. To 0.2 ml of washed packed IgG-coated test RBCs add 0.8 ml of chloroquine diphosphate solution. Similarly treat the control sample.
2. Mix, and incubate at room temperature for 30 to 60 minutes, depending on the strength of the DAT result.
3. Remove a small aliquot (e.g., 1 drop) of the treated RBCs, and wash four times with saline.

4. Test the washed cells with anti-IgG.
5. If nonreactive with anti-IgG, wash the entire sample of treated test RBCs and the control sample three times in saline, and use for phenotyping with antiglobulin-reactive antisera. Use an anti-IgG reagent when testing these cells.
6. If the treated RBCs react with the anti-IgG after the 30- to 60-minute incubation, repeat steps 3 and 4 at 30-minute intervals (for a maximum incubation of 2 hours), until the RBCs are nonreactive with anti-IgG; then proceed as described in step 5.

NOTES

1. Chloroquine diphosphate does not dissociate complement components from RBCs. If cells are coated with both IgG and C3 in vivo, tests should be done after chloroquine treatment using anti-IgG.
2. Incubation of RBCs in chloroquine diphosphate should not be extended beyond 2 hours. Prolonged incubation at room temperature, or incubation at 37°C, may result in hemolysis and damage to or loss of RBC antigens.
3. Some denaturation of Rh antigens may occur. This is most often noted when RBCs have hemolyzed following incubation with chloroquine diphosphate, or when saline-reactive or chemically modified anti-Rh typing antisera are used. Use high-protein antisera and control reagent when Rh typing chloroquine-treated cells.
4. Include an inert control reagent when phenotyping chloroquine-treated RBCs.

E. Digitonin-Acid Elution[18]*

APPLICATION

Removal of antibodies bound to RBC antigens is used in investigation of a positive DAT result associated with warm reactive IgG autoantibodies or alloantibodies, and for the separation of mixtures of IgG antibodies.

MATERIALS

1. Digitonin (0.5 percent weight of solute per volume of solution [w/v]), prepared by dissolving 0.5 g of digitonin in 100 ml of distilled water. Store at 4°C.
2. Glycine (0.1 M, pH 3.0), prepared by dissolving 3.754 g of glycine in 500 ml of distilled water. Adjust pH to 3.0 with 12 N HCl. Store at 4°C.
3. Phosphate buffer (0.8 M, pH 8.2), prepared by dissolving 109.6 g of Na_2HPO_4 and 3.8 g of KH_2PO_4 in approximately 600 ml of distilled water. Adjust pH, if necessary, with either 1 N NaOH or 1 N HCl. Dilute to a final volume of 1 liter with distilled water. Store at 4°C.
4. Bovine serum albumin, 30 percent.
5. Packed RBCs (1 ml), washed six times in saline.
6. Supernatant saline from last wash.

METHOD

1. Warm reagents to 37°C before use, and mix well.
2. Mix 1 ml of packed RBCs and 9 ml of saline in a 16 × 100 mm test tube.
3. Add 0.5 ml of digitonin, and mix by inversion until all RBCs are hemolyzed (at least 1 minute).
4. Centrifuge the tube at 1000*g* for 5 minutes, and discard the supernatant.

---

*From Jenkins, DE and Moore, WH: A rapid method for the preparation of high-potency auto- and alloantibody eluates. Transfusion 17:110, 1977, with permission.

5. Wash the RBC stroma at least five times, or until it appears white. Centrifuge for at least 2 minutes during the washing process.
6. Discard the final supernatant wash solution, and add 2 ml of glycine to the stroma.
7. Mix by inversion for at least 1 minute.
8. Centrifuge the tube at 1000g for 5 minutes.
9. Transfer the supernatant eluate to a clean test tube and add 0.2 ml of phosphate buffer.
10. Mix and centrifuge at 1000g for 2 minutes.
11. Transfer the supernatant eluate into a clean test tube and add one-third volume of 30 percent bovine serum albumin. Test in parallel with the last wash saline.

NOTES

1. The low pH of the acid buffer enhances elution of antibody from the RBC stroma. Phosphate buffer is added to restore neutrality to the acidic eluate. Persisting acidity may cause lysis of RBCs added to the eluate. Adding bovine albumin to the eluate protects against hemolysis.
2. Ensure digitonin is well mixed and warmed to 37°C before use.
3. Use centrifugation times of at least 2 minutes when washing stroma.
4. Phosphate buffer will crystallize on storage at 4°C. Redissolve at 37°C before use.

F. Autologous Absorption of Warm Reactive Antibodies Application

Warm reactive autoantibodies may mask the presence of coexisting alloantibodies in a serum. Absorbing the serum with autologous RBCs can remove autoantibody from the serum, permitting detection of underlying alloantibodies. Circulating autologous cells, however, are already coated with autoantibody. Some of the autoantibody must be removed from the surface of the autologous RBCs in order to achieve maximum of removal of autoantibody by the absorption process.

Autoabsorption should not be performed if a patient has been recently transfused because the circulating transfused cells may absorb out alloantibodies.

1. Heat and Enzyme Method[†]

MATERIALS

1. 6 percent bovine albumin, prepared by diluting 22 percent or 30 percent bovine albumin with saline
2. 1 percent ficin or 1 percent cysteine-activated papain
3. Blood sample containing warm reactive autoantibodies

METHOD

1. Wash 2 ml of RBCs four times in saline, and discard the final supernatant.
2. Add an equal volume of 6 percent albumin to the packed RBCs. Mix and incubate at 56°C for 3 to 5 minutes. Gently agitate the mixture during this time.
3. Centrifuge at 1000g for 2 minutes and harvest the supernatant. This may be used for eluate if the patient's cells are in short supply.
4. Wash the cells three times in saline and discard the final supernatant.

[†]Morel, PA, Bergren, ML, and Frank, BA: A simple method for detection of alloantibody in the presence of autoantibody. (Abstract) Transfusion 18:388, 1978, with permission.

5. Add 1 ml of 1 percent ficin or papain to the RBCs. Mix and incubate at 37°C for 15 minutes.

6. Wash the RBCs three times in saline. Centrifuge the last wash for at least 5 minutes at 1000g. Use suction to remove as much of the supernatant as practical.

7. Divide the RBCs into two equal aliquots.

8. To one aliquot, add 2 ml of patient's serum. Mix and incubate at 37°C for 30 minutes.

9. Centrifuge at 1000g for 2 minutes and transfer the serum to the second aliquot of enzyme-treated RBCs. Mix and incubate at 37°C for 30 minutes.

10. Centrifuge at 1000g for 2 minutes, and harvest the absorbed serum.

11. Test the absorbed serum for antibody activity using an indirect antiglobulin technique.

2. ZZAP Method[‡]

MATERIALS

1. 1 percent cysteine-activated papain.
2. PBS at pH 6.5.
3. 0.2 M DTT prepared by dissolving 1 g of DTT in 32.4 ml of pH 6.5 PBS. Dispense into 2.5 ml aliquots and store at or below −20°C.
4. Blood samples containing warm reactive autoantibodies.

METHOD

1. Prepare ZZAP reagent by mixing 0.5 ml cysteine-activated papain with 2.5 ml DDT and 2 ml pH 6.5 PBS. Alternatively, use 1 ml ficin, 2.5 ml DTT, and 1.5 ml pH 6.5 PBS.

2. To two tubes, each containing 1 ml of packed RBCs, add 2 ml of ZZAP reagent. Mix and incubate at 37°C for 30 minutes.

3. Wash the RBCs three times in saline. Centrifuge the last wash at least 5 minutes at 1000g. Use suction to remove as much of the supernatant as practical.

4. Proceed as from step 8 in Procedure A, shown previously.

INTERPRETATION

A twofold autologous absorption usually removes sufficient autoantibody from the serum so that alloantibody, if present, is readily apparent. Occasionally, two absorptions are insufficient. If the patient's RBCs can be shown to have a negative DAT result after heat treatment (Procedure 1), ZZAP treatment (Procedure 2), or treatment with chloroquine diphosphate, such RBCs may be used to check the efficacy of the absorption process. For example, if Procedure 1 was used and the heat-treated cells obtained after step 4 yield a negative DAT result, the autoabsorbed serum should be tested against them and two group O RBC samples (screening cells).

Results can be interpreted as follows:

1. When there is no reactivity against the group O reagent RBCs, alloantibody is probably not present.

2. If there is reactivity against both the patient's heat-treated RBCs and the group O cells, further absorptions are necessary to remove the autoantibody.

3. When the absorbed serum reacts with one or both of the group O reagent RBCs and not with the autologous RBCs, the serum contains alloantibody, and antibody identification studies should be undertaken on the absorbed serum.

[‡]Branch, DR and Petz, LD: A new reagent (ZZAP) having multiple applications in immunohematology. Am J Clin Pathol 78:161, 1982.

NOTES

1. ZZAP reagent is stable for at least 3 months if kept at 4°C.
2. ZZAP treatment destroys all Kell system antigens except Kx, in addition to other antigens, including M, N, S, s, Fy^a, Fy^b, and other receptors that are destroyed by protease.
3. There is no need to wash RBCs before ZZAP treatment.

G. Demonstration of Immune Complex Formation Involving Drugs[18,37]

APPLICATION

Immune complexes formed between certain drugs and their respective antibodies attach weakly and nonspecifically to RBCs. The bound immune complex activates complement, which may lead to hemolysis in vivo. This procedure provides an in vitro means to demonstrate immune-complex formation associated with drug-antidrug interactions.

MATERIALS

1. Drug under investigation, in the same form that the patient is receiving (tablet, solution, capsules)
2. PBS at pH 7.0 to 7.4
3. Patient's serum
4. Fresh normal serum known to lack unexpected antibodies, as a source of complement
5. Group O RBCs, both untreated and treated with a proteolytic enzyme

METHOD

1. Prepare a 1 mg/ml suspension solution of the drug in PBS. Centrifuge and adjust the pH of the supernatant fluid to 7.0 with either 1 N NaOH or 1 N HCl, as required.
2. Using 0.2 ml of each reactant, prepare the following test mixtures:
   a. Patient's serum plus drug
   b. Patient's serum plus complement (normal serum) plus drug
   c. Patient's serum plus complement (normal serum) plus PBS
   d. Normal serum plus drug
   e. Normal serum plus PBS
3. To 3 drops of each test mixture, add 1 drop of a 5 percent saline suspension of group O RBCs. To another 3 drops of each test mixture, add 1 drop of a 5 percent saline suspension of enzyme-treated group O reagent RBCs.
4. Mix, and incubate at 37°C for 1 to 2 hours with periodic gentle mixing.
5. Centrifuge and examine for hemolysis.
6. Wash the RBCs four times in saline, and test with a polyspecific antiglobulin reagent.

INTERPRETATION

Hemolysis, agglutination, or coating can occur. Such reactivity in any of the tests containing patient's serum to which the drug was added, and absence of reactivity in the corresponding control tests containing PBS instead of the drug, indicates a drug-antidrug interaction.

NOTES

1. The use of a mortar and pestle (if the drug is in tablet form), incubation at 37°C, and vigorous shaking of the solution may help dissolve the drug.
2. Many drugs will not dissolve completely, but enough may be dissolved to react in

serologic tests. Other methods, obtained from the manufacturer or other publications, may be needed to dissolve adequate quantities of some drugs.

H. Detection of Antibodies to Penicillin or Cephalothin[18,37]

APPLICATION

This procedure can be used to investigate positive DAT results associated with penicillin or cephalothin antibodies.

MATERIALS

1. Barbital-buffered saline (BBS) at pH 9.6, prepared by dissolving 20.6 g of sodium barbital in 1 liter of saline. Adjust to pH 9.6 with 0.1 N HCl. Store at 4°C.
2. Penicillin (approximately 1×10^6 units per 600 mg)
3. Cephalothin sodium (Keflin)
4. Washed, packed group O RBCs
5. Serum or eluate to be studied

METHOD

1. Prepare penicillin-coated RBCs by incubating 1 ml of RBCs with 600 mg penicillin in 15 ml BBS for 1 hour at room temperature. Wash three times in saline and store in Alsever's solution at 4°C.
2. Prepare cephalothin-coated RBCs by incubating 1 ml of RBCs with 400 mg cephalothin sodium in 10 ml BBS for 2 hours at 37°C. Wash three times in saline and stored in Alsever's solution at 4°C.
3. Mix 2 or 3 drops of serum or eluate with 1 drop of a 5 percent suspension of drug-coated cells. Dilute serum 1 : 20 with saline for tests with cephalothin-coated cells.
4. Test in parallel uncoated RBCs from the same donor.
5. Incubate the tests at room temperature for 15 minutes. Centrifuge, and examine the RBCs macroscopically for agglutination. Grade and record results.
6. Incubate the tests at 37°C for 30 to 60 minutes. Centrifuge, and examine macroscopically for agglutination. Grade and record results.
7. Wash the RBCs four times in saline, and test by the indirect antiglobulin technique using polyspecific or anti-IgG reagent.

INTERPRETATION

Antibodies to penicillin or cephalothin will react with drug-coated cells but not with uncoated cells. Antibodies to either drug may cross-react with RBCs coated with the other drug (i.e., antipenicillin antibodies cross-react with cephalothin-coated RBCs, and vice versa).

NOTES

1. Phosphate-buffered saline at pH 7.3 may be substituted for BBS in the preparation of cephalothin-coated RBCs.
2. All normal sera react with cephalothin-coated RBCs because such RBCs absorb all proteins nonimmunologically. This reactivity does not occur if incubation times are as short as 15 minutes or if the serum is diluted 1 : 20 with saline before testing.
3. Eluates do not contain enough protein to be absorbed nonimmunologically by cephalothin-coated RBCs. Reactivity of an eluate with cephalothin-coated RBCs indicates antibody to cephalosporins, which may cross-react with penicillin-coated RBCs.

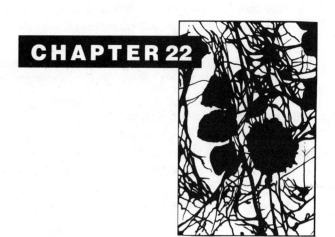

CHAPTER 22

Polyagglutination

Phyllis S. Walker, MS, MT(ASCP)SBB

OBJECTIVES

Upon completion of this chapter, the learner should be able to:

Microbially Associated Forms of Polyagglutination: T, Tk, and Acquired B

1. List the bacterial organism(s) associated with T, Tk, and acquired-B forms of polyagglutination.
2. Describe the mechanism, including the specific microbial product that produces each polyagglutinable state.
3. List the clinical conditions associated with each form of polyagglutination.
4. Discuss the clinical significance of the polyagglutinable state.
5. List the laboratory results that are expected in each form of polyagglutination (e.g., ABO grouping, reactions following enzyme treatment, reactions with various lectins).

Nonmicrobially Associated Polyagglutination: Tn

1 Describe the alternation that characterizes the polyagglutinable state.

2 Discuss the clinical significance of the polyagglutinable state.

3 List the laboratory results that are expected in this form of polyagglutination (e.g., ABO grouping, reactions following enzyme treatment, reactions with various lectins).

Inherited Polyagglutination: Cad and Hereditary Erythroblastic Multinuclearity with a Postive Acidified Serum (Ham's) Test (HEMPAS)

1 State the form of inheritance.

2 Describe the alternation that is seen in the condition.

3 Discuss the clinical significance of the polyagglutinable state.

4 List the laboratory results that are expected (e.g., li antigenic expression, reactions following enzyme treatment, reactions with various lectins).

Polyagglutination is the agglutination of altered red blood cells (RBCs) by a large proportion of ABO-compatible adult human sera. Alterations in the RBC membrane may be acquired following microbial (bacterial or viral) activity, associated with certain forms of aberrant erythropoiesis, or inherited. In the microbially induced forms of polyagglutination, microbial enzymes alter the structure of the normal RBC membrane by removing carbohydrate residues, thus exposing cryptic (hidden) antigens. Naturally occurring immunoglobulin M (IgM) antibodies (polyagglutinins) found in normal adult human sera react with these cryptantigens, causing the altered cells to be polyagglutinable. Cryptantigen exposure can be detected before polyagglutination by testing the RBCs in vitro with specific lectins.[1] Polyagglutination, which requires significant cryptantigen exposure, is a rare condition; however, detectable cryptantigen exposure is not. Microbially induced polyagglutination may occur in vitro or in vivo. When polyagglutination occurs in vivo, the condition is usually transient. The microbial organisms may be present in the bloodstream, or the enzymes may enter the bloodstream from an extravascular site of infection. For polyagglutination to occur, the enzymes must be present in excess of the amount required to neutralize normal plasma enzyme inhibitors.[1] Microbially induced forms of polyagglutination include T, Th, Tk, Tx, acquired B, and acquired microbial polyagglutination due to passive adsorption and probably Vienna (VA). A nonmicrobial form of acquired polyagglutination, Tn, is caused by the somatic mutation of a faulty hemopoietic stem cell clone. This form of polyagglutination is persistent. Finally, some forms of polyagglutination are inherited, including Cad, hemoglobin M-Hyde Park, hereditary erythroblastic multinuclearity with a positive acidified serum (Ham's) test (HEMPAS) and NOR. The inherited forms of polyagglutination are permanent.

Historically, polyagglutination was first described as an in vitro phenomenon caused by bacterial contamination of RBC suspensions. The first report, by Hübener,[2] appeared in 1925. Later, polyagglutination was described by Thomsen and Friedenreich,[3] and it became known as the Hübener-Thomsen-Friedenreich phenomenon. The crypt antigen exposed by the action of the bacterial enzyme became known as the T-receptor (in honor of Thomsen). Over the past 30 years, other forms of polyagglutination have been described. Recognition and classification of polyagglutinable cells may be complicated by variations in the strength of the antigens and antibodies. Also, it is not uncommon to find several forms of polyagglutination existing simultaneously in vivo. This chapter discusses the most common types, including the serologic recognition of polyagglutination and the classification of polyagglutinable RBCs using lectins.

Categories of Polyagglutinable Cells

MICROBIALLY ASSOCIATED

T Polyagglutination

T transformation is a transient, acquired form of polyagglutination usually found in patients with septicemia, gastrointestinal lesions, or wound infections. Occasionally T transformation has been observed in apparently healthy blood donors;[4] however, it is usually considered a pathologic finding, possibly an early symptom of a latent disease condition. It has been more frequently observed in infants and children than in adults. T activation of RBCs is caused by the action of neuraminidase, which is produced by bacteria such as pneumococci, *Clostridium perfringens*, *Vibrio cholerae*, and viruses such as the influenza virus.[5] Neuraminidase cleaves terminal *N*-acetylneuraminic acid (NeuNAc) residues from RBC membrane glycoproteins and glycolipids, exposing the subterminal T receptor.[6] One structure on the RBC membrane that can be altered to express the T receptor is the alkalilabile tetrasaccharide of Thomas and Winzler.[7] These

Alkali-labile tetrasaccharide of Thomas and Winzler:

$$\begin{array}{ccc} \text{Gal-}\beta(1-3)\text{-GalNAc} & \!\!\!\!\!----\alpha---- & \text{Serine or} \\ | & | & \text{Threonine} \\ \alpha(2-3) & \alpha(2-6) & \\ | & | & \\ \text{NeuNAc} & \text{NeuNAc} & \end{array}$$

T receptor:

$$\text{Gal-}\beta(1-3)\text{-GalNAc}----\alpha----\begin{array}{l}\text{Serine or}\\ \text{Threonine}\end{array}$$

Gal = Galactose
GalNAc = N-acetylgalactosamine
NeuNAc = N-acetylneuraminic acid

FIGURE 22-1 Structure of the alkali-labile tetrasaccharide of Thomas and Winzler and the neuraminidase-modified structure that expresses the T receptor in the terminal position.

tetrasaccharides are found on the MN sialoglycoprotein (MN-SGP), the Ss sialoglycoprotein (Ss-SGP), other minor RBC SGPs, and gangliosides.[8] See Figure 22-1 for the biochemical structures of the tetrasaccharide of Thomas and Winzler and the neuraminidase-modified structure that expresses the T receptor.

T activation may occur in vitro or in vivo. In vitro, T activation may be produced by bacterial contamination of blood samples or by the deliberate addition of neuraminidase to RBC suspensions. When T receptors on RBCs are exposed, the cells are agglutinated by almost all normal adult sera that contain naturally occurring anti-T. Patients who have T polyagglutination generally lack anti-T in their sera, and, therefore, they are expected to have negative autologous controls. The degree of T activation or cryptantigen exposure depends on the amount of neuraminidase that gains access to the bloodstream, the amount of inhibitor present in the patient's plasma, and the number of NeuNAc residues that are removed by the enzymes.[9] In addition to being found on RBCs, T receptors may be found as cryptantigens on leukocytes,[10] platelets,[10] and tissue cells,[11] and in body fluids.[12] T activation is a transient condition in vivo. When the microbial organism is eliminated, the polyagglutinable property of the RBCs usually disappears.

Th Polyagglutination

Th polyagglutination is probably another microbially induced form of polyagglutination. This form of polyagglutination was first observed in septic patients by Bird et al. in 1978.[13] Several microbial organisms were isolated from these patients, including clostridia, bacteroides, Escherichia coli, and proteus. Because the polyagglutinins anti-T and anti-Tk were found in normal amounts in the sera of these patients, it was apparent that Th polyagglutination is different from T and Tk polyagglutination. In an in vitro experiment, Sondag-Thull and associates[14] produced Th-transformed RBCs using the neuraminidase produced by Corynebacterium aquaticum. They showed that the neuraminidase associated with Th transformation is weaker than the

neuraminidase that produces T transformation, and they concluded that Th-transformed RBCs express a weakened expression, or an early stage of the T transformation.

Tk Polyagglutination

Like other forms of microbially associated polyagglutination, Tk transformation is a transient, acquired form of polyagglutination usually found in patients with septicemia, gastrointestinal lesions, and wound infections. Initially, enzymes produced by certain strains of Bacteroides fragilis were associated with Tk polyagglutination.[15] Later, cultures of Serratia marcescens, Aspergillus niger, and Candida albicans were also shown to produce endo- and exo-β-galactosidases that are capable of producing Tk transformation. The enzymes cleave a galactose residue from the paragloboside structure, exposing GluNAc, the Tk receptor.[16,17] Paragloboside is a precursor in the biosynthetic pathways of the ABH, Lewis, Ii and P_1 antigens. Thus, Tk-polyagglutinable RBCs may have altered expressions of these antigens, resulting in decreased antigen expression.[18] Figure 22-2 illustrates the biochemical structures of paragloboside and the Tk receptor.

Tk transformation can be produced in vitro or in vivo.[16] When Tk receptors on RBCs are exposed, the cells are agglutinated by almost all normal adult sera that contain naturally occurring anti-Tk. When the microbial organism is eliminated, the polyagglutinable property of the RBCs usually disappears.

Tx Polyagglutination

Tx transformation was first described in children who had pneumococcal infections.[19] The mechanism of Tx transformation has not been explained. A second report of Tx transformation described a child with acute hemolytic anemia.[20] Tx transformation of the child's RBCs was observed, but no direct association with the anemia could be proved. Examination of family members showed Tx polyagglutination of the RBCs of two siblings. The polyagglutination was transient, lasting 4 to 5 months. The Tx transformation could have been caused by an unidentified bacterial or

Paragloboside:

$$\text{Gal-}\beta(1-4)\text{-GluNAc-}\beta(1-3)\text{-Gal-}\beta(1-3)\text{-Glu-Ceramide}$$

Tk receptor:

$$\text{GluNAc-}\beta(1-3)\text{-Gal-}\beta(1-3)\text{-Glu-Ceramide}$$

Gal = Galactose
GluNAc = N-acetylglucosamine
Glu = Glucose

FIGURE 22-2 Structure of paragloboside and the enzymatically modified structure that expresses the Tk receptor in the terminal position.

viral infection; however, blood cultures, nasopharyngeal cultures, and urine and rectal cultures were all negative.

Acquired B Polyagglutination

Like T activation, acquired B polyagglutination is considered transient and is usually found in patients with septicemia, gastrointestinal lesions, and wound infections. Also, like T activation, acquired B polyagglutination has been found in apparently healthy blood donors[21] but is considered pathologic. The acquired B antigen is caused by enzymes produced by certain strains of *E. coli*,[22] *Clostridium tertium*,[22] and probably certain strains of *Proteus vulgaris*.[23] The microbial enzyme causes deacetylation of α-N-acetyl-D-galactosamine (group A determinant) with the production of α-D-galactosamine. α-D-galactosamine is similar to α-D-galactose (group B determinant) and can cross-react with human anti-B typing sera and some monoclonal anti-B typing reagents.[24,25] Figure 22–3 shows the biochemical structures of α-N-acetylgalactosamine and α-D-galactosamine, the acquired B determinant.

Acquired B may be produced in vitro or in vivo. In vitro, acquired B can be produced by coating group A or O RBCs with lipopolysaccharides from *E. coli* O_{86} or *P. vulgaris* 0X19. In vivo, acquired B is a transient condition, occurring only on RBCs that have the A antigen. When the microbial organism is eliminated, the cross-reactivity with anti-B typing reagent usually disappears.

Passive Adsorption of Bacterial Products

Very rarely polyagglutination may be caused by the passive adsorption of bacterial products onto RBCs. Such coated cells can be polyagglutinable because human sera sometimes contain antibodies to the bacteria. Chorpenning and Dodd[26] reported a severe transfusion reaction that was probably caused by this mechanism.

VA Polyagglutination

VA polyagglutination is rare and has not been well characterized. It was first described in a 20-year-old

man from Vienna (hence the name "VA") who had had hemolytic anemia most of his life.[27] The H antigens of VA polyagglutinable RBCs are significantly depressed. The action of a microbial α-fucosidase could account for the depressed H antigens; however, the presence of a microbial enzyme has not been proved.[9] VA polyagglutinability appears to be a persistent condition.

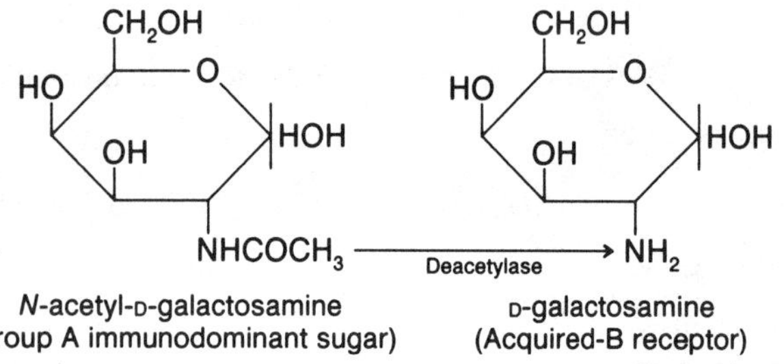

NONMICROBIALLY ASSOCIATED

Tn Polyagglutination

Tn polyagglutinability is believed to be caused by a mutation in the hemopoietic tissue. The mutation gives rise to a clone of cells that lack β-3-D-galactosyl-transferase,[28] the transferase that is needed to complete the biosynthesis of the normal structure of the alkali-labile tetrasaccharide of Thomas and Winzler.[7] This tetrasaccharide structure is found on the MN-SGP and the Ss-SGP.[29] Because this form of polyagglutination is caused by a mutation, it is considered permanent and irreversible. The mutant clone coexists with normal hemopoietic tissue; therefore, this form of polyagglutination is characterized by a mixed-field appearance.[30] Only the cells produced by the mutant clone are agglutinated by the naturally occurring anti-Tn found in normal adult sera. Tn polyagglutination occurs only in vivo, and it may occur in apparently healthy people. When the transferase is absent, the crypt Tn antigen (α-GalNAc) is exposed. The Tn antigen is biochemically similar to the group A determinant; therefore, people with Tn polyagglutination may show mixed-field agglutination with anti-A typing reagent. In addition to being found on RBCs, the Tn-receptor may occur as a cryptantigen on leukocytes,[31] platelets,[31] and tissue cells.[11] Figure 22–4 shows the biochemical structures of the tetrasaccharide of Thomas and Winzler and the incomplete structure that expresses the Tn-receptor.[32]

INHERITED FORMS OF POLYAGGLUTINATION

Cad

Cad polyagglutination was first described in 1968 by Cazal et al.[33] Cad is an inherited autosomal dominant condition that leads to a permanent polyagglutinable state. The amount of Cad antigen on RBCs varies, and, based on the amount of Cad antigen present, RBCs can be divided into four Cad phenotypes.[34] In 1971, Sanger et al.[35] reported that Cad-positive RBCs are agglutinated by anti-Sd^a. It is known that the structure that includes the Cad determinant is a potent inhibitor of anti-Sd^a; however, it is not clear whether this means that Cad and Sd^a are the same thing or whether a concentrated isolate of a structure similar to Sd^a, with GalNAc as the terminal residue, has the ability to cross-react with anti-Sd^a.[36] Inasmuch as anti-Sd^a is present as an autoantibody in most normal adult sera, Cad cells can be classified as polyagglutinable. Cad

N-acetyl-D-galactosamine
(Group A immunodominant sugar)

D-galactosamine
(Acquired-B receptor)

FIGURE 22–3 Structure of the Group A determinant (N-acetyl-D-galactosamine) and the enzymatically modified structure (D-galactosamine) that expresses the acquired-B receptor.

Alkali-labile tetrasaccharide of Thomas and Winzler:

Gal-β(1-3)–GalNAc------α-------Serine or Threonine
　　　|　　　　　|
　α(2-3)　　α(2-6)
　　|　　　　　|
　NeuNAc　　NeuNAc

Tn-receptor:

GalNAc------α-------Serine or Threonine
　|
α(2-6)
　|
NeuNAc

Gal = Galactose

GalNAc = *N*-acetylgalactosamine

NeuNAc = *N*-acetylneuraminic acid

FIGURE 22-4 Structure of the alkali-labile tetrasaccharide of Thomas and Winzler and the incomplete structure that expresses the Tn receptor in the terminal position.

Alkali-labile tetrasaccharide of Thomas and Winzler:

Gal-β(1-3)-GalNAc----α----Serine or
　　　|　　　　　|　　　　　Threonine
　α(2-3)　　α(2-6)
　　|　　　　　|
　NeuNAc　　NeuNAc

Cad receptor:

GalNAc-β(1-4)-Gal-β(1-3)-GalNAc----α----Serine or
　　　　　　　　　　|　　　　　|　　　　　Threonine
　　　　　　　α(2-3)　　α(2-6)
　　　　　　　|　　　　　|
　　　　　　NeuNAc　　NeuNAc

Gal = Galactose
GalNAc = *N*-acetylgalactosamine
NeuNAc = *N*-acetylneuraminic acid

FIGURE 22-5 Structure of the alkali-labile tetrasaccharide of Thomas and Winzler and the modified structure that expresses the Cad receptor.

polyagglutination, however, is quite uncommon. This form of polyagglutination appears to have little clinical significance; however, Cad-positive cells show considerable resistance to invasion by merozoites of *Plasmodium falciparum*.[37] Cad-polyagglutinable RBCs have normal sialic acid levels. The Cad determinant on the RBC membrane and the Sd[a] antigen isolated from Sd(a +) urine share a nonreducing trisaccharide.[38-40] The Cad receptor, a pentasaccharide, is produced when an additional sugar is added to the alkali-labile tetrasaccharide of Thomas and Winzler.[38] Figure 22-5 shows the biochemical structures of the tetrasaccharide of Thomas and Winzler and the modified structure that expresses the Cad receptor.

Hemoglobin M-Hyde Park

Polyagglutination associated with hemoglobin M-Hyde Park was initially reported in a South African family of mixed race.[41] The RBCs of 12 members of the family were weakly agglutinated, often with mixed-field pattern, by many ABO-compatible human sera. All 12 family members who had hemoglobin M-Hyde Park had polyagglutinable RBCs; however, polyagglutination was absent in 23 other family members who had normal hemoglobin. Because all of the family members were apparently healthy, it is unlikely that the polyagglutinability was caused by in vivo bacterial or viral activity. King et al.[42] reported that the polyagglutinability associated with hemoglobin M-Hyde Park RBCs is caused by two unrelated abnormalities. They found heterogeneity in the molecular size of

SGPs and a mild reduction in the sialylation of O-linked oligosaccharide chains on the hemoglobin M-Hyde Park membrane components. Also, these RBCs showed incomplete biosynthesis with exposure of terminal GluNAc on polylactosamine-type, *N*-linked carbohydrate chains of band 3.

HEMPAS

HEMPAS is also known as congenital dyserythropoietic anemia type II (CDA II). HEMPAS is an autosomal recessive condition that is characterized by abnormal RBC membranes, multinucleated erythroblasts in the bone marrow, and RBCs that have a second membrane internal and parallel to the external membrane.[43,44] HEMPAS RBCs have increased amounts of i antigen, decreased amounts of H antigen and sialic acid, and show increased susceptibility to lysis by anti-i and anti-I in the presence of complement. Many normal human sera contain a naturally occurring, IgM, complement-binding, alloantibody that reacts with HEMPAS cells. For this reason, HEMPAS cells are considered polyagglutinable.[9] A specific HEMPAS determinant has not been described.

NOR

NOR, an inherited dominant form of polyagglutination, was discovered when the RBCs of a 19-year-old blood donor from Norfolk, Virginia, were unexpectedly incompatible with the majority of adult sera tested. NOR cells were compatible with cord sera. Tests with lectins and other reagents ruled out other known forms of polyagglutination, and this donor's serum contained the expected naturally occurring antibodies to other forms of polyagglutination. No lectin has been found that agglutinates NOR cells. NOR-polyagglutination may be related to the P blood group, as it has been observed that anti-NOR is inhibited by hydatid cyst fluid and avian P_1 substance. Anti-

NOR is a naturally occurring IgM antibody found in approximately 75 percent of normal adult sera.[45] The NOR determinant has not been described.

Laboratory Testing

DETECTION

It is a common error to expect most forms of polyagglutination to be detected during routine ABO grouping. Only strong examples of polyagglutination are detected by commercially prepared typing sera because the manufacturing process tends to destroy the naturally occurring polyagglutinins. Also, these antibodies are usually present in relatively low titer, and they may be diluted out when typing reagents are prepared from hyperimmune sera. However, ABO discrepancies may be important in the detection of the forms of polyagglutination that are associated with acquired antigens. Acquired B cells may vary in reactivity from strongly positive to very weak with anti-B sera. Individuals who have acquired B polyagglutination regularly produce a potent alloanti-B that does not agglutinate their autologous cells. Monoclonal reagents may also produce discrepant ABO typing results. Monoclonal anti-B reagent prepared from clone ES4 detects acquired B more readily than polyclonal anti-B.[46] Similarly, Tn polyagglutination, which is produced by a mutant clone of hemopoietic cells, may appear as a mixed-field population of A cells in a group O individual or as a weak subgroup of AB in a group B individual. The Tn receptor found on the polyagglutinable cells is *N*-acetylgalactosamine, which cross-reacts with anti-A typing reagent. Tn polyagglutinable cells may be distinguished from weak subgroups of A because they react the same with anti-A and anti-A,B reagents, whereas they react strongly with anti-A_1 lectin (*Dolichos biflorus*). Table 22–1 is an example of ABO discrepancy caused by polyagglutination.

Rh typing discrepancies caused by polyagglutination are very rare because Rh typing reagents are usually prepared from hyperimmune sera, and, as already mentioned, the manufacturing process tends to destroy or dilute the polyagglutinins. Also, the polyagglutinins usually react better at room temperature than at 37°C.

False-positive direct antiglobulin test (DAT) results have occurred because of polyagglutinins in the antiglobulin reagent. Antiglobulin reagents prepared from hyperimmunized rabbit sera contain naturally occurring polyagglutinins; however, again, the manufacturing process usually destroys or dilutes these antibodies.

Polyagglutination is rarely detected by compatibility testing. The major crossmatch, performed to detect antibodies in the patient's serum that react with antigens on the donor's RBCs, is occasionally incompatible owing to polyagglutination. If donor samples become bacterially contaminated in vitro, the samples may become polyagglutinable. Sometimes, apparently healthy donors may have Tn or one of the inherited forms of polyagglutination. When a donor's cells are incompatible with several patients, a DAT should be performed. If the result of the DAT on the donor's cells is negative and the cells are compatible with cord serum, polyagglutination should be suspected. Although the minor crossmatch is not recommended, it is probably more likely to detect polyagglutination than any other test. The minor crossmatch, performed to detect incompatibility between the donor's serum and the patient's RBCs, may detect the bacterially induced forms of polyagglutination in septic patients. Finally, it is important to remember that the ability of the compatibility test to detect polyagglutination depends on the number of receptors on the RBCs, the amount of antibody in the serum, and the conditions of the test. If crossmatch techniques are not designed to detect antibodies that react below 37°C by direct agglutination, polyagglutination may not be observed.

CONFIRMATION

When polyagglutination is suspected, the RBCs should be tested with several cord blood sera and with several normal group AB adult sera. If the RBCs are agglutinated by most of the adult sera and are not agglutinated by the cord sera, polyagglutination has been established. The cord sera used for polyagglutination studies must be pretested to determine that they lack maternal alloantibodies, which might produce misleading results. The adult sera must be pretested to determine that they are free of other unexpected antibodies. Polyagglutinins are naturally occurring anti-

TABLE 22–1 ABO DISCREPANCY CAUSED BY POLYAGGLUTINATION

| | FORWARD TYPING | | | | REVERSE TYPING | | | |
| | REAGENTS | | | | CELLS | | | |
	Anti-A	Anti-A_1 Lectin	Anti-B	Anti-A,B	A_1	A_2	B	Interpretation
Normal cells	0	+++	0	0	++++	++++	++++	Type O
Polyagglutinable cells (Tn)	++mf	+++	0	+++mf	++++	++++	++++	? (further work needed)

mf = mixed field.

bodies in adult serum; however, the amount of antibody varies from one individual to another. For this reason, several adult sera should be used. Polyagglutinins usually react best at lower temperatures by direct agglutination. Because polyagglutinins are unstable, it is important to use fresh adult sera.

N-acetylneuraminic acid (sialic acid) is a normal component of the RBC membrane. Certain forms of polyagglutination (T and Tn) show decreased amounts of sialic acid. It is possible to quantitate sialic acid levels, but such testing is not practical in routine serology laboratories. Instead, sialic acid levels are usually determined qualitatively with polybrene and *Glycine soja* lectin. Polybrene, a positively charged polymer, acts by neutralizing the negative charge on normal RBCs and causing them to aggregate nonspecifically. Because the negative charge is almost entirely due to sialic acid groups, cells that lack sialic acid (T and Tn) are not aggregated by polybrene. Conversely, *G. soja* lectin does not react with normal cells but strongly agglutinates sialic acid–deficient RBCs (T and Tn) as well as Cad cells.

CLASSIFICATION

Enzymes may be useful in the classification of polyagglutinable RBCs. Generally, agglutination of Tk-, Cad-, and NOR-polyagglutinable cells is enhanced following enzyme treatment. HEMPAS-, VA-, and T-polyagglutinable cells show no change in their agglutination by normal adult sera and typing reagents following enzyme treatment. Tn- and Th-polyagglutinable cells show decreased agglutinability following enzyme treatment. Table 22–2 summarizes the findings in normal versus polyagglutinable cells.

Lectins are routinely included in the classification of polyagglutinable RBCs. Lectins are proteins present in plants (usually seeds), invertebrate animals, and lower vertebrates. Lectins bind specifically to carbohydrate determinants, agglutinating erythrocytes through their cell surface oligosaccharide determinants. Highly concentrated lectins may react nonspecifically with all RBCs; however, with careful standardization, a battery of lectin reagents will permit the accurate classification of most forms of polyagglutination. Table 22–3 summarizes the differentiation of polyagglutinable cells using lectins.

Laboratory Methods

Typing polyagglutinable RBCs may be difficult if the cells are strongly polyagglutinable. Several approaches to typing such cells are available.[47]

Adsorption Some polyagglutinable cells (T, Th, Tk, Tx, and acquired B) can be prepared in vitro, and these cells may be used to adsorb the polyagglutinins from typing reagents.

Enzymes Some polyagglutination receptors (Tn and Th) are destroyed by enzymes. In these forms of polyagglutination, the polyagglutinable cells may be enzyme-treated before typing. This approach would be limited to typing the cells for antigens that are not destroyed by enzymes, and careful control must be used to avoid false interpretations caused by unexpected, enzyme-reactive antibodies in the typing sera.

Cord Sera ABO-compatible cord sera that contain the desired antibody specificity may be used as typing reagents. Polyagglutinins are expected to be absent from cord sera.

Aged Sera Polyagglutinins are unstable, and time-expired or aged sera often lack the polyagglutinins. Such sera may be used as typing reagents if the desired antibodies are still demonstrable.

Dilution Hyperimmune sera may be diluted beyond the endpoint of the polyagglutinins and still retain the desired specificity.

Sulfhydryl Compounds 2-mercaptoethanol (2-ME) or dithiothreitol (DTT) may be used to treat typing reagents. These compounds destroy IgM antibodies, such as the polyagglutinins, without affecting IgG antibodies.

Adsorption and Elution Adsorption and elution

TABLE 22–2 NORMAL VERSUS POLYAGGLUTINABLE CELLS

| | SCREENING METHODS | | | | Agglutination After Papain Treatment | Duration |
	Fresh Adult Sera	Cord Sera	Polybrene	Glycine Soja		
Normal group O	0	0	+	0	Usually enhanced	—
T	+	0	0	+	No effect	Transient
Tn	+	0	0/+mf	+	Decreased	Persistent
Tk	+	0	+	0	Enhanced	Transient
Cad	Sometimes +	0	+	0/+w	Enhanced	Permanent
Acquired B	+	0				Transient
VA	+w	0	+	0	No effect	Persistent
Th	+	0	+	0	Decreased	Transient
NOR	+	0	+	0	Enhanced	Permanent

0 = no reactivity; + = reactivity/aggregation; +w = weak reactivity/aggregation; +mf = mixed-field reactivity; Transient = cells revert to normal state after primary condition is resolved; Persistent = essentially permanent, but rare cases have been reported in which the cells returned to normal; Permanent = cells remain permanently altered and polyagglutinable.

TABLE 22–3 **DIFFERENTIATION OF POLYAGGLUTINABLE CELLS USING LECTINS**

	Arachis Hypogaea	Dolichos Biflorus	Saliva Sclarea	Salvia Horminum	Griffonia Simplicifolia (GS II)*	Vicia Graminea (N$_{VG}$ Receptor)
Normal group O	0	0	0	0	0	—
T	+	0	0	0	0	Enhanced
Tn	0	+	+	+	0	Depressed
Tk	+	0	0	0	+	No effect
Cad	0	+	0	+	0	
Acquired B	0	0	0	0	0	
VA	0	0	0	0	0	
Th	+	0	0	0	0	
NOR	0	0	0	0	0	

*Previously known as *Bandeiraea simplicifolia* (BS II).

techniques may be used to determine the blood type of polyagglutinable RBCs. After incubating the polyagglutinable RBCs with typing serum, an elution is performed. If the specificity of the typing serum is demonstrable in the eluate, the cells are considered positive for the antigen.

Clinical Significance

Polyagglutination has both serologic and clinical significance. When cells are altered to expose cryptantigens, they are susceptible to agglutination by most adult sera. The reaction between the cryptantigens and the naturally occurring polyagglutinins produces antibody-coated cells that may be clinically significant. In addition to sepsis, polyagglutination has been associated with hemolytic anemia; hemolytic uremic syndrome; and leukemia, breast cancer, and other malignancies.

SEPSIS

Polyagglutination has been reported in patients with sepsis, upper respiratory infections, wound infections, intestinal infections, and malignancies. A partial list of bacterial and viral organisms that have been associated with polyagglutination include *A. niger, B. fragilis, Candida albicans, Clostridum perfringens,* C. *tertium, Corynebacterium aquaticum,* E. *coli,* pneumococci, *P. vulgaris,* S. *marcescens,* V. *cholerae,* and the influenza virus. Bird[9] pointed out that microbes do not have to be in the bloodstream to cause polyagglutination and that an extravascular site of infection can produce enzymes that enter the bloodstream in amounts greater than those that can be neutralized by normal serum inhibitors.

HEMOLYTIC ANEMIA AND HEMOLYTIC UREMIC SYNDROME

When cryptantigen exposure occurs in vivo, the patient's own IgM, complement-binding polyagglutinins can initiate intravascular hemolysis by binding to the transformed cells. In addition, the transfusion of plasma products containing normal levels of polyagglutinins may intensify the hemolysis. In rare cases, disseminated intravascular coagulation (DIC) and hemolytic uremic syndrome have been reported.[48,49] Hemolytic anemia has been more commonly reported in T polyagglutination,[50–53] however, Th polyagglutination[54] has also been implicated in severe intravascular hemolysis and DIC. The presence of cryptantigens on RBCs, white blood cells (WBCs), platelets, and tissue cells accounts for the anemia, thrombocytopenia, and renal dysfunction. Hemolysis is not seen in newborn infants with neonatal necrotizing enterocolitis (NNE) or other cryptantigen-exposing conditions unless they are transfused with plasma products. The naturally occurring polyagglutinins are absent in newborn infants, and because these antibodies are IgM, they do not cross the placenta.[55]

LEUKEMIA, BREAST CANCER, AND OTHER MALIGNANCES

Tn polyagglutination has been found in apparently healthy people; however, it has also been reported in patients with acute myelocytic leukemia.[56–58] One apparently healthy person who was found to have Tn polyagglutination later developed acute leukemia. Chemotherapy, in two of the leukemia patients, resulted in a clinical remission of the leukemia and the disappearance of the Tn-polyagglutinable RBCs.[57] Thus, it could be concluded that the presence of Tn polyagglutination may be a preleukemic state. Although several healthy individuals are known to have had Tn polyagglutination for a number of years, Ness et al.[57,58] recommend that these individuals be hematologically monitored. The cryptantigens T and Tn have been found on malignant tissue cells from breast, colon, urinary bladder, and in metastatic lesions.[11,59] The presence of these cryptantigens on malignant tissue has been attributed to the incomplete synthesis of MN glycoproteins.[60] The amount of the expressed antigen usually parallels the cancer malignancy and invasiveness.[61] The finding of T and Tn cryptantigens or a decrease in their respective serum antibodies, or both, may serve as an immunologic marker, with diagnostic and therapeutic implications. Because T cryptantigens are commonly found on malignant cells, efforts have been made to use anti-T antibodies in the treatment of breast cancer.[59] Unfortunately, human anti-T is usually too low-titered to be useful, and the lectin anti-T (*Arachis hypogaea*) is a foreign protein that would induce antipeanut antibodies in the recipient.

CRYPTANTIGENS IN THE ABSENCE OF APPARENT INFECTION

Two cases of transient Tn polyagglutination were described in apparently healthy neonates.[62] Delayed maturation of the sialosyltransferase system was postulated as the cause of the cryptantigen exposure. Similarly, both Tn and Th cryptantigens were detected in a patient with myelodysplasia.[63] These cryptantigens were detectable over a 5-year period, and the patient showed no apparent bacterial or viral infection. In a study of maternal and cord bloods, Wahl et al.[64] reported that a significant number of normal mothers and their newborn infants had Th-activated RBCs without polyagglutination. This study suggested that Th activation could represent a normal change in pregnancy, and that the Th antigen could be a marker for fetal hemopoiesis that is enhanced by some conditions during pregnancy and in utero development. Similarly, Herman et al.[65] reported that Th activation may be a RBC developmental marker present in congenital hypoplastic anemias. This study suggested that Th is a more specific marker for congenital hypoplastic anemia than i antigen expression or other fetal RBC characteristics.

BLOOD TRANSFUSION

In conclusion, polyagglutination is a rare condition; however, cryptantigen exposure is not. Cryptantigen exposure can be detected before polyagglutination develops by testing the patient's RBCs in vitro with specific lectins. A screening test using a two-lectin panel of *A. hypogeaea* and *G. soja* is simple to perform and detects most of the causes of polyagglutination: T, Th, Tk, Tn, and Tx.[52] Patients with a potential risk of developing cryptantigen exposure and polyagglutination (i.e., patients with various infections, malignancies, and unexplained anemias) should be screened for cryptantigen exposure using the two-lectin panel. If cryptantigen exposure is detected, these individuals should be tested for polyagglutination using ABO-compatible adult and cord sera. When patients are identified who have polyagglutinable RBCs, they should be evaluated for the possible use of washed RBC products before transfusion.[66–68] When plasma-containing products are required for transfusion, a minor crossmatch between the patient's RBCs and potential donors' plasma should be performed to select plasma for transfusion that lacks the specific polyagglutinin.

Review Questions

1. Polyagglutinable cells are agglutinated by the majority of adult human sera, regardless of:
   A. Temperature
   B. pH
   C. Incubation time
   D. Blood group
   E. Serum-to-cell ratio

2. T activation is:
   A. A preleukemic state
   B. Bacterially induced
   C. Persistent and irreversible
   D. An increased amount of i antigen
   E. An inherited condition

3. T receptor:
   A. Is nonreactive with cord blood sera
   B. Is an *N*-acetyl-galactosamine
   C. Cross-reacts with anti-B typing serum
   D. Cross-reacts with anti-A typing serum
   E. Is exposed by deacetylase

4. T receptor:
   A. Reacts with *Dolichos biflorus*
   B. Reacts with *Salvia sclarea*
   C. Is destroyed by enzymes
   D. Reacts with *Salvia horminum*
   E. Reacts with *Arachis hypogaea*

5. T activation is a form of polyagglutination caused by microorganisms that produce _____ as a metabolic byproduct.
   A. Fucosidase
   B. Deacetylase
   C. Galactosidase
   D. Bromalase
   E. Neuraminidase

6. Th polyagglutination:
   A. Reacts with *Glycine soja*
   B. Is persistent and irreversible
   C. Is considered clinically benign
   D. Is produced by neuraminidase
   E. Is enhanced by enzymes

7. Tk polyagglutination:
   A. Is of autosomal dominant inheritance
   B. Is caused by mutation in the hemopoietic tissue
   C. Shows altered expression of ABH, Lewis, Ii, and P_1
   D. Is of autosomal recessive inheritance
   E. Is permanent and irreversible

8. Tx polyagglutination is associated with:
   A. *Vibrio cholerae*
   B. *Clostridium perfringens*

C. *Candida albicans*
D. Pneumococcus
E. *Serratia marcescens*

9. Acquired B polyagglutination:
   A. Is a mutation in the hemopoietic tissue
   B. Is bacterially induced
   C. Is permanent and irreversible
   D. Shows increased hemolysis with anti-I in the presence of complement
   E. Cross-reacts with anti-A typing serum

10. VA polyagglutination was found in a patient with:
    A. Pneumococcal infection
    B. Leukemia
    C. Breast cancer
    D. Thrombocytopenia
    E. Hemolytic anemia

11. Tn polyagglutination is:
    A. A preleukemic state
    B. Bacterially induced
    C. An inherited condition
    D. Found in vitro and in vivo
    E. Enhanced by enzymes

12. Tn receptor:
    A. Cross-reacts with anti-A typing serum
    B. Cross-reacts with anti-B typing serum
    C. Is exposed by the action of bacterial metabolites
    D. Is galactose
    E. Reacts with *Arachis hypogaea*

13. From the following list, select a form of polyagglutination that is genetically inherited:
    A. Cad
    B. T-activation
    C. Acquired B
    D. Tn polyagglutination
    E. Tk polyagglutination

14. Cad polyagglutination:
    A. Is of autosomal recessive inheritance
    B. Reacts with anti-Sd^a
    C. Is associated with hemolytic anemia
    D. Is associated with hemolytic uremic syndrome
    E. Is associated with breast cancer

15. HEMPAS is:
    A. An autosomally dominant inherited condition
    B. An autosomally recessive inherited condition
    C. Bacterially induced
    D. A mutation in the hemopoietic tissue
    E. Occurs in vitro and in vivo

16. HEMPAS red blood cells are characterized by:
    A. Increased amounts of i antigen
    B. Increased amounts of H antigen
    C. Resistance to lysis

D. Resistance to *Plasmodium falciparum*
E. Increased amounts of sialic acid

17. NOR polyagglutination is caused by:
    A. Bacterial infection
    B. Viral infection
    C. Mutation in the hemopoietic tissue
    D. Autosomally dominant inheritance
    E. Autosomally recessive inheritance

18. Lectins are:
    A. Antibodies
    B. Plant extracts
    C. Enzymes
    D. Bacterial metabolites
    E. Antigens

19. Sialic acid is decreased in which of the following polyagglutinable states?
    A. T and Tn
    B. Acquired B and T
    C. Tk and Tn
    D. Cad and Tk
    E. Acquired B and Tk

20. Patients with in vivo polyagglutination should be transfused with:
    A. Whole blood
    B. Packed cells
    C. Washed RBCs
    D. Fresh frozen plasma
    E. Platelets

Answers to Review Questions

1. D (p 434)
2. B (p 434)
3. A (pp 438–439)
4. E (Table 22–3)
5. E (p 434)
6. D (p 435)
7. C (p 435)
8. D (p 435)
9. B (p 436)
10. E (p 436)
11. A (p 440)
12. A (p 436)
13. A (p 436)
14. B (p 436)
15. B (p 437)
16. A (p 437)
17. D (p 437)
18. B (p 439)
19. A (Table 22–2)
20. C (p 441)

References

1. Bird, GWG: Clinical aspects of red blood cell polyagglutinability of microbial origin. In Salmon, CH (ed): Blood Groups and Other Red Cell Surface Markers in Health and Disease. Masson, New York, 1982.
2. Hübener, G: Untersuchungen über Isoagglutination mit besonderer Berücksichtigung scheinbarer Abweichungen vom Gruppenschema. Z Immun Forsch 45:223, 1926.
3. Friedenreich, V: Production of a Specific Receptor Quality in Red Cell Corpuscles by Bacterial Activity. The Thomsen Hemagglutination Phenomenon. Levin and Munskgaard, Copenhagen, 1930.
4. Stratton, F: Polyagglutinability of red cells. Vox Sang 4:58, 1954.
5. Levene, C, et al: Red cell polyagglutination. Transfus Med Rev 2:176, 1988.
6. Uhlenbruck, G, et al: On the specificity of lectins with broad agglutination spectrum. II. Studies on the nature of the T antigen and the specific receptors for the lectin Arachis hypogaea (ground nut). Z Immun Forsch Allergie Klin Immunol 138:423, 1969.
7. Thomas, DB and Winzler, RJ: Structural studies on human erythrocyte glycoproteins. Alkali-labile tetrasaccharides. J Biol Chem 244:5943, 1969.
8. Anstee, DJ: Blood group MNSs—active sialoglycoproteins of the human erythrocyte membrane. In Sandler, SG, et al (eds): Immunobiology of the Erythrocyte. Progress in Clinical Biological Research. Alan R Liss, New York, 1980.
9. Bird, GWG: Lectins and red cell polyagglutinability: History, comments, and recent developments. In Beck, ML and Judd, WJ (eds): Polyagglutination. A Technical Workshop. American Association of Blood Banks, Washington, DC, 1980.
10. Hicklin, BL and Beck, ML: Latent polyagglutinable receptors on leukocytes and platelets (abstr). Transfusion 14:508, 1974.
11. Anglin Jr., JH, et al: Blood group-like activity released by human mammary carcinoma cells in culture. Nature 269:254, 1977.
12. Kline, WE and Issitt, CH: T substance in body fluids (abstr). Transfusion 16:527, 1976.
13. Bird, GWG, et al: Th, a "new" form of erythrocyte polyagglutination. Lancet i:1215, 1978.
14. Sondag-Thull, D, et al: Characterization of a neuraminidase from Corynebacterium aquaticum responsible for Th polyagglutination. Vox Sang 57:193, 1989.
15. Inglis, G, et al: Effect of Bacteroides fragilis on the human erythrocyte membrane: Pathogenesis of Tk polyagglutination. J Clin Pathol 28:964, 1975.
16. Doinel, C, et al: Tk polyagglutination produced in vitro by an endo-beta-galactosidase. Vox Sang 38:94, 1980.
17. Judd, WJ: The role of exo-β-galactosidases in Tk-activation (abstr). Transfusion 20:622, 1980.
18. Andreu, G, et al: Induction of Tk polyagglutination by Bacteroides fragilis culture supernatants. Associated modifications of ABH and Ii antigens. Rev Fr Transfus Immunohematol 22:551, 1979.
19. Bird, GWG, et al: Tx, a "new" red cell cryptantigen exposed by pneumococcal enzymes. Blood Transfus Immunohematol 25:215, 1982.
20. Wolach, B, et al: Tx polyagglutination in three members of one family. Acta Haematol 78:45, 1987.
21. Kline, WE, et al: Acquired-B antigen and polyagglutination in a healthy blood donor. Transfusion 19:648, 1979.
22. Gerbal, A, et al: Immunologic aspects of the acquired-B antigen. Vox Sang 28:398, 1975.
23. Garratty, G, et al: Acquired-B antigen associated with Proteus vulgaris infection. Vox Sang 21:45, 1971.
24. Salmon, C and Gerbal, A: The acquired-B antigen. In Seligson, D, Greenwalt, TJ, and Steane, EA (eds): Handbook of Clinical Laboratory Science. Vol 1, Sect D. CRC Press, Cleveland, 1977, p 193.
25. Judd, WJ: Review: Polyagglutination. Immunohematol 8:58, 1992.
26. Chorpenning, FW and Dodd, MC: Polyagglutinable erythrocytes associated with bacteriogenic transfusion reactions. Vox Sang 10:460, 1965.
27. Graninger, W, et al: "VA": A new type of erythrocyte polyagglutination characterized by depressed H receptors and associated with hemolytic anemia. I. Serological and hematological observations. Vox Sang 32:195, 1977.
28. Dahr, W, et al: Cryptic A-like receptor sites in human erythrocyte glycoproteins: proposed nature of Tn-antigen. Vox Sang 27:29, 1974.
29. Lee, LT, et al: Immunochemical studies on Tn erythrocyte glycoprotein. Blood 58:1228, 1981.
30. Myllylä, G, et al: Persistent mixed-field polyagglutinability: electrokinetic and serological aspects. Vox Sang 20:7, 1971.
31. Beck, ML, et al: Observations on leucocytes and platelets in six cases of Tn-polyagglutination. Med Lab Sci 34:325, 1977.
32. Dahr, W, et al: Molecular basis of Tn-polyagglutinability. Vox Sang 29:36, 1975.
33. Cazal, P, et al: Polyagglutinabilitié héréditaire dominate: antigène privé (Cad) correspondent à un anticorps public et à une lectine de Dolichos biflorus. Rev Fr Transfus Immunohematol 11:209, 1968.
34. Cazal, P, et al: Les antigenes Cad en 1976. Rev Fr Transfus Immunohematol 20:165, 1977.
35. Sanger, R, et al: Plant agglutinin for another human blood group. Lancet i:1130, 1971.
36. Herkt, F, et al: Structure determination of oligosaccharides isolated from Cad erythrocyte membranes by permethylation analysis and 500-MHz ^{1}H-NMR spectroscopy. Eur J Biochem 146:125, 1985.
37. Issitt, PD: The antigens Sd^a and Cad. In Moulds, JM and Woods, LL (eds): Blood Groups: P, I, Sd^a and Pr: A Technical Workshop. American Association of Blood Banks, Arlington, VA, 1991.
38. Blanchard, D, et al: Comparative study of glycophorin A derived O-glycans from human Cad, Sd(a +), and Sd(a −) erythrocytes. Biochem J 232:813, 1985.
39. Donald, ASR, et al: The human blood group Sd^a determinant: A terminal nonreducing carbohydrate structure in N-linked and mucin type glycoproteins. Biochem Soc Transact 12:596, 1984.
40. Williams, J, et al: Structural analysis of the carbohydrate moieties of human Tamm-Horsfall glycoprotein. Carbohydr Res 134:141, 1984.
41. Bird, AR, et al: Haemoglobin M-Hyde Park associated with polyagglutinable red blood cells in a South African family. Br J Haematol 68:459, 1988.
42. King, MJ, et al: Enhanced reaction with Vicia graminea lectin and exposed terminal N-acetyl-D-glucosaminyl residues on a sample of human red cells with Hb M-Hyde Park. Transfusion 28:549, 1988.
43. Crookston, JH, et al: Red cell abnormalities in HEMPAS (hereditary erythroblastic multinuclearity with a positive acidified serum test). Br J Haematol 23:83, 1972.
44. Gockerman, JP, et al: The abnormal surface characteristics of the red blood cell membrane in congenital dyserythropoietic anemia type II (HEMPAS). Br J Haematol 30:383, 1975.
45. Harris, PA, et al: An inherited RBC characteristic, NOR, resulting in erythrocyte polyagglutination. Vox Sang 42:134, 1982.
46. Beck, ML, et al: High incidence of acquired-B detectable by monoclonal anti-B reagents (abstr). Transfusion 32:17S, 1992.
47. Issitt, PD: Applied Blood Group Serology, ed 3. Montgomery Scientific Publications, Miami, 1985, pp 456–476.
48. Fischer, K, et al: Neuraminidase-induzierte Alteration der Erythrozyten und Gefässendothelium-eine Ursache des hämolytische urämischen Syndroms. Proc 16 Kongr Dtsch Ges Hämat, Bad Neuheim, 1972.
49. Rumpf, KW, et al: Hemolytic-uremic syndrome in an adult with T-cryptantigen liberation. Dtsch Med Wochenschr 115:1270, 1990.
50. van Loghem, Jr, JJ, et al: Polyagglutinability of red cells as a cause of a severe haemolytic transfusion reaction. Vox Sang 5:125, 1955.
51. Moores, P, et al: Severe hemolytic anemia in an adult associated with anti-T. Transfusion 15:329, 1975.

52. Levene, C, et al: Intravascular hemolysis and renal failure in a patient with T polyagglutination. Transfusion 26:243, 1986.

53. Judd, WJ, et al: Fatal intravascular hemolysis associated with T-polyagglutination. Transfusion 22:345, 1982.

54. Levene, NA, et al: Th polyagglutination with fatal outcome in a patient with massive intravascular hemolysis and perforated tumor of colon. Am J Hematol 35:127, 1990.

55. Novak, RW: The pathobiology of red cell cryptantigen exposure. Pediatr Pathol 10:867, 1990.

56. Bird, GWG, et al: Erythrocyte membrane modification in malignant disease of myeloid and lymphoreticular tissues. I. Tn-Polyagglutination in acute myelocytic leukemia. Br J Haematol 33:289, 1976.

57. Ness, PM, et al: Tn Polyagglutination preceding acute leukemia. Blood 54:30, 1979.

58. Ness, PM: The association of Tn and leukemia. Haematologia (Budap) 16:93, 1983.

59. Springer, GF, Murthy, MS, Desai, PR, et al: Human carcinoma-associated Thomsen-Friedenreich (T) antigen and the host's immune response to it. In Protides of Biological Fluids, 27th Colloquium, 1979. Pergamon Press, Oxford, 1980, p 211.

60. Buskila, D, et al: Exposure of cryptantigens on erythrocytes in patients with breast cancer. Cancer 61:2455, 1988.

61. Springer, GF: T and Tn, general carcinoma autoantigens. Science 224:1198, 1984.

62. Rose, RR, et al: Transient neonatal Tn-activation: Another example (abstr). Transfusion 23:422, 1983.

63. Janvier, D, et al: Concomitant exposure of Tn and Th cryptantigens on the red cells of a patient with myelodysplasia. Vox Sang 61:142, 1991.

64. Wahl, CM, et al: Th activation of maternal and cord blood. Transfusion 29:635, 1989.

65. Herman, JH, et al: Th activation in congenital hypoplastic anemia. Transfusion 27:253, 1987.

66. Buskila, D, et al: Polyagglutination in hospitalized patients: A prospective study. Vox Sang 52:99, 1987.

67. Sigler, E, et al: Polyagglutination: A rare mechanism for intravascular hemolysis (letter). Am J Med 92:113, 1992.

68. Adams, M, et al: Exposure of cryptantigens on red blood cell membranes in patients with acquired immune deficiency syndrome or AIDS-related complex. J Acq Immun Defic Synd 2:224, 1989.

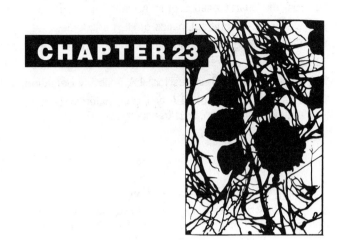

CHAPTER 23

The HLA System

Donna L. Phelan, BA, CHS(ABHI), MT(HEW)

OBJECTIVES

Upon completion of this chapter, the learner should be able to:

1 Define the abbreviations HLA, MLR, MLC, and MHC.
2 Define the standard method used for HLA typing.
3 Describe the three regions of the HLA complex located on the short arm of chromosome 6.
4 List the important characteristics of the HLA genes.
5 List the three exceptions to the practice of naming all serological specificities on the basis of correlation with an identified sequence that eliminates the need for a provisional "w" designation.
6 Describe the current nomenclature for HLA genes.
7 List two clinical situations in which HLA typing is important.
8 Define the term *haplotype*.
9 Describe the difference between HLA phenotype and HLA genotype.

10 List the characteristics of HLA class I and class II gene products.
11 Describe the characteristics of HLA antibodies.
12 Define linkage disequilibrium, a characteristic of HLA antigens.
13 Describe the techniques used for HLA antigen detection.
14 Describe the techniques for HLA antibody detection.
15 Describe the role of HLA typing in: paternity testing, disease association, platelet transfusion, and transplantation.

Human leukocyte antigen (HLA), or human histocompatibility, testing is a specialized division of immunology. The laboratory discipline supports a number of clinical specialties in transplantation, transfusion, and immunogenetics. Because of its specialized nature, HLA is given relatively little attention in most training programs such as nursing or medical technology.

This chapter introduces basic concepts of HLA and clinical applications of HLA testing. It is written for the reader with some training in the biomedical sciences and familiarity with general immunology concepts.

The emphasis of the chapter is on principles and concepts of HLA structure and function, HLA procedures, and the clinical application of HLA testing to immunogenetics (paternity and disease association), transfusion practices, and transplantation. As it is an overview of a technologically complex area, it lacks a great deal of detail. References are provided that will introduce a path to further information.

Evidence for human leukocyte blood groups was first advanced in 1954 by Dausset,[1] who observed that patients whose sera contained leukoagglutinins had received more blood transfusions than other patients. He observed that these agglutinins were not autoantibodies as had been thought previously but, rather, alloantibodies produced by the infusion of cells bearing alloantigens not present in the recipient.

Dausset[2] also observed that the sera from seven polytransfused patients agglutinated leukocytes from about 60 percent of the French population, but not the leukocytes of the seven patients. He termed the leukocyte antigen defined by leukoagglutination techniques MAC, and family studies showed that leukocyte antigens were genetically determined. At about the same time, Payne[3] showed that the sera of patients with febrile nonhemolytic transfusion reactions often contained leukoagglutinins.

The microdroplet lymphocytotoxicity test was introduced by Terasaki, McClelland, et al.,[4,5] at the First International Histocompatibility Workshop as a means to define MAC specificity clearly. The microdroplet technique was adopted as the standard method of typing, owing to the unreliability of the leukoagglutination test. In various modifications this test is still the major HLA-typing serologic technique. The development of HLA typing was further aided by the introduction of computer analysis programs by van Rood and van Leeuwen[6] to study the serologic complexities. Despite numerous false-positive and false-negative serologic reactions, certain specificities could be discerned by computer analysis.

Van Rood applied computer analysis techniques to define specific HLA alleles. He tested approximately 66 sera containing leukoagglutinating antibodies against a random panel of 100 cells. Using two-by-two chi-square analysis, he compared reactivity of each serum with that of every other serum. In this way he was able to identify several groups of sera that were detecting common specificities. In addition, one group of sera having high chi-square values with each other but low values with other serum groups suggested products of allelic genes. Van Rood called this diallelic system 4, with 4^a and 4^b as alleles.

Following the discovery of the first leukocyte antigens and a suitable test system, the number of defined serologic specificities increased rapidly. By 1967 they were all clearly shown to belong to the same genetic system, and the term "human leukocyte antigen" (HL-A or HLA [the hyphen has since been deleted]) was approved by the World Health Organization (WHO) Committee on Nomenclature.[7] The WHO Committee was formed to establish worldwide uniform nomenclature for the HLA antigens. The committee meets after each international workshop and uses the data from the workshop to update and assign new names for antigens. These workshops, which are collaborative efforts to advance the field of histocompatibility, are held approximately every 2 to 3 years (Table 23–1). Standardized name assignments aid the rapid but orderly development in this field.

By 1967, it was generally accepted that the HLA antigens were coded for by two closely linked loci, each coding for several alleles.[8,9] Antigens were assigned to one of the loci, based on large population studies and segregation analysis within families. In 1970, the existence of a third locus was defined that codes for only 10 different alleles to date.[10] Additional research disclosed that the lymphocytes from two different individuals would undergo blast transformation and divide when mixed and cultured in vitro. This cellular response is known as the mixed-lymphocyte reaction (MLR).[11,12] In 1967, Bach and Amos[13] discov-

TABLE 23-1   **INTERNATIONAL WORKSHOPS**

Year	Location	Advances
1964	Durham, North Carolina, USA	Test Techniques
1965	Leiden, The Netherlands	Antigens and Transplantation
1967	Turin, Italy	Family Typing Studies
1970	Los Angeles, California, USA	Common Serum Sets
1972	Evian, France	Population Studies
1975	Arhus, Denmark	MLC, Class II Antigens
1977	Oxford, United Kingdom	Class II Genetics
1980	Los Angeles, California, USA	DR Serology, Haplotype Analyses
1984	Munich, Germany and Vienna, Austria	HTC, DNA Technology
1987	Princeton, New Jersey and New York, New York, USA	RFLP, Cellular Typing
1991	Yokohama, Japan	DNA Technology

ered that the MLR was negative when leukocytes from a pair of HLA-identical siblings were mixed together, indicating that HLA gene products were responsible for the MLR activity. The technique used to test for MLR activity is the mixed-lymphocyte culture (MLC). Data from the MLC revealed that there might be a fourth locus (D) very closely linked with the HLA complex. The Seventh International Histocompatibility Workshop in 1977 clearly established the D locus and also a new D-related (DR) locus* defined by serologic methods.[14] Most significantly, the typing of B lymphocytes for their DR specificities was accomplished.

Recent evidence suggests that a separate HLA-D locus, defined only by MLR, may not exist. HLA-D assignments may be the result of the combined effect of the HLA-DR, HLA-DQ, and HLA-DP determinants, subregions on the class II molecule.

Nomenclature

The HLA genetic region is a series of closely linked genes that determine major histocompatibility factors; that is, surface antigens or receptors that are responsible for the recognition and elimination of foreign tissues. The region is also referred to as the major histocompatibility complex (MHC). The HLA complex contains an estimated 35 to 40 genes physically grouped into three regions located on the short arm of chromosome 6 (Fig. 23-1). The class I region encodes genes for the classic transplantation molecules, HLA-A, -B, and -C. It also encodes for additional nonclassic genes including HLA-E, -F, and -G. The

---

*This locus was found to be identical or similar to the D locus identified by the MLC technique.

HUMAN CHROMOSOME 6

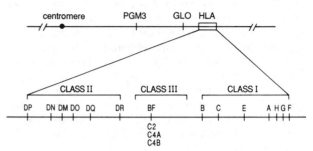

FIGURE 23-1 The HLA complex on the short arm of chromosome 6.

class II region encodes genes for the molecules HLA-DR, -DP, and -DQ composed of both α and β chains. DP molecules are the product of DPA1 and DPB1 alleles (Fig. 23-2) as DPB2 and DPA2 are pseudogenes, genes with mutations that prevent gene activation or transcription. DQ molecules are the product of DQA1 and DQB1 alleles. Last, DR molecules use DRA, but can use alleles coded by DRB1 (the classic DR specificities), DRB3 (DR52 molecules), DRB4 (DR53), and DRB5 (DR51).

The class III region encodes structurally and functionally diverse molecules including C2, C4, Bf (the complement factors), 21-hydroxylase, and tumor necrosis factor. In addition, two other genes, glyoxalase-1 (GLO) and phosphoglucomutase-3 (PGM-3), are linked with the HLA complex.

One very important characteristic of the HLA genes is that they are highly polymorphic, several alleles existing at each locus. The allelic specificities are designated by numbers following the locus symbol (e.g., HLA-A1, HLA-A2, HLA-B5, HLA-B7, etc.). Provisionally identified or tentative specificities, before the 1991 International Workshop, carried the initial letter "w" (for workshop) inserted between the locus letter designation and the temporary allele specificity number. The "w" specificities required further definition and confirmation. For example, HLA-Bw53 indicated that the definition of the Bw53 specificity was not fully agreed on by the WHO Committee on HLA nomen-

CLASS II

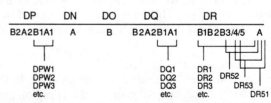

FIGURE 23-2 The loci that code for the major categories of HLA class II gene products. (From Rodey, GE: HLA Beyond Tears. De Novo, Atlanta, 1991, p 12, with permission.)

clature. After the 1991 workshop, however, the WHO Committee agreed that all serologic specificities with "w" indicating provisional status would, with three exceptions, drop the "w."[15] In the future, all serologic specificities will be named on the basis of correlation with an identified sequence, eliminating the need for a provisional "w" designation. The three exceptions are (1) Bw4 and Bw6, to distinguish them as epitopes different from other B locus alleles; (2) the C locus specificities, to maintain distinction between HLA-C locus alleles and the complement components; and (3) the D and DP specificities defined by MLR and primed lymphocyte typing (PLT).

Table 23–2 lists the current specificities of the HLA system recognized by the WHO Committee. Note that specificities within the A and B loci are not numbered consecutively, as are those within the C, DR, DQ, and DP loci. This is because many of the A and B specificities were established before the discovery of the latter loci, and, to avoid renumbering, the existing numbers for the A and B loci were retained.

Also note that many of the broad specificities in Table 23–2 are subdivided into two or more different specificities owing to the detection of discrete gene products by monospecific antisera. Monospecific antisera by definition react only with antigenic determinants unique to the specific antigen. This process of "splitting" previously recognized antigens is still going on.

Table 23–3 lists the broad specificities and their designated split specificities. Also listed are associated antigens (designated with #), which are variants of the original broad specificity and not splits as previously defined.

There are no 4 or 6 allelic assignments within the A and B loci, because these numbers are reserved for the leukocyte antigen systems under active investigation at the time the nomenclature was established. The antigens originally called 4 and 6 are now termed Bw4 and Bw6. Every HLA-B locus and some HLA-A locus molecules carries either the Bw4 or the Bw6 antigenic determinant. The distribution of Bw4 and Bw6 determinants on HLA-A and -B locus gene products is found in Table 23–4.

Current nomenclature was recommended during the 10th International Histocompatibility Workshop in 1987; minor modifications were made in 1990 with total implementation after the 11th International Histocompatibility Workshop in 1991. Many HLA allelic variants were discovered by nucleotide and amino acid sequence data that are not detectable by traditional serologic techniques. This complexity necessitated the development of the following nomenclature for HLA genes:

1. HLA- designates the MHC.
2. A capital letter indicates a specific locus (A, B, C, D, . . .) or region. All genes in the D region are preceded by the letter D and followed by a second capital letter indicating the subregion (DR, DQ, DP, DO, DN, . . .).

3. Loci coding for the specific class I peptide chains are next identified (A1, A2, B1, B2).
4. Specific alleles are designated by an asterisk followed by a two-digit number defining the unique allele. For example, the serologically defined HLA-B27 specificity actually comprises seven distinct allelic variations. These alleles are now defined as HLA-B *2701 through *2707. The nomenclature of certain alleles contains a fifth digit, like HLA-Cw *02021 and *02022. The fifth digit indicates that the two variants differ by a silent nucleotide substitution, but not in amino acid sequence.

Some examples of current HLA genetic nomenclature are given in Table 23–5.

Antigens and Antibodies

It is necessary to evaluate the HLA antigen composition in prospective donor-recipient pairs before organ transplantation and in candidates for platelet therapy who are refractory to random donor platelets. Even more important is the evaluation and identification of HLA antibodies in the serum of recipients before transplantation and transfusion. Evidence clearly indicates that presensitization to HLA antigens may cause rapid rejection of transplanted tissue or poor platelet survival after transfusion.[16] HLA-antigen testing is also used in disease correlation, paternity testing, and anthropologic studies.

Each person has two alleles for each locus. Both alleles or gene products of a locus are expressed codominantly; that is, there is equal expression of both alleles. The presence of one allele does not suppress the expression of the other. If there are two different alleles on one locus, the person is heterozygous. If both alleles on that locus are the same, the person is homozygous.

The entire set of A, B, C, DR, and DP antigens located on one chromosome is called a haplotype. Genetic crossovers and recombination in the HLA region are uncommon (less than 1 percent), and thus a complete set of antigens located on a chromosome is usually inherited by children as a unit (haplotype).

Figure 23–3 illustrates the segregation of HLA haplotypes in a family. The two haplotypes of the father are labeled a and b, and those of the mother c and d. Each offspring inherits two haplotypes—one from each parent. Thus, only four possible haplotypes—ac, ad, bc, and bd—can be found in the offspring. It can be calculated that 25 percent of the offspring will have identical HLA haplotypes, 50 percent will share one HLA haplotype, and 25 percent will share no HLA haplotypes. An important corollary is that a parent and child can share only one haplotype, making an identical match between the two unlikely. It should also be apparent that uncles, grandparents, and cousins are very unlikely to have identical haplotypes

TABLE 23-2 **HLA SPECIFICITIES OFFICIALLY RECOGNIZED FOLLOWING THE 11th INTERNATIONAL HISTOCOMPATIBILITY WORKSHOP**

A	B	C	D	DR	DQ	DP
A1	B5	Cw1	Dw1	DR1	DQ1	DPw1
A2	B7	Cw2	Dw2	DR103	DQ2	DPw2
A203	B703	Cw3	Dw3	DR2	DQ3	DPw3
A210	B8	Cw4	Dw4	DR3	DQ4	DPw4
A3	B12	Cw5	Dw5	DR4	DQ5(1)	DPw5
A9	B13	Cw6	Dw6	DR5	DQ6(1)	DPw6
A10	B14	Cw7	Dw7	DR6	DQ7(3)	
A11	B15	Cw8	Dw8	DR7	DQ8(3)	
A19	B16	Cw9(w3)	Dw9	DR8	DQ9(3)	
A23(9)	B17	Cw10(w3)	Dw10	DR9		
A24(9)	B18		Dw11(w7)	DR10		
A2403	B21		Dw12	DR11(5)		
A25(10)	B22		Dw13	DR12(5)		
A26(10)	B27		Dw14	DR13(6)		
A28	B35		Dw15	DR14(6)		
A29(19)	B37		Dw16	DR1403		
A30(19)	B38(16)		Dw17(w7)	DR1404		
A31(19)	B39(16)		Dw18(w6)	DR15(2)		
A32(19)	B3901		Dw19(w6)	DR16(2)		
A33(19)	B3902		Dw20	DR17(3)		
A34(10)	B40		Dw21	DR18(3)		
A36	B4005		Dw22			
A43	B41		Dw23	DR51		
A66(10)	B42					
A68(28)	B44(12)		Dw24	DR52		
A69(28)	B45(12)		Dw25			
A74(19)	B46		Dw26	DR53		
	B47					
	B48					
	B49(21)					
	B50(21)					
	B51(5)					
	B5102					
	B5103					
	B52(5)					
	B53					
	B54(22)					
	B55(22)					
	B56(22)					
	B57(17)					
	B58(17)					
	B59					
	B60(40)					
	B61(40)					
	B62(15)					
	B63(15)					
	B64(14)					
	B65(14)					
	B67					
	B70					
	B71(70)					
	B72(70)					
	B73					
	B75(15)					
	B76(15)					
	B77(15)					
	B7801					
	Bw4					
	Bw6					

TABLE 23-3 **BROAD SPECIFICITIES, THEIR SPLITS, AND ASSOCIATED ANTIGENS**

Original Broad Specificities	Splits and Associated Antigens (#)
A2	A203#,A210#
A9	A23,A24,A2403#
A10	A25,A26,A34,A66
A19	A29,A30,A31,A32,A33,A74
A28	A68,A69
B5	B51,B52
B7	B703#
B12	B44,B45
B14	B64,B65
B15	B62,B63,B75,B76,B77
B16	B38,B39,B3901#,B3902#
B17	B57,B58
B21	B49,B50,B4005#
B22	B54,B55,B56
B40	B60,B61
B70	B71,B72
Cw3	Cw9,Cw10
DR1	DR103#
DR2	DR15,DR16
DR3	DR17,DR18
DR5	DR11,DR12
DR6	DR13,DR14,DR1403#,DR1404#
DQ1	DQ5,DQ6
DQ3	DQ7,DQ8,DQ9
Dw6	Dw18,Dw19
Dw7	Dw11,Dw17

with any given child. These are important factors when looking for a well-matched organ or blood donor.

The HLA phenotype, then, represents the surface markers or antigens detected in histocompatibility testing of a single individual. The HLA genotype represents the association of the antigens on the two C6 chromosomes as determined by family studies, and the HLA haplotype is the antigenic makeup of a single C6 chromosome, illustrated in Figure 23-4.

HLA GENE PRODUCTS

Structure

HLA gene products are globular glycoproteins, each composed of two noncovalently linked chains. Class I (HLA-A, HLA-B, and HLA-C) molecules consist of a heavy chain of 45,000 dalton (d) molecular weight associated noncovalently with β-2 microglobulin, a nonpolymorphic protein of 12,000 d molecular weight found in serum and urine. The heavy chain folds into three domains and is inserted through the cell membrane via a hydrophobic sequence.[17]

Class II (HLA-DR, HLA-DQ, and HLA-DP) molecules consist of two similar-size chains of 33,000 (alpha) and 28,000 (beta) d molecular weight associated noncovalently throughout their extracellular portions. In these molecules, both chains are inserted through the membrane via hydrophobic regions. The extracellular portions of these chains fold into two domains.[18,19]

Class I molecules are present on all nucleated cells and platelets, whereas class II molecules have a much more restricted distribution. They are found only on B lymphocytes, macrophages, monocytes, and endothelial cells. Although class I and II molecules have some obvious structural differences, they are thought to be very similar in overall three-dimensional configuration (Fig. 23-5). Class I and II molecules are also alike in that most of the polymorphism is expressed in the portion of the molecule farthest from the cell membrane.[20]

Early structural models of class I molecules indicated that the α_1 and α_2 domains consisted of stretches of amino acids that were arranged into helical structures rather then sheets typical of globular proteins. The crystallography studies of Bjorkman et al.[21] elucidated the three-dimensional structure of the class I, HLA-A2 molecule. The α_1 and α_2 domains form a platform overlaid by two helical structures to form the peptide binding site (Fig. 23-6). This groove holds processed peptides for presentation to T cells.

The surface topography, created by the folding of globular proteins into three-dimensional configurations, is large and irregular, containing multiple, nonrepeating sites (antigenic determinants or epitopes) that are potentially immunogenic. It is possible that the entire surface of the HLA molecule consists of these multiple, overlapping epitopes. An epitope is estimated to involve a minimum of five to six amino acid residues, but larger sequences are often necessary to construct the appropriate conformation.

Epitopes that differ among individual members of the same species are alloepitopes. HLA alloepitopes are defined with well-characterized alloantibodies and cloned T lymphocytes. Serologically defined epitopes are located primarily in and around the peptide groove. The epitopes recognized by T lymphocytes are less precisely mapped but are probably distinct from the serologically defined ones.[22]

Function

The primary role of the adaptive arm of the immune system is to recognize and eliminate foreign antigens. An essential feature of this specific function is the

TABLE 23-4 **Bw4 and Bw6 ASSOCIATED SPECIFICITIES**

Bw4:	B5,B5102,B5103,B13,B17,B27,B37,B38(16),B44(12),B47,B49(21),B51(5),B52(5),B53,B57(17),B58(17),B59,B63(15),B77(15) and A9,A23(9),A24(9),A2403,A25(10),A32(19)
Bw6:	B7,B703,B8,B14,B18,B22,B35,B39(16),B3901,B3902,B40,B4005,B41,B42,B45(12),B46,B48,B50(21),B54(22),B55(22),B56(22), B60(40),B61(40),B62(15),B64(14),B65(14),B67,B70,B71(70),B72(70),B73,B75(15),B76(15),B7801

TABLE 23-5   **EXAMPLES OF CURRENT HLA NOMENCLATURE**

Serologic Specificity	Gene Locus	Allelic Variation			Number of Gene Products
HLA-A11	HLA-A	A*1101,A*110?			2
HLA-B7	HLA-B	B*0701,B*0702, B*0703			3
HLA-DR11	HLA-DRB1 HLA-DRA	DRB1*11011 DRB1*11012 DRB1*1102 DRB1*1103	DRB1*11041 DRB1*11042 DRB1*1105		7
HLA-DR52	HLA-DRB3 HLA-DRA	DRB3*0101 DRB3*0201	DRB3*0202 DRB3*0301		4
HLA-DQ2	HLA-DQB1 HLA-DQA1	DQB1*0201 DQA1*0201			1

immune system's ability to discriminate between self and nonself (or "foreign") antigens. MHC class I and II molecules play a crucial role in the process of discrimination at the molecular, cellular, and species levels between self and nonself elements.

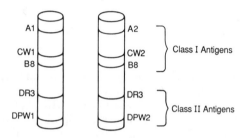

Phenotype: A1,2; B8,-; CW1, W2; DR3,-; DPW1, W2

Genotype: A1,2; B8,8; CW1, W2; DR3, 3; DPW1, W2

Haplotype: A1, B8, CW1, DR3, DPW1/A2, B8, CW2, DR3, DPW2

FIGURE 23-4 Schematic representation of the HLA loci on the short arm of chromosome 6. (From Miller, MV, and Rodey, G: HLA Without Tears. American Society of Clinical Pathologists, Chicago, 1981, p 10, with permission.)

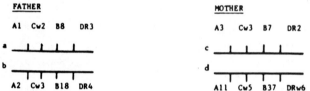

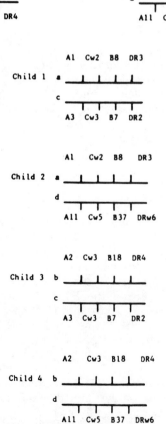

FIGURE 23-3 Segregation of HLA haplotypes in a pedigree. (From Tiwari and Terasaki,[54] p 8, with permission.)

ANTIBODIES

The majority of HLA alloantibodies are immunoglobulin G (IgG). Antibodies to HLA molecules can be divided into two groups: (1) those that detect a single HLA gene product ("private" antibodies binding to an epitope unique to one HLA gene product), and (2) those that detect more than one HLA gene product. These may be "public" (binding to epitopes shared by more than one HLA gene product) or cross-reactive (binding to structurally similar HLA epitopes).[23]

Monoclonal HLA antibodies (moabs) are produced by fusing HLA antibody-producing B cells with plasmacytoma lines.[24] Plasmacytoma cells arise from the malignant transformation of plasma cells or differentiated B cells. These cells continue to secrete antibody after transformation. Moabs detect a broader range of epitopes because they are derived through xenoimmunization, or immunization across different species.

CROSSING OVER

An event that infrequently complicates HLA-typing interpretation and haplotype determination is crossing over, or recombination. During meiosis, material can be exchanged between the paired chromosomes. During chromosomal replication, replicated chromosomes

CLASS I CLASS II

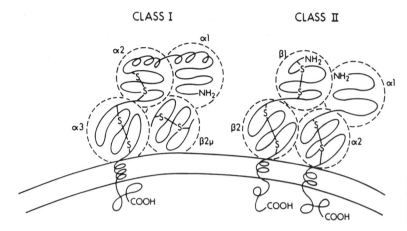

FIGURE 23-5 Three-dimensional configurations of class I and II molecules. (From Rodey, GE: HLA Beyond Tears. DeNovo, Atlanta, 1991, p 17, with permission.)

often overlay each other, forming X-shaped chiasmata (Fig. 23-7). When the chromosomes are pulled apart during meiotic division, breaks can occur at the crossover site, resulting in complementary exchange of genetic material. The farther apart two loci are on a given chromosome, the more likely genetic exchanges will occur. For example, recombination between HLA-A and HLA-DP occurs commonly, whereas recombination between HLA-DQ and HLA-DR is rare. Crossing over has the effect of rearranging the genes on the chromosome to produce new haplotypes in the general population.

LINKAGE DISEQUILIBRIUM

An important characteristic of HLA antigens is the existence of linkage disequilibrium between the alleles of the loci. Linkage disequilibrium is the occurrence of HLA genes more frequently in the same haplotype than would be expected by chance alone. In the Rh system, the blood groups C, D, and e are found together more often than one would expect based on their individual gene frequencies. This is commonly found within the HLA system. In a randomly mating population at Hardy-Weinberg equilibrium,[25] the oc-

currence of two alleles from closely linked genes will be the product of their individual gene frequencies. If the observed value of the joint frequency is significantly different from the expected frequency (the product of the individual allele frequencies), the alleles are said to be in linkage disequilibrium. For example, if HLA-A1 and HLA-B8 gene frequencies are 0.16 and 0.1, respectively, in a population, the expected occurrence of an HLA haplotype bearing both A1 and B8 should be $0.16 \times 0.1 \times 100$, or 1.6 percent. In certain white populations, however, the actual occurrence of this haplotype is as high as 8 percent, far in excess of the expected frequency. The HLA alleles frequently associated through disequilibrium are listed in Table 23-6. Disequilibrium between the B and DR loci alleles may account for problems in correlating B-locus serotyping with allograft survival and disease associations, inasmuch as matching or typing for B-locus alleles would, by disequilibrium, often result in matching or typing for D-locus alleles as well. D-/DR-locus matching has been found to be clinically significant to allograft survival.

CROSS-REACTIVITY

Cross-reactivity is a phenomenon in which an antiserum directed against one HLA antigenic determinant reacts with other HLA antigenic determinants as well. Cross-reactive antigens share important structural elements with one another but retain unique, specific elements. HLA serologists recognized very quickly that many of the HLA alloantibodies were serologically cross-reactive with HLA specificities.[26-28] Legrand and Dausset[29] suggested in 1967 that these antibodies might detect public specificities shared by multiple HLA gene products. The broadly reactive antibodies used in van Rood and von Leeuwen's original computer-derived HLA clusters[6] also defined many of the currently defined major cross-reactive groups (CREGs).

The majority of cross-reactive alloantibodies detect HLA specificities of allelic molecules coded by the

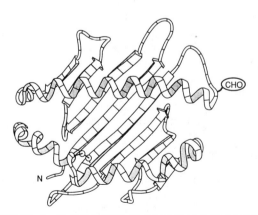

FIGURE 23-6 Peptide binding groove of an HLA class I molecule. (Illustration courtesy of Dr. Peter Parham.)

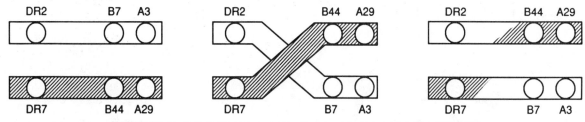

FIGURE 23-7   Schematic of a recombination event between HLA-B and HLA-DR.

same locus. On the basis of these reactions, most specificities can be grouped into major CREGS (Figs. 23-8 and 23-9).[30,31] For example, the HLA-A locus antigens A2, A23, A24, and A28 share a common determinant and therefore make up the A2-CREG, or A2c. HLA-A28 also shares a common determinant with A26, A33, and A34, defining the A28-CREG. There are also at least three interlocus cross-reactions detected by alloantisera and moabs that occur between the HLA-A and HLA-B loci: HLA-A23, HLA-A24, HLA-A25, and HLA-A32 with HLA Bw4;[32-35] HLA-A11 with HLA-Bw6;[36] and HLA-A2 with HLA-B17.[37-39]

Techniques of Histocompatibility Testing

The principles employed in histocompatibility testing are basically similar to those used for red blood cell

TABLE 23-6   HLA ALLELES FREQUENTLY ASSOCIATED THROUGH DISEQUILIBRIUM IN DIFFERENT POPULATIONS

HLA-A,-C,-B	HLA-A,-B,-DR
White	
A1,Cw7,B8	A1,B8,DR3
A3,Cw7,B7	A3,B7,DR2
A2,Cw5,B44	A29,B44,DR7
A1,Cw6,B57	A3,B35,Dr1
A11,Cw4,B35	A1,B17,DR7
A30,Cw6,B13	A30,B13,DR7
Black	
A36,Cw4,B53	A1,B8,DR3
A1,Cw7,B8	A30,B42,DR3
A11,Cw2,B35	A28,B64,DR7
A24,Cw4,B35	A2,B58,DR11
A2,Cw2,B72	A28,B58,DR14
A2,Cw7,B58	A3,B7,DR3
Asian	
A30,Cw6,B13	A24,B52,DR2
A2,Cw1,B46	A33,B44,DR14
A24,Cw1,B54	A24,B7,DR1
A33,Cw3,B58	A33,B44,DR13
A24,Cw7,B7	A30,B13,DR7
A11,Cw4,B62	A24,B54,DR4

(RBC) testing; that is, known sera are used to type HLA antigens on test cells, recipient serum is screened for the presence of HLA antibodies, and crossmatching of donor cells and recipient sera is performed to determine compatibility.

Preformed antibodies to tissue of both donor and recipient may cause significant complications in transplantation or transfusion. Recipient lymphocytotoxic HLA antibodies to donor antigens have been associated with accelerated graft rejection and with poor response to platelet transfusion. Antibody in donor plasma to recipient leukocytes has been associated with severe pulmonary infiltrates and respiratory distress following transfusion.

Crossmatching involves both serologic and cellular procedures. Serologic crossmatching is performed by cytotoxicity and flow cytometric techniques.[39] Lymphocyte-defined compatibility is determined by the MLR or one of its modifications.

Over the past 10 years, practical techniques have been developed to characterize gene structure and specific alleles. The techniques of molecular genetics have revolutionized the field of molecular biology.

HLA Antigen Detection

The agglutination methods initially used to define the HLA complex have given way to a precise microlymphocytotoxicity test.[40] Cytotoxicity techniques require only 1 to 2 μl of serum and are sensitive and reproducible.

Acid-citrated dextrose (ACD) or phenol-free heparinized blood is used for testing. A purified lymphocyte suspension is prepared by layering whole blood on a Ficoll-Hypaque gradient and centrifuging. Residual RBCs and granulocytes are forced to the bottom of the gradient, and platelets remain in the supernatant. Lymphocytes collect at the gradient's interface and can be harvested, washed, and adjusted to appropriate test concentrations (Fig. 23-10). HLA-A, HLA-B, and HLA-C typing is performed on this lymphocyte suspension. HLA-DR typing requires a purified B-lymphocyte suspension.

B-lymphocyte suspensions are generally prepared in two ways: (1) nylon wool separation[41,42] and (2) fluorescent labeling.[43] The nylon wool separation of B lymphocytes is based on the observation that B cells adhere preferentially to nylon wool, from which they can be eluted, whereas T lymphocytes do not adhere

HLA-A LOCUS CREGS

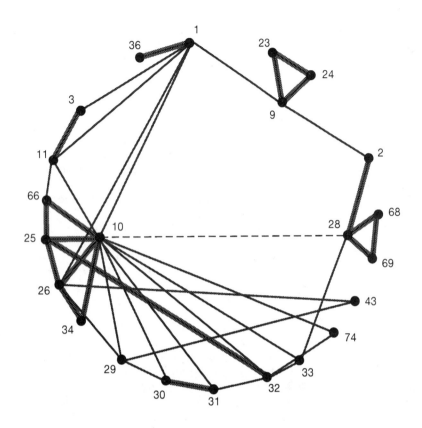

FIGURE 23-8 Cross-reactions within the HLA-A locus. (From Bender, K: The HLA System. Biotest Diagnostics, 1991, p 21, with permission.)

▬▬▬ very frequent ——— frequent – – – – rare

to the wool. Fluorescent labeling involves the incubation of lymphocytes with fluorescein isothiocyanate (FITC)–labeled anti-Ig. B lymphocytes develop distinct fluorescent caps owing to the binding of the labeled anti-Ig to the cell surface Ig found on B cells and not on T cells. A major advantage of the fluorescent labeling technique is that it does not involve the physical separation of T and B cells, in contrast to nylon wool separation.

Techniques have been developed using immunomagnetic beads to positively select (target cells rosetted on beads) lymphocyte subpopulations for use in HLA typing, for both class I and class II antigens.[44] These techniques provide for rapid isolation of cells with a high degree of purity and employ immunofluorescence lymphocytotoxicity. The technique for isolation of either T or B cells depends upon the moab for bead coating.

HLA testing is performed in 60- or 72-well microtiter trays. Antiserum test trays are prepared by dispensing 1 μl of serum into the bottom of each well, which contains mineral oil. Mineral oil is used to prevent evaporation of antisera during test incubations. Antiserum trays are frozen at $-70°C$ until just before use. Upon use, they are removed from the freezer and thawed for 3 to 5 minutes.

Every laboratory performing HLA typing uses some form of complement-dependent microlymphocytotoxicity (CDC) (Fig. 23–11). In this procedure 1 μl of antisera is mixed with 1 μl of cells and incubated at room temperature for 30 minutes. Rabbit serum (5 μl) is added as a source of complement, and the cells are further incubated at room temperature for 60 minutes. Complement-mediated cell membrane injury that is induced in cells binding HLA antibody is visualized by the uptake or release of eosin Y or trypan blue dye. The test is a tertiary binding assay that depends heavily on many factors (e.g., time, temperature, antibody strength) that influence the efficiency with which the antibodies will activate the complement cascade.

Trays are usually read on inverted phase-contrast

HLA-B LOCUS CREGS

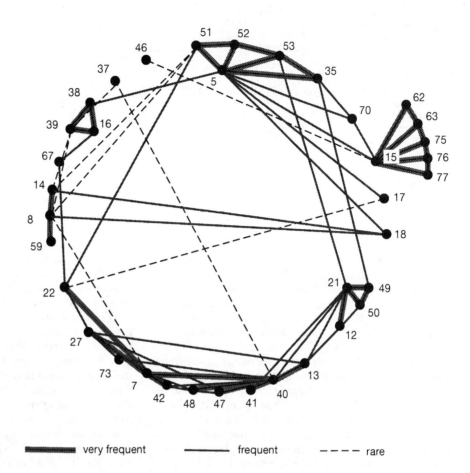

FIGURE 23-9 Cross-reactions within the HLA-B locus. (From Bender, K: The HLA System. Biotest Diagnostics, 1991, p 22, with permission.)

very frequent ——— frequent ---- rare

microscopes. Under properly adjusted phase, cells that have not been injured appear small, bright, and refractile. Injured cells that have taken up eosin Y or trypan dye owing to the antibody and complement flatten and appear large, dark, and nonrefractile. The percent of cell death is coded numerically: 8 is used for a strong positive with essentially all cells killed; 1 is used for a negative reaction in which cell viability is the same as in the negative control. By scoring the reaction of each known serum with test cells, a phenotype can be assigned. Antigen assignment is made by looking at the specificity of the defined HLA antibody in the positive wells. For example, if all wells containing HLA-A3 antibody are positive (eight reactions), the A3 antigen is assigned to the phenotype.

HLA-D Typing

Because allografted tissue is rejected by a lymphocyte-mediated immune response, as well as by antibody response, tests have been developed that use a biologic response of lymphocytes to foreign antigens as a measure of histocompatibility. The MLR test is especially important because it provides an in vitro model in which lymphocytes can be used both as responders (recipient cells) to foreign HLA-alloantigens and as stimulators (donor cells) carrying those antigens.[11] For example, lymphocytes of the recipient are mixed with lymphocytes of the donor, after the donor lympho-

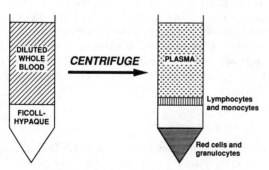

FIGURE 23-10 Lymphocyte separation.

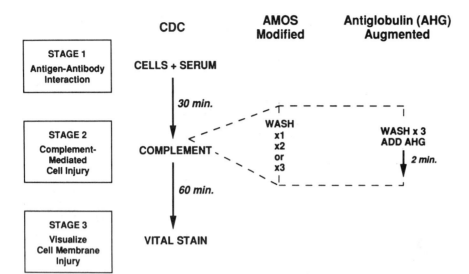

FIGURE 23-11 Complement-dependent microlymphocytotoxicity assay with two variations; three wash amos and antiglobulin.

cytes have been treated with mitomycin C or x-irradiation to inhibit DNA synthesis. The response of the recipient cells to these treated donor cells in the MLR is measured by the incorporation of radioactive thymidine into the responding cells during cell division. If the responding cells have been stimulated, large amounts of labeled thymidine are incorporated into the newly synthesized DNA. This incorporation can be quantitated in a liquid scintillation counting device. Appropriate controls and replicate samples must be tested. The MLR recognizes the antigenic differences on stimulator cells; therefore, it follows that cells bearing the same antigens as the responding cell will cause no stimulation. This indicates that the stimulator and the responder cells have the same HLA-D type.

In order to type for HLA-D antigens, stimulator cells from individuals known to be homozygous for HLA-D series antigens are used. Initially, these homozygous D-typing cells were obtained from HLA-identical children of first-cousin marriages. More recently, similar cells have been found, although infrequently, in the general population. Cells of both types are referred to as homozygous-typing cells (HTC). To perform D typing, homozygous-typing cells of each known phenotype are set up in MLR as stimulators against the test cells. Lack of response in MLR to specific cell types indicates the test cell bears the same antigen as those homozygous-typing cells.

HLA Antibody Detection Techniques

Detection and identification techniques of HLA antibodies are similar to those of RBC antibodies. The unknown serum is tested against a panel of cells of known HLA phenotype. Cells from a large panel of donors must be selected if antibodies to all HLA specificities are to be detected. A panel of at least 30 carefully selected cells is required for initial screening in the determination of panel reactive antibody (PRA), and a panel of at least 60 cells is required for accurate antibody identification. Serum can be screened using

freshly prepared lymphocytes or lymphocytes frozen in bulk or in trays. Lymphocytes frozen in trays have the advantage of rapid preparation, enabling serum to be screened in just a few hours.

The test serum is evaluated by a microlymphocytotoxicity technique. The method depends on the purpose of the screen. When looking for alloantisera to be used as typing reagents, it is essential to screen using the same method that will be used in the typing procedure, the standard CDC being the most common. When screening recipient serum samples, a more sensitive technique—Amos-modified, extended incubation, or antihuman globulin—should be employed. The Amos-modified technique introduces a wash step after the initial serum-cell incubation. The wash step removes anticomplementary activity and aggregated immunoglobulin in the serum, which can activate complement, making it unavailable for binding on the cell membranes. Standard CDC tests rarely detect 100 percent of the antigen-binding specificities of crossreactive antibodies.[45,46] CDC test sensitivity can be greatly enhanced by the addition of an antihuman globulin reagent following serum and cell incubation.[45] The addition of goat antihuman kappa chain increases the likelihood of complement binding and subsequent cell injury, especially in circumstances in which the amount of HLA-antibody binding is below the threshold of detection in the standard technique. The antihuman globulin test functions like a complement-independent technique with respect to HLA alloantibodies. If antibodies to class II molecules (DR and DQ) are to be identified, then separated or labeled B-lymphocyte suspensions of known phenotype must be used.

HLA Crossmatch Techniques

Numerous techniques have been described and applied as crossmatch procedures for transplantation and transfusion. Lymphocytotoxicity is the most widely used technique because the assays are rapid and reproducible and use small volumes of recipient antisera and small numbers of donor cells. The primary purpose of crossmatching before transplantation or transfusion is to identify antibodies in the serum of the potential recipient to antigens present on donor tissues.

To facilitate detection of low levels of antibodies in potential recipients, sensitive techniques must be used, as in recipient serum screens. The correlation between hyperacute rejection and the presence of serum antibody against donor tissue is well established.[16] Cases of irreversible rejection during the first days after transplantation may be due to low levels of antibody undetected by less sensitive techniques.[47,48] Thistlethwaite et al.[49] have observed that T-cell crossmatches performed with an immunofluorescence flow cytometric technique are highly sensitive in detecting donor HLA antibodies in potential allograft recipients, which were undetected by standard serologic techniques (Amos and antihuman globulin). The flow cytometry crossmatch is performed by incubating donor cells with recipient sera followed by a fluoresceinated (FITC) goat antihuman globulin. A phycoerythrin (PE)–labeled antibody to detect either T or B cells is used to discriminate between the two subpopulations of lymphocytes. Cells are analyzed and results expressed as positive or negative based on the shift in fluorescence intensity of the test serum with respect to negative serum (Fig. 23–12). In order to achieve good graft survival rates, centers are investigating more sensitive crossmatch techniques for the detection of donor-specific HLA alloantibodies.

HLA Typing by DNA

HLA class II (-DR, -DQ, -DP) typing is being performed in many laboratories by DNA hybridization techniques.[50] These procedures currently supplement and may well replace serologic typing within the next few years.

Two of the more common techniques used are restriction fragment length polymorphism (RFLP) and oligonucleotide typing (allele specific [ASOP] and sequence specific [SSOP]). Both use the polymerase chain reaction (PCR), an in vitro technique to amplify specific DNA sequences of interest. PCR provides a rapid and sensitive method to identify specific allelic genes when the sequence of the gene is known. Figure 23–13 illustrates a basic strategy for allele-specific oligonucleotide typing.

Direct nucleotide sequencing of HLA genes may be the next step in molecular typing techniques. Since detection is not based on the use of a sequence-specific oligonucleotide probe and prior knowledge of the nucleotide sequences,[51,52] previously undefined alleles could be detected.

Clinical Significance of the HLA System

The identification of HLA antigens was fueled by their potential clinical application to transplantation. The HLA system is still of primary clinical importance in transplantation, but it has recently become of great interest to individuals in the field of human genetics and to investigators of disease associations. HLA antigens are associated with disease susceptibility to a greater extent than any other known genetic marker in humans, and the HLA system has the highest exclusion probability of any single system in resolving cases of disputed paternity.[53]

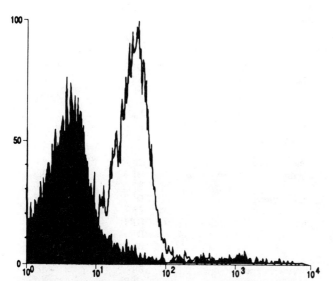

FIGURE 23–12 Flow cytometry histogram illustrating the shift in fluorescence light intensity emitted by a cell population coated with fluorescein-labeled antibody. The vertical ordinate is increasing cell numbers, and the horizontal abscissa represents increasing fluorescence. (From Rodey GE: HLA Beyond Tears. De Novo, Atlanta, 1991, p 56, with permission.)

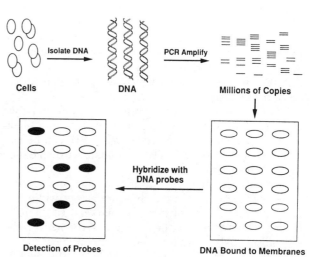

FIGURE 23–13 Strategy for allele-specific oligonucleotide typing.

PATERNITY

HLA polymorphism has provided the genetic tool not previously available to study population migrations and ethnic divergence. With the increase in identifiable HLA markers through standardization of test methods and reagents, courts and attorneys realize that HLA typing is a precise means of resolving cases of disputed paternity. By employing HLA-A and HLA-B locus typing alone, the exclusion rate of falsely accused fathers is as high as 90 percent. In combination with RBC antigen typing or RBC enzymes and serum proteins, exclusion rates as high as 95 percent are achieved. An example of an exclusion follows:

Mother's phenotype	A1,A30;B7,B18
Child's phenotype	A1,A32;B18,B35
Child's maternal haplotype	Al,B18
Child's obligatory paternal haplotype	A32,B35
Excluded putative father's phenotype	A1,A24;B7,B8
Excluded putative father's possible haplotypes	Al,B8/A24,B7 or A1,B7/A24,B8

In this case, the putative father is excluded because his phenotype could not have produced the obligatory haplotype. An example of nonexclusion follows:

Mother's phenotype	A1,A2;B7,B13
Child's phenotype	A1,A11;B7,B27
Child's maternal haplotype	A1,B7
Child's obligatory paternal haplotype	A11,B27
Putative father's phenotype	A2,A11;B13,B27
Putative father's possible haplotypes	A2,B13/A11,B27, or A2,B27/A11,B13

In this case the father cannot be excluded because he could have produced a required haplotype (A11,B27). Inasmuch as A11,B27 is a relatively rare haplotype, the probability that the child and the putative father shared it by chance alone is relatively low —less than 1 percent.

Exclusionary tests are widely accepted and can be either direct or indirect. A direct exclusion, in which the child has a genetic marker absent in both of the parents, is almost absolute evidence of nonpaternity. When the tested man and child are homozygous for different markers in the same system, this constitutes an indirect exclusion.

Confirmation of paternity is more difficult to prove than exclusions. When there is no exclusion, a likelihood of paternity, or paternity index (PI), can be calculated; however, it is only an estimate of the chance that the tested man is the father.

Current advances in chromosomal mapping and molecular genetic typing techniques are providing alternative non-HLA polymorphic markers. In the near future HLA typing may be only one of the many polymorphisms used to detect genetic uniqueness.

DISEASE ASSOCIATION

Recently it has been determined that HLA antigens are associated with disease susceptibility to a greater extent than any other known genetic marker.[54] Many genetic markers have been suspected to be associated with disease, the most extensively studied being blood groups, enzymes, and serum proteins. Data from these studies[55] show weak association of disease and a relative risk of less than 2. Relative risk indicates how many times more frequent the disease is in individuals positive for the marker than in individuals negative for the marker. In contrast, the association between HLA-B27 and ankylosing spondylitis has a relative risk ranging from 60 to 100, depending on the population studied. Although many diseases associated with HLA have a relative risk value greater than 2, none exceed the strength of the association of HLA-B27 with ankylosing spondylitis. To date, 530 diseases have been studied.[54] A list of the most significant HLA and disease associations is given in Table 23-7.

TABLE 23-7 SIGNIFICANT HLA DISEASE ASSOCIATIONS

Disease	HLA	Relative Risk*
Narcolepsy	DR2	129.8
Ankylosing spondylitis	B27	69.1
Reiter's syndrome	B27	37.1
Dermatitis herpetiformis	DR3	17.3
	B8	9.8
Pemphigus vulgaris	DR4	14.6
	A26	4.8
	B38	4.6
Goodpasture's syndrome	DR2	13.8
Celiac disease	DR3	11.6
	DR7	7.7
	B8	7.6
Acute anterior uveitis	B27	8.2
Psorias vulgaris	Cw6	7.5
	B17	5.3
	B13	4.1
	B37	3.9
	DR7	3.2
Idiopathic hemochromatosis	A3	6.7
	B7	2.9
	B14	2.7
Sjögren's syndrome	Dw3	5.7
	B8	3.3
Juvenile rheumatoid arthritis	B27	3.9
	DR5	3.3
Behçet's disease	B5	3.8
Rheumatoid arthritis	DR4	3.8
	B27	2.0
Graves' disease	DR3	3.7
	B8	2.5
Juvenile diabetes mellitus	DR4	3.6
	DR3	3.3
	B8	2.5
	B15	2.1
Myasthenia gravis	B8	3.3
Multiple sclerosis	DR2	2.7
	B7	1.8

*Relative risk of the disease in the white population. Frequencies for other races can be found in Tiwari and Terasaki,[54] p 33.

The exact cause for the association of HLA to disease is unclear. There is no question that genetic factors coded within or near the HLA complex confer susceptibility for a variety of diseases. This susceptibility may somehow be related to altered immunologic responsiveness in many cases. It is also probable that the diseases in question may be a result of both multiple gene interactions and environmental factors. Although the study of HLA and disease associations is very important in understanding disease susceptibility and manifestation, HLA alone is not clinically useful as a diagnostic tool.

PLATELET TRANSFUSION

Bone marrow transplantation and more aggressive use of chemotherapy in the treatment of malignancies have led to a dramatic increase in platelet transfusions in the past decade. HLA class I antigens are expressed variably on platelets.[56-60] Alloimmunization to the HLA antigens results in refractoriness to random donor platelet transfusions. Refractoriness is manifested by the failure to achieve a rise in circulating platelet count 1 hour after infusion of adequate numbers of platelets. The refractory state is often associated with lymphocytotoxic HLA antibodies.

Considering the highly polymorphic nature of the HLA system, it is impossible to obtain sufficient numbers of HLA-typed donors to provide HLA-matched platelets for all alloimmunized patients. Duquesnoy et al.[61] have demonstrated that platelet transfusions from donors mismatched only for cross-reactive antigens can effectively provide hemostasis for refractory patients. For example, an HLA A1,B7;A11,B22 recipient might benefit from the platelets of an A1,B7;A3,B27 donor because A3 and A11 and B27 and B22 are cross-reactive. Table 23–8 lists the major cross-reactive groups and the private specificities associated with each. As a result of these observations, the donor pool necessary to sustain an HLA-matched platelet program can be reduced from 8000 to 10,000 to manageable numbers of 2000 to 5000.

Good platelet survival and HLA matching is not absolute. For example, poor transfusion results are sometimes obtained despite a perfect HLA match. Poor recovery may be a result of sensitization to non-HLA antigens such as platelet-specific antigens. In contrast, excellent transfusion results are sometimes obtained in the presence of complete HLA mismatch. Good recovery may be a function of (1) a restricted pattern of alloimmunization (private versus public antibodies), and (2) variable expression of HLA antigens on the platelet surface.

Leukocytes are more immunogenic than platelets, and refractoriness is probably initiated by HLA antigens on the contaminating leukocytes. Evidence for this is based on a study by Brand et al.,[62] in which they demonstrated a decreased rate of alloimmunization to random donor platelets when contaminating leukocytes were removed before transfusion. Herzig et al.[63] were also able to improve the transfusion response to HLA-matched platelets by removing the leukocytes. This type of approach might be useful for those patients who are unable to produce a response to HLA-matched platelets.

TRANSPLANTATION

Clinical transplant immunology is a difficult field. Unlike animal experimentation, in which studies are performed under controlled conditions in selected inbred strains, transplant immunology deals with actual patients with different medical histories and backgrounds. Individuals working in transplant immunology must determine how best to select recipients and donors, when to increase or to decrease immunosuppressive treatment, and how to precondition potential recipients so that their immune systems will accept a graft. Decisions are based on the relative merits of laboratory findings, which are viewed against complex medical histories. Differences of opinions exist from center to center about the significance of immunologic test results and their considerations in clinical treatment protocols.

Bone Marrow

Bone marrow transplantation is used to treat patients with severe aplastic anemia, immunodeficiency disease, and various forms of leukemia. Since 1980 there has been a change in the proportion of patients treated with bone marrow transplantation for malignant versus nonmalignant diseases.[64] Before 1980, 72 percent of bone marrow transplants were performed for nonmalignant diseases. Since 1980, 77 percent have been performed for malignant diseases.

Pre-1980 bone marrow transplantation was performed only between HLA-identical siblings. This restricted transplantation to 35 to 40 percent of those individuals eligible for transplant. Since then an increasing number of transplants has been performed using family members or unrelated donors who are fully or partially HLA matched with the recipient when no HLA-identical sibling is available. Beatty et

TABLE 23–8   MAJOR CREGs AND THEIR PRIVATE SPECIFICITIES

Major CREG	Associated Private Specificities
A1-CREG	A1, 36, 3, 9(23,34), 10(25,26,34,66), 11, 19(29,30,31,32,33), 28(68,69), 74
A2-CREG	A2, 9(23,24), 28(68,69), B17
B5-CREG	B5(51,52), 15(62,63,75,76,77), 17(57,58), 18, 35, 49, 53, 70(71,72)
B7-CREG	B7, 42, 22(54,55,56), 27, 40(60,61), 13, 41, 47, 48
B8-CREG	B8, 14(64,65), 16(38,39), 18, 55
B12-CREG	B12(44,45), 21(49,50), 13, 40(60,61), 41, 48
4c-CREG	A9(23,24), A25, A32, Bw4
6c-CREG	Bw6, Cw1, Cw3, Cw7

al.[65] recently reported an important application of mismatching for cross-reactive antigens in bone marrow recipients who receive one haplotype-mismatched donor marrow. These investigators observed a significantly lower incidence of graft-versus-host disease (59 percent) in patients receiving donor marrow with compatible class I cross-reactive public antigens compared with patients receiving public antigen-incompatible donor marrow (89 percent). Another study performed by Hows et al.[66] has revealed 58 percent patient survival with unrelated HLA-identical donor transplantation versus 25 percent with related HLA-nonidentical siblings.

The single most important factor for the potential increase of bone marrow transplantation is expanding the donor pool to include both related and unrelated individuals. To meet the needs of patients who do not have a matched, related donor, the US Congress authorized a federal contract in 1986 to establish a national marrow donor registry.

In response to a request for proposal, the National Marrow Donor Program (NMDP) was formed with cosponsorship of the American Association of Blood Banks (AABB), American Red Cross (ARC), and the Council of Community Blood Centers (CCBC). The goals were to recruit a large number of informed HLA-typed volunteers to be listed as potential marrow donors, to combine all available donor HLA data into a centralized registry, and to establish a national coordinating center for facilitating donor searches and communication between donor and transplant centers. As of November 1992, 1428 transplants with unrelated donors were performed and 711,600 donors were HLA-A, -B, -DR, and -DQ phenotyped.

Kidney

Kidney transplantation is used to treat end-stage renal disease (ESRD). Transplantation is preferred over dialysis in treating patients with chronic renal failure because it is more cost effective and it usually returns patients to a state of relatively normal health. The best graft survival rates are obtained when kidneys are obtained from HLA-identical, ABO-compatible siblings, but such donors are available for relatively few patients.[67,68] Three general strategies are employed by transplantation surgeons and immunologists to minimize the graft rejection process: (1) the use of immunosuppressive agents, (2) the reduction of graft "foreignness," and (3) the induction of tolerance.

Immunosuppressive agents such as azathioprine, prednisone, antilymphocyte globulin, and cyclosporin are used to diminish the destructive immunologic responses to the graft. These agents are nonselective and carry risks of serious side effects, especially life-threatening infection.[69]

Extensive efforts are used to minimize graft "foreignness" through matching of donor and recipient antigens. Antigen disparities that most influence graft rejection include the ABO blood group antigens and the HLA antigens. Although it is still not clear what combinations of HLA gene product matching promotes optimal graft survival, it appears that HLA-DR is the most critical for good graft survival.[70-72] In highly sensitized recipients, it is necessary to match for HLA-A and HLA-B owing to the presence of class I HLA antibodies. Sanfilippo et al.[73] have found that matching based on public cross-reactive antigens can provide the same association with graft outcome as private antigens. When matching for highly sensitized recipients, by either private or public antigens, identification of HLA serum antibodies is important. Oldfather et al.[74] have observed that crossmatch results can be predicted in highly sensitized recipients based on careful analysis of serum HLA-antibody specificities.

The third strategy is based on the induction of tolerance to donor-specific antigens. The evidence that transfusion of blood products before transplantation promotes graft acceptance suggests that tolerance induction may be feasible. In 1973, Opelz et al.[75] reported that blood transfusion might promote renal allograft survival in patients receiving kidneys from crossmatch-negative donors. In their retrospective study, graft survival rates at 1 year were significantly improved in patients who had received more than 10 transfusions (66 percent) compared with patients who had received 1 to 10 units (43 percent) or no transfusions (29 percent). Salvatierra et al.[76] applied this observation to the potential benefits of donor-specific blood transfusions and transplants between living related individuals. The effects of blood transfusion on the success of renal transplantation are complex and paradoxic. Transfusion of blood usually leads to HLA alloimmunization, and when this leads to HLA antibody production, it is difficult to find compatible donors. Yet, graft survival rates are improved when pretransplant blood is given to the recipient with no resulting sensitization. Data on the blood transfusion effect were obtained from recipients treated with azathioprine. There is a question as to whether blood transfusion is or will be necessary with therapies using new drugs such as cyclosporine and FK506. Indications are that the transfusion effect will be lost with the newer immunosuppressive agents.

Heart

Heart transplantation is used to treat cardiomyopathies and end-stage ischemic heart disease. Because of the organ's extremely short total ischemic time (3 hours for hearts, compared with 72 hours for kidneys), HLA matching is not feasible. Total ischemic time is the amount of time there is no blood flow through the organ. The single most important HLA test performed pretransplant is the HLA-antibody screen. Recipients with no preformed HLA antibodies are given transplants without crossmatching. Those with preformed HLA antibodies require pretransplant crossmatches to determine recipient-donor compatibility.

In a retrospective study by Yacoub et al.,[77] the effect of class I and II matching on graft survival was observed to be additive. Matching for class II antigens had a marked influence on increased graft survival, whereas matching for class I antigens alone had no influence on the outcome. More data must be analyzed to judge the effect of HLA matching on graft survival. Once conclusive data are found that HLA matching is beneficial to graft outcome, it will be necessary to study methods for increasing the total ischemic time or decreasing the time of test procedures.

Liver

Liver transplantation is now performed with good 1-year graft survival rates (75 percent) owing to the benefits of cyclosporine, the principal immunosuppressive agent. A newcomer drug, FK506, may increase the success of liver transplantation with reported 1-year survivals exceeding 90 percent.[78]

Immunologic factors in recipient-donor matching for liver transplantation and recipient presensitization have largely been ignored in the past. The consequences of HLA presensitization or ABO incompatibility were recently underlined in two reports.[79,80] In the first report, a retrospective analysis of preformed HLA antibodies demonstrated 1-year graft survivals of 40 percent in the presensitized individuals (27) as compared with 83 percent in the nonsensitized individuals. In the second, survival of emergency ABO-incompatible transplants was 30 percent compared with 76 percent in emergency ABO-compatible grafts and 80 percent in elective ABO-compatible grafts.

It is hoped that advances in organ storage will eliminate the need for ABO-incompatible transplantation and increase cold ischemia times allowing for histocompatibility testing, especially for those presensitized patients.

Lung

An overall review of the indications for lung transplantation during the past several years reveals that emphysema and cystic fibrosis account for the majority of double-lung transplants. The major indications for single-lung transplantation include pulmonary fibrosis (33 percent) and emphysema (41 percent). In addition, more patients are now undergoing single-lung transplants for primary hypertension, previously treated by heart-lung transplantation.

Short cold ischemic times for lungs, as with hearts, preclude prospective histocompatibility testing. However, HLA matching between donor and recipient may play an important role in live-donor lung transplantation in an attempt to improve posttransplant conditions and graft survival rates.[81]

Pancreas and Islet Cell

The primary indication for pancreas transplantation is diabetes. The majority of pancreas transplants performed are simultaneous pancreas and kidney transplants (66 percent), with equal numbers of pancreas following kidney (17 percent) and pancreas alone (17 percent).

HLA matching, as reported by two large pancreas transplant centers, has a major effect on graft survival.[82,83] Pirsch et al.[82] reported increased long-term survival rates with HLA-DR matching, significant differences demonstrated between two mismatches and no mismatches. So et al.[83] observed improved graft survivals in all types of pancreas transplants based on the number of HLA mismatches, 80 percent survival with zero to one mismatch versus 44 percent with four to six mismatches.

Due to increased risks of myocardial complications with pancreas transplantation, islet cell transplantation has been actively pursued. Although islet cell transplantation is technically simple, difficulty has been encountered in the achievement of sustained engraftment in humans. Scharp et al[84] reported on their first 9 intraportal islet grafts. The first 6 functioned early, but were all rejected within 2 weeks despite heavy immunosuppression. The last three, transplanted with pooled islet cells, achieved insulin independence ranging from 15 to 184 days. New in vivo systems can now support islet function for greater than 6 months, an important area for continued technologic development.

United Network for Organ Sharing

In an effort to provide a rare commodity, solid organs, equitably, the United Network for Organ Sharing (UNOS) was established in 1986. UNOS received the federal contract to operate the National Organ Procurement and Transplantation Network (OPTN) and develop an equitable scientific and medically sound organ allocation system. The OPTN is charged with developing policies that maximize use of organs donated for transplantation ensuring the quality of care for transplant patients and addressing medical and ethical issues related to organ transplantation in the United States.

Review Questions

1. The HLA genes are located on chromosome number:
   A. 2
   B. 4
   C. 6
   D. 8
   E. 10

2. The majority of HLA antibodies are:
   A. IgA
   B. IgD
   C. IgE

D. IgG

E. IgM

3. The test of choice for HLA antigen testing is:
   A. Agglutination
   B. Inhibition
   C. Cytotoxicity
   D. Fluorescent antibody test
   E. Enzyme-linked immunosorbent assay

4. Of the following diseases, which one has the highest relative risk in association with an HLA antigen?
   A. Ankylosing spondylitis
   B. Dermatitis herpetiformis
   C. Juvenile diabetes
   D. Narcolepsy
   E. Rheumatoid arthritis

5. Why is HLA matching not feasible in heart transplantation?
   A. No HLA antigens are present on cardiac cells.
   B. No donors ever have HLA antibodies.
   C. Total ischemic time is too long.
   D. Total ischemic time is too short.
   E. None of the above

6. DR52 molecules are the product of:
   A. DRA and DRB1
   B. DRA and DRB2
   C. DRA and DRB3
   D. DRA and DRB4
   E. DRA and DRB5

7. In the future, testing of DNA will probably be performed by what technique?
   A. Restriction fragment length polymorphism
   B. Allele-specific oligonucleotide typing
   C. Sequence-specific primer typing
   D. Sequence-specific oligonucleotide typing
   E. Direct nucleotide sequencing

8. The association of the antigens on the two C6 chromosomes as determined by family studies is represented by the:
   A. Haplotype
   B. Genotype
   C. Phenotype
   D. Allotype
   E. Xenotype

Answers to Review Questions

1. C (p 447)
2. D (p 451)
3. C (p 453)
4. A (p 458)
5. D (p 460)
6. C (p 447)
7. E (p 457)
8. B (p 450)

References

1. Dausset, J: Leukoagglutinins. IV. Leukoagglutinins and blood transfusion. Vox Sang 4:190, 1954.
2. Dausset, J: Iso-leuco-anticorps. Acta Haematol 20:156, 1958.
3. Payne, R: The association of febrile transfusion reactions with leukoagglutinins. Vox Sang 2:233, 1957.
4. Terasaki, PI and McClelland, JP: Microdroplet assay of human serum cytotoxins. Nature 204:998, 1964.
5. Terasaki, PI, et al: Microdroplet testing for HLA-A, -B, -C, and -D antigens. Am J Clin Pathol 69:103, 1978.
6. van Rood, JJ and van Leeuwen, A: Leukocyte grouping: A method and its application. J Clin Invest 42:1382, 1963.
7. World Health Organization: Nomenclature for factors of the HL-A system. Bull WHO 39:483, 1968.
8. Dausset, J, et al: Le deuxieme sublocus du systeme HL-A. Nouv Rev Fr Hematol 8:861, 1968.
9. Singal, DP, et al: Serotyping for homo-transplantation. XVII. Preliminary studies of HL-A subunits and alleles. Transplantation 6:904, 1968.
10. Sandberg, L, et al: Evidence for a third sub-locus within the HLA chromosomal region. In Terasake, PI (ed): Histocompatibility Testing 1970. Munksgaard, Copenhagen, 1970, p 165.
11. Bach, FH and Hirshhorn, K: Lymphocyte interaction: A potential histocompatibility test in vitro. Science 143:813, 1964.
12. Bain, B and Lowenstein, L: Genetic studies on the mixed leukocyte reaction. Science 145:1315, 1964.
13. Bach, FH and Amos, DB: Hu-1: Major histocompatibility locus in man. Science 156:1506, 1967.
14. Bodmer, WF, et al (eds): Histocompatibility Testing 1977. Munksgaard, Copenhagen, 1977.
15. Bodmer, JG, et al: Nomenclature for factors of the HLA system. Hum Immunol 34:4, 1992.
16. Kissmeyer-Nielson, F, et al: Hyperacute rejection of kidney allografts associated with preexisting humoral antibodies against donor cells. Lancet 1:662, 1966.
17. Orr, HT, et al: Complete amino acid sequence of a papain-solubilized human histocompatibility antigen, HLA-B7. 2. Sequence determination and search for homologies. Biochemistry 18:5711, 1979.
18. Kaufman, JF and Strominger, JL: Both chains of HLA-DR bind to the membrane with a penultimate hydrophobic region and the heavy chain is phosphorylated at its hydrophilic carboxy terminus. Proc Natl Acad Sci U S A 76:6304, 1979.
19. Kaufman, JF and Strominger, JL: The extracellular region of light chains from human and murine MHC class II antigens consists of two domains. J Immunol 130:808, 1983.
20. Figueroa, F and Klein, J: The evolution of class II genes. Immunol Today 7:78, 1986.
21. Bjorkman, PJ, et al: Structure of the HLA class I histocompatibility antigen, HLA-A2. Nature 329:506, 1987.
22. Bjorkman, PJ, et al: The foreign antigen binding site and T cell recognition regions of class I histocompatibility antigens. Nature 329:512, 1987.
23. Rodey, GE and Fuller, TC: Public epitopes and the antigenic structure of HLA molecules. CRC Crit Rev Immunol 7:229, 1987.
24. Kohler, G and Milstein, C: Derivation of specific antibody producing tissue culture and tumor lines by cell fusion. Eur J Immunol 6:611, 1976.
25. Lee, CC: Population Genetics. University of Chicago Press, Chicago, 1955.
26. Dausset, J, et al: Un nouvel antigene du systeme HL-A (Hu-1), 1' antigene 15 allele possible des antigenes 1, 11, 12. Nouv Rev Fr Hematol 8:398, 1968.
27. Kissmeyer-Nielsen, F, Svejgaard, A, and Hange, M: Genetics of the HL-A transplantation system. Nature 291:1116, 1968.
28. Svejgaard, A and Kissmeyer-Nielsen, F: Crossreactive human HL-A iso-antibodies. Nature 219:868, 1968.

29. Legrand, L and Dausset, J: Histocompatibility Testing 1972. Munksgaard, Copenhagen, 1972, p 441.
30. Rodey, G, et al: ASHI HLA class I public epitope workshop: Phase I report. Transplant Proc 19:872, 1987.
31. Colombani, J, Colombani, M, and Dausset, J: Crossreactions in the HL-A system with special reference to Da 6 crossreacting group. In Terasaki, PI (ed): Histocompatibility Testing 1970. Munksgaard, Copenhagen, 1970, p 79.
32. Legrand, L and Dauset, J: The complexity of the HLA gene product. II. Possible evidence for a "public" determinant common to the first and second HLA series. Transplantation 19:177, 1975.
33. Scalamogne, M, et al: Crossreactivity between the first and second segregant series of the HLA system. Tissue Antigens 7:125, 1976.
34. Kostyu, DD, Cresswell, P, and Amos, DB: A public HLA antigen associated with HLA-A9, Aw32 and Bw4. Immunogenetics 10:433, 1980.
35. Muller, C, et al: Monoclonal antibody (Tu 48) defining alloantigenic class I determinants specific for HLA-Bw4 and HLA-Aw23, -Aw24 as well as -Aw32. Hum Immunol 5:269, 1982.
36. Belvedere, M, Mattiuz, PL, and Curtoni, ES: An antibody crossreacting with LA and FOUR antigens of the HLA system. Immunogenetics 1:538, 1975.
37. McMichael, AJ, et al: A monoclonal antibody that recognizes an antigenic determinant shared by HLA-A2 and B17. Hum Immunol 1:121, 1980.
38. Ahern, AT, et al: HLA-A2 and HLA-B17 antigens share an alloantigenic determinant. Hum Immunol 5:139, 1982.
39. Claas, F, et al: Alloantibodies to an antigenic determinant shared by HLA-A2 and B17. Tissue Antigens 19:388, 1982.
40. Troup, CM and Walford, RL: Cytotoxicity test for the typing of human lymphocytes. Am J Clin Pathol 51:529, 1969.
41. Eisen, SA, Wedner, HJ, and Parker, CW: Isolation of pure human peripheral blood T-lymphocytes using nylon wool columns. Immunol Commun 1:571, 1972.
42. Lowry, R, et al: Improved B cell typing for HLA-DR using nylon wool column enriched B lymphocyte preparations. Tissue Antigens 14:325, 1979.
43. van Rood, JJ, van Leeuwen, A, and Ploem, JS: Simultaneous detection of two cell populations by two-color fluorescence and application to the recognition of B cell determinants. Nature 262:795, 1976.
44. Vartdal, F, et al: HLA class I and II typing using cells positively selected from blood by immunomagnetic isolation—a fast and reliable technique. Tissue Antigens 28:301, 1986.
45. Fuller, TC, et al: Antigenic specificity of antibody reactive in the antiglobulin-augmented lymphocytotoxicity test. Transplantation 34:24, 1982.
46. Fuller, TC and Rodey, GE: Specificity of alloantibodies against antigens of the HLA complex. In Hackel, E and Mallory, D (eds): Theoretical Aspects of HLA: A Technical Workshop. American Association of Blood Banks, Arlington, VA 1982, p 51.
47. Lucas, ZG, et al: Early renal transplant failure associated with subliminal sensitization. Transplantation 10:522, 1970.
48. Patel, R and Briggs, WA: Limitation of the lymphocyte cytotoxicity crossmatch test in recipients of kidney transplants having preformed anti-leukocyte antibodies. N Engl J Med 284:1016, 1971.
49. Thistlethwaite, JR, et al: The T cell immunofluorescence flow cytometric crossmatch: Correlation of results with rejection and graft loss in cadaveric donor renal transplant recipients (abstr). XI Intl Cong Transpl Soc 1:S2.3, 1986.
50. Tiercy, JM, Jannet, M, and Mach, B: A new approach for the analysis of HLA class II polymorphism: HLA oligo typing. Blood Rev 4:9, 1990.
51. Zemmour, J and Parham, P: HLA class I nucleotide sequences. Hum Immunol 31:195, 1991.
52. Marsh, SGE and Bodmer, J: HLA class II nucleotide sequences. Hum Immunol 31:207, 1991.
53. Polesky, HF: New concepts in paternity testing. Diagn Med 1981.
54. Tiwari, JL and Terasaki, PI: HLA and Disease. Springer-Verlag, New York, 1985.
55. Mourant, AE, Kopec, AC, and Domaniewska-Solczak, K: Blood Groups and Diseases. Oxford University Press, New York, 1978.
56. Colombani, J: Blood platelets in HL-A serology. Transplant Proc 3:1078, 1971.
57. Svejgaard, A, Kissmeyer-Nielson, F, and Thorsby, E: HL-A typing of platelets. In Terasaki, PI (ed): Histocompatibility Testing 1970. Munksgaard, Copenhagen, 1970, p 160.
58. Leibert, M and Aster, RH: Expression of HLA-B12 on platelets, on lymphocytes and in serum: A quantitative study. Tissue Antigens 9:199, 1977.
59. Aster, RH, Szatkowski, N, and Liebert, M: Expression of HLA-B12, HLA-B8, W4 and W6 on platelets. Transplant Proc 9:1965, 1977.
60. Duquesnoy, RJ, Testin, J, and Aster, RH: Variable expression of W4 and W6 on platelets: Possible relevance to platelet transfusion therapy of alloimmunized thrombocytopenic patients. Transplant Proc 9:1827, 1977.
61. Duquesnoy, RJ, Filip, DJ, and Rody, GE: Successful transfusion of platelet "mismatched" for HLA antigens to alloimmunized thrombocytopenic patients. Am J Hematol 2:219, 1977.
62. Brand, A, van Leeuwen, A, and Eernisse, JG: Platelet immunology with special regard to platelet transfusion therapy. Excerpta Medica International Congress 415:639, 1978.
63. Herzig, RH, Herzig, GP, and Biell, MI: Correction of poor platelet transfusion responses with leukocyte poor HLA-matched platelet concentrates. Blood 46:743, 1975.
64. Bortin, MM and Rimm, AA: Increasing utilization of bone marrow transplantation. Transplantation 42:229, 1986.
65. Beatty, PG, et al: Correlation between acute graft versus host disease (GVHD) and matching for public class I epitopes in patients receiving one-locus incompatible haploidentical bone marrow transplants (abstr). Hum Immunol 17:150, 1986.
66. Hows, JM, et al: Histocompatible unrelated volunteer donors compared with HLA non-identical family donors for marrow transplantation (abstr). XI Intl Cong Transpl Soc 1:S8.1, 1986.
67. Siegler, HF, et al: Comparisons of mixed leukocyte reactions with skin graft survival in families genotyped for HL-A. Transplant Proc 3:115, 1971.
68. Hamburger, J, et al: The value of present methods used for the selection of organ donors. Transplant Proc 3:260, 1971.
69. Alexander, JW: Impact of transplantation on microbiology and infectious diseases. Transplant Proc 12:593, 1980.
70. Goeken, NE, Thompson, JS, and Corry, RJ: A 2-year trial of prospective HLA-DR matching: Effects on renal allograft survival and rate of transplantation. Transplantation 32:522, 1981.
71. Opelz, G: Effect of HLA matching, blood transfusions, and presensitization in cyclosporine-treated kidney transplant recipients. Transplant Proc 17:2179, 1985.
72. Joysey, VC, Thiru, S, and Evans, DB: Effect of HLA-DR compatibility on kidney transplants treated with cyclosporine A. Transplant Proc 17:2187, 1985.
73. Sanfilippo, F, Vaughn, WK, and Spees, EKL: The effect of HLA-A, -B matching on cadaver renal allograft rejection comparing public and private specificities. Transplantation 38:483, 1984.
74. Oldfather, JW, et al: Prediction of crossmatch outcome in highly sensitized dialysis patients based on the identification of serum HLA antibodies. Transplantation 42:267, 1986.
75. Opelz, G, et al: Effect of blood transfusions on subsequent kidney transplants. Transplant Proc 5:253, 1973.
76. Salvatierra, O Jr, et al: Deliberate donor-specific transfusions prior to living related renal transplantation: A new approach. Ann Surg 192:543, 1980.
77. Yacoub, M, et al: The influence of HLA matching in cardiac allograft recipients receiving CyA and Imuran (abstr). XI Intl Cong Transpl Soc 1:S7.1, 1986.
78. Fung, J, Abu-Elmagd, A, and Jain, A: A randomized trial of primary liver transplantation under immunosuppression with FK506 versus cyclosporine. Transplant Proc 23:2977, 1991.
79. Karuppan, S, Ericzon, BG, and Moller, E: Relevance of a positive crossmatch in liver transplantation. Transplant Int 4:18, 1991.
80. Gugenheim, J, Samuel, D, and Reynes, M: Liver transplantation across ABO blood group barriers. Lancet 336:519, 1990.

81. Shaw, LR, Miller, JD, and Slutsky, AS: Ethics of lung transplantation with live donors. Lancet 338:461, 1991.

82. Pirsch, JD, et al: The effect of donor age, recipient age and HLA match on immunologic graft survival in cadaver renal transplant recipients. Transplantation 53:55, 1992.

83. So, SKS, et al: Matching improves cadaveric pancreas transplant results. Transplant Proc 22:687, 1990.

84. Scharp, DW, Lacy, PE, and Santiago, JE: Results of our first nine intraportal islet allografts in type 1, insulin-dependent diabetic patients. Transplantation 51:76, 1991.

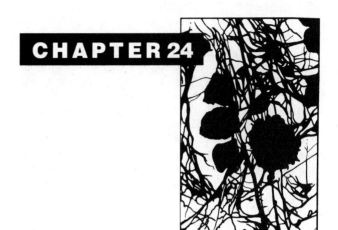

Paternity Testing

Margaret A. Brooks

OBJECTIVES

Upon completion of this chapter, the learner should be able to:

1 State the important reasons for establishing paternity.

2 Discuss the various criteria for determining the suitability of a genetic marker.

3 Define and describe the significance of power of exclusion figures.

4 List the methods of identification, drawing, and transport that comprise the chain of custody that will stand scrutiny in court.

5 Explain the power of HLA testing in determination of paternity.

6 Describe the advantages of DNA testing in determination of paternity.

7 Define a first order exclusion.

8 Describe the situations that comprise a second order exclusion.

9 Relate various phenotypes to the implied genotype for ABO, MNSs, and HLA systems.

10 Calculate a genotype frequency.

Sociolegal Aspects

Our complex society presents many problems requiring the identification of individuals and determination of biologic relationship. Examples include the missing children of Argentina, newborn infants kidnapped from hospital nurseries, children abducted by noncustodial parents or strangers, applicant immigrants and their familial sponsors, participants in surrogate parenting contracts, heirs to disputed estates, and cases of disputed parentage. Paternity cases constitute the majority of investigations. The increasing number of children born out of wedlock has created problems at many levels of society.

The Uniform Parentage Act,[1] which has been adopted by most states, comments in a prefatory note that the concept "substantive legal equality of children regardless of the marital status of their parents" seemed revolutionary if one considered existing state laws on the subject. This act addressed many of the problems associated with illegitimacy. The simple concept of illegitimacy was set aside, and alternate ways of being legitimate were defined.

Beginning in 1968, the status of the illegitimate child was addressed by the Supreme Court.[2] Decisions based on the Equal Protection Clause of the federal Constitution established the principle that a nonmarital child has the same legal rights as a "legitimate" child. Supreme Court decisions have addressed problems on child support, inheritance, custody, birth records, and welfare laws.

In 1975, the federal government enacted Public Law 93-647 Title IV-D, providing for the following.[2]

1. States are to establish plans for child-support enforcement, including establishment of paternity when necessary.
2. An elaborate process is established for the Department of Health, Education and Welfare (HEW) to monitor state's performance and compliance.
3. General incentives are provided for effective performance; conversely, penalties are exacted for decreased support.
4. Absent fathers are traced through Social Security records and other federal bureaus (except the census).
5. Debt of an absent father is assigned to the state for collection.
6. Enforcement by the Internal Revenue Service is used as a last resort.
7. States can save the money collected over and above their Aid to Families of Dependent Children (AFDC) payment.
8. There is legal requirement that mothers must cooperate in ascertaining paternity.

Once paternity has been established, the following happens:[2]

1. Child support should be determined on the same level as the legitimate children in a divorce case.
2. The illegitimate child has some inheritance rights given by a 1977 Supreme Court decision.
3. The father may be awarded custody in some situations.
4. Birth records may be reissued or amended with reference to illegitimate status removed.
5. A nonmarital child may make claims and be compensated as a dependent.

Selecting Test Systems

As the number of paternity cases increases, so has the frequency of genetic testing, using blood group systems to help determine parentage. A blood group system is a set of markers encoded by allelic genes that occupy a locus or a set of closely linked loci on either of a pair of homologous chromosomes. A gene is the basic unit of inheritance that determines the production or nonproduction of specific markers (antigens).

Genetic markers can be defined as recognizable characteristics inherited from parents and controlled by alleles on a pair of chromosomes. Recognizable characteristics can be gross physical qualities such as hair and eye color, or the serologically detectable properties of blood components. Chromosomes are structures located within the cell nucleus that carry genes in a linear order as a part of the DNA molecule. Each egg cell from a mother and each sperm cell from a father (the gametes) carries one chromosome of each pair. When egg and sperm unite, the developing child normally carries 46 chromosomes (i.e., 23 pairs). To be suitable for paternity testing, the genetic markers must follow Mendel's basic rules of inheritance:

1. **Unit inheritance.** The unit of inheritance (gene) is transmitted through generations intact.
2. **Allelic segregation.** A pair of genes (one obtained from each parent and found on separate chromosomes) is never found in the same gamete but is always separate and passes to two different gametes.
3. **Independent assortment.** Different pairs of genes are assorted independently of each other, unless the different genes are closely linked on the same chromosome.

Suitability for genetic study of a marker is determined by:[3]

1. A single and unequivocal pattern of inheritance
2. Accurate classification of different phenotypes by reliable techniques
3. Relatively high frequency of each of the common alleles
4. Reliability of markers (i.e., absence of effect of age, environmental factors, interaction with other genes, or other variables in the expression of the trait)

From a laboratorian point of view, other considerations could be simplicity of test procedures and the number of cases that a technologist can efficiently and accurately process at one time.

When choosing which genetic markers to include in a routine testing format, it is necessary to be selective. The cost of testing for all available genetic markers would be prohibitive. Some reagents (antisera used in test procedures) are extremely rare and can be obtained only for selected studies. One criterion to examine is the usefulness or "power" of a system to exclude. The power of exclusion (PE) depends on several factors (e.g., the number of possible alleles per locus, the number of loci in a haplotype, and the frequency with which those alleles occur in the population).

The PE can be calculated for each test system by:

1. Listing phenotypes of all possible trios (mother, child, possible father) that will result in an exclusion of the alleged father
2. Calculating the frequencies of these possible matings, assuming random matings, using genotype and phenotype frequency charts for a given racial group
3. Combining the results for all possible trios in a system
4. Combining the results for all systems used

The greater the power of the combined test systems, the less likely that a falsely accused man will remain unexcluded by the tests. This is referred to as prior probability of exclusion (PPE).[4]

Laboratories have been performing blood tests for cases of disputed parentage for more than 45 years. The earlier efforts in paternity testing included only the analysis of the red blood cell (RBC) systems ABO, MN, and Rh. The PPE using these systems is about 50 percent, and they were considered informative by the courts only when the putative father was excluded.

Technology has expanded the usefulness of the original systems and added other systems as more knowledge and reagents have become available. In 1976, the American Medical Association (AMA) and the American Bar Association (ABA) published a joint report[5] listing more than 60 blood group systems suitable for use in paternity testing. These systems include RBC antigens, RBC enzymes, serum proteins, and HLA. The development of HLA testing in the early 1970s was a highly significant advance. HLA testing is a very powerful tool in parentage determination and has enabled laboratories to respond to the request for the ascertainment of paternity. RBC enzymes and serum proteins, used for many years in European countries, have been added to test batteries in this country using conventional electrophoresis, isofocusing methods, or both. DNA testing, not available in 1976, is replacing conventional methods and becoming a regular member of test batteries. Table 24–1 lists typical PE figures for the most commonly used systems.

The results of these calculations may differ from study to study because of variation in the number of alleles considered for the system and because genotype and phenotype frequencies vary for the population group or geographic area.

Phlebotomy of Blood Samples

Paternity cases are generally referred to the laboratory by the county court system or agencies for the court. Often cases will not be resolved until a trial is held and a judge or jury renders a decision based on evidence presented by prosecutors and defense attorneys. Generally, when a trial occurs considerable time has elapsed between drawing and testing of samples. It

TABLE 24–1 **PE OF THE MOST COMMONLY USED SYSTEMS**

System	DYKES[13]		AMA-ABA[5]	
	Whites	Blacks	Whites	Blacks
ABO	0.17	0.20	0.1342	0.1174
MNSs	0.31	0.15	0.3095	0.3206
Rh	0.22	0.20	0.2746	0.1859
Duffy	0.18	0.14	0.1844	0.0420
Kidd	0.19	0.16	0.1869	0.1545
Kell	0.04	0.01	0.0354	0.0049
HLA	0.87	0.87	—	—
GC	0.16	0.11	0.1661	0.0731
Tf (IEF)	0.18	0.11	0.0064	0.0410
GM	0.21	0.19	0.2275	0.2071
AcP	0.22	0.17	0.2323	0.1588
PGM	0.15	0.14	0.1457	0.1344
EsD	0.09	0.07	0.0913	

DNA Probes	Whites	Blacks
YNH24	0.903	0.925
TBQ7	0.925	0.937

AcP = acid phosphatase; EsD = esterase D; GC = group specific component; GM = globulin marker; PGM = phosphoglucomutase; Tf(IEF) = transferrin.

is essential to have documentation to verify what occurred at the time of collection and analysis. The laboratory must take precautions to ensure the identity of persons and samples and must be able to assure the courts that unauthorized persons cannot have access to sample tubes or test results. A description of these measures constitutes documentation of a chain of custody.

Parentage testing laboratories may provide service to local agencies or to agencies in other sections of the country. With overnight delivery services routinely available, distance is not a deterrent to providing service. Whether drawn in the laboratory's home office or on the other side of the country, the laboratory must take responsibility for the entire procedure. Samples may be drawn directly from the involved individuals (i.e., mother, child, alleged father) at the same time and at the same place, or they may be drawn from each individual at different times in different places. Establishing an adequate chain of custody is accomplished by adopting suitable procedures for use by laboratory staff in house or by subcontracted laboratories or phlebotomists in remote areas, so that the audit trail is unbroken. The documentation of identification, drawing, and transport must be complete from the point of origin and the chain of custody picked up at the test site in a manner that will stand scrutiny in court.

Drawing procedures begin with positive identification of the parties to be tested. It may be desirable to consider use of more than one method of identification, such as those enumerated here:

1. Confrontation by all parties present at the same time to identify each other (precautions may be necessary, however, if the parties are hostile)
2. Identification sheets to record name, address, birthday, race, transfusion history, personal identification (driver's license, employment identification, social security numbers), and patient signature
3. Information taken during interview may be checked against information provided by the referring agency
4. Taking of individual or group (involved trio) photographs
5. Taking fingerprints of adults and heel prints of infants

Documentation begins with the foregoing identification procedures and continues (audit trail) with phlebotomy of samples. When drawing samples for parentage testing, the tubes used should be clearly labeled with the following information:

1. Name of laboratory
2. Date of sample drawing
3. Patient's name
4. Patient's initials
5. Phlebotomist's initials
6. Case designation

Case designation is often not included but becomes important if several cases are under study at the same time. It is possible for two persons in two different cases to have the same name. Case designation, which is the last name of each party (e.g., Smith versus Jones), will help ensure the correct alleged partners are grouped together. Labels should be correctly prepared and placed on the tubes before blood is drawn. After drawing, the patient should be asked to verify and initial the tube label. The phlebotomist should also check and initial tubes after drawing to verify that labels have been checked and attached correctly. It may be helpful if the mother's, alleged father's, and child's labels are color coded to provide for spot identification.

Written notations (documentation) concerning the following items should be made immediately upon receipt of samples:

1. **Delivery.** Was a common carrier, US Post Office, or delivery service used; or was sample picked up by laboratory personnel at an airport, bus station, and so forth? Record signature of person receiving samples, shipping numbers, date, time, and how the shipping container was sealed.
2. **Opening the shipping container.** Record initials of person opening the container, date, time, condition of samples, and whether tubes were correctly sealed and labeled.

Adopting procedures such as those outlined here as standard operating procedures should ensure the integrity of blood samples drawn for parentage testing.

Technology

The ABO blood group system was discovered in 1901, the MNSs system in 1927. The Rh system has been in use since the 1940s; and the Kell, Duffy, and Kidd systems have been defined in the last 40 years. The serologic technology required to demonstrate the presence of RBC antigens is, therefore, quite familiar to medical technologists, particularly those in blood banking in which the ABO and Rh types of patients requiring blood transfusions must always be determined. If a patient presents no crossmatch problems, these are usually the only blood groups studied. When problems are encountered other antigens in the Rh system or in the MNSs, Kell, Duffy, Kidd, and a host of other blood group systems may be evaluated. Suitable testing reagents, knowledge of appropriate test procedures, and knowledge of expected patterns of reaction for each of these systems are required to enable blood bankers to transfuse "problem patients" safely. The antigen testing in parentage studies is similar to that in blood bank procedures.

Human leukocyte antigen (HLA) was discovered by Dausset and Ivanyi in 1954. Although each of the RBC systems is defined by differing numbers of antigens, none demonstrates the polymorphism (great number of alleles) of the HLA system. The technology developed rapidly once it became apparent that HLA antigens were to play an important role in the transplantation of solid organs and the transfusion of blood components. HLA antigens are present on most body tissues other than red cells and trophoblasts.

Electrophoresis is the technology employed to demonstrate the presence of allelic variants of RBC enzymes and serum proteins. It is the movement of charged particles through some medium (e.g., paper, starch, agar) under the influence of an applied electric field.

DNA is the molecular basis of inheritance. The sequence of the four DNA bases (units) encodes the instructions (genes) by which most large molecules of the body are constructed. DNA is a major constituent of chromosomes. Molecular biologists, by applying the methods of quantitation and reductionism from physics, created the tools by which inheritance could be studied at the molecular level. Ham Smith made a significant contribution in 1972 while studying enzymes that break down DNA in bacteria. Mr. Smith identified an extract that could cut DNA, creating the same fragments every time from the same purified piece of DNA. Progress was made again in 1975, when E.M. Southern demonstrated a method that allowed DNA that had been cut and separated by size in an agarose gel to be bound to a membrane by blotting the buffer out of the gel through the membrane.[6]

The American Association of Blood Banks (AABB) has established standards that must be observed in test procedures and has accredited laboratories to perform testing using the different technologies.[7] Standards require duplicate testing for RBC and HLA antigens and independent reading of electrophoresis results by two technologists. When standards are followed, reliability of test results is usually ensured. Standards have also been formulated for DNA testing using single-locus probes.

Present laboratory procedures for RBC antigens require presenting the test RBCs to a specific antibody (reagent) under optimal conditions for the reaction of the antigen indicated by the known antibody. The absence or presence of the antigen is decided according to the absence (negative reaction) or the presence (positive reaction) of agglutination (clumping). It is possible to determine whether a reaction has occurred by examination of the antigen antibody mixture in the test tube over a magnifying mirror. In some instances, it is desirable to confirm a negative reaction by examining the mixture microscopically.

Red blood cell reagents are available from commercial manufacturers regulated by the Food and Drug Administration (FDA). These companies, of their own accord, use various quality control measures and claim to be even more stringent than the FDA in ensuring antisera of specificity, avidity, and titer, as well as freedom from interference and contamination. Even though AABB standards do not require reagents to be

licensed, it can be helpful as a quality control measure to use commercial products.

The HLA serologic test procedures designate the lymphocyte as the test cell of choice. Present technology requires the harvesting of T lymphocytes and the presenting of these cells to a panel of test sera containing reagent antibody specific for antigens of the HLA system. Testing is performed using a microtiter tray and microliters of test sera. Cells and sera are added to the wells of the trays in measured amounts using a microtiter syringe and capillary pipettes modified to deliver very small, uniform drops of reagents.

The antibody-antigen mixture is maintained at conditions expected to enhance the reaction. If any antibody-antigen reaction occurs, the addition of complement will result in loss of cell membrane integrity. The cytotoxic effect is detected by the use of a vital stain (e.g., trypan blue or eosin). Positive reactions are indicated by stained cells. In the absence of an antibody-antigen complex, the cell wall remains intact and the living cell excludes the dye. The cell remains clear and glistening; absence of staining represents a negative reaction (**see Color Plate 18**).

If RBC and HLA technology are compared, few similarities are found in equipment, procedures, or test results. However, the principles of the testing for paternity rely on the same basic principles of using known antibody to detect the presence of an antigen (genetic marker) on the test cell followed by the application of genetic rules and logic.

Electrophoresis, as previously stated, is used to demonstrate the presence of allelic variants of RBC enzymes and serum proteins. Isoelectric focusing, a related technology, is electrophoresis of proteins in semisolid medium containing ampholytes (artificially manufactured peptides of known size and charge). The ampholytes are prefocused (electrophoresed) to set up a gradient of acidity in the semisolid medium (pH gradient).

Subsequent electrophoresis of an individual's protein mixture (serum or RBC contents) is then carried out. An antigen, moving through a limited pH gradient, reaches its isoelectric point (the pH at which the protein is not charged) and is immobilized. Overlaying the medium with antibody allows for detection of the protein. Fixed antigen-antibody complex can be stained. If the antigen is an enzyme (a protein catalyst), it can be overlaid with specific substrate, incubated, and visualized by production of colored or fluorescent product.

Testing of DNA isolated from peripheral white cells now makes it possible to look directly at variations in the nucleic acid sequence at various genetic loci in order to visualize genetically inherited differences among individuals.

DNA testing is accomplished by the following:

1. Isolate DNA from human samples.
2. Fragment the purified DNA with a restriction enzyme.

3. Electrophorese DNA through an agarose gel to separate fragments based on length (shorter fragments travel farther through gel).
4. Transfer DNA from gel onto membrane (Southern blot).[6]
5. Label cloned (copied) human DNA fragment homologous to the genomic region of interest.
6. Hybridize labeled DNA (probe) to transferred DNA (blot).
7. Generate image of banding pattern.

Interpretation of Test Results

Once accurate test results are compiled, the next step is to determine whether an exclusion of the alleged father has occurred.[8] Exclusions are characterized as first-order (direct) or second-order (indirect). It may be readily apparent after inspection of test results that a contradiction to the expected pattern of inheritance has occurred. If the child's blood type exhibits an antigen lacking in both parents, a first-order exclusion is demonstrated. If neither parent can contribute one of the two allelic genes that appear in the child's phenotype, it must be assumed that a child of the given phenotype could not result from a mating of the adults tested.

Inasmuch as maternity is not in question, in first-order exclusion nonpaternity is assumed. With proper testing procedures, it is rare that a first-order exclusion can be false, and for many years one first-order exclusion has been considered sufficient for a determination of nonpaternity. Although the possibility of mutation is rare, in recent years it has become the practice of most laboratories to require two exclusions.

Second-order exclusions can be explained in one of the three ways:[9]

1. The child is negative for two different allelic antigens, both of which are present in the alleged father. For example:

Alleged father AB Probable genotype *A/B*
Child O Probable genotype *O/O*

A/B genotype indicated the A antigen from one parent and the B antigen from the other. One antigen or the other must be present in offspring. Group O type indicates the absence of both A and B antigens.

2. The child appears homozygous for an antigen demonstrated in the mother but not present in the alleged father. For example:

Alleged father N Probable genotype *N/N*
Mother M Probable genotype *M/M*
Child M Probable genotype *M/M*

3. The alleged father appears homozygous for an antigen not present in the child:

Alleged father CCDe Probable
genotype *CDe/CDe*

Mother ccdee Probable
genotype *cde/cde*
Child ccdee Probable
genotype *cde/cde*

The second and third explanations can be used interchangeably, with the choice depending on traditional use and clarity of expression. The weakness of second-order, or indirect, exclusions is that it is necessary to assume that phenotype denotes genotype. This is not always a correct assumption. Low-frequency alleles, unidentified alleles, and amorphs are found in most blood group systems. Recombination of DNA and interference by events at other loci also can be problematic.

PHENOTYPE INTERPRETATION

Problems may be encountered when making the assumption that a given phenotype represents a specific genotype. For example, before it can be ensured that the following test results indicate a homozygous genotype, it is necessary to test for the low-frequency allele Mg.

Test Sera	M	N	Possible Genotype
Alleged father	−	+	*N/N*
Child	+	−	*M/M*

If Mg testing is included:

Test Sera	M	N	Mg	Possible Genotype
Alleged father	−	+	+	*N/Mg*
Child	+	−	+	*M/Mg*

Not only would it be incorrect to conclude that there is an exclusion, but if calculations for probability of paternity were made, with Mg as the paternal obligatory gene (necessary from the biologic father), the results would undoubtedly be in the "practically proven" category. If Mg typings are negative, it is still not appropriate to base a conclusion of nonpaternity on this system alone, because of the possibility of other, even less-frequent, alleles or amorphs. In black patients, it is not appropriate to make assumptions that S + s − or S − s + phenotypes represent homozygous genotypes of S/S or s/s. The amorph Su (frequency of 0.11) must be considered (i.e., S/su or s/Su).

In the Rh system the most common "low-frequency" allele to consider is Cw. Whenever test results of C + c − suggest the genotype *C/C*, Cw typings are indicated. This system has many possible complications. The pitfalls and cases cited are only a few examples of the many complications and problems encountered when test results are interpreted. It may be necessary to employ other technology, such as adsorption and elution, in order to confirm the presence of a weakened or suppressed antigen and to do titrations for additional evidence of dosage. Although these techniques may resolve some situations, others may require use of additional test systems. In order to guard against false exclusions, it is desirable to demonstrate two second-order exclusions before concluding nonpaternity. (The probability that two such exclusions occur simultaneously is very low.)

MULTIPLE FAMILY MEMBERS

Not all cases consist of three people (i.e., mother, father, and child). Some cases may involve more than one child. When this occurs, additional information may be available for determining genotypes and must be used to interpret results. Consider the following:

Case	Major Blood Group	Possible Genotype
Mother	O	0/0
Alleged father	A1	A1/O,A1/A1,A1/A2
Child 1	O	0/0
Mother	O	0/0
Alleged father	A1	A1/O,A1/A1,A1/A2
Child 2	A1	A1/O
Mother	O	0/0
Alleged father	A1	A1/O,A1/A1,A1/A2
Child 3	A2	A2/O

In each individual case no exclusion would be indicated; however, if all three children were tested as a family group, we would see the following:

	Major Blood Group	Possible Genotype
Mother	O	0/0
Alleged father	A1	
Child 1	O	0/0
Child 2	A1	A1/O
Child 3	A2	A2/O

The three phenotypes of the children could not result from the union of a mother of group O and a father of group A1. The genotypes of a man who types A1 may be A1/O, and he could be the father of child 1 and child 2 but not of child 3. If his genotype is A1/A2, he could father child 2 and child 3, but not child 1. Only additional systems or family studies would help determine paternity for the three children.

LINKAGE

Linkage in some test systems must be taken into consideration. Consider a case study of dizygotic twins in which the MNSs system phenotypes are as follows:

Mother	MNSs
Alleged father	Ns
Twin A	Ns
Twin B	NSs

If each twin is considered individually or if only phenotypes are considered, an exclusion is not apparent. Because the genotype of twin A is most likely Ns/Ns, it can be determined that the mother's genotype is MS/Ns. This child must receive Ns from each of the parents. Twin B's genotype is NS/Ns. The mother and twin B have only Ns in common. The discernible Ns/Ns genotype of the alleged father could not produce an NS child. Because both children were tested at the same time and genotypes of the mother could be determined, it is possible to know how the MN and Ss antigens are linked. Therefore, it is possible to exclude the alleged father as the biologic father of twin B. An additional exclusion in the HLA system confirmed this finding.

The HLA system involves linked loci too, but interpretation presents other considerations. Paternity exclusion cannot be ascertained if two HLA alleles that are believed to be coupled on the same chromosome appear to have segregated. This is because recombination may have occurred during meiosis. (A rare crossing over between the closely linked HLA-A and HLA-B locus alleles can separate them during gametogenesis.)

	Phenotypes	Possible Genotypes
Mother	A01,A29,B12,B37	A01,B12/A29,B37
Alleged father	A02,A03,B18,B22	A02,B18/A03,B22
		A02,B22/A03,B18
Child 1	A01,A02,B12,B18	A01,B12/A02,B18
Child 2	A02,A29,B22,B37	A29,B37/A02,B22

A phenotype of HLA-A02,A03,B18,B22 is consistent with paternity if crossing over occurred.

PROBABILITY

To calculate probability of paternity it is necessary to know the races of the persons in the nonexcluded paternity case and to have the phenotype frequencies for the racial group or groups to which they belong. If phenotype frequencies are available, it is possible to calculate gene frequencies. Gene frequencies may be determined by a direct count if the system has codominant alleles (i.e., no amorphs or recessive genes). Because amorphs exist in all blood group systems and are not always rare, it is usually more appropriate to use a method based on the Hardy-Weinberg principle assuming random mating (selection of mates is independent of blood types and therefore is random). The genetic markers passed by parents to an offspring are also random. This method assumes that in a two-allele system with gene frequencies of p and q, $(p + q)2 = 1$. By squaring both sides of the equation, it can be expanded to $p2 + 2pq + q2$, where $p2$ or $q2$ would represent individuals homozygous for the gene represented by p or q; $2pq$ would stand for the heterozygotes. The same principle may be used to accommodate systems with more than two alleles and is one of the most useful tools in population genetics. Gene-frequency charts are available, and if the phenotype frequency of a given group agrees with the phenotype frequency the gene frequencies were derived from, it is appropriate to use those charts.

The attempt to determine paternity begins with the assumption that the mother is the biologic mother of the child. Consequently, the child's phenotype is, in part, the result of the mother's genetic makeup. For example, if the mother's phenotype is MNS and the child's type is MSs, the list of possible genotypes would be as follows:

	Mother	Child
Phenotype	MNS	MSs
Genotypes	MS/NS	MS/Ms
	MS/Nu	
	Mu/NS	
Genes	MS,NS,Mu,Nu	MS,Ms

The biologic mother is obliged to pass one of the genes in her genotype to her child; it is referred to as the maternal obligatory gene (MOG). As a result, any maternal genotype not bearing a possible MOG can be dropped from consideration. In the foregoing example, the only gene mother and child have in common is MS; therefore, the mother's genotype is either MS/NS or MS/Nu, not Mu/NS. The identification of possible MOGs enables the determination of possible paternal obligatory genes (POGs). To this end, listings of the child's possible genotypes in MOG/POG ordered combinations must be constructed:

	Phenotype	Genotype	
		MOG	POG
Child	MSs	MS	Ms

Note that any accused man whose phenotype could not represent, in part, one of the possible POGs can be excluded from paternity. In the example, the biologic father must be able to pass the Ms gene.

In the event the alleged father cannot be excluded, two probabilities are of interest: (1) the probability that the child resulted from the mating of the mother and alleged father, and (2) the probability that the child resulted from the mating of the mother and a random man.

The probability that a child was the result of the mating of the mother and alleged father is the summation of the probabilities that the following two events occurred simultaneously: (1) the mother passed the MOG to her child, and (2) the alleged father passed the POG to his child. Owing to the independence of the two events, the probability of their simultaneous occurrence is the probability that the mother passed the MOG times the probability that the alleged father passed the POG. Furthermore, the probability that either event occurred is the relative frequency of its occurrence in the set of genotypes that express the mother's and alleged father's phenotypes, respectively. Consequently, the probability of the simultaneous occurrence of MOGs and POGs is the product of the frequencies with which the mother would pass the MOG to her child, and the frequency with which the alleged father would pass the POG to his child.

Given a set of genotypes, the frequency with which a particular gene will be passed to an offspring depends on the following elements: (1) genotype frequency, (2) relative genotype frequency of all genotypes belonging to the set, and (3) the probability that the particular gene will be passed from the genotype. The first ele-

ment, the genotype frequency, is the probability with which the two genes occur simultaneously times the number of ways the genotype could occur. Because the genes were inherited independently, this product is simply the product of the two gene frequencies times the number of ways the genotype could occur. Recall from our example that the mother's genotype is either MS/NS or MS/Nu. Given the gene frequencies listed here, genotype frequencies are computed as follows:

Gene Frequencies	Genotype Frequencies
MS: 0.2578	MS/NS: 2(0.2578)(0.0628) = 0.0324
NS: 0.0628	MS/Nu: 2(0.2578)(0.0004) = 0.0002
Nu: 0.0004	TOTAL 0.0326

The second element or the relative genotype frequency indicates the frequency with which the genotype occurs in the set of genotypes. It is easily computed by dividing the genotype frequency by the sum of the genotype frequencies:

Genotypes	Relative Genotype Frequencies
MS/NS	0.0324/0.0326 = 0.9939
MS/Nu	0.0002/0.0326 = 0.0061
	TOTAL 1.0000

Finally, the probability with which a particular gene is passed from a genotype depends on whether the genotype is heterozygous or homozygous. In the event of homozygosity, the gene appearing in the genotype will be passed 100 percent of the time. On the other hand, in the heterozygous state, each gene of the genotype has a 50 percent chance of being transmitted. Consequently, the frequency with which a gene is passed from a set of genotypes is the sum of the products of the probability that a particular gene will be passed from the genotype and the relative genotype frequency. Continuing with the example, the frequency with which the mother will pass the MS, NS, or Nu gene to her child is computed as follows:

MOG	Frequency
NS	0.5(0.9939) + 0.5(0.0061) = 0.5000
NS	0.5(0.9939) = 0.4970
Nu	0.5(0.0061) = 0.0030
	TOTAL 1.0000

The frequency with which the alleged father will pass the POGs is computed in a similar fashion; however, in this case the alleged father is not assumed to be the biologic father of the child. Consequently, all genotypes indicating the alleged father's phenotype must be considered.

Suppose the alleged father's phenotype is MNSs and the gene frequencies are MS = 0.2578; NS = 0.0628; Ms = 0.2907; Ns = 0.3877. Then:

Phenotype	Genotype Frequencies
MNSs	MS/Ns: 2(0.2578)(0.3877) = 0.1999
	Ms/NS: 2(0.2907)(0.0628) = 0.0365
	TOTAL 0.2364

Phenotype		Relative Genotype Frequencies
MS/Ns:		0.1999/0.2364 = 0.8456
Ms/NS:		0.0365/0.2364 = 0.1544

	Gene	Frequency
	MS	0.5(0.8456) = 0.4228
	NS	0.5(0.1544) = 0.0772
	Ms	0.5(0.1544) = 0.0772
	Ns	0.5(0.8456) = 0.4228

Recall that the probability that the child has resulted from the mating of the mother and alleged father is the sum of the products of the frequency with which the mother passed the MOG and that with which the alleged father passed the POG. The resulting number is referred to as X.

Child

MOG	POG	
MS	Ms	(0.5) (0.0772) = 0.0386 (X = 0.0386)

In a similar fashion, the probability that a child was the result of the mating of a mother and a random man can be computed. Once again it is the summation, over all possible genotypes, of the probability that the following pairs of events occurred simultaneously: (1) the mother passed the MOG to her child; and (2) a random man passed the POG to his child. The two events are independent; therefore, the probability of their simultaneous occurrence is the probability that the mother passed the MOG times the probability that a random man passed the POG. Furthermore, the probability that the mother passed a possible MOG is its relative frequency of occurrence in her set of possible genotypes, whereas the probability that a random man passed the POG is simply the frequency with which the gene is found in the population. As a result, the probability of the simultaneous occurrence of MOG and POG is the product of the frequency with which the mother passed the MOG and the gene frequency of the corresponding POG. The resulting probability is referred to as gene frequency of the corresponding POG. The resulting probability is referred to as Y. Recall that the gene frequency of *MS* is 0.2578.

Child

MOG	POG	
MS	Ms	(0.5) (0.2578) − 0.1289 (Y = 0.1289)

The foregoing logic is used to calculate X and Y values for each blood group system, and the final results must be combined. Recall that the systems appropriate for use in paternity testing adhere to Mendel's rules of inheritance. If each system is inherited independently of the other systems tested, the probability with which a specific set of phenotypes results from the mating of a mother and an alleged father or a mother and a random man is the product of the corresponding probabilities for each system. In other words, the probability that the mother and alleged father pro-

duced the child is the product of all X values, and the probability that the mother and a random man produced the child is the product of all Y values.

The final step is to calculate the two values that are of primary interest. The first is the paternity index or the genetic odds in favor of paternity, which is calculated by dividing the cumulative X by the cumulative Y. The paternity index represents the odds that a mating of the mother and alleged father would result in a child of the given phenotype as compared with the same event occurring through a mating of the mother and a random man. The second value is the relative probability of paternity. The relative probability of paternity is the probability stated as a percent value. It is calculated using the equation X\X + Y or X(pr)/X(pr) + Y(pr), where pr stands for prior probability, which is inherent in the equation. The prior probability allows the nongenetic information in the case or the prior experience of the laboratory or of a judge to be integrated with the blood test results. Most laboratories use a prior probability of 0.5 for one side of the equation, which then means that 1 minus 0.05 is used on the other side of the equation. This gives equal weight to the mother's contention that the alleged father is the father of the child and to the alleged father's contention that he is not the father, but that the true father is someone else (a random man).

Figure 24–1 presents a paternity testing flow diagram.

REPORTING

The reporting of test results should be undertaken only by knowledgeable and experienced workers with a clear understanding of the scientific content as well as the emotional and social consequences of their report. The care given in analyzing the test results of a parentage study should be the same as in any other medical report. One should recognize that these test results can be just as consequential for the involved parties.

When testing includes only conventional testing, approximately 30 percent of cases are resolved by exclusion. In the remaining 70 percent of cases, the calculated probabilities can be categorized as follows:[10,11]

Probability Category	Percent Cases Not Excluded (%)
99.75–99.99	30.9
99.00–99.74	28.7
95.00–98.99	27.8
90.00–94.99	6.0
80.00–89.99	2.6
70.00–79.99	0.9
50.00–69.00	0.7
25.00–49.99	0.8
10.00–24.99	1.6

It is expected that probabilities will be high when the genetic profile of the biologic father is clear and definitive. This is possible when there are specific obliga-

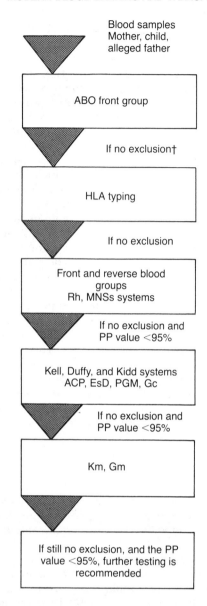

Blood samples
Mother, child,
alleged father

ABO front group

If no exclusion†

HLA typing

If no exclusion

Front and reverse blood
groups
Rh, MNSs systems

If no exclusion and
PP value <95%

Kell, Duffy, and Kidd systems
ACP, EsD, PGM, Gc

If no exclusion and
PP value <95%

Km, Gm

If still no exclusion, and the PP
value <95%, further testing is
recommended

ACP = acid phosphatase	PGM = phosphoglucomutase
EsD = esterase D	Gc = group-specific component

†When one primary or two secondary exclusions are found,
 no further testing is necessary

PP = Plausibility of Paternity

FIGURE 24-1 Paternity testing flowchart. (Adapted from the laboratory's role in a case of disputed paternity. Medical Laboratory Products, 1986.)

tory genes for all or most of the systems studied and when the obligatory genes or combination of obligatory genes are not commonly found in the random population. Low probabilities usually result when the following situations occur:

1. Obligatory genes are not rare (i.e., occur often in the random population).

2. Multiple obligatory genes exist for some or most of the systems tested.
3. Mother or alleged father, or both, have a phenotype that would rarely represent a genotype compatible with paternity.

The use of additional markers may allow for an unqualified statement of exclusion or may produce additional information that will result in an informative probability. Probability statements are often accompanied by verbal predicates,[12] values expressed as subjective statements that describe how likely it is that the alleged father is the biologic father (Table 24-2).

Because of the medicolegal importance of the data involved in parentage testing, a laboratory should follow a strict protocol for written reports. Guidelines on content and format of reports have been established by accreditation groups such as the AABB Parentage Testing Committee.[7] Based on the test data, a written report of findings and conclusions should be sufficiently detailed to minimize questions concerning its content. Reports of parentage testing should contain the following items:

1. Identification of numbers: court case number, laboratory number, etc.
2. Reference to the individuals tested
3. Relative dates: when samples were drawn and testing performed
4. Racial information used in interpretation and calculations
5. Summary of phenotypes: results of all systems tested
6. Interpretation of results
   a. Exclusionary: listing of reasons
   b. Inclusionary: listing of paternity index and probability
7. Definition of terms

The agencies receiving written reports of parentage testing results may use them to resolve excluded cases, in counseling the involved parties, or in negotiating out-of-court settlements. Many hours of court time and thousands of tax dollars can be saved, and justice may be better served in such settlements.

Approximately 1 percent of disputed parentage cases using blood tests require a trial. When this happens, the child may already be 2 or 3 years old. The legal scenario often runs as follows: The mother will

TABLE 24-2 PROBABILITY STATEMENTS

PI	Percentage	Chance of Paternity
>399	99.8-99.9	Practically proven
>99	99.1-99.8	Extremely likely
>19	95-99	Very likely
>9	90-95	Likely
>4	80-90	Hint
>2.3	70-80	Merely suggestive
>1.2	50-70	On the positive side
>1	<50.0	On the negative side

testify she gave birth to the child on a specific date. She will try to determine the date of conception and verify that a relationship existed between her and the alleged father at that critical time. Witnesses may be called to confirm whether and when the relationship existed. The alleged father may testify that there never was a relationship or that it did not exist at the critical time. Events that can verify happenings during the critical period become important. Because it is not customary to keep records to document romantic relationships, it is often difficult to establish the true course of events.

The attitude of the legal community regarding the use of blood tests in this kind of situation was expressed by Justice Brennan while he was a member of the Appellate Division of the New Jersey Superior Court: "In the field of contested paternity . . . the truth is often obscured because social pressures create a conspiracy of silence or worse, induce deliberate falsity. The value of blood tests as a wholesome aid in quest for truth in the administration of justice in these matters cannot be gainsaid in this day. Their reliability as an indicator of the truth has been fully established. The substantial weight of medical and legal authority attests their accuracy, not to prove paternity, and not always to disprove it, but they can disprove it conclusively in a great many cases provided they are administered by specially qualified experts."

Review Questions

1. Which of the following is *not* used in paternity testing?
   A. ABO system
   B. Duffy system
   C. Lewis system
   D. MNS system
   E. Rh system

2. Which of the following may be used to verify patient identification?
   A. Photograph
   B. Fingerprints
   C. Demographic information (name, address, race, etc.)
   D. All of the above
   E. None of the above

3. Which of the following systems exhibits the greatest polymorphism?
   A. ABO
   B. Duffy
   C. HLA
   D. Kell
   E. MNS

4. A first-order exclusion is when:
   A. An antigen is present in the child, present in the mother, not present in the father

B. An antigen is present in the child, not present in the mother, present in the father
C. An antigen is present in the child, present in the mother, present in the father
D. An antigen is present in the child, not present in the mother, not present in the father
E. None of the above

5. Which of the following does not fit the criteria to be used as a genetic marker?
   A. Unit inheritance
   B. Allelic segregation
   C. Independent assortment
   D. Only two alleles
   E. All of the above

Answers to Review Questions

1. C (p 467)
2. D (p 468)
3. C (p 469)
4. D (p 470)
5. D (p 466)

References

1. National Conference of Commissioners on Uniform State Laws: Uniform Parentage Act. 1973.
2. Krause, HD: Legal considerations. In Paternity Testing. American Association Blood Banks, Washington, DC, 1978.
3. Thompson, JS and Thompson, MW: Genetics in Medicine. WB Saunders, Philadelphia, 1973.
4. Walker, RH: Probability in the analysis of paternity test results. In Paternity Testing. American Association of Blood Banks, Washington, DC, 1978.
5. Joint AMA-ABA Guidelines: Present status of serologic testing in problems of disputed parentage. Family Law Quarterly 10:247, 1976.
6. Southern, EM: Detection of specific sequences among DNA fragments separated by gel electrophoresis. J Molec Biol 98:503, 1975.
7. AABB Parentage Testing Committee: Standards for Parentage Testing Laboratories. 1986.
8. Race, RR and Sanger, R: Blood Groups in Man, ed 6. Blackwell Scientific Publications, London, 1975.
9. Hubbell, C, Dracker, R, and Davey, F: Paternity testing. In Henry, JB, et al: Clinical Diagnosis and Management by Laboratory Methods, ed 18. WB Saunders, Philadelphia, 1991, pp 1012–1020.
10. Wenk, RE, Houtz, T, and Brooks, M: Maryland law, disputed paternity and blood tests. Md Med J 32:448, 1983.
11. Wenk, R, Houtz, T, and Brooks, M: Paternity probabilities of biologic fathers and unexcluded falsely accused men using blood group markers. Transfusion 28:316, 1988.
12. Hummell, Von K: Biostatistical Opinion of Parentage. Gustav Fischer Verlag, Stuttgart, Germany, 1971.
13. Dykes, DD: The use of frequency tables in parentage testing. In Probability of Inclusion in Paternity Testing. American Association of Blood banks, 1982.

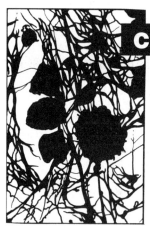

CHAPTER 25

Blood Bank
Information Systems

Chloe M. Scott, MT(ASCP), CLS(NCA)

OBJECTIVES

Upon completion of this chapter, the learner should be able to:

1 Describe the purpose of an information system in the blood bank.
2 Define the components of a blood bank information system.
3 List the responsibilities of operating and maintaining a blood bank information system.
4 Identify the various regulatory and accrediting organization's requirements for information systems.

476

TABLE 25-1 **COMMON ABBREVIATIONS**

CRT: Cathode ray tube
CPU: Central processing unit
HIS: Hospital information system
LIS: Laboratory information system
PC: Personal computer
SOP: Standard operating procedure

Blood banks generate tremendous volumes of information relating to patients and blood products, which must be maintained for extended periods of time. Donor and patient historic information, blood component manufacturing and testing, issuance of appropriate components to patients with special transfusion requirements, and collecting data to support management decisions are just some of the information requirements of the blood bank. The ability to manage the information is crucial to providing quality patient care efficiently. In today's healthcare environment, computers are the most effective means for handling the proliferation of information that is generated in the blood center and transfusion service. Blood bank information systems are computer systems that have been developed specifically to assist blood bank professionals in the management of the patient, donor, and blood component information.

As in any specialized field, there are abbreviations and terms used by the professionals within that specialty. For assistance with the reading of this chapter, the common abbreviations used by information systems personnel are listed in Table 25-1.

System Components

Information systems consist of three components: hardware, software, and users. The hardware components are the tangible, physical pieces of equipment that can be seen and touched. Software is the programmed instructions for the computer that store, manipulate, and retrieve information. Users are individuals who use the information system. Without the third component, the user, an information system is of no value to a blood bank. Individuals within a transfusion service or blood center are trained in the operation of the information system to enter data into the system, update the data, and retrieve the data to assist them in their daily functions. Special users, called system managers, are trained to maintain the information system just as individuals are specially trained to maintain other laboratory instruments.

HARDWARE

The types of hardware that can be combined to make a blood bank system vary widely. In this section the most common types currently available are discussed. Within the field of information technology, hardware is the area where the most rapid advances

and changes are occurring to improve information systems. The central processing unit (CPU) is the core of the information system. Within the CPU are the semiconductor chips that process the instructions of the computer programs. It is through the CPU that the other hardware devices, such as terminals or printers, operate. Other hardware devices, often referred to as "peripherals," serve one or more of three functions: input information, output information, and storage of information. The physical layout and design of the CPU and peripheral devices is the system configuration. Peripheral devices are attached with cables into slots or ports on the CPU. Some devices, such as tape drives and modems, may be incorporated into the CPU cabinet, so that all of the devices in the system may not be readily visible. A schematic of an example hardware configuration is shown in Figure 25-1.

Another common type of configuration is a network. In this type of configuration personal computers (PCs) are linked together with cables. Network software is then used to allow all PCs to access common data and software located on a fileserver. The fileserver is a CPU that stores application software, such as result entry programs, and the product and patient information.

A disk is a thin piece of metal or plastic that is coated with a thin metallic layer on which information can be stored electromagnetically in a format that is easily accessible by the computer programs. Disks are held in a disk drive that can quickly access information stored on a disk, thus making the information readily available to users on the system. Information that is readily available on the information system is said to be available "on-line." Information stored on the disks has a system address that assists in the quick retrieval of the data. Technologic advances have had a tremendous impact on these disks and disk drives, resulting in the ability to store enormous volumes of data in compact spaces and to retrieve the information rapidly. Information that once required devices the size of a washing machine for storage can now be contained in the typical personal computer.

The length of time it takes the computer to respond to a user request is called the response time. An effective system has a very quick response time. The length of response time can depend on the capabilities of the hardware, the number and types of tasks the system is performing, and the efficiency of the software.

After predetermined periods of time, some information may no longer need to be stored on-line. At that point, information can be moved from the disks to magnetic tape for storage. A tape drive is the peripheral device used to perform this data transfer from a disk drive to the tape. Information moved to tape can be retrieved using programs developed specifically for this task. The information retrieved from the tape may be reloaded into the system or printed in a report format. Reports may also be archived by microfiche and optical disk technologies, which provide an exact replica of the original report.

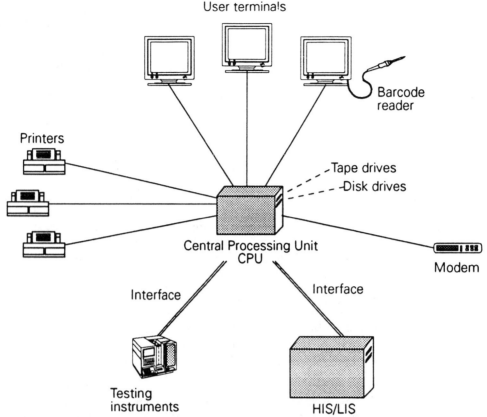

FIGURE 25–1 Example of a blood bank information hardware configuration.

Computer terminals are the devices used by the majority of users on an information system for data entry and data retrieval. Terminals actually consist of two components, a cathode ray tube (CRT) display unit and a keyboard. Through the keyboard, a user enters information or makes requests for data retrieval. Conversations between the user and computer occur on the CRT.

As the computer programs run, they require information from the user. Therefore, the programs request information from the user by displaying sentences or prompts on the CRT screen. The user types in the information using the keyboard, and the entered information is displayed on the CRT for confirmation by the user. When the entered information is correct, the user responds by pressing the appropriate key on the keyboard.

The CRT also serves as a device for data output. A program's request for information on a patient or donor may result in the display of information and reports on the CRT screen.

Another hardware device for data input frequently used in the blood bank is a barcode reader, either an optical or a laser type. The barcode reader is usually attached to the CRT. Blood component labels contain many pieces of information in a barcoded format. This information includes the unit number, product type,

facility identification, blood type, and expiration date. The barcoded format provides for easy, accurate, and efficient data entry. Figure 25–2 shows an example of a blood component label with the barcoded information. As unit information is entered into the system, the technologist can easily scan the required areas of the label to enter the data for each unit.

Printers are included in the system configurations to print the reports, forms, and labels needed by the blood center and transfusion services. Printers vary widely in their characteristics such as their speed of printing and the quality of the print. The type of printer used depends on the specific needs of the application. For example, donor recruitment letters would need to be printed on a printer with high-resolution quality print, but a routine department log could be printed on a printer with lower-quality print.

Modems provide a mechanism for connecting one computer system to another through a telephone line. The ability to attach by this communications mechanism allows remote laboratory facilities to function on a common system. Other uses for modem communications are for the transfer of files (such as data or programs) between two computer systems and the ability of technical support personnel to access the blood bank's information system to investigate and fix any system problems that occur.

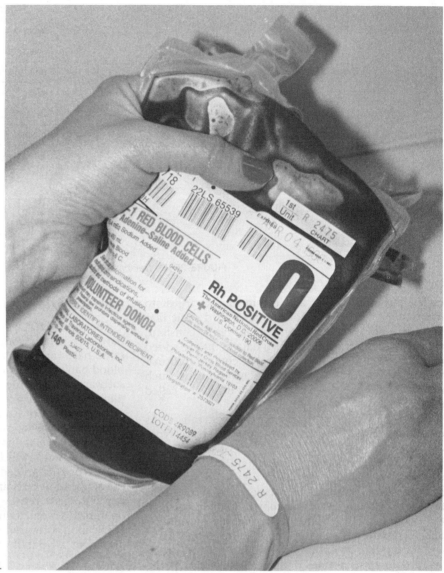

FIGURE 25-2 Barcodes on unit label.

SOFTWARE

Software is the set of instructions that tells the computer what to do with the entered or stored information. The software consists of many different programs, which are written in a computer language. Information systems contain three types of software: application software, operating system software, and interface software.

Application Software

Application software consists of the programs that give the information system the specific feature functionality for being a blood bank system. What makes the blood bank information systems unique is the application software that is specific for the needs of the users. Some of the applications specific for the blood bank include result entry of infectious disease test results, available inventory searches, antigen testing entry, and issuing products for transfusion.

The application software by itself cannot directly write or retrieve data to the system disks. The application software communicates with the operating system and gives the appropriate information to the operating system so it can store or retrieve data on the system disks.

The database is the application software function that stores, modifies, or retrieves many types of data in the information system. The database is organized into files, similar to those you might find in a file cabinet, to make the information data easy to find on the system disks. When an information system is initially installed, many files need to be established to provide an information foundation for the system. These files are basic definition files that establish the terminology that will be used to identify such things as product codes, user identification codes, antigen-antibody

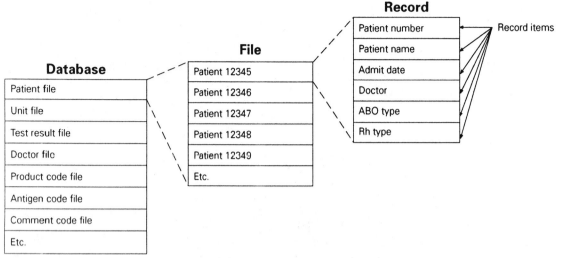

FIGURE 25–3 Database components.

codes, physician codes, and comment codes, just to name a few. These types of files are called static files because once created they remain fairly constant, changing only occasionally when data items are added or modified to the system. Files that contain information that is continuously growing and changing, such as unit history data or patient test data, are called dynamic files.

Figure 25–3 illustrates the parts of a database. As mentioned earlier, the database consists of many types of files, each holding a specific type of information. For example, the product code file might define each of the abbreviated codes used for blood products. Each file is made up of many records. A record contains a set of data items that constitute the record. In the example of the product code file, there would be one record to define WBC, another to define RBC, and yet another to define FFP. Within each record, a set of data items defines the item represented by the record. For example, data items in a product code record could include:

1. Full product name for printing on reports
2. Lifespan of the product for calculating expiration dates
3. Indicator of the product being a red cell product, plasma product, or platelet product
4. ABO/Rh type compatibilities required between the patient and the product
5. Indicator of the product being a pooled type product

Some blood bank information systems are part of an overall information system for the laboratory or the hospital. In this situation, all of the systems will use the same hardware and share database files and software. Other blood bank information systems are independent, with their own hardware, database, and software. This type of system is called a stand-alone system. The stand-alone system is usually interfaced with other information systems to share information.

Operating System Software

The operating system software is specific for the hardware an individual system operates; thus, the same hardware can be used for a banking, hotel, or blood bank information system. The operating system software controls the communication between the application software and all of the hardware components of the system. For example, when the application software gives instructions for data to be stored on the disks, it is actually passing the data to the operating system software, which then writes the data onto the disk. When data need to be retrieved from the disk, the application software sends a request to the operating system to retrieve the data from the disk. The operating system then passes the information to the application software to create output, such as a screen display or a printed report.

Interface Software

In today's information environment it is rare to find a computer system that is completely independent. Many different systems share information by special communications software called interfaces. Most commonly, the blood bank system will be interfaced with either a hospital information system (HIS) or a laboratory information system (LIS). As patient demographic information is entered into these other systems, that information is transmitted into the blood bank system.

This type of interface eliminates the need for blood bank personnel to duplicate the entry of patient data. As patient test results and component information are entered on the blood bank system, the results are automatically transmitted to the LIS or HIS. Additionally, when test results are completed or blood products are available for a patient, this information can be sent from the blood bank system to an HIS for notification of the nursing station.

Interfaces may also be implemented between a blood center information system and a transfusion service system. Information about components in a shipment to the transfusion service could be transmitted through an interface from the blood center computer. Conversely, information on the final disposition of components could be transmitted to the blood center system from the transfusion service system.

Another common interface is between the information system and laboratory instruments. These interfaces transmit the results of tests performed on the instruments into the blood bank system, which then stores the results in the result records for the appropriate unit of blood or patient. As the test results are received from the interface, the data are stored in the database, where they can then be processed by the blood bank system applications that determine the suitability of a component for transfusion. The interface linkage to other information systems or instruments is included in the configuration illustration in Figure 25–1.

USERS

The individuals who use and interact with the information system are known as end-users of the system. Anyone interacting with the system should be appropriately trained in the functionality of those portions of the system with which they will interact. When an information system is installed in a blood bank, the blood bank's technical procedures will be combined with the functionality of the computer to record data as they occur on a real-time basis. Periodically, individual technical competence should be evaluated to ensure continued competence in the combined use of the computer applications and the laboratory's technical procedures.

As the information system is enhanced with new features or changes to existing features, the end-user needs to be continuously trained in the functionality of the system. Anytime new software is added to the system a training plan should be created for the end-users.

An information system will also require at least one individual who is responsible for the system and is intricately familiar with the database and system maintenance procedures. This specialized user is called a system manager. The system manager is also responsible for implementation of new software enhancements, training new users, adding new data items to the database, and other system maintenance. Ideally, several individuals should share this responsibility.

Blood Bank Software Applications

The overall purpose of a blood bank information system is to track a blood product from the time of donation to the point of final distribution. In addition, the system should hold patient historic data for test results and transfusion information for the length of time required by federal or local regulations. Finally, the system should assist the blood bank professionals in selecting and issuing blood products that are safe for patient transfusion.

In the use of the information system, there are many times when evaluations can be made about the appropriateness of the actions taking place. When the system detects inappropriate actions, such as the incorrect labeling of a product or a discrepancy between the ABO/Rh type of a unit of blood and that of the patient, a noticeable warning should be given to the user at the time the problem is detected. In addition, the system should maintain a record of the incident, which can be included on a report.

The blood bank information systems offer many programs or applications to record the data activities in the blood bank. This section presents many, but not all, of the major applications that can be found in a system. As the requirements and needs of blood banks change, the applications in information systems will also change. For a comprehensive listing of applications, please refer to the report of the Information Systems Committee of the American Association of Blood Banks, "Responsibilities in Implementing and Using a Blood Bank Computer System," Appendix A: Functional Characteristics of a Blood Bank Computer System.

SECURITY

A crucial part of any information system is the security applications available to limit access to the system to only authorized individuals. The first level of security determines that a person is allowed access to the information system. A user at this point should be required to have both a user code and an individual password. The system should require users to change their password periodically to optimize the security of the system.

The second level of security is implemented within the software application itself. At this level, each user is allowed access only to specified applications for which they have been authorized by the system manager. For example, technologists would be allowed access to enter test results on a patient. Clerical staff would not be allowed access to these programs, but they could inquire about patient information to answer questions received in a phonecall.

BLOOD DONOR CENTER

Blood donation centers have information requirements that range from the scheduling of blood donors, to the evaluation of donor eligibility, determining what products should be prepared, and checking for the correctness of component labeling. This section describes some of the functional applications that could be found in a blood bank information system for a donor center.

To provide for the safety of our blood supply, the first steps must be taken when a unit is donated. When a donor registers at a donation facility, the first information collected is demographic data such as the donor's name, address, phone number, birth date, and social security number. When this information is entered, the computer system will search the donor records in the system for previous donations by this individual. If a record is not found, a new record is created for the donor that will contain information for this donation. If the donor has previously donated at the center, the information should be retrieved for review by the donor screening personnel and for updating of the demographic data. Computerized systems can also alert or warn the donor room personnel of any items in the donor's history or current donation criteria that indicate that the donor should not be accepted. This could mean a permanent deferral due to previous hepatitis infection or a temporary deferral due to medications currently taken or due to an interval less than 8 weeks since the last donation.

Donations do not always occur at the blood center's main facility but may occur at other fixed-site and mobile locations that are more convenient for the donors. At these donation centers, access to the donor records on the system is required. The mobile unit could review a printed report of deferred donor names that has been printed from the information systems. Another option to accessing the donor records from the information system is to transfer (download) a copy of the donor records from the system to portable PCs. Thus, when the donors come to the mobile facility, their previous histories are available. Upon return to the main facility, the information from the day's donations is then transferred (uploaded) from the PC to the information system and added to the database.

When a donor registers at a donation center, a donor card is printed containing the donor's demographic data. The donor cards are preprinted paper stock with the donor questions, places to record the donor screening information, consent statements, donor signature, and donor room personnel signature. Current blood bank regulations require the completed donor card to be maintained.

Information entered during the donation can be used to calculate the donor's next eligible donation date and the type of products to be created from the unit, and it can be used for future donor recruitment.

Donor confidentiality should be maintained in all areas of an information system; therefore, sensitive information relating to a donor should be accessible only to users such as a medical director, infection control personnel, or supervisors.

As the required testing is performed on the unit samples, the testing results are entered in the system either manually or through an interface with the testing instruments. Ideally, results should be entered via an instrument interface to avoid the possible errors that can occur when results are entered manually.

After all required results are entered into the system the determination is made as to whether or not the unit meets the requirements for release into the inventory for distribution.

If any of the testing for a unit does not meet the standard requirements, the system should place the unit into a quarantine status and not allow the unit to be moved into the available inventory. In addition, once confirmed, the result of the testing should be linked back to the donor's donation record with the appropriate action being taken to notify the donor of testing results.

Testing for antigens is also commonly performed on donated units. The antigen-typing results are added to the component information and also to the donor record. If specific antigen-typed units are requested, an inquiry of the system can locate inventory that meets the specified type requirement. Addition of the typing results to the donor record allows for targeted recruitment efforts when donors of specific blood and antigen types are required to meet special patient transfusion needs.

Based on the donation information and the inventory needs of the blood center, the drawn units are processed into the needed blood components. The information about each component prepared from the original unit should be recorded on the system. After the products are prepared and labeled, the blood bank can check the label by scanning the units with a barcode reader. The system then verifies the scanned information against the information stored in the system. The system can also review the testing results to make sure that the unit is qualified for release. If the unit is incorrectly labeled or should not be moved into the inventory, the system will give a warning notification to the operator and record the incident for reporting on an audit report.

After blood components have been tested and labeled and are determined to be acceptable for administration to patients, the units are placed into the available inventory for distribution to transfusion services or other blood centers. The information system in a blood center must be able to identify the location of all products at any given time. It also must be able to monitor product availability based on the age of components that will be outdated. As products are transferred to other facilities, the system will create shipping invoices and eventually bill the receiving facilities for the products they receive. If the blood center provides blood components to many facilities, the information system must be able to track where all of the components that originated at the blood center are distributed.

Once donors have donated units of blood that have been found to be acceptable for transfusion, recruitment efforts must be made to have these donors return for future donations. The information system provides an invaluable tool to assist in the donor recruitment efforts of the blood center by providing donor mailing labels or listings of donors who are eligible for another donation. For example, a list of donors in a certain zipcode area could be compiled for a mailing of information about when the blood center's mobile units would be in their area.

In some cases, donors with specific blood types and antigen types may have to be recruited for special patient needs. In these cases, the information system can search through the donor records and print a list of eligible donors who meet the special typing requirements.

TRANSFUSION SERVICE

The information system in the transfusion service revolves around the two main files in the system: the blood unit records and the patient records. The majority of the work done in the blood bank involves one or both of these files. When patient records are entered into the system, tests such as the ABO/Rh type and the antibody screen are ordered, and later results are entered. When units of blood are ordered on the patient, a link is created between the patient records and the blood unit records.

If the blood center and the transfusion service are operated jointly, they can share a single information system. In this situation, information about the blood components will be available to the transfusion service as soon as the units are given "available" status. The information system also has application programs that allow the transfusion service to enter units received from a Blood Center into the information system's product inventory.

When a patient specimen is received for testing, a review for previous testing and transfusion must be done by the transfusion service. Patient records are required to be maintained for 5 years, and if the patient has a history of antibodies or transfusion-related problems the records should be maintained indefinitely.

The information system should provide for quick retrieval of a patient history. Besides demographic information, the patient record should include any special requirements the patient has for transfusion. Examples of special transfusion requirements include antibodies that require antigen-negative products or special product requirements such as autologous, cytomegalovirus-negative, or irradiated products.

Ideally, all test results should be entered into the information system at the time when the results are being read. When results are entered, the system should review the past testing and notify the technologist of any discrepancies between the current test results and the previous results, so that potential problems can be investigated.

When compatibility testing is required for a patient, the system can assist in the selection of products that are appropriate for the patient. From the available inventory, products can be selected that match the patient's blood type and meet the special transfusion requirements recorded in the patient record. The sys-

tem may select units for the technologist, or the technologist may actually select the units and then enter the selected units into the system. Whenever the technologist selects and enters units into the system to be associated with a patient, the program should perform a comparison of the patient's record with the unit record. If a selected unit does not match the patient's requirements, a warning notification should be given to indicate the discrepancy. These same checks should be made when a component is issued for transfusion.

The products in a transfusion service continually change as they are modified to meet the requirements for patient transfusion. The information system must continuously track all changes made to a blood component. If the unit is divided into many smaller aliquots, each aliquot should be considered a new component and the history of that component should be traceable to the original unit. A new component is also created when components such as single-donor platelets are pooled. The history of the newly formed pooled product should identify each of the components included in the pool. In addition, it is also essential to be able to trace back each of the individual products to the original donor.

At any time, whether the information system is being used by a blood center or a transfusion service, an inquiry about a unit should produce details of all transactions involving the unit, from the time it is drawn or received to its final disposition. Figure 25–4 is a flowchart depicting the various statuses that a blood component passes through in its lifetime. When

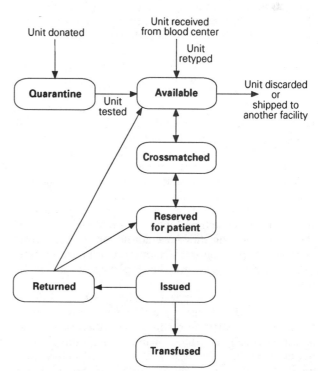

FIGURE 25–4 Various statuses of a blood component on a blood bank information system.

units are first drawn, they are placed in a "quarantine" status until all of the required testing is completed. Acceptable completion of the testing allows a unit to be moved to an "available" status, when it can be selected for transfusion to a patient. In the case of red cell components, crossmatch testing may be completed before the component is moved into the next status of being reserved for the patient. As the unit is placed into a "reserved" status, labels or facility-specific tags, or both, are usually attached to the component to identify the intended recipient of the product. The computer system can generate these labels and tags to contain all of the required information. When the unit is needed for the patient, either at a nursing station or in surgery, the unit is assigned an "issued" status when it is moved from the blood bank to the point of patient care. If the patient receives the unit, it is given a final status of "transfused." In some cases, the unit may be returned to the blood bank for future use on this patient or another one, and thus is returned to a "reserved" or available status. After predefined periods of time, a component can no longer be reserved for a patient. At this point, the component is returned to "available" status in the inventory, and then it can once again be crossmatched and reserved for another patient. Units that become outdated or are returned to the blood bank in unusable condition are disposed of and moved in the information system to a "disposed" status, the final disposition for the unit. Units may also be transported to another blood center or transfusion service and would then be given a status of "transferred," which could be considered a final disposition for the original facility.

In addition, the testing information, which includes all ABO typing, antibody screening, antigen testing, and infectious disease testing, should be available for the unit.

When patients have donated autologous units of blood or when units have been given for direct donation to a specific patient, the information must accommodate the special requirement that these units be transfused only to the patient for which they are intended. Special flags will be defined in the database record for these units and the patient to indicate such special situations. The application software will recognize these flags in the database records and have a different functionality in the handling of these patients and products. For example, in the selection of units for crossmatching blood for a patient, who has a flag set, indicating they have autologous units, if routine inventory products are entered for crossmatching, an alert message will be displayed for the technologist.

Reporting of patient test results and the products reserved or transfused to patients is routinely performed for incorporation into the patient's hospital medical record. The blood bank information for the patient can be included in the patient's electronic medical record through the interfaces between the HIS and LIS. In some facilities, either the HIS, LIS, or blood bank information system may print reports of the cumulative patient information to store in the patient's medical record.

MANAGEMENT ASSISTANCE

A definite advantage of using an information system in a blood center and transfusion service is that information is gathered that can be evaluated to make informed management decisions. By evaluating the numbers, procedures such as donors drawn, tests performed, components prepared, or recruitment activities, managers can evaluate data that indicate productivity of personnel, the use of instruments, or the effectiveness of donor recruitment programs. In addition, more accurate information can be gathered to determine the cost of testing. Accurate billing information is also captured for the billing of patients or institutions receiving components. One of the most common justifications for purchasing a blood bank information system is that use of the system will increase revenue by more accurately capturing charges for all of the procedures done in the blood bank.

Regulatory and Accreditation Requirements

In the late 1980s, it was found that many units of blood were inappropriately released into the available blood supply owing to computer software that was not functioning properly. Because of these findings, the Food and Drug Administration (FDA) focused its attention on the use of information systems in blood centers and transfusion services. As a result of its findings, the FDA issued memoranda in 1988 and 1989 to remind blood establishments of their responsibilities in the use and maintenance of information systems. Areas emphasized by the FDA were data security (particularly donor confidentiality), maintenance requirements such as standard operating procedures (SOP) for backups, manual operations during computer downtimes, data error correction, and validation of software and system functionality.

Besides the FDA, the voluntary accrediting organizations of the American Association of Blood Banks (AABB) and the College of American Pathologists (CAP) include within their inspections specific standards for computer systems that emphasize the responsibilities of the laboratories toward the implementation, use, and maintenance of an information system.

In addition to the requirements specifically for the computer systems, blood banks must also evaluate regulations and accreditation standards that apply to all records maintained by a laboratory. A laboratory that is using an information system must be sure that all requirements for records are met by the information system or a combination of their manual procedures and the information system.

System Responsibilities

As with any automation in the laboratory, responsibilities must be taken for the operation and maintenance of the information system. The first responsibility occurs when the system is first purchased. The blood center or transfusion service must define the specific requirements that an information system should have to meet the needs of their facility. After it defines its needs and requirements, the next step is a thorough evaluation of the information systems available in the market place and selection of the one that most closely fits the identified needs.

STANDARD OPERATING PROCEDURES

Just as standard operating procedures (SOPs) are written for the technical procedures in the laboratory, they must also be written for the procedures of the information system. The basic information for maintenance procedures for the information system is provided by the manufacturer of the information system. However, some options exist that must be incorporated into the specific blood center or transfusion service's SOPs. In addition to the system maintenance SOPs, the technical procedures such as antibody screening or antigen testing should be written to include the use of the information system.

MAINTENANCE

Information systems have maintenance requirements that include both hardware and software components. For the software, periodic programs may need to be run to purge data from the system to prevent the disks from becoming full. The database integrity may also be monitored with special utility programs, which will notify the system manager of problems to be corrected. Hardware devices have preventative maintenance schedules to ensure the proper functionality of the devices. The recommendations for hardware maintenance are made by the hardware vendor.

The software and database should routinely be copied onto a tape media or another set of discs to serve as a backup for the system data. The frequency for creating the backup depends on the volume of data entered and the vendor recommendations. The backup copies should be stored in a safe area to prevent damage of the media. Copies should be stored in a location away from the computer system to ensure that if the computer area met with a disaster such as a flood or fire, the backup copies would not be destroyed. The usual recommendation is that a periodic backup should be placed in an off-site storage location. In the event of such a disaster, the backup copies could be used to recreate the information system database and software.

Error Reporting

In the routine maintenance and monitoring of an information system, any problems or errors should be recorded in a log. The information recorded in this log should include the date and time of the problem, the person identifying the problem, the steps that occurred before the problem, the corrective action taken to resolve the problem, and, if indicated, to whom the problem may have been escalated for resolution.

DOWNTIME PROCEDURE

Periodically the information system may be unavailable for use ("down") when hardware maintenance is performed, system backups are being done, or software enhancements are loaded. This type of system downtime can be scheduled and planned for in advance. Unscheduled downtime can occur unexpectedly during power outages or natural disasters. The facility should have an established procedure for operating in a manual mode during the downtime, whether scheduled or unscheduled, and for data recovery once the system is again functional.

During downtime, some mechanism should be available for checking donor deferrals and identifying patients with a history of antibodies or special transfusion requirements. Periodic reports or cards from the information system could be printed or information could be transferred, or downloaded, to a PC for access to the needed information during the downtime.

Downtime procedures should also include the availability of any forms or labels needed during the downtime. Once the procedure is developed and individuals are trained, the procedure should be tested for its effectiveness. After the test, modifications should be made to correct any noted problems. Periodic testing of the procedure is advisable because daily routines can change, and the procedure should change also to meet the current needs of the facility.

VALIDATION

Validation is a systematic process of testing the components of an information system—hardware, software, and user—to ensure that they are functioning correctly for their intended purposes. Information systems constitute an invaluable tool that assists blood bank professionals in providing quality care to patients. Therefore, every step must be taken to guarantee that the system is functioning as it should. When system validation is done, thorough documentation of the process should be maintained as the validation process is conducted.

Control Points

During the operation of a software application, the software will either make a decision based on the data it has accumulated or it may display the data and request the user to make the decision before it can further process the data. A point at which a decision is made is called a control point. These control points vary depending on the criticality of the decision to be made and how that decision will affect the patient. An example of a critical control point in a blood bank information system is the issuance of compatible products to a patient, based on the patient's blood type and special transfusion requirements. Even though the system may not actually make a decision, because it supplies information for a technologist to make a decision, the software is considered to be a part of a critical control point.

Types of Validation

Through the life cycle of an information system, different types of validation can be performed. If the system has been in use but has never been formally validated, retrospective validation would be performed on the system. This type of validation was required by the FDA in 1989 for blood bank systems that had never been previously validated.

Prospective validation is performed before implementing a new system. Periodically, after an information system has been implemented, new software, hardware, or database items may be added to the system to enhance existing applications or add new features. Any changes made to the system should be validated for correct functionality. This type of validation is referred to as change control.

The final type of validation is periodic. Periodic validation can be part of a quality assurance program that monitors the functionality of the system when no changes are being made to the system. Examples of periodic validation might include quarterly checks of calculations made by the system, monthly accuracy checks of donor deferral lists, or annual competency testing of users.

Testing Procedures

An SOP should be created for validating the information system. This SOP procedure should contain various requirements for different types of validation and for the breadth of testing that is required for each type. The SOP should identify the individuals responsible for the development of the test plans, conducting the testing, and evaluating the test results for acceptable performance, as well as the approval process for placing the software into operation in the routine system functionality.

Before testing the software, a written test plan that considers all of the application functionality should be created. This test plan should consider the following items:

Control points
Security

Conditions that trigger warning messages and alerts
Methods of data entry (keyboard, barcode reader, instrument interface)
Valid data versus invalid data (alphabetic data in numeric fields, numeric data in alphabetic fields)
Data storage
Data retrieval

The test plan should also identify the acceptable test results.

Testing should occur under conditions that will not affect the current system data. Ideally, a test database that is separate from the live database should exist for testing. As testing is conducted, documentation should be maintained of the testing process. Documentation can include test results noted in written logs, prints of the screen information, or printed reports. Testing forms could be created to record testing and provide a standard format of documentation.

Upon completion of testing scenarios, the test results should be reviewed for acceptable performance. An unacceptable result should be reviewed to determine the criticality of the problem. Some situations will require software changes, whereas others may require database or procedural changes. After corrective actions have been made, testing should again be performed and reviewed for acceptance. A record of all corrective actions should be maintained with the validation documentation.

Completion of the testing process results in the changes being incorporated into the live information system. The individual responsible for making the decision to add the changes to the system should formally document his or her approval. The date and time of the implementation of the changes should also be included with the documentation.

Review Questions

1. Components of an information system consist of all of the following, *except*:
   A. Hardware
   B. Software
   C. Validation
   D. Users

2. Which of the following does *not* have specific requirements for blood bank information systems?
   A. FDA
   B. JCAHO
   C. AABB
   D. CAP

3. The type of validation performed when a new information system is installed is called:
   A. Retrospective validation
   B. Change control validation
   C. Quality assurance validation
   D. Prospective validation

4. An example of interface software functionality is:
   A. The entry of blood components into the blood bank database.
   B. The transmission of patient information from the HIS to the blood bank system.
   C. The printing of a workload report at a printer.
   D. Disallowing a person access to the system.

5. Backup copies of the information system:
   A. Can be used to restore the information system data and software if the live information system is damaged.
   B. Are used to maintain hardware components.
   C. Are performed once a month.
   D. Are created any time changes are made to the information system.

6. When new software enhancements are received from an information system vendor, which procedure should be used?
   A. Change control
   B. Backup
   C. Downtime
   D. Crossmatch

7. The combined hardware component design of the information system is called the system:
   A. Peripheral
   B. Database
   C. Interface
   D. Configuration

8. Information data are stored in a collection of many different files, which is called the:
   A. Database
   B. Configuration
   C. Hardware
   D. Disk drive

9. Application software communicates with this type of software to retrieve data from the system disks:
   A. Interface
   B. Operating system
   C. Security
   D. Program

10. Validation testing for software should consider all of the following items, *except*:
    A. Methods of data entry
    B. Control points
    C. Performance of testing in live system
    D. Invalid data

Answers to Review Questions

1. C (p 477)
2. B (p 484)
3. D (p 486)
4. B (p 481)
5. A (p 485)
6. A (p 486)
7. D (p 477)
8. A (p 479)
9. B (p 481)
10. C (p 486)

Bibliography

American Association of Blood Banks: Control Function Guidelines (draft). Letter to all institutional members, November 25, 1991.

American Association of Blood Banks: User Validation Guidelines (draft). Letter to all institutional members, November 25, 1991.

Butch, SH: Computer software quality assurance. Lab Med 22:18, 1991.

Elevitch, FR and Aller, RD: The ABCs of LIS: Computerizing Your Laboratory. American Society of Clinical Pathologists Press, Chicago, 1986.

Food and Drug Administration: Recommendations for implementation of computerization in blood establishments. Memo to all registered blood establishments, April 6, 1988.

Food and Drug Administration: Requirements for computerization of blood establishments. Memo to all registered blood establishments, September 8, 1989.

Leavitt, J and Steane, S (directors): Technical Workshop on Standards for Computer Systems in Blood Banking. American Association of Blood Banks Annual Meeting, New Orleans, October, 1989.

Responsibilities in Implementing and Using a Blood Bank Computer System. American Association of Blood Banks, Washington, DC, 1989.

Wilson, JK and Elliott, DM: Computers in the Blood Bank. American Association of Blood Banks, Washington, DC, 1984.

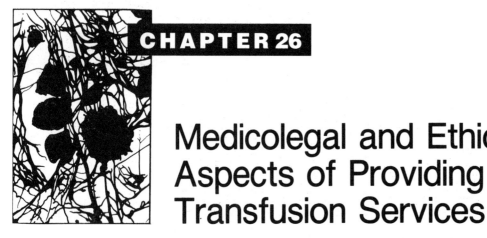

CHAPTER 26

Medicolegal and Ethical Aspects of Providing Transfusion Services

Kathleen Sazama, MD, JD, MT(ASCP)

OBJECTIVES

Upon completion of this chapter, the learner should be able to:

1 Understand the legal and ethical implications of provision of transfusion services.

2 Discuss the legal bases for liability for providing transfusion medical services.

3 Define the necessity for establishing and following standard operating procedures similar to other comparable facilities throughout the United States.

4 Identify and list the evolving legal and ethical concerns likely to accompany the increasing complexity of providing blood during the 1990s.

5 List two reasons patients sue for transfusion injury.

6 List the steps blood bank professionals can take to avoid litigation.

7 Describe the legal issues related to transfusion-transmitted diseases in laboratory medicine.

Legal issues involving transfusion medicine in the 1990s continue to center on transfusion-transmitted acquired immunodeficiency syndrome (TTAIDS), first reported in 1983. However, even before TTAIDS became the basis for numerous lawsuits against blood centers, hospitals, and physicians (probably more than 500 since 1985), there was litigation because of death and serious injury due to transfusion-transmitted hepatitis (TTH) (*Perlmutter v Beth David Hospital*, 123 NE2d 792, [NY 1954])* and a few because of donor injury.[1] The TTH cases stimulated nearly every state legislature to enact protection for blood banks through so-called blood shield statutes.[2] (California was the first state to enact such protection for blood banks in 1955; only New Jersey lacks such a law, but similar protection is available through judicial decisions.) Because of these blood shield statutes, most of which extended protection without amendment or modification for TTAIDS as well as for TTH, many TTAIDS lawsuits have been either dismissed or unsuccessful for the person suing (the plaintiff). Recently, however, these blood shield statutes have come under new challenge in the courts.

Although blood shield statutes protect against application of strict liability, other civil bases of liability defined in tort and, to a limited extent, contract law exist. In this chapter, following a brief discussion of source of law, theories of liability are discussed with practical hints for reducing likelihood of being found liable, when possible. Emerging concerns for the 1990s are also identified. This chapter is not intended to substitute for legal advice necessary in particular situations but rather to provide the reader with some general principles and definitions so that ethically and legally sound practices may continue within transfusion medicine.

Sources of Law

Laws are created by society, either through legislation called statutes (passed by either the US Congress or by individual state legislatures) or through court decisions (in federal courts including the US Supreme

Court or in state courts through the highest state court).

STATUTES AND REGULATIONS

Frequently, federal law (enacted by the US Congress or by decision in federal courts, including the US Supreme Court) supersedes state law, but both can be and often are applied in particular instances. The details of how laws will be put into action are provided in regulations. Regulations, both federal and state, can be applied only if they have been established according to a formal process detailed in the Administrative Procedure Act (APA).[3] Federal regulations that apply specifically to blood banking are found in Title 21, Code of Federal Regulations, Parts 600 to 699 and, to some extent, Parts 200 to 299, published annually on April 1.[4] Blood banks are also federally regulated by provisions of the Clinical Laboratories Improvement Act of 1988 and the Medicare provisions of the Social Security Act.

State legislatures also enact laws and publish explanatory regulations about blood banking, clinical laboratories, and transfusion practices, principally covering licensure of facilities and personnel.

CASE LAW

Law is also established by court decisions, sometimes related to interpretations and applications of statutes and regulations. Patients usually believe that medical treatment administered to them (with their consent, it is hoped) will, on balance, be beneficial. When transfusion causes harm (e.g., TTAIDS), patients have understandably reacted by seeking redress in the courts. The legal bases for such lawsuits are generally civil (not criminal) actions for tort and sometimes contract liability.

United States civil law depends on each adult person in our society behaving reasonably (i.e., not negligently and not aggressively) toward every other person, respecting other persons' rights. Civil lawsuits arise because someone disrespects another's rights by (1) striking or threatening to strike another person (battery and assault), (2) being careless or reckless (negligence), (3) failing to complete an agreement (breach of contract), (4) intruding on another's property or privacy, or (5) misbehaving in other similar ways. Civil suits can also arise because of violation of specific statutes or regulations that require certain types of actions.

---

*The court decided that transactions involving blood were not sales but were incidental to the provision of medical services. The effect of this decision was to preclude application of commercial law, particularly that of warranties, to blood transfusions.

Basis of Liability: Torts

INTENTIONAL TORT: BATTERY

Any unconsented touching (including deliberate blows and intentional striking) is legally defined as battery. For transfusion medicine, this concept is used when a donor or a patient claims that he or she never agreed to have the needle placed into his or her arm.

DOCTRINE OF INFORMED CONSENT

Particularly in the special circumstances of the practice of medicine, the issue of whether a patient (or, in the case of a blood collection organization, a donor) agreed to undergo the procedure actually performed with full knowledge of the possible benefits and harm that accompany it has come to be known as the doctrine of informed consent. This doctrine protects the patient (or donor) by requiring that information be provided in a manner understandable to the patient under circumstances that permit the patient to ask and receive answers to any questions or concerns he or she may have (*Canterbury v Spence*, 464 F2d 772 [DC Cir 1072]).

For TTAIDS transfusion recipients this issue came into sharp focus in the case of *Kozup v Georgetown University Hospital* (663 F Suppl 1048 [DC 1987]; 851 F2d 437 [DC Cir 1988]; 906 F2d 783 [DC Cir 1990]). In this case, an infant brought by his parents to Georgetown University Hospital for medical care contracted TTAIDS and died. His parents argued that they were insufficiently informed about the potential harm of the transfusions and did not specifically agree to transfusions among other care given their child. The District of Columbia Court ruled that their actions in bringing the child to the hospital and not objecting to transfusions at time of infusion amounted to tacit consent. However, this issue of whether specific consent is required for transfusion and who should obtain such consent (usually physicians have been held responsible [*Ritter v Delaney*, 790 SW2d 29 (Tex App—San Antonio 1990) and *Howell v Spokane*, 785 P2d 815 (Wash 1990)]) remains controversial (*Hoemke v New York Blood Center*, 90-7182 2d [New York 1990] and *Gibson v Methodist Hospital*, 01-89-00645-CV [Tex Ct App 1991]) except in some states such as California where specific requirements have been enacted.

Another arena in which the doctrine of informed consent will be key to resolving disputes is that of donor rights. With the onset of AIDS the language of donor histories has been subjected to continuing revision and updating to include information about the disease, how it is acquired, and under what circumstances a person should donate blood. Federal and voluntary requirements for how the history is obtained have emphasized more face-to-face oral questioning, not just self-administration of these questionnaires. One part of the donation process has always been for donors to sign a statement of consent to donate.

Until the late 1980s, donors were protected from subpoena in cases of transfusion-transmitted diseases. However, an increasing number of plaintiffs in state courts are insisting that for TTAIDS cases the donor be subject to questioning regarding his or her donation. This questioning may completely or partially protect a donor's identity or may require that donor to appear in open court. Because no donor donates blood expecting to have to defend that altruistic act at some future date, the impact of these decisions on the future availability of blood for transfusion is uncertain.

INTENTIONAL INFLICTION OF EMOTIONAL DISTRESS

As the phrase suggests, a plaintiff must show that what the defendant did to cause actual and severe emotional distress was intentional, usually some extreme or outrageous conduct that was calculated deliberately to cause real harm to the plaintiff. This can take the form of a claim for wrongful death of the plaintiff's relative, particularly in some TTAIDS cases.

NEGLIGENCE

Elements

Liability for negligence is found when all of the following factors are satisfied:

1. There was a duty owed to the injured party.
2. The duty was not met by the injuring party.
3. Because the duty was not met, the injured party was harmed.
4. Failure to meet the duty owed was directly responsible for or could have been predicted to cause the harm suffered by the injured party.
5. Some measurable (compensable) harm occurred (called "damages") (Table 26–1).

To be successful in a negligence action, the plaintiff is responsible for proving all of these factors against the person being sued (the defendant).

Standard of Care

When the negligence involves ordinary things that everyone encounters such as traffic accidents, for example, a jury (or judge) can consider the facts and decide whether the behavior of the defendant was reasonable; that is, did the defendant meet the standard of care required in the situation? For ordinary or usual negligence, this standard of care depends on

TABLE 26–1 ELEMENTS OF NEGLIGENCE

Duty owed
Breach of duty
Causation
Damages

what the average person, such as a juror, believes is acceptable in our society. Thus, the jury decides whether a reasonable person, in the same circumstances as the defendant was in, would have acted the same as (or differently than) the defendant did. If the defendant acted reasonably in the circumstances, the plaintiff will be unsuccessful in the lawsuit, and vice versa.

In situations in which larger organizations are involved, the question of who is liable for the actions of employees has been resolved under the doctrine of respondent superior. Under this doctrine, the actions of employees are attributable to the employer or other person who directs their actions. This responsible person for transfusion services has been defined by federal regulation and general practice to be a physician, a definition that has been reinforced by judicial decision in many states for blood centers as well as for hospitals. The advantage of having a physician as the responsible employer is that the principles and regulations related to medical malpractice usually apply, including the requirement for establishing a professional standard of care.

Professional Standard of Care

When the negligence lawsuit involves professionals such as physicians and scientists, including laboratory professionals, nurses, or other allied health practitioners, the definition of what's reasonable, the standard of care, depends on expert testimony from other physicians or scientists about what should have been done by other reasonable practitioners (usually of the same specialty). The law makes the extra requirement that, in discharging his or her duty to the plaintiff, the defendant must apply the special knowledge and ability he or she possesses by virtue of the profession. This increased professional standard of care is not just what the judge or jury would have done but what other professionals (so-called expert witnesses) testify should have been done. For the complex scientific, technical, and medical issues involved in TTAIDS litigation, this distinction has been of great significance in protecting blood bankers.

VOLUNTARY AND MANDATORY STANDARDS

The testimony of experts generally should be supportable by authorities such as statutes, regulations, or other bodies of published knowledge, including published scientific articles and texts. The existence of voluntary standards—particularly that provided by the American Association of Blood Banks (AABB),[5] but also those from the College of American Pathologists, the American Association of Tissue Banks, the American Society for Histocompatibility and Immunogenetics, the Joint Commission on Accreditation of Healthcare Organizations, and other organizations— are helpful in establishing the professional standard of practice for transfusion medicine. In fact, some state

and federal regulations cross-reference the AABB standards specifically. Blood banks and transfusion services that can show that they acted in conformance with these standards are much less likely to be found negligent than those who do not follow such guidelines.

IS BLOOD BANKING A MEDICAL PROFESSION?

The question of whether blood banking is a medical profession is being relitigated in courts today, with conflicting results.[6] One possible chilling result is that the collection, processing, and distributing of blood may be considered differently than the crossmatching, issuance, and transfusion of blood to individual patients. Redefining blood banking as not a medical practice will remove the extra protection provided by the requirement for expert medical testimony to establish the standard of care, leaving defendants to be judged by the ordinary negligence standard. There is little dispute that loss of medical professional stature would significantly alter the practice of blood banking. None of the protections of medical malpractice reform will be available, and blood centers may even find themselves subject to strict liability.

Case 1

A 26-year-old woman is critically injured in a two-car collision. She is rushed via helicopter to the nearest trauma center, where 10 units of uncrossmatched O-negative red blood cells, 12 units of crossmatch-compatible B-negative red blood cells, 4 apheresis platelet packs, and 4 jumbo units of fresh frozen plasma are administered within the first 24 hours of her care. Soon after her admission, she is taken to the operating room where splenectomy is performed, liver and left kidney lacerations are repaired, numerous fractures of both lower extremities are reset, and a chest tube is placed for a collapsed left lung. She requires only 4 more units of packed red blood cells during the next several days and recovers sufficiently to be discharged home to recuperate 15 days after the accident. Two years later, in 1986, during her first prenatal visit for a second pregnancy, she tests positive for the human immunodeficiency virus (HIV). Two weeks later she is told by her obstetrician that the blood center reported that one of the units she received came from a donor who recently tested positive for HIV.

QUESTIONS:

1. Was the blood center negligent?

2. Was the physician who transfused the patient negligent?

3. Would using an "ordinary" versus a "professional" standard of care yield a different answer?

STRICT LIABILITY

Manufacturers and distributors of goods used in everyday life have been defined by law to have certain responsibilities in their activities to protect consumers. Among other requirements, certain warranties exist that a bought product (e.g., a television set) will actually work and will continue to do so for some fixed period of time, with small risk of harm to the purchaser from such things as electric shock or explosion. These warranties, actual or implied, exist for virtually anything a consumer buys and uses. If a product fails to perform as expected or creates harm when none was expected, the consumer has the right to have a replacement or, if the manufacturer denies responsibility, to sue for negligent manufacturing or distribution.

In addition, for some items (such as dynamite), the danger from its proper use is so great that manufacturers are legally liable for *all* harm that occurs—so-called strict liability. This means that anyone harmed when properly using dynamite does not have to prove that the manufacturer or distributor was negligent, they only have to show that they were injured while properly using it. Imagine how rare and expensive blood transfusions would become if these theories were allowed to be applied. Instead, states enacted specific protection, the blood shield statutes described earlier, to exclude harm from blood transfusions from suit under these legal theories. It is important that blood bankers avoid implying or stating that blood transfusion is completely safe because such statements may be construed as creating a warranty, invoking these theories of liability.

INVASION OF PRIVACY

Healthcare providers, including blood bankers, are required to respect personal privacy and maintain patient and donor confidentiality. Plaintiffs may claim remuneration for loss of privacy under four theories:

1. Intrusion upon plaintiff's seclusion or solitude or into his or her private affairs
2. Public disclosure of embarrassing facts
3. Placing plaintiff in a "false light" in public
4. Appropriation of plaintiff's name or likeness for defendant's benefit.

These categories protect a patient or donor from illegal or inadvertent disclosure of his or her personal information, of particular concern with HIV because of the lack of appropriate safeguards to prevent loss of employment, housing, insurance, and other benefits of society. When information is exciting or noteworthy, the media may become aware of and publish private information. Blood banks and transfusion services will be involved in such suits if they are responsible (through negligence or by intention) for release of the data. Great care should be exercised by blood banking professionals to ensure that private information (whether about donors, patients, or relatives) be kept confidential and not released without written authorization. Procedures to safeguard such release should include proper use of photocopying and facsimile machines as well as direct electronic transfer via information systems.

Case 2

A 32-year-old man who was a frequent blood donor has a positive result on a new HIV test, having repeatedly tested HIV negative on prior donations. Before confirmatory testing is completed, he returns to the blood collection center to donate HLA-matched platelets. Before questioning begins, the registering staffperson notices that his prior record indicates his deferral status. The staffperson informs the donor he is not eligible to donate the platelets. The donor is shocked and embarrassed by the news and storms out of the center. Two weeks later, the donor sues the blood center for intentional infliction of emotional distress.

QUESTIONS

1. Will the donor likely be successful?
2. Are there other bases on which suit can be brought?
3. Are there established standards for preventing such an occurrence?

Basis of Liability: Contract

Contracts arise by agreement between at least two parties, both of whom promise to do (or refrain from doing) something of value in exchange for the other doing (or not doing) something else. In transfusion medicine, the donation and transfusion relationships have sometimes been alleged to be a contract, even though, for donors, the collecting facility rarely provides anything of value to the altruistic donor, and, for recipients, the patient-physician relationship has long been denied status as a contract. (There is a contract between the patient and hospital, but that relationship does not usually involve blood banks.) Because breaches of contract center on existence of a valid contract, as well as interpretations of the language of the agreement and whether one party satisfied its responsibility, the lack of a valid contract negates further review. When donors are paid to donate, however, the theories of breach of contract liability are easier to apply. The profession's insistence on a totally altruistic blood supply has been instrumental in avoiding contract liability.

Restrictions on Plaintiff Suits and Recovery

STATUTES OF LIMITATIONS

Some protection arises in TTAIDS and other transfusion cases because of a statutorily defined limit of time during which a lawsuit can be filed. However, until the issue of blood banking as a medical profession or as the provision of medical services is finally decided, states will continue to make conflicting determinations. Statutes of limitations are usually shorter (approximately 2 years from date that the injury should have been discovered in adults) than those for other kinds of negligence (2 to 6 years is common).

DOCTRINE OF CHARITABLE IMMUNITY

Historically, courts provided immunity for nonprofit organizations like hospitals from excess liability because they performed charitable acts. Many state legislatures have enacted and continue to support statutes to provide protection for boards of directors or volunteers or both, using this common law rationale. However, many healthcare institutions rely less on this doctrine and more on insurance for protection.

TORT REFORM

With skyrocketing costs of malpractice in some states, physicians have been leaving the inhospitable states to practice in kinder climes. State legislatures, recognizing the need to protect some specialties such as obstetrics, have been active in seeking limits on damages against physicians, protecting them from abusive litigation. It is vital that these protections be afforded for transfusion practices.

Risk Management and Quality Performance

Avoiding liability for TTAIDS and other possible harm from practicing transfusion medicine whether in hospitals or blood centers depends on having well-established policies and procedures that comply with recognized authorities, regulations, and statutes and on having some way of measuring whether persons engaged in all activities actually follow those procedures. To avoid being negligent, behavior must be reasonable. Reasonable behavior for transfusion medicine practice includes continually obtaining and applying new knowledge from all possible sources that will safeguard the donor during collection, the component during handling and delivery, and the patient before and during transfusion.

DONOR ISSUES

Screening

What the AIDS epidemic has taught us is that every person who volunteers to donate blood does not have an unqualified right to do so. In fact, for several years before March 1985, when the first test for HIV in blood was made available, the best safeguard against TTAIDS was improved donor education and more pertinent questioning regarding behaviors that might put that donor at risk for acquiring HIV. Although numerous lawsuits have been filed against blood collection agencies for improper donor screening, few have been successful when collecting facilities could show that they had written procedures, properly trained employees who followed those procedures, and proper documentation of each screen. Problems occurred only when breaches in procedure, typically failures to follow or properly document actual practice, were discovered. However, with several state courts now demanding release of donor identity or access to donor for questioning, further attention to the process of donor screening, including consideration of adding information for donors that they may be subject to subpoena if transfusion harm occurs, will be required. Balancing the real threat of lack of availability of blood with the serious nature of TTAIDS- or TTH-related litigation is a constant challenge to blood banking professionals in the 1990s.

Donations Requested by Patients

Several monetary settlements in the hundreds of thousands to millions of dollars have resulted from either failing to offer directed donor services or for improperly characterizing them.

Untimely Notification of TTAIDS or TTH

When recipients received notification years after blood centers knew (or should have known) the recipient had received an HIV-reactive unit, many of them or their families were angry enough to file suit on the basis that they should have been informed sooner. Procedures for lookback and recipient notification were not well established for several years following application of specific testing in most blood collection organizations. Despite efforts by knowledgeable and concerned scientists, no consensus was reached until late in the TTAID epidemic about notification of either donors or recipients (or their sexual contacts). The broader public health issues in this epidemic continue to elude concrete rules.

Case 3

A 67-year-old woman crippled by degenerative arthritis requests her own blood and blood from members of her family to be used for her hip replacement. The blood center describes their donation procedures that do not permit directed donations. Although she is disappointed, she agrees to donate for herself. Her first unit is tested and is repeatedly reactive for HIV. The patient-donor is advised that she may no longer donate and that the unit she has already donated will not be available for her surgery. Surgery proceeds. She received 4 units of volunteer blood and develops AIDS 3 years later. She sues the blood-collecting organization.

QUESTIONS

1. On what legal grounds can this suit be brought?

2. What is the current standard of care regarding directed donations?

3. Can healthcare organizations deny autologous donor-patients access to their own test-reactive blood?

Component Collection

Occasionally lawsuits have occurred from injury to donors during the collection process. Usually these injuries are more severe than a simple bruise at the needlesite and involve such things as nerve damage, slip-and-fall incidents, and severe reactions. The continuing problem of microbial contamination during collection, though infrequent, remains a more serious concern. Donor deaths continue to be reported at a rate of approximately two each year, and these infrequently result in litigation.

PROCESSING, LABELING, AND DISTRIBUTION

No Standard Protocol for Implementing Testing

Several successful TTAIDS lawsuits awarded millions of dollars against blood collecting organizations (*Belle Bonfils Memorial Blood Bank v Denver District Court*, 723 P2d 1003 [Colo 1988]) because they had no standard protocol for implementing new testing to ensure that all available components (including those distributed or in active inventory) tested negative before transfusion, once the test kits and equipment were received by the collection facility. The lack of a written plan to implement such testing, including training of personnel, validating instrumentation and reagents, and establishing the necessary information service support, was seen as negligent by the jury (even *with* expert testimony to the contrary).

Failure to Perform Surrogate Testing

Despite concerted efforts, rarely has a plaintiff prevailed for alleging that blood collection facilities should have performed more or different surrogate tests between 1983 and 1985 when a specific test was first available (*Baker v JK and Susie Wadley Research Institutes and Blood Bank, dba The Blood Center at Wadley*, 86-2728-C [Tex Jud Dist Ct 1988] and *Clark v United Blood Services*, CV 88-6981 [Nev 2nd Jud Dist Ct 1990]).

Failure to Perform Testing Properly

Testing personnel should be constantly alert to proper performance and documentation of all required testing of blood components. Failure to document is as damning as failure to perform at all and must be avoided. Considerable effort has been expended by the Food and Drug Administration (FDA) to inform and enforce requirements for proper testing for virally transmissible diseases in blood components. Private accrediting organizations likewise emphasize proper performance and documentation of these activities.

Informed Consent

In TTAIDS cases arising in the early 1980s it was frequently alleged that patients were insufficiently warned of the hazards of transfusion because transfusion experts failed to warn hospitals and ordering physicians about them. Few cases were successful because the state of scientific knowledge, established by expert testimony relying on published data, was limited. Also, the early TTH cases had established a record that supported the defense position that transfusions were already known by hospitals and other physicians to be unavoidably unsafe, particularly for transfusion-transmitted viral diseases. Some states (e.g., California) enacted specific legislation about informed consent for transfusion.

MEDICAL MALPRACTICE

Several multimillion-dollar suits, decided in favor of the plaintiff, resulted from successful allegations that the patient did not need a transfusion at all, could have waited until test-negative blood was available before being transfused, or required transfusion solely because of something the physician did. In all of these cases, the basis for fault was negligence by the treating physician.

Case 4

A 43-year-old man received a 1-unit transfusion of red blood cells during an emergency coronary artery bypass operation. Three years later, just before his second marriage, he was found to be HIV positive. He sued his cardiologist and the blood center.

1. Which issues are likely to be successful for this plaintiff?

2. Would the result be different if ordinary rather than professional standard of care were applied?

Emerging Concerns

Among the other concerns listed previously there are new ones surrounding changing practices of transfusion medicine such as responsibilities for out-of-hospital (specifically at home) transfusions, issues surrounding provision of autologous services (cross-over of unused units, transfusion of reactive components, freezing of unused reactive units, informed consent, etc.), new therapies such as red blood cell substitutes and use of recombinant erythropoietin, standards for provision of perioperative blood collection and re-infusion, and control over use of gene therapy to treat certain transfusion-dependent illnesses. In the TTAIDS area, suits have been filed for reporting false AIDS test results and for fear of AIDS because of exposure through transfusion or via a healthcare worker, plus ongoing concerns over handling of look-back. New concerns about bacterial contamination, fueled by the still-unexplained upsurge in *Yersinia* growth in red blood cells, and newer issues surrounding hepatitis C and other non-A, non-B hepatitis viruses will surface.

Conclusions

The lessons learned from the spate of TTAIDS and other litigation underscore that every blood bank and transfusion service needs complete, comprehensive, and current written procedures and policies. When such procedures and policies conform to federal and state statutes and regulations as well as meeting private voluntary standards, such as those of the College of American Pathologists (CAP), AABB, and Joint Commission of Accreditation of Hospitals (JCAHO), the organization can have a higher assurance that it will meet the standard of care required to avoid being found negligent and thus liable for the damages the patient or donor suffered. Pending and future issues will redefine legal and ethical aspects of transfusion medicine in the future.

Review Questions

1. Transfusion-transmitted diseases can result in lawsuits for which of the following reasons?
   A. Battery
   B. Invasion of privacy
   C. Negligence
   D. A and B
   E. A, B, C

2. Laws applicable to blood banking and transfusion medicine can arise:
   A. In state and federal courts
   B. In US Congress, state legislatures, and state and federal courts
   C. In state legislatures and courts
   D. In state legislatures and US Congress

3. The reasons patients have sued for transfusion injury include:
   A. Failure to perform surrogate testing
   B. Failure to test blood components properly
   C. Failure to screen donors properly
   D. Unnecessary transfusion
   E. All of the above

4. Blood banking professionals can minimize liability from litigation by:
   A. Knowing the legal bases for liability
   B. Following published regulations and guidelines
   C. Disclosing all information about patients and donors
   D. Practicing good medicine
   E. None of the above

5. All issues about transfusion-transmitted diseases:
   A. Have already been litigated
   B. Always result in plaintiff verdicts
   C. Never have provided for any protection for defendants
   D. Are known and avoidable
   E. Are evolving and will continue to result in litigation in the foreseeable future.

Answers to Review Questions

1. E (pp 490, 492, 493)
2. B (p 489)
3. E (p 494)
4. B (p 493)
5. E (p 493)

References

1. Randall, CH, Jr: Medicolegal Problems in Blood Transfusion. Joint Blood Council, Washington, DC, 1962. Reprinted by the Committee on Blood, American Medical Association, Chicago, 1963.
2. Rabkin, B, and Rabkin, MS: Individual and institutional liability for transfusion-acquired diseases. An update. JAMA 256:2242, 1986.
3. Administrative Procedure Act, 60 Statutes 237–244, 5 USC Sections 551–559, 1988.
4. Code of Federal Regulations: Food and Drug Administration, Title 21, Parts 200–299 and 600–699. US Government Printing Office, Washington, DC, 1992.
5. Standards for Blood Banks and Transfusion Services, ed 14. American Association of Blood Banks, Arlington, VA, 1990.
6. Kelly, C and Barber, JP: Legal issues in transfusion medicine: Is blood banking a medical profession? Clinics Lab Med 12:819, 1992.

Bibliography

Clark, GM: Legal Issues in Transfusion Medicine. American Association of Blood Banks, Arlington, VA, 1985.
Cooper, JS and Rodrigue, JE: Legal issues in transfusion medicine. Lab Med 23:794, 1992.
Holland, PV: Standards for Blood Banks and Transfusion Services, ed 14. American Association of Blood Banks, Arlington, VA, 1990.
Informed Consent. American Association of Blood Banks, Arlington, VA, 1991.
Prosser, WL, Wade, JW, and Schwartz, VE: Torts—Cases and Materials. ed 7. Foundation Press, Mineola, NY, 1980.
Rabkin, B and Rabkin, MS: Individual and institutional liability for transfusion-acquired disease: An update. JAMA 256:2242, 1986.

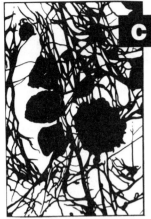

CHAPTER 27

Technologic Advances and Future Trends in Blood Banking

Chantal Ricaud Harrison, MD

OBJECTIVES

Upon completion of this chapter, the learner should be able to:

1 Describe the principles and applications of recombinant DNA technology.

2 Describe how plasma proteins are produced by recombinant DNA technology.

3 Name proteins that are produced by DNA technology and their use in diagnostics or therapeutics.

4 Describe the techniques of dot blot and restriction fragment length polymorphism testing and list the types of diagnostic use they are best suited for.

5 Define the polymerase chain reaction.

6 Define oligonucleotide typing.

7 Describe how monoclonal antibodies are made.

8 Name some diagnostic and therapeutic uses of monoclonal antibodies.

9 Name some lymphokines and identify their functions and the cells that produce them.

10 Define lymphokine-activated killer cell therapy.

11 Describe how antithymocyte and antilymphocytic globulins are prepared.

12 Name some diseases in which intravenous immunoglobulin therapy is effective.

13 Identify the special requirements of the transfusion support of patients who received a bone marrow transplantation.

14 List some of the advantages that peripheral blood stem cell collection has over bone marrow harvest.

15 Name some of the types of processing that may be done on bone marrow.

16 Name some of the types of tissues that are transplanted.

17 List advantages that autologous blood has over allogeneic blood.

18 Define directed donation.

19 List some of the problems that must be resolved in designing a home transfusion program.

We are undergoing a period of rapid evolution in transfusion medicine. Recent developments on both the scientific and socioeconomic fronts are driving this evolution. Owing to the availability of specific blood components and massive education efforts, there has been an almost complete acceptance by physicians of more and more specific therapy in transfusion medicine. Whole blood transfusions now represent a minimal fraction of transfusion therapy. The occurrence of a new disease, acquired immunodeficiency syndrome (AIDS), has heightened the patients' awareness of the risks of transfusion-transmitted diseases. The concept of limiting donor exposures in order to lessen the risk of transfusion-transmitted disease has gained acceptance. This has been instrumental in the amazing growth in use of single-donor apheresis platelets instead of multiple-platelet units derived from whole blood. The Tax Equity and Fiscal Responsibility Act (TEFRA) was passed in 1982 in response to uncontrolled inflation of health care costs. This led to the subsequent establishment of the prospective payments system for reimbursement of Medicare services based on diagnosis-related groups (DRGs). Concerns about the quality of health care are being addressed by the establishment of quality-assurance committees and the requirement by the Joint Commission on Accreditation of Healthcare Organizations (JCAHO) that every blood component transfused be evaluated for appropriateness and justification of use. In 1988 Congress enacted a Clinical Laboratory Improvement Act (CLIA '88) to be implemented by the Health Care Financing Administration (HFCA). This will have considerable impact on the management of blood banks and transfusion services. These forces all converge toward a more specific and rational application of transfusion practices and prepare the way for acceptance of specific substitutes of nonhuman origin as they gradually appear on the market. Synthetic substitutes for almost every component of blood are currently being developed, and as a result of recent discoveries and technologic advances, some of these have recently become available as safe, cost-effective products. In addition, new therapies such as bone marrow and organ transplantation and immunotherapy that are currently restricted to a few specialized research centers will become more widespread. The impact of all these factors on the practice of blood banking, and particularly on independent blood centers, will be great. Blood centers will need to diversify and to adapt to these changes if they are to survive.

In this chapter the technologic advances that may influence the practice of blood banking are reviewed in detail, and possible ways of preparing for anticipated changes are discussed.

Technologic Advances

The rapid progress of research in recombinant DNA and hybridoma technology in the last few years has brought a revolution in the production of therapeutic plasma components and laboratory diagnostic tools. Better understanding of the physiology of the immune system is leading to novel therapeutic approaches to certain cancers and aplastic anemia. Immunoglobulin preparations made to be injected intravenously have become available and been shown to be effective in the treatment of a variety of diseases. The following sections describe the technical background and current applications of genetic engineering, monoclonal antibody production, and immunotherapy.

GENETIC ENGINEERING TECHNOLOGY

Genetic engineering, also referred to as recombinant DNA technology, relies on the ability to isolate fragments of DNA from different sources and to splice them together. These DNA fragments may originate from two different organisms within the same species or from different species. The ability to isolate a specific gene and to transfer it into a different host leads to two types of application: (1) the gene can be expressed in the host cell and the cell turned into a factory of the protein coded by that gene, or (2) the gene can be cloned to produce large quantities of identical fragments of DNA, which, once labeled with radioactive or nonradioactive tracers, can be used as a diagnostic tool to detect complementary strands of DNA or RNA in diagnostic material. The introduction to basic molecular genetics and its terminology, which follows, aids in the understanding of the recombinant DNA technology applications.

Description of Recombinant DNA Technology

The duplication of a length of DNA occurs by the process of unwinding the two strands of the double helix and adding complementary bases to each strand through the action of the enzyme DNA polymerase. When a gene is to be expressed, a complementary RNA strand, called a messenger RNA (mRNA), is produced through the process of transcription with the enzyme RNA polymerase. This RNA, through the process of translation, will direct the formation of a polypeptide by cytoplasmic organelles called ribosomes. An enzyme, reverse transcriptase, which allows the formation of complementary DNA from RNA, was described in 1977.[1] The functions of these enzymes are illustrated in Figure 27–1. Other enzymes that allow manipulation of the DNA are restriction endonucleases, exonucleases, and ligases. Restriction endonucleases, first described in 1970,[2] are bacterial enzymes that cleave the DNA whenever a specific sequence between four and six base pairs is encountered. Each enzyme has a characteristic sequence that it recognizes. A diagram of the recognition of a specific sequence by the restriction endonuclease Eco R1, a restriction enzyme derived from *Escherichia coli,* is shown in Figure 27–2. An exonuclease is an enzyme that attaches to one end of a DNA fragment and clips off bases one by one continuously until an area pro-

```
         ↓
---AGCTTACCG GAATTC GTAATGA---
                                        + Eco RI
---TCGAATGGC CTTAAG CATTACT---
         ↑

---AGCTTACCGG          AATTCGTAATGA---
                  and
---TCGAATGGCCTTAA          GCATTACT---
```

FIGURE 27–2 The recognition site of the restriction endonuclease Eco R1 is boxed. When cutting DNA, Eco R1 produces fragments with "sticky" ends that can be religated easily with other fragments cut with the same restriction enzyme.

tected by a protein is found. A ligase is an enzyme that attaches two DNA fragments.

Genes can be introduced into host cells through the means of vectors such as bacteriophages, plasmids, or cosmids (Fig. 27–3). A library of all of the genes of a single organism can be created by introducing all the genes into a population of bacteria. There are two types of libraries: the genomic library and the complementary DNA (cDNA) library. A genomic library is produced by cutting all the DNA in a single cell with a restriction endonuclease and inserting it into a population of bacteria. A cDNA library is produced by isolating all mRNA from a cell and synthesizing the cDNA complementary to all the mRNA through the use of reverse transcriptase. These cDNA are then introduced into the bacterial population. A genomic library will contain all the genes of the particular cell involved, whereas a cDNA library will contain only the genes that are expressed, because the source of the genetic material is the mRNA. In addition, the cDNA sequence in eukaryotic cells is different from the genomic DNA. Eukaryotic cells are cells in which the DNA is contained within a nucleus and separated from the cytoplasm by a nuclear membrane. Most multicellular organisms and some unicellular organisms, such as

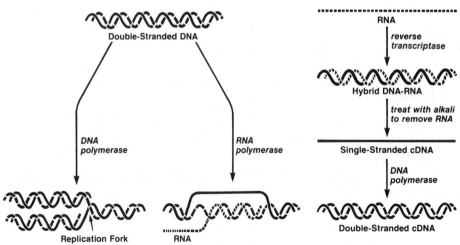

FIGURE 27–1 Enzymes involved in DNA and RNA replication: DNA polymerase produces two double-stranded DNA from one double-stranded DNA by gradually unwinding the strands and pairing nucleotides with each strand. RNA polymerase produces single-stranded RNA from double-stranded DNA by unwinding a small length of DNA and pairing nucleotides with one strand. Reverse transcriptase creates hybrid RNA-DNA from an RNA template. After alkali treatment to remove the RNA strand, DNA polymerase will convert the single-stranded cDNA into a double-stranded cDNA.

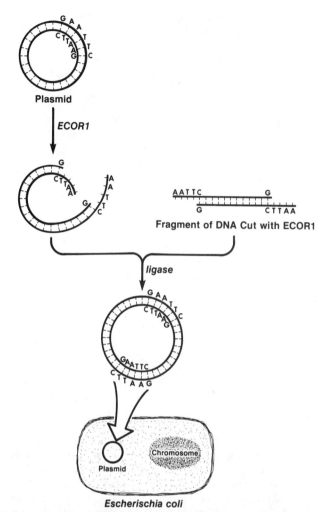

FIGURE 27–3 A fragment of foreign DNA, which was cut with Eco R1, is ligated to a plasmid that has been cut open with Eco R1. The chimeric plasmid is then introduced into the bacteria *Escherichia coli.*

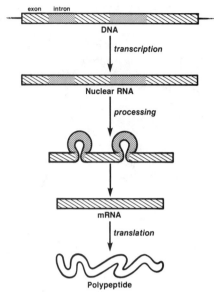

FIGURE 27–4 Production of mRNA in eukaryotic cells: The DNA contains noncoding sequences called introns. The initial RNA contains corresponding sequences to the introns and is processed to remove these sequences and to form mRNA.

yeast and fungi, are eukaryotes. On the other hand, bacteria and blue-green algae are prokaryotes; their DNA is not separated from the cytoplasm. In eukaryotic cells the genes contain noncoding regions, called introns, and coding regions, called exons. The original RNA produced from the DNA, called heteronuclear RNA, is a copy of all the introns and all the exons. This RNA is then processed, and the introns are spliced out to produce the functional mRNA that will leave the nucleus and be the information source to produce the polypeptide (Fig. 27–4). Thus, a cDNA library contains only the exons of the original cellular DNA, and a genomic library contains both the exons and the introns.

The critical step in the definition of a gene library is the identification of the specific gene cloned in a bacterial colony. This is called screening. Screening can be performed by direct detection of the gene through hybridization with a natural DNA fragment or a synthetic DNA fragment, or even an mRNA. Screening can also be done, if the gene is expressed, through detection of the biologic activity of the expression

protein or through an immunologic method. Once the gene of interest has been identified and characterized, it can be amplified by growing the host cell in which it has been transferred, a process called cloning. It can then be introduced into an appropriate host for expression and protein production or labeled for the production of probes for diagnostic use. The general scheme of the different aspects of recombinant DNA technology and their applications is depicted in Figure 27–5.

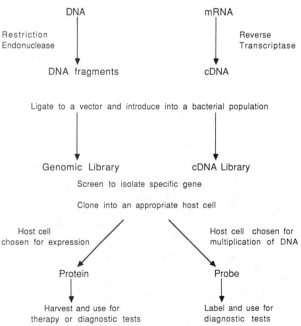

FIGURE 27–5 General scheme of recombinant DNA technology.

Plasma Protein Production by Recombinant DNA Technology

Once a gene for a specific protein of interest has been isolated, the crucial step is to select the appropriate host for expression. Some bacteria, such as *E. coli*, will produce the protein but not secrete it. To harvest the protein, the bacteria must be lysed and the protein purified to remove bacterial contaminants. Other bacteria, such as *Bacillus subtilis*, will secrete the protein into the culture medium, which makes purification much simpler. The function of some proteins depends on posttranslational modifications such as glycosylation, proper folding of the protein, and cross-linking with disulfide bonds. The intracellular environment of bacteria is not conducive to the formation of disulfide bonds, and bacteria do not have the enzymatic ability to glycosylate. Mammalian cells, on the other hand, are difficult and expensive to grow but provide advantages such as secretion of the desired protein, disulfide bond formation, and complex glycosylation. Table 27-1 describes the relative advantages and disadvantages of the different expression systems.

Albumin The gene for albumin was first cloned in 1981 by identifying the appropriate cDNA from a cDNA library produced from human liver cells.[3] Albumin has been synthesized experimentally from bacterial and yeast expression systems. A British brewing company is apparently scaling up the process for production of human albumin in yeast and expects to introduce a therapeutic albumin in the 1990s. It is unclear at this time whether this method will produce an albumin that will be competitive in price with the albumin produced by conventional fractionation methods from human plasma. Inasmuch as the albumin produced by fractionation is pasteurized and is well known not to transmit diseases, albumin produced by recombinant DNA technology will not offer additional safety advantages. Thus, production costs will be the only factor determining the market share of the recombinant DNA technology albumin.

Factor VIII The gene for factor VIII was isolated and cloned in 1984 by two groups independently. Wood et al. and Gitschier et al.[4,5] identified the gene for factor VIII from a human genomic library prepared from cells of an individual who had four X chromosomes. On the other hand, Toole et al.[6] first identified human liver as the site of synthesis for factor VIII and then constructed a human liver cDNA library

and isolated a cDNA clone for the factor VIII gene. Recently two different recombinant DNA factor VIII, based on the two cloning methodologies described earlier, have been licensed in the United States. One preparation is produced in Chinese hamster ovary cells, the other in baby hamster kidney cells. The two products differ only by one amino acid and appear to be equally effective and well tolerated. Both products are as effective as the human-derived factor VIII, and early concerns that they might be more antigenic appear unfounded.[7,8] Human-derived factor VIII has been fraught with a serious drawback owing to the transmission of viral diseases, especially hepatitis and human immunodeficiency virus (HIV) infections. Modifications in the production of factor VIII from human plasma, such as affinity purification, slow heat treatment, solvent-detergent inactivation, and screening of donors for anti-HIV have apparently successfully addressed the transmission of HIV infection and possibly of hepatitis C.[9] Recent reports, however, suggest that hepatitis A may be transmitted by human-derived factor VIII.[10] The possibility of transmission of viruses resistant to the inactivation processes or the inadvertent failure of these processes during manufacturing will remain. Factor VIII produced by recombinant DNA technology will probably rapidly replace human-derived factor VIII, if priced competitively.

Other Coagulation Factors Factor IX is a serine protease, the deficiency of which causes hemophilia B. It is a much smaller and simpler protein than factor VIII, and its gene has been cloned by multiple groups by both the genomic DNA and the cDNA methods. Although several companies are developing factor IX production by recombinant DNA technology, this production has low priority owing to the much lower demand for factor IX than for factor VIII. In effect, hemophilia B is much less common than hemophilia A and usually much less severe, so specific factor therapy is in less demand.

Tissue plasminogen activator, a thrombolytic agent, has been produced by recombinant DNA technology. It may have a significant impact on the therapy of coronary heart disease and affect the overall demand of blood for open-heart surgeries.

Although the genes for factor X, prothrombin, fibrinogen, and antithrombin III have been cloned, commercial production is not contemplated at this time owing to the lack of demand.

Erythropoietin The gene for erythropoietin was cloned and expressed in mammalian cells in 1985,[11] and recombinant human erythropoietin (rHuEPO) is currently available. Clinical trials have demonstrated the effectiveness of this recombinant DNA produced hormone in the correction of anemia in patients with end-stage renal disease.[12,13] This therapy has almost completely replaced red cell transfusions in patients receiving renal dialysis. It appears that rHuEPO is also effective in treating anemia secondary to zidovudine therapy in patients with AIDS. Another application of

TABLE 27-1 RELATIVE ADVANTAGES AND DISADVANTAGES OF DIFFERENT EXPRESSION SYSTEMS

	Bacteria	Yeasts	Mammalian Cells
Ease of growth	++++	+++	+
Secretion of protein	+/-	+	+
Glycosylation	-	+/-	+
Disulfide bond formation	-	-	+

erythropoietin therapy may be in the context of the anemia of prematurity.[14] Erythropoietin is being considered in the management of patients undergoing certain elective surgery to allow for the collection of large quantities of autologous blood.

Colony-Stimulating Factors Other hematologically active hormones, such as granulocyte colony-stimulating factor (G-CSF) and granulocyte macrophage colony-stimulating factors (GM-CSF), have been produced by recombinant DNA technology. Therapy with G-CSF or GM-CSF or both has successfully reduced the granulocytopenic period induced by chemotherapy in patients with certain cancers or during bone marrow transplantation. This therapy has great potential for reducing hospitalization and transfusion requirements of oncology patients. It also plays a role in increasing the yield of peripheral blood stem cell collection.

Miscellaneous Plasma Proteins and Vaccines Insulin, growth hormone, and interferon-alpha produced by recombinant DNA technology are currently marketed. Several recombinant DNA–derived hepatitis B vaccines have been introduced since 1986, and these have entirely replaced the human-derived vaccine. The future holds great potential with respect to the production of vaccines by recombinant DNA technology.

Diagnostic Use of Recombinant DNA Technology: Techniques

The ability to isolate, characterize, and amplify a gene by cloning may lead to great diagnostic advances. If the DNA fragments can be labeled with radioactive material such as ^{32}P or ^{35}S or with a nonisotopic marker, as in a biotin-avidin technique, then they can be used as probes to detect the corresponding gene or mRNA by hybridization in diagnostic material.

Dot Blot There are two different approaches in using DNA probes for diagnostic purposes. The first approach will detect the presence or absence of a specific DNA or RNA fragment through hybridization or lack of hybridization with a labeled probe and is usually performed as a spot or dot blot technique. This technique is particularly well suited to the detection of viral DNA or RNA or to the detection of a gene deletion such as in alpha-thalassemia.

Restriction Fragment Length Polymorphism The second technique, called restriction fragment length polymorphism (RFLP) analysis, can detect strategically located point mutations in DNA. First the DNA material to be tested is cut into fragments with a restriction endonuclease; then the DNA fragments are separated according to size by gel electrophoresis. The DNA fragments are then transferred or blotted onto a membrane and denatured to render them single stranded. Next, hybridization is performed with a labeled probe, and the DNA fragments containing complementary sequences to the probe will appear as

bands in a specific location representing their size. When a point mutation has occurred within or near a gene and has created either a new cleavage site for the restriction endonuclease used, or the disappearance of a cleavage site, the gene will be associated with a different DNA fragment size. Figure 27–6 illustrates the general principle behind RFLP analysis. This technique, called Southern blotting, is particularly suited for the detection of polymorphism in DNA and is very valuable in genetic screening and parentage testing.

Polymerase Chain Reaction Described in 1986, polymerase chain reaction (PCR) is an in vitro method of amplification of a targeted segment of DNA.[15] It greatly increases the sensitivity of detection of the targeted DNA segment. Polymerase chain reaction is based on the fact that DNA polymerase cannot initiate DNA replication. It can only add deoxyribonucleotides to an already started fragment of DNA. These initiating fragments are called primers. The originality of the concept of PCR lies in the use of a set of primers that flank the DNA segment of interest and allow DNA synthesis to proceed from both DNA strands at the same time in opposite directions. A diagram of PCR is depicted in Figure 27–7. The DNA in the diagnostic material is heated to between 95°C and 100°C to separate the DNA strands; then the temperature is lowered to between 45°C and 55°C to allow annealing of the primers. The primers are added at a high concentration, so that the original DNA will preferentially anneal to the primers, rather than back to each other. The temperature is then raised to around 72°C to maximize the efficiency of DNA polymerase in extending the primers. These heating and cooling cycles are repeated, with each cycle approximately doubling the number of DNA segments present. Each cycle takes approximately 2 minutes and the duplication occurring over 30 cycles is theoretically a billionfold (2^{30}). The discovery of thermostable DNA polymerase, which is stable at high temperature, simplified the methodology by obviating the need to add fresh polymerase at each cycle. Automated thermal cycling machines are now available. Once PCR is performed, the PCR product, if present (i.e., if the targeted DNA segment was present in the original diagnostic material), can be detected by a dot blot technique. Alternatively, because the PCR product consists of DNA fragments of identical size, it can be detected after electrophoresis and ethidium bromide staining as a single bright band.

Oligonucleotide Typing Also referred to as the sequence-specific oligonucleotide probe (SSOP) technique, oligonucleotide typing is the use of synthetic probes of approximately 20 bases in length. These probes are used under hybridization conditions with high stringency; that is, conditions such that they will only bind to DNA sequences that are a perfect match. These probes are used as a set of allele-specific oligonucleotide probes with a dot blot technique, often after PCR amplification of the gene of interest.

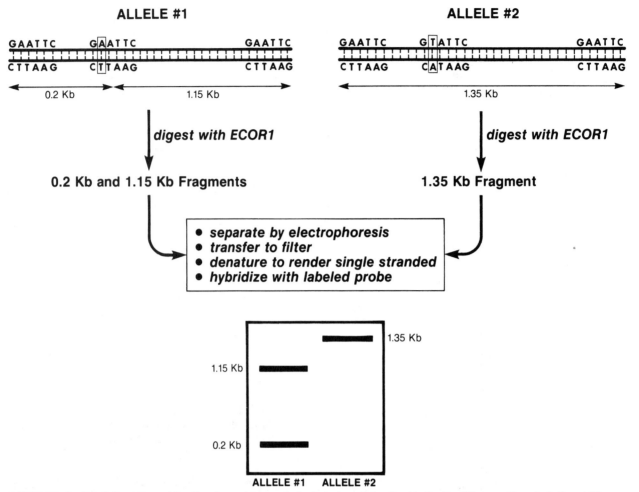

FIGURE 27–6 Restriction fragment length polymorphism analysis: A single mutation (box) in the Eco R1 recognition site in the middle area of allele #1 results in a noncutting area in allele #2. Digestion of the DNA with Eco R1 gives two fragments (0.2 Kb and 1.15 Kb) with allele #1 and only one fragment (1.35 Kb) with allele #2. After Southern blot analysis with a labeled DNA probe complementary for the gene studied, the different alleles can be identified from the pattern of the bands.

Diagnostic Use of Recombinant DNA Technology: Applications

Viral Infection Screening The use of hybridization techniques with specific viral nucleic acid probes is increasing steadily in the study of viral infectious diseases. Of interest to blood banking are mostly hepatitis B virus, hepatitis C virus, HIV, and cytomegalovirus (CMV) infections. The use of a DNA probe for hepatitis B virus DNA (HBV DNA) using dot blot hybridization is as sensitive, if not more so, than the conventional method of detecting hepatitis B surface antigen (HB$_s$Ag) in the sera of individuals infected with hepatitis B. In effect, several studies have demonstrated the presence of HBV DNA by dot blot hybridization in HB$_s$Ag-negative patients with chronic liver disease.[16,17] In addition, HB$_s$Ag and hepatitis B core antigen (HB$_c$Ag) have been produced from recombinant DNA sources, and tests for hepatitis B markers based on these recombinant antigens are widely available, bringing an improved specificity to the testing.

The detection of hepatitis C viral RNA after PCR amplification has become the "gold standard" for the diagnosis of active infection with hepatitis C.[18] The testing for anti-HCV by enzyme immunoassay is based on the availability of recombinant DNA to produce hepatitis C antigens.

A very small proportion of helper T cells infected by HIV can be detected following viral gene amplification by PCR.[19] If the method can be applied to mass screening, it may have great implications in the detection of carriers during the latency period before HIV antigen or HIV antibody is produced. It is too early to say whether this will be applicable to blood screening. HIV antigens produced by recombinant DNA are now available and are taking their place as a more specific reagent for the detection of anti-HIV.

Cytomegalovirus DNA probes are very specific and sensitive and can detect CMV in the urine or buffy coats of patients in 2 to 3 days, whereas cultures require at least 3 weeks. It does not appear, at this time, that this technique is capable of providing a practi-

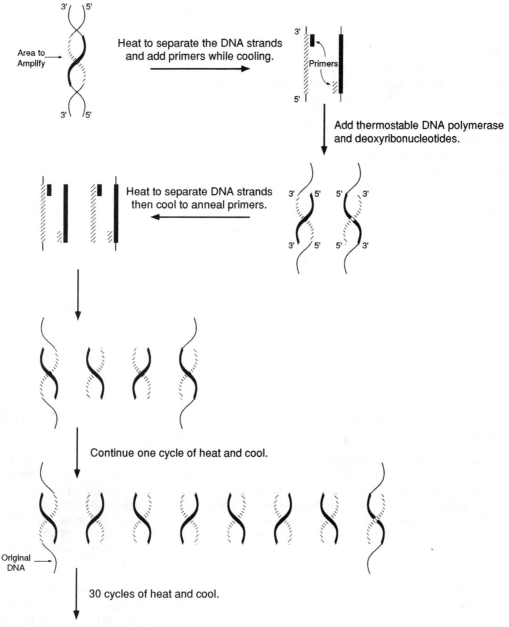

FIGURE 27–7 Diagram of the principle of polymerase chain reaction: Each heat and cool cycle results in the doubling of the DNA segment that is amplified. The primers are selected to limit the amplification segment, one on each end. After 30 cycles, the original DNA segment will have been amplified 2^{30} or one billionfold. All amplified segments will have the same size.

cal alternative to CMV-antibody testing for blood screening.

Genetic Screening The number of genetic diseases that can be diagnosed by DNA analysis is continuously increasing. Those of particular interest to blood bankers are the hemoglobinopathies, mostly sickle cell anemia and thalassemia, and hemophilias A and B. All these diseases can now be diagnosed prenatally during the ninth to 10th weeks of pregnancy by testing samples obtained by chorionic villi sampling. If widely applied for prenatal counseling, this technique has the potential to affect greatly the blood needs in

areas where these genetic diseases occur frequently. Indeed, this has already occurred in certain areas of the world, such as Sardinia.[20]

HLA Typing Sequence-specific oligonucleotide probes, in conjunction with PCR amplification, are widely used in identifying alleles at the DQ_α and DR_β loci. These techniques are more specific than the classic lymphocytotoxicity method and have become the reference method for the HLA antigens nomenclature. The national marrow donor program is embarking on a project of typing marrow donors with molecular biology techniques. SSOP will uncover mismatches at the gene level that are not detected by immunologic methods. The actual clinical significance of these mismatches in organ and bone marrow transplantation is yet to be determined.

Parentage Testing Restriction fragment length polymorphism analysis has a great future in the determination of parentage. New polymorphic sites identified by a specific probe and a specific restriction endonuclease are continuously being described. Work still needs to be done in standardization of the methods, availability of the probes, family studies to define the inheritance pattern, population studies to obtain frequencies of the different alleles at each polymorphic site, and calculation methods.

Cancer Diagnosis Diagnostic molecular pathology is now a recognized tool in the diagnosis of certain cancers. The clonality of a lymphoid proliferation can be ascertained through the detection of a clonal rearrangement of the immunoglobulin (Ig) chain genes in B-cell tumors and of the T-cell receptor β gene for T-cell tumors. The bcr:abl gene detection in chronic myelogenous leukemia is more sensitive and specific than the classic detection of the Philadelphia chromosome by karyotyping. These two examples of the application of recombinant DNA technology to the diagnosis of cancer are only the "tip of the iceberg" in this rapidly developing field.

IMMUNOGLOBULIN PRODUCTION BY HYBRIDOMA TECHNOLOGY

The description by Kohler and Milstein[21] in 1975 of a method to produce monoclonal antibodies by fusing a myeloma cell with lymphocytes from an immunized animal has brought a profound change in the production of antibodies for diagnostic and therapeutic purposes. Until then, antibodies were obtained by purifying serum from immunized animals or humans and consisted of a mixture of antibodies with different affinities and biologic activities, dependent on the immune responses of the source. Each animal or human source represented a unique reagent that could not be exactly duplicated. With hybridoma technology, all the antibody molecules in the preparation derive from a single clone of B lymphocytes and are identical.

Description of Hybridoma Technology

Myeloma cells are neoplastic plasma cells and can be grown in culture indefinitely. By fusing B lymphocytes from immunized animals with a myeloma cell, one can obtain a hybrid cell that can be grown in culture and will secrete the antibody produced by the original B lymphocyte. Most plasma cell myelomas secrete their own monoclonal antibody of unknown specificity. A hybrid cell thus would make two types of heavy chains and two types of light chains, which could lead to a mixed population of antibodies, inasmuch as the chains from the two different cells of origin could associate with each other. However, nonsecreting variants of myeloma cells exist and make an ideal fusing partner, because the hybrid cell can secrete only the antibody from the fused B lymphocyte. To produce hybrid cells, one mixes the myeloma cells with spleen, lymph node, or peripheral blood mononuclear cells from the immunized animal in the presence of polyethylene glycol, an agent that promotes membrane fusion. The myeloma cell lines used for fusion have been selected so that they are unable to grow in a medium containing hypoxanthine, aminopterin, and thymidine (HAT medium). They lack the enzyme hypoxanthine-guanine phosphoribosyltransferase (i.e., they are HPRT$^-$). This enzyme is part of a salvage pathway for the production of nucleic acids from exogenous purines and is necessary for survival if aminopterin, an inhibitor of the de novo synthesis of nucleic acids, is present in the medium. By growing the cell mixture in the HAT medium after fusion, unfused myeloma cells will not survive. Only the fused cells, which are complemented for the HPRT enzyme by the lymphocyte partner, will survive. The HPRT$^-$ cells, also called drug-marked myeloma cells, are first selected by adding a cytotoxic purine analog such as 6-thioguanine (6-TG) or 8-azaguanine (8-AG) to the culture media. HPRT$^+$ cells will convert these purine analogs to substituted nucleic acids, which will kill them, and only HPRT$^-$ cells will survive. After fusion the cells are distributed into multiple-well cell culture plates at such a dilution that no more than one fused cell will be present in a well. After several weeks of culture, the supernatant is assayed for the presence of antibody. If a desirable antibody is found, the hybrid cell can then be propagated to produce a continuing source of monoclonal antibody. Although the final reward is high, when a hybrid producing a good antibody is found, only a fraction of the hybrid cells formed, less than 1 per 1000, may be productive. This technique, first developed with mouse myeloma cells, has been readily extended to rat myeloma cells. The majority of monoclonal antibodies available are made in rodents. An additional advantage offered by mouse monoclonal antibodies is that they can be made in large quantities by injecting the hybrid cell into the peritoneal cavity of a mouse from the same inbred mouse strain that provided the immunizing lymphocyte. The hybrid cell will grow in the mouse as a tumor and secrete large quantities of monoclonal antibody in the ascitic fluid. A diagram of the different steps involved in the production of monoclonal antibodies is depicted in Figure 27–8.

Extension of these techniques to produce human monoclonal antibodies has been difficult. There are currently no good nonsecreting human myeloma cell lines available as a fusion partner. A successful alternative has been to use lymphoblastoid cells — cells that have been immortalized by infection with the Epstein-Barr virus (EBV) — as a fusion partner or to immortalize B lymphocytes from an immunized human with EBV to serve as the source of a continuous production of human monoclonal antibody.

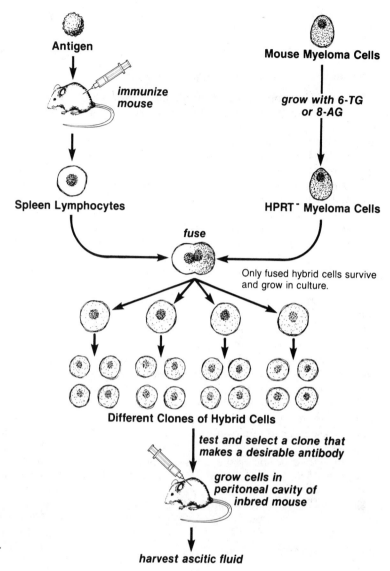

FIGURE 27-8 Production of monoclonal antibodies.

Monoclonal Antibodies for Diagnostic Purposes

Reagents derived from monoclonal antibodies have great advantages over their polyclonal counterpart. They are not contaminated with nonimmunoglobulin serum proteins, they have a consistently reproducible affinity and specificity, and they can theoretically be produced in unlimited quantities over an indefinite period of time. Several monoclonal reagents have been successfully introduced in routine blood groupings such as anti-A, anti-B, anti-D, anti-Le[a], anti-Le[b], anti-M, and antihuman globulin. Monoclonal antibodies with more esoteric specificities toward red cell antigens have also been developed. One can predict a future in which all red cell typing antisera will be originated from monoclonal antibodies. When using monoclonal antisera, one must become familiar with their characteristics. They often have higher affinities than polyclonal reagents and are difficult to elute after absorption.

Numerous monoclonal antibodies to HLA antigens have been produced. At this time their greatest application has been in the investigation of the biochemistry and function of the HLA system. Monoclonal antibodies probably will be soon introduced into routine HLA serotyping. Currently available monoclonal antibodies have high affinities toward small epitopes and detect cross-reactive antigens too readily. Serotyping methods may need to be modified to correct this problem.

Monoclonal antibodies to lymphocyte markers have been an invaluable tool in the dissection of the different functions of the T-lymphocyte subsets and their differentiation. In conjunction with the advent of flow cytometry technology, the availability of standardized monoclonal antibodies has had a major impact in the routine clinical evaluation of a patient's immune status and in the phenotyping of leukemias and lymphomas.

A wide variety of application for monoclonal antibodies exists, from the detection of viral antigens such as Hb$_s$Ag to the immunoassays of hormones and the diagnoses of certain human cancers.

Monoclonal Antibodies for Therapeutic Purposes

Therapeutic applications of monoclonal antibodies are still experimental at this point. Monoclonal antibodies have been produced that are specific for antigens present on some cancer cells, particularly melanomas, breast cancers, leukemias, and colon, pancreas, lung, kidney, ovarian, and testicular cancers. In some cases, remission or decrease in tumor size was obtained after injecting the patient with monoclonal antibodies reacting against their tumor. The cell-killing activity was either directly mediated by the antibody or through toxins such as ricin, diphtheria toxin, or radioisotopes that had been conjugated with the antibody. In the latter case, the antibodies served as a way to deliver the toxic agent directly to the tumor cells. Monoclonal antibodies have been used successfully to treat, in vitro, bone marrow collected from patients with leukemia, in order to kill the leukemic cells before reinfusing the marrow as part of an autologous bone marrow transplantation protocol. In another application to bone marrow transplantation, monoclonal antibodies with specificity against mature T cells have been used to kill the mature T cells from a donor bone marrow preparation, resulting in a striking decrease in graft-versus-host (GVH) disease in the recipient.

All these therapeutic applications of monoclonal antibodies are still in their infancy. Much work still remains to be done in defining effective dosage, treatment protocols, and newer antibody specificities.

IMMUNOTHERAPY

The existence of soluble factors secreted by mononuclear cells, lymphocytes, monocytes, or macrophages that regulate the immune response (cellular and humoral), hemopoiesis, and tumor cell cytotoxicity has long been recognized. Cell culture media "conditioned" by leukocytes were often the magic ingredient in the in vitro demonstration of a variety of immune responses. However, the exact characterization of these soluble factors, now termed lymphokines, has just recently become a reality, mostly as a result of the powerful tool offered by recombinant DNA technology. The lymphokine family includes several interferons, interleukins, tumor necrosis factors, and colony-stimulating factors. Table 27–2 summarizes the cell origin and known activities of the different lymphokines that are currently well characterized. The availability of large quantities of pure preparations, from recombinant DNA origin, of each lymphokine has opened the way to a much greater understanding of immune regulation and to newer therapies that involve modulation of the immune response.

Lymphokine-Activated Killer Cell Therapy

Lymphokine-activated killer (LAK) cell therapy has evolved from the serendipitous finding that human peripheral blood lymphocytes, after incubation with interleukin-2 (IL-2), had a very potent antitumor activity.[22] Previously known as T-cell growth factor (TCGF), IL-2 is a 15,000-dalton glycoprotein secreted by activated helper T cells in response to various stimuli such as bacteria, alloantigens, and lectins. It stimulates the clonal expansion of certain T-cell subpopulations and enhances cytotoxic T-cell activity. It is a necessary factor in the long-term culture of T cells. The LAK cells have been shown to be different from other cells involved in the killing of tumor cells, such as natural killer (NK) cells and cytotoxic T lymphocytes (CTLs). After establishing a successful protocol in the treatment of a variety of cancers in mice, Rosenberg et al.[23] extended the therapy to humans with metastatic or advanced unresectable cancer. The treatment consists of infusions of large doses of IL-2 (100,000 U/kg every 8 hours) for 4 to 5 days, followed by daily lymphocytopheresis for 5 days. The lymphocytes collected are incubated with IL-2 for 3 to 4 days and transfused back to the patient with additional intravenous IL-2 infusion. Complete or partial response is obtained in a significant number of patients. The tumors that seem most sensitive to this therapy are renal cell carcinoma, melanoma, non-Hodgkin's lymphoma, and colorectal carcinoma. However, the toxicity of the therapy is high. Patients experience fever, chills, nausea, diarrhea, diffuse erythematous rash with desquamation, liver dysfunction, capillary leakage leading to fluid retention and sudden weight gain, and occasionally life-threatening hypotensive episodes. The mortality rate of LAK cell therapy is approximately 2 percent. The collection of lymphocytes from areas surrounding the tumor itself as a source for LAK cells, along with other methods for improvement, is currently being investigated.

Antithymocyte Serum and Aplastic Anemia

Both antithymocyte globulin (ATG) and antilymphocyte globulin (ALG) have been effective in the modulation of the immune response in organ and bone marrow transplantation. Their use as a conditioning regimen for HLA-incompatible bone marrow transplantation in some patients with aplastic anemia unexpectedly resulted in autologous marrow recovery. This led to the use of ATG or ALG as the sole mode of therapy for aplastic anemia. Both ATG and ALG are polyclonal antibodies raised in horses. For ALG the horses are immunized with intact human thoracic duct lymphocytes,[24] and the recovered serum is absorbed with human placenta and human red cell stroma. To produce ATG, homogenized fragments of human thymus removed during pediatric surgery are injected into the horses, and the serum is absorbed with human red cell stroma and human plasma and further puri-

TABLE 27–2 **LYMPHOKINES: GENE LOCATION, CELLS OF ORIGIN, AND FUNCTIONS**

Lymphokine (Previous Names)	Chromosome	Cells of Origin	Functions
IL-1α and β (lymphocyte-activating factor, endogenous pyrogen)	2	Macrophages, astrocytes, antigen-presenting cells, endothelial cells	Fever and acute phase response, release of neutrophils from bone marrow, helper T-cell activation, IL-6 production, B-cell differentiation
IL-2 (T-cell growth factor)	4	Activated helper T cells	T-cell proliferation, induction of LAK cells
IL-3 (multi-CSF burst-promoting activity, CFU-stimulating factor)	5	Activated helper T cells	Stem cell differentiation into all blood cell lines, induction of 20α hydroxysteroid dehydrogenase, mast cell proliferation
IL-4 (B-cell growth factor I, mast cell growth factor II)	5	Activated helper T cells	B-cell growth and differentiation, IgG$_1$ and IgE production, mucosal mast cell proliferation, T-cell proliferation
IL-5 (B-cell growth factor II, eosinophil differentiation factor)	5	Activated helper T cells	Eosinophil proliferation
IL-6 (interferon β2, B-cell stimulatory factor 2, hepatocyte-stimulating factor)	7	Macrophages, T cells, fibroblasts, endothelial cells	B-cell differentiation, fever and acute phase response, enhancement of activity of IL-3, M-CSF, and GM-CSF
IL-7 (lymphopoietin-1)	8	Bone marrow stromal cells	Proliferation of B-lymphocyte precursors, T-cell proliferation
Interferon α and β (IFN-α/β)	9	All virus-infected cells	Antiviral activity, enhancement of MHC class I antigen expression
Interferon γ (IFN-γ) (macrophage-activation factor)	12	Activated T cells, large granular lymphocytes	Antiviral activity, enhancement of MHC class I and II antigen expression, macrophage activation
Tumor necrosis factor α (TNF-α) (cachectin) Tumor necrosis factor β (TNF-β) (lymphotoxin)	6	Macrophages (TNF-α), activated T cells (TNF-β)	Fever and acute phase response, hemorrhagic necrosis of tumors, delayed hypersensitivity reactions, IL-1 production, induction of septic shock, induction of weight loss and muscle wasting
G-CSF	17	Macrophages, endothelial cells, fibroblasts, T cells	Differentiation and activation of neutrophils
GM-CSF	5	Macrophages, endothelial cells, activated T cells	Stimulates production of macrophages, neutrophils, eosinophils, and megakaryocytes
M-CSF	5	T cells	Production and activation of macrophages

CFU = colony-forming unit; CSF = colony stimulating factor; IL = interleukin; LAK = lymphocyte activated killer; MHC = major histocompatibility complex.

fied to recover the IgG fraction by passage through an ion exchange resin.[25] Patients receiving ALG often will develop a positive direct antihuman globulin test result with a positive eluate mimicking an autoantibody, and occasionally a positive indirect antihuman globulin test result causes difficulties in crossmatching. This has been attributed to cross-reactive antihorse antibody in the antihuman globulin reagents and can be resolved by absorbing the antihuman globulin reagent with ALG-coated red blood cells[26] or neutralizing the antihorse activity by adding a small amount of horse serum to the antihuman globulin reagent.

In aplastic anemia, therapy with ALG or ATG re-sults in a response rate of approximately 50 percent. The overall ultimate survival of patients with aplastic anemia is similar with ALG or ATG therapy as with allogeneic bone marrow transplantation. However, when only patients less than age 20 are compared, allogeneic bone marrow transplantation is clearly superior to ALG or ATG therapy with respect to overall survival. Although most patients receiving ALG or ATG develop serum sickness within 2 to 3 weeks of therapy, this side effect is minor compared with the morbidity associated with bone marrow transplantation. Thus, ALG or ATG is considered as the initial therapy for patients older than 20 years of age with severe aplastic anemia and for those younger than 20 years of age who do not have an HLA-identical sibling.[27]

Although the mechanism of action of ALG or ATG in aplastic anemia classically has been attributed to its lymphocytotoxicity, there is evidence that it has direct stimulatory activity on certain lymphocytes, which results in the production of lymphokines that enhance erythroid progenitor cells.[28] Abnormal lymphokine production has been demonstrated in patients with aplastic anemia.[29,30] Further refinements in the immunotherapy of aplastic anemia may involve more specific antibody therapy with monoclonal antibodies directed toward a specific mononuclear cell or a lymphokine receptor or specific lymphokine replacement therapy.

Intravenous Immunoglobulin Therapy

Therapy using intravenous immunoglobulin (IVIg) was originally licensed as replacement therapy for patients with primary immunodeficiency. Its use was extended to patients with secondary immunodeficiency and is effective in reducing the number of infections in patients with chronic lymphocytic leukemia or who have received bone marrow transplants. The unexpected finding that IVIg was effective in the treatment of patients with idiopathic thrombocytopenic purpura[31] has led to its use in a wide variety of autoimmune disorders and some diseases of unknown etiologies. These trials have met with a variable degree of success. A Consensus Development Conference on the safe and effective use of IVIg was held by the National Institutes of Health in 1990. A summary of this conference is available.[32] Adverse reactions with IVIg infusions are minimal. However, a potential deleterious effect may result from the erroneous diagnosis of an infectious disease based on the detection of an antibody to an infectious agent, when this antibody may have been passively acquired through IVIg infusion. Spurious clusters of hepatitis C infections have been reported, which were traced to IVIg infusion.[33]

Future Trends

When the applications of these new technologies have been fully developed and incorporated into routine therapy, synthetic substitutes for human red cells and plasma proteins will replace much of the blood components currently provided by blood banks. The demand for human platelets will last longer, because synthetic substitutes for platelets are not as far in development at this time. One can predict that a shift from whole blood toward apheresis collection will occur. The demand for specially selected blood components to fulfill specific needs will increase. To survive, blood banks will have to diversify their products and their services.

DIVERSIFICATION OF PRODUCTS

Special Support for Bone Marrow Transplantation

The first attempt at bone marrow transplantation in order to restore hemopoiesis in a human occurred in France in 1959. The modern era of bone marrow transplantation dates back to 1969, when basic concepts such as the need for histocompatibility between donor and recipient, the need to prepare the recipient by total body irradiation and immunosuppression, and the minimal dose of nucleated bone marrow cells needed were understood and applied, resulting in the survival of patients through the acute period following the transplantation. Since then the number of bone marrow transplantations has increased every year to total more than 10,000 throughout the world, greater than 50 percent of which are performed in the United States. The list of diseases for which bone marrow transplantation is considered is growing steadily (Table 27–3). Currently the majority of the transplantations are carried out in patients with either aplastic anemia or malignant hematologic disorders such as acute leukemia, chronic myelogenous leukemia, advanced Hodgkin's disease, and non-Hodgkin's lymphomas. These usually consist of a syngeneic or allogeneic transplant; that is, from an identical twin or from a sibling matched for HLA antigens. A few centers will perform transplantations from family members with one or two mismatched HLA antigens or from a fully matched unrelated donor, identified through the Bone Marrow Donor Registry. In addition, autologous bone marrow transplantation has become a mode of therapy for certain advanced solid tumors such as melanoma, breast cancer, testicular cancer, neuroblastoma, and lymphoma. Bone marrow is obtained from the patient and stored, usually frozen in liquid nitrogen, while the patient is receiving high-dose chemotherapy and radiotherapy that otherwise could not be tolerated because of marrow toxicity. The marrow is then infused back to the patient and will repopulate the bone marrow space.

Patients undergoing bone marrow transplantation, whether allogeneic or autologous, require special blood bank support. As a result of the total body irradiation and chemotherapy required in the preparation for transplantation, these patients are immuno-

TABLE 27–3 DISEASES TREATABLE BY BONE MARROW TRANSPLANTATION

Congenital	Acquired
Thalassemia major	Aplastic anemia
Severe combined immunodeficiency	Acute leukemia
Osteopetrosis	Chronic myelogenous leukemia
Gaucher's disease	Hodgkin's disease
Other inborn errors of metabolism	Non-Hodgkin's lymphoma

suppressed and susceptible to GVH disease, if transfused with blood components that contain live lymphocytes capable of dividing. To prevent this, all blood components must be irradiated. The recommended dose is 25 grey (Gy) (1 Gy is equivalent to 100 rads). This is usually accomplished with a special blood irradiator that contains a cesium radiation source and can deliver such a dose in a few minutes.

Until the donor marrow engrafts, red blood cells and platelets will be needed to keep the hemoglobin level above 9 g/dl and the platelet count above $20,000/\mu l$. Engraftment takes place in 2 to 4 weeks but may be delayed if complications occur. The total red blood cells transfused is not usually very high (6 to 20 units), but the need for platelet support ranges in the hundreds if one considers only random-donor platelets. Platelets are better provided by apheresis. Occasionally a patient will become refractory to platelet therapy owing to HLA antibodies and will require HLA-matched platelets. Blood centers serving bone marrow transplantation services should participate in an HLA-typed platelet donor program. To prevent white cell–mediated febrile transfusion reactions and to minimize the risk of CMV transmission, patients should receive leukoreduced blood components. This can be achieved through the use of specialized filters at the bedside or at the collection facility. Some experimental evidence suggests that alloimmunization to white cell antigens may be avoided if the patient receives only leukoreduced components.

The immunosuppression also results in great susceptibility to infectious diseases. Most patients will routinely receive antibiotics, antifungal agents, and IVIg. Viral infections are of great concern, particularly CMV infection, which results in a serious, often fatal, interstitial pneumonitis during the second to fourth month after the transplant. CMV infection may be caused by a reactivation of a latent infection or acquired by blood transfusion. If both the patient and the bone marrow donor have no evidence of a previous CMV infection (i.e., they demonstrate no antibodies to CMV), then all blood components transfused should be negative for CMV antibodies.

Peripheral Blood Stem Cell Collection

The demonstration in 1975 that stem cells circulated in the blood of humans[34] opened the door for the idea of collecting stem cells through apheresis instead of bone marrow harvest. In 1986 multiple cases of successful hematopoietic reconstitution from peripheral blood stem cells (PBSCs) that had undergone cryopreservation were reported in patients with a variety of oncologic disorders such as acute nonlymphocytic leukemia,[35] Burkitt's lymphoma,[36] and breast cancer.[37] Peripheral blood stem cell transplantation (PBSCT) has several advantages over bone marrow transplantation: (1) the harvesting of peripheral stem cells is less traumatic than bone marrow harvest and

does not require general anesthesia; (2) the engraftment after PBSCT appears to be more rapid; and (3) in some cases PBSCs are less contaminated with tumor cells than bone marrow.

Peripheral stem cells are collected through multiple apheresis sessions lasting 3 to 4 hours each. A number of interventions have been shown to increase the yield of the PBSCs collection process: optimal timing of the collection after chemotherapy or cyclophosphamide therapy; pretreatment with G-CSF, GM-CSF, IL-3, or a combination of these (see Table 27–3 for additional information on these lymphokines). A convenient and reproducible quality control method for the yield of a PBSC collection, which correlates satisfactorily with the likelihood of engraftment, still needs to be devised. Among the methods being investigated are total mononuclear cell counts in conjunction with colony-forming units granulocytes-macrocytes (CFU-GM) or stem cell counting by immunofluorescence flow cytometry targeting the CD33 and CD34 differentiation antigens.[38] Techniques for processing and preservation of PBSC collections are similar to those for bone marrow described subsequently. Various neoplastic disorders have been treated with autologous PBSCT including chronic granulocytic leukemia, acute leukemia, Hodgkin's disease, non-Hodgkin's lymphoma, multiple myeloma, breast cancer, small cell carcinoma of the lung, and neuroblastoma.[39] Allogeneic PBSCT has great potential that has yet to be explored.

Bone Marrow Storage and Processing

The field of bone marrow storage and processing offers great opportunity for expansion to blood banks. Familiarity with blood handling and component separation under aseptic conditions, quality control, accurate identification and record keeping, and inventory control make blood banks a natural site for the processing and storage of bone marrow.

The amount of processing needed is variable and depends on the extent of blood type and HLA matching between the donor and recipient. In addition, in the case of autologous marrow, some processing may be necessary to rid the marrow of tumor cells.

Bone marrow is aspirated from multiple punctures in both iliac crests into syringes, anticoagulated with heparin, and filtered through a stainless-steel mesh screen to remove bone and particulate fragments. The aspirated material constitutes a mixture of peripheral blood and marrow, and a volume corresponding approximately to 10 to 12 percent of the total blood volume is procured, containing 2 to 5×10^8 nucleated bone marrow cells per kilogram of body weight. If no additional processing is needed, the marrow is filtered and transferred into a plastic bag and transfused into the recipient intravenously. The marrow stem cells will travel in the recipient circulation and home to the bone marrow spaces.

The volume aspirated may represent 1 to 2 liters,

and volume reduction by centrifugation and plasma removal may be necessary if the recipient is too small to tolerate the volume. When donor and recipient have different ABO blood types, further processing may be involved. If a major incompatibility is present (e.g., a type O recipient with a type A donor), the majority of the red cells can be removed by sedimentation in the presence of hydroxyethyl starch (HES).[40] For minor incompatibility the plasma is removed by centrifugation.

The major hurdle to widespread application of bone marrow transplantation is the occurrence of GVH disease. This may occur in some patients in spite of a complete HLA match between the donor and the recipient, but it will occur systematically if there is an HLA mismatch. The majority of patients that could benefit from bone marrow transplantation do not have an HLA-matched sibling. Because it is felt that the acute GVH disease is caused by the mature T lymphocytes from the donor, there has been a great interest in marrow-processing methods that would remove mature T lymphocytes while preserving the stem cells. Different methods have been investigated. Treatment with monoclonal antibodies OKT3 to OKT11, recognizing antigens on mature T cells and complement, has been successful in removing over 80 percent of the T lymphocytes.[41] Other techniques using soybean lectin agglutination and E-rosette depletion[42] or immunotoxins[43] have had equal success in removing mature T cells. Although early results were encouraging and demonstrated significant decrease in GVH disease, concerns have surfaced that grafts may be more easily rejected, especially in patients with aplastic anemia, and that in patients with leukemia, leukemia relapse may have an increased frequency. GVH disease may have some antileukemic activity that is negated by its prevention.

In the case of autologous bone marrow transplantation, additional processing may involve the removal of tumor cells, and storage is crucial. The purging of the marrow is done by treatment with monoclonal antibodies against tumor antigens in conjunction with complement or bound to toxins such as ricin or to magnetic beads. An alternate method is the treatment of the marrow with a drug such as cyclophosphamide, which has antitumor activity.

Storage of bone marrow is done in the frozen state. The most popular method uses dimethyl sulfoxide (DMSO) in a concentration of 10 percent as the cryopreservative agent. The marrow is frozen in a rate-controlled freezer at a rate of 1°C to 2°C per minute and stored in liquid nitrogen at −196°C. Thawing is done rapidly in a 37°C water bath followed by dilution with tissue culture media.

Bone and Tissue Banking

The field of tissue banking offers another opportunity for expansion to blood banks. The demand for a wide variety of human tissues—including cornea, skin, bone, semen, dura mater, veins, nerves, fascia lata, amnion, cartilage, tendons, and temporal bones—is greatly exceeding the supply. New therapeutic procedures based on human tissue graft are continuously devised. The American Association of Tissue Banks (AATB) is attempting to organize a field consisting of 300 to 400 small programs centered on a local hospital or an individual surgeon and of 30 to 40 larger regional or institutional programs. AATB has developed standards, a technical manual, and an accreditation program for bone and tissue banking.

The risk of disease transmission through human tissue has been highlighted by reports of transmission of AIDS from skin graft and semen, hepatitis B from semen and cornea, and Creutzfeldt-Jakob disease from cornea and dura. A recent case has involved an HIV-seronegative donor, apparently in the window phase, whose organs (heart, liver, and kidneys) transmitted HIV infection to all four recipients.[44] In addition, three of the four patients who received fresh frozen bone from this donor also developed HIV infection. When it concerns the risk of disease transmissions, donor selection should be as strict as that for blood donation. Additional criteria may apply for each specific tissue to ensure the efficacy of the product. For example, persons with osteoporosis are not suitable bone donors. Donor testing should include all tests required on blood, except possibly for alanine aminotransferase (ALT) level, which may not be meaningful in potential donors owing to the underlying medical or surgical condition. Informed consent should be obtained from the donor or from the legal next of kin. Records of donors and recipients should be kept in as strict a fashion as kept for blood. In the case alluded to earlier, six recipients of tissues from this particular donor could not be accounted for by the hospitals. Specific aspects of bone, skin, cornea, and semen banking will be discussed subsequently.

Bone grafts are used in many orthopedic reconstructive surgeries and in the repair of nonunion fractures. The grafted bone will be resorbed and replaced slowly. The bone graft may originate from the patient's own iliac cancellous bone or from living or cadaveric donor. Living donor bone is obtained during surgery such as total hip replacement (femoral head), total knee replacement (tibial plateau), or thoracotomy (rib). These bones are collected under sterile conditions and stored in a double container (the inner container remains sterile) in a −70°C freezer. Cultures are taken of small chips from the outer surface or from a swabbing of a large area at the time of collection. When needed, the bone is thawed at room temperature and shaped according to the patient's need, usually in the form of cancellous bone chips. Alternatively, the bone may be stored freeze dried. Cadaveric donors supply long bones for replacement of large segments of bones that have been resected for the treatment of tumors or traumatic injuries.

Split-thickness skin grafts are used in the treatment of burns. They provide for wound coverage and decrease the rate of sepsis and the evaporative water loss. Skin grafts are obtained from cadavers up to 18 hours postmortem. The skin is removed from the back and the legs at a thickness of 0.3 to 0.5 mm and is placed on a nylon net with the dermis side up. It is then placed in a double-bag wrapper, sealed in a mylar foil bag, and stored in liquid nitrogen or stored at $-70°C$.

Cornea transplants have long been used to treat keratoconus, corneal dystrophy, corneal ulcers, and traumatic injuries. A new technique, epikeratophakia, for the treatment of severely myopic or aphakic patients, will increase the demand for human cornea. In 17 states corneas can be removed from individuals whose cause of death places them under the jurisdiction of a medical examiner or a justice of the peace, without obtaining consent from the legal next of kin. Cornea collection, storage, and distribution are performed by eye banks, which are organized through the Eye Bank Association of America (EBAA). They represent the greatest number in tissue grafts.

Semen banking in the management of infertility may involve the storage of semen for future use when a patient may become sterile as a result of therapy for a malignant disease or the provision of semen for artificial insemination from an anonymous donor. In the latter case, recent recommendations are that the donor be tested for HIV at the time of donation and again 3 months later before the semen is released. This is to prevent transmission of HIV during the window period, when a donor is infected but has not yet produced an antibody. Medical history screening for semen donors is more extensive and includes a two- to three-generation family history to rule out the transmission of genetic diseases. An attempt is made to match the physical characteristics of the husband, such as race, hair and eye color, and body build, and the blood type should be compatible with that of the wife, particularly in the Rh system. Semen is cryopreserved, with glycerol as the cryoprotective agent, in liquid nitrogen.

DIVERSIFICATION OF SERVICES

Autologous and Directed Donations

The safety of transfusion using autologous blood has long been recognized, but this option was markedly underused until the last few years. The appearance of AIDS and the realization in 1983 that it could be transmitted by blood transfusion was highly publicized by the media. Patients and physicians requested safer blood, and autologous donations in advance of elective surgery became increasingly popular. In addition, patients believed that blood from family and friends would be safer and demanded to receive blood only from donors that they themselves would recruit, a practice called directed donation. Because there is no scientific evidence that directed donation blood is safer than volunteer blood, and because the rate of positivity for any of the infectious disease markers

routinely performed on blood donation is similar in both groups, the American Association of Blood Banks (AABB) does not encourage directed donations. However, the almost hysterical fear of blood transfusion generated in the patients created such pressure that most blood centers and hospital blood banks have established a directed donation program. In some states this was mandated by law.

Autologous blood transfusion has clear advantages over transfusion using homologous blood: it eliminates the transmission of infectious diseases and carries no risk of alloimmunization to cellular or plasma protein antigens. In addition, preoperative phlebotomy stimulates erythropoiesis, which may accelerate the postoperative normalization of the hemoglobin level. An autologous blood program may involve four types of procedures:

1. Preoperative phlebotomy, also called predeposit, in which 1 to 6 units of blood may be collected over the 6 weeks preceding surgery.
2. Immediate preoperative phlebotomy with hemodilution, in which up to 2 units may be collected in the operating room with simultaneous volume restoration.
3. Intraoperative blood salvage, in which blood is suctioned from the wound, washed, and reinfused in the patient.
4. Postoperative blood salvage, in which blood is collected from a chest tube and washed before reinfusion.

Blood banks are directly concerned only with the first option. Most patients can safely donate once a week up to 72 hours before surgery, when receiving iron and folic acid replacement. Criteria for selection of autologous donors are much less strict than those for homologous donors, inasmuch as disease transmission is of no concern. In addition, medical conditions, such as slightly abnormal blood pressure, low hematocrit, or presence of chronic disease, would not be cause for automatic deferral. It would be the medical director's decision whether it would be safe to phlebotomize the patient. The standards of the AABB allow for the hematocrit and hemoglobin to be as low as 33 percent or 11 g/dl. AABB standards require that an ABO and Rh type be performed, and if the blood is transfused outside the collecting facility, the first unit from a given patient during a 30-day period must be tested for HB_sAg, anti-HIV, and anti–hepatitis C virus. Many institutions elect to complete all volunteer blood testing because it is usually safer not to vary from the routine processing procedure. The only drawback to an autologous blood program is the marked increase in clerical work necessary to implement a system of records and identification, to ensure that the patient will receive the autologous blood and not homologous blood at the time of surgery. In general, autologous blood cannot be released to other patients, even when the donor meets all the criteria for a homologous donation, unless the donor-patient has been an allogeneic blood donor in the past. It is felt by some, and specifically by the Food and Drug Administration (FDA), that autologous donors are not volunteer donors and cannot adequately self-defer.

A directed donation program requires even more clerical support because the donors may be incompatible with the intended recipient. The units must be checked after processing to determine whether they can be held for the patient or released to stock. Directed donors are allogeneic donors and must meet all the donor-selection criteria and have all tests completed before the blood is transfused. Directed donation from a husband to a wife is not recommended because it would expose her to antigens that may result in alloimmunization with a high risk for hemolytic disease of the newborn (HDN) in the future. Cellular components of directed donations from blood relatives should be irradiated to prevent the possibility of GVH disease, which could occur if the donor was homozygous for an HLA haplotype possessed by the recipient. In general, components will be prepared and only the red blood cells will be reserved for the patient. If the patient needs platelets, these are better prepared by apheresis from the directed donor. Once implemented, a directed donor program may increase the blood supply by bringing donors that would otherwise not be recruited. It certainly serves a role in relieving psychologic stress in some patients.

Outpatient and Home Transfusions

With the shift of healthcare delivery from hospital inpatient to hospital outpatient and to the home setting, requests for outpatient and home transfusions have been increasing. Patients with a wide variety of disorders require long-term transfusion: chronic gastrointestinal bleeding, aplastic anemia, thalassemia, sickle cell anemia, anemia or thrombocytopenia associated with a malignancy, myelofibrosis, AIDS, and so forth. For many of these patients, it is less time consuming and less costly to receive blood transfusions as an outpatient. For others, transportation would be difficult, may require an ambulance, and would result in a very taxing effort to go to an outpatient facility; these patients may be candidates for home transfusion. Problems posed in delivering such a service include securing a blood sample within 72 hours of the transfusion; identification of the patient, blood specimen, and blood units, inasmuch as the patient does not have a hospital identification wristband; delivery of blood to the place of transfusion; record keeping and documentation of the transfusion; therapy of possible transfusion reactions; monitoring of possible delayed reactions; disposal of transfusion materials; and follow-up on the effect of the blood transfusion. With careful planning, each problem can be resolved and the procedure can still meet the AABB transfusion standards and maintain safety.

In the outpatient setting, the patient must come the day before the transfusion to have a blood sample drawn. In the home setting, a nurse from a home healthcare agency can visit the patient the day before the transfusion to draw the blood sample. A wristband can then be placed on the patient with his or her name and social security number to serve as the identifying link between the patient, the blood sample, and the blood units. A special documentation form for the transfusion episode can be designed. The problem of a transfusion reaction occurring in the home setting is worrisome, but its likelihood can be minimized by transfusing washed blood and carefully screening patients so that they are alert and cooperative, have no previous history of transfusion reaction, and have appropriate indication for transfusion. An emergency kit should be available to the nurse-transfusionist, there should be immediate access to a physician by telephone, and a responsible adult should be present during and after the transfusion. AABB standards require that written instructions be given to patients on recognizing signs and symptoms of possible transfusion reaction, particularly symptoms of delayed reactions, and instructions should be given regarding whom to contact if such symptoms are experienced.

Conclusions

Many of the issues discussed in this chapter have been speculative. It is evident that changes will occur in blood banking practices. Only the future will tell how soon and how far the trends that are foreseen will be established. Blood banks must stay abreast of the new developments and be flexible to adapt to these changes.

Review Questions

1. Which of the following best describes genetic engineering?
   A. Isolating fragments of DNA from different sources and splicing them together
   B. Isolating fragments of RNA from different sources and splicing them together
   C. Isolating fragments of DNA from the same source and splicing them together
   D. Isolating fragments of RNA from the same source and splicing them together
   E. None of the above

2. All of the following enzymes are used in recombinant DNA technology, *except:*
   A. DNA polymerase
   B. Reverse transcriptase
   C. Glutathione synthetase
   D. Restriction endonuclease
   E. Ligase

3. Which of the following statements about a cDNA library is true?
   A. It originates from the cellular mRNA.
   B. Reverse transcriptase was used to synthesize the cDNA.
   C. It contains only the exons of the original cellular DNA.
   D. It contains only the genes that are expressed in the cell of origin.
   E. All of the above

4. Which of the following statements about the use of mammalian cells in the production of proteins by recombinant DNA technology is true?
   A. Mammalian cells are easier to grow in large batches than yeast.
   B. Mammalian cells will perform post translational modification such as glycosylation and disulfide bond cross-linking.
   C. Mammalian cells do not secrete the proteins and must be lysed to harvest the proteins.
   D. Mammalian cells are less expensive to grow than *B. subtilis.*
   E. All of the above

5. All of the following products have been produced by recombinant DNA technology, *except:*
   A. Antihemophilic factor (factor VIII)
   B. Erythropoietin
   C. Glycogen
   D. Granulocyte-macrophage colony-stimulating factor
   E. Hepatitis B vaccine

6. Which of the following statements about RFLP analysis is true?
   A. The DNA in the diagnostic material must be cut by restriction endonucleases.
   B. An electrophoresis step is involved.
   C. Hybridization with a labeled probe locates a specific DNA fragment.
   D. The location of the band identified by the probe represents the size of the DNA fragment identified.
   E. All of the above

7. Which of the following best describes the elements of the PCR technique?
   A. Primers, thermostable RNA polymerase, deoxyribonucleotides, heat and cool cycles
   B. Primers, thermostable RNA polymerase, ribonucleotides, heat and cool cycles
   C. Primers, thermostable reverse transcriptase, deoxyribonucleotides, heat and cool cycles
   D. Primers, thermostable DNA polymerase, deoxyribonucleotides, heat and cool cycles
   E. Primers, thermostable DNA polymerase, ribonucleotides, heat and cool cycles

8. Advantages of monoclonal antibodies over polyclonal antibodies include all of the following, *except:*
   A. Not contaminated with nonimmunoglobulin proteins
   B. Easy to elute
   C. Consistent reproducibility
   D. Consistent specificity
   E. Producible in unlimited quantities

9. The majority of monoclonal antibodies are produced in which of the following animals:
   A. Cow
   B. Horse
   C. Rodent
   D. Dog
   E. Goat

10. Which of the following proteins has been effective in treating aplastic anemia?
    A. Antithymocyte globulin
    B. Antipituitary globulin
    C. Antipancreatic globulin
    D. Antimarrow globulin
    E. Antigranulocytic globulin

11. Intravenous immunoglobulin therapy can cause the false diagnosis of which of the following diseases?
    A. Hepatitis C infection
    B. Systemic lupus erythematosus
    C. Acute leukemia
    D. Idiopathic thrombocytopenic purpura
    E. Myasthenia gravis

12. Until a bone marrow transplant engrafts, which two components are the ones most needed?
    A. Whole blood and platelets
    B. Red blood cells and fresh frozen plasma
    C. Red blood cells and platelets
    D. Red blood cells and cryoprecipitate
    E. Whole blood and cryoprecipitate

13. All of the following statements comparing PBSC collection to bone marrow harvest are true, *except:*
    A. PBSC collection gives a greater yield of cells than bone marrow harvest.
    B. PBSC collection is less contaminated with tumor cells in patients with bone marrow tumor involvement.
    C. PBSC collection does not require general anesthesia.
    D. The engraftment after PBSC collection transplantation is more rapid than after bone marrow transplantation.
    E. PBSC collection is less traumatic than bone marrow harvest.

14. The banking of which of the following products involves a multigenerational history of donor?
    A. Bone
    B. Bone marrow
    C. Cornea
    D. Semen
    E. Skin

15. Which of the following statements applies to directed blood donation?
    A. Blood from directed donation is safer than volunteer donor blood.
    B. The rate of positivity for infectious disease markers is lower in directed donation blood than in volunteer donor blood.
    C. In general, there is no contraindication for a husband to give blood for his wife.
    D. Directed donation blood from a first-degree blood relative of a patient must be irradiated.
    E. Directed donation blood should always be leukoreduced.

Answers to Review Questions

1. A (pp 497–498)
2. C (p 498)
3. E (pp 498–499)
4. B (p 500; Table 27–1)
5. C (pp 500–501)
6. E (p 501)
7. D (p 501; Fig. 27–7)
8. B (p 505)
9. C (p 504)
10. A (pp 506–507)
11. A (p 508)
12. C (p 509)
13. A (p 509)
14. D (p 511)
15. D (p 512)

References

1. Verma, IM: The reverse transcriptase. Biochim Biophys Acta 473:1, 1977.
2. Kelly, TJ and Smith, HO: A restriction enzyme from Hemophilus influenzae. II. Base sequence of the recognition site. J Mol Biol 51:393, 1970.
3. Lawn, RM, et al: The sequence of human serum albumin cDNA and its expression in *E. coli*. Nucleic Acids Res 9:6103, 1981.
4. Wood, WI, et al: Expression of active human factor VIII from recombinant DNA clones. Nature 312:330, 1984.
5. Gitschier, J, et al: Characterization of the human factor VIII gene. Nature 312:326, 1984.
6. Toole, JJ, et al: Molecular cloning of a cDNA encoding human antihaemophilic factor. Nature 312:342, 1984.
7. Sharrer, I: Current status of a recombinant antihemophilic factor VIII clinical trial organized by Baxter. Annals of Hematology 63:172, 1991.
8. Schwartz, RS, et al: Human recombinant DNA-derived antihemophilic factor (factor VIII) in the treatment of hemophilia A. Recombinant factor VIII study group. N Engl J Med 323:1800, 1990.
9. Schimpf, K, et al: Absence of hepatitis after treatment with a pasteurized factor VIII concentrate in patients with hemophilia and no previous transfusions. N Engl J Med 316:918, 1987.
10. Normann, A, et al: Detection of hepatitis A virus RNA in commercially available factor VIII preparation (letter). Lancet 340:1232, 1992.
11. Jacobs, K, et al: Isolation and characterization of genomic and cDNA clones of human erythropoietin. Nature 313:806, 1985.
12. Winearls, CG, et al: Effect of human erythropoietin derived from recombinant DNA on the anemia of patients maintained by chronic haemodialysis. Lancet ii:1175, 1986.
13. Eschbach, JW, et al: Correction of the anemia of end-stage renal disease with recombinant human erythropoietin. N Engl J Med 316:73, 1987.
14. Carnielli, V, et al: Effect of high doses of human recombinant erythropoeitin on the need for blood transfusions in preterm infants. J Pediatr 121:98, 1992.
15. Mullis, K, et al: Specific enzymatic amplification of DNA in vitro: The polymerase chain reaction. Cold Spring Harbor Symp Quant Biol 51:263, 1986.
16. Brechot, C, et al: Hepatitis B virus DNA in patients with chronic liver disease and negative test for hepatitis B surface antigen. N Engl J Med 312:270, 1985.
17. Scotto, J, et al: Detection of hepatitis B virus DNA in serum by a simple spot hybridization technique: Comparison with results for other viral markers. Hepatology 3:279, 1983.
18. Garson, JA, Ring, CJA, and Tuke, PW: Improvement of HCV genome detection with "short" PCR products (letter). Lancet 338:1466, 1991.
19. Ou, C-Y, et al: DNA amplification for direct detection of HIV-1 in DNA of peripheral blood mononuclear cells. Science 239:295, 1988.
20. Zorcolo, G, et al: Beta-thalassemia control (letter). Lancet ii:103, 1986.
21. Kohler, G and Milstein, C: Continuous cultures of fused cells secreting antibody of predefined specificity. Nature 256:495, 1975.
22. Grimm, EA, et al: Lymphokine-activated killer cell phenomenon: Lysis of natural killer-resistant fresh solid tumor cells by interleukin 2-activated autologous human peripheral blood lymphocytes. J Exp Med 155:1823, 1982.
23. Rosenberg, SA, et al: Observation on the systemic administration of autologous lymphokine-activated killer cells and recombinant interleukin-2 to patients with metastatic cancer. N Engl J Med 313:1485, 1985.
24. Gluckman, E, et al: Treatment of severe aplastic anemia with antilymphocyte globulin and androgens. Exp Hematol 6:679, 1978.
25. Wechter, WJ, et al: Manufacture of antithymocyte globulin (ATGAM) for clinical trials. Transplantation 28:303, 1979.
26. Swanson, JL, et al: Resolution of cross matching problems associated with patients receiving anti-lymphocyte globulin (abstract). Transfusion 22:415, 1982.
27. Hunter, RF and Huang, AT: Antithymocyte globulin: A realistic approach to therapy for severe aplastic anemia. S Med J 79:1121, 1986.
28. Mangan, KF, D'Alessandro, L, and Mullaney, MT: Action of antithymocyte globulin on normal human erythroid progenitor cell proliferation in vitro: Erythropoietic growth enhancing factors are released from marrow accessory cells. J Lab Clin Med 107:353, 1986.
29. Gascon, P, et al: Lymphokine abnormalities in aplastic anemia: Implications for the mechanism of action of antithymocyte globulin. Blood 65:407, 1985.
30. Mangan, KF: Immune disregulation of hematopoiesis. Annu Rev Med 38:61, 1987.
31. Imbach, P, et al: High dose intravenous gammaglobulin for idiopathic thrombocytopenic purpura in childhood. Lancet i:1228, 1981.
32. Intravenous Immunoglobulin: Prevention and treatment of disease. Summary of the NIH Consensus Conference. Transfusion Med Rev 5:171, 1991.

33. Kudesia, G, Price, C, and Clewley, J: Passively transfused hepatitis C antibody (letter). Lancet 340:1291, 1992.
34. Barr, RD, Whang-Peng, J, and Perry, S: Hemopoietic stem cells in human peripheral blood. Science 190:284, 1975.
35. Reiffers, J, et al: Successful autologous transplantation with peripheral blood hemopoietic cells in a patient with acute leukemia. Exp Hematol 14:312, 1986.
36. Korbling, M, et al: Autologous transplantation of blood-derived hemopoietic stem cells after myoablative therapy in a patient with Burkitt's lymphoma. Blood 67:529, 1986.
37. Kessinger, A, et al: Reconstitution of human hematopoietic function with autologous cryopreserved circulating stem cells. Exp Hematol 14:192, 1986.
38. Siena, S, et al: Flow cytometry for clinical estimation of circulating hematopoietic progenitors for autologous transplantation in cancer patients. Blood 77:400, 1991.
39. Inwards, D and Kessinger, A: Peripheral blood stem cell transplantation: Historical perspectives, current status, and prospects for the future. Transfusion Med Rev 6:183, 1992.
40. Lasky, LC, et al: Hemotherapy in patients undergoing blood group incompatible bone marrow transplantation. Transfusion 23:277, 1983.
41. Herve, P, et al: Removal of marrow T cells with OKT3-OKT11 monoclonal antibodies and complement to prevent acute graft-versus-host disease. Transplantation 39:138, 1985.
42. O'Reilly, RJ, et al: Transplantation of marrow-depleted T cells by soybean lectin agglutination and E-rosette depletion: Major histocompatibility complex–related graft resistance in leukemia transplant recipients. Transplant Proc 17:455, 1985.
43. Filipovich, AH, et al: Ex vivo T cell depletion with immunotoxins in allogeneic bone marrow transplantation: The pilot clinical study for the prevention of graft-versus-host disease. Transplant Proc 17:442, 1985.
44. Simonds, RJ, et al: Transmission of human immunodeficiency virus type I from a seronegative organ and tissue donor. N Engl J Med 326:726, 1992.

Bibliography

Allen, KA and Jackson, JB: New testing approaches in transfusion medicine. In Cooper, ES (ed): Selected Topics in Transfusion Medicine. Clin Lab Med 12:759, 1992.
Aubuchon, JP and Sacher, RA (eds): Marrow Transplantation: Practical and Technical Aspects of Stem Cell Reconstitution. American Association of Blood Banks, Bethesda, MD, 1992.

Beverley, PCL (ed): Monoclonal Antibodies. Churchill Livingstone, Oxford, 1986.
Bollon, AP: Recombinant DNA Products: Insulin, Interferon and Growth Hormone. CRC Press, Boca Raton, FL, 1984.
Dawson, MM: Lymphokines and Interleukins. CRC Press, Boca Raton, FL, 1991.
Edwards-Moulds, J and Lasky, LC (eds): Clinical Applications of Genetic Engineering. American Association of Blood Banks, Arlington, VA, 1987.
Edwards-Moulds, J and Masouredis, S (eds): Monoclonal Antibodies. American Association of Blood Banks, Arlington, VA, 1989.
Edwards-Moulds, J and Tregallas, WM (eds): Introductory Molecular Genetics. American Association of Blood Banks, Arlington, VA, 1986.
Fawcett, K and Barr, AR (eds): Tissue Banking. American Association of Blood Banks, Arlington, VA, 1987.
Fenoglio-Preiser, CM and Willman, CL (eds): Molecular Diagnostics in Pathology. Williams & Wilkins, Baltimore, 1991.
Fukui, H and Aronson, DL (chairs): First International Symposium on Recombinant Factor VIII. Semin Hematol 28(Suppl 1):1, 1991.
Garner, RJ and Silvergleid, AJ: Autologous and Directed Blood Programs. American Association of Blood Banks, Arlington, VA, 1987.
Klingeman, HG, et al: The role of erythropoietin and other growth factors in transfusion medicine. Transfusion Medicine Reviews 5:33, 1991.
Lewin, B: Genes IV. John Wiley & Sons, New York, 1990.
Murawski, K and Peetoom, F (eds): Transfusion medicine: Recent technological advances. Proceedings of the XVIIth Annual Scientific Symposium of the American Red Cross. Alan R Liss, New York, 1986.
Sacher, RA, et al (eds): Cellular and Humoral Immunotherapy and Apheresis. American Association of Blood Banks, Arlington, VA, 1991.
Sacher, RA, McCarthy, LJ, and Smit Sibing, CT (eds): Processing of Bone Marrow for Transplantation. American Association of Blood Banks, Arlington, VA, 1990.
Snyder, EL and Menitove, JE (eds): Home Transfusion Therapy. American Association of Blood Banks, Arlington, VA, 1986.
Stehling, L (ed): Perioperative Autologous Transfusion. American Association of Blood Banks, Arlington, VA, 1991.
Strelkauskas, AJ (ed): Human Hybridomas: Diagnostic and Therapeutic Applications. Marcel Dekker, New York, 1987.
Thomson, A (ed): The Cytokine Handbook. Academic Press, San Diego, 1991.
Westphal, RG and Kasprisin, DO (eds): Current Status of Hemapheresis: Indications, Technology and Complications. American Association of Blood Banks, Arlington, VA, 1987.

Glossary

Abruptio placentae: Premature detachment of normally situated placenta.

Absorbed anti-A₁: If serum from a group B individual that contains anti-A plus anti-A₁ is incubated with A₂ cells, the anti-A will adsorb onto the cells. Removal of the cells then yields a serum containing only anti-A₁; thus, absorbed anti-A₁.

Absorption: Removal of an unwanted antibody from a serum; often used interchangeably with adsorption.

Acid-citrate-dextrose (ACD): An anticoagulant and preservative solution that once was used routinely for blood donor collection but is now used only occasionally.

Acid phosphatase (ACP): A red cell enzyme used as an identification marker in paternity testing and criminal investigation.

Adenosine deaminase (ADA): A red cell enzyme used as an identification marker in paternity testing and criminal investigation.

Adenosine triphosphate (ATP): A compound composed of adenosine (nucleotide containing adenine and ribose) and three phosphoric acid groups, which, when split by enzyme action, produces energy that can be used to support other reactions.

Adenylate kinase (AK): A red cell enzyme used as an identification marker in paternity testing and criminal investigation.

Adjuvant: One of a variety of substances that, when combined with an antigen, enhance the antibody response to that antigen.

Adsorption: Providing an antibody with its corresponding antigen under optimal conditions so that the antibody will attach to the antigen, thereby removing the antibody from the serum; often used interchangeably with absorption.

Agammaglobulinemia: A rare disorder in which gamma globulin is virtually absent.

Agglomeration: The reversible aggregation of red cells in the presence of a high sugar concentration.

Agglutination: The clumping together of red blood cells or any particulate matter resulting from interaction of antibody and its corresponding antigen.

Agglutinin: An antibody that agglutinates cells.

Agglutinogen: A substance that stimulates the production of an agglutinin, thereby acting as an antigen.

Agranulocytosis: An acute disease in which the white blood cell count drops to extremely low levels and neutropenia becomes pronounced.

Albumin: Protein found in the highest concentration in human plasma; used as a diluent for blood typing antisera and a potentiator solution in serologic testing to enhance antigen-antibody reactions.

Aldomet: *See* Methyldopa.

Alkaline phosphatase (ALP): A red-cell enzyme used as an identification marker in paternity testing and criminal investigation.

Allele: One of two or more different genes that may occupy a specific locus on a chromosome.

Allo-: Prefix indicating differences within a species (e.g., an alloantibody is produced in one individual against the red cell antigens of another individual).

Allograft: A tissue transplant between individuals of the same species.

Allosteric change: A change in conformation that exposes a new reactive site on a molecule.

Alpha-adrenergic receptor: A site in autonomic nerve pathways wherein excitatory responses occur when adrenergic agents such as norepinephrine and epinephrine are released.

Alum precipitation: A method for obtaining an enhanced response when producing antibody; *see also* Adjuvant.

Amniocentesis: Transabdominal puncture of the amniotic sac, using a needle and syringe, in order to remove amniotic fluid. The material may then be studied to detect genetic disorders or fetomaternal blood incompatibility.

Amniotic fluid: Liquid or albuminous fluid contained in the amnion.

Amorph: A gene that does not appear to produce a detectable antigen; a silent gene, such as Jk, Lu, O.

Anamnestic response: An accentuated antibody response following a secondary exposure to an antigen. Antibody levels from the initial exposure are not detectable in the patient's serum until the secondary exposures, when a rapid rise in antibody titer is observed.

Anaphylaxis: An allergic hypersensitivity reaction of the body to a foreign protein or drug.

Anastomosis: A connection between two blood vessels, either direct or through connecting channels.

Anemia: A condition in which there is reduced oxygen delivery to the tissues; may result from increased destruction of red cells, excessive blood loss, or decreased production of red cells. **Aplastic a.:** Anemia caused by aplasia of bone marrow or its destruction by chemical agents or physical factors. **Autoimmune hemolytic a.:** Acquired disorder characterized by premature erythrocyte destruction owing to abnormalities in the individual's own immune system. **Hemolytic a.:** Anemia caused by hemolysis of red blood cells resulting in reduction of normal red cell life span. **Iron-deficiency a.:** Anemia resulting from a greater demand on stored iron than can be met. **Megaloblastic a.:** Anemia in which megaloblasts are found in the blood. **Sickle cell a.:** Hereditary, chronic hemolytic anemia characterized by large numbers of sickle-shaped red blood cells occurring almost exclusively in blacks.

Angina pectoris: Severe pain and constriction about the heart caused by an insufficient supply of blood to the heart.

Anion: An ion carrying a negative charge.

Antecubital: In front of the elbow, at the bend of the elbow; usual site for blood collection.

Antenatal: Occurring before birth.

Anti-A₁ lectin: A reagent anti-A₁ serum produced from the seeds of the plant *Dolichos biflorus;* reacts with all A₁ cells

516

but not with A subgroup cells such as A_2, A_3, and so on; reacts weakly with A_{int} cells.

Anti-B lectin: A reagent anti-B serum produced from the seeds of the plant *Bandeiraea simplicifolia.*

Antibody: A protein substance secreted by plasma cells that is developed in response to, and interacting specifically with, an antigen. In blood banking, it is found in serum, from either a commercial manufacturer or a patient. **Cross-reacting a.:** Antibody that reacts with antigens functionally similar to its specific antigen. **Fluorescent a.:** Antibody reaction made visible by incorporating a fluorescent dye into the antigen-antibody reaction and examining the specimen with a fluorescent microscope. **Maternal a.:** Antibody produced in the mother and transferred to the fetus in utero. **Naturally occurring a.:** Antibody present in a patient without known prior exposure to the corresponding red cell antigen.

Antibody screen: Testing the patient's serum with group O reagent red cells in an effort to detect atypical antibodies.

Anticoagulant: An agent that prevents or delays blood coagulation.

Anticodon: A sequence of three bases that is found on transfer RNA, which also carries an amino acid residue; recognizes its complementary codon on messenger RNA at the ribosome and deposits the amino acid on the ribosome, generating the amino acid sequence of the protein.

Anti-dl: An antibody implicated in warm autoimmune hemolytic anemia, which reacts with all Rh cells including Rh_{null} and Rh-deleted cells.

Antigen: A substance recognized by the body as being foreign, which can cause an immune response. In blood banking, antigens are usually, but not exclusively, found on the blood cell membrane.

Antihemophilic factor: *See* Hemophilia A.

Antihemophilic globulin: *See* Hemophilia A.

Antihistamine: Drug that opposes the action of histamine.

Anti-H lectin: A reagent anti-H produced from the seeds of the plant *Ulex europaeus.*

Antihuman globulin: *See* Antihuman serum.

Antihuman globulin serum: *See* Antihuman serum.

Antihuman globulin test (AGT): Test to ascertain the presence or absence of red cell coating by immunoglobulin G (IgG) or complement or both; uses a xenoantibody (rabbit antihuman serum) to act as a bridge between sensitized cells, thus yielding agglutination as a positive result. Also referred to as antiglobulin test. **Direct antihuman globulin test (DAT):** Used to detect in vivo cell sensitization. **Indirect antihuman globulin test (IAT):** Used to detect antigen-antibody reactions that occur in vitro.

Antihuman serum: An antibody prepared in rabbits or other suitable animals that is directed against human immunoglobulin, complement, or both; used to perform the antihuman globulin or Coombs' test. The serum may be either polyspecific (anti-IgG plus anticomplement) or monospecific (anti-IgG or anticomplement).

Anti-M lectin: A reagent anti-M serum produced from the plant *Iberis amara.*

Anti-nl: An antibody implicated in warm autoimmune hemolytic anemia, which reacts with all normal Rh cells except Rh_{null} cells and deleted Rh cells.

Anti-N lectin: A reagent anti-N serum produced from the plant *Vicia graminea.*

Anti-pdl: An antibody implicated in warm autoimmune hemolytic anemia, which reacts with all normal Rh cells and deleted Rh cells but not with Rh_{null} cells.

Antipyretic: An agent that reduces fever.

Antiserum: A reagent source of antibody, as in a commercial antiserum.

Antithetical: Referring to antigens that are the product of allelic genes (e.g., Kell [K] and Cellano [k]).

Apheresis: A method of blood collection in which whole blood is withdrawn, a desired component separated and retained, and the remainder of the blood returned to the donor. *See also* Plateletpheresis and Plasmapheresis.

Aplasia: Failure of an organ or tissue to develop normally.

Arachis hypogaea: A peanut lectin used to differentiate T polyagglutination from Tn polyagglutination.

Asphyxia: Condition caused by insufficient intake of oxygen.

Asthma: Paroxysmal dyspnea accompanied by wheezing caused by a spasm of the bronchial tubes or by swelling of their mucous membrane.

Atypical antibodies: Any antibody other than anti-A, anti-B, or anti-A,B.

Australia antigen: Old terminology referring to the hepatitis B–associated antigen.

Auto-: Prefix indicating self (e.g., an autoantibody is reactive against one's own red cell antigens); usually associated with a disease state.

Autoabsorption: A procedure to remove a patient's antibody using the patient's own cells.

Autologous control: Testing the patient's serum with his or her own cells in an effort to detect autoantibody activity.

Autosome: Any chromosome other than the sex (X and Y) chromosomes.

Bactericidal: Destructive to or destroying bacteria.

Bandeiraea simplicifolia: *See* Anti-B lectin.

Barcode reader: An optical input device that reads and interprets data from a barcode for entry into a computer system.

Bilirubin: The orange-yellow pigment in bile carried to the liver by the blood; produced from hemoglobin of red blood cells by reticuloendothelial cells in bone marrow, spleen, and elsewhere. **Direct b.:** The conjugated water-soluble form of bilirubin. **Indirect b.:** The unconjugated water-insoluble form of bilirubin.

Bilirubinemia: Pathologic condition in which excessive destruction of red blood cells occurs, increasing the amount of bilirubin found in the blood.

Binding constant: The "goodness of fit" in an antigen-antibody complex.

Biphasic: Reactivity occurring in two phases.

Blood bank information system: Computer system that has been developed specifically to assist blood bank professionals in the management of the patient, donor, and blood component information.

Blood gases: Determination of pH, P_{CO_2}, P_{O_2}, and HCO_3 performed on a blood gas analyzer.

Blood group–specific substances (BGSSs): Soluble antigens present in fluids that can be used to neutralize their corresponding antibodies; systems that demonstrate BGSSs include ABO, Lewis, and P blood group systems.

Bombay: Phenotype occurring in individuals who possess normal A or B genes but are unable to express them because they lack the gene necessary for production of H antigen, the required precursor for A and B. These persons often have a potent anti-H in their serum, which reacts with all cells except other Bombays. Also known as O_h.

Bovine: Pertaining to cattle.

Bradykinin: A plasma kinin.

Bromelin: A proteolytic enzyme obtained from the pineapple

Buffy coat: Light stratum of a blood clot seen when the blood is centrifuged or allowed to stand in a test tube. The red blood cells settle to the bottom and between the plasma and the red blood cells is a light-colored layer that contains mostly white blood cells.

Burst-forming unit committed to erythropoiesis (BFU-E): A primitive stem cell committed to erythropoiesis and thought to be a precursor to the CFU-E.

C3a: A biologically active fragment of the complement C3 molecule that demonstrates anaphylactic capabilities upon liberation.

C3b: A biologically active fragment of the complement C3 molecule that is an opsonin and promotes immune adherence.

C3d: A biologically inactive fragment of the C3b complement component formed by inactivation by the C3b inactivator substance present in serum.

C4: A complement component present in serum that participates in the classic pathway of complement activation.

C5a: A biologically active fragment of the C5 molecule, which demonstrates anaphylactic capabilities as well as chemotactic properties upon liberation. This fragment is also a potent aggregator of platelets.

Cardiac output: The amount of blood discharged from the left or right ventricle per minute.

Catecholamines: Biologically active amines, epinephrine and norepinephrine, derived from the amino acid tyrosine. They have a marked effect on nervous and cardiovascular systems, metabolic rate, temperature, and smooth muscle.

Cathode ray tube (CRT): A display device in an information system.

Cation: An ion carrying a positive charge.

Central processing unit (CPU): The part of a computer that contains the semiconductor chips that process the instructions of the computer programs.

Central venous pressure: The pressure within the superior vena cava reflecting the pressure under which the blood is returned to the right atrium.

Chemically modified anti-D: IgG anti-D reagent antisera in which the immunoglobulin has been chemically modified to react in the saline phase of testing by breaking disulfide bonds at the hinge region of the molecule, converting the Y-shaped antibody structure to a T-shaped form through the use of sulfhydryl-reducing reagents.

Chemotaxis: Movement toward a stimulus, particularly that movement displayed by phagocytic cells toward bacteria and sites of cell injury.

Chimera: An individual who possesses a mixed cell population.

Chloroquine: White crystalline powder used for its antimicrobial action, especially in the treatment of malaria and lupus erythematosus.

Chromogen: Any principle that may be changed into coloring matter.

Chromosome: The structures within a nucleus that contain a linear thread of DNA, which transmits genetic information. Genes are arranged along the strand of DNA and constitute portions of the DNA.

Cis position: The location of two or more genes on the same chromosome of a homologous pair.

Citrate: Compound of citric acid and a base; used in anticoagulant solutions.

Citrate-phosphate-dextrose (CPD): The anticoagulant preservative solution that replaced ACD in routine donor collection. It has been replaced by CPD-A1 in routine use.

Citrate-phosphate-dextrose-adenine (CPD-A1): The anticoagulant preservative solution in current use. It has extended the shelf life of blood from 21 days (ACD and CPD) to 35 days.

Clone: A group of genetically identical cells.

Codominant: A pair of genes in which neither is dominant over the other; that is, they are both expressed.

Codon: A sequence of three bases in a strand of DNA that provides the genetic code for a specific amino acid. The complementary triplets are found on messenger RNA, which is synthesized from the DNA and then proceeds to the ribosomes for protein synthesis.

Colloid: A gluelike substance such as protein or starch whose particles, when dispersed in a solvent to the greatest possible degree, remain uniformly distributed and fail to form a true solution.

Colony-forming unit—culture (CFU-C): Generation of stem cells using tissue culture methods. Current synonym is CFU-GM, which is a colony-forming unit committed to the production of myeloid cells (granulocytes and monocytes).

Colony-forming unit committed to erythropoiesis (CFU-E): A stem cell that is committed to forming cells of the red blood cell series.

Colostrum: Thin yellowish breast fluid secreted 2 to 3 days after birth but before the onset of true lactation; it contains a great quantity of proteins and calories as well as antibodies and lymphocytes.

Compatibility testing: All pretransfusion testing performed on a potential transfusion recipient and the appropriate donor blood, in an attempt to ensure that the product will survive in the recipient and induce improvement in the patient's clinical condition; the crossmatch between recipient's serum and donor's cells.

Complement: A series of proteins in the circulation that, when sequentially activated, causes disruption of bacterial and other cell membranes. Activation occurs via one of two pathways, and once activated, the components are involved in a great number of immune defense mechanisms including anaphylaxis, chemotaxis, and phagocytosis. Red cell antibodies that activate complement may be capable of causing hemolysis.

Complement fixation (CF): An immunologic test.

Component therapy: Transfusion of specific components (e.g., red blood cells, platelets, plasma) rather than whole blood to treat a patient. Components are separable by physical means such as centrifugation.

Compound antibody: An antibody whose corresponding antigen is an interaction product of two or more antigens.

Compound antigen: Two or more antigens that interact and are recognized as a single antigen by an antibody.

Configuration: The physical layout and design of the central processing unit and the peripheral devices of an information system.

Conglutinin: A substance present in bovine serum that will agglutinate sensitized cells in the presence of complement.

Constant region: The portion of the immunoglobulin chain that shows a relatively constant amino acid sequence within each class of immunoglobulin. Both light and heavy chains have these constant portions, which originate at the carboxyl region of the molecule.

Convulsion: Involuntary muscle contraction and relaxation.

Coombs' serum: *See* Antihuman serum.

Coombs' test: *See* Antihuman globulin test (AGT).

Cord cells: Fetal cells obtained from the umbilical cord at birth; may be contaminated with Wharton's jelly.

Coumarin (Coumadin): A commonly employed anticoagulant that acts as a vitamin K antagonist that prolongs the partial thromboplastin time.

Counterelectrophoresis (CEP): An immunologic procedure.

Crossmatch: Testing a patient and prospective donor for compatibility. **Major c.:** Recipient serum tested with donor cells. **Minor c.:** Recipient cells tested with donor serum or plasma.

Cryoprecipitate: A concentrated source of coagulation factor VIII prepared from a single unit of donor blood; it also contains fibrinogen, factor XIII, and von Willebrand factor.

Cryopreservation: Preservation by freezing at very low temperatures.

Cryoprotectant: A substance that protects blood cells from damage caused by freezing and thawing. Glycerol and dimethyl sulfoxide are examples.

Cryptantigens: Hidden receptors that may be exposed when normal erythrocyte membranes are altered by bacterial or viral enzymes.

Crystalloid: A substance capable of crystallization; opposite of colloid.

Cyanosis: Slightly bluish or grayish skin discoloration resulting from accumulations of reduced hemoglobin or deoxyhemoglobin in the blood caused by oxygen deficiency or carbon dioxide buildup.

Cytomegalovirus (CMV): One of a group of species-specific herpesviruses.

Cytopheresis: A procedure performed using a machine by which one can selectively remove a particular cell type normally found in peripheral blood of a patient or donor.

Cytotoxicity: Ability to destroy cells.

Cytotoxicity testing: Procedure commonly used in HLA typing and crossmatching.

Dane particle: Hepatitis B virion.

Database: An organized group of files in which information is stored in an information system.

Deglycerolization: Removal of glycerol from a unit of red cells after thawing has been performed; required to return the cells to a normal osmolality.

Deletion: The loss of a portion of chromosome.

Deoxyribonucleic acid (DNA): The chemical basis of heredity and the carrier of genetic information for all organisms except RNA viruses.

Dexamethasone: A topical steroid with anti-inflammatory, antipruritic, and vasoconstrictive actions.

Dextran: A plasma expander that may be used as a substitute for plasma; can be used to treat shock by increasing blood volume. Rouleaux may be observed in the recipient's serum or plasma.

Diagnosis-related group (DRG): Classification system that organizes short-term, general hospital inpatients into statistically stable groups based on age and illness.

Diaphoresis: Profuse sweating.

Diastolic pressure: The point of least pressure in the arterial vascular system; the lower or bottom value of a blood pressure reading.

Dielectric constant: A measure of the electrical conductivity of a suspending medium.

Differential count: Counting 100 leukocytes to ascertain the relative percentages of each.

2,3-Diphosphoglycerate (2,3-DPG): An organic phosphate in red blood cells that alters the affinity of hemoglobin for oxygen. Blood cells stored in a blood bank lose 2,3-DPG, but once infused, the substance is resynthesized or reactivated.

Diploid: Having two sets of 23 chromosomes, for a total of 46.

Disk drive: A hardware device in an information system that contains a disk(s) on which data are stored; provides for quick access to storing or retrieval of data.

Disseminated intravascular coagulation (DIC): Clinical condition of altered blood coagulation secondary to a variety of diseases.

Dithiothreitol (DTT): A sulfhydryl compound used to disrupt the disulfide bonds of immunoglobulin M, yielding monomeric units rather than the typical pentameric molecule.

Diuresis: Secretion and passage of large amounts of urine.

Diuretic: An agent that increases the secretion of urine, either by increasing glomerular filtration or by decreasing reabsorption from the tubules.

Dizygotic twins: Twins who are the product of two fertilized ova (also called fraternal twins).

DNA polymerase: Also known as the HB$_e$Ag of the hepatitis B virion.

Dolichos biflorus: *See* Anti-A$_1$ lectin.

Domain: Portions along the immunoglobulin chain that show specific biologic function.

Dominant: A trait or characteristic that will be expressed in the offspring even though it is only carried on one of the homologous chromosomes.

Donath-Landsteiner test: A test usually performed in the blood bank to detect the presence of the Donath-Landsteiner antibody, which is a biphasic immunoglobulin G antibody with anti-P specificity found in patients suffering from paroxysmal cold hemoglobinuria.

Donor: An individual who donates a pint of blood.

Dopamine: A catecholamine synthesized by the adrenal gland, used especially in the treatment of shock.

Dosage: A phenomenon whereby an antibody reacts more strongly with a red cell carrying a double dose (homozygous inheritance of the appropriate gene) than with a red cell carrying a single dose (heterozygous inheritance) of an antigen.

Dyscrasia: An old term now used as a synonym for disease.

Ecchymosis: A form of macula appearing in large irregularly formed hemorrhagic areas of the skin; originally blue-black, then changing to greenish brown or yellow.

Edema: A local or generalized condition in which the body tissues contain an excessive amount of tissue fluid.

Electrolyte: A substance that in solution conducts an electric current; common electrolytes are acids, bases, and salts.

Electrophoresis: The movement of charged particles through a medium (paper, agar gel) in the presence of an electrical field; useful in the separation and analysis of proteins.

Eluate: *See* Elution.

Elution: A process whereby cells that are coated with antibody are treated in such a manner as to disrupt the bonds between the antigen and antibody. The freed antibody is collected in an inert diluent such as saline or 6 percent albumin. This antibody serum then can be tested to identify its specificity using routine methods. The mechanism to free the antibody may be physical (heating, shaking) or chemical (ether, acid), and the harvested antibody-containing fluid is called an eluate.

Embolism: Obstruction of a blood vessel by foreign substances or a blood clot.

Embolus: A mass of undissolved matter present in a blood or lymphatic vessel, brought there by the blood or lymph circulation.

Endemic: A disease that occurs continuously in a particular population but has a *low* mortality; used in contrast to epidemic.

Endogenous: Produced or arising from within a cell or organism.

Endothelium: A form of squamous epithelium consisting of flat cells that line the blood and lymphatic vessels, the heart, and various other body cavities; derived from mesoderm.

Endotoxemia: The presence of endotoxin in the blood; endotoxin is present in the cell of certain bacteria (e.g., gram-negative organisms).

Engraftment: The successful establishment, proliferation and differentiation of transplanted hematopoietic stem cells.

Enzyme: A substance capable of catalyzing a reaction; proteins that induce chemical changes in other substances without being changed themselves.

Enzyme-linked immunosorbent assay (ELISA): An immunologic test.

Enzyme treatment: A procedure in which red blood cells are incubated with an enzyme solution that cleaves some of the membrane's glycoproteins, are then washed free of the enzyme, and used in serologic testing. Enzyme treatment cleaves some antigens and exposes others.

Epistaxis: Hemorrhage from the nose; nosebleed.

Epitope: The portion of the antigen molecule that is directly involved in the interaction with the antibody; the antigenic determinant.

Equivalence zone: The zone in which antigen and antibody concentrations are optimal and lattice formation is most stable.

Erythroblast: Any form of nucleated red corpuscles, containing hemoglobin, which are not normally seen in the circulating blood.

Erythroblastosis fetalis: *See* Hemolytic disease of the newborn (HDN).

Erythrocyte: The blood cell that transports oxygen and carbon dioxide; a mature red blood cell.

Ethylenediaminetetraacetic acid (EDTA): An anticoagulant useful in hematologic testing and preferable when direct antihuman globulin testing is indicated.

Euglobulin lysis: Coagulation procedure testing for fibrinolysins.

Exogenous: Originating outside an organ or part.

Extracorporeal: Outside of the body.

Extravascular: Outside of the blood vessel.

Factor assay: Coagulation procedure to assay the concentration of specific plasma coagulation factors.

Factor VIII concentrate: A commercially prepared source of coagulation factor VIII.

Febrile reaction: A transfusion reaction caused by leukoagglutinins that is characterized by fever; usually observed in multiple transfused or multiparous patients.

Fibrin: A whitish filamentous protein or clot formed by the action of thrombin on fibrinogen, converting it to fibrin.

Fibrinogen: A protein produced in the liver that circulates in plasma. In the presence of thrombin, an enzyme produced by the activation of the clotting mechanism, fibrinogen is cleaved into fibrin, which is an insoluble protein that is responsible for clot formation.

Fibrinolysin: The substance that has the ability to dissolve fibrin; also called plasmin.

Fibrinolysis: Dissolution of fibrin by fibrinolysin caused by the action of a proteolytic enzyme system that is continually active in the body but that is increased greatly by various stress stimuli.

Fibroblast: Cells found throughout the body that synthesize connective tissue.

Ficin: A proteolytic enzyme derived from the fig.

Ficoll: A macromolecular additive that enhances the agglutination of red cells.

Ficoll-Hypaque: A density-gradient medium utilized for the separation and harvesting of specific white blood cells, most commonly lymphocytes.

Formaldehyde: A disinfectant solution.

Forward grouping: Testing unknown red cells with known reagent antisera to determine which ABO antigens are present (cell type).

Fresh frozen plasma (FFP): A frozen plasma product (from a single donor) that contains all clotting factors, especially the labile factors V and VIII; useful for clotting factor deficiencies other than hemophilia A, von Willebrand's disease, and hypofibrinogenemia.

Freund's adjuvant: Mixture of killed microorganisms, usually mycobacteria, in an oil-and-water emulsion. The material is administered to induce antibody formation and yields a much greater antibody response.

Furosemide (Lasix): An oral diuretic.

G6PD (glucose-6-phosphate dehydrogenase): A liver enzyme used to monitor liver function.

Gamete: A mature male or female reproductive cell.

Gamma globulin: A protein found in plasma and known to be involved in immunity.

Gamma marker: Allotypic marker on the gamma heavy chain of the IgCG immunoglobulin.

Gene: A unit of inheritance within a chromosome.

Genotype: An individual's actual genetic makeup.

Gestation: In mammals, the length of time from conception to birth.

Globin: A protein constituent of hemoglobin. There are four globin chains in the hemoglobin molecule.

Glomerulonephritis: A form of nephritis in which the lesions involve primarily the glomeruli.

Glutamic pyruvate transaminase: A live enzyme used to monitor liver function; also called serum glutamic pyruvate transaminase (SGPT).

Gluten enteropathy: A condition associated with malabsorption of food from the intestinal tract.

Glycerol: A cryoprotective agent.

Glycerolization: Adding glycerol to a unit of red cells for the purpose of freezing.

Glycine soja: Soybean extract or lectin used to differentiate different forms of polyagglutination.

Glycophorin A: A major glycoprotein of the red cell membrane. MN antigen activity is found on it.

Glycophorin B: An important red cell glycoprotein; SsU antigen activity is found here.

Glycosyl transferase: A protein enzyme that promotes the attachment of a specific sugar molecule to a predetermined acceptor molecule. Many blood group genes code for transferases, which reproduce their respective antigens by attaching sugars to designated precursor substances.

Goodpasture syndrome: A disease entity that represents a rapidly progressive glomerulonephritis associated with pulmonary lesions. Usually the patients possess an antibody to the basement membrane of the renal glomeruli.

Graft-versus-host (GVH) disease: A disorder in which the grafted tissue attacks the host tissue.

Granulocytopenia: Abnormal reduction of granulocytes in the blood.

Hageman factor: Synonym for coagulation factor XII.

Half-life: The time that is required for the concentration of a substance to be reduced by one half.

Haploid: Possessing half the normal number of chromosomes found in somatic or body cells; seen in germ cells (sperm and ova).

Haplotype: A term used in HLA testing to denote the five genes (HLA-A, -B, -C, -D, -DR) on the same chromosome.

Haptene: The portion of an antigen containing the grouping on which the specificity depends.

Haptoglobin: A mucoprotein to which hemoglobin released into plasma is bound; it is increased in certain inflammatory conditions and decreased in hemolytic disorders.

Hardware: Components of an information computer system that are the tangible, physical pieces of equipment that one can see and touch such as the central processing unit, cathode ray tube, and keyboard.

HB$_c$Ag: Hepatitis core antigen, referring to the nucleocapsid of the virion.

HB$_e$Ag: Hepatitis DNA polymerase of the nucleus of the virion.

HB$_s$Ag: Hepatitis B surface antigen.

Hemangioma: A benign tumor of dilated blood vessels.

Hemarthrosis: Bloody effusion into the cavity of a joint.

Hematinic: Pertaining to blood; an agent that increases the amount of hemoglobin in the blood.

Hematocrit: The proportion of red cells in whole blood, expressed as a percentage.

Hematoma: A swelling or mass of blood confined to an organ, tissue, or space and caused by a break in a blood vessel.

Hematuria: Blood in the urine.

Heme: The iron-containing protoporphyrin portion of the hemoglobin wherein the iron is in the ferrous (Fe^{++}) state.

Hemodialysis: Removal of chemical substances from the blood by passing it through tubes made of semipermeable membranes, which are continually bathed by solutions that selectively remove unwanted material; used to cleanse the blood of patients in whom one or both kidneys are defective or absent and to remove excess accumulation of drugs or toxic chemicals in the blood.

Hemodilution: An increase in the volume of blood plasma, resulting in reduced relative concentration of red blood cells.

Hemoglobin: The iron-containing pigment of the red blood cells whose function is to carry oxygen from the lungs to the tissues.

Hemoglobinemia: Presence of hemoglobin in the blood plasma.

Hemoglobin-oxygen dissociation curve: The relationship between the percent saturation of the hemoglobin molecule with oxygen and the environmental oxygen tension.

Hemoglobinuria: The presence of hemoglobin in the urine freed from lysed red blood cells, which occurs when he-moglobin from disintegrating red blood cells or from rapid hemolysis of red cells exceeds the ability of the blood proteins to combine with the hemoglobin.

Hemolysin: An antibody that activates complement leading to cell lysis.

Hemolysis: Disruption of the red cell membrane and the subsequent release of hemoglobin into the suspending medium or plasma.

Hemolytic disease of the newborn (HDN): A disease characterized by anemia, jaundice, enlargement of the liver and spleen, and generalized edema (hydrops fetalis) that is caused by maternal IgG antibodies crossing the placenta and attacking fetal red cells when there is a fetomaternal blood group incompatibility (usually ABO or Rh antibodies). Synonym is erythroblastosis fetalis.

Hemolytic transfusion reaction (HTR): A reaction from red cell destruction caused by patient's antibody(ies) directed to donor red cell antigen(s).

Hemophilia A: A hereditary disorder characterized by greatly prolonged coagulation time. The blood fails to clot and bleeding occurs; caused by inheritance of a factor VIII deficiency, it occurs almost exclusively in males.

Hemophilia B: "Christmas disease," which is a hemophilia-like disease caused by a lack of factor IX.

Hemopoiesis: Formation of blood cells. Synonym is hematopoiesis.

Hemorrhage: Abnormal internal or external bleeding; may be venous, arterial, or capillary; from blood vessels into the tissues or out of the body.

Hemorrhagic diathesis: Uncontrolled spontaneous bleeding.

Hemosiderin: An iron-containing pigment derived from hemoglobin from disintegration of red blood cells; a method of storing iron until it is needed for making hemoglobin.

Hemostasis: Arrest of bleeding; maintaining blood flow within vessels by repairing rapidly any vascular break without compromising the fluidity of the blood.

Hemotherapy: Blood transfusion as a therapeutic measure.

Heparin: An anticoagulant used for collecting whole blood that is to be filtered for the removal of leukocytes.

Hepatitis: Inflammation of the liver.

Hepatitis-associated antigen (HAA): Older terminology currently replaced by HB$_s$Ag.

Hepatitis B immunoglobulin (HBIg): An immune serum given to individuals exposed to the hepatitis B virus.

Heterozygote: An individual with different alleles for a given characteristic.

Heterozygous: Possessing different alleles at a given locus.

High-frequency antigen: Also known as high-incidence antigen; antigen whose frequency in the population is 98 to 99 percent.

Histocompatibility: The ability of cells to survive without immunologic interference; especially important in blood transfusion and transplantation.

HLA: Human leukocyte antigen.

Homeostasis: State of equilibrium of the internal environment of the body that is maintained by dynamic processes of feedback and regulation.

Homozygote: An individual developing from gametes with similar alleles and thus possessing like pairs of genes for a given hereditary characteristic.

Homozygous: Possessing a pair of identical alleles.

Hormone: A substance originating in an organ or gland that is conveyed through the blood to another part of the body, stimulating it chemically to increase functional activity and increase secretion.

Hyaluronidase: An enzyme found in the testes; present in semen.

Hybridoma: A hybrid (cross) between a plasmacytoma cell and a spleen (or Ab-producing) cell that produces a monoclonal antibody, resulting in a malignant cell line that can grow indefinitely in culture and can produce high quantities of Ab. This antibody is monoclonal because only one Ab-producing cell combined with the plasmacytoma cell is present.

Hydatid cyst fluid: Source of P_1 substance.

Hydrocortisone: A corticosteroid with anti-inflammatory properties.

Hydrops fetalis: *See* Hemolytic disease of the newborn (HDN).

Hydroxyethyl starch (HES): A red cell sedimenting agent used to facilitate leukocyte withdrawal during leukapheresis.

Hypertension: Increase in blood pressure.

Hyperventilation: Rapid breathing that results in carbon dioxide depletion and accompanies hypotension, vasoconstriction, and fainting.

Hypogammaglobulinemia: Decreased levels of gamma globulins seen in some disease states.

Hypotension: Decrease in blood pressure.

Hypothermia: Having a body temperature below normal.

Hypovolemia: Diminished blood volume.

Hypoxia: Deficiency of oxygen.

Iberis amara: *See* Anti-M lectin.

Icterus: A condition characterized by yellowish skin, whites of the eyes, mucous membranes, and body fluids caused by increased circulating bilirubin resulting from excessive hemolysis or from liver damage due to hepatitis. Synonym is jaundice.

Idiopathic: Pertaining to conditions without clear pathogenesis, or disease without recognizable cause, as of spontaneous origin.

Idiopathic thrombocytopenic purpura (ITP): Bleeding owing to a decreased number of platelets; the etiology is unknown, with most evidence pointing to platelet autoantibodies.

Idiothrombocythemia: An increase in blood platelets of unknown etiology.

Idiotype: The portion of the immunoglobulin variable region that is the antigen-combining site, which interacts with the antigenic epitope.

Immune response: The reaction of the body to substances that are foreign or are interpreted as being foreign. Cellmediated or cellular immunity pertains to tissue destruction mediated by T cells, such as graft rejection and hypersensitivity reactions. Humoral immunity pertains to cell destruction response during the early period of the reaction.

Immune serum globulin: Gamma globulin protein fraction of serum-containing antibodies.

Immunoblast: A mitotically active T or B cell.

Immunodeficiency: A decrease from the normal concentration of immunoglobulins in serum.

Immunodominant sugar: In reference to glycoprotein or glycolipid antigens, the sugar molecule that gives the antigen its specificity (e.g., galactose, which confers B antigen specificity).

Immunogen: Any substance capable of stimulating an immune response.

Immunogenicity: The ability of an antigen to stimulate an antibody response.

Immunoglobulin (Ig): One of a family of closely related though not identical proteins that are capable of acting as antibodies: IgA, IgD, IgE, IgG, and IgM. IgA is the principal immunoglobulin in exocrine secretions such as saliva and tears. IgD may play a role in antigen recognition and the initiation of antibody synthesis. IgE, produced by the cells lining the intestinal and respiratory tracts, is important in forming reagin. IgG is the main immunoglobulin in human serum. IgM is formed in almost every immune response during the early period of the reaction.

Immunologic memory: The development of T and B memory cells that have been sensitized by exposure to an antigen and respond rapidly under subsequent encounters with the antigen.

Immunologic unresponsiveness: Development of a tolerance to certain antigens that would otherwise evoke an immune response.

Immunoprecipitin: An antigen-antibody reaction that results in precipitation.

Incubation: In vitro combination of antigen and antibody under certain conditions of time and temperature to allow antigen-antibody complexes to occur.

Initiation: The deposition of *N*-formylmethionine on the ribosome, which begins the synthesis of all proteins.

In Lu: A rare dominant gene that inhibits the production of all Lutheran antigens as well as i, P_1, and Au^a (Auberger). The quantity of antigen on the red cell is markedly reduced in the presence of In Lu; it may be virtually undetectable.

Interface: Software that allows a computer system to send data to or receive data from another computer system.

Intraoperative salvage: A procedure to reclaim a patient's blood loss during an operation by reinfusion.

Intravascular: Within the blood vessel.

In utero: Within the uterus.

Inv: Light-chain marker on the kappa light chains of IgG.

Inversion: The breaking of a chromosome during division with subsequent reattachment occurring in an inverted or upside-down position.

In vitro: Outside the living body, as in a laboratory setting.

In vivo: Inside the living body.

Ion exchange resin: Synthetic organic substances of high molecular weight. They replace certain positive or negative ions, which they encounter in solutions.

Ionic strength: Refers to the number of charged particles present in a solution.

Ir genes: Immune response genes found within the region of the major histocompatibility complex. *Ir* genes in humans are likely to exist; preliminary evidence shows genes at the D-related locus may be analogous to the *Ir* genes of mice.

Ischemia: Local and temporary deficiency of blood supply caused by obstruction of the circulation to a cell, tissue, or organ.

Isogglutinins: The ABO antibodies anti-A, anti-B, and anti-A,B.

Isoimmune: An antibody produced against a foreign antigen in the same species.

Isotype: The subclasses of an immunoglobulin molecule.

Jaundice: *See* Icterus.

Karyotype: A photomicrograph of a single cell in the metaphase stage of mitosis that is arranged to show the chromosomes in descending order of size.

Kernicterus: A form of icterus neonatorum occurring in

infants, developing at 2 to 8 days of life; prognosis poor if untreated.

Kinin: A group of polypeptides that have considerable biologic activity (e.g., vasoactivity).

Kleihauer-Betke technique: Quantitative procedure used to determine the amount of fetal cells present in the maternal circulation.

Km: Light chain marker on the kappa light chains of IgG.

Labile: Capable of deteriorating rapidly upon storage.

Lectin: Proteins present in plants (usually seeds), which bind specifically to carbohydrate determinants and agglutinate erythrocytes through their cell surface oligosaccharide determinants.

Leukemia: Malignant proliferation of leukocytes, which spill into the blood, yielding an elevated leukocyte count.

Leukoagglutinins: Antibodies to white blood cells.

Ligature: Process of binding or tying; a band or bandage; a thread or wire for tying a blood vessel or other structure in order to constrict it.

Linkage: The association between distinct genes that occupy closely situated loci on the same chromosome, resulting in an association in the inheritance of these genes.

Linkage disequilibrium: Genes associated in a haplotype more often than would be expected on the basis of chance alone.

Locus: The site of a gene on a chromosome.

Low-frequency antigen: Also known as low-incidence antigen; antigen whose frequency in a random population is very low—less than 10 percent.

Low ionic–polycation test: A compatibility test that incorporates both glycine (low ionic) and protamine (polycation) in an effort to obtain maximal sensitivity and to minimize the need for antibody screening.

Low ionic strength solution (LISS): A type of potentiating medium in use for serologic testing. Reducing the ionic strength of the red cell suspending medium increases the affinity of the antigen for its corresponding antibody such that sensitivity can be increased and incubation time decreased. LISS contains glycine or glucose in addition to saline.

Lymphocyte: A type of white blood cell involved in the immune response. Lymphocytes normally total 20 to 45 percent of total white cells. T lymphocytes mature during passage through the thymus or after interaction with thymic hormones; these cells function both in cellular and humoral immunity. Subsets include helper T cells (T_h), which enhance B-cell antibody production, and suppressor T cells (T_s), which inhibit B-cell antibody production. B-lymphocyte cells are not processed by the thymus. Through morphologic and functional differentiation, they mature into plasma cells that secrete immunoglobulin.

Lymphoma: A solid tumor of lymphocyte cells.

Lysosomes: Part of an intracellular digestive system that exists as separate particles in the cell. Even though their importance in health and disease is certain, all the precise ways lysosomes effect changes are not understood.

Macroglobulinemia: Abnormal presence of high molecular weight immunoglobulins (IgM) in the blood.

Macrophage: End-stage development for the blood monocyte; these cells can ingest (phagocytose) a variety of substances for subsequent digestion or storage and are located in a number of sites in the body (e.g., spleen, liver, lung), existing as free mobile cells or as fixed cells. Func-

tions include elimination of senescent blood cells and participation in the immune response.

Major crossmatch: Compatibility testing procedure using recipient's serum and donor red cells.

Major histocompatibility complex (MHC): Present in all mammalian and ovarian species; analogous to HLA complex. HLA antigens are within the MHC at a locus on chromosome 6.

Malaria: An acute and sometimes chronic infectious disease caused by the presence of a parasite within red blood cells. The parasite is *Plasmodium* (*P. vivax, P. falciparum, P. malariae, P. ovale*), which is introduced through bites of infected female *Anopheles* mosquitoes or through blood transfusion.

Meiosis: Type of cell division of germ cells in which two successive divisions of the nucleus produce cells that contain half the number of chromosomes present in somatic cells.

Menorrhagia: Excessive menstrual bleeding, in number of days or amount of blood or both.

2-Mercaptoethanol (2-ME): A sulfhydryl compound used to disrupt the disulfide bonds of immunoglobulin M, yielding monomeric units rather than the typical pentameric units.

Metastasis: Movement of bacteria or body cells, especially cancer cells, from one part of the body to another; change in location of a disease or of its manifestations or transfer from one organ or part to another not directly connected. Spread is by the lymph or blood circulation.

Methemoglobin: An abnormal form of hemoglobin wherein the ferrous (Fe^{++}) iron has been oxidized to ferric (Fe^{+++}) iron.

Methyldopa (Aldomet): Common drug used to treat hypertension; frequently the cause of a positive direct Coombs' test result.

Microaggregates: Aggregates of platelets and leukocytes that accumulate in stored blood.

Microglobulin (β_2): A protein of unknown function; thought to be the light chain of the HLA molecule with structural similarities to the light chain in immunoglobulins.

Microspherocytes: Red blood cells, small and spherical, in certain kinds of anemia.

Minor crossmatch: Compatibility testing procedure using recipient's red cells and donor's serum.

Mitosis: Type of cell division in which each daughter cell contains the same number of chromosomes as the parent cell. All cells except sex cells undergo mitosis.

Mixed field: A type of agglutination pattern in which numerous small clumps of cells exist amid a sea of free cells.

MLC: Mixed lymphocyte culture.

MLR: Mixed lymphocyte reaction.

Modem: Hardware device that provides the ability to attach to a computer system via telephone communication lines.

Monoclonal: Antibody derived from a single ancestral antibody-producing parent cell.

Monocytes: *See* Macrophage.

Monozygotic twins: Two offspring that develop from a single fertilized ovum.

Mosaic: An antigen composed of several subunits, such as the $Rh_0(D)$ antigen. A mixture of characteristics that may result from a genetic cross-over or mutation.

Multiparous: Having borne more than one child.

Multiple myeloma: A neoplastic proliferation of plasma cells, which is characterized by very high immunoglobulin levels of monoclonal origin.

Mutation: A change in a gene potentially capable of being transmitted to offspring. **Point m.:** A change in a base in DNA that can lead to a change in the amino acid incorporated into the polypeptide; identifiable by analysis of the amino acid sequences of the original protein and its mutant offspring. **Frameshift m.:** A change in which a message is read incorrectly either because a base is missing or an extra base is added, which results in an entirely new polypeptide because the triplet sequence has been shifted one base.

Myelofibrosis: Replacement of bone marrow by fibrous tissue.

Myeloproliferative: An autonomous, purposeless increase in the production of the myeloid cell elements of the bone marrow, which includes granulocytic, erythrocytic, and megakaryocytic cell lines as well as the stromal connective tissue.

N-acetyl neuraminic acid (NANA): *See* Sialic acid.

Neonate: A newborn infant up to 6 weeks of age.

Network: Configuration of personal computers linked together with cables; allows all of the personal computers to access common data and software located on a fileserver.

Neuraminidase: An enzyme that cleaves sialic acid from the red cell membrane.

Neutralization: Inactivating an antibody by reacting it with an antigen against which it is directed.

Neutrophil: A leukocyte that ingests bacteria and small particles and plays a role in combating infection.

Nondisjunction: Failure of a pair of chromosomes to separate during meiosis.

Nonresponder: An individual whose immune system does not respond well in antibody formation to antigenic stimulation.

Normal serum albumin: *See* Albumin.

O$_h$: *See* Bombay phenotype.

Oligonucleotide: A short, approximately 20 nucleotides in length, synthetic segment of DNA used as a probe.

Oliguria: Diminished amount of urine formation.

Opsonin: A substance in serum that promotes immune adherence and facilitates phagocytosis by the reticuloendothelial system.

Orthostatic: Concerning an erect position.

Osmolality: The osmotic concentration of a solution determined by the ionic concentration of dissolved substances per unit of solvent.

Ouchterlony diffusion: An immunologic procedure in which antibody and antigen are placed in wells of a gel medium plate and allowed to diffuse in order to visualize the reaction by a precipitin line.

Oxyhemoglobin: The combined form of hemoglobin and oxygen.

P$_{50}$: The partial pressure of oxygen or oxygen tension at which the hemoglobin molecule is 50 percent saturated with oxygen.

Pallor: Paleness; lack of color.

Panagglutinin: An antibody capable of agglutinating all red blood cells tested, including the patient's own cells.

Pancytopenia: A reduction in all cellular elements of the blood, including red cells, white cells, and platelets.

Panel: A large number of group O reagent red cells that are of known antigenic characterization and are used for antibody identification.

Papain: A proteolytic enzyme derived from papaya.

Paragloboside: The immediate precursor for the H and P antigens of the red cell.

Paroxysm: A sudden, periodic attack or recurrence of symptoms of a disease.

Paroxysmal cold hemoglobinuria (PCH): A type of cold autoimmune hemolytic anemia usually found in children suffering from viral infections in which a biphasic immunoglobulin G antibody can be demonstrated with anti-P specificity. *See also* Donath-Landsteiner test.

Paroxysmal nocturnal hemoglobinuria (PNH): An intrinsic defect in the red blood cell membrane rendering it more susceptible to hemolysins in an acid environment; characterized by hemoglobin in the urine following periods of sleep.

Perfusion: Supplying an organ or tissue with nutrients and oxygen by passing blood or another suitable fluid through it.

Perioral paresthesia: Tingling around the mouth occasionally experienced by apheresis donors, resulting from the rapid return of citrated plasma, which contains citrate-bound calcium and free citrate.

Peroxidase: An enzyme that hastens the transfer of oxygen from peroxide to a tissue that requires oxygen; this process is essential to intracellular respiration.

Phagocytosis: Ingestion of microorganisms, other cells, and foreign particles by a phagocyte.

Phenotype: The outward expression of genes (e.g., a blood type). On blood cells, serologically demonstrable antigens constitute the phenotype, except those sugar sites that are determined by transferases.

Phenylthiocarbamide (PTC): A chemical used in studying medical genetics to detect the presence of a marker gene. About 70 percent of the population inherit the ability to taste PTC, which tastes bitter; the remaining 30 percent find PTC tasteless. The inheritance of this trait is due to a single dominant gene of a pair.

Phlebotomy: The procedure used to draw blood from a person.

Phosphoglyceromutase: A red cell enzyme.

Phototherapy: Exposure to sunlight or artificial light for therapeutic purposes.

Plasma: The liquid portion of whole blood containing water, electrolytes, glucose, fats, proteins, and gases. Plasma contains all the clotting factors necessary for coagulation, but in an inactive form. Once coagulation occurs, the fluid is converted to serum.

Plasma cell: A B lymphocyte–derived cell that secretes immunoglobulins or antibodies.

Plasmapheresis: A procedure using a machine to remove only plasma from a donor or patient.

Plasma protein fraction (PPF): Also known as Plasmanate; sterile pooled plasma stored as a fluid or freeze dried and used for volume replacement.

Plasminogen: A protein in many tissues and body fluids important in preventing fibrin clot formation.

Plasmodium: *See* Malaria.

Plasmodium knowlesi: A parasite that causes malaria in monkeys.

Platelet: A round or oval disc, 2 to 4 μm in diameter, that is derived from the cytoplasma of the megakaryocyte, a large cell in the bone marrow. Platelets play an important role in blood coagulation, hemostasis, and blood thrombus formation. When a small vessel is injured, platelets adhere to each other and to the edges of the injury, forming a "plug" that covers the area and stops the blood loss.

Platelet concentrate: Platelets prepared from a single unit of whole blood or plasma and suspended in a specific volume of the original plasma; also known as random-donor platelets.

Plateletpheresis: A procedure using a machine to remove only platelets from a donor or patient.

PRP: Platelet rich plasma.

Polyacrylamide gel: A type of matrix used in electrophoresis upon which substances are separated.

Polyagglutination: A state in which an individual's red cells are agglutinated by all sera regardless of blood type.

Polyagglutinins: Naturally occurring immunoglobulin antibodies that are found in most normal human adult sera.

Polybrene: A positively charged polymer that causes normal red cells to aggregate spontaneously by neutralizing the negative surface charge contributed by sialic acid.

Polyclonal: Antibodies derived from more than one antibody-producing parent cell.

Polycythemia vera: A chronic life-shortening myeloproliferative disorder involving all bone marrow elements, characterized by an increase in red blood cell mass and hemoglobin concentration.

Polymer: Combination of two or more molecules of the same substance.

Polymerase chain reaction (PCR): An in vitro method of amplification of a specific DNA segment.

Polymorphism: A genetic system that possesses numerous allelic forms, such as a blood group system.

Polyspecific Coombs' sera: A reagent that contains antihuman globulin sera against immunoglobulin G and C3d.

Polyvinylpyrrolidone (PVP): A neutral polymeric substance used to increase blood volume in patients with extensive blood loss; also used to enhance antigen-antibody reactions in vitro.

Portal hypertension: Increased pressure in the portal vein as a result of obstruction of the flow of blood through the liver.

Postpartum: Occurring after childbirth.

Potentiator: A substance that, when added to a serum and cell mixture, will enhance antigen-antibody interactions.

Precipitation: The formation of a visible complex (precipitate) in a medium containing soluble antigen (precipitinogen) and the corresponding antibody (precipitin).

Precipitin: An antibody formed in the blood serum of an animal by the presence of a soluble antigen, usually a protein. When added to a solution of the antigen, it brings about precipitation. The injected protein is called the antigen and the antibody produced, the precipitin.

Precursor substance: A substance that is converted to another substance by the addition of a specific constituent (e.g., a sugar residue).

Primer: A short segment of single-stranded DNA, usually 17 to 25 nucleotides long, used to initiate DNA replication in PCR.

Private antigen: An antigenic characteristic of the red blood cell membrane that is unique to an individual or a related family of individuals and, therefore, is not commonly found on all cells (usually less than 1 percent of the population).

Probe: A fragment of DNA which is labeled and hybridized to diagnostic material to locate a complementary strand of DNA.

Prodrome: A symptom indicative of an approaching disease.

Propositus: The initial individual whose condition led to investigation of a hereditary disorder or to a serologic evaluation of family members. Feminine form is proposita. Synonyms are proband and index case.

Prospective validation: Validation testing of software; done before implementation of the computer system.

Prosthesis: An artificial substitute for a missing part, such as an artificial extremity.

Protamine: A polycation with applications similar to those of polybrene.

Protamine sulfate: A substance used to neutralize the effects of heparin.

Prothrombin complex: A concentrate of coagulation factors II, VII, IX, and X in lyophilized form.

Prozone: Incomplete lattice formation caused by an excess of antibody molecules relative to the number of antigen sites, resulting in false-negative reactions.

Public antigen: An antigenic characteristic of the red blood cell membrane found commonly among individuals, usually greater than 98 percent of the population.

Pulmonary artery wedge pressure: Pressure measured in the pulmonary artery at its capillary end.

Pulse pressure: The difference between the systolic and the diastolic pressures.

Radioimmunoassay (RIA): A very sensitive method for determination of substances present in low concentrations in serum or plasma by using specific antibodies and radioactively labeled or tagged substances.

Rapid passive hemagglutination assay (RPHA): A third-generation procedure used in hepatitis testing.

Rapid passive latex assay (RPLA): A second-generation procedure used in hepatitis testing.

Raynaud's disease: A peripheral vascular disorder characterized by abnormal vasoconstriction of the extremities upon exposure to cold or emotional stress. A history of symptoms for at least 2 years is necessary for diagnosis.

Recessive: A type of gene that, in the presence of its dominant allele, does not express itself; expression occurs when it is inherited in the homozygous state.

Recipient: A patient who is receiving a transfusion of blood or a blood product.

Refractory: Obstinate; stubborn; resistant to ordinary treatment; resistant to stimulation (said of a muscle or nerve).

Respiratory distress syndrome (RDS): A condition, formerly known as hyaline membrane disease, accounting for more than 25,000 infant deaths per year in the United States. Clinical signs, including delayed onset of respiration and low Apgar score, are usually present at birth.

Reticulocyte: Also known as neocyte, the last stage of development before becoming a mature erythrocyte. The reticulocyte has lost its nucleus but retains some residual RNA in its cytoplasm, which is stainable by special techniques. It may be slightly larger than the mature red cell.

Reticuloendothelial system (RES): The fixed phagocytic cells of the body, such as the macrophage, having the ability to ingest particulate matter.

Retrospective validation: Validation testing of software, which is done after the computer system has been implemented.

Reverse grouping: Testing a patient's serum with commercial or reagent A and B red blood cells to determine which ABO antibodies are present.

Rh immunoglobulin (RhIg): A concentrated, purified anti-$Rh_0(D)$ prepared from human serum (of immunized donors), which is given to $Rh_0(D)$-negative mothers after they have given birth to an $Rh_0(D)$-positive baby or after abortion or miscarriage. It acts to prevent the mother from becoming immunized to any $Rh_0(D)$-positive fetal cells that may have entered her circulation and thereby prevents formation of anti-Rh$_0$(D) by the mother.

Rh$_{null}$: A rare Rh phenotype in which no Rh antigens are expressed on the red blood cell; may result from the action of an inhibitor gene that is inherited independently from the *Rh* genes or caused by the rare genotype $\overline{r}\,\overline{r}$, which is the *Rh* amorphic gene.

Ribonucleic acid (RNA): A nucleic acid that controls protein synthesis in all living cells. There are three different types, and all are derived from the information encoded in the DNA of the cell. Messenger RNA (mRNA) carries the code for specific amino acid sequences from the DNA to the cytoplasm for protein synthesis. Transfer RNA (tRNA) carries the amino acid groups to the ribosome for protein synthesis. Ribosomal RNA (rRNA), which exists within the ribosomes, is thought to assist in protein synthesis.

Ribosome: A cellular organelle that contains ribonucleoprotein and functions to synthesize protein. Ribosomes may be single units or clusters called polyribosomes or polysomes.

Rickettsia: Any of the microorganisms belonging to the genus *Rickettsia*.

Ringer's lactated injection: An aqueous solution suitable for intravenous use.

Rouleaux: Coinlike stacking of red blood cells in the presence of plasma expanders or abnormal plasma proteins.

Saline anti-D: A low-protein (6 to 8 percent albumin) immunoglobulin M anti-D reagent.

Salvia horminum: Plant lectin used in the differentiation of various forms of polyagglutination.

Salvia sclarea: Plant lectin with anti-Tn activity, used in the differentiation of various forms of polyagglutination.

Screening cells: Group O reagent red cells that are used in antibody detection or screening tests.

SD: Serologically defined antigens.

Secretor: An individual who is capable of secreting soluble, glycoprotein ABH-soluble substances into saliva and other body fluids.

Sensitization: A condition of being made sensitive to a specific substance (e.g., an antigen) after the initial exposure to that substance. This results in the development of immunologic memory that evokes an accentuated immune response with subsequent exposure to the substance.

Sepsis: Pathologic state, usually febrile, resulting from the presence of microorganisms or -heir poisonous products in the blood stream.

Septicemia: Presence of pathogenic bacteria in the blood.

Serologic test for syphilis (STS): First developed in 1906 by Wassermann, present tests are of three main types based on complement fixation, flocculation, and detection of specific antitreponemal antibodies.

Serotonin: A chemical present in platelets that is a potent vasoconstrictor.

Serum: The fluid that remains after plasma has clotted.

Sex chromosome: Chromosomes associated with determination of sex.

Sex linkage: A genetic characteristic located on the X or Y chromosome.

Shelf life: The amount of time blood or blood products may be stored upon collection.

Shock: A clinical syndrome in which the peripheral blood flow is inadequate to return sufficient blood to the heart for normal function, particularly transport of oxygen to all organs and tissues. Shock may be caused by a variety of conditions, including hemorrhage, infection, drug reac- tion, trauma, poisoning, myocardial infarction, or dehydration. Symptoms include paleness of skin (pallor), a bluish gray discoloration (cyanosis), a weak and rapid pulse, rapid and shallow breathing, or blood pressure that is decreased and perhaps unmeasurable.

Sialic acid: A group of sugars found on the red cell membrane attached to a protein backbone; the major source of the membrane net negative charge.

Sickle trait: Blood that is heterozygous for the gene coding for the abnormal hemoglobin of sickle cell anemia.

Siderosis: A form of pneumoconiosis resulting from inhalation of dust or fumes containing iron particles.

Single-donor platelets: Platelets collected from a single donor by apheresis.

Sodium dodecyl sulfate (SDS): An anionic detergent that renders a net negative charge to substances it solubilizes.

Software: Written instructions for a computer, which result in information being stored, manipulated, and retrieved.

Specificity: The affinity of an antibody and the antigen against which it is directed.

Splenomegaly: Enlargement of the spleen.

Steatorrhea: Increased secretion of the sebaceous glands.

Stem cell: An unspecialized cell that gives rise to a group of differential cells such as the hematopoietic cells.

Steroid hormones: Hormones of the adrenal cortex and the sex hormones.

Stertorous: Pertaining to laborious breathing.

Storage lesion: A loss of viability and function associated with certain biochemical changes that are initiated when blood is stored in vitro.

Stroma: The red cell membrane that is left after hemolysis has occurred.

Subgroup: Antigens within the ABO group that react less strongly with their corresponding antisera than do A and B antigens.

Survival studies: A measure of the in vivo survival of transfused blood cells; usually performed with radioactive isotopes. Normal red cells survive approximately 100 to 120 days in circulation.

Syngeneic: Possessing identical genotypes, as monozygotic twins.

Synteny: Genes that are closely situated on a chromosome but cannot be shown to be linked.

System manager: A specially trained person who is responsible for the maintenance of an information system.

Systemic lupus erythematosus (SLE): A disseminated autoimmune disease characterized by anemia, thrombocytopenia, increased immunoglobulin G levels, and the presence of four immunoglobulin G antibodies: antinuclear antibody, antinucleoprotein antibody, anti-DNA antibody, and antihistone antibody; believed to be caused by suppressor T cell dysfunction.

Systolic pressure: Maximum blood pressure that occurs at ventricular contraction; upper value of a blood pressure reading.

Tachycardia: Abnormally rapid heart action, usually defined as a heart rate greater than 100 beats per minute.

Tachypnea: Abnormally rapid respirations.

Template bleeding time: The elapsed time a uniform incision made by a template and blade stops bleeding, which is a test of platelet function, assuming a normal platelet count.

Tetany: A nervous affection characterized by intermittent spasms of the muscles of the extremities.

Thalassemia major: The homozygous form of deficient

beta-chain synthesis, which is very severe and presents itself during childhood. Prognosis varies; however, the younger the child at disease onset, the less favorable the outcome.

Thermal amplitude: The range of temperature over which an antibody demonstrates serologic and/or in vitro activity.

Thrombin: An enzyme that converts fibrinogen to fibrin so that a soluble clot can be formed.

Thrombocytopenia: A reduction in the platelet count below the normal level, which is associated with spontaneous hemorrhage.

Thrombotic thrombocytopenic purpura (TTP): A coagulation disorder characterized by (1) increased bleeding owing to a decreased number of platelets, (2) hemolytic anemia, (3) renal failure, and (4) changing neurologic signs. The characteristic morphologic lesion is thrombotic occlusion of small arteries or capillaries in various organs.

Thymidine: An essential ingredient used in DNA synthesis and incorporated by T lymphocytes undergoing blast transformation in response to foreign HLA-D antigens in the mixed lymphocyte culture test.

Titer: A measure of the strength of an antibody by testing its reactivity at increasing dilutions against the appropriate antigen.

Titer score: A method used to evaluate more precisely than simple dilution by comparing the titers of an antibody. Agglutination at each higher dilution is graded on a continuous scale; the total is the titer score.

Trait: A characteristic that is inherited.

Trans: The location of two or more genes on opposite chromosomes of a homologous pair.

Transcription: The process of RNA production from DNA, which requires the enzyme RNA polymerase.

Transferase: An enzyme that catalyzes the transfer of atoms or groups of atoms from one chemical compound to another.

Transfuse: To perform a transfusion.

Transfusion: The injection of blood, a blood component, saline, or other fluids into the bloodstream. **Cadaver blood t.:** Using blood obtained from a cadaver within a short time after death. **Direct t.:** Transfer of blood directly from one person to another. **Exchange t.:** Transfusion and withdrawal of small amounts of blood, repeated until blood volume is almost entirely exchanged; used in infants born with hemolytic disease. **Indirect t.:** Transfusion of blood from a donor to a suitable storage container and then to a patient. **Intrauterine t.:** Transfusion of blood into a fetus in utero.

Transfusion reaction: An adverse response to a transfusion.

Translation: The production of protein from the interactions of the RNAs.

Translocation: Transfer of a portion of one chromosome to its allele.

Transposition: The location of two genes on opposite chromosomes of a homologous pair.

Trypsin: A proteolytic enzyme formed in the intestine.

Type and screen: Testing a patient's blood for ABO group, Rh type, and atypical antibodies. The sample is then retained in the event that subsequent crossmatching is necessary.

Ulex europaeus: See Anti-H lectin.

Ultracentrifugation: Rapid and prolonged centrifugation used to separate by density gradients substances of various specific gravities.

Urticaria: A vascular reaction of the skin similar to hives.

User: A person who uses a computer information system.

Vaccine: A suspension of infectious organisms or components of them that is given as a form of passive immunization to establish resistance to the infectious disease caused by that organism.

Validation: A systematic process of testing the hardware, software, and user components of an information system to ensure that they are functioning correctly for their intended purpose.

Valvular: Relating to or having a valve.

Variable region: That portion of the immunoglobulin light and heavy chains where amino acid sequences vary tremendously, thereby permitting the different immunoglobulin molecules to recognize different antigenic determinants. In other words, the variable region determines the antigen against which the antibody will react, thus providing each antibody molecule with its unique specificity. The variable region is located at the amino terminal region of the molecule.

Vasculitis: Inflammation of a blood or lymph vessel.

Vasoconstriction: Constriction of blood vessels.

Vasodilatation: Dilatation of blood vessels, especially small arteries and arterioles.

Vasovagal syncope: Syncope resulting from hypotension caused by emotional stress, pain, acute blood loss, fear, or rapid rising from a recumbent position.

Venesection: *See* Phlebotomy.

Venipuncture: Puncture of a vein for any purpose.

Venule: A tiny vein continuous with a capillary.

Viability: Ability of a cell to live or to survive for a reasonably normal life span.

Vicia graminea: See Anti-N lectin.

Virion: A complete virus particle; a unit of genetic material surrounded by a protective coat that serves as a vehicle for its transmission from one cell to another.

von Willebrand factor: Coagulation factor VIII.

von Willebrand's disease: A congenital bleeding disorder.

WAIHA: Warm autoimmune hemolytic anemia. A hemolytic anemia caused by the patient's autoantibody that reacts at 37°C.

Wharton's jelly: A gelatinous intercellular substance consisting of primitive connective tissue of the umbilical cord.

X chromosome: The chromosome that determines female sex characteristics. The normal female has two X chromosomes, and the normal male an X and a Y chromosome.

Xeno-: Prefix indicating differing species. For example, a xenoantibody is an antibody produced in one species against an antigen present in another species. Synonym is hetero-.

Yaws: An infectious nonvenereal disease caused by a spirochete, *Treponema pertenue*, and found mainly in humid equatorial regions.

Zeta potential: The difference in charge density between the inner and outer layers of the ionic cloud that surrounds red cells in an electrolyte solution.

Index

Numbers followed by an *f* indicate figures; numbers followed by a *t* indicate tabular material.

529